PROFESSIONAL PARAMEDIC

TRAUMA CARE & EMS OPERATIONS

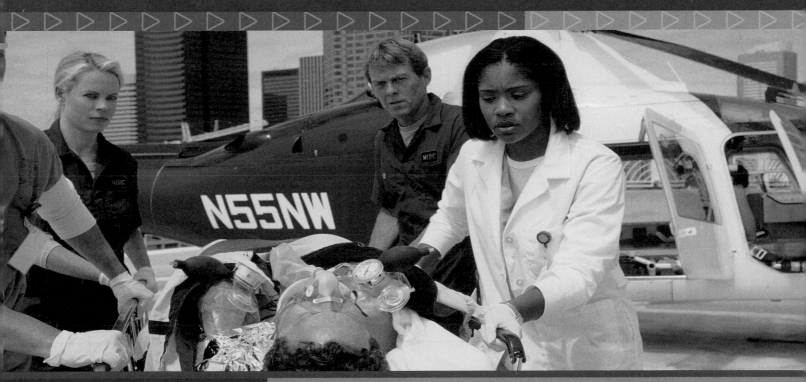

VOLUME III | RICHARD BEEBE | JEFFREY MYERS, DO

D0071385

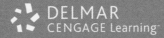

DELMAR
CENGAGE Learning

Australia • Brazil • Japan • Korea • Mexico • Singapore • Spain • United Kingdom • United States

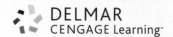

Professional Paramedic:
    Trauma Care & EMS Operations
Richard Beebe and Jeffrey Myers, DO

Vice President, Career and Professional
    Editorial: Dave Garza

Director of Learning Solutions: Sandy Clark

Senior Acquisitions Editor: Janet Maker

Managing Editor: Larry Main

Senior Product Manager: Jennifer A. Starr

Editorial Assistant: Amy Wetsel

Vice President, Career and Professional
    Marketing: Jennifer Baker

Marketing Director: Deborah S. Yarnell

Senior Marketing Manager: Erin Coffin

Associate Marketing Manager: Shanna Gibbs

Production Director: Wendy Troeger

Production Manager: Mark Bernard

Senior Content Project Manager:
    Jennifer Hanley

Art Director: Benjamin Gleeksman

For product information and technology assistance, contact us at
Cengage Learning Customer & Sales Support, 1-800-354-9706
For permission to use material from this text or product,
submit all requests online at **www.cengage.com/permissions.**
Further permissions questions can be e-mailed to
permissionrequest@cengage.com

Library of Congress Control Number: 2010938210

ISBN-13: 978-1-4283-2348-3

ISBN-10: 1-4283-2348-1

Delmar
5 Maxwell Drive
Clifton Park, NY 12065-2919
USA

Cengage Learning is a leading provider of customized learning solutions with office locations around the globe, including Singapore, the United Kingdom, Australia, Mexico, Brazil, and Japan. Locate your local office at:
international.cengage.com/region

Cengage Learning products are represented in Canada by Nelson Education, Ltd.

To learn more about Delmar, visit **www.cengage.com/delmar**

Purchase any of our products at your local college store or at our preferred online store **www.cengagebrain.com**

NOTICE TO THE READER

Publisher does not warrant or guarantee any of the products described herein or perform any independent analysis in connection with any of the product information contained herein. Publisher does not assume, and expressly disclaims, any obligation to obtain and include information other than that provided to it by the manufacturer. The reader is expressly warned to consider and adopt all safety precautions that might be indicated by the activities described herein and to avoid all potential hazards. By following the instructions contained herein, the reader willingly assumes all risks in connection with such instructions. The publisher makes no representations or warranties of any kind, including but not limited to, the warranties of fitness for particular purpose or merchantability, nor are any such representations implied with respect to the material set forth herein, and the publisher takes no responsibility with respect to such material. The publisher shall not be liable for any special, consequential, or exemplary damages resulting, in whole or part, from the readers' use of, or reliance upon, this material.

Printed in the United States of America
1 2 3 4 5 6 7 15 14 13 12 11

DEDICATION

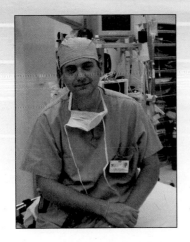

Dedicated to the memory of John Pryor: Paramedic, surgeon, father, husband, brother, and son.

On Christmas Day, 2008, while serving his country in Iraq, Dr. Pryor was tragically killed in the line of duty. Dr. Pryor felt compelled to join the U.S. Army Reserve after witnessing the effects of September 11, 2001, from the rubble pile at Ground Zero. As a member of the U.S. Forward Army Surgical Unit, Dr. Pryor volunteered for not one, but two tours of duty in Iraq, believing that he needed to be there to help others, especially his fellow soldiers. Dr. Pryor's history as a volunteer in medical service started at age 17 with the Clifton Park-Halfmoon Volunteer Ambulance Corp., where he became an Emergency Medical Technician and later a Paramedic. These early beginnings in EMS may have led Dr. Pryor to a career as a widely respected trauma surgeon in Philadelphia.

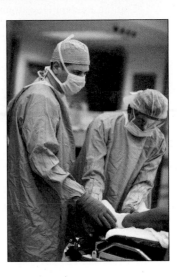

Dr. Pryor often wrote eloquently about his view of the human condition, whether he observed it in war-torn Iraq or the streets of Philadelphia. In one letter he wrote to the family of a mortally wounded Marine, he described his struggle to save the soldier. He expressed that he, his fellow physicians, and especially the Paramedics and EMTs who had the honor of serving with the dead Marine "more than anyone else, know he was a true American hero."

The life of service, love for others, and spirit of devotion of Dr. John Pryor is an example for us all. We, his fellow Paramedics, more than almost anyone else, know he was a true American hero.

TABLE OF CONTENTS

29. WILDERNESS SEARCH AND RESCUE   558

30. TECHNICAL ROPE RESCUE   576

31. MASS-GATHERING MEDICINE   592

32. TACTICAL EMERGENCY MEDICAL SUPPORT   604

FOREWORD

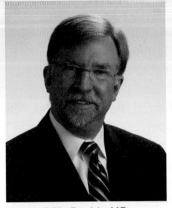

Edward M. Racht, MD

EMS is a practice of medicine....

In medicine, there is an art and a science to everything. The science is *what* we need to do to improve our patient's condition. In its purest form, *what* we do is based on rigorous scientific scrutiny and all the available evidence applicable to the conditions we treat. The art of medicine is *how* we apply the science to our patients in a way that maximizes the potential for an improved outcome. Ironically, the science is often much easier to master than the art. This is perhaps no more pronounced than in the ever-changing, often unpredictable world of EMS.

One thing is very clear: A good practitioner must be accomplished at both the art and the science of medicine.

This is a fascinating time to work in emergency health care. EMS is undergoing tremendous evolution. Not only do we know more about the conditions we treat, but more and more of our clinical practices are now based on sound scientific evidence that applies specifically to our patient population. In the early days of EMS, we adapted evidence from inpatient studies or the laboratory environment and applied it to what we did in the field. While that was certainly appropriate for much of what we did, the challenges of the field and the unique environment of medical care outside the hospital created the need for very targeted research in out-of-hospital medicine. Fortunately, we have more academic initiatives focused on the field than ever before in our brief history. The more we study, the more we learn.

We also understand much more about the seemingly insignificant details that can have a dramatic impact on patient outcomes. Paying attention to those details and focusing on what's truly important in the field practice of medicine is another characteristic of the EMS evolution. For example, there are major changes in the way we attempt to resuscitate our patients. A very consistent, focused attention to perfusion is at the core of everything we do during resuscitation attempts. While many would say we've always believed that to be true, the fact is we didn't always focus on those details during patient care. During those critical moments of assessing and repairing altered physiology and broken anatomy, paying attention to details can often mean the difference between life and death.

As we learn more about the amazing science of the human body and how it behaves when it's "broken," we appreciate that the best approach to management of illness and injury requires more than just memorizing facts. It requires us to put together everything we know, use all our available resources, and develop a plan of action that incorporates clinical care, different modes of transport, and different receiving facilities that have different capabilities. EMS, as a unique practice of medicine, is charged with making complex decisions in short periods of time, often with only limited data. The educational toolbox you hold in your hand will follow you throughout your career and guide you in making the tough calls.

Our role in the Big Picture of Medicine is also evolving. The devastating and unfortunate events of September 11th and the emerging challenges of terrorism, intentional violence, and newer, unpredictable threats have forever focused the American public's attention on the importance of emergency medical care. EMS providers must have the knowledge and ability to deal with an entire spectrum of out-of-hospital problems, ranging from the simple to the unimaginable. Because of the potential for rapidly changing scenarios, we as Paramedics must now know where to go to get the right information and how to rapidly access data we need to make our decisions. Our ability to rapidly deploy our resources throughout a community has also highlighted the value of using EMS providers and systems to disseminate emergency medications and immunizations in the event of a need for rapid public health interventions.

As economic conditions change, our society is retooling healthcare delivery and our patients are using EMS in different ways than they have historically. While that creates some new stresses on EMS, it's a vitally important part of our EMS culture. We are the safety net for many communities suffering from inadequate healthcare resources. Regardless of the number of facilities, patients still get sick and hurt. We should be very proud of our collective ability to care for our fellow human beings regardless of their ability to afford it or our community's ability to provide it. It's who we are.

The newly promulgated Educational Standards are the result of thousands of hours of work from the most accomplished EMS educators, clinicians, and administrators in the profession. The standards provide us with a new approach to delivering the tools that perfect the out-of-hospital delivery of medical care. Rich Beebe, Jeff Myers, and their colleagues have done a spectacular job of presenting the latest evidence in a very comprehensible manner.

As you embark on your educational journey to master the art and science of field medicine, you will continuously discover the valuable educational approach of the *Professional Paramedic Series*. Volume I provides a solid foundation in the knowledge and clinical skills a Paramedic needs to expertly assess and treat patients. In Volumes II and III, the clinical material is presented in a unique way that facilitates the development of critical thinking skills (remember the art?). These volumes use an interrupted case format that narrows a patient's chief concern into a paramedical diagnosis. Volume III also discusses the wide range of operational issues faced by the Paramedic and presents students with the many niches within EMS. In addition, the accompanying student resources and instructor curriculum provide additional cases and avenues to test student knowledge, further refine critical thinking skills, and enhance the teaching and learning experience. Throughout the learning process, students will not only understand what's important, they will also learn how to think their way into the diagnosis and develop an approach that has the best opportunity to improve a patient's condition. *That* is critical thinking.

Enjoy. Enjoy this part of your journey. Enjoy taking care of people when they need you the most. Enjoy learning about the fascinating intricacies of the human body, and enjoy the impact you will have on people's lives every day.

Always remember how important your knowledge, skills, and compassion are for those at the other end of the 9-1-1 call.

Edward M. Racht, MD

PREFACE

THE INTENT OF THIS BOOK

Volume III: Trauma Care and EMS Operations, the final volume in the *Professional Paramedic Series*, applies the knowledge and skills learned in Volumes I and II to both trauma and special response situations.

With a focus on both future Paramedics *and* the Paramedics of today, the *Professional Paramedic Series* was designed as a comprehensive resource for Paramedic students during their education and as a source for life-long learning. This series seeks to prepare aspiring Paramedic students in community colleges, universities, and other educational programs with not only the knowledge to become a Paramedic, but also the ability to think critically and decisively when seconds count. Beyond the basic foundation of paramedical knowledge and skills, this series helps the Paramedic student reach a higher level of understanding. For this reason, the *Series* is also an essential resource for practicing Paramedics who are studying for recertification and continuing education.

In January 2009, the new National EMS Education Standards were released to the EMS community. This document serves to set an academic standard for all Paramedic education programs. The *Professional Paramedic Series* was specifically developed with the National EMS Education Standards in mind, yet can also be used in Paramedic programs that have not yet transitioned to the new standards. Each of the three volumes within this series meets *and exceeds* these new education standards by not only teaching the essential knowledge and skills, but also by preparing each student to *think* like a Paramedic. As Paramedics who started in the streets and who continue to practice there, we support the vision of the National EMS Education Standards, and have created this series, aptly named *Professional Paramedic*.

WHY WE WROTE THIS SERIES

As educators, we *challenge* our learners—the students of this series—to be the best Paramedics possible. Although other Paramedic textbooks are available, we felt that the evolving nature of the Paramedic field demanded a fresh approach. We wanted our textbook to challenge Paramedic students to think about the application of medical knowledge to field practice. This approach changed the focus of a Paramedic textbook from being the center of a Paramedic's education to one in which it serves as an authoritative resource that implores the student to explore the current state of the science.

As part of our vision in writing this series, we wanted to recognize the practice of *paramedicine*. What is paramedicine? Paramedicine is a unique practice of emergency medicine that happens in the out-of-hospital setting. First described in the *EMS Agenda for the Future* in 1996, paramedicine is the result of the growth of EMS over almost one-half of a century. It encompasses the complete roles and responsibilities of the Paramedic within the domains of health care, public health, and public safety systems. We offer this series as a guide to prehospital emergency medical care and the practice of paramedicine, providing learners with a reference for the often complex, at times ambiguous, and always challenging field of emergency medicine.

We understand that often the best Paramedics are those who start with a natural curiosity about emergency medicine and inquisitiveness about how that medical knowledge could be practically applied in the streets. These students know it is important to be *street smart* as well as *book smart*. This book seeks to help answer their questions through a conversation with the student.

THE *PROFESSIONAL PARAMEDIC SERIES*

This series is designed to follow a logical progression of learning, in which knowledge and skills are presented first in Volume I, followed by the application of those skills in emergency situations in Volume II, and then trauma and special response considerations in Volume III. The framework of each book is practical in approach: introducing principles, skills, and terminology; presenting a typical case; walking through critical response steps; and again reviewing key concepts to ensure understanding for successful application on the job.

The series is inclusive of all of the content areas listed in the National EMS Education Standards and contains material on most of the critical and emergent disorders listed in the EMS core content as well as many of the lower acuity conditions. This coverage helps ensure the student's preparation for the National Registry or state Paramedic certification examinations. More importantly, the series helps prepare the Paramedic student for professional Paramedic practice.

VOLUME I: FOUNDATIONS OF PARAMEDIC CARE

ISBN: 978-1-14283-2345-2

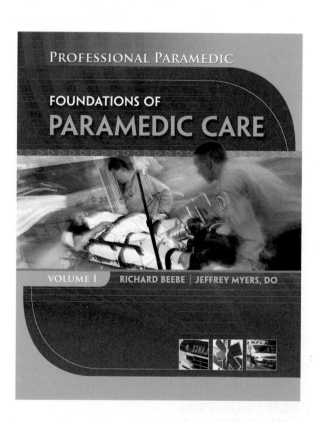

To be able to make a Paramedical diagnosis, the Paramedic must be well-grounded in the basics of medicine: anatomy and physiology, as well as pathophysiology. *Volume I: Foundations of Paramedic Care* begins with the basics. This first volume in the series initiates this learning by introducing the fundamental knowledge and skills needed for success,

as well as the necessary tools to begin developing a professional approach to emergency medicine and Paramedic care.

Volume I is divided into six sections:

- ■ **Section I:** Framework for Paramedic Practice
- ■ **Section II:** Ethics and Law in EMS
- ■ **Section III:** EMS and Public Health
- ■ **Section IV:** Scientific Principles
- ■ **Section V:** Principles of Clinical Practice
- ■ **Section VI:** Clinical Essentials

VOLUME II: MEDICAL EMERGENCIES, MATERNAL HEALTH, AND PEDIATRICS

ISBN: 978-1-4283-2351-3

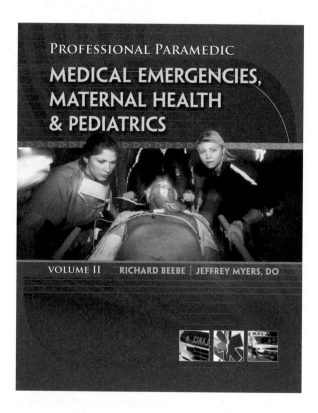

Volume II of the series introduces an *interrupted case* approach to discuss medical, maternal, and pediatric emergencies, as well as emergencies in special patient populations. This book walks the reader through a wide range of emergency response situations: from cardiac emergencies to various diseases and disorders, from gynecological concerns to neonatal resuscitation, from the chronically ill to the victims of domestic violence and sexual assault. Utilizing a typical emergency that a Paramedic might encounter in the field, each chapter includes a Case Study that relates to the subject of the chapter and presents critical information, leading the reader to develop a Paramedic's diagnosis from the information provided.

Volume II is divided into four sections:

- ■ **Section I:** Medical Emergencies
- ■ **Section II:** Maternal Health and the Newly Born
- ■ **Section III:** Pediatrics
- ■ **Section IV:** Special Patients

VOLUME III: TRAUMA CARE AND EMS OPERATIONS

ISBN: 978-1-4283-2348-3

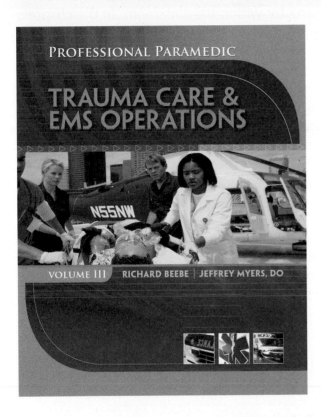

Volume III highlights the care of patients with traumatic and environmental emergencies. Additionally, it presents special response considerations and a broad range of operational medical topics to prepare readers with the complete spectrum of knowledge required to succeed as a Paramedic. These aspects of Paramedic practice help to make paramedicine a unique profession with its own unique body of knowledge.

In addition, Volume III is a unique blend of the typical case approach that is found in Volume I (as pertaining to special response considerations) as well as the *interrupted case* approach found in Volume II (as pertaining to the trauma chapters). As with Volume II, it should be understood that the interrupted cases present only one potential patient presentation for that chief concern. To that end, we have included additional cases in the accompanying *Study Guide*. It is the responsibility of both the student and the instructor to explore these other cases, as well as other real world examples, to fully appreciate other potential patient presentations.

SAFETY NOTICE

The technical rescue chapters included in this volume are intended to raise the Paramedic's *awareness* of various techniques utilized in rescue operations. They are *not* intended to serve as complete, comprehensive training on the subject. Extensive training and a separate certification in these specialized fields is required before Paramedics may perform these technical rescue techniques on-scene.

This volume is divided into four sections.

SECTION I: TRAUMA CARE

Providing care for an injured patient is one of the foundations of EMS, and stems from the 1966 white paper, "Accidental Death and Disability: The Neglected Disease of Modern Society." Trauma care is considered one of the essential aspects of paramedicine, as a significant percentage of the calls requiring a Paramedic response will be due to trauma. In this section, trauma care is presented as it relates to various body systems, with each chapter covering the care of life-threatening injuries as well as minor trauma related to that system. The section culminates in a discussion of pediatric trauma considerations and an overview of trauma resuscitation. This overview combines data from all of the individual chapters to create a comprehensive approach to the treatment of the critically injured patient.

SECTION II: ENVIRONMENTAL MEDICINE

This section on environmental medicine discusses conditions requiring outdoor care, such as heat and cold emergencies, mountain medicine, water emergencies, and envenomations.

SECTION III: EMS OPERATIONS

Maintaining an attitude of safety first is important in EMS operations. If Paramedics do not operate in a safe manner, they risk injury, thus rendering themselves unable to care for patients. This section leads off with a comprehensive chapter on EMS safety considerations. The next two chapters focus on aeromedical considerations and specialty care transport, respectively, and examine the provision of paramedicine in these specialized environments.

SECTION IV: EMERGENCY INCIDENT MANAGEMENT

Since Paramedics operate in a variety of conditions and situations, the Paramedic must be able to integrate medical care into a variety of special circumstances. This section begins with a general review of Incident Command and management, discussion of triage of patients in multiple-casualty situations, and review of paramedicine in the support of different operational situations, such as hazardous materials and Tactical Emergency Medical Services. These operational chapters provide the basics for the new Paramedic, but also demonstrate the breadth of paramedicine. During her career, a Paramedic may choose to specialize in one or more of these operational areas, deepening her knowledge and allowing her to serve as an expert for her agency.

FEATURES

Along with an appealing design, the *Professional Paramedic Series* has many features intended to motivate the student to read and learn the knowledge and skills presented in each volume.

COMPREHENSIVE COVERAGE

The complex depth and comprehensive breadth of information required for a working knowledge of Paramedic practice, for Paramedic certification, and ultimately for success on the job are all provided in an engaging and reader-friendly manner. Students will be properly prepared for these challenges with evidence-based information presented within the content that meets and *exceeds* National EMS Education Standards.

KEY CONCEPTS

Presented in the beginning of each chapter, the Key Concepts set learning goals for students and preview both the didactic and psychomotor skills presented in the chapter that they are expected to learn.

ANATOMY CONCEPTS

Following the Key Concepts at the beginning of each medical chapter, Anatomy Concepts outline the anatomy and physiology topics that students should be familiar with in order to gain a complete understanding of the subject matter discussed in the chapter.

CASE STUDIES

The case studies included in each chapter facilitate the *conversation*, both the internal dialogue within the student and the dialogue between the student and instructor within the classroom. In the chapters containing *interrupted cases*, the Case Study is carried through the entire chapter—with each new section providing further details on the medical emergency in order to encourage students to develop critical thinking skills. By portraying realistic emergency situations related to chapter content, the book introduces the student to the material in a meaningful manner. This presentation also encourages the decision-making process involved in making a field diagnosis, and outlines a plan of treatment that meets the standard of care within the scope of practice for the patient for prehospital care and transport to the hospital. Each case is designed to encourage a Paramedic's thought process and includes follow-up questions.

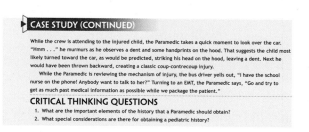

CASE STUDY (CONTINUED)

While the crew is attending to the injured child, the Paramedic takes a quick moment to look over the car. "Hmm . . ." he murmurs as he observes a dent and some handprints on the hood. That suggests the child most likely turned toward the car, as would be predicted, striking his head on the hood, leaving a dent. Next he would have been thrown backward, creating a classic coup-contrecoup injury.

While the Paramedic is reviewing the mechanism of injury, the bus driver yells out, "I have the school nurse on the phone! Anybody want to talk to her?" Turning to an EMT, the Paramedic says, "Go and try to get as much past medical information as possible while we package the patient."

CRITICAL THINKING QUESTIONS
1. What are the important elements of the history that a Paramedic should obtain?
2. What special considerations are there for obtaining a pediatric history?

CHEATED METHOD

This method follows the Paramedic's standard medical intelligence (sometimes called "medic think") and encourages students to engage in the critical-thinking process needed for a proper Paramedical diagnosis and treatment—Chief concern, History, Examination, Assessment, Treatment, Evaluation, and Disposition. Each is discussed, as applicable, within the chapter and follows the presentation of each case so that learners can think logically about these critical response steps.

PROFESSIONAL PARAMEDIC

Integrated throughout the book, this feature highlights the professional attitudes that signify the difference between a competent Paramedic and an expert Paramedic—one whom fellow Paramedics respect and look to as a leader.

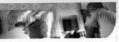

PROFESSIONAL PARAMEDIC

The corollary to the heat index is the wind chill chart. Paramedics consult the wind chill chart to determine the risk of frostbite, prompting people to respond by wearing extra thick gloves. Paramedics should consult the heat index to determine the risk of heat illness and respond accordingly as well.

STREET SMART

Consisting of lessons learned by the authors while in practice in the field, Street Smart tips focus on practical information that can help new Paramedic students perform in less-than-ideal or unusual situations.

STREET SMART

Football players—particularly linemen who have repeated impacts to their head—have experienced traumatic brain injury, despite the use of helmets. In some cases, the injuries have resulted in death.

CULTURAL/REGIONAL DIFFERENCES

Important considerations are noted for responding to patients of different cultural backgrounds. This prepares students to serve the diverse patient population that the Paramedic will encounter in emergency situations. Understanding these cultural/regional differences will increase the Paramedic's effectiveness in the field.

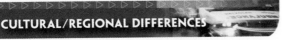

CULTURAL/REGIONAL DIFFERENCES

The Dead category has also been the basis of misinterpretation by the public. The deaths of a number of patrons at a night club in a predominantly ethnic neighborhood caused a public uproar following reports that the fire department was refusing to treat patients because of their ethnic origins. In reality, it was a misunderstanding based on terminology.

STEP-BY-STEP SKILLS

Photos and descriptions are combined to present critical information on the fundamental skills of Paramedic practice. Each Skill is included at the end of the chapter to avoid interrupting the flow of learning, and is referenced in the applicable discussion within the chapter.

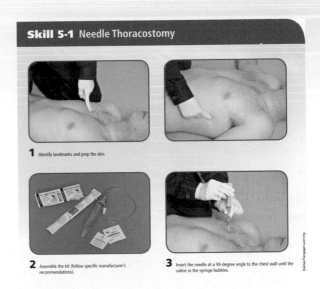

Skill 5-1 Needle Thoracostomy

1 Identify landmarks and prep the skin.

2 Assemble the kit (follow specific manufacturer's recommendations).

3 Insert the needle at a 90-degree angle to the chest wall until the saline in the syringe bubbles.

CONCLUSION AND KEY POINTS

Critical points included in the chapter are covered and provide a basis of review for the student. Whereas the Conclusion provides an overall summary of the chapter's main theme, the Key Points provide a bulleted list of important information that is helpful for study or review.

REVIEW QUESTIONS

Questions at the end of each chapter are helpful for evaluating student knowledge of the concepts presented in the chapter.

CASE STUDY QUESTIONS

Following the Review Questions at the end of each chapter, the Case Study Questions focus on the Case Study that is presented within each chapter. The Case Study Questions encourage learners to take a step back and review the entire case from chief concern to disposition.

REFERENCES AND AN EVIDENCED-BASED APPROACH

Validation is essential to ensure the content discussed is substantiated by science and medicine. Each thoroughly researched chapter includes documentation of references that support the content presented in the chapter.

REFERENCES:

1. Davis DP, Hoyt DB, Ochs M, et al. The effect of Paramedic rapid-sequence intubation on outcome in patients with severe traumatic brain injury. *J Trauma.* 2003;54:444–453.
2. Robertson C. Desaturation episodes after severe head injury: influence on outcome. *Acta Neurochirurgica Supplementum.* 1993;59:98–101.

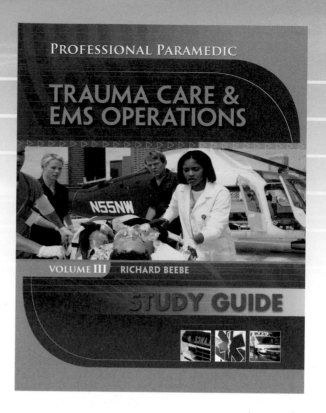

THE *PROFESSIONAL PARAMEDIC SERIES* CURRICULUM PLAN

We are proud to present a robust curriculum plan for the Paramedic student and instructor. As part of this plan, we offer resources that work hand-in-hand with each volume in the series, serving to further enhance both the teaching and the learning experience. For the students, resources are available that will help them review important concepts through practical application, develop and practice critical-thinking skills, and guide them toward further research and discovery. For the instructors, we offer tools that will help them efficiently prepare for classroom instruction, manage and track student progress of didactic and skill requirements, keep informed of new advances in the EMS field, and overall, engage students in learning both in and out of the classroom.

FOR THE STUDENT

STUDY GUIDES

Bridging the gap between knowledge and application, one *Study Guide* accompanies each volume to offer students additional case studies for each chapter, along with multiple types of practice questions and activities required for comprehension of the material.

- Volume I Study Guide, ISBN: 978-1-4283-2346-9
- Volume II Study Guide, ISBN: 978-1-4283-2352-0
- Volume III Study Guide, ISBN: 978-1-4283-2349-0

ONLINE COMPANIONS

Students are provided with FREE access to our website with an Online Companion that accompanies each volume. This website invites students to further study and explore the concepts presented in each volume. The Online Companion includes articles and up-to-date information on the EMS field, related links to important industry organizations and resources, information related to national guidelines, illustrated glossaries, and bonus content. Each Online Companion is uniquely designed to the corresponding volume in the series, and contains information relevant to the topics covered within that volume.

Visit http://www.cengage.com/community/ems to access these Online Companions!

FOR THE INSTRUCTOR

INSTRUCTOR RESOURCES (CD-ROM)

Our Instructor Resources for each volume are designed to help you effectively prepare students to become well-rounded, street-smart Paramedics within the guidelines of the new National EMS Educational Standards. The Instructor Resources on the CD-ROM include tools that help instructors and administrators prepare their Paramedic program

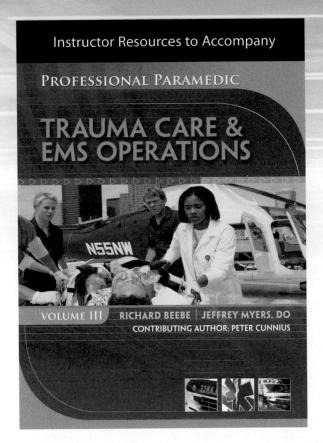

Instructor Resources to Accompany

PROFESSIONAL PARAMEDIC

TRAUMA CARE & EMS OPERATIONS

VOLUME III   RICHARD BEEBE | JEFFREY MYERS, DO
CONTRIBUTING AUTHOR: PETER CUNNIUS

in a timely and efficient manner. Each CD-ROM includes the following features:

■ **Administration:** This section includes information on setting up the program, as well as practical advice for transitioning your program to the new National EMS Educational Standards. In addition, it includes the following tools:

● **Equipment Checklist:** The Equipment Checklist provides a resource for instructors to ensure that they have the necessary tools for classroom instruction and for setting up and running skill sequences.

● **Concept Maps:** Highlighting the decision-making process, these Concept Maps offer a way for instructors to help students conceptualize ideas in the classroom and help them develop the critical-thinking skills necessary for determining a field diagnosis. Each Concept Map, utilizing a typical emergency scenario, walks students through the critical-thinking steps used during an EMS response.

● **Correlation to National EMS Education Standards and D.O.T. Paramedic Curriculum:** These guides map out Paramedic content and indicate the volume, chapter, and pages where this content is covered in the *Professional Paramedic Series*.

■ **Lesson Plans:** These Lesson Plans—which include an outline of each chapter, with correlations to the accompanying PowerPoint© presentations, skill sheets, and helpful teaching tips—provide a helpful guide for classroom instruction. These are provided in Word format so that instructors may revise them according to local practice variations and regional/state medical protocols.

■ **PowerPoint© Presentations:** Correlated to the accompanying Lesson Plans, these presentations combine key points with photos, graphics, and video to serve as a basis for either interactive classroom instruction or as augmentation of an asynchronous distance learning program.

■ **Computerized Test Banks:** Containing over 1,000 questions and covering the content in each chapter, these Test Banks in ExamView format allow instructors to manage test administration in the classroom. Instructors may create or edit tests based on existing questions, edit questions, and add or delete questions to fit local practice variations and regional/state medical protocols—all in this user-friendly program.

■ **Teaching Sheets:** Highlighting the Paramedic skills necessary for Paramedic practice, these Teaching Sheets provide a baseline for skills learning. Each Teaching Sheet provides a breakdown of the critical principles for the skill, and is included in Word format to allow instructors to add specifics based on their local requirements and/or regional/state protocols and procedures.

■ **Clinical Logs:** Based on the Teaching Sheets, these Clinical Logs provide forms for tracking student accomplishment of prehospital (field) and in-hospital (clinical) skills. These forms, complete with a signature page, are provided in Word format to allow instructors to edit them in order to meet local requirements.

■ **Research and Discovery-Instructor Reference Guide:** Paramedicine, like medicine, has an ever-changing body of knowledge. To remain current, the Paramedic must be a life-long learner. In addition to the listing of references that appears at the end of chapters in each volume in the series, this Instructor Reference Guide provides additional resources—including articles, websites, organizations, and other reference materials—to find information on specific topics. This ensures that instructors remain informed of current practices in the EMS field.

ONLINE COMPANIONS

Linked to the student Online Companions, these resources provide instructors FREE access to bonus content, articles on new information and technology, links to EMS community websites, information related to national guidelines, and additional classroom materials. Each Online Companion is uniquely designed to the corresponding volume in the series, and contains information relevant to the topics covered within that volume.

WEBTUTOR ON WEBCT AND BLACKBOARD

Providing a content-rich, Web-based teaching and learning aid, this tool helps to emphasize and clarify complex concepts, provides a forum for discussion, and offers a venue for tracking course syllabus and other program-related activities.

The WebTutor on Blackboard Course allows instructors to quickly and easily jump-start their on-line course development. Whether you want to Web-enable your class or put an entire course on-line, WebTutor delivers!

ABOUT THE AUTHORS
RICHARD BEEBE, MSED, BSN, RN, NREMT-P

Richard Beebe started his EMS career as an Explorer Scout with the Moyers Corners Volunteer Fire Department in upstate New York in 1974. Since obtaining his Emergency Medical Technician certification in 1975, Mr. Beebe has continuously maintained his certification and his practice. During his career, Mr. Beebe has served in fire/EMS, commercial EMS, volunteer EMS, and as a municipal Paramedic. During that time, he has served as a volunteer crew chief, a squad captain, and a Paramedic supervisor. Mr. Beebe currently serves as a civilian Paramedic for the Guilderland Police Department, outside of Albany, New York.

Mr. Beebe has also been a critical care nurse since 1985, having practiced for 10 years in both the Emergency Department and the Intensive Care Unit. During these years, Mr. Beebe developed his knowledge of medicine and—perhaps more importantly—an appreciation of the potential impact that prehospital advanced life support can have on patient morbidity and mortality.

Consistent with that belief, Mr. Beebe became a Paramedic in 1988 and, in hopes of advancing the practice of his fellow Paramedics, started his career as a Paramedic Educator.

During his tenure as a Paramedic Educator, Mr. Beebe has served in the capacity as lecturer, instructor-coordinator, and Paramedic program director. He continues to speak at local, regional, state, and national conferences on topics of importance to both the EMT and the Paramedic.

Mr. Beebe is presently Associate Director of Education at Mohawk Ambulance Training and Education Center, located in the New York capital district, and owner of MedicThink, LLC, a private education and consulting firm.

Mr. Beebe has been published in several journals, including the *Journal of Emergency Medical Services and Fire-Engineering*, as well as being a co-author for Delmar/Cengage Learning's *Fundamentals of Basic Emergency Care*, now in its third edition.

Mr. Beebe has contributed to the previous editions of the National Standard Curriculum for Paramedic, Intermediate, and Basic; contributed to the national EMS Education Agenda for the Future; contributed to the national EMS Scope of Practice; and served as content leader for the National EMS Education Standards. Mr. Beebe is also a charter member of the National Association of EMS Educators.

For questions or inquiries, please go to Mr. Beebe's website (http://medicthink.com) or e-mail him at MedicThink@gmail.com.

JEFF MYERS, DO, EDM, NREMT-P, FAAEM

Dr. Myers has been involved in EMS for more than 20 years, including 12 years of active duty in the prehospital environment and over 18 years as an EMS educator. Dr. Myers began his EMS journey in 1988 in upstate New York by volunteering for his college ambulance (RPI Ambulance) and a local community ambulance (North Greenbush Ambulance Association). He began teaching in 1990 for the Rensselaer County Ambulance and Rescue Association, eventually becoming a state-certified instructor coordinator. Dr. Myers ran the EMT-Basic original course in Rensselaer County for three years before leaving to attend medical school. During the early 1990s, he also served as a Deputy County EMS Coordinator in Rensselaer County for four years, responding to multi-ambulance and multi-agency incidents. His field experience includes volunteer, commercial, and combination paid-volunteer agencies as a Paramedic in upstate New York and in southern Maine.

Dr. Myers attended medical school at the University of New England College of Osteopathic Medicine in Biddeford, Maine. While in medical school, he continued to teach fellow students, ACLS and BCLS classes through the local hospital, and Paramedic students.

Dr. Myers then moved to Buffalo, New York, completing his residency in Emergency Medicine at the State University of New York at Buffalo in 2004. In his final year of residency he served as Chief Resident. He stayed in Buffalo for a two-year EMS Fellowship through the Erie County Medical Center and completed a Masters in Education at the University at Buffalo. He is board certified in Emergency Medicine and a Fellow of the American Academy of Emergency Medicine.

He is currently on faculty at the State University of New York at Buffalo as a Clinical Assistant Professor and serves as the Associate System EMS Medical Director and EMS Fellowship Director at the Erie County Medical Center. Dr. Myers is an active member of the Specialized Medical Assistance Response Team, western New York's physician response team, which is called upon to augment local EMS in MCIs, assist in special situations, and provide tactical medical support. He recently became the Medical Director for the Paramedic program at the Erie Community College and is also Director of the Behling Simulation Center at the University at Buffalo, an interprofessional simulation center that brings together students from all health professions.

Dr. Myers has several publications in peer-reviewed journals and is an author for Delmar/ Cengage Learning, writing *Automated Defibrillation for Professional and Lay Rescuers* and *Principles of Pathophysiology and Emergency Care*. He also produced and directed the *Techniques in Airway Management* DVD series. Dr. Myers has spoken at several regional and national conferences on a variety of topics.

For more information on topics or to provide feedback on the textbook, please check out Dr. Myers' website at http://www.photoemsdoc.com.

ACKNOWLEDGMENTS

As with all of our projects, the *Professional Paramedic Series* would not have been possible without the support, guidance, and participation of the contributors, reviewers, and advisory board members. We owe these individuals our sincere thanks.

CONTRIBUTORS

For the development of *Volume III: Trauma Care & EMS Operations*, we were honored to have the following contributors participate in researching, writing, editing, and reviewing materials to ensure a comprehensive and accurate Paramedic guide.

Zachary Bair, DO, Attending Physician, Emergency Department, Banner Desert Medical Center, Mesa, AZ

Kyle David Bates, MS, NREMT-P, CCEMT-P, FP-C, Paramedic, Town of Tonawanda Police Emergency Medical Unit, Tonawanda, NY

Anthony Billittier IV, MD, Commissioner of Health, Erie County, NY; Assistant Professor Emergency Medicine, Department of Emergency Medicine, School of Medicine and Biomedical Sciences; Assistant Professor, Department of Social and Preventative Medicine, School of Public Health and Health Professions, State University of New York at Buffalo

Paul Bishop, MPA, NREMT-P, CIC, Program Coordinator, Monroe Community College, Rochester, NY

John Bray, BS, NREMT-P, CCEMT-P, EMS Operations Manager, New York Downtown Hospital, New York, NY

Kerry Cassel, MD, Clinical Assistant Professor Emergency Medicine, Erie County Medical Center and Buffalo General Hospital; Associate Director, Ultrasound Fellowship

Sonia Chacko, MD, Albert Einstein Medical Center, Department of Emergency Medicine, Division of Disaster and Prehospital Medicine, Philadelphia, PA

Dave Dalrymple, Executive Educator, Roadway-Rescue LLC, Clinton, NJ

Col. (ret) William Dice, MD, Clinical Assistant Professor of Emergency Medicine, University at Buffalo, State University of New York, Buffalo, NY

Deborah Funk, MD, FACEP, Assistant Professor/ Attending Physician, Department of Emergency Medicine, Albany Medical Center Hospital, Albany, NY

Abigail Harning, EMT-P, MEd, Associate Professor, Erie Community College, State University of New York, Buffalo, NY

Clark E. Hayward, EMT-P, AWLS, Director, Founder, Adirondack Wilderness Medicine, Wilderness, EMS, Rescue Medicine Training

Nadine Levick, MD, MPH, Research Director, EMS Safety Foundation; Chair, National Academies Transportation Research Board, EMS Safety Subcommittee; Chief Executive Officer, Objective Safety

Mike McEvoy, PhD, NREMT-P, RN, CCRN, EMS Coordinator, Saratoga County, NY; Clinical Care Associate Professor, Critical Care Medicine, Albany Medical College, Albany, NY

Kevin R. McGee, DO, EMT-P/FF, Clinical Assistant Professor of Emergency Medicine, University at Buffalo, School of Medicine and Biomedical Sciences

John Pryor, MD (Deceased), Assistant Professor of Surgery, University of Pennsylvania, Division of Trauma, Philadelphia, PA

Tammi Schaefer, DO, FAAEM, Assistant Professor of Emergency Medicine, University of Colorado-Denver, School of Medicine, Aurora, CO; Rocky Vista University College of Osteopathic Medicine, Parker, CO; Attending and Core Faculty, Medical Toxicology, Rocky Mountain Poison and Drug Center-Denver Health, Denver, CO

Jeffrey Thompson, MD, Attending Physician, Professional Emergency Services and Clinical Instructor of Emergency Medicine, State University of New York at Buffalo, Buffalo, NY

Captain Steve Treinish, Lead Instructor, Dive and Rescue Team, Columbus Ohio Fire Department, Fairfield County Special Operations Dive Unit, Columbus, OH

Robert Waddell, II, BS, BA, EMT-P (ret), Vice President, Think Sharp, Inc., Cheyenne, WY

For the development of the art program in this volume—the countless hours spent in preparation, set up, and shooting of the photography appearing in this book, as well as the extensive research, persistence, and acquisition of those "hard to find" photos and graphics—we express our gratitude to the following individuals:

Jon Behrens, AAS, EMT-P, Paramedic Instructor, State University of New York at Cobleskill

Liana Dypka, Art Manuscript Development

Mike Gallitelli, Photographer, Metroland Photo, Inc.

Dawn Jacobson, Photo Acquisition and Permission Coordinator

REVIEWERS

To the reviewers, who provided an honest evaluation of the content in the book and continual guidance throughout development of this volume, we express our appreciation:

Greg LaMay
Education Coordinator, ETMC-EMS, Tyler, TX

Mike McLaughlin
Director of Health Occupations, Kirkwood Community College, IA

M. Jane Pollock
Extension Education Training Specialist, Emergency Medicine, East Carolina University, NC

Jason Segner
Program Director, EMS Education, Blinn College, TX

Mike Ward
Director of Emergency Health Services, George Washington Medical Center, Washington DC

EMS ADVISORY BOARD

We offer special thanks to our Advisory Board Members, who take time out of their schedules to advise us on our training materials, the status of the EMS field, and to work with us as partners in striving to meet the needs of the students and instructors of today—and those of the future.

Scott Bourn, National Director of Clinical Programs, National Resource Center, American Medical Response, CO

Deb Cason, Associate Professor, University of Texas Southwestern Medical Center, TX

Don Collins, Captain, Massport Fire-Rescue, Logan International Airport, Boston, MA

Stephen Dean, Director, Corporate Training, Paramedic Plus, OK

Joe Grafft, President, Customized Safety Training

Art Hsieh, Chief Executive Officer and Director of Education, San Francisco Paramedic Association, CA

Mike Kennamer, Director of Workforce Development, Northeast Alabama Community College, AL

Guy Piefer, Paramedic Program Coordinator, Borough of Manhattan Community College, City of Yonkers Fire Department, NY

Ed Racht, Chief Medical Officer, American Medical Response

Karla Rickards, EMS Training Coordinator, Unified Fire Authority, Salt Lake County

John Rinard, Training Coordinator, TEEX, Texas A&M University

John Sinclair, Fire Chief, Kittitas Valley Fire Rescue; Emergency Manager, City of Ellensburg, WA; Immediate Past Chair and International Director, International Association of Fire Chiefs, Emergency Medical Services Section

Mike Ward, Director of Emergency Health Services, George Washington Medical Center, Washington DC

FROM THE AUTHORS

BEEBE

First, I would like to acknowledge my friends and family, and particularly my wife Laura, whose support has sustained me over the 10 years that it took to write this book. Thank you for your love.

I would also like to thank the professionals at Delmar/Cengage Learning who have helped support this idea from its onset and continue to encourage me to greater accomplishments. I would like to thank Sandy, Benj, Erin, and, particularly, Jennifer, the backbone of this excellent team.

Finally, I would like to thank my students who, each and every year, challenge me to be the best Paramedic that I can be and the best educator that I can be and who, even to this day, continue to inspire me. In the 30-plus years I have been involved in EMS and EMS education I have truly seen EMS in general—and Paramedics in particular—evolve into a caring profession that we all can be proud of.

MYERS

Thanks and love to my family. This textbook (and all my life's projects) would not be possible without their support.

DELMAR/CENGAGE LEARNING TEAM

For the team that always finds a way, every day, to turn an idea into a reality, we thank these extraordinary people for their hard work, dedication, support, and creativity:

Janet Maker, Senior Acquisitions Editor

Jennifer Starr, Senior Product Manager

Amy Wetsel, Editorial Assistant

Jennifer Hanley, Senior Content Project Manager

Benjamin Gleeksman, Art Director

Erin Coffin, Senior Marketing Manager

Shanna Gibbs, Associate Marketing Manager

CLOSING THOUGHTS

In a time when the importance of quality improvement is understood and appreciated, we encourage students and instructors alike to communicate with us. Via these conversations, all parties can improve their understandings. We are all enriched through this communication.

Richard W. O. Beebe
MedicThink@gmail.com

Jeffrey W. Myers
http://www
.photoemsdoc.com

SECTION 1

TRAUMA CARE

Providing care for an injured patient is one of the foundations of EMS, and stems from the 1966 white paper, "Accidental Death and Disability: The Neglected Disease of Modern Society." Trauma care is considered one of the essential aspects of paramedicine, as a significant percentage of the calls requiring a Paramedic response will be due to trauma. In this section, trauma care is presented as it relates to various body systems, with each chapter covering the care of life-threatening injuries as well as minor trauma related to that system. The section culminates in a discussion of pediatric trauma considerations and an overview of trauma resuscitation. This overview combines data from all of the individual chapters to create a comprehensive approach to the treatment of the critically injured patient.

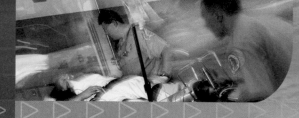

CHAPTER 1

TRAUMA OVERVIEW

KEY CONCEPTS:

Upon completion of this chapter, it is expected that the reader will understand these following concepts:

- That trauma is a devastating and potentially preventable condition
- The dramatic impact trauma systems can have on morbidity and mortality
- The ways field triage optimizes a patient's chance of survival
- How mechanism of injury and kinematics lead to a predictable injury pattern
- How laws of physics affect kinematics

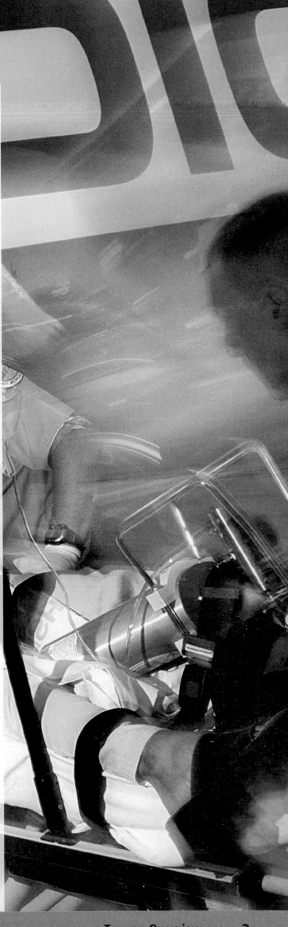

CASE STUDY:

The explosion that came from the port was deafening and could be heard for miles around. Almost as deafening is the sound of sirens, bells, and pager tones. It seems like everyone from the fire chief to the postal carrier is being called to respond.

The explosion came from inside the building that controlled the catalytic "cracking" process at the petroleum plant. Somewhere something failed, placing the rows of gas tanks in the "tank-farm" in danger. Nevertheless, the scene is deemed "safe for now," and EMS is being dispatched for a reported man down.

As the Paramedic approaches the scene and witnesses the chaos unfold, she stops to think, "If someone can survive a blast this big, what kind of injuries will he have?"

CRITICAL THINKING QUESTIONS

1. What are some of the possible injuries that may be suspected based on the mechanism of injury?
2. Are any of these injuries potentially life-threatening injuries?

OVERVIEW

Trauma is defined as an injury caused by exposure to excessive physical forces such as mechanical forces, heat and cold, electricity, chemicals, and ionizing radiation.[1,2,3] Trauma also occurs when essential substances are withheld from the body. An example is when a person is deprived of oxygen as in drowning, strangulation, and carbon monoxide poisoning.[1,4] Although many do not think of cold as something that causes trauma, hypothermia results in injuries such as frostbite.[1,4,5] Chemicals can cause injury via liquefaction necrosis or coagulation. In addition, the effects of electricity and radiation on the body are well known.

Injuries can be caused intentionally or unintentionally, and wounds produced by trauma can be either penetrating or blunt.[4,5,6] Penetrating injuries are caused when a projectile or other sharp object breaks the skin's integrity and enters the body, making contact with internal organs and tissues. The object sometimes becomes impaled or is retained as a foreign body. In other cases, the object creates an exit wound as it leaves the body.[4,6] Blunt trauma is defined as an internal injury caused by any force that does not result in penetration through the skin and into the body.[4,6]

According to the federal Centers for Disease Control (CDC), unintentional injuries are currently the leading cause of death for people under the age of 35 in the United States, and remains within the leading nine causes of death throughout a person's lifetime.[1,2] Homicide ranks within the top nine causes of death for ages 1 to 64, peaking as the second leading cause of death in people ages 15 to 24.[2,6] Suicide is the third-leading cause of death for people ages 10 to 24 and remains in the top eight-leading causes of death through age 64.[2] To demonstrate the prevalence of trauma, as many as 40% of emergency transports to the emergency department are for injured patients.[3]

In addition to the suffering caused by injury- and trauma-related deaths, trauma causes heavy financial burdens that are passed on to taxpayers.[4,5,6] These costs not only include patient care and rehabilitation, but also lost productivity when injuries make it impossible for the patients to provide for themselves and their families.[4,5,6] The loss of productivity accounts for as much as 70% of society's cost for trauma, with total annual costs estimated at over $200 billion.[4,5]

Injury Prevention

Over 50% of trauma deaths occur outside of the hospital, before EMS arrives on-scene or during treatment and transport to the emergency department. Although injuries have historically been perceived as an act of God or as unpreventable accidents due to bad luck, those assumptions don't hold true.[4,5,6] In actuality, like other conditions such as infection, injuries are impacted by demographic distributions, predictable seasonal patterns, epidemic episodes, and risk factors.[4,5,6] As with diseases, trauma injury is preventable (Figure 1-1). The best opportunity to save trauma patients is through the delivery of effective injury prevention programs.

A risk factor is a behavior or condition that increases an individual's likelihood of developing a condition, such as an injury.[4] Evaluation of risk factors brings awareness of the causes of injuries and allows people to prevent injuries in two ways. The first is through better engineering of products and roadways, using these engineering safety modifications to reduce the risk of injury. Examples of engineering designs that have dramatically reduced injuries include vehicle crumple zones designed to dissipate energy during an impact and automatic shutoff systems for lawnmowers and tractors in the event the operator falls off.[4,7,8] The second way is through alteration of behaviors that place individuals at higher risk.

Some examples of behavior modification techniques include public education to reduce driving while impaired by

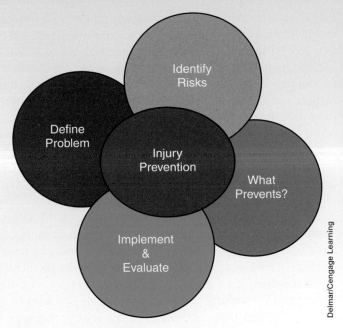

Figure 1-1 Trauma is preventable.

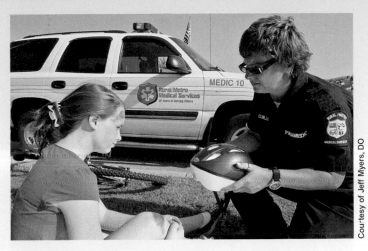

Figure 1-2 Take advantage of teachable moments after close calls.

alcohol, improving compliance with the use of safety devices such as seat belts or protective devices designed for use while operating machinery, and using protective gear before participating in extreme sports.[4] A recent study showed that helmet use during motorcycle accidents dramatically reduced the cost of trauma and the severity of injuries suffered.[9] This highlights the importance of helmet legislation, as well as other injury prevention programs, in reducing healthcare costs to society.[9] These are just a few examples from a long list of compelling problems.

STREET SMART

Despite evidence to the contrary, several states have repealed their helmet laws for motorcyclists. Undoubtedly those states will see an increase in the costs of trauma-related health care for motorcycle crash patients.

Paramedics are given the opportunity to assess risk factors in the patient's environment that can lead to serious trauma. Paramedics enter the patient's home during an emergency, providing the Paramedic an opportunity to observe the patient's ordinary living conditions.[4,6] Threats inside the home a Paramedic may recognize include a lack of smoke detectors, throw rugs that increase the risk for geriatric falls, and inadequate childproofing.[5]

Although patients are often evaluated for their risk of medical conditions (e.g., hypertension for stroke or cigarette smoking for heart attack), their environment is rarely assessed for risks that may lead to serious injury.[4] Paramedics responding to the home, for example, have narrowly escaped personal injury.[4,6]

The Paramedic can assess the patient's use of situation-specific safety devices, such as helmets while bicycling, protective padding while playing sports, occupant restraints while riding in a motor vehicle, and body armor when in a tactical situation.[4,5] When an injury occurs, the Paramedic can take advantage of this teachable moment to instruct the recently injured patient and his family about injury prevention. A discussion at that particular moment might leave a greater lasting impact on the patient than a random lecture (Figure 1-2).[4,6]

Trauma often results when someone performs a task poorly.[4,5,6] Small children often attempt to do tasks they are not physically prepared to safely accomplish. Therefore, they must have adequate supervision to reduce the risk of injury.[4,5,6] Patients who have neuromuscular diseases, those who have had a stroke, or those with diminished motor skills from other causes are at risk of injury from a fall.[4,5,6] Impaired mental status due to the use of alcohol or drugs can also result in poor task performance and lead to injury (e.g., drunk driving resulting in motor vehicle collisions).[4,5,6]

The environment in which an activity takes place can contribute to the risk of injury. Poorly maintained roads, sharp curves, inadequate lighting, and rough terrain increase the risk of crashes and subsequent injuries while operating a motor vehicle. Injuries due to motor vehicle collisions (MVCs) have been reduced through improved road design and engineering.[5] One example is the use of rumble strips. In Delaware, the Department of Transportation installed centerline rumble strips on Route 301, a rural route two-lane highway with a notoriously high accident fatality rate. The year after they installed rumble strips, the accident rate on that highway decreased by 90% with no traffic fatalities (Figure 1-3).[7,8] The New York State Thruway experienced an 88% reduction in "run off the road accidents" and a 95% reduction in fatalities after installing rumble strips along the shoulders.[8] Virginia experienced a reduction of over 50%

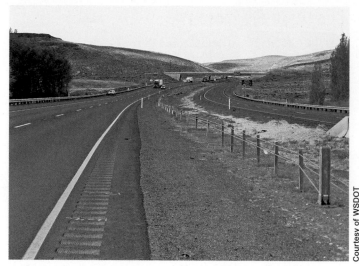

Figure 1-3 Centerline and shoulder rumble strips have dramatically reduced the number of highway fatalities.

Courtesy of WSDOT

in "run off the road" accidents and estimated the rumble strips saved 52 lives between 1997 and 2000. These examples show that simple and inexpensive structural changes in road construction can dramatically reduce the rate of serious collisions.[8]

The **Haddon matrix** (Table 1-1) is used to illustrate factors contributing to the outcome of an event that leads to an injury and illustrate that injuries are a result of many factors, not just random events.[4] In the Haddon matrix, three rows list the phases of an event: pre-event, event, and post-event.[4,10] Four columns contain information concerning the host, vector or agent, physical environment, and sociocultural environment.[4,10]

The pre-event evaluation can reveal factors that inhibit or contribute to an accident, such as incapacitation by alcohol or drugs, poor maintenance of roads or vehicles, or environmental conditions such as poor weather and rough terrain.[4,10] Pre-event factors that may reduce or prevent injury include the use of occupant restraints, wearing protective garments and helmets, and developing better engineering with safety as a goal.[4,10] During the event, safety engineering such as the use of guard rails and vehicle crumple zones are designed to dissipate energy and reduce injury.[4,10] Post-event factors include knowledge of first aid, extent of injuries, and ability to rapidly access emergency medical services.[4,10] Results of the event include environmental damage, property damage, physical injury, lost productivity, and costs due to the incident.[4,10] The host is the person at risk of injury.[10] The agent is energy that is transmitted to the host through a vehicle (inanimate object) or vector (person or animal).[10] The physical environment includes characteristics of the setting where the accidents take place; for instance, a road, building, or playground.[10] The social environment refers to social and legal norms and practices as they relate to the accident.[10] In other words, if an organization fails to comply with the latest OSHA standards because they've always worked a certain way, and that contributed to the injury, that would create a social environment. Some other examples are police departments that are reluctant to wear body armor and fire departments that are reluctant to use self-contained breathing apparatus and full turnout gear during some fire operations (Figure 1-4).

Information gathered in the Haddon matrix is invaluable when developing prevention strategies tailored to specific epidemiologic problems.[4,10] Primary injury prevention is aimed at stopping the event from ever occurring.[4,5] Primary prevention strategies include public education and legislation aimed at altering behaviors such as making drunk driving a crime and encouraging seat belt use.[4,5] Secondary injury prevention is aimed at minimizing further injury or death following an injury event.[4,5] Airway management and immobilization of potential injuries are examples of secondary injury prevention carried out by Paramedics.[4]

There are three modes for primary prevention: education, enforcement, and engineering.[4,5] Education programs are aimed at changing behaviors by making individuals aware of risks and actions they can take in their home, workplace, and

Table 1-1 The Haddon Matrix for Near Drowning

	Host	Agent	Physical Environment	Social Environment
	Person	Water	Pool, lake, or beach	Community or home
Pre-event: Before submersion	Pool safety education; swimming lessons; feet-first programs	Water depth	Pool cover; four-sided pool fence; swimming warning signs at beaches	Boating and swimming regulations; adult supervision; lifeguard actions
Event: Submersion	Host's physical condition; wearing a life jacket; alcohol consumption	Water temperature; water currents	Dual pool drains; pool depth; pool alarm	Buddy swimming; lifeguard present
Post-event: Near drowning	Physical condition of the host; alcohol intoxication	Temperature, depth, and clarity of the water	Location of life preservers, boats, ropes, resuscitation equipment, cellular phone	Emergency medical services; community cardiopulmonary resuscitation (CPR); 9-1-1 services; cellular services

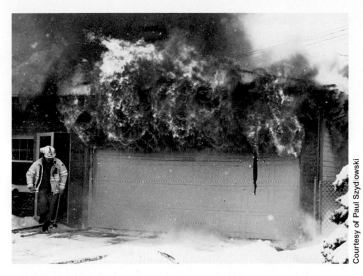

Courtesy of Paul Szydowski

Figure 1-4 Workplace patterns of behavior can promote risk taking, but those cultures can be changed.

while in transit to decrease the risk of injury.[5] The downside of education is that it relies on individuals to change habits that are sometimes difficult to break; for example, staying dedicated to medication compliance or post-MI rehabilitation.[5] Fines, penalties, and even imprisonment can be used to elicit a greater and more rapid change in behavior.[5] Although some people argue that this infringes on individual rights, the justification for such laws may lie largely in financial burden on society when serious injuries or death occur.[5]

Engineering may be the most effective form of injury prevention because it does not rely on individuals to change personal behavior patterns.[5] The downside is that engineering changes can potentially add sizable cost to products.[5] Examples of innovations designed to prevent injury include the automatic shutoff for tractors and riding lawnmowers in the event the operator falls off; automatic shutoff and blade guards for power tools; rumble strips and reflective dividing line markers for roadways; and needleless drug injection systems. Other safety mechanisms include airbags, three point seat belts, and properly installed child restraint devices. Today, even playgrounds are built with both fun and safety in mind, with safety engineered into swings, slides, and the like.[4,6]

Prehospital care providers have the opportunity to play a vital role in injury prevention as respected and credible members of the healthcare system.[4,6] This can be done through public education at safety booths at fairs, ambulance tours at schools, and safety awareness demonstrations during public events. The time spent providing care for patients who are not severely injured is an ideal time to counsel the patient and family members about safety. Paramedics can also become spokespersons for injury prevention at community events. By providing accurate documentation of the events surrounding an injury, Paramedics are taking part in injury surveillance.

Trauma Systems

Early in the history of modern EMS, people recognized that patients would be better cared for in hospitals that specialized in trauma care. In order to accomplish this goal, the federal government took a regional approach to develop systems whereby an injured patient could move rapidly from anywhere in the region to a trauma center.

Trauma System Development

The 1966 report "Accidental Death and Disability: The Neglected Disease of Modern Society," also known as "The White Paper," resulted in the passage of the Highway Safety Act of 1966.[5,11] The focus of this act was to guide the development of emergency services; improve equipment, communication, and transportation; and develop training standards.[11] "The White Paper" recognized accidental death as an epidemic requiring action on the part of public health officials and the development of an emergency medical response system.[5,11] As emergency systems started to evolve in the 1960s and 1970s, ambulances transported seriously injured trauma patients to the nearest hospitals.[11] Unfortunately, many trauma patients died due to a lack of consistent trauma services at the nearest receiving hospital.[12] That would later change with the development of trauma care systems.

The Trauma Care Systems Planning and Development Act of 1990 defined the components of a trauma system and designated funding between 1992 and 2005 for the development of trauma systems.[13–17] A **trauma system** integrates local, regional, and state resources for preventing injury, treating trauma patients, providing rehabilitation services, collecting data on trauma for research, and improving quality. All of these efforts set a goal of improving patient outcomes.[11,13–17] The Trauma Care Systems Planning and Development Act of 2007 restored the funding provided by the 1990 act. It also expanded reporting requirements, authorized allocation of funding with grants aimed at projects that may improve rural EMS communications systems and integration with the state EMS systems, promoted data collection in a more standardized manner, and ensured the timely dissemination of information.[13,15]

The 2007 act gave funding priority to nonprofit and public agencies that were compliant with required reporting and that used the grants to focus on improving access to trauma care systems.[13,15] Preference was given to applicants whose system used national standards for designating trauma centers, recognized protocols for the delivery of seriously injured patients to trauma centers, had a process for evaluating the performance of the trauma system, and agreed to participate in specified information systems by collecting, providing, and sharing information.[13,15]

Trauma Center Designation

As a component in the development of trauma systems, the American College of Surgeons (ACS) has published national standards for **trauma center** designation.[18,19] Many states have adopted the ACS criteria, although others have developed their own criteria, and others still lack established trauma center designation criteria.[18,19] The ACS has defined criteria for trauma center designation in four center levels—Levels I–IV. The following is not a comprehensive description, as the criteria required is too detailed to cover here.[18,19] Level I Trauma Centers must be able to provide 24-hour in-house general surgical intervention as well as specialty care in orthopedic surgery, neurosurgery, emergency medicine, radiology, internal medicine, and critical care.[18,19] In addition, the Level I Trauma Center must be prepared to handle most specialty trauma, including burns, eye injuries, hand injuries, and vascular injuries.[18,19] In addition to patient care, the Level I Trauma Center must provide leadership in injury prevention and public education, continuing medical education for all members of the emergency medical team, comprehensive quality assessment, data collection, and research.[18,19]

The Level II Trauma Center criteria include 24-hour immediate care by trauma surgeons, as well as specialty care in orthopedic surgery, neurosurgery, emergency medicine, radiology, internal medicine, and critical care.[18,19] Tertiary care such as cardiac surgery, microvascular surgery, and hemodialysis may be referred to a Level I Trauma Center.[18,19] The Level II Trauma Centers' role in providing education and research as a teaching hospital may be more limited than at a Level I facility. However, a commitment to injury prevention and dedication to improving trauma care through a comprehensive quality assessment program must be present.[18,19]

Level III Trauma Centers must have 24-hour coverage by emergency medicine physicians with prompt availability of general surgeons and anesthesiology.[18,19] Level I and II Trauma Centers must have surgical capability within 15 minutes, with compliance at least 80% of the time.[18] Level III Trauma Centers are allowed a 30-minute surgical response with 80% or more compliance.[18] Level III Trauma Centers must be involved in injury prevention and outreach education, and must participate in a comprehensive quality assessment program.[18,19] A transport plan and agreement must be in place to rapidly provide for the transfer of patients requiring additional services at a Level I or Level II Center.[18,19]

Level IV Trauma Centers provide 24-hour emergency department facilities with the ability to implement Advanced Trauma Life Support (ATLS) protocols and 24-hour laboratory coverage, with transfer protocols and formal transfer agreements for patients requiring a higher level of care.[18,19] A Level IV Trauma Center must participate in injury prevention and outreach education within its community, demonstrate a commitment to continued improvement, and maintain a formal quality assessment program including prehospital quality improvement.[18,19]

The Pediatric Trauma Center Designation is defined for Level I and Level II Trauma Centers dedicated to the special needs of pediatric patients and caring for a large population of pediatric patients on a routine basis.[18,19] Criteria for Pediatric Trauma Centers is similar to criteria for other trauma centers; however, they more specifically address the unique needs of the pediatric population.[18,19]

Trauma Registry and Prehospital Trauma Research

Trauma registries provide trauma-related data from prehospital care records and hospital trauma data.[4,6,20] Today, through the use of data captured by the trauma registries, continuous quality improvement processes and clinical research are occurring that will allow for refinements of, and improvements in, the field triage process.[5] Trauma registries are vital to the advancement of trauma triage, trauma system planning, and medical research.[4,6,20] The ACS has developed the National Trauma Data Bank® (NTDB), which contains over two million cases from over 600 U.S. trauma centers.[21] The NTDB is believed to be the largest aggregation of trauma registry data ever assembled.[21] Trauma data is vital to epidemiology, injury prevention, research, education, acute care, and resource allocation.[20,21]

A 2006 paper by Dr. Henry, the New York State EMS Medical Director, highlighted the difficulty in evaluating trauma triage criteria with data provided from prehospital care reports. He stated the mechanism of injury was often underreported or unreported.[22] Dr. Henry pointed out the need to develop structured trauma data fields with trauma center criteria to improve reporting by prehospital providers and increase the amount of useful, quality data available for research and system quality improvement.[22] On the surface, the completion of additional data fields may seem to be burdensome to field providers, However, there are far reaching benefits of data collection, including the validation of EMS system contributions to overall trauma patient survival and recovery.[4,6,21]

It is vital that data is accessible from all phases of trauma care, including prehospital EMS, hospital care, rehabilitation, discharge, and medical examiner reports.[21] The data needs to be readily linked to create a trauma system registry of data.[21] To achieve this, software solutions are being developed and field tested to allow widespread linkage of data sets.[4,6,21] Electronic patient care reports may enhance rapid and effective data collection in the future while lessening the documentation burden for Paramedics.[4,6,21] The **National Emergency Medical Services Information System (NEMSIS)** is establishing standards for EMS data collection to maintain a national EMS dataset collected from all states on a limited number of data elements.[20,21] This data will be housed at the National Center for Statistics and Analysis.[20]

Field Triage

Triage is defined as the process of sorting patients to prioritize their need for care when resources are limited.[4,6] During the triage process, patients are not treated on a "first come first serve" basis, but instead in the order determined to be most appropriate based on available resources.[4,6] Field triage is also used to determine the most appropriate destination hospital for the patient.[4,6] Local protocols should address appropriate destination facilities within the region and transport decision criteria.[4,6]

The goal of getting the highest priority patients to the nearest appropriate facility as expeditiously as possible is best met when the region's resources are clearly defined within the EMS protocols.[23,24] The primary goal of field triage is to decrease disability and death resulting from injuries by determining the best way to "get the right person to the right place at the right time."[12,25]

In the late 1700s, Baron Jean Dominique Larrey (Figure 1-5) said, "Those who are most dangerously wounded should receive the first attention, without regard to rank or distinction," contrary to the custom of the day.[25] This may be the first documented recognition for the need to develop a medically based field triage system.[25] Since then various schemes using physiologic parameters, anatomical assessment findings, and mechanism of injury have historically served to aid in field triage. These triage schemas were historically developed from opinions based on anecdotal experience.[12,22,25] Today, with the application of scientific knowledge, the parameters used for field triage criteria are being refined and improved.[12,22,25,26] A discussion of triage systems utilized for multiple-casualty events and disasters can be found in Chapter 23. The remainder of this discussion will focus on determining the most appropriate destination for an injured patient.

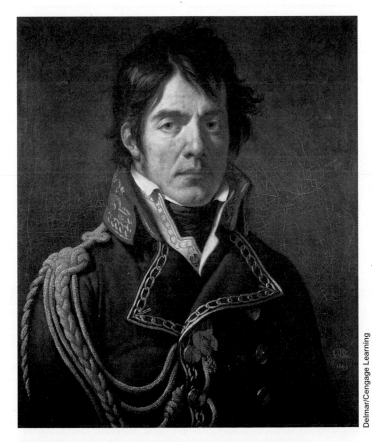

Figure 1-5 Baron Jean Dominique Larrey documented the first known triage efforts during the Napoleonic Wars.

Information applied to field triage decisions must include the initial exam findings, baseline vitals, mechanism of injury, and availability of resources.[23,27] Combining these parameters improves predictability significantly over the use of any one parameter alone.[23,27–29] Special considerations that must be weighed in triage decisions for the trauma patient include the patient's age, general health, and coexisting conditions such as pregnancy and burns.[4,6,30] Patients with these conditions have a greater risk of a poor outcome and therefore demand higher prioritization.[4,6] In 1987, the ACS first published a **field triage criteria**, an algorithm that included anatomical issues, physiological issues, and mechanism of injury as decision parameters designed to aid Paramedics in making treatment and transportation decisions for injured patients.[3,5,12,25,26] Additionally, this is the first field triage algorithm known to have addressed comorbid factors such as geriatric and pediatric age groups.[25,26]

Changes in field triage schemes have been introduced in response to advances in medical treatment as well as evolving trauma systems.[25,26] During the Civil War, gunshot wounds to the extremities were prioritized whereas abdominal wounds were deemed a lower priority due to a lack of capability to care for abdominal trauma and the realization that abdominal wounds were mortal.[25] Although mortality from extremity wounds during the Civil War was also high, amputation was a common life-saving procedure, making patients with limb injuries high priority for that era.[25] Certainly these priorities are no longer followed today. Field triage protocols must be dynamic and responsive to clinical research findings, advancements in medical care, and an awareness of organized and coordinated local and regional trauma resources.[25] Paramedics need to be prepared to embrace change as advancements in medical care come about.

Triage is an art that requires a great deal of clinical judgment. **Undertriage**, or underestimating the severity of trauma patients, is detrimental because seriously injured trauma patients will not receive vital trauma care services in a timely fashion.[12,22,25] The consequences of undertriage include increased morbidity and mortality.[12,22,25]

Overtriage, or overestimating the seriousness of a patient's injuries, may have similar negative effects on the provision of trauma care.[12,22,25] Overtriage results in an overwhelmed trauma system that becomes depleted of trauma resources, contributing to emergency department overcrowding, and resulting in unnecessary delays in patient care, especially for patients with non-life-threatening wounds.[12,22,25] Overtriage also results in greater out-of-service time for ambulances as they bypass nearer facilities to deliver their patients to trauma centers.[3,12]

Overtriage has economic implications as well. Overtriage causes local hospitals to be bypassed in favor of the trauma centers. These bypassed hospitals suffer negative economic consequences. As a result, small rural hospitals become less economically viable as more and more patients are transported to other facilities.[3,12] When patients with non-life-threatening wounds experience long delays before receiving treatment, recovery is often delayed, disabilities are more likely to result, and the quality of pain management often suffers.[12,22] Despite the problems associated with overtriage, the ACS states that an overtriage rate of 30% to 50% may be necessary to avoid otherwise preventable fatalities.[22]

In response to evolving trauma systems, expansion of air medical coverage, expanded EMS scope of practice, testing of existing field triage criteria, advancement of medical technology, and changes in law and policies (e.g., the Emergency Medical Treatment and Active Labor Act [EMTALA] and the Health Insurance Portability and Accountability Act [HIPAA]), the ACS implemented revisions to the field triage criteria in 2006.[26] The 2006 recommendations break field triage into a three-step process that addresses physiological findings, anatomical regions affected, and mechanism of injury (Figure 1-6).[26] Special considerations such as age and general health are also addressed in the ACS field triage criteria.[26]

Step one provides physiologic findings that should be given priority. The physiologic criteria include a Glasgow Coma Scale less than 14, systolic blood pressure less than 90, or a respiratory rate less than 10 or greater than 29 (less than 20 in an infant less than 1 year of age).[26] If any of the physiologic criteria listed is present, transport the patient to the highest level of care within the regional trauma system.[26] If none of the criteria are present, move to step two and assess the anatomical location of the injury.[26]

Anatomical criteria indicating the need to transport the patient to the highest level trauma center within the trauma system include penetrating trauma of the head, neck, torso, or extremities proximal to the elbow or knee; flail chest; two or more proximal long-bone fractures; a crushed, degloved, or mangled extremity; amputation proximal to the wrist or ankle; pelvic fractures; open or depressed skull fracture; and paralysis.[26]

Patients who do not meet the criteria for step one or two of the ACS field triage protocol should then be evaluated for the mechanism of injury criteria before the Paramedic determines the most appropriate facility for transport.[26] The following mechanism of injury criteria are considered indications for transport to the nearest appropriate trauma center, which may or may not be the highest level trauma center for the particular trauma system: falls of greater than 20 feet for an adult or 10 feet (or three times the child's height) for a child (one story of a house or floor of a building is typically about 10–12 feet high.); high-risk automobile crashes with greater than 12 inches of intrusion into the passenger compartment where the patient was seated or 18 inches of intrusion at any other site; partial or complete ejection from the vehicle; death of another occupant in the same passenger compartment; automobile versus pedestrian or bicyclist when the patient was thrown, run over, or faced a significant impact defined as greater than 20 mph; and motorcyclist crashes at greater than 20 mph.[26] Note that the rollover mechanism is not included in the mechanism of injury criteria because no correlation was found between rollover alone and the need

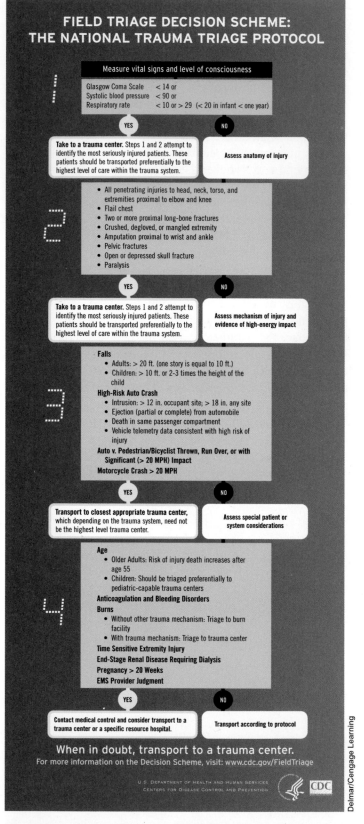

Figure 1-6 Centers for Disease Control (CDC) field triage criteria, 2006.

for trauma surgical intervention in the absence of confounding physiologic or anatomic criteria.[31]

Although mechanism of injury alone can be a determinant in the need to transport a patient to a trauma center, serious injury can occur in the absence of significant mechanism of injury.[4,6,26,27,32] Do not trivialize exam findings or patient complaints due to a seemingly insignificant mechanism of injury.[4,6,26,32] Remember to consider all field triage criteria before making a final triage decision.[4,6,26] Significant mechanism of injury alone requires transport to a trauma center, but if the findings of the initial exam and baseline vitals are within normal limits and there are no apparent life-threatening injuries, the patient should be transported to the closest appropriate hospital and not necessarily to the highest level trauma center in the system.[26]

In addition to considering physical exam findings and mechanism of injury, other special considerations should weigh in the field transport decision.[4,6,26] For example, older patients and very young patients are at greater risk of injury with less ability to compensate.[4,6,26] Risk of injury and death increases after the age of 55 due to a number of physiologic changes including decreased pulmonary function and loss of tissue elasticity.[4,6,26] Infants do not have fully developed compensatory mechanisms, and their disproportionately large head makes them more susceptible to head trauma.[4,6,26,29,33] Pediatric patients should be triaged to a pediatric-capable trauma center.[4,6,26,29,33] Other special considerations include the patient's general health, such as the use of anticoagulants or the presence of bleeding disorders and end-stage renal disease requiring dialysis.[4,6,26] Coexisting factors, including pregnancy greater than 20 weeks' gestation and trauma associated with burns, can threaten the patient's outcome.[4,6,26] Patients with significant burns should be triaged to a burn center. However, patients who have sustained burns in addition to significant traumatic injury must be triaged to the nearest trauma center.[4,6,26] Local or regional protocols should address appropriate facilities for transport when dealing with these special circumstances.

Initial field triage is always aimed at identifying potentially life-threatening conditions.[4,6,26] However, less seriously injured patients may also benefit from transport to a trauma center as it may improve their chances of recovery.[24,34] Time-sensitive extremity injuries, especially injuries resulting in neurovascular compromise, should be prioritized to follow immediately life-threatening injuries.[4] Unfortunately, transporting all patients to trauma centers would overburden Level I and Level II Trauma Centers and diminish outcomes for all patients.[6,24] If unsure about the proper destination, the Paramedic should contact medical control and discuss appropriate transport destinations.[4,6,26]

After immediate life threats have been identified and addressed, the second priority must be to prevent long-term disability due to injuries that require specialty care such as burns, musculoskeletal injuries with neurovascular compromise, and ocular injuries.[4,6,23,27] Neurological compromise should be suspected when a patient complains of paresthesia or paralysis.[4,6] Paresthesia is abnormal sensations such as tingling, numbness, burning sensation, and jolting pains caused by nerve injury.[4,6] Vascular compromise is a state of inadequate perfusion that can affect the entire body or localized regions of the body.[4,6] Cool, pale, or cyanotic skin, as well as weak or absent peripheral pulses, indicate inadequate perfusion to the region of the body affected.[4,6]

There is a need for more studies to determine how to improve outcomes from minimal injuries at receiving facilities other than trauma centers.[24] Triage schematics that triage non-life threatening injuries that can most benefit from trauma center treatment also need to be developed.[23] When faced with a transport decision for minimally injured patients, other considerations that must also be weighed include the patient's age, general health, and injuries requiring specialty care.[4,6,23,27]

The 2006 edition of the Centers for Disease Control trauma triage guideline reflects updated knowledge about the effect of the mechanisms that create injury, the consideration of comorbid factors, de-emphasis of medical control, and increased emphasis for relying on the judgment of Paramedics.[26] The 2006 revision also addresses the need to transport the patient to the nearest appropriate trauma center, which is not necessarily a Level I Trauma Center. These revisions are a reflection of improved injury surveillance data and analysis of data collected by trauma registries, making it the first trauma triage protocol to be published using clinical evidence.[26] Despite the incorporation of clinical research data into this algorithm, there is an acknowledgement for the need to continue clinical research to validate the protocol and to allow for future advancements.[26]

The final parameter is the Paramedic's gut instinct. A small subset of patients won't meet the criteria discussed in the algorithm. However, the Paramedic may be concerned about underlying injury, perhaps because the patient does not look well. If there is reason for doubt, err on the patient's side and transport to the trauma center or contact medical control for advice.[4,6,23,27,28]

Mechanism of Injury

Mechanism of injury (MOI) is the study of how specific forms of energy transferred to a patient can create predictable injury patterns (PIP).[5,6] The term "mechanism of injury" describes a group of principles that can be applied to predict the presence of life-threatening injuries, even when the injuries are not apparent externally.[4,6,23,27,28,30,35] Mechanism of injury is most relevant and accurate when it is applied as part of the entire clinical picture that includes physical findings such as vital signs, level of responsiveness, and other obvious physical exam findings. Inclusion of MOI in the assessment may lead the Paramedic to suspect internal injuries that are catastrophic and can lead to rapid deterioration of the patient's condition.[4,27] Principles described in this chapter will aid the Paramedic in identifying patients who are at risk of internal injuries when no external clues are evident.[4,6]

A growing knowledge of mechanism of injury can also be applied to the development of injury prevention programs and improvement of personal protection gear.[4,6] Documenting and reporting mechanism of injury serves two purposes: it helps to identify patients who require frequent reassessment and transport to a trauma center, and it can be applied in research used to prevent similar future traumatic events.[4,6]

Mechanism of injury is, and will remain, a vital part of the patient assessment, but it can no longer be looked at alone without other significant anatomical and physiological considerations.[4] Paramedics must understand the limitations of stand-alone assessment of mechanism of injury, as well as the benefits that come from considering MOI in the trauma patient's assessment.[4]

Although mechanism of injury is a critical tool in predicting the possible presence of occult life-threatening injuries, a seemingly insignificant mechanism of injury can also produce critical and life-threatening injuries.[4] Combining the assessment findings of the scene size-up, primary assessment, and secondary assessment allows critical clinical decision making before the patient's condition precipitously deteriorates.[4,6,36] The lack of significant mechanism of injury cannot be used to rule out the need for advanced life support (ALS) transport to the trauma center.[4] In fact, falls are the leading cause of accidental death in the elderly, with most fatal falls occurring from the standing position.[32]

Physics and Trauma

Mechanical, chemical, thermal, electrical, and barometric sources of energy produce different kinds of injury.[4,6] There are two forms of mechanical energy: kinetic energy and potential energy.[36] **Kinetic energy** refers to movement, as in the example of a vehicle driven down a road.[36] **Potential energy** is energy stored within a mechanical system ready to become kinetic energy. For falls, the potential energy depends on an object's mass and its distance above the ground (Figure 1-7).[36] As an example, a penny held over the edge of a tall building has greater potential energy than a penny lying on the ground.[36] Chemical energy is energy stored in the chemical bonds between molecules.[36] Explosions create pressure waves (i.e., shock waves) as a result of energy release when chemical bonds are broken.[36] Lightning strikes and electrocution are examples of injuries caused by electrical energy.[36] Barometric energy results from a change in pressure which can cause high altitude sickness and scuba-diving injuries.[36] Barometric energy is also responsible for injury caused by the pressure wave formed as high velocity bullets pass through tissue.[4,6,36]

A basic knowledge of physics is vital in understanding mechanism of injury. These basic principles, developed by Sir Isaac Newton, assist in understanding what happens when a body is subjected to falls, collisions, and other forces. Sir Isaac Newton's observations led him to develop three statements describing the movement of objects now known as **Newton's laws of motion**.[4,36] His first law of motion, called the law of inertia (Figure 1-8), states that *all objects remain in their state of rest, or in motion in a straight line, unless acted upon by an outside force.*[4,6] For example, a bullet is acted upon first by being propelled by a weapon, then by gravity as it travels through the air, and by objects it strikes along its

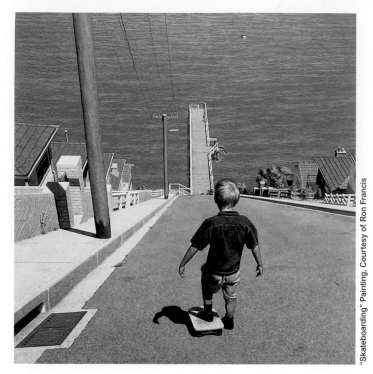

"Skateboarding" Painting, Courtesy of Ron Francis

Figure 1-7 The child in this picture has a significant amount of potential energy due to the height difference in the street.

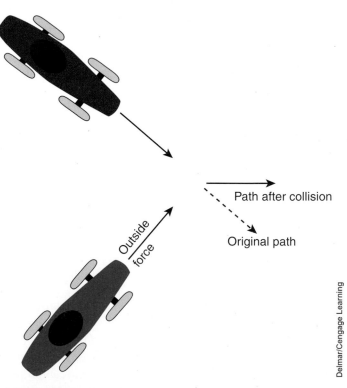

Delmar/Cengage Learning

Figure 1-8 The law of inertia observes that *all objects remain in their state of rest, or in motion in a straight line, unless acted upon by an outside force.*

path.[4,6] The motor vehicle demonstrates this law of motion when a stationary vehicle is struck from behind, propelling it forward until friction from the brakes stops it, or it is thrust against a stationary object.[4,6,36]

Newton's second law of motion states that *force is equal to the product of mass and acceleration* (Figure 1-9).[4,6,36] Force is defined as the amount of push or pull exerted on an object.[36] If a person is thrown through the air by a motor vehicle, the patient experienced greater force than a patient who was simply knocked to the ground and not thrown.[36] The force required to move the body a greater distance is the product of greater mass and greater acceleration.[36]

Newton's third law of motion states that *for each action there is an equal and opposite reaction.*[36] The third law of motion can be demonstrated by coup-contrecoup head injuries.[4,6,36] The force of the patient's head striking the windshield exerts force on the windshield, causing it to break. The windshield exerts an equal and opposite force on the skull, stopping forward motion of the brain, causing the brain to strike the opposite side of the skull.[4,6,36]

When force is applied to the body, the energy is dissipated among the body's tissues.[5,6] Younger patients and athletic patients have a greater ability to dissipate energy due to their improved flexibility and strength. Elderly patients have less tissue elasticity, less bone density, and decreased muscle mass, making them more susceptible to serious injury.[4,6] Very young children have greater flexibility of bone tissue, which is not fully calcified. This makes complete fractures less common, but provides less structural protection for organs in the chest and upper abdomen.[4,6] Exchanges of force and energy are external factors contributing to the severity of trauma.[4,6]

Velocity is the distance an object travels over time in a specified direction.[4,6,36] Acceleration is the rate of change in velocity. Although this term can mean any change in the velocity rate, both positive and negative, it is commonly used to refer to increasing velocity.[4,6,36] The term "deceleration" describes a reduction in rate of velocity.[36] Common causes of mechanical injury include rapid acceleration or deceleration that cause shearing forces on the body.[4,6] Gravity is downward acceleration due to the effects of Earth's mass, also referred to as a field of force.[9,36]

Kinetic energy is energy associated with movement of an object and is equal to one-half the object's mass multiplied by the velocity squared.[4,6,36] Increases in velocity are exponential and have a greater effect on kinetic energy than proportional changes in mass (Figure 1-10).[4,6,36]

Example 1:
vehicle mass = 3,000 lbs; vehicle speed = 30 mph
Kinetic energy = $3,000/2 \times 30 \text{ mph}^2 = 1,350,000 \text{ lbs} * \text{mph}^2$

Example 2:
vehicle mass = 6,000 lbs; vehicle speed = 30 mph
$6,000/2 \times 30 \text{ mph}^2 = 2,700,000 \text{ lbs} * \text{mph}^2$

Example 3:
vehicle mass = 3,000 lbs; vehicle speed = 60 mph
$3,000/2 \times 60 \text{ mph}^2 = 5,400,000 \text{ lbs} * \text{mph}^2$

This relationship of velocity to kinetic energy explains a small bullet's ability to cause lethal damage.[4,6] It is unlikely someone would be seriously injured if struck by a penny traveling at 15 mph. However, a bowling ball traveling at 15 mph could certainly cause devastating injuries. In terms of proportionate changes in mass versus velocity, an increase in speed results in a greater increase in kinetic energy than an increase in the object's mass.[4,6] The more massive an object and the faster it is moving in a direction, the greater the kinetic energy.[4,6] In comparison, a slow moving truck and a rapidly moving bullet could potentially have an equivalent amount of kinetic energy.[4,6]

Kinetic energy of a moving object must dissipate for the object to come to rest.[4,6,36] The more sudden that dissipation occurs, the more likely one is to incur an injury.[4,6] An example of slowing the dissipation of energy is laying a motorcycle down during an accident, dropping the bike horizontal to the

$$KE = \frac{\text{Mass} \times \text{Velocity}^2}{2}$$

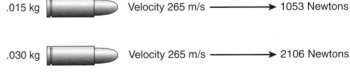

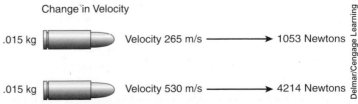

Figure 1-10 Effects of a change in mass and a change in velocity on kinetic energy.

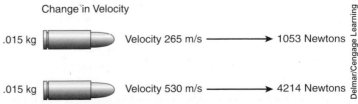

Force = Mass × Acceleration

Figure 1-9 Force equals mass × acceleration.

road to increase surface area to slow the bike.[4,6,36] Hypothetically, riders who are able to lay the bike down often suffer much less injury than riders who are ejected from the motorcycle.[4,6,36] Braking dissipates kinetic energy in a process that produces heat.[4,6] Crumple zones in cars are designed to allow energy to dissipate as steel bends.[4,6]

In a vehicle collision, the occupant's body is traveling at the same rate of speed as the vehicle.[4,6,36] When the vehicle is abruptly stopped by a collision with another object, such as a cement wall, the unrestrained body will continue to move forward until striking an object in its path.[4,6] Energy from the vehicle is transferred to the body as it impacts the vehicle's interior.[4,6] Specific types of body collisions produce predictable injury patterns and must be evaluated as part of the overall patient assessment to determine the possibility for severe internal injuries.[4,6,23,27,36] The vehicle's interior must be assessed for damage, which is important in identifying significant forces involved during the collision. During the collision, body organs continue to move within the body's cavities, producing overstretching and shearing forces that result in internal injuries.

The direction of impact can greatly influence outcomes as well.[4,6] Rear-end collisions are typically not as deadly as head-on collisions, for one because front-end collisions with another vehicle often combine speeds whereas rear-end collisions do not.[4,6] During a blast, the position of the patients in reference to ground zero contributes to their probability of severe injuries and survival.[4,6] Patients who are facing away from the blast and parallel with the ground receive less energy because less surface area of their bodies is facing the pressure wave.[4,6]

The duration of exposure to energy is best illustrated in terms of the length of exposure time to a thermal, chemical, or electrical energy source.[4,6] During mechanical energy exchanges, the more surface area energy is dissipated across, the less likely it is to cause serious injury or penetrating trauma.[4,6] If a woman is wearing narrow heels, the heel of her shoe is more likely to sink into the ground and leave an indentation as energy dissipates downward than if she were wearing flat-soled footwear.[4,6] This principle is applied to many devices designed to protect people from injury.[4,6] Crumple zones, airbags, and seat belts allow the vehicle to absorb and dissipate energy to objects other than the vehicle's occupants and slow the transfer of energy to the body.[4,6] Body armor dissipates a bullet's energy and slows its speed while causing the bullet to expand and increase surface area contact, decreasing the likelihood of penetrating trauma.[4,6] Helmets, sport pads, turnout gear, and earplugs are all examples of devices used to dissipate energy, slow the transfer of energy, and prevent injury.[4,6]

Exposure to energy can be acute (immediate) or chronic (repetitive over time). In an acute exposure, a single event (such as a bomb blast) leads to injury. An example of chronic energy is a stress fracture. Stress fractures are caused by cumulative exposure to repetitious energy on the legs over time, such as running or jumping on a hard surface. Many work-related injuries suffered by Paramedics are related to chronic exposure to energy that stresses the body over an extended period of time until symptoms of injury occur.

The density of body organs is also a factor and is related to the organ's consistency (i.e., if it is gas filled, fluid filled, or solid).[4,6] Lungs and intestines are gas-filled organs, which makes them more susceptible to tearing and shearing from compression forces of a pressure wave but more forgiving of penetrating trauma.[4,6] Liquid-filled organs are less compressible and more likely to rupture than air-filled spaces.[4,6] Solid density in the human body is present mostly in bones such as the cranium.[4,6] If a bullet penetrates the cranium, but does not exit the other side, its energy will dissipate only as the bullet travels inside the cranium, causing further tissue damage.[4,6]

The density of organs fluctuates with bodily functions.[4,6] If blunt force is applied to the lower abdomen, the urinary bladder is at much greater risk of rupture when it is full compared to when it is empty.[4,6] If a patient reflexively takes a deep breath just before sustaining blunt trauma to the chest, there is an increased risk of pneumothorax or bronchial tree injury due to the sudden increase in intrathoracic pressure that occurs as the force is applied to the chest.[4,6] This mechanism is similar to expanding a brown paper bag with a breath, closing the bag tightly, and then striking it with the other hand, causing the bag to rupture as the pressure within the bag suddenly increases.[4]

Although mechanism of injury alone cannot definitively determine the severity of injury, it raises the index of suspicion that serious injury may have occurred when high amounts of energy are exchanged with the body.[4,6]

Certain injuries may prove to be associated with a greater risk of life-threatening injuries.[4,6,23,27–30,32–34,37,38] In one study, 44% of patients with serious hand injuries also had life-threatening injuries, with the most common associated organ injuries being to the head and chest.[34] Unbelted vehicle occupants who used arm resistance during the crash had an increased risk of significant cervical spine injuries and associated hand, arm, and shoulder injuries.[35] Paramedics must consider how energy is transferred and dissipated through the patient's body.[4,6,27,28] By following the path of energy exchange, signs of occult life-threatening injuries may be detected sooner, with more appropriate triaging of the patient.[4,6]

Blunt Trauma

As mentioned previously, **blunt trauma** is defined as an internal injury caused by any force that does not result in penetration through the skin and into the body.[4,6] Because injuries due to blunt mechanisms often leave the skin intact, external evidence of internal injuries is frequently absent in the first minutes and hours following an accident.[4,6] Periorbital ecchymosis (raccoon eyes) and occipital ecchymosis (Battle's signs) are signs of a basilar skull fracture that typically do not develop for several hours following an accident.[4,6] Recognizing that the patient suffered significant force to the head helps Paramedics keep a high index of suspicion for significant head trauma, and directs the Paramedic to reassess the patient frequently for changes in clinical status that indicate a possible basilar skull fracture.[4,6]

Automobile accidents account for the greatest number of unintentional fatalities due to blunt trauma.[4,6] Assessment of a motor vehicle collision scene should begin by observing damage to the exterior and interior of the vehicles and other objects struck by the vehicles involved.[4,6] It is also important to determine if occupant safety devices (i.e., seat belts and airbags) were used correctly, as they are designed to dissipate energy from the collision and prevent the secondary impact of the patient striking against the inside of the vehicle.[4,6]

The road and the vehicle's exterior should be evaluated.[4,6] The longer the skid marks, the more energy was dissipated before the collision—although this estimation is less accurate than in the past due to the development of anti-skid braking systems and vehicle stability control systems.[4,6] Debris along the road may indicate multiple collisions.[4,6] Determine how much deformity to the vehicles occurred from the collision and whether the damage clearly indicates the type of collision.[4,6] For example, damage to the roof and hood and blown out windows suggest the vehicle rolled over.[4,6]

When assessing the vehicle's interior for damage that can be related to potential patient injuries (Figure 1-11), look for a starred/spider or outwardly bowed windshield to alert you to possible head trauma and cervical spine injuries.[4,6] A bent steering wheel or column is often associated with soft-tissue neck trauma, chest trauma, and abdominal trauma.[4,6] Dashboard damage may indicate pelvic fractures, hip and knee dislocations and fractures, and femur fractures.[4,6] A collapsed seat can indicate lumbar spine trauma and intra-abdominal injuries.[4,6] The patient's position in relation to the vehicle's damage may also provide an indication as to the potential for injury.

Common Injury Patterns by Type of Collision

Motor vehicle collisions are classified by the angle of impact as head-on collisions, rollovers, lateral collisions, rotational collisions, or rear impact collision.[4,6] Motor vehicle collisions are additionally described as occurring with ejection or without ejection.[4,6] The injury patterns described in the following collision classifications are consistent with that of an unrestrained occupant.[4,6]

Head-On Collisions

In instances where a head-on collision occurs between two moving vehicles, kinetic energy is calculated using the sum of the velocity for both vehicles.[4,6] In a rear-end collision of two vehicles, the kinetic energy of the collision is determined using the difference between the velocities of both vehicles.[36] By observing injury patterns and the vehicle's interior damage as well as determining the use of occupant restraint systems, it is possible to determine the pathway the patient's body traveled during the collision.[4,6,33,35] Unbelted occupants or occupants wearing only a shoulder harness without a lap belt often take the down-and-under pathway or the up-and-over pathway.[4,6]

In the **down-and-under pathway**, the occupant's lower body travels under the dashboard (Figure 1-12).[6,30] The occupant's face, head, neck, and chest are susceptible to injuries when colliding with the steering wheel and column.[4,6] Pelvic fractures, hip and knee dislocations and fractures, femur fractures, and lower extremity trauma are common due to this pathway.[4,6] Knee imprints in the dashboard often indicate life- or limb-threatening pelvic, hip, and femur injuries.[4,6]

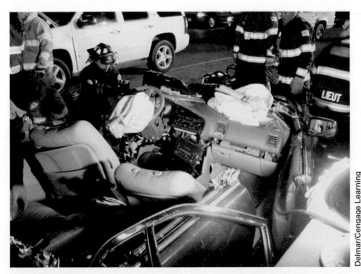

Figure 1-11 The vehicle's interior must be assessed for damage to determine energy transfer during the body collision.

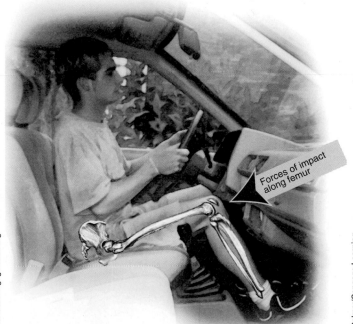

Forces of impact along femur

Figure 1-12 Down-and-under pathway injuries occur when a patient's body travels under the dashboard.

In the **up-and-over pathway**, the patient's head leads as the body travels toward the windshield, steering column, and dashboard (Figure 1-13).[4,6] As the head impacts the vehicle's interior, injury occurs to the head and frequently to the spine due to axial loading, hyperextension, or hyperflexion of the neck (Figure 1-14). Other injuries due to the up-and-over pathway include soft-tissue injury of the anterior neck, potentially leading to airway compromise; chest trauma; and abdominal trauma.[4,6] Chest injuries include tension pneumothorax, hemothorax, pulmonary contusion, flail chest, rib and sternal fractures, ruptured aorta, myocardial contusion, and pericardial tamponade.[4,6] The kidneys, liver, and spleen are at risk of vascular injury due to rapid deceleration and compression forces.[4,6]

Rollovers

An unrestrained occupant in a rollover collision is subjected to multiple angles of impact within the car and an increased risk of ejection from the vehicle.[4,6] In contrast, restrained occupants are protected from most impacts and are not likely to be ejected when the lap belt and shoulder harness are used correctly.[4,6,30]

There is no single predictable injury pattern for rollover events.[4,6] Assuming the vehicle's roof has adequate structural support to prevent collapse, occupants sometimes escape the crash with minor injuries because the vehicle dissipates the energy without transferring it to the occupant as the vehicle rolls to a stop.[27] Internal organs are subjected to shearing forces, even in restrained occupants.[4,6] Axial loading, compression along the long axis of the body, occurs when the vehicle's roof collapses, leading to head and spinal trauma (Figure 1-15).[4,6]

Lateral Impact

Lateral impact, also called T-bone or side impact, delivers the most energy to the same-side occupant.[4,6] Seat belts are designed to protect the occupant from forward movement due to rapid deceleration, but provide little protection during a lateral impact. Crumple zones allow for energy to dissipate

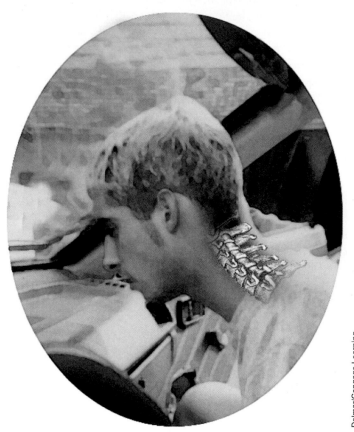

Figure 1-14 Head injury due to impact with the windshield frequently causes axial loading to the cervical spine.

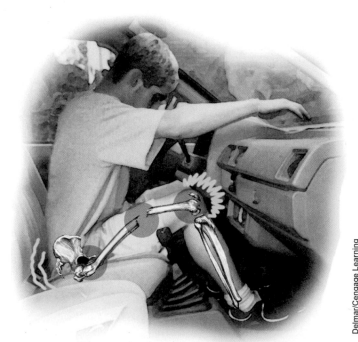

Figure 1-13 Up-and-over pathway injuries result from the body moving toward the windshield and steering column.

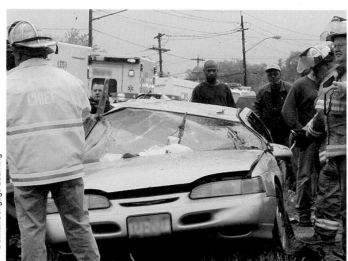

Figure 1-15 Look for signs of vehicle rollover that may indicate axial loading injuries.

into the front end of vehicles, but side impacts do not obtain the same protection.[4,6]

The force of lateral impact pushes the car out from under the occupant, causing rotation or hyperextension of the neck.[4,6] Intrusion of the vehicle door more than 12 inches has the potential to cause serious injuries to the occupant of that compartment due to a lack of crumple zones or side door protection.[4,6] Injuries are predominantly on the ipsilateral, or same, side of the impact and injure organs on the same side as the impact.[4,6] Passenger-side occupants are at risk of liver injury, whereas driver-side occupants are at risk of spleen injury. The kidneys are susceptible either way.[4,6] Occupants on either side of the vehicle are also at risk of impact side injuries to the extremities, clavicle, chest, and pelvis.[4,6] Contralateral, or opposite, side injuries occur when the occupants collide with each other, or objects, within the vehicle.[4,6]

Lateral collision fatalities are most often due to head and chest injuries, with head injuries due to impact with the vehicle's B-pillar (Figure 1-16).[38] Deformity of the B-pillar should be specifically documented along with any additional indication that the head was struck on the B-pillar.[4,6,38]

Vehicles equipped with side curtain airbags provide greater protection from lateral impacts; however, not all cars have this feature.[4,6,37] Side curtain airbags are located on the outboard edge of the seatback, door, or roof rail above the door.[37] They provide upper body protection, as well as head protection in models with extended airbags.[37] However, close proximity to a deploying airbag can result in injury.[4,6,37] Occupants should not lean against the door or lean against the seat when in the front seat.[30,37]

Rotational Collisions

Rotational collisions occur when a vehicle is struck on one of four corners, causing it to spin.[4,6] The greatest occupant injuries will be suffered when the vehicle suddenly decelerates.[4,6] The vehicle's continued motion dissipates energy without transferring energy to the occupants. However, secondary collisions are common as the vehicle spins out of control.[4,6] Occupants are subjected to shearing injuries due to rapid acceleration–deceleration forces.[4,6] Diagonal movement of the occupants can result in collision with the rearview mirror, sun visor, or the A-post, which is the windshield's support structure.[4,6] Three-point restraints are often effective in preventing injury during rotational collisions.[4,6,30]

Rear Impact

When a vehicle that is stationary or traveling at a slow rate of speed is struck from behind, the impact causes sudden acceleration force.[4,6] If the occupants are properly restrained and headrests are positioned at the occiput of the occupant's head, the chances of fatalities and serious injuries are greatly reduced.[4,6,30] However, unrestrained occupants and occupants whose heads are not supported by the headrest are subjected to substantial forces.[4,6] The patient's head will hyperextend as the body moves forward, then snap forward with hyperflexion of the neck.[4,6] As the chest moves forward, the head can hyperextend again.[4,6] This type of injury is referred to as whiplash.[4,6,35] During rear impact, the seat may collapse, increasing the risk of lumbar spine and intra-abdominal injuries.[4,6] It is vital to document the use of occupant restraints, the position of the headrest, and the condition of the seatback when caring for patients who were involved in rear-end collisions.[4,6,35]

Ejection

Partial or complete ejection from a vehicle is one of the most catastrophic types of MOI.[4,6,39] In fact, ejection was the cause of death for 25% of all vehicular fatalities in 2002.[6,39] During 2003, SUVs were the vehicle type with the highest rate of ejection fatalities, with a 65% fatality rate.[39] During and after ejection, the patient is subjected to multiple secondary impacts, and is often crushed by the vehicle before being thrown against terrain or becoming susceptible to impact with oncoming traffic.[4,6] When partial ejection occurs, limbs or sections of the body can be pinned or crushed beneath the overturning vehicle.[4,6] Due to multiple impacts, ejection has a significantly greater fatality rate than other MOI.[4,6] However, ejection is easily preventable with the proper use of occupant restraints.[4,6,39] In 2003, only 6% of fatal ejection patients were using occupant restraints at the time of collision.[39]

To reduce ejections, medians are placed on highways. Medians between opposing directions of traffic are designed to prevent front-end collisions, which are typically more deadly than other types of collisions, due to the increased risk of ejection and combined velocities of both vehicles.

Occupant Restraint Systems

Vehicle occupant restraints hold the patient in the seat within the vehicle compartment throughout a collision as energy dissipates, significantly reducing the risk of serious injury or death.[4,6,40] Occupant restraints reduce the risk of ejection and

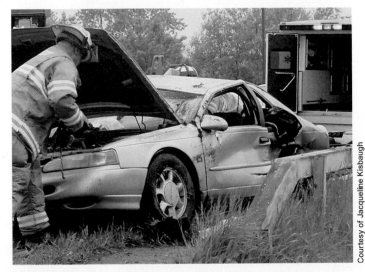

Figure 1-16 Document a deformity to the B-pillar.

Courtesy of Jacqueline Kisbaugh

significantly reduce the number of fatalities and serious injuries.[4,6] When a three-point restraint system is correctly used, life-threatening injuries are less common.[4,6,40] In 2003, 57% of all traffic fatalities were unrestrained within their vehicles at the time of the collision.[39] In restrained patients, clavicle fractures are one of the most common injuries and occur at the point where the shoulder harness crosses over the clavicle.[4,6] Unfortunately, serious injuries can still occur, even when restraints are used properly.[4,6,30,33]

Organ collision will occur in a high energy deceleration crash regardless of the use of occupant restraint systems, and can result in life-threatening internal injuries even when restraints are worn correctly.[4,6] It is always important to determine if occupant safety restraints were used and whether the restraints were used correctly since these do dramatically change anticipated injury patterns.[4,6,39-41]

Lap belts must be worn directly over the iliac crests.[4,6] If worn too high or too loosely, they contribute to abdominal and lumbar spine injuries and rupture of the diaphragm.[4,6] If worn too low, lap belts can contribute to dislocated hips and fractured femurs.[4,6] A lap belt worn without a shoulder harness causes the body to bend forward at the hips after impact, leading to facial, neck, and head injuries.[4,6] Some occupants place the shoulder belt underneath their arm instead of across the clavicle.[30] This disperses the energy directly into the chest and increases the risk of pulmonary and cardiac injury.[4,6]

Headrests should be raised or lowered to a height that supports the occiput, especially during a collision (Figure 1-17).[4,6,30] An improperly adjusted headrest increases the risk of whiplash injuries.[30,40] If the headrest is positioned too low, the head will hyperextend over the headrest, causing shearing and overstretching of ligaments and the spinal cord (Figure 1-18).[4,6] Double impacts, in which the impacted car is thrown forward following a rear-end collision and collides with another vehicle or object, have an even greater risk of injuries.[4,6]

Airbags are designed to provide additional protection to a belted adult driver or occupant.[4,6,37,40,41] They are extremely effective during the first collision, but do not provide protection for subsequent or secondary collisions because they deflate instantaneously.[4,6,41] Although airbags prevent major trauma, they are associated with common minor injuries that may require a Paramedic's attention.[4,6,41] Common injuries include abrasions on the arms, chest, and face; foreign bodies to the face and eyes, especially when eyeglasses are damaged; and superficial burns.[4,6] More serious injuries and fatalities can also occur, especially if seat belts are not used, the occupant is not in the correct seated position at the time of the collision, or if a small statured occupant is seated too close to the airbag when it deploys.[4,6,37] A distance of 10 inches or more between the occupant's sternum and the airbag cover plate is recommended by the National Highway Traffic and Safety Administration.[40,41] Occupants who fail to wear three-point restraints may follow the down-and-under pathway and experience blunt trauma as their body impacts the deploying airbag.[4,6,37,40,41] In the latter situations,

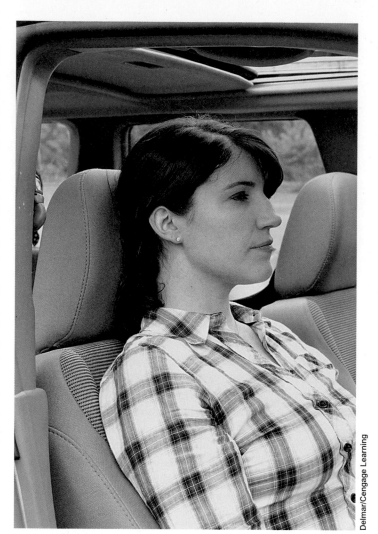

Figure 1-17 The proper headrest position will support the occiput during a collision.

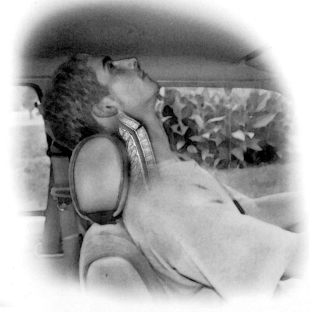

Figure 1-18 Headrests positioned too low or too distant from the occiput do not provide adequate protection from cervical spine injuries.

significant—and sometimes fatal—head, chest, and abdominal trauma have been documented.[4,6,37]

The Paramedic should lift up and look under the deployed airbag to assess the steering wheel's condition.[4,6,37] A deformed steering wheel is a sign that the patient may have serious internal injuries.[4,6,37] Injuries can also occur indirectly when the occupant is displaced from the seat by the airbag and strikes the vehicle's interior.[4,6,37]

The patient's position in the vehicle at the time the collision occurred is vital to document when it is possible to determine.[4,6,40,41] This is a common problem with children who have outgrown their safety seats, but have difficulty sitting still, even for short rides.[4,6,30,40,41] Occupants who are positioned improperly in their seat are more susceptible to injury because restraint systems are designed to best protect occupants who are properly seated.[4,6,30,41]

In children, there is an increased risk of abdominal and spinal injuries when seat belts are poorly fitted or not correctly positioned.[4,6,37,40] Due to the risk of ambulance collision during transport, pediatric patients should be transported in appropriate safety seats when possible. It is important that the ambulance and stretcher are designed for the safe transport of pediatric patients (Figure 1-19).[4,6,30,37]

Tractor Accidents

Tractors have a high center of gravity and are at higher risk of overturning compared with other vehicles.[4] Most tractor overturns occur to the side (85%), giving the occupant an opportunity to jump away and thus decrease the risk of getting pinned (Figure 1-20).[4] Rear overturns are more likely to trap the occupant since there is little opportunity to jump away from the tractor's path.[4] Crush injuries are common in tractor accidents. Crush syndrome is likely to result because the lone driver is unable to signal for help and remains trapped until found some time later.[4] Chemical and thermal burns may also occur due to gasoline or diesel fuel leaks, hydraulic fluid leaks, and battery acid in combination with hot engine surfaces.[4]

Small Vehicle Crashes

Many smaller motorized vehicles are used on land, on the snow, and in the water. These small vehicles present unique mechanisms and considerations when caring for injured patients from these collisions.

Motorcycles

Injuries to motorcyclists are affected by the same types of impact as occur in automobile collisions.[4,6] In a head-on impact, the motorcycle will tip forward as it rapidly decelerates, causing the occupant to travel into or over the handlebars.[4,6] This mechanism results in trauma to the body parts that impact the handlebars, pavement, or other objects.[4,6] If the feet remain on the pegs of the motorcycle as the occupant's body moves forward, bilateral femur fractures can occur as the thighs strike the handle bars.[6] Angular impact typically results in the occupant becoming pinned under the motorcycle, causing upper and lower extremity trauma.[6] Because the rider is unrestrained, there is a high risk of ejection from the vehicle.[4,6] This results in secondary impacts with the pavement, guardrails, on-coming traffic, and any other objects in the occupant's path.[6]

The Paramedics should document the type of collision, known secondary impacts, distance of skids, motorcycle deformity, deformity of objects the motorcycle collided

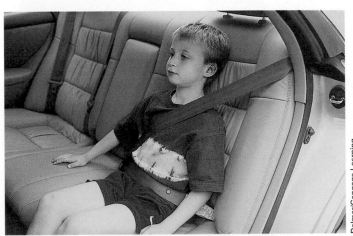

Figure 1-19 Proper seat belt positioning optimizes safety for children.

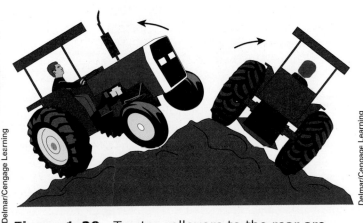

Figure 1-20 Tractor rollovers to the rear are more likely to cause entrapment than rollovers to the side.

with, and use of protective equipment.[4,6] Boots, leather clothing, and helmets offer limited protection to motorcyclists (Figure 1-21).[4,6]

By laying the motorcycle down before striking an object, the motorcyclist can separate from the bike and the object in an attempt to avoid collision.[4,6] Bone fractures on the side of the body that made contact with the roadside and massive abrasions are common injuries resulting from this evasive driving technique. In this situation, the Paramedic should transport damaged protective equipment with the patient to the emergency department.[4,6] Airbag vests and jackets are now available for motorcyclists (Figure 1-22).[4,6,37] These airbag garments are tethered to the motorcycle and trigger deployment if the motorcyclist is ejected.[4,6,37] These garments are intended

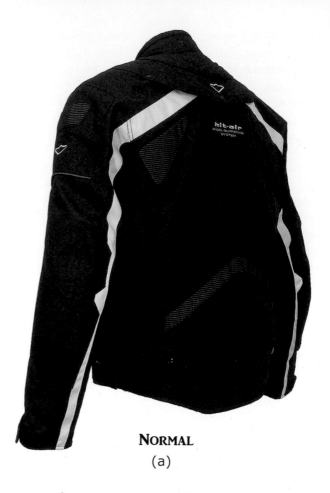

NORMAL

(a)

Courtesy of Bikebone.com

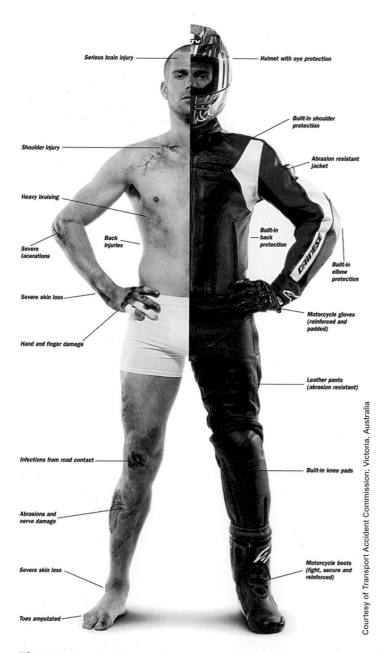

Courtesy of Transport Accident Commission; Victoria, Australia

Figure 1-21 Protective gear reduces the number and severity of injuries.

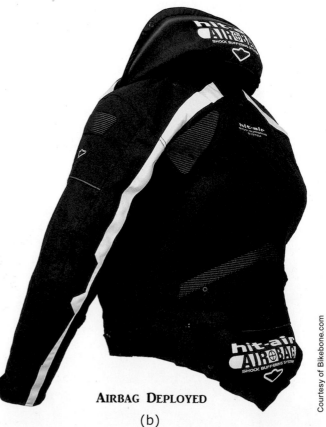

AIRBAG DEPLOYED

(b)

Courtesy of Bikebone.com

Figure 1-22 Airbag-equipped protective garments are now available.

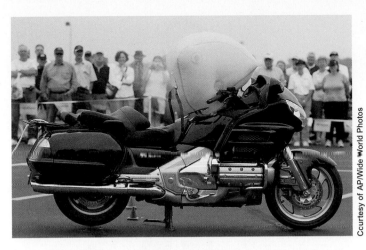

Figure 1-23 Motorcycles equipped with airbags may help to prevent ejection and reduce injuries.

to be reusable and are expensive.[4,6,37] Some motorcycles are currently being marketed with a front airbag (Figure 1-23).[37] Crash testing shows promise that the front airbag will prevent ejection and improve survival in head-on collisions.[37]

All-Terrain Vehicles

The three-wheeler has a high center of gravity and is prone to rollovers that pin the occupants.[4,6] Other types of injuries result from falling off the back of the all-terrain vehicle, injuries from forward deceleration and impact with other objects, and trauma to the rider's head and extremities when passing too close to other objects causes them to impact against those objects.[4,6] If the rider instinctively puts his foot on the ground to stabilize the vehicle or to help stop it, the foot may get caught by the rear wheel, throwing the rider forward off the vehicle. In this case, head and spine injuries, soft-tissue neck trauma, and extremity injuries are common.[4,6] Injuries due to environmental exposure may occur when the rider becomes stranded at the scene outdoors for an extended period of time before being found.[4,6]

Personal Watercraft

Injuries that occur while using personal watercraft cause 8.5 times the number of emergency department visits as the use of motorboats, and the death rate for personal watercraft collisions is about 3 times greater than for motorboats.[4,6] Injury patterns are similar to motorcycle injuries since the occupant in a watercraft is unrestrained and unprotected from ejection and secondary impacts.[4,6] When occupants fall backwards off the personal watercraft, rectal and vaginal trauma can occur.[4,6] An additional secondary injury risk is drowning.[4,6] Drowning can occur even with the use of a personal flotation device, particularly if the occupant loses consciousness.[4,6] However, the use of helmets and personal floatation devices may reduce the risk of drowning.[4,6]

Snowmobiles

Injuries due to snowmobile accidents are similar to those linked to all-terrain vehicles. However, the compact weight distribution of the snowmobiles makes crush injuries more likely.[4,6] Snowmobiles are lower to the ground, and thus increase the risk of hangman-type injuries that result from running into fence wires or clotheslines.[4,6] The Paramedic should be alert for soft-tissue injury to the neck, cervical spine injuries, and potential airway compromise.[4,6] Hypothermia is commonly associated with snowmobile crashes.[4,6]

Pedestrian Injuries

Vehicle impact speed is the single most important variable influencing the severity of injury in vehicle–pedestrian accidents.[4,33] Young children are more likely to suffer severe head, pelvis, and upper leg injuries and older children are more likely to suffer head and lower extremity injuries.[33] Bumper and hood height relative to the patient's height are factors affecting the mechanism of injury.[6,33] High vehicles impacting short pedestrians are more likely to result in the pedestrian being knocked to the ground and subsequently driven over, dragged, or pinned.[6]

Taller pedestrians struck by lower vehicles are more likely to be thrown onto the hood or clear of the vehicle (Figure 1-24).[4,6] Head injury, chest trauma, and lateral compression pelvic fractures are common when a pedestrian is thrown onto or over a vehicle.[4,6] When the bumper contacts a patient's legs, limb-threatening injuries may occur, including knee dislocation.[4,6] When a shorter pedestrian is struck, the injury pattern moves upward to include the abdomen, chest, arms, and head and spine (Figure 1-24).

Factors concerning the mechanism of injury that should be documented include the approximate speed the vehicle was traveling at when the pedestrian was struck; whether the pedestrian was thrown, dragged, or run-over; and the distance the pedestrian was dragged or thrown.[4,6] If the patient was thrown, it is also valuable to determine what type of surface the pedestrian landed on. Softer material (e.g., damp dirt, grass, or bushes) deform under impact and dissipate some of the kinetic injury, resulting in less severe injury than if the pedestrian landed on concrete or pavement.

Falls

The four factors that affect the severity of injury from a fall are the distance of the fall, the landing surface, the patient's position at impact, and the general health of the patient.[4,6] Injuries due to falls are caused by compression forces and rapid deceleration. It is uncommon for a patient to survive falls of greater than five stories. Falls from greater than three times the individual's height are most likely to cause serious injury or death, although seemingly insignificant falls, such as from a standing position, can also result in serious injury.[4,6]

Adults most commonly land on their feet after falling from a height. This mechanism has a predictable injury pattern of bilateral calcaneus fractures, leg fractures, hip and pelvic fractures, axial loading of the lumbar and cervical spine, and wrist fractures (Figure 1-25).[4,6] Vertical deceleration forces to the organs cause injury to the spleen and kidneys.[4,6] Infants and toddlers are more likely to fall head first

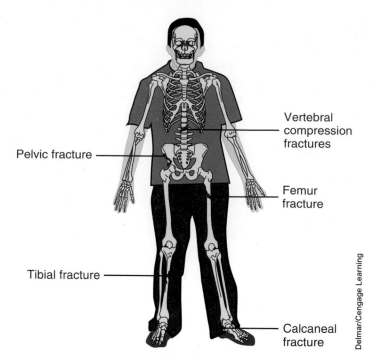

Figure 1-25 Fractures are commonly associated with a fall when the patient lands on both feet.

Vertebral compression fractures

Pelvic fracture

Femur fracture

Tibial fracture

Calcaneal fracture

Delmar/Cengage Learning

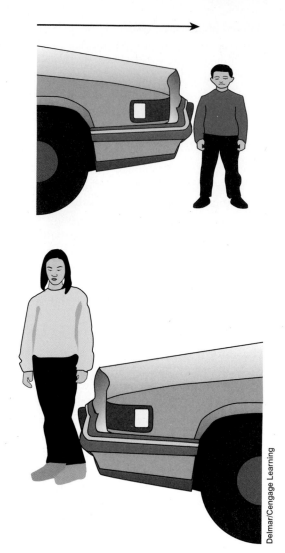

Figure 1-24 A struck pedestrian's injury patterns vary based on bumper height and the patient's age and height.

Delmar/Cengage Learning

because their head is proportionately larger than the head of an older child or an adult.

In diving injuries, the point of impact is typically the head, leading to head injuries. They can also cause spinal trauma due to axial loading combined with hyperextension or hyperflexion injuries of the cervical spine (Figure 1-26). Diving injuries are frequently complicated by near drowning due to altered mental status or loss of mobility.[4,6]

If patients survive falls from dramatic heights, their survival can often be attributed to gradual dissipation of energy. This occurs by landing on a pliable surface that can absorb energy, or by drag created during the fall due to a partially opened parachute, tree branches, or friction while sliding down a steep slope.[4,6,42] The larger the surface area of the body impacted, the greater the dissipation of force. To reduce the chances of injury, stunt designers use devices that stretch out the time it takes to stop a body's momentum.[42] The longer the period of time used in slowing the momentum, the less

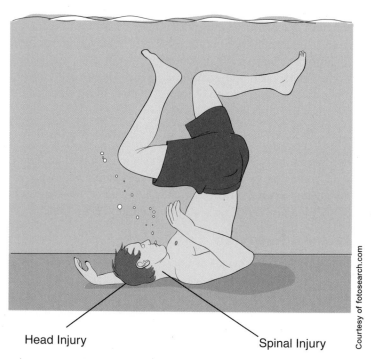

Figure 1-26 Diving injuries typically impact the head and spine.

Head Injury

Spinal Injury

Courtesy of fotosearch.com

force will be exchanged upon impact.[42] Tucking and rolling techniques used by stuntmen are useful in preventing injury because they help to gradually dissipate energy.[4,6,42] Airbags and elastic ropes are also used to dissipate energy more gradually and soften the impact.[42]

Hip fractures can occur in elderly patients without significant mechanism of injury due to decreased bone density.[4,6,32]

Penetrating Trauma

In **penetrating trauma**, the skin is disrupted with entry of a penetrating object into, or passage through, underlying tissue (Figure 1-27).[4,6] Penetrating injuries are frequently caused by firearms, knives, or projectiles from malfunctioning machinery, shrapnel due to an explosion, and impalements.[4,6] Injuries caused by weapons may have been inflicted intentionally or unintentionally.[4,6] In 2001, about 39% of fatalities resulting from firearm injuries were homicides, 57% were suicides, 3% were unintentional, and in 1% of the cases the intent was unclear.[43]

According to the U.S. Bureau of Justice, in 2006, about 68% of all murders, 42% of all robberies, and 22% of all aggravated assaults that were reported to the police were committed with a firearm.[43] Nonfatal firearm violence peaked in 1994 at 1,286,860 and has steadily declined; in 2005, there were only 477,040 nonfatal patients.[43]

There are few reports on the treatment of penetrating trauma to the thoracic vessels before the twentieth century because of the absence of survivors.[44] It wasn't until 1934 that an American physician named Alfred Blalock successfully repaired an aortic injury with the assistance of his colleague, Vivien Thomas.[44] The first documented guidelines for the surgical treatment of penetrating thoracic trauma were not established until World War II.[44] The number of penetrating trauma patients in large metropolitan areas of the United States rose so rapidly in the 1970s and 1980s that the military sent its medical personnel to train caregivers in the management of penetrating trauma wounds at many major medical centers serving urban areas.[44]

Objects that penetrate the skin can become impaled in underlying connective tissue and bone, and can carry debris deep inside the wound.[4,6] As a general rule, impaled objects should always be stabilized in place, unless the object is in the cheek and interfering with the airway.[4,6] When a projectile enters the body, its path of travel is not always clear

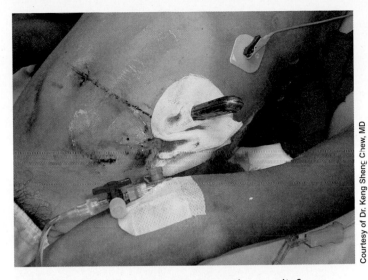

Courtesy of Dr. Keng Sheng Chew, MD

Figure 1-27 Penetrating wounds result from a missile or other object penetrating the skin and entering the body, sometimes passing through the body or becoming embedded or impaled.

and predictable.[4,6,44] Consider the possibility of projectiles ricocheting and deflecting in unexpected directions. Wounds produced by bullets can penetrate all regions of the body regardless of the point of entry.[45] Projectiles may also pass through the body, producing an entrance and exit wound.[4,6,44]

The entrance wound is usually smaller and typically more symmetrical than the exit wound (Figure 1-28).[4,6] The entrance wound may also be encircled with gunpowder tattoo marks, muzzle burns, or dark discolored skin if a bullet is fired from close range (Figure 1-29).[4,6] Subcutaneous emphysema may be present as it is produced when a vacuum is created by ammunition traveling at high velocity.[4,6] Not all entry wounds have associated exit wounds. It is also possible to have multiple exit wounds from a single projectile entering the body due to bullet and bone fragmentation.[4,6] Exit wounds are typically

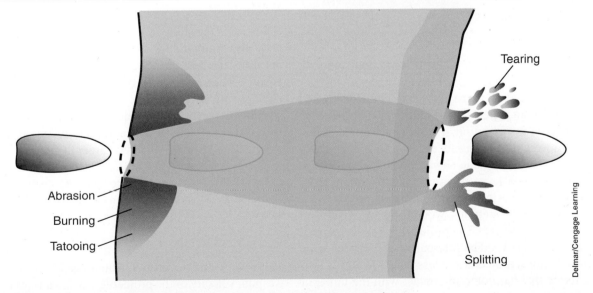

Tearing

Abrasion

Burning

Tatooing

Splitting

Delmar/Cengage Learning

Figure 1-28 General characteristics of entrance and exit wounds.

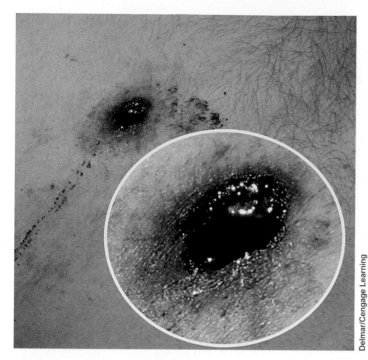

Figure 1-29 An example of a gunshot entrance wound that shows tattooing from the gunpowder when the firearm is discharged at close range.

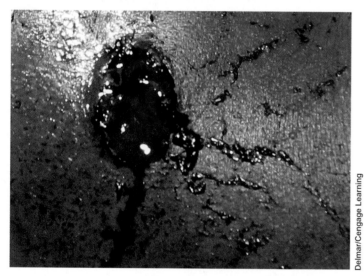

Figure 1-30 An example of a gunshot exit wound.

larger and more jagged in shape than entrance wounds and often have a blown out appearance (Figure 1-30).[4,6] On-scene and in the midst of a resuscitation, it may be difficult to definitively identify a wound as an entrance or an exit wound due to multiple factors. The Paramedic should document a description of the wound and leave definitive identification of an entrance and exit point to the forensic investigators.

The path between the entrance wound and the exit wound is not always a straight line.[4,6] The projectile's path is referred to as the internal wound.[4,6] The internal wound produced by low velocity weapons, projectiles at less than 300 m/s, is limited to the tissue that has come in contact with the bullet or fragment.[4,6]

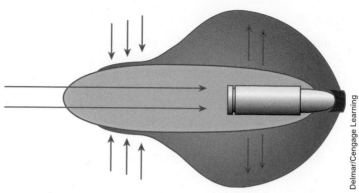

Figure 1-31 High-velocity projectiles can cause significant tissue damage due to the pressures that result in cavitation.

High-velocity weapons produce a shock wave that can create a temporary cavity that is as much as 30 to 40 times the projectile's diameter.[4,6] Upon entering, the projectile's speed causes a vacuum that pulls tissue toward the projectile's path. Shortly after entering, the projectile produces a shock wave that causes an immense pressure that pushes tissue in front of and lateral to the projectile. This shock wave is capable of causing tissue damage to areas surrounding the direct path of the projectile and may be transmitted by body fluids to distant parts of the body.[4,6] The internal wound is characterized by a permanent cavity and the surrounding tissue affected by the temporary cavity, a phenomenon known as cavitation (Figure 1-31).[4,6]

Tissue damage is affected by the density and elasticity of tissue that is penetrated.[4,6] Highly dense tissue, such as bone, and the less elastic tissue of the brain, liver, and spleen sustain more permanent damage in the zone of the temporary cavity.[4,6] Air is less dense, and lung tissue is very elastic, making the lungs more resilient than other tissue.[4,6] Bowel, muscle, and lung tissue are very elastic and more resilient to temporary cavitation as well.[4,6]

Ballistics

Ballistics is the study of motion as it affects projectiles, typically ammunition such as bullets, bombs, and rockets.[4,6] As discussed earlier, the kinetic energy from the projectile is equal to ½ mass × velocity². Injury caused by projectiles is most greatly affected by the projectile's velocity upon impact with the tissue.[4,6,44] High-velocity projectiles produce a pressure wave that creates cavitation and results in a temporary wound that can be significantly larger than the permanent cavity.[4,6,44] Low-velocity weapons, defined as producing velocities of less than 2,000 feet per second, cause a smaller amount of cavitation.[4,6] Most handguns and some rifles are low-velocity weapons.[4,6]

Gunshot Wounds

The severity of a gunshot wound depends on the type of weapon, velocity of the projectile when it strikes tissue, physical properties of the projectile, and type of tissue impacted.[4,6]

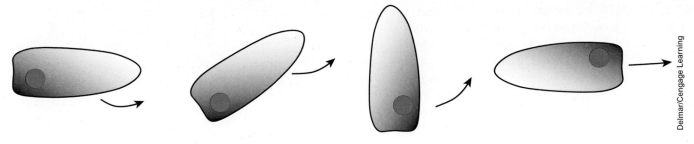

Delmar/Cengage Learning

Figure 1-32 Tumbling increases surface area.

There are literally thousands of brands of firearms in the United States, but most fall into one of three broadly defined classes: handguns, shotguns, and rifles.[4,6]

Handguns generally produce the lowest velocity of the three categories when firing a bullet.[4,6] Revolvers and pistols are both types of handguns.[44] Revolvers can hold up to 10 rounds of ammunition in a cylinder.[44] Pistols have a separate magazine that can hold as much as 17 rounds of ammunition or more.[44] Handguns can have rifled barrels designed to put spin on the bullet and improve its accuracy.[44] Because the barrel of a handgun is much shorter than a rifle's, it is less accurate at a distance than a rifle.[44] The ammunition used in handguns is generally less devastating than that of rifles because it travels at a lower velocity.[4,6,44]

Shotguns fire rounds of pellets, also called shot.[4,6] As many as several dozen pellets can be loaded in a shotgun shell and be fired each time.[4,6] A sabot is a large pellet that can be loaded into a shotgun shell and is capable of causing much more damage than smaller pellets.[44] The barrel of a shotgun is generally smooth bore and does not put spin on the shell or pellets.[44] As the pellets leave the barrel, they disperse.[4,6] The distance between a target and the shotgun can be estimated by shot density.[44] Shot density describes the distance of the pellets from one another as they present on the target.[44] Close range shotgun wounds are not only subjected to greater projectile velocity, but also to greater surface area damage due to shot density.[44]

Rifles fire a single projectile at a time at greater velocity than handguns or shotguns.[4,6] Rifle barrels are grooved to put a spin on the projectile, which adds to its stability and accuracy (i.e., the barrel is "rifled").[4,6] Automatic and semi-automatic rifles can fire multiple rounds of bullets without releasing and re-pulling the trigger, giving these weapons a greater ability to cause lethal wounds when compared with handguns and shotguns.[4,6]

Other factors that affect the severity of injury due to a projectile include projectile size, projectile deformity, tumbling, and yaw.[4,6] Larger projectiles produce a larger permanent cavity.[4,6] Some projectiles are designed to deform on contact with the target to increase the size of the permanent cavity (i.e., hollow nose bullets).[4,6] Hollow nose and soft point bullets flatten out on impact and increase the impact's surface area.[4,6] The semi-jacketed bullet is likewise designed to expand on impact.[4,6] As the projectile tumbles, it causes a wider path of destruction.[4,6] Yaw is an oscillating motion

vertically and horizontally about its axis.[4] The horizontal oscillation is also called wobble.[4] Yaw results in a larger surface area when it has contact with tissue (Figure 1-32).[4]

The projectile material can also affect the damage produced in the tissue. Rubber bullets have been used as an alternative to more lethal bullets in situations where killing is not the goal, such as riot control.[46] Although rubber bullets are safer than other ammunition, they can still penetrate the body and produce lethal wounds, particularly at close range.[46] The full metal jacket round is designed to limit mushrooming and increase its ability to penetrate body armor.[46]

Body Armor

Body armor is used to protect against penetrating wounds from bullets and other sharp objects.[46] It can also offer limited protection from blunt trauma by dispersing forces over a greater surface area.[46] Body armor, often referred to as bulletproof vests, is unable to stop all types of projectiles, however.[46] High-velocity weapons can produce enough energy to penetrate armor, especially when bullets designed to pierce body armor are used.[46] At close range, velocity is greatest, increasing the risk of body armor penetration.[46]

Hard body armor is made of a thick ceramic or metal plate hard enough to deflect the force of a projectile.[46] It provides much more protection than soft body armor, but it also is much more cumbersome to wear.[46] Police officers and military personnel wear hard body armor primarily during high-risk activities when attack with a deadly weapon is anticipated.[46] **Soft body armor**, made of Kevlar or some other fabric, is worn during more routine activities due to its increased flexibility and decreased weight in comparison to hard body armor.[46]

Soft body armor works very much like a net.[46] Nets used for sports such as hockey and soccer are made with many long lengths of tether, woven together and fastened to a frame.[46] The forward energy of a ball or puck pushes the tethers and extends the tethers from one side of the frame to the other.[46] The energy transfer continues horizontally and vertically due to the net's weave pattern.[46] This disperses the energy across the net and away from the point of impact.[46] Regardless of where the ball hits, the net will absorb its forward inertia.[46]

Kevlar is a strong fabric woven to disperse energy in a similar fashion as a sports net, but much tighter.[46] To make soft body armor, several layers of Kevlar are sandwiched between layers of plastic film.[46] Spectra and Vectran are newer materials that are used in armor.[46] Vectran is reported to be lighter than Kevlar but to have twice its strength.[46]

In addition to stopping the bullet from reaching the body, a piece of body armor also has to protect against blunt trauma caused by the force of the bullet.[46] Body armor is designed to optimize the dispersal of energy across the entire piece of armor.[46] If the energy is too focused, bullets may penetrate the armor or focused energy may cause internal injuries due to blunt forces.[46] Because each additional layer of armor material disperses more energy, the more layers, the more protection—assuming the layers in the armor are comparable.[46]

A bullet does not have to pierce body armor to cause serious injuries or death.[4,46] The Paramedic must assess areas posterior to the impact point on the body armor for signs of both penetrating and blunt injury.[4,46] High-speed weapons fired at close range can penetrate body armor. Some bullets can also pierce body armor, and blunt injuries can occur when energy is dissipated over the greater surface area.[4,46] Before removing body armor in the field for assessment purposes, weigh the benefit of removal against the risk of repeated attacks.

If the type of weapon and ammunition used is known, it should be documented and reported to the emergency physician. However, that information is often not readily available on-scene.[4,6] Weapons may have been taken from the scene by the perpetrator, ammunition is often lodged in the patient's body and thus is not visible, or it may have passed through the patient and will need to be located by crime investigators.[4,6] Even when weapons or ammunition are observed by Paramedics at the scene, they should not be handled in an effort to identify them because they are part of the crime scene.[4] It is far more important to assess and treat the patient with an understanding of the unpredictable path bullets can take through the body, and the effects of both the permanent and temporary cavity caused by high-velocity weapons.[4,6] Paramedics should report the use of body armor and whether penetration of the missile was prevented by the armor.[46]

Stabbings

The severity of a stab wound is not easily predictable by observing the external injury.[4,6] Factors to consider include the potential depth of injury if the type of weapon is known, the angle of the weapon during penetration, and the anatomical area involved.[4,6] Stab wounds may involve cutting, hacking, twisting, or jabbing motions as the weapon is impaled in tissue, causing greater internal injury than can be perceived from the external wound. Larger, heavier weapons such as machetes and power tools can result in musculoskeletal injuries and amputation.

Wounds involving the neck and torso are typically most critical.[4,6] In the neck, vital structures such as the airway, large blood vessels, and the cervical spine may be injured.[4,6] Depending on the diaphragm's location during the assault, abdominal wounds may involve the thoracic cavity and thoracic wounds may involve abdominal organs (Figure 1-33).[4,6] On full exhalation, the anterior diaphragm can ascend as high

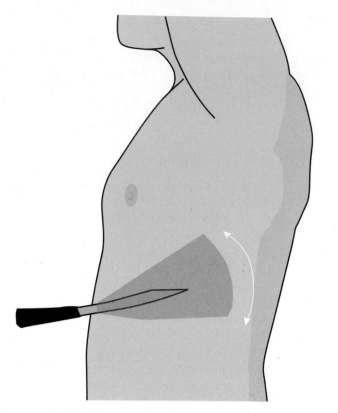

Figure 1-33 The stab wound path of injury may not be immediately apparent based on the wound's location.

as the fourth intercostal space.[4,6] Wounds to the back and wounds caused by female perpetrators are typically downward. Wounds to the anterior of the body and wounds caused by male perpetrators are more typically angled upward.[4,6]

Blast Injuries

Explosions occur in warfare, but they also occur in industrial settings and homes.[47] Wherever combustible or explosive materials can be found, such as natural gas leaks, meth labs, and so on, blasts may occur.[47] Incidents may be accidental or intentional and can have a magnitude as small as that produced by a firecracker or as catastrophic as that produced by a nuclear detonation.[47] Explosions in closed spaces or those that result in structural collapse have higher mortality and injury rates than open-air bombings.[47] In terrorist bombings that produced 30 or more casualties, 1 out of 4 patients died immediately in structural collapse, 1 of 12 in confined space bombings, and 1 in 25 in open air bombings.[47] Bus bombings in the Israeli experience resulted in the highest mortality rate.[47] Blasts that occur in confined spaces are the most lethal because the energy is magnified within the closed space; however, they often produce a smaller number of patients due to the confinement of the area involved.[4,6,47,48]

Primary blast injuries are wounds caused by the direct effects immediately after the explosion. Explosions produce a blast wave that results from changes in atmospheric pressure and moves outward from the epicenter.[47,48] The overpressurized "wave" is caused by a rapid increase, immediately followed by a sudden decrease, in pressure.[46-48] It is a focused force that causes compression followed by rapid decompression of gas-containing organs when it strikes the body.[47,48] If the patient is standing near a reflecting surface or is in a confined space, energy is reflected back at the patient, thus increasing the severity of his injuries.[47,48] Underwater detonation causes an increased risk of injury or death because water is more dense than air and transmits the blast wave three times more effectively than air.[4,6,47,48]

Most injuries caused by the pressure wave affect air-filled organs.[4,6,47,48] Ruptured eardrums are common.[4,6,47,48] Injury to the lungs, abdominal injury, and bowel perforation may also occur.[4,6,47,48] Energy release from the blast produces heat that can cause burns.[4,6,47,48]

Pulmonary blast injury is the most common cause of death due to the primary blast.[4,6,47,48] The blast typically affects the side of the body facing the blast wind; however, in confined spaces energy is reflected back, causing bilateral or both anterior and posterior injuries (Figure 1-34).

Secondary blast injuries, or fragmentation injuries, are caused as the patient is struck by debris propelled by the blast wind, causing lacerations, penetrating wounds, and fractures.[4,6,47,48] Conventional military explosives can propel shrapnel and other debris nearly 3,000 mph.[47] Many of the principles that apply to penetrating trauma also apply to secondary blast injury (Figure 1-34).

Tertiary blast injuries occur when patients are thrown to the ground or against objects.[4,6,47,48] Structures may collapse,

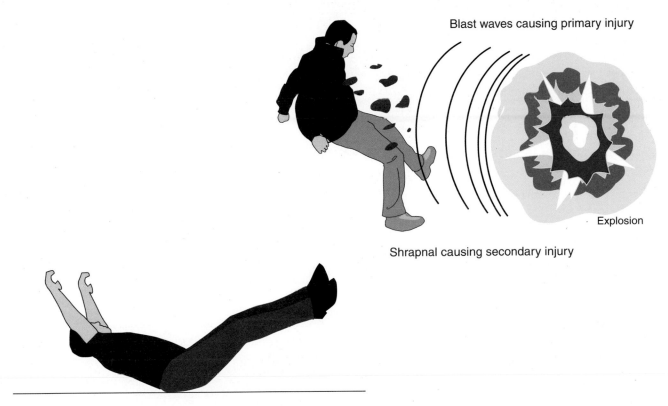

Blast waves causing primary injury

Explosion

Shrapnal causing secondary injury

Tertiary injury from secondary collisions

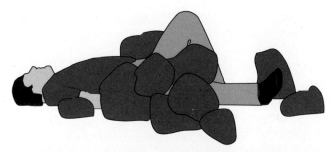

Quaternary injury from entrapment, burns, brain injury, respiratory complications

Figure 1-34 Primary, secondary, tertiary, and quaternary blast injuries.

Delmar/Cengage Learning

causing multisystem trauma similar to that of a rollover motor vehicle crash or fall from a height.[4,6,47,48] Crush injuries and entrapment may further complicate the injuries (Figure 1-34).[4,6,47,48]

Quaternary blast injuries are described as injuries and illnesses that occur which are not due to the primary, secondary, or tertiary injuries.[6,47,48] Quaternary blast injuries include burns, crush injuries due to prolonged entrapment, hypoxic brain injury, and complications of asthma and COPD due to inhalation of fumes, dust, and toxins (Figure 1-34).[6,47,48]

The concept of **quinary blast injuries** is relatively new when discussing blast injuries.[6,47,48] After blast injury, some individuals develop a hyperinflammatory state with an excessive and unusual rise in body temperature, sweating, decreased central venous pressure, and a significant positive fluid balance during treatment.[47,48] This syndrome of symptoms is not explained by the apparent physical injuries directly related to the blast.[6,47,48] Quinary injuries are thought to be caused by additives to bombs such as bacteria, radiation, and chemicals.[6,47,48] Fragments of human remains can become impaled or embedded in another person with devastating psychological and physical effects and have been added to the definition of quinary blast injuries.[6,48]

CASE STUDY CONCLUSION

With the patient loaded, the Paramedic turns and thinks to herself, "He was hurt badly but he could have been killed!" Her muse is disturbed by the radio: "All EMS prepare for incoming wounded. Standby for unit roll call."

CRITICAL THINKING QUESTIONS

1. What are some of the possible soft-tissue injuries that may be suspected based on the mechanism of injury?

2. Are any of these soft-tissue injuries potentially life-threatening injuries?

CONCLUSION

Paramedics can play a vital role in injury prevention by encouraging safer practices, taking advantage of teachable moments when close calls occur, and documenting factors that affect the severity of injury, such as use of protective gear.

Field triage criteria incorporates information gathered from the scene size-up, primary assessment, baseline vitals, and past/present medical history to determine what resources will best meet the patient's needs without overburdening the EMS or hospital trauma system with patients not in need of a trauma center's resources. Effective field triage improves the quality and speed of access to definitive care, improves survival rates of multisystem trauma patients, and utilizes resources in a more cost-effective manner, making those resources more accessible to patients most in need of special trauma resources. An understanding of the physics of trauma allows the Paramedic to predict the injuries associated with the many different types of trauma.

KEY POINTS:

- Trauma is injury caused by multiple forces impacting the body's homeostasis and impairing physiologic processes.

- Trauma strikes people at any time and creates a heavy financial burden for the patient, the patient's family, and society as a whole.

- Trauma is preventable by mitigating circumstances.

- The Haddon matrix illustrates factors involved in trauma and where trauma can be reduced by simple measures.

- The three modes of injury prevention are education, enforcement, and engineering.

- Trauma systems were established to prevent death from trauma. Different levels of trauma centers provide care not otherwise available at local or community hospitals.

- Trauma registries provide data of all aspects of trauma care, from the streets to the morgue. Using the National EMS Information System (NEMSIS), they provide physicians, planners, and scientists the information needed to make systematic changes to reduce trauma morbidity and mortality.

- Starting with Baron Jean Dominique Larrey, triage has been used to sort the casualties and organize patient care to provide optimal outcomes for the greatest numbers.

- The order of trauma transport triage is abnormal physiologic parameters, anatomical criteria, mechanism of injury, and special considerations.

- Assessment of the mechanism of injury, coupled with knowledge of kinematics, can help ascertain the predictable injury pattern.

- The key to kinematics is energy: actual (i.e., kinetic) energy and potential energy.

- Newton's laws of motion are key to understanding kinematics: objects at rest will stay at rest unless acted upon by an outside force, objects in motion will stay in motion unless acted upon by an outside force, and for every action there is an equal and opposite reaction.

- In the kinetic energy formula of mass and velocity, velocity is more important.

- Current safety research and development is developing means to dissipate and slow the transfer of energy to prevent injury.

- External signs of blunt trauma can provide clues to internal damage.

- Common motor vehicle collisions have predictable injury patterns: the up-and-over pathway and down-and-under pathway of frontal collisions, rollovers, lateral impact, rotational, rear impact, and ejection.

- Occupant restraint systems, such as seat belts and airbags, dissipate energy and reduce injury.

- Special vehicles, such as all-terrain vehicles and snowmobiles, have injury patterns as well.

- Penetrating trauma creates both a permanent and a temporary cavity.

- Ballistics, the study of the motion of projectiles, uses the speed and mass of a projectile to predict the injury pattern.

- Blast injuries have five phases of injury, each with a predictable injury pattern.

▶ REVIEW QUESTIONS:

1. Name three of the five physical forces that can cause trauma.
2. What four phases of trauma are listed in the Haddon matrix?
3. What is meant by the term "undertriage" and what are its consequences?
4. What are Newton's three laws of motion?
5. What are the predictable injury patterns in a down-and-under pathway during a front-end collision? From an up-and-over pathway?

▶ CASE STUDY QUESTIONS:

Please refer to the Case Study in this chapter, and answer the questions below:

1. What are the predictable injuries for each phase of a blast injury?
2. What are the scene safety concerns for the Paramedic responding to a reported explosion?
3. Would body armor be helpful in preventing injury to the Paramedic?

▶ REFERENCES:

1. Anderson RN, Minino AM, Fingerhut LA, Warner M, Heinen MA. Deaths: injuries, 2001. *Natl Vital Stat Rep.* 2004;52(21):1–3.
2. Anderson RN, Smith BL. Deaths: leading cause for 2002. *Natl Vital Stat Rep.* 2005;53(17):13–14.
3. Lerner EB. Studies evaluating current field triage: 1966–2005. *Prehosp Emerg Care.* 2006;10(3).
4. Campbell JE. Ed: *International Trauma Life Support for Prehospital Care Providers* (6th ed.). Upper Saddle River, NJ: Pearson Education Incorporated; 2008:1–26, 391–399.
5. American College of Surgeons Subcommittee on Injury Prevention and Control. Injury prevention. Available at: **http://www.facs.org/trauma/injuryprevent.pdf.** Accessed March 1, 2009.
6. McSwain N, Salomone JP, et al. (eds.). *Prehospital Trauma Life Support* (6th ed.). St. Louis, Missouri: Mosby Elsevier; 2007.
7. Persaud BN, Retting RA, Lyon CA. Crash reduction following installation of centerline rumble strips on rural two-lane roads. September 2003. Available at: **http://www.dot.state.mn.us/trafficeng/safety/rumble/IIHS_report.pdf.** Accessed August 29, 2008.
8. Oklahoma Department of Transportation. Shoulder treatments—rumble strips. Available at: **http://www.okladot.state.ok.us/oshsp/pdfs/ld-shouldertreatments.pdf.** Accessed June 10, 2009.
9. Eastridge BJ, Shafi S, Minei JP, Culica D, McConne C, Gentilello L. Economic impact of motorcycle helmets:

from impact to discharge. *J Trauma-Injury, Infect Crit Care.* 2006;60(5):978–984.

10. Queenlands Government. Haddon's matrix. Available at: **http://www.health.qld.gov.au/chipp/what_is/matrix.asp.** Accessed March 5, 2009.

11. Cooper G, Laskowski-Jones L. Development of trauma care systems. *Prehosp Emerg Care.* 2006;10(3):328–331.

12. Hunt RC, Jurkovich GJ. Field triage: opportunities to save lives. *Prehosp Emerg Care.* 2006;10(3).

13. American College of Emergency Physicians. 2007 ACEP Press Releases. Nation's emergency physicians herald passage of Trauma Care Act of 2007. Available at: **http://www.acep.org/pressroom.aspx?id=25694.** Accessed February 29, 2009.

14. National Highway Traffic and Safety Administration. Trauma system agenda for the future. Available at: **http://www.nhtsa.dot.gov/people/injury/ems/emstraumasystem03/index.htm.** Accessed February 29, 2009.

15. Trauma Care Systems Planning and Development Act of 2007, H.R. 272, PUBLIC LAW 110–23—MAY 3, 2007. Available at: **http://www.govtrack.us/congress/billtext.xpd?bill=h110-727.** Accessed February 29, 2009.

16. U.S. Department of Health and Human Services, Health Resources and Services Division (released February 2006). Model Trauma System Planning and Evaluation.

17. Nathens AB, et al. Committee on Trauma, American College of Surgeons, Trauma System Evaluation and Planning Committee. Regional trauma systems: optimal elements, integration, and assessment. Systems consultation guide; 2008. Available at: **http://www.facs.org/trauma/consultationguide-prq.pdf.** Accessed August 30, 2008.

18. American College of Surgeons. Trauma Programs: New verification site visit outcomes; June 7, 2007. Available at: **http://www.facs.org/trauma/verifivisitoutcomes.html.** Accessed August 31, 2008.

19. American College of Surgeons. Resources for optimal care of the injured patient, 2006. Available at: **http://www.facs.org/trauma/hospitallevels.pdf.** Accessed March 12, 2009.

20. Dawson DE. National Emergency Medical Services Information System (NEMSIS). *Prehosp Emerg Care.* 2006;10(3):314–316.

21. American College of Surgeons. National Trauma Data Bank; 2009. Available at: **http://www.facs.org/trauma/ntdb/index.html.** Accessed March 12, 2009.

22. Henry MC. Trauma triage: New York experience. *Prehosp Emerg Care.* 2006;10(3).

23. Cherry R, King TS, Carney DE, et al. Trauma team activation and the impact on mortality. *J Trauma.* 2007;63(2):326–330.

24. Nirula R, Brasel K. Do trauma centers improve functional outcomes: a national trauma data bank analysis. *J Trauma: Injury, Infect Crit Care.* 2006;61(2):268–271.

25. Mackersie RC. History of trauma field triage development and the American College of Surgeons criteria. *Prehosp Emerg Care.* 2006;10(3):287–294.

26. Wang SC. Upcoming revisions to field trauma triage criteria, 2006. Available at: **http://www.nhtsa.dot.gov/staticfiles/DOT/NHTSA/NRD/Featured%20Services/CIREN/2006%20Presentations/Michigan0906.pdf.** Accessed March 3, 2009.

27. Chapleau W. Mechanism of injury & outcomes. JEMS.com Web site. 2007. Available at: **http:www.jems.com/news_and_articles/columns/Mechanism_of_Injury_Outcomes.** Accessed December 7, 2007.

28. Demetriades D, Kuncir E, Brown CV, et al. Early prediction of mortality in isolated head injury patients: a new predictive mode. *J Trauma, Injury, Infect Crit Care.* 2006;61(4):868–872.

29. McNett M. A review of predictive ability of Glasgow Coma Scale scores in head-injured patients. *J Neurosci Nurs.* 2007;39(2):68–75.

30. Lapner PC, McKay M, Howard A, et al. Children in crashes: mechanism of injury and restraint systems. *Can J Surg.* 2001;44(6):445–449.

31. Sasser SM, Hunt RC, Sullivent EE, et al. Guidelines for field triage of injured patients: recommendations of the national expert panel on field triage. *MMWR.* January 23, 2009;58(RR01):1–35.

32. The Ohio State Extension. Falls in the home; April 2002. From National AG Safety Database. Available at: **www.cdc.gov/nasd/docs/d000101-d000200/d000131/d000131.html.** Accessed October 10, 2007.

33. Liu X, Yang J. Velocity and front-end structure on dynamic responses of children pedestrians. *Traffic Inj Prev.* 2003;4(4):337–344.

34. Vossoughi F, Kranz B, Fann F. Hand injuries as an indicator of other associated severe injuries. *Am Surg.* 2007;73(7): 706–708.

35. Jakobsson L, Norin H. Whiplash-associated disorders in frontal impacts: influencing factors and consequences. *Traffic Inj Prev.* 2003;4(2):153–161.

36. DePree C. *No Nonsense Knowledge: Physics Made Simple.* New York, NY: Broadway Books of Random House Incorporated; 2004.

37. Department of Transportation. What you should know about airbags, DOT HS 809 575. Available at: **http://www.nhtsa.dot.gov/people/injury/airbags/.** Accessed April 7, 2009.

38. Nirula R, Mock C, Kaufman R, et al. Correlation of head injury to vehicle contact points using crash injury research and engineering network data. *Accid Anal Prev.* 2003;53(2): 201–210.

39. National Center for Statistics and Analysis. Passenger vehicle occupant fatalities by restraint use and ejection status, 2003. September 2004. Available at: **http://www-nrd.nhtsa.dot.gov/Pubs/809782.PDF.** Accessed January 19, 2009.

40. NHTSA. The need to promote occupant restraint use for children, youth, and 16- to 20-year-olds. Available at: **http://www.nhtsa.dot.gov/people/injury/airbags/OccupantProtectionFacts/restraint.htm#adult.** Accessed January 19, 2008.

41. Safercar.gov. Air bags safety. Available at: **http://www.safercar .gov/portal/site/safercar/menuitem.13dd5c887c7e1358fefe0a2 f35a67789/?vgnextoid=bc4f3613ffffe110VgnVCM1000002fd1 7898RCRD.** Accessed January 20, 2009.

42. *Newton's Apple. Hollywood Stunts*. Produced by KTCA Twin Cities Public Television. Available at: **http://www.darylscience .com/Demos/StuntMen.html.** Accessed January 1, 2009.

43. United States Bureau of Justice, Bureau of Justice Statistics. After peaking in 1993, the number of gun crimes reported to police declined and then stabilized at levels last seen in 1988. Available at: **http://www.ojp.usdoj.gov/bjs/glance/guncrime.htm.** Accessed January 1, 2009.

44. Shahani R, Galla J. Penetrating chest trauma. EMedicine. October 8, 2008. Available at: **http://emedicine.medscape.com/ article/425698-overview.** Accessed January 17, 2009.

45. United States Bureau of Justice, Bureau of Justice Statistics. Nonfatal firearm-related violent crimes, 1993–2005. Available at: **http://www.ojp.usdoj.gov/bjs/glance/tables/ firearmnonfataltab.htm.** Accessed January 1, 2009.

46. Discovery Communications, LLC. How body armor works. Available at: **http://www.howstuffworks.com/body-armor.htm.** Accessed January 29, 2009.

47. MedScape Today. Mechanisms of injury and injury patterns in explosions. 2005. Available at: **http://www.medscape.com/ viewarticle/516117_4.** Accessed February 28, 2009.

48. DePalma R, Burris D, Champion H, Hodgson M. Blast injuries. *N Engl J Med*. 2005;352(13):1335–1342.

CHAPTER 2

TRAUMATIC BRAIN INJURY

KEY CONCEPTS:

Upon completion of this chapter, it is expected that the reader will understand these following concepts:

- Epidemiology of traumatic brain injury
- Classifications of traumatic brain injury
- Pathophysiology of increased intracranial pressure
- Types of herniation syndromes
- Examination of the patient with suspected head injury
- Treatment of the suspected increased intracranial pressure

ANATOMY CONCEPTS:

Prior to reading this chapter the Paramedic student should be familiar with the following anatomy and physiology concepts:

- Anatomy of the skull, the brain, and the meninges
- Neuroreflexes
- Physiology of intracranial pressure

The call came in as: "Runner versus bicyclist." Dispatch reported the two had collided with one another but both were conscious and breathing. The runner was complaining of a headache. Bystanders, probably other runners, saw the calamity and called 9-1-1. The Paramedic discusses with his partner how the combined speed of the runner and bicyclist might contribute to the severity of their injuries and the two start to consider suspected injuries as they arrive on-scene.

CRITICAL THINKING QUESTIONS

1. What traumatic brain injuries might be suspected based on the mechanism of injury?

2. Are any of these traumatic brain injuries potentially life-threatening injuries?

OVERVIEW

"The patient may have had a loss of consciousness." When those ominous words are spoken at the scene of a trauma, they suggest a head injury. Head injuries, and subsequent brain injuries, are the leading cause of death in trauma and a leading cause of permanent disability in industrialized countries. Each year traumatic brain injuries occur in approximately one and a half million Americans. To put this into perspective, a traumatic brain injury occurs once every seven seconds in the United States.[1] Approximately one-quarter million Americans with a traumatic brain injury are hospitalized. Over 50,000 patients will die from their traumatic brain injuries.[2]

Traumatic brain injury (TBI) is defined as "a traumatic insult to the brain capable of producing intellectual, emotional, social and vocational changes."[3] As the definition implies, traumatic brain injury can have wide ranging and devastating implications for a patient. Immediate implications may include loss of short-term memory and development of seizure disorders. Long-term implications may include Alzheimer's disease and Parkinson's disease.

A traumatic brain injury can occur due to a variety of traumatic causes (Figure 2-1), including vehicle collisions (the leading cause of traumatic brain injury), falls, and assaults.

A large portion of traumatic brain injuries occur in teenagers and young adults, with a peak incidence occurring between the ages of 15 and 24. These injuries are primarily a result of motor vehicle collisions and assaults. Another major patient population affected by traumatic brain injury is the elderly, who often experience traumatic brain injury from falls. A third major patient population at risk for traumatic brain injury is soldiers injured during explosions from improvised explosive devices (IED) and munitions in war zones.

The most deadly cause of traumatic brain injury is use of a firearm, whether in an assault, homicide, or suicide (which is the most common cause). Mortality from a traumatic brain injury caused by a firearm is approximately 90%.[1]

With over five million patients afflicted with TBI in the United States, the care of the brain-injured patient, either immediately following the trauma or for the years afterwards, is an important aspect of the Paramedic's practice.[3]

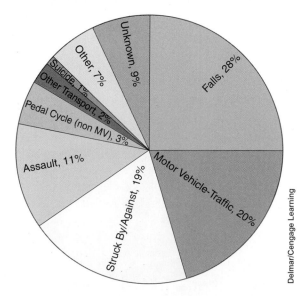

Figure 2-1 Causes of traumatic brain injury.

Delmar/Cengage Learning

Football players—particularly linemen who have repeated impacts to their head—have experienced traumatic brain injury, despite the use of helmets. In some cases, the injuries have resulted in death.

Chief Concern

The brain is literally central to who and what we are. It is the source of our consciousness and what makes humans sentient (i.e., able to sense and perceive the world). Therefore, it can be argued that the brain is the most important organ in the body. Although the brain only weighs approximately three pounds,

Table 2-1 Classifications of Traumatic Brain Injury

- Primary brain injury
  - Soft-tissue injury
    - Concussion
    - Diffuse axonal injury
  - Intracerebral hemorrhage
    - Cerebral contusion
    - Cerebral laceration
  - Extracerebral hemorrhage
    - Subarachnoid
    - Subdural
    - Epidural
- Secondary brain injury
  - Metabolic
    - Hypoxia
    - Hypoperfusion/ischemia
    - Hypoglycemia

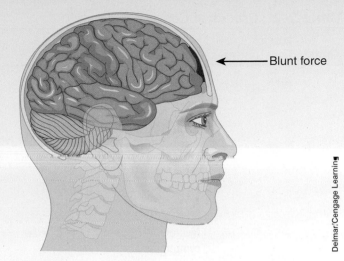

Blunt force

Delmar/Cengage Learning

Figure 2-2 Concussion is the most common type of TBI.

which is less than 2% of the total body weight, it demands the greatest portion of metabolic resources. The brain uses 20% of cardiac output, 25% of the blood glucose, and 20% of the blood's oxygen.

Any interruption in the flow of these metabolic substrates (such as by hypoxia, hypoglycemia, or hypoperfusion) can impair brain function. Although trauma, specifically chest trauma, can adversely affect oxygenation, cerebral perfusion is most affected by traumatic brain injury. There are various classifications of traumatic brain injuries (Table 2-1).

Soft-Tissue Injury

Brain injuries are categorized as **primary brain injury** (i.e., damage that occurs at the time of the trauma) and **secondary brain injury** (damage secondary to extracranial etiology that impairs brain function). Primary brain injury can further be divided into soft-tissue injuries, those involving the gray and white matter, and vascular injury that results in intracranial hemorrhage.

The majority of traumatic brain injuries impact the soft tissues and are simple concussions. Paramedics will likely encounter a patient with a concussion at one point or another. However, other traumatic brain injuries, such as subdural hematomas, are more life-threatening conditions. The crux of the problem is trying to distinguish a minor concussive episode from a more problematic intracranial hemorrhage.

Concussion

A transient loss of consciousness may result from a mild TBI. One example of a mild TBI—the most common example—is a concussion. "Concussion" comes from the Latin *concussus,*

meaning "striking together." A concussion results when the tissues of the brain violently strike against one another (Figure 2-2).

The signs and symptoms associated with a concussion include a loss of consciousness, especially if it is a witnessed loss of consciousness of greater than 30 seconds. Although the patient may be unsure if she was unconscious, retrograde amnesia—an inability to remember the traumatic event—should suggest to the Paramedic that the patient suffered a concussion. Other signs of concussion include perseverating (repeating the same questions or phrases despite being given an answer) and a headache. The headaches are considered "secondary" headaches (i.e., originating from other disease, in this case trauma). The patient may describe the headache as being "unusual" for him.

Other symptoms of concussion include a blank or vacant stare when asked a question, confusion or an inability to focus on the task at hand (easily distracted), and delays in verbal and/or motor responses (failure to follow commands). Additional symptoms are disorientation, displayed by walking in the wrong direction; emotions that are out of proportion to the circumstances; and slurred/incoherent speech. The Glasgow Coma Scale is often used to evaluate a person's mental awareness.[4]

Not all experts agree that loss of consciousness should be the clinical marker for a concussion. Some patients with a concussion may instead present with a short period of confusion and a feeling of being "dazed" or having their "bell rung." This may or may not be associated with retrograde amnesia.[5] Research indicates that the concussion's severity is related more to the duration of the altered mental status than the loss of consciousness. Various grades of concussion are identified by the American Academy of Neurology (Table 2-2). Many sports are commonly associated with concussion (Table 2-3).

Evaluation of the patient with a suspected concussion should include tests of orientation (person, place, and time),

Table 2-2 Grades of Concussion

Grade	Loss of Consciousness	Symptoms	Return to Sport
1	None	Resolves in less than 15 minutes	Repeat assessment every 5 minutes–return in 15 minutes if symptoms resolve
2	None	Greater than 15 minutes	No return to game Follow-up with physician Possible return in 1 week
3	Yes	Neurological symptoms persist	Transport to the ED

Table 2-3 Sports Associated with Concussion

- Football: 10% of college and 20% of high school players per season
- Soccer: 5% of all players
- Ice hockey
- Skiing
- Sledding

memory (using three-object recall at five-minute intervals), and concentration (ability to perform serial seven subtractions or reverse order months of calendar). The neurological examination should include papillary response and cerebellar tests (for example the, Romberg test) for coordination. (A simple balance test is walking a line with heel to toe or running the heel of one foot against the shin of the other leg.)

Diffuse Axonal Injury

In the past, a concussion was dismissed as a minor head injury that did not cause permanent physical harm to the patient. However, current research suggests that rather than sustaining a concussion, a patient may in fact have a mild form of diffuse axonal injury (DAI), which may lead to permanent impairment that may be prevented with appropriate diagnosis and treatment.[6]

Diffuse axonal injury (DAI) occurs as a result of the rapid acceleration–deceleration of the brain within the skull. This movement of tissues over and away from other tissues results in shearing forces that disrupt neural connections. This damage is greatest at the interface between areas of varying density, such as the gray matter–white matter junction or the basal ganglia (Figure 2-3). The basal ganglia is the area where the cerebral cortex connects with the thalamus and the brainstem. Examples of items within the basal ganglia are the caudate and the nucleus accumbens that connect to the frontal lobe and the limbic areas; the origins of short term memory and emotions.

One person who exemplifies the long-term consequences of concussion is Muhammad Ali. During his boxing career, Ali suffered many minor concussions. As a result of these repeated concussions, he developed a syndrome known as dementia pugilistica (DP). However, these repeated concussions led Muhammad Ali to a form of chronic traumatic brain injury.

The immediate effects of these repeated cerebral insults can include speech problems, such as slurred speech; an

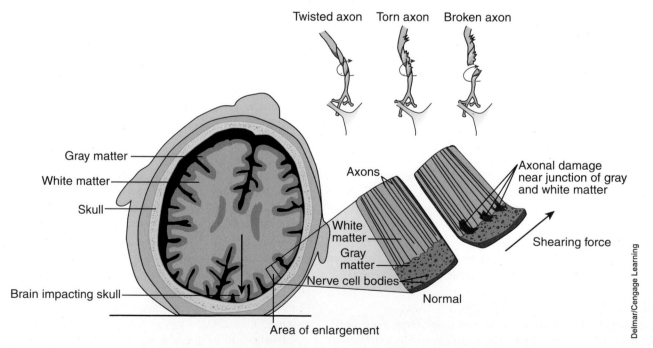

Figure 2-3 Diffuse axonal injury can lead to severe neurological issues over time.

unsteady gait, or ataxia, similar to the stagger of an intoxicated person; and abnormal behaviors such as explosive personality disorders (i.e., being "punch drunk"). The long-term effects of the chronic TBI, also called chronic traumatic encephalopathy, include dementia, Parkinsonism, and a decline in both mental and physical ability.

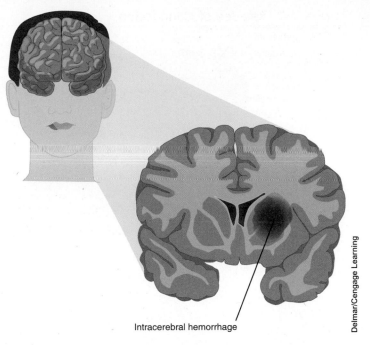

Figure 2-4 Intracerebral hemorrhage is bleeding within the brain's soft tissues.

STREET SMART

The first sign of mild concussion (i.e., grade 1) may be when the athlete forgets the play or the position that she is supposed to play. Listening to teammates as well as the player may lead the Paramedic to suspect a concussion.

The consequences of a second concussion immediately following an initial concussion, within days or weeks, can be deadly. Referred to as **second impact syndrome (SIS)**, this syndrome is thought to occur because the brain loses its ability to autoregulate cerebral perfusion. The second concussion triggers a cascade of events that include cerebral edema, increased intracranial pressure, and, eventually, herniation. These events will be described in detail shortly.

Part of the basal ganglia includes the substantia nigra pars reticulate (SNpr). Injury in this area leads to Parkinson-like syndromes that present with tremors while at rest, rigidity in the extremities, and bradykinesia, or slow movements of the extremities.

STREET SMART

A study of fatal head injuries in high school and college football players over a 13-year period attributed 94 cases of death to second impact syndrome.[7]

Intracerebral Hemorrhage

Intracerebral hemorrhage, also called intraparenchymal bleeding, is bleeding that occurs within the brain's soft tissues (i.e., the cerebral cortex) (Figure 2-4). Bleeding within the cerebral cortex is relatively uncommon and usually occurs due to either a rupture of an aneurysm or arteriovenous malformation (AVM) or, alternatively, from bleeding within a tumor. Trauma-induced intracerebral hemorrhage can occur as a result of either a cerebral contusion or a cerebral laceration.

STREET SMART

When a Paramedic encounters a patient who has fallen and who presents with a neurological deficit, the Paramedic may suspect a stroke. However, traumatic intraparenchymal hemorrhage, bleeding into the soft tissues of the brain, is also a possibility.

Cerebral Contusion

A cerebral contusion, literally a brain bruise, is an intraparenchymal hemorrhage that results from acceleration–deceleration forces. These forces cause the brain to strike the inner surface of the skull, resulting in a coup injury (the word "coup" is French for "strike"). Often the brain rebounds, causing the opposite brain surface to strike the inner surface of the skull, causing a **contrecoup injury** (Figure 2-5).

Cerebral contusions often occur in motor vehicle collisions. Around 50% of patients with a cerebral contusion experience loss of consciousness. The cerebral contusion often involves the most anterior portions of the brain: the temporal lobe and the lower frontal lobe.

The ability to develop and execute a plan, called executive functions, is a function of the frontal lobe. Patients

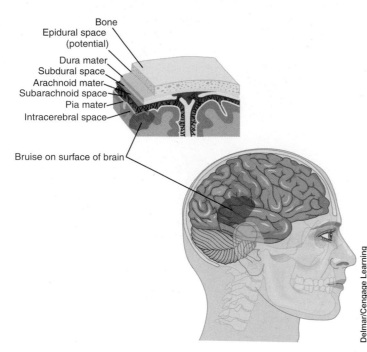

Figure 2-5 Cerebral contusion results from acceleration–deceleration forces.

with moderate cerebral contusions to the frontal lobe may have impaired executive functions. They may appear confused or disorganized, and even more so as stress increases. Injury to the frontal lobe also has an impact on a patient's affect and, more specifically, her emotional control. These patients often display anger but also have difficulty with concentration.

Patients with cerebral contusions to the temporal lobe have a slightly different presentation that includes disturbances of hearing and perception. The speech of these patients may also be disorganized and incoherent, and the patient's answers to questions may be nonsensical. The Paramedic can use the Glasgow Coma Scale (GCS) to help detect and track the progression of these pathological changes secondary to a cerebral contusion.

Cerebral Laceration

The soft tissue in the cerebral cortex can also become torn and lacerated. These "white matter tears" can be the result of a penetrating projectile, such as a gunshot wound (GSW), or bony fragments from a skull fracture.

Unlike cerebral contusions, the meninges is usually torn when a cerebral laceration occurs. This compounds the problem by adding vascular bleeding. A cerebral laceration can generate substantial amounts of blood. Like a cerebral hemorrhage, it can also lead to herniation.

Extracerebral Hemorrhage

Bleeding can occur outside of the cerebral cortex but below the cranium. Three layers of tissues, called the meninges, surround the cerebral cortex. The outermost layer is called the dura mater, which is Latin for "tough mother." The dura mater is a tough and relatively inflexible sheath around the brain that helps to protect it and extends the length of the entire central nervous system. Below the dura mater lays the arachnoid mater and pia mater. These three membranes are separated by the thinnest amount of cerebral spinal fluid. Above, below, and within these membranes are numerous blood vessels, both arterial and venous, that supply the brain with blood.

Injury to any one of these blood vessels that lie within the meninges can result in hemorrhage and a significant collection of blood. As the skull has a limited space, this collection of blood acts as a space-occupying lesion which competes with the brain for space. This bleeding, outside of the brain but within the skull, is called extra-axial bleeding. It consists of three types: subarachnoid hemorrhage, subdural hemorrhage, and epidural hemorrhage.

Traumatic Subarachnoid Hemorrhage

A **traumatic subarachnoid hemorrhage (SAH)** is an extracerebral hemorrhage of the small corticomeningeal blood vessels within the arachnoid space. The blood often mixes with the cerebral spinal fluid (CSF) that is present and quickly spreads over the brain's surface. The hemoglobin released from the red blood cells in the blood causes localized vasospasm and creates the characteristic "thunder clap" headache the patient experiences. Typically, the patient complains of a headache that started at one point and then spread over a portion of the hemisphere. The patient generally complains that the headache is like none other experienced and that it is the worst headache in the patient's life.

To some degree, a SAH occurs in most traumatic brain injuries. However, a SAH is generally not problematic. When a SAH occurs, the blood mixes with the CSF, which prevents it from clotting. Unless the bleeding is massive, the blood does not have the ability to organize into a clot and become a space-occupying lesion on the brain's surface.

One of the perplexing questions that a Paramedic must consider is whether the patient experienced a sudden SAH and fell or whether he first fell and that event caused a traumatic SAH. Both situations present with neurological deficits and in both cases the Paramedic should take trauma precautions.

Subdural Hematoma

Between the dural sinus and below the dura mater, emissary or bridging veins connect the dura mater with the surface of the cerebral cortex. When a sudden force such as an acceleration–deceleration occurs, these fragile veins can tear and cause bleeding within the subdural space. The resultant **subdural hematoma (SDH)** is a rapidly expanding collection of blood into an organized clot that exerts downward pressure onto the already damaged cerebral cortex and increases intracranial pressure in the process (Figure 2-6).

Although there are nontraumatic forms of SDH, secondary to rupture of cerebral aneurysm or arteriovenous malformation (AVM), most SDH occur as a result of trauma. Based partially on their appearance on a CT scan, these traumatic SDH are divided into three classifications: acute, subacute, and chronic SDH.

An acute SDH occurs in less than 72 hours and is often associated with cerebral contusion (82% of the time, according to one study).[8] An SDH is present in about 12% to 29% of severe TBI and can have a mortality rate of 40% to 60%.[9]

In minor cases, the low-pressure venous bleeding clots and the damage is localized and minimized. However, the presence of anticoagulants or liver disease can prevent blood

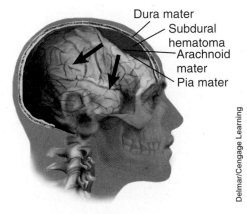

Figure 2-6 Subdural hematoma is a space-occupying lesion that exerts downward force on the cerebral cortex.

Dura mater
Subdural hematoma
Arachnoid mater
Pia mater

Delmar/Cengage Learning

clotting, leading to a more significant "bleed." Other factors that impact the morbidity and mortality associated with a SDH include age, alcoholism, and hemophilia. The brain of an elderly patient is atrophied, stretching the bridging veins and making them more susceptible to tearing in even minor trauma. Alcoholic patients have prolonged bleeding times, secondary to decreased liver-produced coagulation factors, and a tendency toward thrombocytopenia. And, as would be expected, the patient with hemophilia does not have the capacity to stop the bleeding. Even a trivial trauma in the patient with hemophilia can be a medical emergency.

In some cases, the patient with an SDH may lose consciousness, probably secondary to a concurrent concussion. However, in many cases the patient does not lose consciousness. Whenever a trauma patient has a Glasgow Coma Scale of less than 15, and especially in the absence of intoxication, the Paramedic should suspect a SDH. If the intoxicated patient sobers but his neurological deficits, or a GCS less than 15, remains, then the Paramedic should suspect a SDH that warrants medical evaluation, including a CT scan.

The patient with a subacute subdural hematoma may present to the Paramedic three days to three weeks after the inciting trauma. Initially, the SDH is "clinically silent" until the gradual accumulation of blood leads to a shift in the brain, called a mass effect, and the patient becomes symptomatic with complaints of headache, drowsiness, confusion, and so on. Although at first one might tend to be dismissive of the patient's complaints, because the trauma occurred days or weeks prior, the fact that the process of increasing intracranial pressure has progressed and the patient is symptomatic makes the situation no different than if the trauma had occurred that day.

A chronic SDH is older than 21 days and represents another pathological process. When a subdural hemorrhage occurs, a clot forms and stops the bleeding. As the clot organizes and matures it undergoes the natural process of liquefaction; the assumption is that healing has gone on underneath the clot. If the clot dissolves prematurely, or healing has not occurred (secondary to nutrient deficiency, for example), then rebleeding will occur. This rebleeding can be significant if the patient lacks clotting factors that permit reclotting.

The result is that the patient experiences another subdural hematoma weeks after the original insult. Populations at risk for chronic subdural hematomas include alcoholic patients and those with liver disease.

When bleeding occurs in the subdural space, some of the blood is mixed with cerebral spinal fluid. If sufficient blood clots form to occlude CSF circulation, and particularly impair the outflow tracts for CSF to the dural sinus, the resulting buildup of CSF can create a form of hydrocephalus (water on the brain) called a **subdural hygroma**. The localized mass effect of this fluid collection can cause neurological deficits that mimic a stroke.

The very old—patients greater than 75 years of age are at greater risk for a subdural hygroma that is secondary to brain atrophy. These patients may experience a subdural hygroma from relatively minor falls. Therefore, it is important for a Paramedic to ascertain if the elderly patient with stroke-like symptoms may have recently struck his head, even in a fall from a standing position. The resulting symptoms may be secondary to a subdural hygroma rather than a stroke.

Shaken Baby Syndrome

Similar to the elderly patient's brain, the infant's brain does not fill the cranial vault. The resulting large subarachnoid space stretches the emissary or bridging veins, leaving them vulnerable to tearing. However, unlike the elderly patient's brain, the infant's brain is unmyelinated, has greater water content, and is generally softer. Therefore, any violent shaking to and fro can literally cause the brain to slush within the skull. These rotational forces can cause diffuse axonal injury as well as the creation of subdural hematoma. These forces are 50 times greater if the head strikes a surface during the process of being shaken.

The combination of SDH and DAI that occurs during this type of assault is called **shaken baby syndrome**. The population at risk for shaken baby syndrome is generally less than 2 years of age, although shaken baby syndrome has also been documented in children up to age 5. Additionally, the patients are generally male.

Indicators that may lead a Paramedic to suspect shaken baby syndrome include persistent crying, inconsolability, a refusal to nurse or feed, and vomiting, especially vomiting that is not proceeded by nausea. The perpetrators of this type of assault are generally males, either spouses or paramours of the mother (in some 90% of cases) or a babysitter.

Infants have weak neck muscles and are prone to cervical spine injuries. These cervical spine injuries are notable as they are difficult to detect with medical imaging. They are referred to as SCIWORA, which stands for **S**pinal **C**ord **I**njury **W**ith**O**ut **R**adiological **A**bnormality. In one study, all infants suffering from child abuse experienced SCIWORA.[10] Therefore, spinal precautions should be taken for any infant with suspected shaken baby syndrome.

STREET SMART

The presence of a subdural hematoma and retinal hemorrhage alone are not sufficient in some courts of law for a charge of child abuse as evidenced by shaken baby syndrome. Courts have stated that the clinical picture must be considered. The Paramedic should accurately document scene assessments and parental interaction, as well as the clinical history, to aid the investigation.

Epidural Hematoma

Intracranial bleeding above the dura mater creates an **epidural hematoma**. An epidural hematoma typically occurs in the temporoparietal region, although it can occur anywhere in the central nervous system covered by the dura mater.

Although an epidural hematoma can occur as a result of large rotational forces or sudden acceleration–deceleration forces during massive head trauma, an epidural hematoma is typically secondary to a focused blow from an object such as a club. It is often associated with a cranial fracture. Bleeding is the result of injury to arteries proximal to the fracture. The thin pterion area of the skull—the juncture of the frontal, parietal, temporal, and sphenoid bones—is a particularly vulnerable area that overlies the middle meningeal artery. Between 70% and 80% of epidural hematomas are owed to hemorrhage in this area (Figure 2-7).

Although an isolated epidural hematoma only accounts for 1% to 2% of all head trauma, the morality rate from them can be as high as 43%. This high mortality is owed, in part, to the rapid arterial bleeding that can occur. Although the very young (less than 5 years old) and the aged (greater than 55 years old) have a greater mortality, the greatest number of epidural hematomas occur in persons under 20 years of age, secondary to assault in many cases.

The presentation of the epidural hematoma is similar to all extracerebral hemorrhage. It includes headache, projectile vomiting, and seizures. An assessment finding that has been attributed to epidural hematomas, although it is not unique to epidural hematoma, is the lucid interval. The **lucid interval** occurs when the patient is rendered unconscious, then regains consciousness, only to deteriorate into unconsciousness again. This momentary consciousness is thought to be due to intracranial compensatory mechanisms that temporarily

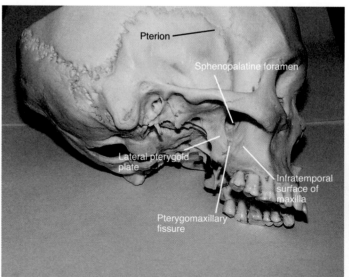

Figure 2-7 The pterion area of the skull is a vulnerable area for epidural hematoma. Note the sutures of the four bone plates connecting in one area.

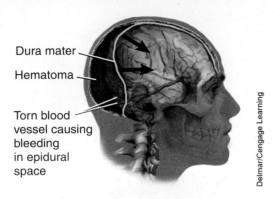

Dura mater

Hematoma

Torn blood vessel causing bleeding in epidural space

Delmar/Cengage Learning

Figure 2-8 Epidural hematomas are often found underlying a skull fracture.

mitigate the effects of rising intracranial pressure. Although the finding of a lucid interval can be helpful when the Paramedic suspects an epidural hematoma, it only occurs in about 20% of cases of epidural hematoma.

Because epidural hematomas are often found underlying a skull fracture, it is important that the fracture be left in order to allow expansion. This will permit the intracranial pressure to dissipate (Figure 2-8). The treatment of choice for an epidural hematoma is trephination, the placement of a Burr hole proximal to the expanding hematoma. Trephination is usually performed at a trauma center by a neurosurgeon.

Pathophysiology of Traumatic Brain Injury

The skull, sometimes referred to as the cranial vault, is a rigid container that holds approximately 1,200 to 1,500 mL of volume. Typically that volume is 80% nervous tissue, 12% cranial blood volume, and the remaining 8% is cerebral spinal fluid (CSF).

The Monroe–Kellie Doctrine states that, as part of the volume–pressure relationship, an increase in one volume must therefore result in a corresponding decrease in another. These volumes—blood, brain, and CSF—are in a constant state of dynamic equilibrium and an attempt to maintain cerebral perfusion at optimal intracranial pressure (approximately 10 to 15 mmHg).

Therefore, an increase in the cranial blood pool (for example, secondary to static hematoma formation) will subsequently increase intracranial pressure (ICP) while decreasing cerebral blood flow, thereby decreasing cerebral perfusion pressures (CPP). In fact, any space-occupying lesion, be it a static hematoma or tumor, or swelling of the brain (cerebral edema) due to inflammation (for example, from an infection or ischemia), will result in increased ICP and decreased CPP. If left untreated, the increased ICP will eventually lead to herniation syndrome, which is described shortly.

Therefore, the key to maintaining intracerebral equilibrium is tied to maintaining sufficient blood pressure and/or intracranial pressure. An increase in ICP compresses cerebral arteries, resulting in decreased cerebral perfusion, which in turn leads

to cellular injury, ischemia, and infarction. Normally a CPP above 70 mmHg, delivering 50 mL of blood to 100 grams of brain per minute (50 mL/100 g/min), is necessary to maintain cerebral perfusion. When the CPP falls below 60 mmHg, cellular injury occurs. When the CPP falls below 50 mmHg (18 to 20 mL/100 g/min), ischemia sets in. Ultimately, with CPP less than 40 mmHg or persistent low CPP, cellular infarction will occur, resulting in permanent brain damage.

Therefore, the therapeutic goal is to maintain the CPP at approximately 60 to 70 mmHg in order to maintain cerebral perfusion and brain viability. Paramedics, however, are unable to measure and monitor CPP in the field. Instead, Paramedics must rely on indirect means. Understanding that cerebral pressure is equal to the mean arterial pressure (MAP) minus the intracranial pressure, and by monitoring the MAP and factoring in the ICP, the Paramedic can estimate the CPP (CPP = MAP − ICP).

The MAP can either be calculated or obtained from readings taken from the noninvasive blood pressure (NIBP). MAP is calculated as the diastolic pressure plus one-third of the pulse pressure: D/P + 1/3 (SP − DP). As an example, a blood pressure of 150/90 would have a MAP of 110 mmHg (90 + 1/3 [150 − 90]) = (90 + 1/3 [60]) = (90 + 20) = 110, and a blood pressure of 90/50 would have a MAP of 63 mmHg. The minimum cerebral perfusion pressure is 60 mmHg.

Understanding the importance of MAP to maintaining CPP, it is imperative that hypotension be corrected and prevented. Uncorrected hypotension may be the single largest cause of secondary injury in cases of traumatic brain injury. A single episode of hypotension has been shown, in at least one study, to increase mortality in traumatic brain injured patients by 50%.

As the ICP is relatively constant, around 10 to 15 mmHg, the Paramedic need only monitor the MAP to help maintain CPP. However, as the ICP increases, the MAP must increase correspondingly to maintain the CPP. The Paramedic will suspect an increased ICP as the patient becomes more and more symptomatic.

Logically, to counter the increased ICP in those cases, the Paramedic should only need to increase the MAP. This can easily be accomplished with intravenous fluids, as the MAP is a function of cardiac output (crudely measured by the systolic pressure) times the systemic vascular resistance (crudely measured by the diastolic pressure) plus the central venous pressure.

This all could be true if the brain was an open system. However, the brain is a closed system. By applying the Monroe–Kellie doctrine, the Paramedic understands that there is a limit to the amount of intravenous fluid that can be administered without risking herniation. The key is maintaining a balance of fluid administration that prevents hypotension without inducing increased intracranial pressure.

Herniation Syndromes

Like the heart and the lungs, the brain is surrounded by a tough and relatively inelastic membrane. This membrane, the dura mater, separates and compartmentalizes the three parts of

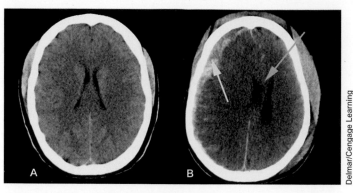

Figure 2-9 (A) Normal head CT scan. (B) CT scan from a patient with a large subdural hematoma indicated by the yellow arrow. The blue arrow indicates the mass effect or pressure on the opposite side of the brain from the subdural hematoma and associated swelling.

Table 2-4 Herniation Syndromes

- Supratentorial
  - Central (transtentorial) herniation
  - Lateral (uncal) herniation
  - Cingulated herniation
- Infratentorial
  - Tonsillar herniation
  - Transcalvarial herniation

the brain—the cerebral cortex, cerebellum, and brainstem—within the skull. The cerebral cortex is separated from the cerebellum by the tentorium cerebella. Furthermore, the falx cerebri, a sickle-shaped dura mater, separates the two hemispheres into right and left.

The only exit from this cranial vault is via the small openings at the base of the skull where the cranial nerves exit or via the foramen magnum, the large opening at the base of the skull where the spinal cord exits the skull. Whenever pressure builds up in one compartment, due to an expanding hematoma or other space-occupying lesion, that compartment compresses the other compartments, creating what is called the **mass effect**. The mass effect is best understood when comparing a normal CT scan to one with a subdural hematoma (Figure 2-9).

As intracranial pressure increases within the compartment, and the mass effect gets greater, the entire brain starts to move toward the foramen magnum, a process called **herniation**. Dependent on the location of the space-occupying lesion, herniation begins either above the tentorium (supratentorial) or below the tentorium (infratentorial) (Table 2-4).

Supratentorial Herniation

Since the tentorium separates the cerebrum from the cerebellum, any expanding hematoma, for example, would either exert a downward pressure and essentially funnel the

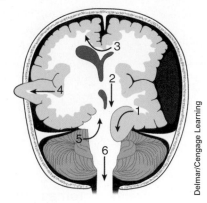

Figure 2-10 Herniation types: 1. Uncal 2. Central 3. Cingulate 4. Transcalvarial 5. Upward 6. Tonsillar.

cerebrum into foramen magnum or would exert horizontal pressure across the brain from one hemisphere to another. As a result, there are three varieties of **supratentorial herniation** (Figure 2-10).

The first supratentorial herniation is called a **central herniation**. During a central herniation, increasing intracranial pressure exerts a force upon the diencephalon (at the midline of the brain above the brainstem), the thalamus, and the hypothalamus, as well as the temporal lobes. Early signs of this increasing intracranial pressure, and subsequent mass effect, include the loss of extraocular movement (EOM), particularly the downward gaze. Then, as the herniation continues unabated, the third cranial nerve (CN III) is compressed and the patient's pupil becomes fixed and dilated.

This downward pressure also stretches the basilar artery to the point that it tears and bleeds. The pooling blood from the bleeding basilar artery, called a duret hemorrhage, exerts pressure on the upper portions of the brainstem, at the level of the pons. The pons, responsible for many essential life functions including consciousness, is thus compromised, leading to death. The classic triad of symptoms of a central herniation is coma, fixed and dilated pupils, and posturing.

The next type of herniation is called an **uncal herniation**. Lateral forces created by the expanding space-occupying lesion created by a blood clot compress the brain in the opposite hemisphere. The expanding lesion obliterates the cerebral ventricles within the core of the cerebral cortex. As a result, the patient may experience contralateral motor signs along with unilateral papillary changes on the ipsilateral side during the early phases of the herniation. When this occurs, the patient may appear to be experiencing a hemorrhagic stroke (a hemorrhagic stroke has the same progression as a traumatic hematoma). Again, without intervention, the lateral herniation will progress to a central herniation and the classic triad of central herniation will present.

The final supratentorial herniation is called **cingulated herniation**. During a cingulated herniation, an accumulation of blood from the expanding hematoma, particularly at the frontal lobe, creates a mass effect that pushes the cerebral cortex at the medial brain, called the cingulated gyrus, under the falx cerebri at the midbrain. This midline shift applies pressures upon the frontal lobe and along the cingulated gyrus, which affects the limbic system, the seat of emotion formation and memory. As a result, the patient experiences problems of memory, particularly short-term memory, as well as problems with emotions such as anger or confusion.

Infratentorial Herniation Syndromes

Intracranial hemorrhage can be the result of trauma low in the skull, toward the base of the skull, and create **infratentorial herniations** (herniations below the tentorium) (Figure 2-10). The first, called **tonsillar herniation**, is the result of expanding hematoma formation proximal to the cerebellum. The cerebellum comes to two points, called the tonsils. Pressure exerted from above on either of these tonsillar points results in compression of the posteroinferior cerebellar artery, compression of the medulla oblongata, and compression of the upper portions of the cervical sign. An early sign of a tonsillar herniation can be neck pain (nuchal rigidity) that progresses to tetraplegia (formerly quadriplegia). The Paramedic might assume that these developments are the result of a cervical spine injury, except for the corresponding changes in level of consciousness and vital signs (particularly the development of Cushing's triad, which will be discussed shortly).

A **transcalvarial herniation** is herniation of the brain through an open fracture. Any time gray matter leaves the skull, the impact can be devastating and may lead to meningitis, encephalitis, and permanent brain damage.[11]

CASE STUDY (CONTINUED)

Witnesses state that the runner was jogging along the pathway encircling the office park when he suddenly and unexpectedly ran into a cyclist, literally. The cyclist went up and over the handlebars and his helmeted head landed square in the middle of the runner's chest. The runner fell backwards, striking his head with a sickening crack. Both parties got up and started to dust themselves off, but the runner seemed a little dazed and complained of a headache. Witnesses were sure that the runner was "knocked out" for at least 30 seconds.

CRITICAL THINKING QUESTIONS

1. What are the important elements of the history that a Paramedic should obtain?
2. What is the symptom pattern for increased intracranial pressure?

History

During a trauma, Paramedics tend to focus on the mechanism of injury and the subsequent kinematics. As a result, the patient's history is often not given the consideration that it should get. However, the history can be very telling. Often patients who have suffered traumatic brain injury will manifest subtle indicators early in the injury. The Paramedic should concentrate on compiling a complete SAMPLE history (**S**igns and symptoms, **A**llergies, **M**edications, **P**ast history, **L**ast oral intake, and **E**vents leading up to the emergency) whenever possible.

Patients with traumatic brain injury may complain of a headache, which may be due to increasing intracranial pressure. Others may complain of neck pain (nuchal rigidity), as blood, irritating the meninges, flows around the brain and down the cervical spine.

The Paramedic should ascertain a history of allergies to medications while the patient is conscious in case the patient requires airway management, sedation or becomes unconscious.

The Paramedic should obtain as comprehensive a medication list as possible. Under normal circumstances, the heart rate of the hypovolemic patient is tachycardiac. Beta blockers, for example, may mask this sign until the more ominous hypotension occurs. Hypotension coupled with traumatic brain injury can lead to worsened outcomes and increased mortality.

One classification of medications, which can have particularly ominous implications, is that of anticoagulants. Anticoagulants can prevent clot formation and make a seemingly innocent mechanism of injury, such as a fall from a standing position, into a potentially life-threatening condition.

The Paramedic should try to get as complete a past medical history as possible. For example, ventilation is an important aspect of treatment of traumatic brain injury. Any comorbid pulmonary disease that affects ventilation, such as emphysema, can have a negative impact on the patient's survivability.

Since many patients with severe traumatic head injury will be intubated to protect the airway and carefully control ventilation, it is important that the Paramedic know when the patient's last meal was eaten. With this foreknowledge, the Paramedic can more properly prepare for the possibility of regurgitation and prevent aspiration.

The last element of a SAMPLE history may be the most important. Difficulty with remembering events that preceded the trauma suggests amnesia and may be indicative of a frontal brain injury.

CASE STUDY (CONTINUED)

The patient is lying supine on the grass with a helpful bystander holding in-line stabilization of the cervical spine. The Paramedic proceeds with his examination, starting with the patient's mental status. Immediately it becomes apparent that the patient's level of consciousness is waning rapidly and his respiratory pattern is starting to change.

CRITICAL THINKING QUESTIONS

1. What are the elements of the physical examination of a patient with suspected herniation syndrome?
2. Why are vital signs a critical element in this examination?

Examination

The nature of the call typically gives the Paramedic clues regarding the mechanism of injury. As previously stated, falls and vehicular crashes are two major causes of blunt trauma that consistently produce traumatic brain injury. A GSW, especially when accompanied with a report of unconsciousness, is suggestive of a penetrating head injury. Sources of combined blunt and penetrating trauma are explosions with both flying fragments and blast overpressure.

Clearly, a diffuse head injury with multiple sites of impact, such as might occur in a rollover motor vehicle crash, is more ominous than the presence of one focal injury site.

Although a head injury may manifest over hours or days, the Paramedic's focus is on the patients who present with signs of traumatic brain injury within minutes of the trauma or, perhaps more importantly, are at risk for secondary injury.

The three major etiologies of secondary head injury can be summed up with the letter H: hypoxia, hypercarbia, and hypoperfusion. The combination of both hypoxia and hypotension can be potentially lethal to the patient with a traumatic brain injury. The Paramedic's primary assessment should be focused on identifying potential sources of secondary brain injury.

Primary Assessment

After reviewing the mechanism of injury and upon approaching the patient, the Paramedic proceeds with a general impression of the patient. This includes the patient's level of consciousness and the level of interaction that the patient is having with the environment and other responders.

Head injuries may have accompanying spine injury. Conversely, a patient with a subdural hematoma may present with upper cervical pain from bleeding into the spinal cord. After establishing manual cervical stabilization, the Paramedic proceeds with the primary assessment, starting with an assessment of the patient's level of consciousness. Early changes in mental status are suggestive of underlying traumatic brain injury.

The AVPU scale (**A**lert, **V**oice, **P**ain, **U**nresponsive) is a quick focused means of assessing the patient's level of consciousness. The most disconcerting finding during the examination of level of consciousness is coma.

Coma is a state of deep unconsciousness that occurs from serious traumatic brain injury and that tends to progress through three stages. In the initial stage, the patient with increasing intracranial pressure may present with **decorticate rigidity** or **flexor posturing**. This flexor posturing is demonstrated by adduct of the shoulders, as the shoulders rotate internally with slight flexion while the forearms pronate and wrist and fingers flex. Simultaneously, the lower extremities will demonstrate "triple flexion" of the hip, knee, and ankles.

Next, the patient may demonstrate **decerebrate rigidity** or **extensor posturing**. Extensor posturing generally indicates upper brainstem injury and is often a premorbid finding. With extensor posturing, both the hips and shoulders extend and internally pronate while the forearms hyperpronate, the most noticeable characteristic of extensor posturing. The Paramedic may also witness plantar flexion with inversion. The Paramedic may note extensor posturing on only one side of the patient's body with flexor posturing on the other, sometimes seen in uncal herniation (Figure 2-11).

In the deepest level of a coma, the patient will be totally areflexic to sustained central painful stimulus. In the deepest coma, only spinal cord reflexes will remain intact (e.g., reflexes such as Babinski's reflex, in which the great toe flares upward).

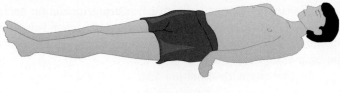

Decerebrate

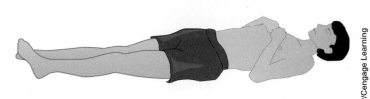

Decorticate

Figure 2-11 Decerebrate and decorticate rigidity.

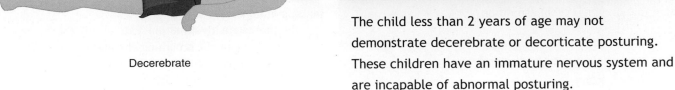
The child less than 2 years of age may not demonstrate decerebrate or decorticate posturing. These children have an immature nervous system and are incapable of abnormal posturing.

A patent airway is a primary objective with every trauma patient. However, it may be even more important in the head injury patient. Beyond the prevention of aspiration, prevention of secondary brain injury from hypoxia and hypercarbia is paramount. Therefore, in the case of any patient with a suspected head injury and an altered mental status, the Paramedic must consider advanced airway management.

Beyond the routine primary assessment performed on every trauma patient, the Paramedic should pay particular attention to the patient's respiratory pattern (Figure 2-12). The brainstem, through reflexive mechanisms located in the pons

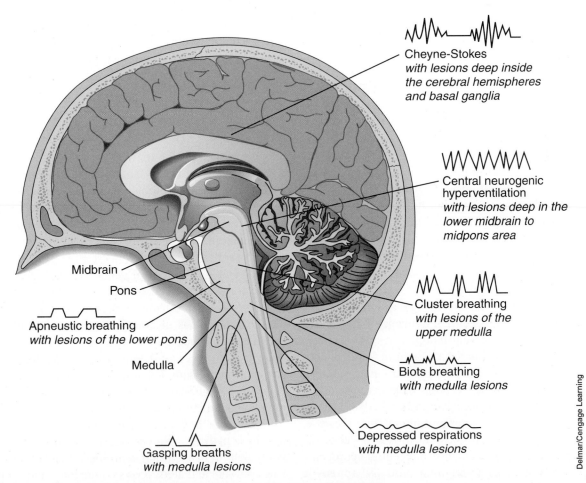

Cheyne-Stokes
with lesions deep inside the cerebral hemispheres and basal ganglia

Central neurogenic hyperventilation
with lesions deep in the lower midbrain to midpons area

Midbrain

Pons

Cluster breathing
with lesions of the upper medulla

Apneustic breathing
with lesions of the lower pons

Medulla

Biots breathing
with medulla lesions

Depressed respirations
with medulla lesions

Gasping breaths
with medulla lesions

Figure 2-12 Abnormal respiratory patterns with increasing ICP.

Table 2-5 Respiratory Patterns and Associated Areas of Brain Injury

- Forebrain damage
  ○ Cheyne–Stokes respiration
- Midbrain damage
  ○ Central neurogenic hyperventilation
- Pons dysfunction
  ○ Apneustic breathing
  ○ Cluster breathing
- Medullary dysfunction
  ○ Ataxic breathing

and medulla, is primarily responsible for respiratory rhythm generation. However, respirations can also be altered by behavioral influences that originate in the forebrain. As ICP increases within the cerebrum (generally) and upon the forebrain (specifically), the patient will start to manifest different patterns of respiration that can be indicative of head trauma.

The normal ebb and flow of respiration is referred to as "eupnea." This regular respiratory pattern is the result of interplay between the lungs and the brain in which the brain tries to maintain a carbon dioxide level within a narrow range. As the carbon dioxide tension builds, the brain stimulates the lungs to breathe. This feedback loop is almost instantaneous and imperceptible. When brain trauma occurs, the increasing ICP causes changes in respiratory patterns according to the level of brainstem dysfunction (Table 2-5).

Following traumatic head injury, increasing ICP compresses the forebrain and causes the first change to Cheyne–Stokes respiration. **Cheyne–Stokes respiration** is described as periods of hyperpnea followed by periods of apnea. During the periods of hyperpnea, the patient's breathing starts out quietly and gradually builds to deep inspiration, which is followed by a decreasing respiratory effort until apnea ensues. Initially, the periods of apnea may be short and almost unnoticeable. However, as the ICP increases the periods increase in duration until they last between 10 and 15 seconds. Eventually, this pattern of crescendo–decrescendo breathing, with periods of apnea, becomes more obvious until increased ICP causes the next change in respiration.

The next change of increasing ICP, and a sign of advancing brainstem dysfunction, is **central neurogenic hyperventilation**. This sustained hyperventilation, at respiratory rates of 40 to 60 breaths a minute, marks a departure from the periods of apnea noted in Cheyne–Stokes respiration. It is caused by pressure on the pulmonary receptors within the brainstem that control respirations and represents midbrain dysfunction.

In the face of unabated increasing intracranial pressure, and when brainstem dysfunction extends to the level of the pons, the patient's breathing changes from central neurogenic hyperventilation to apneustic breathing. Initially, **apneustic breathing** appears as a profound bradypnea with periods of apnea. However, upon closer examination the Paramedic will

note that the patient actually pauses during inhalation, as if to hold the breath, for periods of two to three seconds before exhaling. These breaths are then followed by equal length periods of apnea.

As brainstem dysfunction extends to the level of the medulla oblongata, the breathing changes yet again. This time it changes to cluster and ataxic breathing. Cluster breathing is a pattern of increasing depth of respirations until a sudden period of apnea occurs. Cluster breathing occurs when brainstem dysfunction has progressed to the higher medullary area, proximal to the pons.

Ataxic breathing, also called **Biot's breathing**, is a pattern of irregularly irregular gasping breathing or breathing that is arrhythmic in nature. Biot's breathing is generally a premorbid sign and is often missed by Paramedics who have been assisting respirations before this phenomenon occurred. An abrupt loss of blood pressure is associated with ataxic breathing as well.

Hypotension coupled with traumatic brain injury dramatically increases mortality. When confronted with a hypotensive patient, the Paramedic should aggressively seek to control the bleeding, if possible, and to stabilize the patient with fluid resuscitation. When considering potential sources of hidden bleeding, the Paramedic should exclude the skull. There is insufficient space to hemorrhage into the adult skull before the hemorrhage causes brain herniation. However, this is not true for children. Therefore, other potential etiologies for hypotension should be considered, including spinal cord injury and associated neurogenic shock. Although rare, cardiac contusions, particularly with associated dysrhythmia and internal hemorrhage, can also be a cause.

Disability

As part of the ABCs (**A**irway, **B**reathing, **C**irculation) of the trauma patient's primary assessment, the Paramedic should assess the patient's neurological status (under D for disability). Going beyond the AVPU determination made at the start of the primary survey, the disability step of the primary assessment includes a closer look at the patient's mental status and papillary reactions.

All changes of mental status are on a continuum from awake and alert and cooperative with care to comatose. Early changes of level of consciousness include confusion and disorientation, loss of both judgment and memory, and the presence of a headache. As the intracranial pressure increases there is a progressive deterioration of the patient's level of consciousness from lethargic to stupor to comatose. The Glasgow Coma Scale (Table 2-6) is the best tool for assessing and documenting these changes.

Although the Glasgow Coma Scale is helpful with assessing those patients with obviously altered mental status, it is not as helpful in assessing neurological changes in the patient who is awake and alert, obeys commands, and is conversant.

At the simplest level, the Paramedic may want to use short-term memory as an indicator of neurological function,

Table 2-6 Glasgow Coma Scale

Modified Glasgow Coma Scale		
Eye Opening	Best Verbal Response	Best Motor Response
Spontaneous 4	Oriented, conversing 5	Obeys verbal commands 6
To verbal command 3	Disoriented, conversing 4	Localize to pain 5
To pain 2	Inappropriate words 3	Flexion/withdrawal 4
None 1	Incomprehensible sounds 2	Abnormal flexion (decorticate) 3
	No verbal response 1	Extension (decerebrate) 2
		No response (flaccid) 1

since the frontal lobe is often involved in head injury. To help assess the patient with a mild head injury, the Paramedic may choose to use the six-item recall tool. The Paramedic asks the patient to remember a spoken list of three words and three drawn shapes and then asks the patient to recall that list at regular intervals, often five minutes apart. Alternatively, the Paramedic may ask the patient to perform serial sevens (subtracting seven from 100 backwards). Finally, to check attention span, the Paramedic can ask the patient to repeat a gradually increasing series of numbers; for example, $1 - 2 - 4 - 5$, then $5 - 6 - 8 - 1 - 0 - 3$. Most patients should normally be able to repeat at least seven digits.

Aside from the six-item recall test, there are a few other assessments that the Paramedic can use to assess and document the patient's mental status changes. Modifying its function slightly, the Paramedic can use the Rancho Los Amigos scale of cognitive functioning, a tool used in TBI rehabilitation programs. Like the Glasgow Coma Scale, the Rancho Los Amigos scale of cognitive function was developed to monitor neurological changes and predict eventual outcomes. Although patient outcomes, in terms of rehabilitation, may not be germane to the Paramedic's immediate task of caring for the brain-injured patient in the field, the levels of patient response can be useful in describing the patient presentation to the physician.

The modified Rancho Los Amigos scale is divided into 10 levels with associated clinical presentations. For purposes of Paramedic care, the levels VII through X represent what might be considered a normal initial presentation. Of more value are the descriptions of levels I to VI.

Patients at level VI of the modified Rancho Los Amigos scale are periodically confused as to person, place, or time. Although their long-term memory is intact, their recent memories (for example, of the events surrounding the crash) are inconsistent.

Patients at level V are alert but have problems of focus. Their attention wanders and at times they become agitated with excessive external stimulation. These patients are often not oriented, or must be constantly reoriented to themselves or their situation, often with statements like, "You were just in an accident."

Patients at level IV are agitated and confused. They often manifest a complete lack of short-term memory, as shown by repeated questions. These patients may speak gibberish or make nonsensical statements. More importantly, these patients may be aggressive or demonstrate flight behaviors, such as trying to remove spinal immobilization. Generally speaking, these patients are uncooperative with care.

Patients at level III are awake but unable to respond to simple commands. These patients blink and squint when a penlight crosses over their visual field, as if in pain. These patients will pull at tubes, such as an intravenous line or an endotracheal tube, and against restraints. These patients will turn away from strong auditory stimulation and will withdraw from painful stimuli. These patients may be described as being in a light coma.

Patients at level II demonstrate reflexive behaviors in response to painful stimulus. The response is random and nonpurposeful, neither pushing away the stimulus nor withdrawing from it. These patients are described as comatose.

Patients at level I are without any visible response to any stimulus. Only primitive spinal cord reflexes, such as Babinski's reflex, may be present. The Paramedic observes no opening of the eye or any papillary responses. The patient is completely limp and unresponsive.

The advantage of the Rancho Los Amigos scale of cognitive function is it relates behavioral changes to deteriorating neurological status in patients who presented initially as awake, alert, and oriented. Patients in levels I, II, or III of the Rancho Los Amigos scale generally have a Glasgow Coma Scale of less than eight.

Pupillary Response

Following the mental status exam, the pupils should be examined for the "three S's": size, shape, and symmetry. Pupillary reaction is a function of the third cranial nerve (CN III). The efferent fibers of the third cranial nerve exit the midbrain under the temporal lobe at the uncus. Normally the pupils constrict in response to direct light as well as consensually.

When there is increased ICP (for example, secondary to an uncal herniation), then the pupillary response will be altered. If the compression is unilateral there will be a loss of direct response to a bright light, but the consensual response may be preserved. As the ICP increases, the affected pupil tends to dilate and become nonreactive.

While examining the pupils for reactivity, the Paramedic should also assess the pupil for shape and symmetry. The pupil is typically round, unless altered by surgery. However, during a transtentorial herniation, and with compression of the third cranial nerve, the pupil has been known to take an oval or cat's eye appearance.

The Paramedic may also witness **hippus**, a rapid alternating constriction and dilation to bright light as the pupil tries to adjust. Hippus is an early sign of an uncal herniation.

Finally, the Paramedic should examine the pupils for symmetry. Although a small portion of the population has

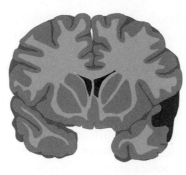

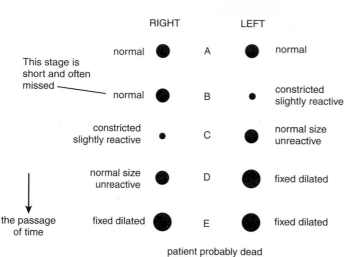

	RIGHT		LEFT	
normal	●	A	●	normal
normal	●	B	•	constricted slightly reactive
constricted slightly reactive	•	C	●	normal size unreactive
normal size unreactive	●	D	●	fixed dilated
fixed dilated	●	E	●	fixed dilated

This stage is short and often missed

the passage of time

patient probably dead

Figure 2-13 Progression of papillary changes associated with increasing ICP and herniation syndromes.

anisocoria (unequal pupils), this difference should be less than 1 mm. Asymmetrical pupils, greater than 1 mm, are abnormal and an early sign of brainstem herniation (Figure 2-13).

Rapid Trauma Examination

A head-to-toe rapid trauma examination may reveal subtle clues to the Paramedic. Starting at the skull, careful palpation and inspection may reveal a skull fracture. It is estimated that one in four skull fractures have an underlying intracranial hematoma and that 80% of fatal head injuries have an associated skull fracture.

Linear skull fractures, which make up 69% of skull fractures, are the most common skull fractures. Linear skull fractures are usually the result of low energy blunt trauma across a broad area. This nondisplaced fracture is not visible and therefore it may only be suspected if the patient has point tenderness in the area and/or soft-tissue injury. Based on examination of the mechanism of injury and the subsequent lines of force, the Paramedic should focus the examination on those areas most likely to have sustained trauma.

The depressed skull fracture, as opposed to a linear skull fracture, is generally due to a focused high-energy blow to the skull (sometimes called a burst fracture). One-third of the fracture fragments penetrate the meninges, and approximately another one-third penetrates the underlying brain.

Like the spider pattern on a broken windshield, they spread out in a centrifugal manner. The thinner pterion area is prone to depressed skull fractures and often has associated underlying bleeding.

STREET SMART

Whenever a laceration overlies a bony deformity, it is assumed that the fracture is an open fracture and should be treated accordingly.

Basilar Skull Fracture

The cerebral cortex sits positioned inside the skull like two boxers' gloves side by side. To the side (the thumb position) sits the temporal lobe and to the center (the mitt) sits the frontal lobe. Between these two lobes is the mastoid process. The mastoid process is a bony projection, found behind the ear, that serves as a point of impact when the brain moves forward during acceleration.

The most common basilar skull fracture, making up about 75% of cases of basilar fracture, is the temporal bone fracture. Basilar skull fracture of the temporal bone, proximal to the thin pterion, occurs proximal to external auditory os and is associated with **otorrhea**, leakage of cerebrospinal fluid from the ear, and Battle's sign. **Battle's sign** is a discoloration behind the ear that represents hematoma formation.

Basilar skull fractures involving the anterior cranial fossa tend to present with **rhinorrhea**, leakage of CSF from the nose, and bilateral periorbital ecchymosis (i.e., raccoon's eyes). As the base of the skull is the origin of many cranial nerves, basilar skull fractures can impact those nerves. Presentations that suggest a possible basilar skull fracture include facial palsy, facial numbness secondary to impingement of the facial nerve, and nystagmus and hearing loss, secondary to injury to the vestibulocochlear nerve.

STREET SMART

In the past, Paramedics depended on the "halo" sign to determine if CSF was in blood draining from the ear. The theory was that if a drop of fluid dropped onto a gauze pad, or the tip of a gauze pad was dipped in the fluid, then the red blood cells would migrate to the outside and form a ring or "halo." This theory has been largely discounted. It has been abandoned in the prehospital environment also because it is time-consuming to perform.

Cranial Nerve Exam

An abbreviated cranial nerve exam is in order for the patient with suspected head injury. As the cranial nerves exit the base of the skull they are sensitive to, and therefore early indicators of, increasing intracranial pressure.

To start, the patient should be asked to perform the cardinal gazes while the Paramedic observes for extraocular movements (EOM). The third, fourth, and sixth cranial nerves control the eye's movements. Any EOM is suggestive of traumatic brain injury. The presence of nystagmus is suggestive of a basilar skull fracture whereas loss of the lateral gaze, secondary to impairment of the abducens nerve (CN VI), is suggestive of uncal herniation.

Next, the Paramedic should examine the trigeminal nerve (CN V) by asking the patient if he can feel his face or forehead being stroked. If the patient is unconscious or semiconscious, the Paramedic should perform a tap between the eyebrows, called a glabellar tap, which will cause the eyes to blink.

Next, the patient should be asked to smile. The Paramedic then checks to see if the forehead wrinkles in the process. Also, the patient should be asked to close his eyelids and to prevent the Paramedic from opening his eyelids against resistance, thereby testing the VII cranial nerve.

The whispered voice is a particularly telling examination, as hearing loss may be indicative of a basilar skull fracture. Hearing is partially a function of the vestibulocochlear nerve, the VIII cranial nerve, which is often disrupted by a basilar skull fracture.

Cerebellar tests, such as alternating pronation and supination of the hands, or a Romberg test (for example, heel to shin), can be used to assess for infratentorial mass effect.

► CASE STUDY (CONTINUED)

The Paramedic suspects, based on the symptom pattern of hypertension, bradycardia, and the Cheyne-Stokes respiratory pattern, that the runner has a traumatic brain injury and impending transtentorial herniation as a result of increasing intracranial pressure.

CRITICAL THINKING QUESTIONS

1. What is the significance of the Cushing's triad?
2. What is the patient's prognosis?

Assessment

The presence of a symptom complex, including **Cushing's triad** (hypertension, bradycardia, and altered respiratory pattern), is suggestive of herniation syndrome. The mechanism of injury leads the Paramedic to have a high index of suspicion that a traumatic brain injury may have occurred. In the presence of a coma, and without benefit of a CT scan, the Paramedic must assume a diffuse vascular injury with impending intracranial catastrophe.

The best indicator of the traumatic brain injury's severity is the Glasgow Coma Scale (GCS). Developed in 1974 by Teasdale and Jennett at the University of Glasgow, the GCS is an assessment of function, not injury, and is only a snapshot in a moment of time. Neurologic function, and therefore the GCS, can be affected by hypoxia, hypotension, acidosis, hearing loss, facial injury, and so on.

As the patient is stabilized, a trend will develop. As a trend develops, from repeated assessments, the GCS begins to have some prognostic value. Patients with a GCS of 13 to 15 have mild injury and less than 3% will deteriorate. This group represents some 80% of head-injured patients and a mortality that approaches zero.

Those patients with a GCS score between 9 and 12 have moderate head injury and often present with altered mental status and/or focal neurological deficits. One in five of these patients will deteriorate into coma, although 60% will progress to a good recovery. The remainder will sustain a moderate disability, defined as an impairment of their ability to perform the activities of daily living (ADL).

One of the key features of moderate head injury is the inability to follow simple commands. Patients with severe head injuries do not follow commands and generally have a GCS score between 3 and 8. Patients within this group have a 30% mortality rate and another 17% will experience moderate to severe disabilities. The remainder of this group will be in a coma.

Coma is a neurological state in which the patient does not respond to sustained (>30 seconds) painful stimuli. Some patients in a coma have eye opening and are said to be in a vegetative state (without cognitive or affective function). Some patients in a "light" coma are minimally responsive (i.e., are higher functioning than coma), but have debilitating neurological complications that leave them totally dependent.

Although not technically a coma, a patient with **akinetic mutism** may present similarly to a patient in coma (i.e., without facial expression, mute but eyes open and able to fix a gaze on a person). Akinetic mutism occurs with frontal lobe trauma, such as contusions or anterior cerebral artery damage, and specifically the destruction of the cingulate gyrus.

Another patient presentation that can occur in trauma is called locked-in syndrome. With **locked-in syndrome**, the entire body is paralyzed with the exception of the eyes. The patient with locked-in syndrome may be conscious and alert but unable to move or speak. The paralysis is not the result of cervical spine injury but a pontine hemorrhage (bleeding within the pons), which can occur with trauma and is seen with basilar skull fractures. Unlike spine-induced tetraplegia,

the patient with locked-in syndrome is unable to move the lower face, extending to the level of the eyeballs. All these patients may be able to do is blink and move their eyes vertically.

STREET SMART

Consider drug toxidromes including alcohol intoxication in differential diagnoses.

CASE STUDY (CONTINUED)

Within what seems like minutes, the patient has gone from unconscious to conscious to unconscious again. When stimulated, the patient seems to moan and curl his arms inward. The Paramedic remembers the triple H's of head injury: prevent hypoxia, reverse hypoglycemia, and treat hypotension. This litany reminds him of a list of tasks to be performed, starting with airway management, all while en route to the hospital. Fortunately, the fire department's first responders arrive, providing plenty of personnel to expedite the patient's packaging.

CRITICAL THINKING QUESTIONS

1. What is the national standard of care of patients with suspected herniation syndrome?
2. What are some of the patient-specific concerns and considerations that the Paramedic should consider when applying this plan of care that is intended to treat a broad patient population presenting with acute herniation syndrome?

Treatment

Although the Paramedic may be focused on the patient's neurological state, particularly the coma, head injury does not happen alone. Therefore, other aspects of assessment must not be ignored. Among patients with severe traumatic head injury, 75% have associated multiple trauma. Therefore, treatment must focus on treating the whole patient and supporting basic life functions. Studies have shown that 30% of patients with traumatic brain injury arrived at the emergency department hypoxic and 15% presented hypotensive. Hypotension with head injury has a 50% increase in mortality. A combination of both hypoxia and hypotension has an associated mortality of 75%.[12]

The first priority of treatment of any trauma patient is proper spinal stabilization and immobilization, as indicated. Improper application of the cervical immobilization device, compressing the jugular veins, or failure to maintain the patient's head in a neutral in-line position can increase ICP, worsening the patient's condition.

To further improve venous outflow in the head-injured patient, after spinal immobilization, the head of the stretcher should be elevated approximately 30 degrees, but no greater,

as elevation above 30 degrees may decrease cerebral perfusion pressures.[13] An added benefit of head elevation in this population is the reduced risk of aspiration.

Patients with suspected spinal cord injury, and associated head trauma, may experience sudden and unannounced projectile vomiting. This vomiting is due to direct pressure on the medulla oblongata. In these cases, nausea may not proceed to vomiting. Therefore, all precautions should be taken to prevent aspiration, including early and aggressive airway control that may include intubation or medication-facilitated intubation.

Prior to intubation, it is customary to use lidocaine intravenously to help blunt sudden increases in intracranial pressure.[14] However, there is some opposition to the routine use of lidocaine prior to intubation of the head-injured patient. Lidocaine is a negative inotropic agent and, as such, can lower blood pressure. Hypotension in the face of traumatic brain injury has been shown to create the worst outcomes. Therefore, the use of lidocaine should be reserved for only those patients who are hemodynamically stable.

The use of paralytics to facilitate intubation of the head-injured patient is an accepted practice that has come under increased scrutiny, specifically by the Brain Trauma

Foundation.[15] One of the concerns raised was the potential induced hypotension that may occur with intubation. In the hypotensive head-injured patient population, the use of ketamine should be considered. The decision whether to use paralytics or any drugs to facilitate intubation of head-injured patients should be a medical control decision.

One of the major concerns raised regarding medication-facilitated intubation is the accidental practice of hyperventilation prior to or during intubation attempts. Careful attention to the ventilatory status of the head-injured patient is critical. The presence of hypoxia, a SpO_2 of < 90% or PO_2 < 60 mmHg, can lead to increased cerebral blood flow, through vasodilation and a subsequent increase in ICP. If the SpO_2 is less than 70% (approximate PO_2 of 30 mmHg), the room air oxygen saturation on top of Mount Everest, the cerebral blood flow will double. (This assumes normal hemoglobin of 15 mg/L. The patient's hemoglobin may be lower if the patient is hemorrhaging as well.)

Similarly, a pCO_2 of greater than 45 mmHg (i.e., hypercarbia) will lead to cerebral vasodilation. Therefore, it is important to try to consistently maintain the pCO_2 within a normal range of 35 to 46 mmHg. This can be accomplished by careful monitoring of the end-tidal CO_2.

STREET SMART

Although use of hyperbaric oxygen therapy for traumatically injured brains may seem intuitive, the evidence appears insufficient to support its routine use at this time, unless complications such as smoke inhalation and carbon monoxide poisoning coexist.[16]

Although intravenous access should be obtained and maintained for medication administration, strict fluid conservation should be observed unless the patient is hypotensive. A single episode of hypotension with blood pressure < 90 mmHg has been shown to double mortality.[17] If hypotension does occur, the patient's mean arterial pressure should be maintained between 60 and 65 mmHg. Alternatively, if the MAP is unavailable, the systolic pressure should be maintained at approximately 90 mmHg using isotonic solutions. Dextrose-containing solutions should be avoided as they can worsen lactic acidosis and increase cerebral edema, further adding to the ICP.

Some studies encourage the use of hypertonic 3% to 7.5% saline solutions (i.e., super saline solution). These hypertonic saline solutions (HTS) can pull up to 2,500 cc from tissues and thereby reduce cerebral edema while increasing the systemic blood volume. However, this may, in turn, increase space for intracranial bleeding. Use of hypertonic saline solutions should only be accomplished with medical direction.

The maintenance of an adequate blood flow cannot be overemphasized. During low flow rates, red blood cells tend to clump and remain in the center of great vessels. The result is that peripheral arterioles have a lower hematocrit, a phenomena known as plasma skimming. This reduced hematocrit in peripheral arterioles results in injury and ischemia that is magnified in the oxygen-dependent brain cells.

The use of dopamine, and other catecholamines, to help maintain blood pressure in the patient with traumatic brain injury is controversial. There are a minimal number of alpha receptors, which cause vasoconstriction, in the brain. Therefore, dopamine should minimally impact cerebral blood flow (CBF). CBF is more likely controlled by local endothelium-derived factors (such as nitric oxide) and local metabolic factors such as increased carbon dioxide and acidosis. Therefore, it may be more important to concentrate on ventilation and elimination of carbon dioxide than the administration of vasopressors, such as dopamine, during a cerebral resuscitation.

Anticonvulsants, such as diazepam, are not routinely given prophylactically to patients with suspected traumatic brain injury. However, 30% to 40% of patients with a penetrating head injury will seize. Such seizures should be aggressively treated as they can increase metabolic demand, worsen hypoxia and hypercarbia, and raise ICP dramatically.

Increased ICP can result in the production of dysrhythmia. It is estimated that 90% of patients who have sustained a traumatic brain injury will have dysrhythmia. These dysrhythmias, including ventricular tachycardia, are secondary to catecholamine release from brainstem compression. As dysrhythmia can have dramatic impacts on cardiac output, treatment of these dysrhythmia may be appropriate.

It has been noted that there is a release of excessive glutamate, an excitatory neurotransmitter, during head injury. Glutamate causes the passage of calcium ions into the cells, forcing potassium out in the process, with a subsequent loss of energy. In the future, Paramedics may possibly use calcium channel blockers as a neuroprotective agent to offset the effects of glutamate.

Another treatment that may have promise is the use of induced hypothermia for traumatic brain injury. The Brain Trauma Foundation task force has given induced hypothermia a level III recommendation for use in selected cases of traumatic brain injury only.[17]

Goal-Driven Therapy

The therapeutic goals for the patient with a traumatic brain injury are to maintain an SpO_2 between 92% and 100%, a $PaCO_2$ between 35 and 45 mmHg, and a MAP of 60 or systolic pressure of 90 to 100 mmHg, assuming the patient is normothermic and normoglycemic.[18]

STREET SMART

Some Paramedics remember the rule of "90-90-9": maintain the systolic blood pressure at or above 90 mmHg, keep the oxygen saturation above 90, and try to maintain the Glasgow Coma Scale above 9.

While loading the backboarded patient into the ambulance, the Paramedic sees the patient struggling. A well-meaning firefighter is encouraging the patient to just relax and not fight when the Paramedic announces that the patient is having a seizure.

CRITICAL THINKING QUESTIONS

1. What are some of the predictable complications associated with acute herniation syndrome?
2. What are some of the predictable complications associated with the treatments for acute herniation syndrome?

Evaluation

The presence of Cushing's triad, either extensor or flexor posturing, or other signs of cerebral herniation (such as dilated, nonreactive, or asymmetric pupils) should be immediately treated with **therapeutic hyperventilation** (faster and deeper respirations than needed) until the symptoms abate. Hyperventilation rids the blood of carbon dioxide, a potent vasoconstrictor, and results in decreased intracerebral bleeding and/or decreased ICP. The goal of hyperventilation is to maintain an $EtCO_2$ between 30 and 35 mmHg.

However, hyperventilation is not without its dangers. The decrease of 1 mmHg of $EtCO_2$ can cause a 3% decrease in cerebral blood flow. Therefore, a drop of $EtCO_2$ from 35 to 30 mmHg could result in a 15% drop in pancerebral circulation, resulting in pancerebral anoxia. For this reason, hyperventilation should not be used prophylactically and its use should be reserved for life-threatening herniation.

Hyperosmolar therapies, such as Mannitol, have been used to reduce intracranial pressure. Mannitol, a hypertonic simple sugar, is effective within 15 minutes. However, its use is not supported in the prehospital setting by the Brain Trauma Foundation.

CASE STUDY CONCLUSION

With the patient's seizure successfully controlled with diazepam, the Paramedic directs his partner to precede to the trauma center with lights and sirens. Although the trip is short—the trauma center is less than five minutes from the scene—the Paramedic elects to have dispatch contact the trauma center and call for a "trauma alert." Even five minutes might give the trauma team time to assemble and to alert medical imaging of the impending arrival of a traumatic brain injury.

CRITICAL THINKING QUESTIONS

1. What is the most appropriate transport decision that will get the patient to definitive care?
2. What are the advantages of transporting a patient with suspected acute herniation syndrome to these hospitals, even if that means bypassing other hospitals in the process?

Disposition

Survival for the patient with traumatic brain injury depends on rapid identification of the hematoma, usually via CT scan, and clot extraction via craniotomy, similar to the ancient practice of trephination, or craniectomy (the creation of a bone flap). These surgical procedures, and subsequent intensive care, are available at a trauma center.

CONCLUSION

With 50% of death secondary to brain injury occurring in the first two hours, the care of the brain-injured patient is an important aspect of the Paramedic's practice.[3] Prehospital treatment of hypoxia, hypercarbia, and hypotension can help prevent secondary brain injury and improve overall survival of this deadly trauma.

KEY POINTS:

- Traumatic brain injury is the most frequent cause of trauma death and has substantial long-term disability.

- Although Paramedics can have little impact on primary brain injury, they can prevent secondary brain injury.

- The most common brain injury is concussion that is characterized by prolonged altered mental status rather than unconsciousness.

- Intraparenchymal hemorrhages, such as cerebral contusion, diffuse axonal injury, and concussion, are likely due to acceleration-deceleration injury and may have associated contrecoup injury.

- Extracerebral hemorrhages, such as traumatic subarachnoid hemorrhage, subdural hematoma, and epidural hematoma, frequently cause an increase in intracranial pressure.

- Shaken baby syndrome is a combination of subdural hematoma and diffuse axonal injury due to acceleration-deceleration of the cerebral cortex during the violent movement of the head.

- Subdural hematomas form slowly as a result of venous bleeding, whereas epidural hematomas can develop rapidly as a result of arterial bleeding.

- Cerebral perfusion pressure is a function of blood pressure and intracranial pressure. As intracranial pressure rises, the blood pressure must rise to compensate until it reaches a tipping point and the patient rapidly decompensates (i.e., Monroe-Kellie hypothesis).

- The effects of increased intracranial pressure are manifest in the herniation syndromes.

- Supratentorial herniations include central herniation, uncal herniation, and cingulated herniation. These three herniation syndromes are the result of increased intracranial pressure.

- Infratentorial herniations result from trauma low to the skull and include tonsillar herniations and transcalvarial herniation.

- Posturing, either decorticate or decerebrate posturing, is a sign of increased intracranial pressure.

- There are discernable patterns in ventilation as well as papillary reaction that accompany increasing intracranial pressure.

- Changes in mental status can be subtle, and tests like the six-item recall can detect these changes.

- Pupillary changes are another indicator of increasing intracranial pressure.

- Cushing's triad is hypertension, bradycardia, and altered respiratory pattern.

- External signs of a basilar skull fracture include otorrhea, rhinorrhea, bilateral periorbital ecchymosis, and Battle's sign.

REVIEW QUESTIONS:

1. What are the three "H's" that can cause secondary brain injury?
2. Which extracerebral hemorrhage is rapid in onset and what symptom is often used to differentiate it?
3. What is the Monroe–Kellie hypothesis?
4. What is the symptom pattern associated with transtentorial central herniation?
5. What are the benefits and risks of therapeutic hyperventilation?

CASE STUDY QUESTIONS:

Please refer to the Case Study in this chapter, and answer the questions below:

1. What are the potential risks and benefits of using medication-facilitated intubation for the patient with a traumatic brain injury?
2. What is the importance of performing a trauma examination for the head-injured patient?
3. The suspected head injury in the case was an epidural hematoma. Suppose the head injury was a simple concussion instead. How would the patient have presented differently or similarly?

REFERENCES:

1. Centers for Disease Control and Prevention. Available at: **http://www.cdc.gov/.** Accessed March 1, 2010.
2. Langlois JA, Rutland-Brown W, Thomas KE. *Traumatic Brain Injury in the United States: Emergency Department Visits, Hospitalizations, and Deaths*. Atlanta, GA: Centers for Disease Control and Prevention, National Center for Injury Prevention and Control; 2006.
3. Brain Injury Association. Available at **http://www.biausa.org/.** Accessed March 1, 2010.
4. Kelly J, Rosenburg J. *Practice Parameters for the Management of Concussion.* St. Paul, MN: American Academy of Neurology; 1997.
5. Lezak M. *Neuropsychological Assessment* (3rd ed.) New York: Oxford University Press; 2004. This book has a comprehensive treatment of this subject beginning at page 178.
6. Bazarian JJ. Diagnosing mild traumatic brain injury after a concussion. *Journal of Head Trauma Rehabilitation.* 2010; 25(4):225-227.
7. Boden BP, Tacchetti RL, Cantu RC, Knowles SB, Mueller FO. Catastrophic head injuries in high school and college football players. *Am J Sports Med.* Jul 2007;35(7):1075-1081.
8. Kotwica Z, Brzezinski J. Acute subdural haematoma in adults: an analysis of outcome in comatose patients. *Acta Neurochir (Wien).* 1993;121(3-4):95-99.
9. Silver J, McAllister T, Yudofsky S. *Textbook of Traumatic Brain Injury.* Arlington, VA: American Psychiatric Publishing, Inc.;2004.
10. Brown RL, Brunn MA, Garcia VF. Cervical spine injuries in children: a review of 103 patients treated consecutively at a level 1 pediatric trauma center. *J Pediatr Surg.* Aug 2001;36(8):1107-1114.
11. Barker E. *Neuroscience Nursing: A Spectrum of Care* (2nd ed.). New York: Elsevier-Mosby; 2002;387-389.
12. American College of Surgeons. *Advanced Trauma Life Support Course* (7th ed.) Chicago: Committee on Trauma, American College of Surgeons; 2006.
13. Durward QJ, Amacher AL, Del Maestro RF, Sibbald WJ. Cerebral and cardiovascular responses to changes in head elevation in patients with intracranial hypertension. *J Neurosurg.* 1983;59:938-944.
14. Reynolds SF, Heffner J. Airway management of the critically ill patient: rapid-sequence intubation. *Chest.* 2005;127:1397-1412.
15. Davis D, Fakhry S, Wang H, Bulger E, et al. Paramedic rapid sequence intubation for severe traumatic brain injury: perspectives from an expert panel. *Prehosp Emerg Care.* 2007;1(1):1-8.
16. *Cochrane Database Systems Review.* Oct 2004;18(4):CD004609.
17. Peterson K, Carson S, Carney N. Hypothermia treatment for traumatic brain injury: a systemic review and meta-analysis. *J Neurotrauma.* 2008;25(1):62-71.
18. Badjatia N, et al. *Prehospital Emergency Care.* January–March 2007;12(1).

NECK AND FACIAL TRAUMA

KEY CONCEPTS:

Upon completion of this chapter, it is expected that the reader will understand these following concepts:

- The origin of most facial and neck trauma
- The problem of disfigurement and functional sensory impairment with facial trauma
- Differentiation and classification of facial fractures
- Potential sight-threatening eye injuries
- Associated underlying injuries associated with facial and neck trauma
- Treatment priorities in facial and neck trauma

ANATOMY CONCEPTS:

Prior to reading this chapter the Paramedic student should be familiar with the following anatomy and physiology concepts:

- Facial bony, vascular, and nervous anatomy
- Anatomy of the eyes and ears
- Structures of the throat

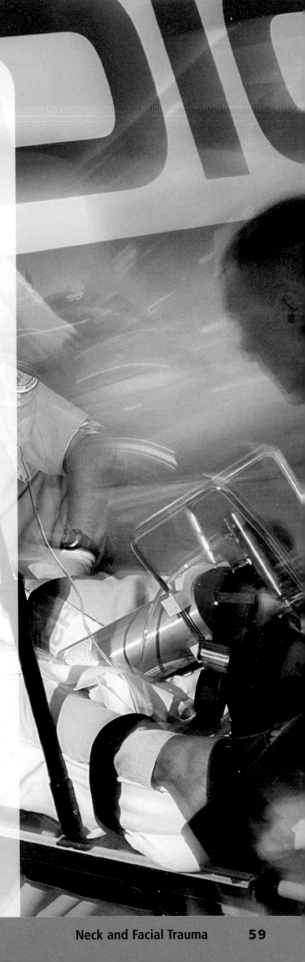

CASE STUDY:

A sea of patrol cars is on-scene. Apparently someone had a disagreement with someone else at a bar, someone pulled out a baseball bat, and the rest is history. The "perpetrator" is being led away in handcuffs. As he is directed to the back step of the pumper by police, the patient can be seen leaning forward, elbows on his knees, and holding his head up with his hands. Between his fingers the Paramedic can see the telltale sign of severe bleeding: long stringy clots and dripping blood.

After carefully putting on gloves and goggles, the Paramedic crouches down in front of the patient to introduce himself. The patient's clear answer at least confirms he is awake, alert, and maintaining an airway for the time being. The Paramedic explains that someone will temporarily be holding his head while they examine him.

CRITICAL THINKING QUESTIONS

1. What are some of the possible facial injuries that would be suspected based on the mechanism of injury?
2. Are any of these facial injuries potentially life-threatening injuries?

OVERVIEW

Injuries to the head, face, and neck occur both as isolated trauma and as part of multisystem trauma. Both blunt and penetrating trauma can cause injury to the head, face, and neck. These injuries range from the minor to the potentially life-threatening. An awareness of the mechanisms that produce these injuries, as well as the pathophysiology of the injuries, allows the Paramedic to assess for and effectively manage them. In this chapter, we will examine traumatic injuries that occur to the face (maxillofacial), the eyes, the ears, and the neck.

Chief Concern

Forces applied above the clavicles can produce injury in the face, eyes, ears, and neck. Injuries to each of these areas have unique characteristics, including disfigurement, impairment of sensory organs, and the need for significant posttrauma care.

Facial Injuries

Facial injuries most commonly occur in the setting of blunt trauma, with assaults, motor vehicle crashes, and falls serving as the major causes of maxillofacial fractures.[1,2] There is also an association between mild head injuries and facial fractures,[2] although a lower association exists between significant ocular injuries and facial fractures.[3] The face is the most injured part of the body when children play baseball.[4] Although these injuries are often not life-threatening, airway compromise is the primary concern when force is applied to the face.

Many small and fragile bones connect together to form the face (Figure 3-1). Fractures of the zygomatic arches and the nasal bones are common, and although they can be disfiguring they are rarely serious. These bones fracture when subjected to less force than other bones of the face.[5] In contrast, fractures of the angle and symphysis of the mandible, the supraorbital rim, and the frontal bone may require significant force in order to develop a fracture and are associated with intracranial and cervical spine injuries.[6]

In the late 1800s, René Le Fort, a French surgeon, performed a series of experiments on cadavers to study fracture patterns of the facial bones.[7] Dr. Le Fort applied forces to the face using various methods including striking the face with a wooden club and a metal shaft, dropping the head against

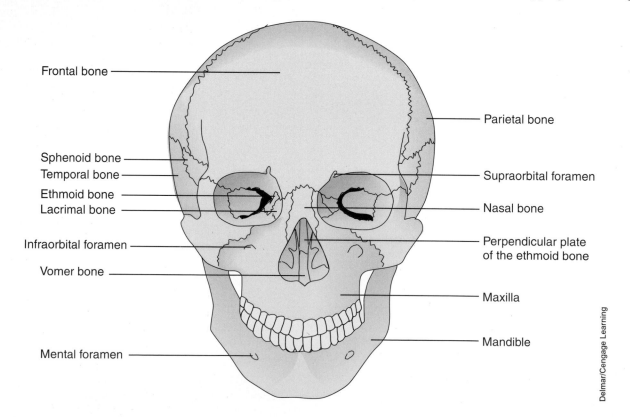

Figure 3-1 Bony structures of the face.

a marble table, and kicking the face.[8] He attempted to allow the cadaver to fall from a standing position; however, he was not able to generate sufficient force against the face using that method. Contrary to popular folklore, Dr. Le Fort did not drop cannonballs on the subjects' faces. Based on the series of experiments reported in his three papers published in 1901,[7] Dr. Le Fort grouped facial fractures into three classifications that later were named Le Fort I, II, and III fractures (Figure 3-2).

The Le Fort I fracture (Figure 3-2a) is a horizontal fracture of the maxilla that causes a separation of the hard palate from the rest of the face. The Paramedic may note that the hard palate and upper teeth float or are mobile when performing airway management procedures on the patient. A Le Fort II fracture occurs slightly posteriorly and involves separation of the nasal bones and maxilla from the rest of the face (Figure 3-2b). A Le Fort III fracture (often called complete craniofacial dysfunction) occurs when the fracture line is along the separation between the cranial bones and the facial bones (Figure 3-2c). All three of these fractures are unstable and require surgical stabilization and repair. These fractures may cause a significant amount of bleeding, generally from the nares due to the vascularity of the nasal and sinus mucous membranes. Bleeding may be significant enough to cause airway compromise or hypotension if not controlled. Patients with fractures that involve the midface, such as those with any of the three types of Le Fort fractures, have a significantly higher risk of death from neurologic injury.[9] This indicates that the forces that cause facial fractures are often transmitted to the brain.

Orbital fractures commonly accompany other facial bone fractures (i.e., Le Fort fractures). The bones that make up the inferior and medial (nasal) walls of the orbit are thin bones that are easily fractured, whereas the superior and lateral (temporal) portion of the orbit tends to be a bit stronger and is thus fractured less often.[10] These fractures are commonly called **orbital blowout fractures** because the force causes an inferior and medial displacement of the orbital walls, or a "blowing out" of the orbit, without fracturing the stronger and thicker orbital rim. Although this physiologically dissipates the forces and prevents globe rupture, up to one-third of blowout fractures have an associated eye injury.

The cause of orbital blowout fractures has been debated since the early 1900s.[11,12] One theory states the forces applied to the orbital rim are transmitted to the weaker bones of the orbit, producing a buckling effect and ultimately fracture (Figure 3-3a). A second theory proposes that the forces applied to the face are transmitted through the somewhat incompressible liquid-filled eye to the weaker bones of the orbit, creating a hydraulic effect and causing the blowout fracture (Figure 3-3b). Although several researchers have attempted to prove one theory over the other, a 1999 study demonstrated that both mechanisms can cause orbital blowout fractures. Lateral wall fractures, in contrast, are more often associated with forces that are applied to the globe.[12] The infraorbital nerve, which takes sensory information from skin over the territory from the maxilla to the inferior orbital rim, is sometimes damaged from the blowout fracture, causing decreased sensation in the area over the cheek on the side of the fracture (Figure 3-4).

In general, orbital fractures are not serious injuries; however, some will require surgical repair. In addition to injury to the eye and damage to the infraorbital nerve, the other significant complication of a blowout fracture is entrapment of the extraocular muscles. The six extraocular muscles surround the eye and provide movement in all directions (Figure 3-5). The two muscles that are most likely trapped are the inferior rectus muscle in orbital floor fractures and the medial rectus muscle in medial wall fractures. If the inferior rectus

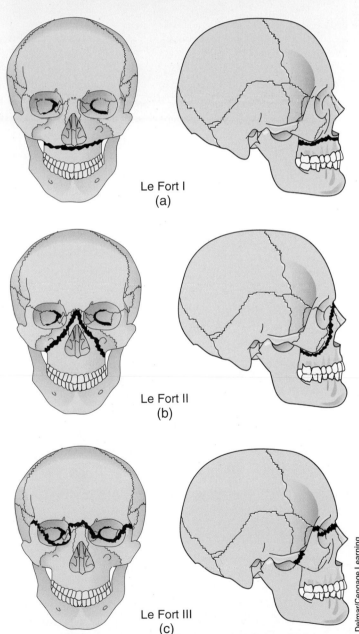

Le Fort I
(a)

Le Fort II
(b)

Le Fort III
(c)

Delmar/Cengage Learning

Figure 3-2 The Le Fort classification of maxillofacial injuries. (a) Le Fort I fracture. (b) Le Fort II fracture. (c) Le Fort III fracture.

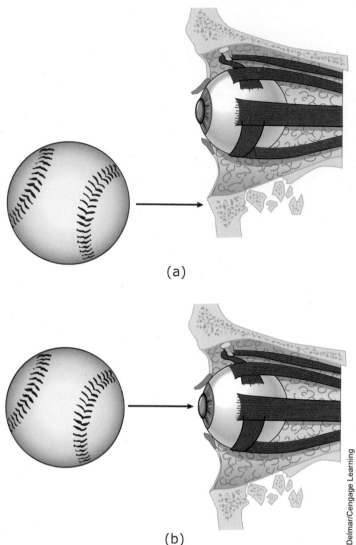

(a)

(b)

Figure 3-3 The two mechanisms thought to produce orbital blowout fractures are (a) the buckle theory and (b) the hydraulic theory.

muscle is trapped in the fracture fragments, the patient will not be able to look upward and may have pain with extraocular movements (EOM). If the medial rectus muscle is trapped in the fracture fragments, then the patient will have difficulty in looking laterally and associated pain.[10]

The mandible is also susceptible to fractures and dislocation, especially when forces are applied obliquely to its lateral aspect. Most often, the mandibular ramus or condyle is fractured, as the mandible is essentially a ring that dissipates forces along the entire circumference of the mandible. For this reason, a fracture on one side of the mandible is often accompanied by a fracture somewhere else along the mandible. The most serious mandibular fracture is a fracture through the mandibular symphysis, or the spot where the right and left halves of the mandible are fused. A fracture at this location disrupts the support structure for the tongue, causing the tongue to be displaced posterior, placing the patient at risk for airway obstruction.[13] The Paramedic may also encounter floating mandibular fractures in which the mandible has

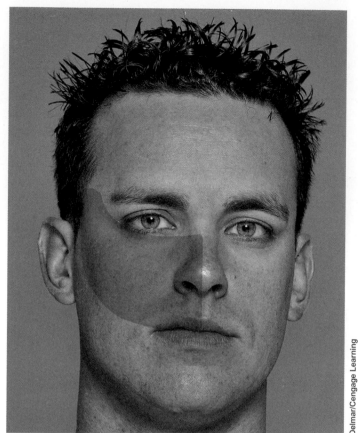

Figure 3-4 Damage to the infraorbital nerve may indicate the presence of an orbital blowout fracture and is noted by decreased sensation in the shaded area.

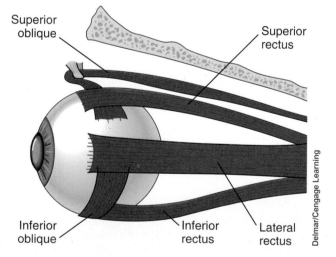

Superior oblique

Superior rectus

Inferior oblique

Inferior rectus

Lateral rectus

Figure 3-5 The extraocular muscles are responsible for moving the eye through its range of motion.

been fractured in two locations and the segment between is free floating. This can also compromise the airway and make laryngoscopy more difficult. Lacerations in the skin or oral mucosa overlying the fracture must be assumed to be open fractures until proven otherwise.

Forces applied to the mouth may also disrupt the teeth and cause **dental malocclusion**. Lost teeth that cannot be found are assumed to have ended up in the airway until proven otherwise by X-ray in the emergency department. Fractures involving the alveolar ridge, or the portion of the maxilla where the teeth are implanted, may result in loose teeth and bleeding at the gum line. A presentation of lower teeth that are loose with blood present on the gums in the area of mandibular tenderness should be assumed to be an open mandibular fracture.

Fractured teeth are classified by the amount of tooth involved using the **Ellis classifications** (Figure 3-6).[14] Ellis I tooth fractures only involve the enamel and tend to not produce significant pain (Figure 3-6a). Ellis II tooth fractures run through the enamel into the dentin, leaving the yellowish colored dentin exposed (Figure 3-6b). A tooth that has sustained an Ellis II fracture tends to be painful to palpation or exposure to the air. Ellis III fractures (Figure 3-6c) extend down to the pulp and can be extremely painful. The pulp can be visualized by observing a centered pink or red spot in the yellow dentin that represents a small amount of bleeding from the blood vessels that supply the tooth.

Ocular Injuries

Ocular injuries can be isolated or may accompany other facial injuries. These injuries are often caused by direct force applied to the globe, causing **globe rupture** (a loss of the eyeball's integrity). In the United States, there are over two million eye injuries per year, with 2% resulting in permanent visual defects, including blindness and orbital paralysis.[15]

As previously discussed, the bony structure of the bones that make up the orbit provides some protection to the globe by giving way and dissipating the energy applied to the globe, much in the way automobile crumple zones are designed to dissipate much of the energy of an automobile crash before it reaches the passenger compartment. When blunt force is applied directly to the globe, it significantly increases the pressure of the fluid within the eye. Rather than rupturing the globe, however, the force displaces the globe against the thin bones of the orbit, which gives way and fractures. At some point, however, the blunt force applied to the eye is significant enough to cause a globe rupture, even with an associated orbital blowout fracture.

More often, globe rupture is subtle, with the patient complaining of eye pain and no other physical findings. On the other end of the spectrum, the rupture may be severe enough for the Paramedic to notice a deformity of the globe. Visual acuity is often decreased or completely absent. A small, dark black spot may be noticeable on the sclera, which occurs when the deeper layers are exposed. In a patient who has also received blunt trauma to the face, globe ruptures may not be immediately noticeable, especially if the patient has altered mental status due to a head injury or intoxication. In motor vehicle crashes, airbags have been implicated as a cause of facial fractures and globe rupture.[16]

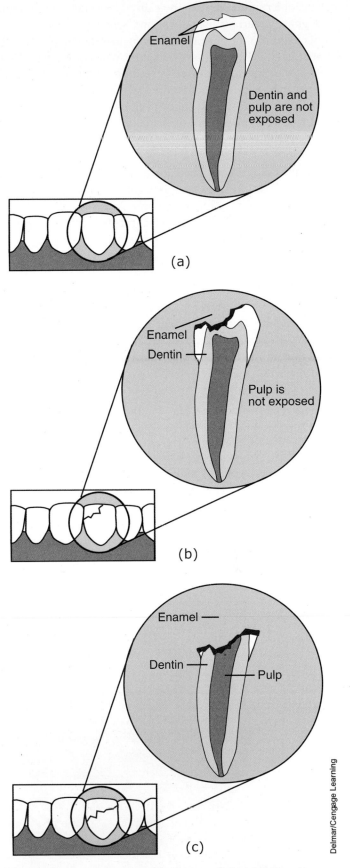

Figure 3-6 Ellis classification of dental fractures: (a) Ellis I, through the enamel; (b) Ellis II, which shows the dentin; and (c) Ellis III, which shows the pulp.

Globe rupture can also be caused by penetrating trauma. BB guns, firearms, fishhooks, and writing instruments are some examples of objects that can penetrate the globe. If the object is still in place, globe rupture will be obvious. However, if the object is removed or falls out, it may not be immediately apparent that a penetrating injury occurred. Generally, in the case of a BB or a higher velocity projectile such as a bullet, it will be apparent to the Paramedic that a globe rupture has occurred.

Another serious ocular injury is a retinal detachment. In a **retinal detachment**, the retina lifts up from the posterior portion of the globe, interrupting its blood supply and causing ischemia. Unless repaired within 24 hours, visual deficits can be permanent.[17] Retinal detachments may occur when a tear develops in the retina, allowing the vitreous fluid in the globe to leak behind and displace the retina (Figure 3-7).

Retinal detachments may also occur if there is buildup of material underneath the retina. This occurs in many chronic diseases (e.g., hypertension). In trauma, a retinal detachment occurs most often due to a tear in the retina.[18] Due to other injuries, along with the possibility of head injury, the retinal detachment may not be detected until it is too late to repair the retina. Retinal detachments often cause a painless loss of vision that some describe as a curtain or blind closing in front of the eye, causing all or part of the eyesight to go black. In some cases, the vision loss is partial or the patient will report the presence of floaters.

Three other ocular injuries often associated with direct trauma are hyphema, traumatic iritis, and subconjunctival hemorrhage. A **hyphema** is blood that collects in the anterior chamber of the eye between the cornea and the iris (Figure 3-8). The force applied or transmitted to the globe causes the small blood vessels in the sclera to rupture and bleed into the anterior chamber. Although not immediately serious, if left untreated a hyphema can cause an increase in the intraocular pressure within the anterior chamber, threatening vision. The iron in the hemoglobin also can stain the lens, potentially impacting vision.[19]

Traumatic iritis occurs in the setting of blunt trauma to the eye and can be extremely painful. In traumatic iritis, the iris is contused and has difficulty contracting. Shining a light in either eye produces pain in the affected eye due to the injured iris's attempt to constrict and decrease the pupil size. In some cases, the pupil may appear paralyzed, either pinpoint or dilated, and minimally reactive to light. Although traumatic iritis usually occurs shortly after injury, it may occur up to three days after the injury.[20]

Finally, a **subconjunctival hemorrhage** occurs due to capillary leaking within the conjunctiva over the sclera (Figure 3-9). This is a benign condition similar to developing

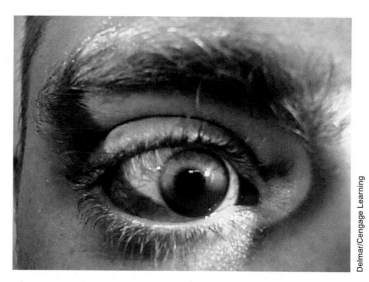

Figure 3-8 A hyphema is seen in the anterior chamber of the eye and may require oblique or tangential lighting in order to be observed.

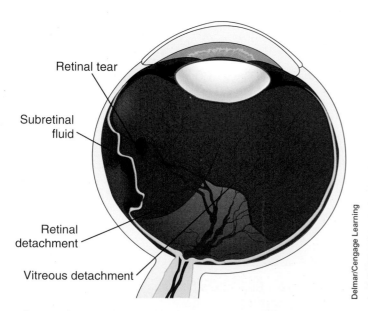

Figure 3-7 Most traumatic retinal detachments are caused by a hole or tear in the retina.

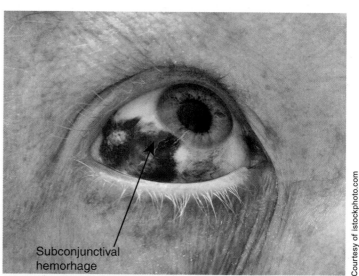

Figure 3-9 Subconjunctival hemorrhage occurs from capillary leaking within the conjunctiva.

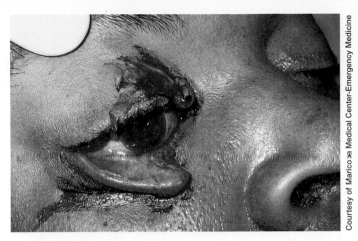

Figure 3-10 Eyelid lacerations extending through the edge of the lid may require repair by a specialist.

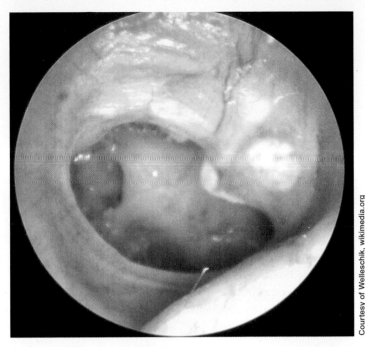

Figure 3-11 A perforated tympanic membrane.

ecchymosis on the skin. Subconjunctival hemorrhage can also occur spontaneously secondary to coughing or straining. The hemorrhage will generally resolve within two to three weeks and not require treatment.[21]

Eyelid lacerations can occur in penetrating trauma due to either a projectile or a sharp edge. Eyelid lacerations occur in blunt trauma primarily due to shearing forces applied to the face. Lacerations that are on the outer surface of the lid can be easily repaired in the emergency department. However, lid lacerations that extend through the edge of lid (Figure 3-10) are more complex and may require a specialist to repair the laceration to prevent eyelid dysfunction. Lacerations that are close to or involve the lacrimal (tear duct) system, located on the medial aspect of the eyelid closest to the nose, should be repaired by an ophthalmologist.

Ear Injuries

As with other facial injuries, the ears can be injured by blunt or penetrating trauma. In many cases, lacerations of the ear involve the cartilage, and repair at the emergency department is usually straightforward.

Tympanic membrane perforation (Figure 3-11) may occur either from direct penetrating trauma to the tympanic membrane (for example, from a projectile or cotton-tipped swab) or can occur from barotraumas, often seen with blast injuries. It is common for blood to be present in the auditory canal from the small capillaries in the tympanic membrane. Patients will report a hearing loss that ranges from a slight decrease in volume to complete absence of hearing. If the injury involves the organs of the inner ear, the patient may experience complete hearing loss, severe vertigo, and intractable nausea and vomiting. These symptoms occur because the inner ear organs are responsible not only for hearing but also for balance.

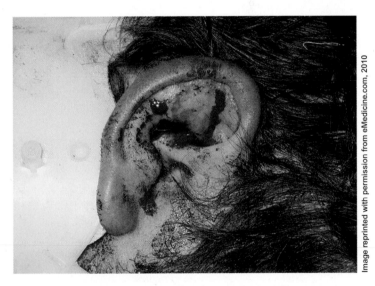

Figure 3-12 An auricular hematoma threatens the viability of the cartilage.

Patients who receive direct blunt trauma to the ear may also develop bleeding within the cartilage and soft tissues that make up the ear. As this bleeding progresses, the patient develops an **auricular hematoma**, commonly referred to as a cauliflower ear (Figure 3-12). Auricular hematomas may occur up to seven days after an injury, although most develop within several hours.[22] Auricular hematomas require drainage at the emergency department to relieve the buildup in pressure from the bleeding. If the hematoma is not drained, the compression of the cartilage by the hematoma may permanently damage and deform the cartilage; this is sometimes seen in wrestlers.

Neck Injuries

Many important structures are located in the soft tissues of the neck. Although trauma to the neck is not common due to the smaller area of the neck compared to the head and torso, neck injuries can threaten the patient's airway or circulatory pathways to the brain with grave consequences. Traditionally, the neck is divided into three zones (Figure 3-13 and Table 3-1), with the ultimate surgical management dependent on the location of the injury. Injuries that penetrate the **platysma**, the sheetlike muscle that superficially covers the anterior portion of the neck from the floor of the mouth to the clavicle, typically undergo surgical exploration. With improved technology, these patients will undergo CT scanning in the emergency department to determine the need for surgery. Given the potential seriousness of the injury, patients who sustain significant neck trauma, with potential for airway compromise or cervical spine injury, are generally transported to a trauma center. The two areas of neck injury that are most concerning to the Paramedic are injuries to the hypopharynx, larynx, and trachea as well as injuries to the vasculature.

Injuries to the mid to lower airways can affect the Paramedic's ability to maintain a patent airway. In penetrating trauma, damage most often occurs from penetration of the larynx or trachea by the projectile or object. In blunt trauma, injury most often occurs from direct force applied to the larynx or trachea or from extension injuries to the vascular structures of the neck. Tracheal rupture may also occur with blunt trauma to the chest if the patient inhales and holds his breath just before impact—this is the so-called paper bag effect. The action of holding one's breath closes the glottis and the force applied to the chest rapidly increases the pressure within the respiratory tree, which may cause the trachea to rupture. Escaping air may cause subcutaneous emphysema that will develop along the neck and upper chest, similar to what occurs when the patient develops a traumatic pneumothorax.

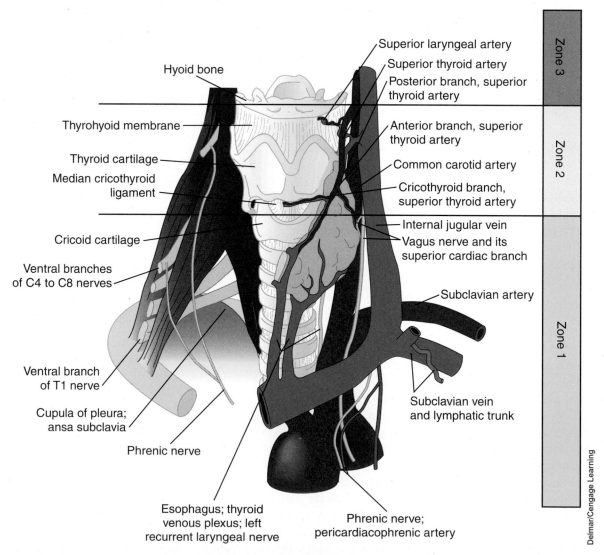

Figure 3-13 There are three anatomical zones used traditionally to classify neck injuries. Zone I is from the clavicle to the cricoid cartilage, Zone II is from the cricoid cartilage to the angle of the mandible, and Zone III is from the angle of the mandible to the base of the skull.

Table 3-1 Selected Contents of the Neck by Zone

- Zone I:
  - Common carotid artery
  - Vertebral artery
  - Subclavian artery
  - Major vessels of the mediastinum
  - Lung apices
  - Esophagus
  - Trachea
  - Thyroid
- Zone II:
  - Carotid artery
  - Vertebral artery
  - Larynx
  - Trachea
  - Esophagus
  - Pharynx
  - Jugular vein
- Zone III:
  - Distal carotid artery
  - Vertebral artery
  - Distal jugular vein
  - Cranial nerves 9 through 12

Laryngotracheal injury occurs infrequently in blunt trauma but is present in up to 10% of penetrating neck trauma.[23] Laryngeal or tracheal disruption can complicate attempts at airway management by disrupting the pathway that an endotracheal tube normally takes into the trachea. Fracture of the cricoid ring can produce acute airway obstruction from swelling.[23]

Penetrating trauma to the neck can also be associated with chest trauma or head trauma depending on the path of the projectile or length of the object. The apices of both lungs extend above the clavicle during inhalation and can be injured by forces applied to the neck.

Vascular injuries can also occur from both penetrating and blunt trauma. The important vascular structures in the neck include the common carotid arteries and jugular veins that travel toward the head on either side of the anterior neck (Figure 3-13). Just superior to the thyroid, the common carotids divide into the internal carotid arteries, which travel into the skull to provide arterial blood to the brain, and the external carotid arteries, which provide blood to the face. The internal carotid arteries form the anterior part of the circle of Willis, supplying much of the brain with arterial blood.

Blunt injury to the carotid arteries often produces a dissection in the inner wall of the vessel. The dissection can either completely or partially occlude the blood vessel, thereby limiting blood flow to the brain. It can also develop a thrombus, which can break off and travel upstream into the brain. Patients who develop a carotid artery dissection will often have signs and symptoms of a stroke. The exact signs and symptoms will vary depending upon the extent of the dissection, but will generally include hemiparesis, aphasia, or sensory deficits.

Penetrating injury to a carotid artery or jugular vein can produce significant bleeding in a very short period of time. If this bleeding has an external exit, the patient can exsanguinate (be drained of blood) within minutes. However, the patient may survive if a nearby bystander quickly intervenes. In 2008, Florida Panthers hockey player Richard Zednik narrowly escaped death when another player's skate struck him in the neck and severed his carotid artery. Due to bystander assistance and Paramedic intervention on-scene, Zednik survived and was able to return to play the following season.[24]

If the bleeding from a carotid or jugular injury is contained within the neck, a rapidly expanding hematoma can develop. The Paramedic may not immediately appreciate hematomas of the neck if the hematoma grows internally rather than externally. Therefore, the Paramedic must maintain a high index of suspicion for an expanding hematoma, as it can distort, compress, or disrupt normal airway anatomy. Hoarseness of the patient's voice, neck swelling, or difficulty swallowing, secondary to compression of cranial nerves, should alert the Paramedic to the possibility of an expanding neck hematoma.

Posteriorly, the vertebral arteries travel along the spinal column, protected by the vertebral canal. The vertebral arteries enter the skull and join together to form the basilar artery, preferentially supplying the cerebellum with arterial blood. At the level of the first and second vertebrae, the vertebral arteries make an "S" shaped turn posteriorly (Figure 3-14)

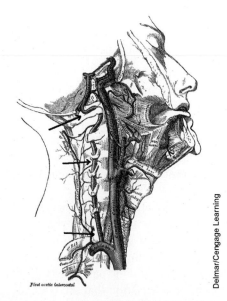

Delmar/Cengage Learning

Figure 3-14 The vertebral arteries are susceptible to injury at the level of the first and second cervical vertebrae by extension and rotational injuries.

before entering the head. This creates a point where the artery can overstretch if the patient's head rotates and extends to the limit of the range of motion.

Injury to the vertebral arteries in blunt trauma often occurs at this level where the artery dissects, disrupting blood supply or showering the brain with blood clots. Patients will exhibit signs and symptoms similar to those of a stroke. The exact signs and symptoms depend on the extent of the injury and can vary from vertigo to imbalance to hemiparesis. The Paramedic should maintain a high index of suspicion of a vertebral artery injury if the patient was exposed to a mechanism of injury that caused the neck to markedly extend and rotate. There is also a high association of vertebral artery injury with midcervical and upper cervical spine fractures.[25] The Paramedic should be aware that the signs and symptoms of vertebral artery injury may not develop for several hours after the injury.

Near hanging (aborted suicide) and strangulation during suicide attempts, for example, also provide a mechanism that potentially can damage the laryngotracheal or vascular structures. Court-ordered judicial hangings, as sentences for a high crime, occur by placing the large rope knot anteriorly underneath the chin and dropping the individual a significant distance. This mechanism produces a vertebral fracture (hangman's fracture—see Chapter 4), distraction of the head from the spine, spinal cord transaction, and disruption of the vascular structures supplying the brain. The combination of these injuries rapidly leads to death. However, the vast majority of patients who attempt suicide by hanging do so in a way that does not produce the same mechanism as judicial hanging. Death in these non-judicial situations typically occurs either through asphyxiation, laryngeal injury, or by disruption of blood flow to the brain by bilateral carotid artery compression.[23]

> ◤ CASE STUDY (CONTINUED)

With manual cervical movement restriction in place, and after performing a primary assessment, the Paramedic starts to question the patient about loss of consciousness and, most importantly, "Where does it hurt?" The patient denies any loss of consciousness but says his face is "busted up" and that he is having trouble breathing. The Paramedic asks him if he has any trouble seeing and if he is nauseous and feels like throwing up.

CRITICAL THINKING QUESTIONS

1. What are the important elements of the history that a Paramedic should obtain?
2. Why would nausea be a problem?

History

Once the Paramedic ensures scene safety and identifies any additional resources required on initial contact, he can obtain a history. The history includes the mechanism of injury, which provides the Paramedic with a litany of potential injuries. The mechanism may also assist the Paramedic in determining the source of bleeding. The scalp and face are highly vascular; as a result, a small laceration or puncture can cause a significant amount of bleeding.

Focusing on traumatic injury to the face, the Paramedic should determine the location of any pain or bleeding. Pain with eye movement may indicate entrapment of one of the extraocular muscles within an orbital fracture. Mandible fractures should be suspected if the patient reports pain with mandible movement or a sensation that the teeth are not aligned. A history of epistaxis may indicate nasal injury.

Focusing on traumatic injury to the neck, the Paramedic should ascertain the location of pain and radiation of pain from the patient. Difficulty swallowing or speaking should also be noted and may indicate laryngotracheal injury. In the situation of penetrating trauma, the Paramedic should attempt to determine the type of weapon, its direction, and either the length of the penetrating object or caliber, distance, and type of firearm. This information will also alert the Paramedic to the potential of an associated chest, facial, or head injury.

Other historical factors important in the setting of neck trauma include the presence of neurological symptoms or deficits. Although these are more commonly associated with either spinal cord or spinal nerve root injury, the Paramedic should suspect a vascular injury if the patient provides a history of hemiparesis, weakness, aphasia, or other symptoms of a cerebrovascular accident.

The timing of the injury and onset of the symptoms may also provide the Paramedic with clues to potential injuries. Initially, an isolated injury to the neck may seem minor and not cause the patient any concern. Symptoms may develop later, especially in isolated blunt injury to the neck (e.g., a clothesline to the anterior neck). Symptoms associated with a cerebrovascular accident often do not begin until several hours after the incident.

Starting in a methodical manner from the top of the patient's head, the Paramedic assesses for DCAP BTLS (Deformity, Contusions, Abrasions, Punctures, Burns, Tenderness, Lacerations, or Swelling). Most of the trauma seems to be focused to the patient's midface. There is no pain or midline tenderness to the midline posterior neck, although cervical immobilization is being placed as a precaution.

Gentle palpation on the midface reveals an obvious broken nose and some point tenderness to the left inferior orbital rim. There is an obvious step-off on the zygoma and crepitus. The eye has already started to swell shut, making it impossible to examine the eye.

CRITICAL THINKING QUESTIONS

1. What are the elements of the physical examination of a patient with suspected Le Fort fractures?
2. Why would a cranial nerve exam be a critical element in this examination?

Examination

As with all trauma patients, the Paramedic should assess for and immediately treat all conditions that compromise the airway, breathing, and circulation. In many patients with injuries to the face and neck, injuries are also present in other body systems. Regardless, the patient must be assessed and treated as a whole.

Once the primary survey is completed and immediately life-threatening issues have been addressed, the Paramedic can turn to the patient's face. The face is inspected for deformities, swelling, and ecchymosis, which may indicate underlying injury. The Paramedic should assess the extraocular movements of the eyes for smoothness and pain on movement. The Paramedic should also assess for pupillary reaction, visual acuity, and presence of a hyphema (Figure 3-15). Mouth opening and closing should also be assessed for smoothness and alignment of the teeth. Missing or fractured teeth should also be noted. If possible, the patient should be asked about the condition of her teeth prior to the injury to confirm if missing teeth were dislodged during this injury.

The Paramedic should palpate the patient's face and generally assess the stability of the midface. The Paramedic should suspect a Le Fort fracture if any instability of the maxilla is felt. Stability of the maxilla can be best appreciated in the compliant patient by placing two gloved fingers into the patient's mouth and grasping hold of the maxilla between the fingers and thumb. The Paramedic applies gentle force and notes any instability. Excessive force should not be used during this maneuver. The remaining facial bones can be thoroughly palpated for stability and tenderness.

The Paramedic should make a thorough inspection of the neck for deformities, ecchymosis, lacerations, and other evidence of trauma. As the majority of patients require spinal motion restriction, the Paramedic should ensure the cervical spine is stabilized throughout this process. The Paramedic

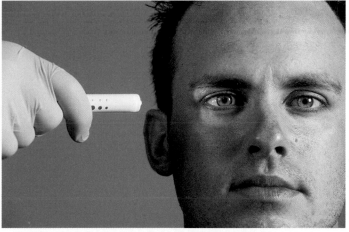

Figure 3-15 The Paramedic should assess for the presence of a hyphema by shining a penlight laterally across the cornea.

can ask the patient to open his mouth to assess the hypopharynx for signs of injury that may be related to neck trauma.

The Paramedic should palpate the neck for masses and deformity. The position of the trachea is assessed at the level of the sternal notch. The Paramedic palpates the carotid arteries to assess for pulse presence and quality. Then she palpates the larynx and hyoid bone (Figure 3-13) for tenderness and stability, especially in cases of blunt trauma to the anterior neck. Finally, she should assess the neck for subcutaneous emphysema, which may indicate a pneumothorax or tracheal leak.

The carotid arteries can also be auscultated for the presence of bruits, which may indicate a carotid dissection. The Paramedic can also auscultate the larynx if he is unsure if airway sounds are originating in the upper or lower airway.

Even if by history the face or neck injury appears to be isolated, the Paramedic should perform an examination on the other body systems that may also be affected. The Paramedic should perform a brief neurologic examination to assess for the likelihood of a vascular injury to the neck. She should also assess the cervical spine and take precautions for potential cervical spine injury. She should assess the thorax for pneumothorax and vascular injury, and the upper extremities for the presence of a vascular injury. In settings of penetrating trauma, the Paramedic should also assess the abdomen as projectiles can take roundabout routes as they travel through the body. The same is true for penetrating wounds to the neck; the projectile may end up in the face or skull. The number of penetrating wounds should be counted and documented without judging which wounds may be entrance and exit wounds.

CASE STUDY (CONTINUED)

The patient complains that he cannot see out of the affected eye. Although the eye is very swollen, there is a chance of eye injury including retinal detachment. The Paramedic is concerned about the latter issue. Although other potentially more life-threatening injuries must be dealt with, such as traumatic brain injury or cervical spine fracture, permanent loss of vision is serious, too.

CRITICAL THINKING QUESTIONS

1. What is the significance of the loss of vision?
2. What is the patient's prognosis?

Assessment

As previously discussed, the Paramedic needs to maintain a high index of suspicion for potentially life-threatening injuries as she assesses the mechanism of injury, the historical information, and information she obtained from a thorough examination.

Any hoarseness of the patient's voice or difficult or painful swallowing should alert the Paramedic to the potential for an impending airway issue. Neurologic symptoms similar to those found with a stroke should suggest to the Paramedic injury to a vascular structure in the neck. Significant midface ecchymosis and epistaxis should suggest to the Paramedic the presence of a Le Fort fracture and the potential for associated head and cervical spine injury. Clear fluid from the nose or ear, ecchymosis around the eyes, or ecchymosis at the base of the skull suggests a basilar skull fracture.

CASE STUDY (CONTINUED)

The Paramedic knows multiple injuries mean multiple priorities. He considers lying the patient supine on the backboard, but is concerned that the patient may be swallowing blood. However, if he keeps the patient seated upright, he risks the patient leaning forward and potentially detaching his retina.

CRITICAL THINKING QUESTIONS

1. What is the national standard of care of patients with suspected midface fractures?
2. What are some of the patient-specific concerns and considerations that the Paramedic should consider when applying this plan of care that is intended to treat a broad patient population presenting with midface fractures?

Treatment

The initial treatment priorities for the Paramedic include addressing issues that affect the airway, breathing, or circulation during the primary assessment. Once these issues are stabilized, the Paramedic can provide treatment for the less serious injuries.

Injuries to both the face and the neck can cause airway issues. Midface instability is often associated with significant intraoral or nasal bleeding which can occlude the airway. Aggressive suctioning may be required in order to prevent aspiration and clear the way for airway management. Bleeding may be heavy enough, or the amount of foreign material may be significant enough, that the Paramedic may elect to go directly to a supraglottic airway or utilize a gum elastic bougie, lighted stylette, or videoscopic-assisted intubation in the obtunded patient to rapidly gain control of the airway. In some cases, the facial and neck deformity is significant and the Paramedic may elect to perform a surgical airway rather than make multiple attempts at intubation. In situations where an expanding hematoma of the neck is suspected, the Paramedic should elect early intubation, if feasible, to ensure the airway is controlled. The Paramedic should anticipate and plan for a difficult airway from the outset as distortion of airway anatomy may not be immediately apparent externally.

Once the airway is addressed, the Paramedic can address breathing issues. From a ventilation standpoint, the Paramedic should treat a tension pneumothorax with needle decompression. Facial instability and foreign material in the airway can affect the Paramedic's ability to adequately ventilate the patient. Suction and airway adjuncts should be utilized appropriately as needed to improve ventilation. Care should also be taken not to worsen facial fractures by unnecessary pressure on the face. From an oxygenation standpoint, the Paramedic should place the patient on high-concentration, high-flow oxygen by nonrebreather mask, bag-valve mask, or invasive airway device.

Hemorrhage from facial injuries can be significant due to the rich blood supply to the face and scalp. Appropriate hemorrhage control measures should be rapidly taken once the airway has been controlled as significant blood loss can occur. In the setting of potential midface fractures, hemorrhage frequently occurs from the nose[26] and may be difficult for the Paramedic to control. Often patients with massive oral or nasal hemorrhage actually have a nasal source and ultimately require nasal packing in order to control the hemorrhage.[26–29] Once the airway is definitively controlled by endotracheal intubation or a supraglottic airway, and an oral source of bleeding is identified, packing the oral cavity with

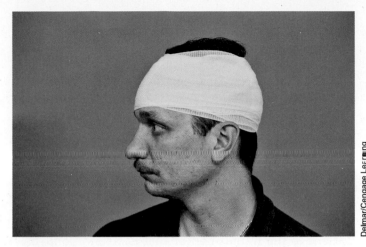

Figure 3-16 Bleeding control of a scalp wound may be accomplished by way of a scalp bandage to maintain pressure on the wound.

gauze may help slow the hemorrhage enough to stabilize the patient until arrival at the emergency department.

Scalp wounds may also require direct pressure or pressure bandaging (Figure 3-16) in order to control bleeding and prevent hemorrhagic shock. Blood loss from scalp lacerations can be significant, even those that continuously ooze, and should be adequately managed with hemorrhage control measures. This is especially true in interfacility transport of a patient from a community hospital to a trauma center.[30]

Once the airway, breathing, and circulation are adequately addressed, the Paramedic can then treat less severe injuries. The majority of the time, care can be limited to supportive measures (for example, dressing of minor lacerations and application of ice) and analgesia. The Paramedic must also perform spinal motion restriction with a cervical collar and long spine board when indicated.

▶ CASE STUDY (CONTINUED)

Suddenly the patient wants to sit upright immediately. He states he is going to "puke." Quickly turning the backboard to the side and grabbing for the suction, the Paramedic anxiously observes the left eye for any signs of protrusion. "If only I had another medic," the Paramedic thinks, "he could have given the Zofran® and prevented the vomiting."

CRITICAL THINKING QUESTIONS

1. What are some of the predictable complications associated with midface fractures?
2. What are some of the predictable complications associated with the treatments for midface fractures?

Evaluation

Continual monitoring of the airway during transport is essential. As the vast majority of patients with facial or neck injuries are transported supine on a long spine board, extra attention is required as the patient cannot manage his own airway as effectively as when seated. Periodic suction may be required in order to keep the airway clear and decrease patient anxiety. As the face and neck have a rich blood supply, vital signs should be assessed frequently in order to detect hypovolemia early. A patient can easily progress from isolated facial hemorrhage into Class III or IV hemorrhagic shock.

▶ CASE STUDY CONCLUSION

Because of the nature of the assault and the obvious multitrauma, the Paramedic elects to transport the patient to the trauma center that is 10 additional blocks away, much to the dismay of the police. Telling the driver to "light it up," the Paramedic starts to formulate his report for the radio.

CRITICAL THINKING QUESTIONS

1. What is the most appropriate transport decision that will get the patient to definitive care?
2. What are the advantages of transporting a patient with suspected midface fractures to these hospitals, even if that means bypassing other hospitals in the process?

Disposition

Patients who have the potential for multiple system injuries should be transported directly to a Level I or Level II Trauma Center, depending upon regional resources and availability. The trauma centers have the resources available to coordinate care between the multiple specialists required to care for the complex trauma patient. If the airway is unstable and the Paramedic is not able to secure an appropriate airway for the patient, then the patient should be brought to the closest capable emergency department to allow airway stabilization before continuing to a trauma center.

Patients who have sustained significant facial injury ideally should be transported to a facility with an available facial surgeon or ophthalmologist, depending on the injuries. Most emergency departments, however, are capable of handling initial patient management and then subsequently transferring the patient to a specialty care center if necessary. The only exception for patients with an isolated facial injury is if a Le Fort fracture is suspected. Due to the high incidence of associated head and cervical spine injuries, these patients should be transported directly to a Level I or Level II Trauma Center.

Most emergency departments are also capable of performing the initial assessment and management of isolated neck injuries. Patients who demonstrate signs or symptoms of a vascular injury should be transported directly to a Level I or Level II Trauma Center or to a facility with an available vascular surgeon.

CONCLUSION

Facial injuries are very common and may be associated with other injuries, especially in the setting of multiple trauma. Fortunately, the vast majority of facial injuries are non-life-threatening, with the more serious injuries associated with airway bleeding and other head and neck injuries.

Although a neck injury is not common, several potentially life-threatening injuries can occur to the neck. The Paramedic needs to maintain a high index of suspicion for life-threatening neck injuries and intervene accordingly to reduce mortality and improve morbidity.

KEY POINTS:

- The majority of facial trauma comes from assault, motor vehicle collisions, and falls.

- Midface fractures can be separated into Le Fort I, II, and III fractures, according to which structures are fractured.

- Eye injuries include blowout fractures, globe ruptures, and retinal detachment.

- The neck is divided into three zones (I, II, III), and injuries in zone I are the most lethal.

- Facial structures should be inspected, then palpated, in a methodical manner from the top of the skull to the top of the clavicle for injuries sustained during trauma.

- Although facial injuries can be awe-inspiring and devastating, underlying injuries such as basilar skull fractures or cervical spine factures can be more life-threatening.

- Treatment focuses around maintaining a patent airway.

- Hemorrhage, particularly from scalp wounds, can be significant and difficult to manage. In some cases the bleeding can be life-threatening.

- As cosmesis and functional impairment are major concerns with facial trauma, significant facial trauma is usually treated at a trauma center where surgeons, particularly plastic and orthopedic surgeons, are available.

REVIEW QUESTIONS:

1. What differentiates Le Fort I from Le Fort II from Le Fort III fractures?
2. What is the implication of a loss of a cardinal gaze (i.e., loss of an EOM)?
3. What are the Ellis classifications?
4. Beyond retinal detachment and globe rupture, what are the other three traumatic ocular injuries?
5. What structures exist in zone I of the neck?

CASE STUDY QUESTIONS:

Please refer to the Case Study in this chapter, and answer the questions below:

1. What is the appropriate response if the patient's initial response was not clear, but hoarse instead?
2. Suppose the patient in this case complained loudly that his eye hurt and refused to let the Paramedic examine his eye. What would the Paramedic suspect?
3. Why is the Paramedic concerned about the patient vomiting?

REFERENCES:

1. Lee KH. Interpersonal violence and facial fractures. *J Oral Maxillofac Surg.* Sep 2009;67(9):1878–1883.

2. Rajendra PB, Mathew TP, Agrawal A, Sabharawal G. Characteristics of associated craniofacial trauma in patients with head injuries: an experience with 100 cases. *J Emerg Trauma Shock.* 2009;2(2):89–94.

3. He D, Blomquist PH, Ellis E. Association between ocular injuries and internal orbital fractures. *J Oral Maxillofac Surg.* 2007;65(4):713–720.

4. Lawson BR, Comstock RD, Smith GA. Baseball related injuries in children treated in the hospital emergency departments in the United States, 1994–2006. *Pediatrics.* 2009;123(6):e1028–e1034.

5. Widell T. Face fractures. E-medicine online Emergency Medicine Textbook, updated March 6, 2008. Available at: **http://emedicine.medscape.com/article/824743-overview.** Accessed September 9, 2009.

6. Mithani SK, St-Hilaire H, Brooke BS, et al. Predictable patterns of intracranial and cervical spine injury in craniomaxillofacial trauma: analysis of 4786 patients. *Plast Reconstr Surg.* 2009;123(4):1293–1301.

7. Le Fort R. Etude experimentale sur les fractures de le machoire superieure. *Revue Chir de Paris.* 1901;23:208–227, 360–379, 479–507.

8. Dyer PV. Experimental study of fractures of the upper jaw: a critique of the original papers published by Rene Le Fort. *Trauma.* 1999;1(1):81–84.

9. Plaisier BR, Punjabi AP, Super DM, Haung RH. The relationship between facial fractures and death from neurologic injury. *J Oral Maxillofac Surg.* 2000;58(7):708–712.

10. Widell T. Orbital fracture. E-medicine online emergency medicine textbook. Updated March 6, 2008. Available at: **http://emedicine.medscape.com/article/825772-overview.** Accessed September 14, 2009.

11. Rhee JS, Kilde J, Yoganadam N, Pintar F. Orbital blowout fractures: experimental evidence for the pure hydraulic theory. *Arch Facial Plast Surg.* 2002;4(2):98–101.

12. Waterhouse N, Lyne J, Urdang L, Garey L. An investigation into the mechanism of orbital blowout fractures. *Br J Plast Surg.* 1999;52(8):607–612.

13. Richards ME, Yeargan A. Chapter 12: Facial and ocular trauma. In: Hubble MW, Hubble JP, eds. *Principle of Advanced Trauma Care.* Clifton Park, NY: Delmar Cengage Learning; 2002:223–246.

14. Thomas JJ, Edwards AR. Fractured teeth. E-medicine online Emergency Medicine Textbook. Updated March 29, 2009. Available at: **http://emedicine.medscape.com/article/82755-overview.** Accessed September 14, 2009.

15. Robson J, Behrman AJ. Globe rupture. E-medicine online Emergency Medicine Textbook. Updated July 16, 2009. Available at: **http://emedicine.medscape.com/article/798223-overview.** Accessed September 14, 2009.

16. Cooper H, Thomas T. Ocular injuries related to airbag use. *Am J Emerg Med.* 2004;22(2):135–137.

17. Larkin GL. Retinal detachment. E-medicine online Emergency Medicine Textbook. Updated April 7, 2008. Available at: **http://emedicine.medscape.com/article/798501-overview.** Accessed September 14, 2009.

18. Arroyo JG. Retinal tear and detachment. Up To Date online. Last updated January 6, 2009. Available at: **http://www.utdol .com/online/content/topic.do?topicKey=priophth/8273& selectedTitle=1~82&source=search_result.** Accessed September 23, 2009.

19. Hodge C, Lawless M. Ocular emergencies. *Aust Fam Physician.* 2008;37(7):506–509.

20. Ehlers JP, Shah CP, eds. Chapter 3: Trauma. In: *The Wills Eye Manual: Office and Emergency Room Diagnosis and Treatment of Eye Disease* (5th ed.). Philadelphia, PA: Lippincott, Williams and Wilkins; 2008.

21. Pavan-Langston D, Colby K. Chapter 5: Cornea and external disease. In: Pavan-Langston D, ed. *Manual of Ocular Diagnosis and Therapy* (8th ed.). Philadelphia, PA: Lippincott, Williams and Wilkins; 2008.

22. McKay MP, Mayersak RJ. Facial trauma. In: Marx JA, Hockberger RS, Walls RM, eds. *Rosen's Emergency Medicine* (7th ed.). Philadelphia, PA: Mosby Elsevier; 2010:333.

23. Newton K. Neck. In: Marx JA, Hockberger RS, Walls RM, eds. *Rosen's Emergency Medicine* (7th ed.). Philadelphia, PA: Mosby Elsevier; 2010:377–386.

24. Gleason B. Zednik made a narrow escape after injury against Sabres. *Buffalo News.* March 12, 2009. Available at: **http://www.buffalonews.com/sports/story/604927.html.** Accessed December 20, 2009.

25. Willis BK, Greiner F, Orrison WW, Benzel EC. The incidence of vertebral artery injury after midcervical fracture or subluxation. *Neurosurgery.* 1994;34(3):435–442.

26. Shimoyama T, Kaneko T, Horie N. Initial management of massive oral bleeding after midfacial fracture. *J Trauma.* 2003;54(2): 332–336.

27. Cogbill TH, Cothren CC, Ahearn MK, et al. Management of maxillofacial injuries with severe oronasal hemorrhage: a multicenter perspective. *J Trauma.* 2008;65(5):994–999.

28. Siritongtaworn P. Management of life threatening hemorrhage from facial fracture. *J Med Assoc Thai.* 2005;88(3):382–385.

29. Dean NR, Ledgard JP, Katsaros J. Massive hemorrhage in facial fracture patients: definition, incidence, and management. *Plast Reconstr Surg.* 2009;123(2):680–690.

30. Fitzpatrick MO, Seex K. Scalp lacerations demand careful attention before interhospital transfer of head injured patients. *J Accid Emerg Med.* 1996;13(3):207–208.

CHAPTER 4

SPINAL TRAUMA

KEY CONCEPTS:

Upon completion of this chapter, it is expected that the reader will understand these following concepts:

- Common spinal column injuries
- Complete and incomplete spinal cord injury
- Mechanism of injury that causes spinal cord injury
- Examination of the patient with suspected spinal cord injury
- Treatment of the patient with suspected spinal cord injury
- Treatment of neurogenic shock

ANATOMY CONCEPTS:

Prior to reading this chapter the Paramedic student should be familiar with the following anatomy and physiology concepts:

- Spinal vertebrae, structure and function
- Spinal cord, structure and function

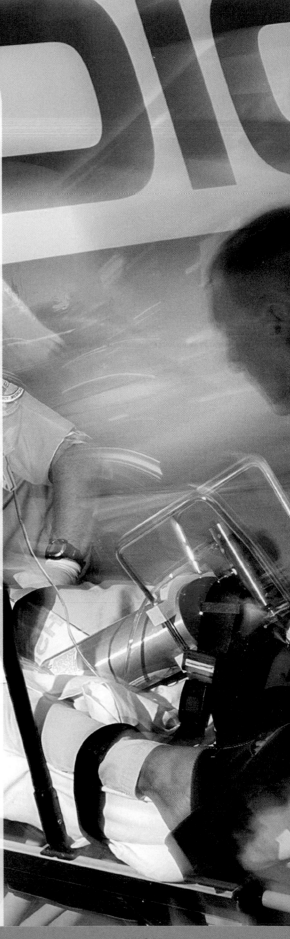

"Medic 78, respond to 35 Pine Valley Circle for a report of a 17-year-old female with trouble breathing and numbness in her hands and feet."

During the 10-minute response, the Paramedic runs through common techniques to diffuse hyperventilation and discusses with her partner how many different causes of anxiety might result in such a nervous reaction. Grabbing only the bare minimum of equipment as they approach the residence, the crew is met at the door by a nervous-looking young woman.

"Come on, she's in the back yard. We were practicing some of our throws for cheerleading. We missed the catch and she hit the ground pretty hard. We tried to help her inside, but she couldn't get up so we called 9-1-1. She's breathing real fast and keeps telling us that she can't move her arms or legs."

The second Paramedic instantly turns around and heads back to the ambulance to get additional equipment while the first Paramedic continues to the back yard to find the patient.

CRITICAL THINKING QUESTIONS

1. What are some of the possible causes of paralysis?
2. How is trouble breathing related to the paralysis?

OVERVIEW

The spinal cord is the portion of the central nervous system that carries continuous messages from the brain to the rest of the body and back. It sits securely inside the structures of the spinal column. When the spinal cord is damaged, the brain and body can no longer effectively communicate. At present, the spinal cord cannot be repaired; however, advances in induced therapeutic hypothermia and stem cell research hold promise for spinal cord recovery.

Chief Concern

Over the course of evolution, the human body has developed ways to manage the trauma associated with everyday life. A healthy person who trips and falls, even while running at full speed, is unlikely to sustain an injury to her spinal cord. Similarly, a fall from a relatively short height (less than twice a person's height) or a punch from a person of similar size is not likely to injure the spinal cord or other important organs. However, once a person experiences a force greater than what he can generate on his own, his risk for significant injury—and especially spinal cord injury—increases.

One hundred years ago, no person had safely traveled at greater than 100 miles per hour. Only a few thousand years ago, our bodies rarely traveled at speeds equal to that of the galloping horse. In short, the human body has not yet evolved to tolerate the energy that it may be subjected to on a daily basis. However, engineering in our society has helped reduce the likelihood that we will be injured during everyday activities. Seat belts keep us restrained in our seats in motor vehicles, harnesses are standard equipment when working at heights, and people use impact-resistant equipment during high-risk activities. When considering the possibility of injury, Paramedics must consider the amount of energy that was transferred to the body during the event (kinematics). It is also important to consider the direction in which the energy was transferred, as the body is prepared to absorb energy in some directions better than others.

Spinal Cord Injury

It is estimated that every year about 12,000 Americans, or about 40 people per million populations, suffer a spinal cord injury. Although large, this number represents only about 0.03% of the 41 million injuries that are seen in the emergency department each year. About a quarter of a million Americans are living with some degree of spinal cord injury (SCI).[1]

Spinal cord injury is generally considered a condition associated with young males. More than 75% of spinal cord injuries occur in men, and their average age at the time of injury is 39.5 years. This average age of injury has increased by more than 10 years since 1980, when it was 28.7 years. One reason for this upward shift is the increase in spinal cord injuries among patients older than 60, from 4.7% to 11.5%—perhaps caused by the increasing numbers of people in this population and their desire to be more active.[1]

Motor vehicle crashes, the leading cause of spinal cord injury, account for an estimated 42% of all spinal cord injuries. Falls are responsible for 27%, violent acts (primarily gunshot wounds) are responsible for 15.3%, and sports cause 7.4% of spinal cord injuries. The remaining 8% or so are from other etiologies. Because spinal cord injuries are rare, it is not unusual for Paramedics to go many years between seeing patients with a spinal cord injury. However, Paramedics must remain vigilant about the possibility of spinal cord injury even when responding to the most innocuous events, as spinal cord injuries can have a dramatic impact on their patients' lives.

Spinal cord injuries are primarily described based on the amount of function that is retained after the injury and the specific vertebrae where the injury occurred. Complete **tetraplegia** is defined as loss of sensation and motor control in the arms and legs as well as the torso after an injury in the cervical spine region. Incomplete tetraplegia describes a patient who has reduced motor control and sensation in all four extremities after an incomplete injury in the cervical spine. Complete tetraplegia accounts for 18% of spinal cord injury patients and incomplete tetraplegia accounts for about 34%. **Paraplegia** describes a thoracic or lumbar spinal cord injury that limits or eliminates motor control and sensation in the lower extremities. Incomplete paraplegia accounts for 18.5% of spinal cord injuries, and complete paraplegia accounts for about 23%. Less than 1% of spinal cord injuries have complete neurological recovery.

A patient with tetraplegia in the area of C1 to C4 has an estimated cost for continued medical care of $775,000 the first year and an annual cost of $139,000 thereafter. The lifetime cost for living and health care expenses for a 40-year-old

STREET SMART

In 1991, the American spinal cord injury classification system was revised. The term "quadriplegia" was replaced with the term "tetraplegia," meaning paralysis of four limbs.

with a C1-C4 tetraplegia is thus estimated at $3.5 million. It must also be noted that the life expectancy for such a 40-year-old is reduced from 39.5 years to 19.9 years.[1]

Anatomy of the Spine

The spine is an intricate structure including bones, nerve tissue, muscles, ligaments, and cartilage. Each component has a vital role in a person's health; therefore, any change to that system will have dramatic effects on the patient.

The vertebrae are 33 uniquely shaped structures that run along the posterior of the torso from the skull to the pelvis and together form the spinal column. In general, the vertebrae are larger if they have more weight they must support. A pair of ligaments—the anterior and posterior longitudinal ligaments—travel the length of the spinal column and provide a significant source of stability. These ligaments help connect the vertebrae with the skull and pelvis.

Additionally, the erector spinae gluteus medius, gluteus maximus, and latissimus dorsi muscles allow for both movement and stability of the spine. These structures can be a source of both traumatic and nontraumatic back pain, although spinal cord injury is not likely if these are the only portions involved.

Each vertebra has several unique features that allow them to provide the needed strength and mobility for physical activity while allowing for the rapid transmission of information in the nervous system (Figure 4-1). The vertebral body is the anterior portion of the vertebrae and is made of cancellous bone (spongy or honeycomb-like structure), which allows for them to be less dense and yet support great weight in comparison to their own weight. The size of the vertebral body varies greatly over the length of the spine. The anterior portion of the vertebrae is smooth and rounded.

The vertebral foramen is the opening in the posterior portion of the bone that holds the spinal cord. The series of openings, called the vertebral forman, exist in the vertebral column referred to as the vertebral canal. The transverse process, which projects laterally from the vertebral column, serves to limit lateral motion and provide for attachment from the various muscles and ligaments. The spinous process is the portion of the spinal column most often examined by the Paramedic provider, as it is proximal to the surface of the skin, and is only a fraction of the mass of the spine.

The spinous process aids in limiting hyperextension of the spine and provides another site for the connection of muscles and ligaments. The transverse and spinous process work in concert to limit the spine's rotation. The intervertebral foramens are formed bilaterally on the inferior portion of the vertebral foramen and allow for spinal nerves to connect to the spinal cord through the spinal canal. Between each set of vertebrae are the fibrocartilaginous discs that provide cushioning and allow for the spine's movement. These discs decrease in size as a person ages and can rupture when too much stress is placed on the spine during a lift. They can also decay over time with repeated motion (Figure 4-2).

The spinal column is divided into five sections. Inside each section, the vertebrae are numbered sequentially as they descend. The seven cervical vertebrae are the most superior and support the head. The top two vertebrae are named the

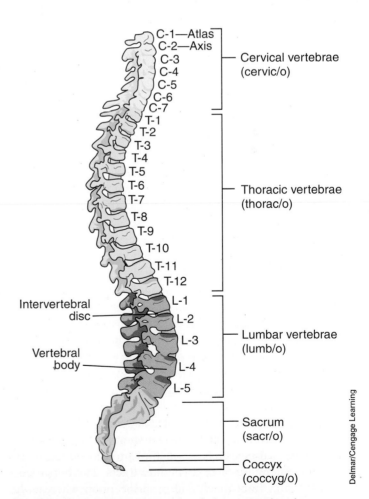

Figure 4-2 The sections of the spinal column.

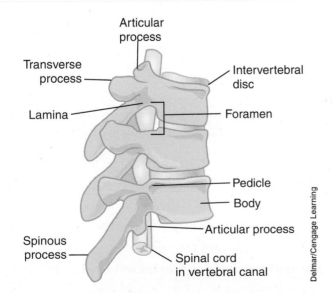

Figure 4-1 Cross-section of vertebrae.

Delmar/Cengage Learning

atlas and the axis. Together, they form the atlanto-axial joint. This joint has a unique structure to allow for the head's rotation. When properly aligned, the cervical spine has a slight posterior curve. There are 12 thoracic vertebrae that form the posterior portion of the rib cage. The ribs join to the vertebrae on the lateral portion and provide support for the spinal column. The five lumbar vertebrae are the largest in the spine. They are susceptible to lifting and moving injuries because they bear a great deal of weight with only the support of muscles and ligaments. The five vertebrae of the sacrum are fused together and form the posterior of the pelvis. The four vertebrae of the coccyx are fused.

The Spinal Cord

The spinal cord is the essential portion of a person's internal communication system. It carries all messages from the brain to the rest of body. The cord is contiguous with the brain and exits the skull at the foramen magnum. It joins the brain at the medulla oblongata and extends inferiorly to the lumbar region, generally L2 in adults. Like the brain, the spinal cord is wrapped in three meninges—the dura mater, arachnoid mater, and pia mater. Cerebrospinal fluid circulates inside the arachnoid mater.

The spinal cord consists of white matter and gray matter. The gray matter forms a butterfly-like shape in the center of the cord. It contains the anterior or ventral horn with motor neurons and the posterior or dorsal horn with sensory neurons. The white matter surrounds the gray matter and contains the major nerve tracts. Damage to any of these tracts can cause isolated loss of motor or sensory messages to the specific area of the body they innervate, but leave nearby tissues intact.

The spinal nerve roots that leave the ventral aspect of the spinal cord conduct motor messages, and the dorsal roots conduct the sensory messages. These messages are conducted to or from the peripheral nervous system to the nerve roots and into the gray matter. In adults, the cord ends at about the level of L1-L2. The cauda equina descends below that level and is descriptively named for the nerves that exit the spinal cord, which have the appearance of a horse's tail.

The spinal cord also has tracts. These tracts are either ascending tracts that send sensory information to the brain or descending tracts that send motor nerve instructions to the muscles. The descending, or **corticospinal tract** (from the cortex to the spine), is found in the anterior portion of the spinal cord. The corticospinal nerve fibers cross over at the level of the medulla. Therefore, an injury to the anterior portion of the spinal cord causes motor dysfunction (paralysis).

Similarly, the ascending sensory nerve tract, called the **spinothalamic tract** (from the spine to the thalamus), transmits sensations such as touch or proprioception to the thalamus. There are three ascending tracts. The dorsal columns transmit light touch and proprioception whereas the lateral spinothalamic tract transmits pain and temperature. The third tract, the anterior spinothalamic tract, transmits light touch.

Vascular Supply

In some cases, the spinal cord injury is the indirect result of interruption of the blood supply to the spinal cord, secondary to compression or laceration of the spinal arteries.

A single anterior artery provides blood to the anterior and central cord. There is a pair of posterior vertebral arteries as well, except in the cervical area. These spinal arteries arise primarily from the aorta and the radicular arteries.

Spinal Column Injuries

Vertebral body fractures are more common than spinal cord injuries. Any amount of energy that can damage the bone might also damage the spinal cord. However, fracture of a vertebra does not mean certain injury to the spinal cord.

For example, damage to the larger vertebrae of the thoracic or lumbar region may occur without damage to the cord. This result is common because the transfer of energy may crack the bone or remove a chip without affecting the alignment of the vertebral foramen. Therefore, the injury is unlikely to damage the spinal cord. A burst fracture may occur during sudden decelerations and may cause the vertebrae to scatter fragments in all directions. Wedge fractures are caused when the front part of the vertebral body is compressed rapidly during flexion and the front of the body cleaves away.

Dislocations and Subluxation

The spinal column is in nearly constant motion and every aspect is designed to remain in alignment. Trauma leading to excessive motion, may cause the vertebrae to lose their correct alignment. If the vertebral foramen becomes misaligned, sharp bony edges can sever the spinal cord (i.e., **spinal transection**), causing nerve conduction and communication to cease at the injury site. Minor incomplete dislocations, often referred to as subluxation, can occur without affecting the spinal cord. Any misalignment of the spine can impact the

STREET SMART

The field of chiropractics is based on keeping the spine in alignment and eliminating subluxation. Although some in the mainstream medical establishment are skeptical of chiropractic care, many Americans seek care for back pain from chiropractors and most insurance companies will pay for the care.

spinal nerves' roots. This misalignment will often present itself along with a neurological deficit.

Ligaments, Tendons, and Muscle Injuries

Injuries to soft tissues in the back account for the vast majority of pain-producing back injuries. During their lifetime, it is estimated that four out of five adults will miss work or have to reduce activities as a result of back pain. Often these injuries are muscle and tendon strains or ligament sprains. These painful injuries must be carefully evaluated regarding the mechanism of injury and presence of any neurological deficits to assess for any involvement of the spinal cord.

Disc Herniation

Intravertebral discs are round rubbery structures that absorb energy and allow for movement of the vertebrae. As we age, the discs decrease in size and flexibility. The discs have a soft gel-like center with a thicker ring on the perimeter. A herniated disc occurs when the center pushes its way out of the perimeter. This action disrupts the structure of the spinal column and can cause pressure on spinal nerves. These injuries are more likely to occur in the lumbar and cervical regions of the spine (Figure 4-3).

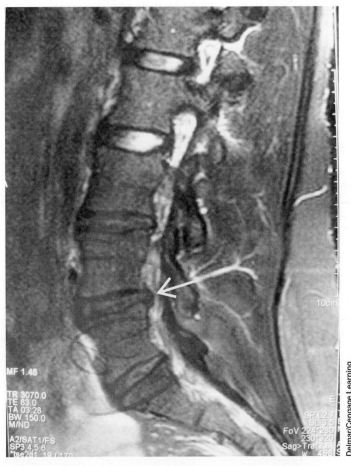

Figure 4-3 Disc herniation is more likely to occur in the lumbar and cervical regions of the spine.

Spinal Cord Injuries

Spinal cord injuries are commonly divided into "complete" and "incomplete" in reference to the amount of the cord that has been transected or severed. Cord injuries are described by the level at which the body retains sensation and everything distal to the level is impaired. For example, a T10 injury indicates that the patient has lost sensation and movement below the level of the umbilicus.

Although Paramedics can assess for deficits, it is important to remember that the initial findings may change as the body reacts to the injury. Primary injuries are defined as the injury to the spinal cord that occurs at the time of the trauma. Secondary injuries occur either from movement of the patient after the initial trauma, bleeding in the spinal cord, or an inflammatory response to the injury. In addition to the cord injury, the body will have a reaction to the injury, particularly if the sympathetic nervous system has been disrupted. As previously discussed, prevention is the key for primary injuries. EMS may have an impact on reducing the severity of secondary injuries and can certainly have an effect on the hypothermia and hypoperfusion that may occur after a spinal cord injury. It is unclear what amount of injury is caused by the patient's movement after the initial insult, but it is the standard practice that all personnel reduce the opportunity for movement unless they are confident that a spinal injury is unlikely.

Complete Cord Transection

Complete cord transection can occur at any level and will eliminate the transmission and reception of all messages below the area of the insult. The bundled nerve cells that travel in the spinal column are severed by a displacement of the vertebra, presence of a foreign object, or potentially by being stretched (distraction). Some patients may have symptoms of a complete transection at the time of the injury, but may regain sensation or motion after a period of time.

Additionally, patients may have sensation at a level below where they retain motor control. Paramedics should focus on accurate assessment and work with the patient to obtain as accurate a description of the neuropathy as possible.

Anterior Cord Syndrome

Anterior cord syndrome refers to damage to the anterior portion of the spinal cord (Figure 4-4). This condition often occurs when there is an obstruction of the artery feeding the anterior of the cord. The finding is characterized on exam by a loss of motor function, pain, and temperature sensation, although the presence of touch, vibration, and position sense remain. This occurs because the latter senses are associated with posterior spinal cord tracts and are fed by arteries in those areas. This can occur at any level of the spinal cord.

Cord Lesion	Area of Cord Injury	Signs and Symptoms	Anatomical Area of Involvment
Complete cord transection	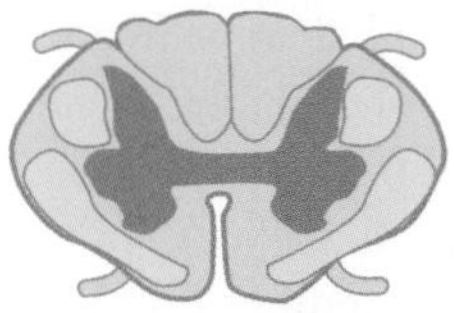	Loss of sensory and motor function below the level of the lesion May result in neurogenic shock Loss of bowel and bladder control	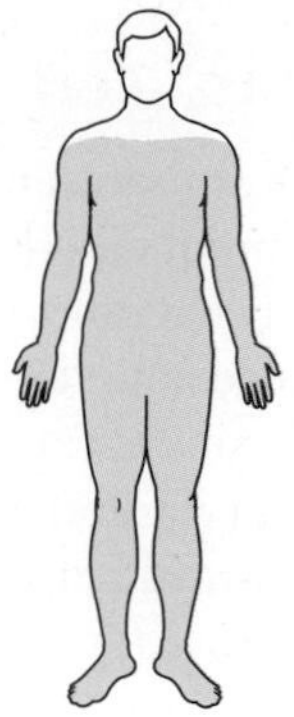
Anterior cord syndrome	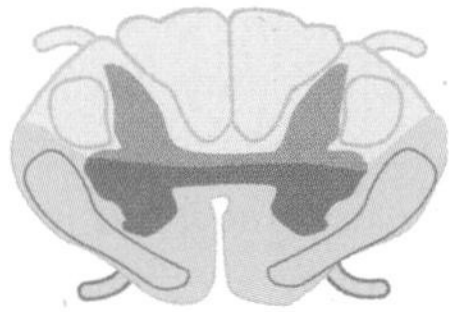	Typically the result of hyperflexion injuries Loss of voluntary and reflex motor activity Loss of pain and temperature sensation Preservation of proprioception, vibratory sense, and ability to sense light pressure	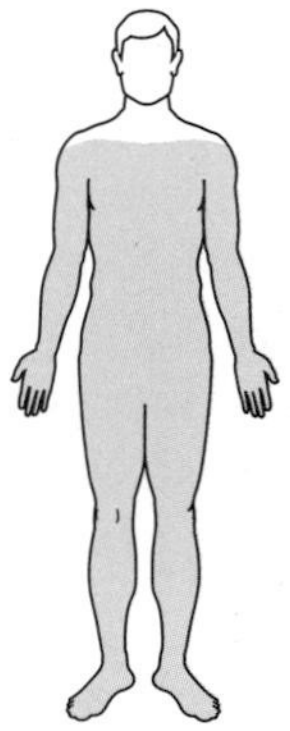
Central cord syndrome	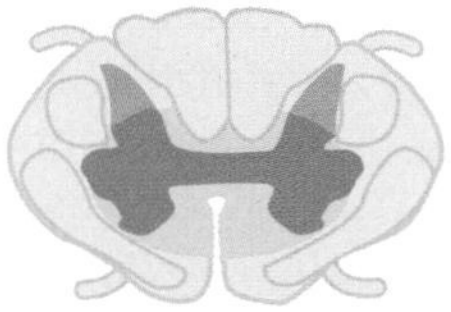	Typically the result of hyperextension injuries Damage to central signal tracts which mainly affect the upper extremities Paralysis or paresis in upper extremities with possible preservation of function in lower extremities Paresis often denser distally in upper extremities than proximal	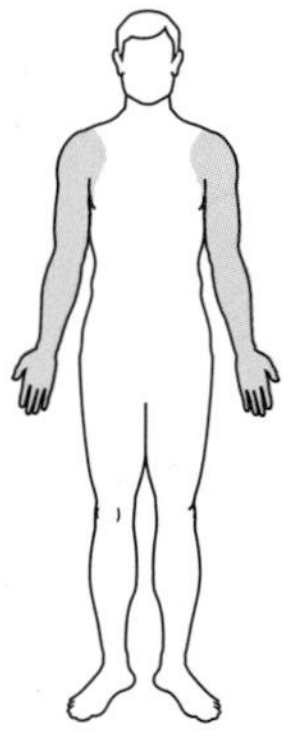
Brown-Sequard's syndrome	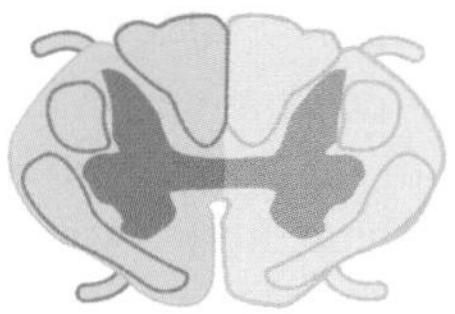	Cord damage limited to one hemisphere. Usually the result of penetrationg trauma Ipsilateral motor loss Ipsilateral loss of proprioception Contralateral loss of pain and temperature sensation	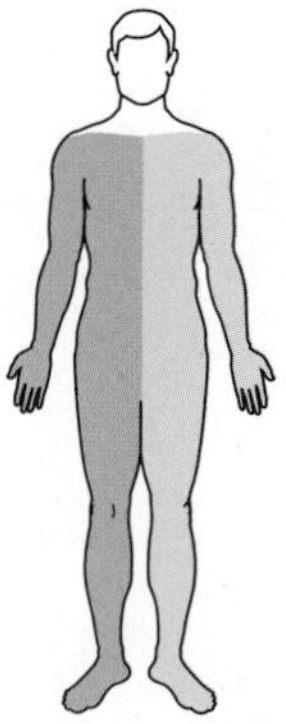

Figure 4-4 Summary of spinal cord injuries.

Delmar/Cengage Learning

Brown-Sequard Syndrome

Brown-Sequard syndrome is a partial transection of the cord which reduces position sense and motor control on the side with the injury (ipsilateral) and reduces pain and temperature sense on the other side (contralateral) (Figure 4-4). Often the contralateral findings begin two or three dermatomes below the site of the injury. The findings occur in this manner because the nerve pathways for pain and temperature cross over and travel up the opposite side of the spinal cord. This syndrome usually occurs with a penetrating traumatic injury such as a knife or gunshot wound in the back.

Central Cord Syndrome

Central cord syndrome usually involves a cervical injury with a mechanism of hyperextension. Central cord syndrome is the most common partial cord syndrome. The populations involved are typically either young adults who have suffered trauma or an older adult with a progressive narrowing of the vertebral canal. In the older population, a relatively minor mechanism of injury may cause the condition. For example, the patient may fall forward onto his chin, referred to as a "deadman's fall," and, upon striking his chin, cause hyperflexion of the neck, thus creating central cord syndrome.

The symptom that usually occurs is a motor weakness in the upper extremities. The weakness is more pronounced distally and is manifest by a weaker-than-normal grasp. It may also be accompanied by loss of pain and/or temperature sensation in the upper extremities (Figure 4-4).

Conus Medullaris and Cauda Equina Syndrome

Patients with sacral injuries (i.e., trauma to the pelvic area) may experience a loss of bladder or bowel control. **Conus medullaris syndrome**, an altered mental status secondary to traumatic brain injury and incontinence associated with this sacral cord injury, may be confused with the incontinence and confusion seen in the post-ictal phase of epilepsy.

Similar to conus medullaris, cauda equina syndrome is associated with incontinence, secondary to injury to the lumbosacral nerve roots. Cauda equina syndrome is seen in cases of lumbar disc herniation.

Spinal Cord Concussion

A spinal cord concussion is described as a temporary reduction in motor and sensation functions without any structural damage to the cord itself. This syndrome is believed to be rare and occurs with a violent impact, such as one would receive in contact sports. It can occur with any range of symptoms including full loss of sensation and motion, mimicking central cord syndrome, or only a decrease in either strength or sensation. Like the cerebral concussion, the spinal cord concussion can resolve within 24 to 72 hours. In the field, since Paramedics will be unable to discern the difference between a concussion and a true spinal cord injury, they should always treat for the spinal cord injury.

▶ CASE STUDY (CONTINUED)

Arriving at the patient's side, and after directing one of her teammates how to manually stabilize the young girl's head, the Paramedic turns to talk to the patient. Visibly distraught, the young girl keeps repeating over and over, "I can't feel my legs." At first a bit shaken by the enormity of the situation, the Paramedic leans down and, in deliberate measured words, whispers into the young girl's ears, "I am here with you. We are going to help you but we need your help, too. Please take a moment, catch your breath, and tell me as clearly as you can what exactly happened."

With tears rolling down her cheek, the girl looks the Paramedic in the eyes and starts to explain that they were practicing for the homecoming game. They wanted to do something special that they had seen on TV. When she was thrown in the air she was supposed to twist and fall into a team member's arms. But the throw went wrong, and she landed off-balance and fell straight down on top of her head. She remembered hearing a snap, then she lost control of her arms and legs. Unwittingly, some of her teammates tried to help her stand up and she collapsed. Shortly thereafter, she started to have trouble breathing.

CRITICAL THINKING QUESTIONS

1. What are the important elements of the history that a Paramedic should obtain?
2. Are transient neurologic signs and symptoms as important as persistent neurologic signs and symptoms?

History

The key to diagnosing a spinal cord injury is the mechanism of injury that may have created the spinal cord injury. However, use of the SAMPLE history should not be ignored. For example, the same medications that increase bleeding in head trauma (anticoagulants) can also cause bleeding in the spinal cord. Another example is diabetes. Patients with diabetes can develop peripheral neuropathy, damage to the peripheral nervous system secondary to diabetes. These peripheral neuropathies can mimic spinal cord injury. Similarly, some HIV drugs can also cause peripheral neuropathy. These examples help to illustrate the importance of a complete SAMPLE history.

Mechanisms of Injury

When considering the type and severity of injury sustained by a patient, the Paramedic must consider several factors (Table 4-1). First, how much kinetic energy was applied to the body and in what direction? Newton's first law of motion states that a body acted upon by a force will continue in motion until acted upon by another force. To illustrate the forces, one can consider a simplified example of a motor vehicle crash. The initial energy is the kinetic energy of the person traveling at a velocity of 62 mph (100 km/h) combined with the person's mass. Speed or velocity is considered as its square and mass is considered at its half. In short, the speed of the object has a much greater impact than its size.

STREET SMART

Medical research indicates that patients who are shot, even those who are shot in the head, do not generally require cervical spinal immobilization unless the patient presents with a neurologic deficit.[3,4]

Table 4-1 High-Risk Mechanisms of Injury

- Falls
  - Adults: > 20 feet (one story is equal to 10 feet)
  - Children: > 10 feet or two to three times the height of the child
- High-risk auto crash
  - Intrusion: > 12 in. occupant seat > 18 in. any site
  - Ejection (partial or complete) from automobile
  - Death in same passenger compartment
  - Vehicle telemetry data consistent with high risk of injury
- Auto vs. pedestrian/bicyclist thrown, run over, or with significant (> 20 mph) impact
- Motorcycle crash > 20 mph[2]

At the time of impact, the patient is acted upon by several forces to bring the kinetic energy to zero. The first force that acts upon the body will likely be the seat belt as it tightens and pushes the person back into the seat. However, the patient's head will continue forward at its previous speed until it strikes something or completes its arc of motion. The airbag is designed to reduce the kinetic energy by transferring it into a cushion of air. Internal organs also continue to move until they meet resistance. If all the energy isn't expended during the initial impact, there will be additional motion and rebound injuries until the energy has been expended.

Rarely is just one vector of energy applied to the body. A motor vehicle crash will have the force from the object the patient struck, which may then cause the vehicle to rotate and strike another object. It is not possible, nor is it very helpful, to focus on all the different forces that may have caused an injury to the patient. However, it is important to understand that certain forces will be more likely to cause certain injuries and are more destructive than others.

Flexion

The spine moves with flexion when it bends forward, such as when touching the chin to the chest or bending to touch the toes. Normal flexion occurs hundreds of times a day. However, abnormal flexion can occur when a force causes the head to move forward with greater speed or acceleration than would be natural or when the upper portion of the torso forces the lumbar spine to bend forward beyond its natural range. Examples of this type of injury include sudden deceleration in a car accident, head first falls during a flip, and being struck in the head from behind with a blunt object. Lifting an object that is too heavy would also be a flexion injury.

Extension

The spine moves with extension when it bends backward, such as when a person looks above or intentionally stretches backwards. It can also be described as extension when the person moves directly laterally, such as when touching an ear to a shoulder. The range of motion is much less in this direction because the spinous processes are designed to give the spine strength when moving this way. Abnormal extension occurs when a force causes the head or torso to bend backwards beyond its natural range of motion. Examples include when a patient's forehead strikes a windshield or someone suffers a blow to the side of the head.

Rotation

The spine moves in circular motion along the longitudinal axis. Rotational injuries can be caused by a blow to the chin, which causes the sudden movement of the spinal column. This mechanism of injury can also occur during a variety of activities such as contact sports, violent crime, or falls from a height.

Distraction

Distraction injuries occur when the cord is stretched beyond its normal length. This elongation is associated with the head being moved forcefully away from the rest of the body, which can occur while operating open vehicles such as snowmobiles and all-terrain vehicles (ATV) when the driver strikes an object such as a wire or a low hanging branch. This injury is also the classic mechanism for death from hanging. The cause of a hangman's fracture (C2) is a distraction injury displacing the vertebrae.

In some cases, the spinal column damage is not apparent on physical examination or X-ray. This can be the result of a distracting injury, such as hanging. Termed **SCIWORA**, meaning spinal cord injury without radiologic abnormality, these spinal cord injuries should be suspected based on mechanism of injury. MRI technologies are able to detect SCIWORA.

Compression

Compression injuries (also referred to as axial loading) occur when force is applied directly to the long axis of the spine. The cord is jolted and the spinal nerve roots may receive a significant injury when the vertebrae are forced together. This mechanism is often found in diving accidents. Compression injuries have been identified as being more likely to have neurological deficits than other mechanisms. Compression injuries are often implicated in burst fractures.

Penetrations

A solid object can also harm the spinal cord as it pierces the cord or becomes lodged in it. Bullets, knives, and shrapnel are external examples of penetrating objects. Pieces of a fractured vertebra or other bone may also enter the spinal cord to cause a disruption in transmission.

Combination

During a traumatic event, the body moves in a variety of directions as it is exposed to numerous forces. The cervical spine may rotate to the left as it is being extended during a motor vehicle crash or a gymnast may flex her head as she compresses her spine. It is not necessary to identify which mechanisms caused the injury, but it is essential to assess a patient properly if there is any suspicion of spinal cord injury.

► CASE STUDY (CONTINUED)

Thankfully, an engine company from the local volunteer fire department arrives. The additional hands will be helpful later when the patient needs to be moved. Right now, however, the fire department is assembling the spinal immobilization and resuscitation equipment.

The Paramedic's first priority is the patient's breathing difficulty. Although her room air oxygen saturation is acceptable, the Paramedic still calls for a bag-valve-mask assembly to be connected to high-flow, high-concentration oxygen at standby. A new first responder agrees to count ventilations every minute and call them out.

CRITICAL THINKING QUESTIONS

1. What are the elements of the physical examination of a patient with suspected spinal cord syndrome?
2. Why is a dermatome-focused neurological examination a critical element in this examination?

Examination

Paramedics should perform a thorough examination before making an assessment whether or not to treat for a spinal cord injury. If there is a suspicion that the patient may have a spinal cord injury at any point during the course of care, the Paramedic should immobilize the patient.

First, the Paramedic should assess the situation and pay particular attention to the mechanism of injury. Patients with a high-risk MOI should be immobilized. The pre-immobilization physical examination in these cases primarily consists of an evaluation of distal motor and sensory function of all extremities.

Second, and barring a high-risk MOI, the Paramedic should identify any pre-existing conditions that may make the patient likely to have a spinal cord injury. These conditions include age of over 65; suspected atlanto-axial instability, such as patients with Down syndrome; and a history of osteoporosis or the taking of medications to prevent osteoporosis, such as the bisphosphonates (alendronate/Fosamax, risedronate/Actonel, and zoledronic acid/Reclast, as well as raloxifene/Evista and hormone therapies).

Third, the Paramedic should assess the patient for examination reliability. Patients must be calm and cooperative for the exam to be accurate. Existence of a language barrier and inability to communicate clearly, patients who are in the midst of an **acute stress reaction** (a psychological response to a traumatic event), or those patients who may be under the influence of alcohol are examples of patients that may not be able to give the Paramedic reliable answers to questions or be aware of their own injuries. To be reliable, the patient must be able to communicate, be calm, and have a mental status unimpaired by alcohol or other substances, including prescription medications.

Finally, the Paramedic should be patient with a patient suffering from a **painful distracting injury** or a circumstance in which a person is not able to participate in a reliable exam. These injuries or circumstances might include a broken limb, trouble breathing, or a significant laceration.

The Paramedic should then evaluate the patient for physical findings that may indicate a spinal cord injury such as an abnormal sensory exam, poor motor response, or pain along the spine. Assuming that the primary assessment has already been performed, this examination can be performed quickly in a head-to-toe fashion starting with level of consciousness.

Primary Assessment

Loss of ventilatory function is probably one of the most devastating consequences of spinal cord injury. When there is a spinal cord injury at C1 or C2 (hangman's fracture or Jeffersonian fracture), the patient may lose 90% of her vital capacity and the ability to cough, suggesting vigilance is needed to prevent aspiration.

If the spinal cord injury is a high cervical injury (i.e., C3-C6), then the patient will only have 20% of her vital capacity and a weak and ineffective cough. High thoracic spinal cord injuries can diminish vital capacity by one-half. The clear implication is that, although the paralysis may be devastating, the loss of ventilatory capacity and airway control is truly life-threatening.

After assuring that the patient's ventilatory function is adequate, the Paramedic may turn to circulation as part of the ABCs. Although neurogenic shock is a possibility, particularly if the spinal cord injury is above T6, it is more likely that any hypotension is the result of hemorrhage. Although the classic triad of hypotension, vasodilation, and bradycardia is suggestive of neurogenic shock, the reality is that this picture is often distorted (i.e., tachycardia exists for other reasons including pain).

Dermatomes

Dermatomes are areas of the body innervated by specific spinal nerves (nerves that leave the spinal cord). In the cervical spine, they are described consecutively in descending order from C1 to C8. The C1 spinal nerves refer to the nerves that leave the spinal cord superior to the C1 (atlas) vertebrae. The C8 spinal nerves leave inferior to C7. For the thoracic and lumbar regions of the spine, the designations describe the vertebrae above the opening from which they exit the spinal cord. Although the spinal cord proper ends at L1-L2, dermatomes are described for the peripheral nerves that exit through the openings in the spinal column below the cauda equina.

Although the actual dermatome is not of great importance in the patient's field assessment, it is crucial for the Paramedic to be aware of where neurological deficits begin and if there is any change in them during care. Regardless of the deficit's location, the presence of any motor or sensory deficits requires full immobilization and very careful movements (Figure 4-5).

Detailed Spinal Examination

Time permitting, the Paramedic may want to complete a thorough neurological examination to establish a baseline. This examination can be performed quickly in a head-to-toe fashion starting at the shoulders and testing motor strength first.

Starting at the shoulders, the Paramedic should assess for motor strength along the shoulders (deltoids), anterior upper arms (biceps), forearms, wrists, and fingers. Motor strength is graded from 0 (total paralysis) to 5 (active movement against full resistance). If there is a visible contraction only, then the muscle function is given a score of 1. If the patient is able to lift an extremity against gravity, then the muscle function is scored a 3 (Table 4-2).

The Paramedic can assess finger strength by asking the patient to spread his fingers and then inserting her fingers between the patient's digits and asking the patient to close his hand. Next, the Paramedic asks the patient to close his fingers. The Paramedic grasps the fingers and asks the patient to

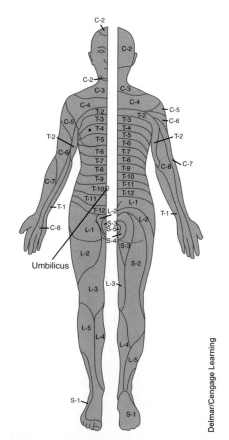

Figure 4-5 Dermatomes are areas of the body innervated by specific spinal nerves.

Table 4-2 Strength Grading System

0 = Total paralysis
1 = Visible muscle contraction
2 = Active movement limited by gravity
3 = Active movement against gravity
4 = Active movement against minimal resistance
5 = Active movement against full resistance

Table 4-3 Spinal Levels for Muscles Tested during Motor Strength Testing

C-5	Elbow flexors (biceps)
C-6	Wrist extensors (extensor carpi radialis longus)
C-7	Finger flexors (triceps)
C-8	Finger abductors (flexor digitorum profundus)
L-2	Hip flexors (iliopsoas)
L-3	Knee extensors (quadriceps)
L-4	Ankle dorsiflexion (tibialis anterior)
L-5	Large toe extensors (extensors hallucis longus)
S-1	Ankle plantar flexion (gastrocnemius)

open the fingers. This tests key muscles and their associated spinal nerve roots by level (Table 4-3).[5]

Next, using the dermatomes, the Paramedic should perform an examination of sensation. Starting at the shoulders, the Paramedic should lightly tap and/or squeeze the shoulders, the upper arm, and the forearm. To test the hands, the Paramedic should utilize "position sense." Grasping the distal pharyngeal joint to stabilize it, the Paramedic then moves the finger upward and downward. With the patient's eyes closed, the Paramedic asks the patient which direction the finger is moving. Although this is a crude test, repeating it several times increases the test's accuracy and improves its reliability.

An appropriate prehospital physical exam should include evaluation of the patient's sensory abilities at a variety of levels. The sensation of a palpation of the posterior head and neck is related to the C2 and C3 dermatomes. The C3 dermatome is tested at the supraclavicular fossa and C4 is tested at the top of the shoulder proximal to the acromioclavicular joint. Next, the Paramedic should test the lateral side of the antecubital fossa. Note that the diaphragm is controlled by the C3 to C5 nerve roots and that injury in the cervical area can lead to respiratory distress/arrest. The thumb generally corresponds with C6, the middle finger with C7, and the pinky with C8.

Moving along the inner aspect of the arm, the Paramedic should test for sensation at the medial side of the antecubital fossa that corresponds with T1. Moving next to the trunk, the Paramedic can poke or pinch the apex of the axilla, T2, and move anterior to the angle of Louis or T3. Each intercostal space corresponds with the same level of the spinal column. T5 is usually identified with the nipple line. The umbilicus is at the T10 area.

Next, the Paramedic should ask the patient if he has any numbness or tingling in the perineal area. This finding is called sacral sparing. The presence of these sensations with paralysis may indicate an incomplete spinal cord injury.

Priapism is a painful sustained erection without apparent stimulation, and may be an indication of sacral nerve injury. Priapism can also be caused by illicit drug use or sickle cell crisis, which can complicate the trauma patient's clinical picture. Priapism is a medical emergency.

Finally, moving to the lower extremities, the Paramedic tests the lumbar spine. L2 is tested on the anterior thigh, L3 is typically tested at the knee, and L5 is tested at the toes. The final assessment is for a plantar reflex.

Grasping the ankle firmly with one hand, the Paramedic should take a pen or similar object and rake the arch of the sole of the foot in a C shape. Normally the toes should curl and the foot will arch. If the big toe should flare upward and the toes fan, called Babinski's reflex, this is the result of a reflex arc from the sacrum. Normally, the plantar reflex overrides Babinski's reflex once the higher functions within the cerebellum take control and the person begins to walk.

Each assessment should include a check of motion and sensation, if possible, as the dermatomes for sensation are slightly different than those for motion. Additionally, a painful stimulus (a pinch or poke with a blunt object) may be felt at a lower level than a gentle touch.

► **CASE STUDY (CONTINUED)**

The Paramedic wants the patient to remain able to communicate as she methodically goes down the dermatomes. The patient lost feeling just below the clavicle, suggesting to the Paramedic that the injury is near C5. Beyond the shoulders, the patient has no feeling and no movement.

CRITICAL THINKING QUESTIONS

1. What is the significance of the loss of feeling at the shoulders?
2. What diagnosis did the Paramedic announce to the patient?

Assessment

When assessing a patient with a potential spinal cord injury, Paramedics must process and apply a great deal of information to arrive at a course of treatment. In certain situations, it is an easy decision to suspect a spinal cord injury. Paramedics can safely suspect that trauma patients that are or were unconscious, suffering paralysis or paresthesia, have pain near the spine, or have a gunshot wound to the thorax have a spinal cord injury.[6]

Conversely, there are certain situations in which a patient is unlikely to have a spinal cord injury. Patients with an isolated extremity injury, those in a low-speed motor vehicle crash, or those who had a short fall are unlikely to have a spinal cord injury unless physical findings indicate one. However, many emergency calls do not fall neatly into either side of the continuum to suspect a spinal cord injury.

Selective Spinal Immobilization

For many years, Paramedics were trained to treat the patient based solely on the mechanism of injury and not account for the patient's physical findings. A patient was treated for suspected spinal cord injury with immobilization even if he had no signs or symptoms of spinal cord injury. However, research such as the NEXUS and the Canadian C-Spine Rules[7] have identified certain physical findings that are much more likely to identify patients without a spinal cord injury than those with an injury. According to the Canadian C-Spine Rules, stable and alert patients are less likely to have a spinal cord injury and do not need to be radiographed if they meet certain signs and symptoms (Table 4-4).

When used in the hospital, these findings allow physicians to bypass radiography based on the very low chance that these patients have a spinal cord injury. This research has been transferred into selective spinal immobilization protocols for EMS systems across the United States. These protocols have been established to help Paramedics accurately decide not to immobilize patients thought to have uninjured spinal cords.

The National Association of EMS Physicians, in its position paper on spinal immobilization, has indicated three contraindications to selective spinal immobilization: altered mental status, evidence of intoxication, and a painful distracting injury such as a long-bone fracture. If any one of these three conditions is met, regardless of the outcomes of the physical examination, and the patient has a significant mechanism of injury, then the Paramedic should receive spinal precautions.

When initially approaching the patient, the Paramedic should automatically expect to treat the patient for a spinal cord injury and only decide against it after a thorough history and physical exam.

Table 4-4 Canadian C-Spine Rules

- High-risk factors
  - Age greater than or equal to 65
  - Dangerous mechanisms
    - Fall from elevation greater than three feet or five stairs
    - Axial load to head
    - MVC with high speed (> 63 mph), rollover, ejection
    - Motorized recreational vehicles
    - Bicycle struck or collision
  - Paresthesia in extremities
- Low-risk factors that allow safe assessment of range of motion
  - Simple rear-end MVC
  - Sitting position
  - Ambulatory at any time
  - Delayed onset of neck pain (not immediate at time of accident)
  - Absence of midline cervical spine tenderness
- Able to actively rotate neck
  - 45 degrees right and left

Paramedics should understand that certain patients are at a higher risk of suffering spinal cord injury. Older patients (age 65 and up) may have a decreased muscle or bone mass. Pediatric patients may not be able to effectively communicate the sensations of pain or paresthesia. Patients with Trisomy 21 (Down syndrome) are at risk of atlanto-axial instability. Instability of the first and second cervical vertebrae affects approximately 17% of patients with Down syndrome. A person with degenerative bone disease or spinal tumors is also at greater risk for a fracture.

Since there is currently no successful treatment for a revitalization of the transected spinal cord, the Paramedic's primary concern should be prevention of the injuries. Proper engineering of the environment can reduce the amount of energy that a person is exposed to during a traumatic event and thus reduce spinal cord injuries. For example, seat belts and airbags help absorb energy during a motor vehicle crash. Bicycle helmets can reduce the energy transferred to the body during a collision. Removal of trip hazards in a home environment can reduce the likelihood of falls. Behavior modifications can also reduce dangerous activities that may lead to spinal cord injury. Education on proper tackling techniques can reduce spear tackling in football. Limiting diving into only deep swim areas or emphasizing spotting during cheerleading and gymnastics can reduce chances for injuries during those activities.

As the patient continues to maintain an adequate oxygen saturation with the high-flow, high-concentration oxygen via nonrebreather mask and the vital signs are stable, the Paramedic calls the engine company together to explain that, first, there is no immediate life-threatening emergency, and therefore the team is going to move slowly and deliberately to ensure that no secondary injury occurs.

CRITICAL THINKING QUESTIONS

1. What is the national standard of care of patients with suspected spinal cord injury?
2. What are some of the patient-specific concerns and considerations that the Paramedic should consider when applying this plan of care that is intended to treat a broad patient population presenting with spinal cord injury?

Treatment

The treatment of the spinal cord-injured patient, like all trauma patients, starts with the airway. Once all life threats have been identified and treated, the Paramedic should immobilize the patient.

Airway Management

A patient with a high cervical injury may lose the ability to control the diaphragm, the intercostal muscles, or both. The phrenic nerve originates from the spinal nerve roots at C3, C4, and C5; the high cervical area.

If these patients experience respiratory distress, the patient will need careful airway management as any additional manipulation of the spine (for example, to intubate) may worsen the injury. An experienced provider should attempt oral trauma intubation if it is required, although careful consideration should be given to maintaining a basic life support (BLS) airway or using a blind insertion airway device that does not require movement of the neck. Maintaining a BLS airway may be the best option if the airway can be managed that way. One technique to improve the success rate of intubating an immobilized patient is to place the patient on a gurney and elevate the head of the stretcher 25 degrees. This allows the patient to be placed into a modified sniffing position and improves the Paramedic's visualization of the glottic opening.

STREET SMART

The saying goes "3-4-5 keeps a guy alive." This reminds Paramedics the phrenic nerve, responsible for diaphragm movement, originates from cervical spine nerves 3, 4 and 5.

In addition, remote-viewing laryngoscopes may also improve the likelihood of successful intubation. The Paramedic should use manual stabilization of the spine during intubation attempts in order to reduce the chance of spinal manipulation. Cervical collars have been demonstrated to markedly reduce mouth opening. "Opening" the collar, with manual stabilization instituted, has been shown to improve visualization by one grade on the Mallampati scale in the majority of cases.[8]

Spinal Motion Restriction

For decades, EMS practice has been to immobilize the patient as soon as a suspicion of a spinal cord injury exists based on mechanism of injury. That practice has been thrown into question recently, as some believe mechanism of injury may not be a reliable predictor of spinal cord injury. However, the general practice of immobilizing patients with suspected spinal injury remains.[9]

It is reasonable to suspect spinal injury whenever there is a relevant mechanism of injury and the patient complains of midline cervical pain, has pain on palpation of the midline cervical area, and/or has neurologic deficits including paresthesia and/or paralysis.[6]

Spinal immobilization begins with a manual stabilization of the cervical spine while reducing movement of the rest of the body until the Paramedic makes an assessment to either treat for the injury by completing immobilization or choosing to not immobilize. It is believed that proper complete body spinal immobilization reduces the chance of a spinal cord injury caused by moving an unstable spinal column.

However, as a treatment, spinal immobilization has potential harmful side effects including lower back pain, creation of pressure sores, and the development of tenderness from being placed in the various devices.[10] When deciding to treat the patient, the Paramedic must first obtain consent, noting the potential consequences of not immobilizing the spinal injury. After the patient is immobilized, the patient must be observed for vomiting. As she is immobile on a long back-board, the patient is at risk for aspiration. Therefore, suction should be readily available for patients that are immobilized.

Cervical Collars

A rigid cervical collar is a part of the generally accepted treatment for spinal trauma, regardless of where the injury is suspected to have occurred. The device must be properly sized and applied to reduce the patient's discomfort. The Paramedic should ensure that the patient's earrings, necklaces, and hair are not pressed against the skin to prevent pressure sores.

Long Board Devices

When immobilizing patients during transportation in the ambulance and transferring them at the hospital, the industry standard is to use a long backboard. Its goal is to limit the movement of the spine by restraining movement from the head to the pelvis, which have been described as the joints above and below the bones of the vertebrae. Patients are moved onto this device using a variety of techniques based on how the patient is found. Regardless of the technique, the spine should be moved as little as possible.

Supine patients are frequently moved with a log-roll maneuver. At least three people are needed to perform this movement properly, and using more is preferable. Even when done with enough help, this motion has been shown to allow a measurable amount of spinal column movement.

An alternative to the log roll is using a split rigid stretcher that can be slid underneath the patient with little movement. The devices still provide adequate support to the spinal column and eliminate much of the motion required to get the patient on the device.[11]

Another accepted method of moving the patient to the backboard is the four-person lift. Although it is manpower intensive, this technique has great promise for limiting cervical spine movement.

A variety of methods have been suggested for properly securing a patient to restrict movement. To secure the body, straps forming an "X" across the shoulders, another "X" across the hips, and a final strap below the knees should be sufficient. If practical, slight padding in the lower back and behind the knees may reduce the pain that is often associated with being on a backboard for a long period of time. Occasionally, large patients may require more straps. Once the body is secured, the head must be secured to the board.

Patients with a kyphosis, an extreme forward curvature of the thoracic spine, may require padding under their head to ensure patient comfort and proper immobilization. Paramedics must also monitor patients for postural dyspnea and adjust the positioning, if possible.

One study suggested that placing approximately 1.5 inches (range 0 to 3.75 inches) of occipital padding under the patient's head would increase the percentage of patients whose head would be in neutral alignment as well as increase patient comfort.[12]

Short Spine Devices

Short spine immobilization devices are recommended when moving a stable patient from a seated position to the long spine devices. There are a variety of devices that Paramedics may have available to use. The concept of each is to restrict movement of the patient's torso and head by securing them with straps to a rigid device. The patient is then moved as a single unit to a long board device. It is accepted practice to forgo these devices in the case of an unstable patient.

PROFESSIONAL PARAMEDIC

The current science in emergency medicine recommends against Paramedics administering steroids for spinal cord injuries. A number of studies have shown that there is no discernable benefit for patients that receive steroids immediately after the incident.

CASE STUDY (CONTINUED)

Carefully lifting the fully immobilized cheerleader, the team moves her to the ambulance. Once on-board, the Paramedic asks for the first responder to take vital signs every 10 minutes. The first responder asks why, stating that if she is stable then vital signs are normally taken every 15 minutes. At least, that was what he was told in school.

Taking a deep breath, the Paramedic explains that a rare form of shock can occur suddenly, finishing the statement by saying, "An ounce of prevention is worth a pound of cure."

CRITICAL THINKING QUESTIONS

1. What are some of the predictable complications associated with spinal cord injury?
2. What are some of the predictable complications associated with the treatments for acute spinal cord injury?

Evaluation

The nerves within the spinal cord largely maintain physiologic stability, and a spinal cord injury can lead to fluctuation in vital signs such as heart rate, temperature, and so on. Therefore, the Paramedic should assess, and then frequently reassess, the patient with a spinal cord injury and be prepared to intervene to help stabilize the patient.

Physiologic Reaction to Spinal Cord Injuries

The tearing or severing of the spinal cord is the beginning of a series of reactions that continue for days. When the cord is damaged, neurotransmitters flood the area, perhaps in an attempt to reestablish communication. However, they have the effect of killing neurons and axons. There is often a decrease in blood flow at the injury site in the spinal cord as a result of injury and/or inflammation. Blood vessels in the gray matter within the spinal cord begin to leak and cause additional swelling.

Several hours to days after the injury, immune system cells arrive at the injury site and create additional swelling and inflammation. This secondary damage begins to exacerbate the damage caused by the primary injury, which can further lead to hypoperfusion and an increase in the severity of neurologic deficits.

Spinal Shock

Spinal shock is the loss of motor control and sensation below the injury site. First described by Dr. Whytt in 1750, spinal shock is the loss of both sensation and motor function (paralysis) below the level of the spinal cord transection. The muscles that are regulated by nerves distal to the cord transection are flaccid. A patient may also lose bowel or bladder control.

The body goes through four stages or phases of spinal shock. However, the Paramedic is likely to only witness the first phase since it occurs within the first 24 hours.[13] The first phase involves loss of all reflexes distal to the spinal cord injury, whereas primitive protective reflex arcs, such as Babinski's reflex, return.

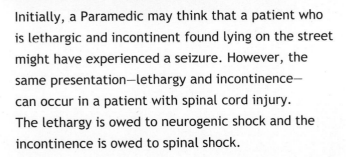

STREET SMART

Initially, a Paramedic may think that a patient who is lethargic and incontinent found lying on the street might have experienced a seizure. However, the same presentation—lethargy and incontinence—can occur in a patient with spinal cord injury. The lethargy is owed to neurogenic shock and the incontinence is owed to spinal shock.

Neurogenic Shock

Whereas spinal shock is localized and affects the spinal nerves, **neurogenic shock** is a systemic manifestation of spinal cord injury. When the spinal cord is transected, the brain loses the ability to control the body distal to the cord disruption. This results in severe autonomic dysfunction and specifically interrupts the sympathetic nervous system. As a result of the sympatholytic effect of spinal cord injury, there is unopposed parasympathetic stimulation that leads to vagally mediated vasodilation and distributive shock, as well as bradycardia. This classic triad—hypotension, bradycardia, and peripheral vasodilation—is suggestive of neurogenic shock.

The body's ability to regulate temperature is also adversely affected. This can result in the characteristic skin pattern of cool and diaphoretic skin above the level of the spinal cord injury and warm and flushed skin below the level of the injury. This vasodilation can lead to loss of core heat and subsequent hypothermia, even in temperate climates. Therefore, all spine-injured patients should be covered with a blanket to help preserve body heat and to prevent hypothermia.

In some cases, the combination of bradycardia and a relative hypovolemia lead to hypotension ($SV \times HR = CO$). Treatment for this vasovagal event typically involves a fluid bolus to maintain a sufficient systolic blood pressure. Significant bradycardias may also need to be treated with atropine.

STREET SMART

In patients with permanent paralysis, a phenomenon called autonomic dysreflexia (sometimes called autonomic hyperreflexia) can occur. As opposed to spinal shock, autonomic dysreflexia results in profound hypertension, diaphoresis, and loss of bladder and bowel control. Autonomic dysreflexia occurs in phase four of spinal shock, and usually occurs in the first year.

Complicating Hemorrhagic Shock

Although hemorrhagic shock is not caused by a spinal cord injury, patients with a spinal cord injury have likely undergone a significant mechanism of injury and need to be carefully evaluated for signs of hemorrhagic shock. The Paramedic needs to rule out all causes of this type of shock before deciding that the patient has neurogenic shock. The injury to the spinal cord may also reduce the patient's ability to compensate for even moderate blood loss through loss of sympathetic response.

Initially, the family insists that their daughter be transported to Memorial Hospital, where her pediatrician works. But they ultimately agree to have their daughter transported to the trauma center in the next city when the Paramedic advises them of the services that are available at the trauma center which are unavailable at the local hospital.

CRITICAL THINKING QUESTIONS

1. What is the most appropriate transport decision that will get the patient to definitive care?
2. What are the advantages of transporting a patient with suspected spinal cord injury to these hospitals, even if that means bypassing other hospitals in the process?

Disposition

The Centers for Disease Control, as part of the National Trauma Triage Protocol,[2] recommends that all patients with paralysis be transported to a trauma center based on the availability of specialists to treat this injury and its sequela. Patients without paralysis should be transported to a trauma center based on their physical findings for other injuries and regional protocols.

The Paramedic should carefully document all physical findings. Patients with spinal cord injuries face massive expenses, particularly in the first year following the injury, and often seek redress in the courts.

CONCLUSION

Spinal cord injuries are relatively infrequent but have profound impacts on patients when they occur, potentially causing life-long paralysis. The spinal column consists of 33 vertebrae, ligaments, intravertebral discs, muscles, and the spinal cord. The spinal nerves connect to the spinal cord between each vertebra until the lumbar region, where the nerves extend down from the cauda equina. The body is divided into regions called dermatomes. These dermatomes indicate which spinal nerves carry messages. The spinal column is susceptible to a variety of injuries; the most serious is a spinal cord injury. Spinal cord injuries may be complete or partial, impacting only certain nerve pathways, depending on how and where the injury occurred. Recent emergency medicine research indicates that patients with a high risk of having a spinal cord injury can be identified with physical findings and risk factors that are common in injured patients. The cause of spinal trauma varies greatly and often involves multiple forces. Prehospital treatment currently focuses on restricting movement and monitoring for the onset of spinal shock. Patients with paralysis should be taken to a trauma center.

KEY POINTS:

- Annual costs associated with spinal cord injury—including medical, social, and personal costs—are high.

- The complete cord transection results in distal paralysis and paresthesia distal to the insult.

- Anterior cord syndrome, a partial cord syndrome, causes loss of pain, temperature sensation, and motor function. However, the patient retains touch, vibration, and position sense.

- Brown-Sequard syndrome, another partial cord syndrome, causes loss of motor control on the side with the insult and loss of pain on the other side of the body.

- Central cord syndrome, the third and most common partial cord syndrome, causes weakness in the upper body, particularly affecting the patient's grasp.

- Mechanism of injury must be considered when assessing for spinal cord injury.

- The mechanism of injury can cause flexion, extension, rotation, distraction, and compression of the spinal column, leading to spinal cord injury.

- Certain patient populations are at greater risk of spinal cord injury, including the elderly, those with atlanto-axial instability (such as persons with Down syndrome), and those with a history of osteoporosis.

- Understanding dermatomes can help the Paramedic estimate the level of the spinal cord injury.

- In certain cases, the Paramedic may decide not to immobilize a trauma patient based on a specific set of protocols called the selective spinal immobilization protocols.

- Three contraindications to selective spinal immobilization are intoxication, altered mental status, and a painful distracting injury.

- Cervical injuries have implications for ventilation.

- The three methods of moving a patient to a backboard/spine board are modified log roll, split rigid stretcher (orthopedic stretcher), and the most effective, a four-person lift.

- Spinal shock is a distal motor control problem, and is not the same as neurogenic shock.

- Neurogenic shock is a systemic manifestation that leads to hypoperfusion because of the misdistribution of blood volume.

▶ REVIEW QUESTIONS:

1. Complete cord transection presents with paralysis below the insult. What condition presents with paralysis on one side of the body and paresthesia on the other?

2. What traumatic spinal cord injury may present like epilepsy?

3. What is the origin of the high-risk mechanisms of injury?

4. To be a reliable patient, what three conditions must be met?

5. Gently tapping or squeezing the shoulders, upper arm, and forearm tests which dermatomes?

▶ CASE STUDY QUESTIONS:

Please refer to the Case Study in this chapter, and answer the questions below:

1. Explain the connection between shortness of breath and spinal cord injury.

2. Assuming a high cervical fracture, with complete cord transection and resultant tetraplegia, what would be the safest means to move the patient from the ground to the backboard for spinal immobilization?

3. What is the difference between spinal shock and neurogenic shock?

▶ REFERENCES:

1. National Spinal Cord Injury Statistical Center, Birmingham, Alabama. Spinal cord injury: facts and figures at a glance. January 2008.

2. Centers for Disease Control and Prevention, National Triage Decision Scheme. Available at: **http://www.cdc.gov/FieldTriage.** Accessed August 2009.

3. Kaups K, Davis J. Patients with gunshot wounds to the head do not require cervical spine immobilization and evaluation. *J Trauma*. 1998;44(5):865–867.

4. Medson R, et al. Stability of cervical spine fractures after gunshot wounds to the head and neck. *Spine*. 2005;30(20):2274–2279.

5. Harris MB, Sethi RK. The initial assessment and management of the multiple-trauma patient with an associated spine injury. *Spine*. May 15, 2006;31(11 Suppl):S9–15.

6. Domeier RM. Indications for prehospital spinal immobilization. National Association of EMS Physicians Standards and Clinical Practice. *Prehosp Emerg Care*. July-September, 1999;3(3):251–253.

7. Stiell I, et al. The Canadian c-spine rule for radiography in alert and stable trauma patients. *JAMA*. 2001;286:1841–1848.

8. Heath KJ, et al. The effect of laryngoscopy of different cervical spine immobilization techniques. *Anaesthesia*. 2007;47(10):843–845.

9. Hauswald M, et al. Out of hospital spinal immobilization: its effect on neurologic injury. *Acad Emerg Med*. 2008;5(3): 214–219.

10. Chan D, et al. Pain and tissue interface pressures during spine-board immobilization. *Ann Emerg Med*. 1995;26(1):31–36.

11. Krell J, et al. Comparison of Ferno scoop stretcher with the long backboard for spinal immobilization. *Prehosp Emerg Care*. 2006;10(1):46–51.

12. Schriger DL, Larmon B, LeGassick T, Blinman T. Spinal immobilization on a flat backboard: does it result in neutral position of the cervical spine? *Ann Emerg Med*. Aug 1991;20(8):878–881.

13. Ditunno JF, et al. Spinal shock revisited: a four phase model. *Spinal Cord*. 2004;42:383–395.

CHAPTER 5

THORACIC TRAUMA

KEY CONCEPTS:

Upon completion of this chapter, it is expected that the reader will understand these following concepts:

- The different mechanisms in blunt and penetrating injuries
- The pathophysiology associated with thoracic trauma injuries
- Using mechanism and patient presentation to identify the leading diagnoses in thoracic blunt and penetrating injuries
- Initiating the proper treatment protocol for each symptom complex
- Transferring patient care to the appropriate facility or transport unit

ANATOMY CONCEPTS:

Prior to reading this chapter the Paramedic student should be familiar with the following anatomy and physiology concepts:

- Thoracic anatomy
- Pulmonary physiology
- Cardiovascular anatomy

CASE STUDY:

The two Paramedics assigned to the ALS ambulance are dispatched to a report of a car accident. Arriving on-scene first, they encounter a 34-year-old male driver who is conscious, alert, and oriented with a chief complaint of chest pain and dyspnea. It appears that his car "submarined" under a pickup truck and the bumper of the pickup truck is in the car's windshield. The Paramedics note that the windshield has heavy damage, the airbag did not deploy, and the patient is pinned behind the steering wheel. Fire department heavy rescue is in the process of establishing extrication.

CRITICAL THINKING QUESTIONS

1. What are some of the possible causes of chest trauma?
2. How is trouble breathing related to chest trauma?

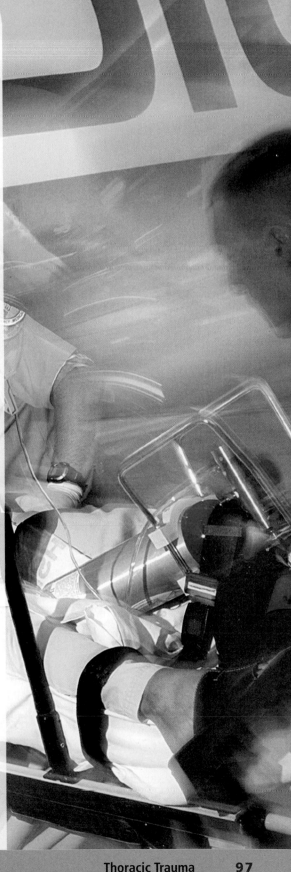

OVERVIEW

Approximately 100,000 Americans die from traumatic injuries each year, and thoracic injuries account for nearly 25% of these trauma deaths.[1] More men and women ages 1 to 44 will die from traumatic injuries than from any other cause. Thoracic injuries also account for lengthy hospital stays and long-term disabilities. Every Paramedic working in EMS is faced with providing care to trauma patients on a regular basis. For the Paramedic, early recognition, appropriate treatment, and transport to the proper receiving facility will improve patient morbidity and survival. This chapter will provide the basis for identifying thoracic trauma injuries and initiating a treatment plan.

Chief Concern

When assessing a patient for the presence of chest injury, the Paramedic starts with the mechanism of injury. Mechanism of injury, and an understanding of kinematics, guides the Paramedic in making potential diagnoses and developing treatment plans. The mechanism provides information about the pattern and force leading to patient injury. In the trauma patient, mechanism of injury is divided into two categories: blunt and penetrating.

Mechanism of Injury for Blunt Trauma

Any outside force that impacts the body across a large area can lead to a blunt traumatic injury. Injuries from blunt trauma are due to transmission of energy rather than transmission of an object. This characteristic defines the difference between blunt and penetrating trauma.

Blunt injury is usually the result of motor vehicle accidents, falls, and assaults. In the case of a motor vehicle accident, airbag deployment, seat belt usage, damage to the car, ejection, cab intrusion, and the patient's location in the car can all influence the forces applied to a patient and the resulting pattern of injury. Airbags and seat belts prevent serious injury in an automobile accident by stopping ejection and preventing impact with the steering wheel. Although these safety devices prevent many injuries, airbag impact on the chest or the force of the body against a seat belt may lead to blunt thoracic injury. In addition, chemical burns on the patient's body from airbag deployment or bruises from a seat belt are signs of potential injury. The patient's location and extent of damage to the car also lead the Paramedic to a high index of suspicion of underlying patient injury. This is especially so if intrusion is noted where the patient was seated or if damage to the car is primarily on the patient's side.

When examining a patient suffering from a fall, the Paramedic should determine the height of the fall, the landing surface, and the point of impact on the patient's body. A patient that has fallen a short distance and lands on a soft surface will likely have a less severe injury than a patient who falls multiple stories and lands on concrete. Remember, however, that elderly individuals who suffer falls, even from a standing position, may have more severe injuries than normally expected (this topic is discussed later in the chapter).

The point of impact is important because forces can be transmitted through the body, leading to indirect injury. For example, although a patient may land on his or her feet, the force involved from a high level fall may cause injury to the cervical spine as the injury is transmitted along the length of the spine.

Specific Traumatic Thoracic Injury

Thoracic trauma can cause injury to the organs and structures within the thoracic cavity including bone, lung, heart and vessels, diaphragm, and esophagus. This section will present the pathophysiology, morbidity and mortality, and mechanism of injury most commonly associated with each category.

Rib Fractures

The thoracic cavity is enclosed both anterior and posterior by bones. The clavicle extends laterally from the sternum and connects to the humerus and scapula. The first seven ribs extend from the spine, attach via individual costal cartilage to the sternum, and are called the "true" ribs. The next three ribs attach to the sternum via the seventh costal cartilage. The last two ribs are known as "floating ribs" and extend posterior from the spine. The ribs that do not attach to the sternum are called the "false" ribs. True ribs cover and protect the lungs, whereas false ribs protect and cover the core organs, liver, spleen, and kidneys.

Ribs four through nine are most commonly fractured from blunt force because of their exposed location (an area known as the center of mass). Underlying organ injuries that may be life-threatening may also be present where rib fractures are found. The Paramedic should suspect lung parenchyma injuries (parenchyma are the essential tissues of an organ) in upper or true rib injuries and abdominal organ injuries (i.e., liver, kidneys, and spleen) in lower or false rib fractures.

Multiple rib fractures leading to separation of one segment of the chest is known as a flail chest. **Flail chest** is defined as at least two ribs broken in two or more places that, more importantly, demonstrate paradoxical movement. When inhalation occurs, the chest wall cavity normally expands to accommodate the increased lung volume. However, the flail chest segment is unable to expand adequately, leading to the **paradoxical motion** (motion opposite the rest of the rib cage) (Figure 5-1).

This paradoxical motion alters the mechanics of breathing. Without the integrity of the chest wall, the thoracic cage is unable to create the negative force required to expand the lungs in the affected area. If the chest wall defect is large enough, systemic hypoxia will occur.

The motion may be subtle or absent even with multiple rib fractures because of the stability provided by muscles and other ribs. Paradoxical motion will also not be evident in obese individuals due to the presence of adipose tissue. Flail chest injuries are not common but are seen with widespread blunt force. This type of injury mostly occurs in motor vehicle crashes but may also be seen in falls from heights and assaults. Of 50,000 trauma patients, only about 75 will be diagnosed with flail chest. Of those with flail chest injuries, 20% to 40% die due to associated injuries.

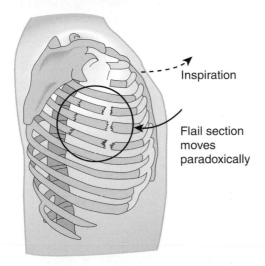

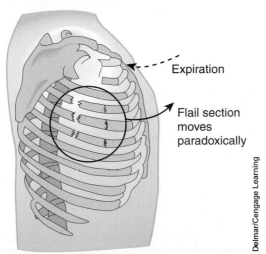

Figure 5-1 Paradoxical motion from flail chest injury alters the mechanics of breathing.

Delmar/Cengage Learning

Other bones of the thoracic cage may also be fractured in a blunt injury to the chest. Sternal fractures require a significant force and may also be indicative of underlying injury, specifically to the heart. The xiphoid process, the inferior pointed end of the sternum, may be fractured and can penetrate the liver. Scapular fractures also require much force; when they are suspected, the Paramedic should consider underlying organ injury. The clavicle is the last thoracic bone that may be injured in traumatic situations. Clavicular fractures are most commonly seen after falls onto a shoulder. The clavicle is easily fractured; however, underlying injury may be present in a high-velocity fall or impact.

Bone injuries in children and the elderly require special consideration. Most bones develop from a cartilage template. This cartilage is gradually replaced by bone throughout childhood development. Bones in young children tend to be "softer" than in adults because this development is still occurring. In pediatric thoracic trauma, a child could have underlying organ damage without necessarily having rib injury because the softer bones are able to absorb more energy after a blunt injury.

Osteoporosis affects about 10 million Americans a year, with women about four times more likely than men to be affected. Although people of any age can be affected, osteoporosis is most commonly observed in the elderly. In patients with osteoporosis, bone mass and structure deteriorate, making these individuals more prone to fractures. In an elderly individual with osteoporosis, a fall from standing position has a higher probability of leading to thoracic bone fractures.

STREET SMART

The presence of a pediatric rib fracture should cause the Paramedic to suspect a significant mechanism of injury with a potentially life-threatening underlying injury to the internal organs. It is very difficult to fracture a child's ribs.

Pulmonary Injuries

Lung injuries occur after both blunt and penetrating injuries. Penetrating injuries cause lung collapse from the accumulation of air (a simple pneumothorax) or blood (a **hemothorax**) in the pleural cavity (the potential space between the covering of the lung and the chest wall). Pulmonary contusions and tracheal injuries also occur with blunt or penetrating injuries. A simple pneumothorax can either be closed, in which air collects in the pleural space and creates a tension pneumothorax (described shortly), or it can be an **open pneumothorax**, in which case the air escapes through an open wound upon exhalation.

Between 10% and 30% of blunt trauma patients will have some form of pneumothorax: a simple pneumothorax, a hemothorax, or a combination called a hemopneumothorax.

A **simple pneumothorax** is a collection of air between the lung and the chest wall that causes the lung on the injured side to collapse. With a simple pneumothorax, the air is trapped in the pleural space.

A **tension pneumothorax** arises when air enters the lung and escapes into the pleural cavity through the damaged section and compresses the heart, lung, and great vessels. The air accumulates in the chest wall and increases pressure in the chest cavity, causing mediastinal and tracheal shifts in severe cases. Until the pressure builds enough to compromise hemodynamics, the pneumothorax is considered a simple pneumothorax. When the great vessels and the heart are compressed, causing the blood pressure to drop, then a simple pneumothorax becomes a tension pneumothorax. Essentially, a tension pneumothorax is a simple pneumothorax with hypotension.

Open pneumothorax, sometimes called a **sucking chest wound** because of the sound that the air makes, occurs when a penetrating injury causes a wound that communicates with the pleural cavity and the outside air. Air enters through the injury but is then able to escape through the same wounds during exhalation. If air cannot exit the chest wall through the communicating wound, a tension pneumothorax may also develop. Death due to pneumothorax is usually the result of delayed treatment. Therefore, any patient who presents with signs and symptoms suggestive of pneumothorax should be promptly evaluated and treated.

A **pulmonary contusion** is an injury to the lung itself and is the most common injury in blunt thoracic trauma. There are three impacts of trauma to the lungs themselves (Figure 5-2): swelling, bleeding, and atelectasis. Atelectasis results from lack of ventilation as well as swelling and bleeding into the alveoli. Fluid accumulates in the injured alveoli and blocks oxygen exchange. Blood is shunted away from the blocked alveoli, leading to hypoxemia. Because these injuries are so common, they should be suspected in any patient with a chest wall injury from blunt forces. Pulmonary contusions have a mortality rate of 14% to 20% because other injuries are often associated. Some patients with a pulmonary contusion may go on to develop acute respiratory distress syndrome (ARDS). ARDS is a life-threatening inflammatory reaction in which the alveoli collapse, shunting occurs, and life-threatening hypoxia progresses to shock.[2]

Vascular Injuries

Blunt injuries can also damage the heart and the vessels in the thorax. Most of these structures are located in the mediastinum. This region is in the medial chest between the two lungs and is composed of the heart, trachea, major vessels, nerves, esophagus, and thymus.

The aorta is the artery that supplies blood to most of the body. This artery extends from the left ventricle and is filled with oxygenated blood. The aortic arch begins behind the cartilage of the second rib and extends into the superior

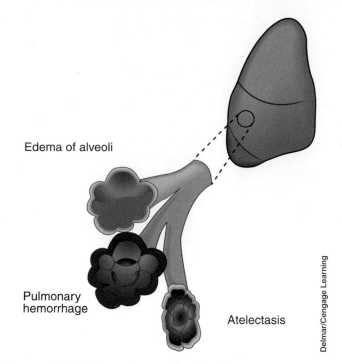

Edema of alveoli

Pulmonary hemorrhage

Atelectasis

Delmar/Cengage Learning

Figure 5-2 Three impacts of pulmonary contusion affect the lungs: swelling, bleeding, and atelectasis.

mediastinum. The arch gives off branches (brachiocephalic trunk, left carotid, and left subclavian) that provide oxygenated blood to the head and arms. The aorta then proceeds inferiorly to supply oxygen to the rest of the body.

Traumatic aortic disruptions are typically seen in rapid deceleration injuries. A speed gradient is established across the arch that pulls on the ligamentum arteriosum, the remnants of fetal circulation, which leads to shearing of the vessel. Between 85% and 95% of these patents die instantaneously.

STREET SMART

The recurrent or inferior laryngeal nerve lies proximal to the ligamentum arteriosum and the aorta. When the ligamentum arteriosum is stretched, the patient may experience a hoarse voice. The Paramedic should suspect injury to the aorta when hoarseness accompanies severe thoracic trauma.

The superior and inferior vena cava (SVC and IVC) drain deoxygenated blood from the body back to the heart. The superior vena cava is formed from the left and right brachiocephalic veins (also known as innominate veins, which drain the head, neck, and arms) and the azygos (which drains the rib cage). The SVC is usually ruptured by penetrating trauma but may also be ruptured by deceleration forces. After a rupture, blood accumulates in the thoracic cavity, leading to exsanguinations and a hemothorax.

The inferior vena cava is formed from the common iliac veins and runs along the right side of the abdominal aorta. Abdominal injuries to this structure will be discussed in Chapter 6; however, because the inferior vena cava also empties deoxygenated blood into the right atrium, it may be injured in the thoracic cavity. Like the aortic rupture, injuries to the superior and inferior vena cava are usually lethal.

Two pulmonary arteries originate from the right ventricle and carry deoxygenated blood to the lungs. Like aortic and vena cava ruptures, if the pulmonary arteries are ruptured, patients may bleed intrathoracically. This bleeding may lead to a hemothorax. Pulmonary veins return oxygenated blood from the lungs to the left atrium of the heart. Two pulmonary veins from each lung return to the left atrium, for a total of four veins returning to the heart. Injuries to the pulmonary veins also bleed into the mediastinum and deprive the heart and systemic circulation of oxygenated blood, leading to profound systemic hypoxia.

Cardiac Injuries

The heart is about the size of a fist and weighs approximately 250 g. The center of the heart is located about 1.5 cm to the left of midline. The apex of the heart is located left of center, between the fifth and sixth ribs, and the superior portion of the heart can extend as high as the second costal cartilage.

Blunt cardiac injuries cause direct structural damage to the heart in the forms of myocardial contusion and rupture. A **myocardial contusion** is a bruising of the heart muscle that can lead to a period of abnormal heart contraction. The most common cause of such an injury is blunt force trauma such as a fall, motor vehicle accident, or cardiopulmonary resuscitation. Patients will usually recover from contusions, although some progress to myocardial infarction over the injured area of muscle. The right ventricle is the most anterior heart chamber behind the sternum and is most likely to be injured in an anterior impact.[3]

A **myocardial rupture** can have a delayed occurrence after a contusion or it can occur immediately after direct blunt impact. The heart ruptures after a rapid deceleration when it may be displaced rapidly into the sternum or the spine. Mortality rates for this injury are high, so early recognition is imperative to patient survival. The heart muscle (myocardium) or the septum wall may be sheared, leading to shunting and a rapid deterioration of the patient. For patients who arrive at the hospital alive, the most commonly affected chamber is the right atrium.

Although myocardial rupture in blunt trauma may or may not involve the pericardium, myocardial rupture in penetrating trauma always involves the pericardium. This may lead to the comorbid conditions cardiac tamponade (discussed shortly) or intrathoracic hemorrhage.[4]

Special Case of Commotio Cordis

Commotio cordis (Latin for commotion of the heart) is a type of sudden cardiac death that involves disruption of the contraction cycle without structural damage. This event is most often observed in young athletes who experience a direct blunt injury to the anterior chest, such as a collision with a baseball or other projectile. Commotio cordis is a rare event because the blunt impact must occur at the correct location on the chest and at the correct time in the heart's depolarization/repolarization cycle (ascending phase of the T wave or the relative refractory period) (Figure 5-3). If these conditions are met, the heart goes into ventricular fibrillation. Save rates for patients with this type of injury are low unless automatic external defibrillators and individuals trained in CPR are on hand at the sporting event.[5]

Diaphragmatic Injuries

The diaphragm is a muscle that extends across the bottom of the rib cage and separates the lungs and heart from the abdominal cavity. During inspiration, the diaphragm contracts inferiorly to increase the volume of the thoracic cavity and reduce the intrathoracic pressure. Air can then move from external higher to internal lower pressure. The liver sits underneath the diaphragm on the right side and the spleen is under the diaphragm on the left. There are several natural openings in the diaphragm that allow for the passage of the aorta, esophagus, and inferior vena cava.

Injuries to the diaphragm are difficult to diagnose in the field. However, the identification of certain injury patterns will allow the Paramedic to suspect diaphragmatic injury.[6] Diaphragmatic injuries are often secondary to lower rib fractures and are the result of blunt and penetrating injuries. Most blunt diaphragmatic injuries occur after motor vehicle accidents, whereas most penetrating diaphragmatic injuries occur after gunshot wounds. Left-sided diaphragmatic injuries from

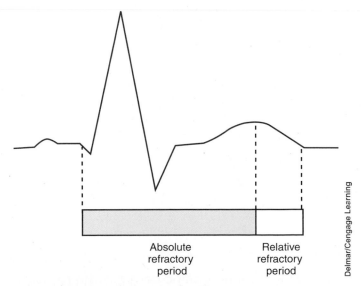

Figure 5-3 Relative refractory period refers to the ascending phase of the T wave.

blunt force trauma most often present to the hospital. Right-sided diaphragmatic injuries tend to be more severe[7] because the liver protects the diaphragm on the right side and more force is required to cause injury.

Diaphragmatic Rupture

Diaphragmatic rupture (i.e., **diaphragmatic herniation**) is the result of the abdominal contents being forced upward into the thoracic cavity. The vast majority of diaphragmatic ruptures, some 80% to 90%, occur in motor vehicle collisions. Lateral side impacts have been specifically implicated. The sideward forces against the false ribs create an upward pressure that shears the ipsilateral diaphragm and forces abdominal contents into the thoracic cavity. One study of diaphragmatic rupture found the left side to be the most commonly affected side.[8] Diaphragmatic rupture can also occur with penetrating knife wounds, particularly upward-thrusting knife attacks. Injuries often associated with diaphragmatic rupture include pelvic fracture (40%) and splenic and liver laceration in about 25% of cases (Figure 5-4).[9]

Traumatic Asphyxia

Traumatic asphyxia is a rare condition that occurs when a massive crushing force causes trauma. This occurs in events such as a landslide or when a vehicle falls off of a jack and onto the patient's chest. First described over 150 years ago by Olivier when he witnessed a stampede in a Paris crowd during an event, traumatic asphyxia is more of a curiosity than it is a potential life-threatening injury. Other associated thoracic traumas tend to be more life-threatening than traumatic asphyxia.

Mechanism of Injury for Penetrating Trauma

Penetrating trauma is typically created by a projectile from a firearm (such as a gunshot wound), shrapnel from a bomb, or a stabbing injury. When examining a patient with a gunshot wound, the Paramedic should determine the type of weapon, caliber or diameter of the firearm chamber, distance from the patient the weapon was fired, number of bullets fired, and entrance and exit wounds. Different types of firearms have different injury patterns. Handgun injuries have a defined bullet path with bone, bullet fragments, and hemorrhage. In most types of handgun injuries, the trajectory is more important than the size or speed of the bullet[10] because as the bullet moves through tissue, it transfers energy in a perpendicular manner to the path of the projectile. This creates both a permanent and a temporary cavity. The temporary cavity, the result of tissue recoil, can be 10 times larger than the permanent cavity.

The Paramedic must identify all entrance and exit wounds on the patient. Bear in mind that these sites may not provide conclusive information about underlying injuries because bullets have rotational forces and do not have to travel in a linear fashion. The bullet may also travel through distant parts of the body, depending on the bullet's trajectory, so a patient shot in the arm may have a penetrating thoracic injury.

Shotguns produce different injury patterns than bullets due to the presence of pellets within a shell, with the exception of the shotgun slug. A shotgun fired at close range will lead to one single, large penetrating wound, whereas a shotgun fired at medium range will lead to deep penetrating pellets throughout the body. In contrast, a long-range shotgun assault victim may have many shotgun pellets, some that only penetrate skin deep.

Stab wounds from sharp objects (e.g., knives, ice picks, and arrows) are considered low velocity wounds, and thus create less tissue damage than a GSW. When examining a patient who has been stabbed, the Paramedic should consider the motion of the stabbing and the length and style of blade. The directional motion of the stabbing leads the Paramedic to suspect additional injuries that may not be obvious from looking at surface wounds. An upward stabbing motion causing an abdominal wound may also penetrate the diaphragm. Longer blades also increase the probability of organ injuries and internal bleeding.

Assaults and blast injuries cause both penetrating and blunt injury. Weapons used in assaults can cause either type of injury. A knife or firearm injury causes penetrating injury, whereas assault with a baseball bat will cause blunt injury.

Diaphragmatic Hernia

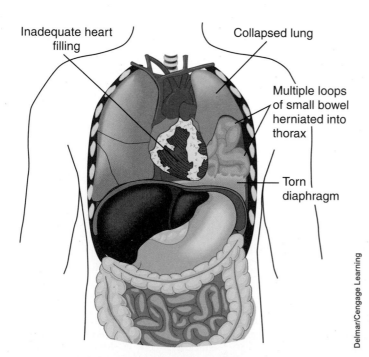

Inadequate heart filling

Collapsed lung

Multiple loops of small bowel herniated into thorax

Torn diaphragm

Delmar/Cengage Learning

Figure 5-4 Diaphragmatic hernia is the result of the abdominal contents being forced upward into the thoracic cavity.

Additional blunt injury may also be caused from a fall after the initial assault.

Blast injuries require special considerations from the EMS provider. Explosion scenes, both intentional and unintentional, can be overwhelming to EMS personnel, so an understanding of the injuries caused by such events will help the Paramedic with triage. Blast injuries from bomb explosions present with a combination of blunt and penetrating injuries. When a device explodes, it creates pressure waves that emanate away from the initial explosion, leading to a blunt injury. This wave transfers energy throughout the body and causes shearing forces that damage internal organs. Although an external injury may not be visible, underlying injuries will be present. Blunt injuries may also be caused if the forces are great enough to throw the patient away from the device. Penetrating injuries are caused from the shrapnel associated with explosions. The shrapnel acts like a projectile, leading to internal injury.

Penetrating Pulmonary Injuries

The trachea and bronchi may be damaged by a penetrating injury. These injuries are rare (less than 3% of all penetrating trauma) but have a high mortality (around 30%). The trachea is composed primarily of cartilage and originates from the larynx. It extends down the neck and into the thoracic cavity where it bifurcates in the mediastinum at the angle of the sternum to form the right and left bronchi. Injuries to the trachea or bronchi, called **tracheobronchial disruption**, can cause a pneumothorax, simple or tension, from air leaking into the chest cavity. An injury to this region can also lead to asphyxia if air is no longer able to pass into the lungs.

A hemothorax is an accumulation of blood from broken vessels in the pleural cavity most commonly caused by a penetrating mechanism. Because a hemothorax is a bleed in the chest that leads to lung collapse, there are both respiratory and hemodynamic consequences that can cause respiratory difficulty, shock, and death. Among those with a great vessel (brachiocephalic veins, common carotid artery, right brachiocephalic artery, left subclavian artery) injury that leads to a hemothorax, 50% will die immediately and another 25% will die in the 5 to 10 minutes immediately after suffering a hemothorax.

A **hemopneumothorax** is an accumulation of air and blood in the pleural cavity leading to lung collapse. The presence of blood and air in the pleural cavity leads to an increase in intrathoracic pressure. A penetrating injury is the most common cause of a hemopneumothorax. A stab wound to the chest, for example, could lead to leaking of air from the injured lung and blood from the damaged blood vessels that the knife cut as it passed into the chest.

Penetrating Cardiovascular Injuries

The outer layer of the heart is known as the epicardium, and the pericardium is a fibrous covering that encases the heart. A potential space exists between the epicardium and the pericardium. This space is normally empty but may become filled with blood or fluid after an injury, leading to a condition called **cardiac tamponade**. Since the pericardium encasing this sac is fibrous, it does not stretch. The accumulation of fluid (as much as 1,000 to 1,500 mL chronically, but as little as 150 mL acutely) does not allow the heart to refill with blood after a contraction because the heart chambers cannot dilate in the compressed space. Cardiac tamponade is seen in penetrating trauma more than blunt trauma.[11]

Esophageal Injuries

The esophagus is situated behind the trachea and runs in the posterior mediastinum. Most esophageal injuries are due to penetrating injury. However, damage to the esophagus will not cause immediate life-threatening injury like injuries to other mediastinal structures. The Paramedic should consider management of injuries to the trachea, heart, and vessels before addressing potential esophageal injury.

CASE STUDY (CONTINUED)

The car was traveling at 65 mph when the vehicle in front suddenly stopped. The patient applied the car's brakes but hit the car in front of him. The Paramedics notice no airbag deployment and major damage to the front of the vehicle. The patient denies loss of consciousness but relates he has severe chest pain and trouble breathing; "I can't seem to catch my breath!"

The Paramedics choose to be conservative with their questions. The patient appears to be a relatively healthy young man in good physical condition, so they quickly run down the SAMPLE mnemonic.

CRITICAL THINKING QUESTIONS

1. What are the important elements of the history that a Paramedic should obtain?
2. What is the symptom pattern for tension pneumothorax?

History

The Paramedic should always attempt to obtain a complete history for a trauma patient. As part of that history, she should determine allergies, past medical history, and medications taken. In the unconscious patient, family, friends, and medical alert bracelets provide some history for the patient. Important past medical history includes the presence of a pacemaker, an automatic internal cardiac defibrillator (AICD), and previous surgeries. Knowledge of the patient's recent procedures provides the Paramedic with insight into potential injuries. For example, a fall from standing position after some surgeries may lead to thoracic injury. Coronary artery bypass grafting (CABG) is a procedure performed when coronary arteries are blocked, jeopardizing blood flow to the heart. Arteries and veins from other regions of the body are taken and used to reroute blood around the occluded portion of the coronary artery. In order to perform this procedure, the sternum must be split. When the operation is completed, the sternum is wired back together. If the patient suffers a fall, the sternum may become separated and cardiac or pulmonary injury may result.

A medication list is important to obtain, especially in elderly patients because most are on multiple medications. For example, warfarin (Coumadin®) and clopidogrel (Plavix®) prevent clotting by inhibiting the production of clotting factors. If an injury occurs to an individual on Coumadin® or Plavix®, that patient will have impaired clotting capabilities, making it difficult to stop the bleeding. This can lead to severe blood loss when injuries occur. Psychotropic medications—such as Zoloft® for depression and anxiety, cardiac medications such as Norvasc® for hypertension, Vasotec® for high blood pressure, Procardia® for angina and hypertension, and a list of analgesic medications—are associated with falling in the elderly, which can lead to blunt injury.

CASE STUDY (CONTINUED)

The patient was not wearing his seat belt and the steering wheel has been pushed back into his chest. The Paramedics immediately expect some type of blunt injury and proceed with the assessment. The Paramedic begins the examination by speaking with the patient in order to assess his airway while his partner takes a set of vitals. The patient has an oxygen saturation of 82% on outside air, blood pressure of 130/90, pulse rate of 96, and respiration rate of 28, shallow and labored. The patient is able to speak but is having difficulty catching his breath to complete sentences. A firefighter starts to apply oxygen, but this does not seem to relieve the patient's respiratory distress.

CRITICAL THINKING QUESTIONS

1. What are the elements of the physical examination of a patient with chest trauma?
2. Why is auscultation a critical element in this examination?

Examination

The physical exam begins with evaluation of the patient's airway after assessing the level of consciousness. The Paramedic can easily assess an intact airway if the patient is awake and talking. If the patient has an altered level of consciousness or is unconscious, however, the Paramedic should ensure that the airway is patent and protected before proceeding with the rest of the assessment. After the airway is opened and secure, she can proceed through the rest of the exam.

The patient's breathing is examined next. The Paramedic auscultates lung sounds to ensure that they are present and equal bilaterally. Absence of breath sounds on one or both sides indicates a hemothorax or pneumothorax. The Paramedic assesses breathing rate and quality in the conscious patient by listening to the patient speak. A patient with dyspnea or tachypnea may have a bone, cardiac, or pulmonary injury. After listening to the patient speak and assessing lung sounds, the Paramedic palpates and inspects the chest. Subcutaneous emphysema occurs when air leaks into surrounding tissues. It indicates a pneumothorax or tracheal injury and feels like crepitus when palpating the chest. Jugular vein distention (JVD) is a visible sign of an increase in intrathoracic pressure. One cause of this increase in pressure is a pneumothorax. Tracheal deviation is only seen in severe cases of tension pneumothorax. Pressure increases from trapped air and pushes the mediastinum in the opposite direction of the collapsed lung.

The Paramedic must identify and address any gross bleeding. This bleeding may be visible on the street or may be internal. Any patient has the potential to internally bleed into the chest, head, abdomen, or joints. Penetrating injuries may damage internal organs, which may subsequently bleed. The Paramedic should address both visible and internal bleeding before continuing with the exam.

If the patient is responsive, the Paramedic should assess neurological status for level of consciousness and intact motor and sensation in all four extremities. In the thoracic trauma patient, damage to the brachial plexus leads to weakness and loss of sensation in the patient's arm. The neurological exam is discussed in depth in Chapter 4.

After completing the initial assessment steps listed previously, the Paramedic should proceed to the secondary assessment. This assessment may not be completed until after the patient is immobilized and placed in the ambulance. The patient is thoroughly examined from head to toe so that subtle injuries are not missed. The Paramedic obtains vital signs and takes blood pressures in both arms if aortic rupture is suspected. Cardiac monitoring is another important component of the secondary assessment and provides information about potential cardiac injury. The secondary assessment should be repeated, time permitting.

Thoracic Cage Trauma

Patients with rib fractures will have pain when taking deep breaths, bruising, and a deformity over the affected area. Severe rib injuries present as a flail chest with paradoxical motion. A first or second rib fracture is indicative of an injury with significant force and may also indicate injuries to the aorta or trachea. Lower left rib fractures may cause an underlying splenic injury, and rib fractures on the right may indicate a liver laceration; these injuries will be presented in more detail in Chapter 6. Patients who previously had rib fractures but returned home may develop complications that the Paramedic will be called to handle. These complications may include atelectasis and pneumonia. Atelectasis, or a collapsed lung from the loss of alveoli, occurs when the patient does not take deep breaths. Patients who do not adequately take deep breaths and who do not cough are also at increased risk of pneumonia because of decreased clearing of bacteria.

Sternal fractures, although rare, do occur in accidents involving significant force. Pain and bruising will be the primary findings in a patient with a sternal fracture. Complete sternal fractures, sometimes called **floating sternum**, will have paradoxical motion. Forces that cause fractures over the body of the sternum also lead to myocardial injury, especially to the right ventricle and specifically to the right atrium; the right heart is responsible for preload.

The clavicle requires little force to break. Fractures usually occur in the middle and distal third of the clavicle and a deformity may be visible, often described as a "handlebar" fracture due to its shape. Since arteries and nerves may be damaged if the clavicle is injured, the Paramedic must assess for the presence of bleeding and neurological deficits. The subclavian artery runs under the clavicle. If the clavicle is fractured, the subclavian artery may also be damaged, leading to bleeding into the thoracic cavity. Damage to the subclavian artery is assessed by looking for a hematoma near the clavicle or noting a diminished or absent radial pulse on the affected side. The radial pulse is decreased because the subclavian artery ultimately terminates as the radial artery. Nerves also pass under the clavicle. The brachial plexus is a group of nerves that control movement and sensation from the proximal arm to the fingers. Determining sensory and motion deficits helps the Paramedic assess for nerve injuries.

Scapular fractures present with pain when moving the arm on the affected side. Pain, swelling, and bruising will be present over the fracture. These injuries require significant force, and patients with them tend to have underlying thoracic injuries. Before focusing on the scapular injury, the Paramedic should rule out life-threatening thoracic injuries.

Cardiopulmonary Trauma

A tension pneumothorax has a variety of signs and symptoms. The patient will have dyspnea and diminished or absent breath sounds of the affected side. Less commonly, JVD and tracheal deviation toward the unaffected side will be present. Other systemic findings include tachycardia; pale, cool, and clammy skin; and hypotension. Subcutaneous emphysema may also be felt on chest palpation because air is able to enter tissues under the skin after the injury.

The presence of an open pneumothorax is suspected on physical exam with the presence of an open chest wound. The term "sucking chest wound" is used to describe this injury because air is heard entering and exiting through the communicating wound. Patients with an open pneumothorax will also have dyspnea and decreased breath sounds on the affected side. Since air can escape through the communicating wound, a tension pneumothorax and tracheal deviation will only develop if the injury is completely sealed.

Pulmonary contusions lead to impaired oxygen exchange and may eventually cause respiratory failure. Patients with pulmonary contusions will present with crackles upon auscultation and low oxygen saturation. Patients with a pulmonary contusion are at increased risk for ARDS approximately 24 hours after the injury occurs. Individuals with this condition have decreased oxygen saturation, signs of shock, and respiratory acidosis. A patient who has recently suffered a traumatic injury but did not seek medical attention at the time may call EMS with acute worsening respiratory distress. Obtaining a thorough history is helpful in recognizing ARDS.

Commotio cordis is a rare condition but does occur in young athletes. This condition can be diagnosed through mechanism of injury, usually a blunt blow to the chest, and the observation of ventricular fibrillation on a cardiac monitor. When responding to an athletic event with an unresponsive patient, the Paramedic should consider commotio cordis as a possible issue. The patient will be found apneic, unresponsive, and pulseless. Bruising may be noted over the anterior chest with or without sternal or rib injury.

The two categories of blunt cardiac injury are contusion and cardiac rupture. Patients with myocardial contusions present with pain and bruising over the sternum and may have a dysrhythmia. However, the dysrhythmia may not be present on ambulance arrival if the injury is minor. Patients with myocardial rupture have a high mortality rate, so they may be found in cardiac arrest on-scene. If not in arrest, these patients will present with bruising, chest pain, dysrhythmias, hypotension, and shock.

Cardiac rupture is more commonly the result of a GSW to the heart, although a weakened ventricular wall (e.g., post-myocardial infarction) can rupture if struck with a severe blunt force. Cardiac tamponade can rapidly develop from cardiac rupture.

Aortic disruptions are often fatal because most patients exsanguinate (bleed out) at the scene. Some patients who survive the initial aortic rupture may have no other external injuries or symptoms, whereas others will present with pain in the neck and chest, scapular fractures, first or second rib fractures, sternal fractures, and steering wheel marks on their chests. Hypertension, hypotension, blood pressure differentials in the upper extremities, and loss of upper extremity pulses are exam findings that indicate aortic disruption.

Hypertension occurs as the body attempts to compensate for the decreased blood flow to the majority of the body. Hypotension is a late finding that occurs when the heart can no longer compensate. If the tear occurs between the brachiocephalic and left common carotid arteries, the patient will have a higher blood pressure in the right arm than in the left arm. The patient will also have a stronger pulse in the right arm. In the hospital, treatment of these injuries includes administration of beta blockers to decrease intra-aortic pressure. After repairing any other life-threatening emergencies, the physician then addresses aortic rupture.

Superior vena cava injuries are also often fatal. Those patients that do survive such an injury will present with chest pain. Upper extremity pulses should still be present until the patient has lost enough blood that inadequate volume remains in the arterial system to circulate to the rest of the body. Patients may present with hypotension and shock, as well as signs and symptoms of a hemothorax from blood loss in the chest. Injuries to the inferior vena cava, pulmonary arteries, and veins will have a similar presentation to those seen in superior vena cava injuries.

Diaphragmatic Rupture

The patient with a suspected diaphragmatic rupture may present with shortness of breath and, in more severe cases, tracheal deviation secondary to a mediastinal shift, as well as the absence of breath sounds on the affected side. A diaphragmatic hernia is often missed; in fact, 10% to 50% of cases of diaphragmatic herniation are missed or misdiagnosed as being a pneumothorax. A telltale sign of diaphragmatic rupture is the presence of bowel sounds in the thoracic cavity above the level of the false ribs.[12]

Patients with a diaphragmatic injury may be symptomatic or have occult injuries that go undiagnosed for months. The Paramedic should suspect a diaphragmatic injury in any patient with a thoracic or abdominal injury. Among diaphragmatic ruptures, 40% are associated with pelvic fractures, 25% with spleen lacerations, 25% with liver lacerations, and 5% to 10% with a thoracic aortic rupture. The most common finding in symptomatic patients is dyspnea.[13]

Patients with a hemothorax will have similar signs and symptoms to those listed for the pneumothorax. They will have decreased breath sounds on the affected side, dyspnea, anxiety, and pain. In addition to the respiratory problems associated with this condition, Paramedics should also keep in mind that the patient is bleeding internally and could develop signs and symptoms of hemorrhagic shock (see the following text).

The signs and symptoms of hemopneumothorax are similar to those seen with pneumothorax and hemothorax. Patients will have difficulty breathing and decreased lung sounds on the affected side. As was the case with the patients with a hemothorax, these patients have respiratory and hemodynamic concerns.

Patients with a rupture of the trachea or bronchi will have difficulty breathing and will cough up secretions or blood. Air escapes through the damaged trachea during inspiration, leading to a pneumothorax and subcutaneous emphysema. Tracheal asphyxia or suffocation occurs if the airway is occluded with fluid or blood. Patients with asphyxia secondary to tracheal trauma will have JVD and appear cyanotic above the neck. If the penetrating injury is midline, expect other mediastinal injuries as well.

Patients with cardiac tamponade will have anxiousness or a "feeling of impending doom." Signs and symptoms of cardiac tamponade include hypotension, JVD (since the heart chambers cannot completely dilate to fill, blood backs up and increases pressure in the neck veins), and muffled heart sounds (fluid muffles the normal sounds); these symptoms making Beck's triad. JVD may not be present if the patient is hypovolemic and heart sounds may be difficult to note in the field, so the mechanism of injury and the exam will provide the Paramedic with a high level of suspicion that the patient has cardiac tamponade. Cardiac monitoring provides additional evidence that a patient may have cardiac tamponade. Possible dysrhythmias include tachycardia, ST elevation, T inversion, right bundle branch block, premature contractions, and atrial fibrillation. Finally, patients with cardiac tamponade may present with a paradoxical pulse (i.e., the pulse becomes weaker as a patient inhales and stronger as a patient exhales). The systolic blood pressure also drops as the patient inhales.

Tension pneumothorax and cardiac tamponade have similar patient presentations, but there are differences between the two. Tension pneumothorax and cardiac tamponade may both be suspected in a patient who has hypotension with no apparent blood loss, JVD, and a significant mechanism of chest trauma. A tension pneumothorax can be differentiated with the absence of breath sounds on one side and tracheal deviation. Patients with cardiac tamponade will have bilateral breath sounds and no tracheal deviation unless they have a comorbid pneumothorax or hemothorax. Those with cardiac tamponade also have a paradoxical pulse.

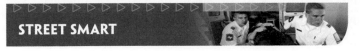
Since the esophagus runs in the midline with the trachea and other mediastinal structures, the Paramedic should evaluate the patient for life-threatening injuries first. Patients with esophageal injuries have difficulty swallowing (dysphagia), hoarseness, respiratory distress, local tenderness, and vomiting. Infections are a consequence of undiagnosed esophageal injury because food and other contents leak into the thoracic cavity. Patients with an infection secondary to esophageal injury will have a history of the previously listed symptoms, previous thoracic trauma, and a fever.

Traumatic Asphyxia

A sudden compressive force that crushes the chest between two surfaces, such as occurs in a building collapse, forces blood rapidly into the upper thoracic area and face. The resulting increased capillary pressures result in capillary rupture. These capillary ruptures produce craniocervical cyanosis, facial edema, and subconjunctival hemorrhage. In one study of 14 cases of traumatic asphyxia, this triad of symptoms was found in 100% of the cases.[14]

Traumatic asphyxia is occasionally associated with loss of hearing, which is thought to be due to edema in the Eustachian tube, and loss of vision due to retinal hemorrhage. Associated injuries, such as head injury and/or pulmonary contusion, are often lethal and should be suspected in cases of traumatic asphyxia.

CASE STUDY (CONTINUED)

The patient is hypotensive and tachycardiac, and the Paramedic notes paradoxical pulses, jugular vein distention, and muffled heart sounds. While the Paramedic waits for his partner to return with the backboard and stretcher, the patient's pulses become weaker. With the findings just presented, the patient appears to have signs consistent with cardiac tamponade.

CRITICAL THINKING QUESTIONS

1. What is the significance of Beck's triad?
2. What are the potential implications of sudden hypotension?

Assessment

The Paramedic should understand how to identify mechanism of injury and form a list of possible field diagnoses based on that mechanism. The Paramedic should also have a foundation for taking a history and examining the trauma patient. Next, potential field diagnoses will be compared to exam findings so that the student can recognize the most likely injury or injuries associated with various symptoms that suggest shock.

The most common cause of shock in the trauma patient is blood loss secondary to hemorrhage. Patients lose blood either externally or internally and no longer have the blood volume to supply the body with oxygenated blood. When assessing a patient with signs and symptoms of shock, the Paramedic should exclude all hemorrhagic causes, both internal and external, before considering other causes of shock. After excluding the possibility of hemorrhagic shock, the Paramedic should consider cardiogenic shock. In thoracic trauma patients, cardiogenic shock is caused because the heart is unable to pump blood either from direct injury (i.e., cardiac contusion) or cardiac tamponade. These patients also present with signs and symptoms of shock because blood volume is not circulated.

With the patient secured to the backboard, the Paramedic elects to withhold further treatment until the patient is in the ambulance and on the way to the trauma center. Once in the ambulance, the Paramedic obtains venous access after assuring continuous high-flow, high-concentration oxygen. The Paramedic elects to try a trial of fluid with the therapeutic goal of keeping a mean arterial pressure of at least 65 mmHg to ensure adequate cerebral perfusion.

CRITICAL THINKING QUESTIONS

1. What is the national standard of care of patients with suspected cardiac tamponade?
2. What are some of the patient-specific concerns and considerations that the Paramedic should consider when applying this plan of care that is intended to treat a broad patient population presenting with suspected cardiac tamponade?

Treatment

The Paramedic's treatment begins with ensuring a patent airway after checking the patient's level of consciousness. If the patient has an altered level of consciousness or is unconscious, the Paramedic must secure the airway before continuing the assessment. Thoracic trauma patients who are conscious and protecting their airway will still benefit from high-flow, high-concentration oxygen via nonrebreather mask while being transported to the hospital. Supplemental oxygen will help patients to remain adequately perfused until they are transferred to definitive care. Some injuries that appear severe do not require intubation if the patient is adequately perfused and protecting his airway. Although a flail chest segment on its own is not an absolute indication to intubate, respiratory rate, volume, and oxygen saturation should all be monitored closely for any changes.

If the patient is not protecting his airway, the Paramedic should perform a jaw-thrust maneuver and provide basic life support; high-flow, high-concentration oxygenation; and ventilation until advanced life support equipment is set up and available. Airway adjuncts such as nasopharyngeal and oropharyngeal airways can be used until intubation equipment is prepared. Patients with a gag reflex will not tolerate the oropharyngeal airway. After advanced airway equipment is prepared, the Paramedic intubates the patient. Remember, the best method for ensuring correct tube placement is to visualize the endotracheal tube passing through the vocal cords. The Paramedic should recheck tube placement by assessing breath sounds, looking for condensation on the tube, and monitoring CO_2 levels. Also, she should listen to epigastric sounds. If endotracheal intubation is unsuccessful, she can utilize rescue airways or bag-valve ventilation until the patient arrives at the hospital. If the patient is not breathing and the Paramedic cannot secure any other airway, either via endotracheal intubation or supraglottic airway, she should perform a cricothyrotomy, provided that this procedure is included in local protocols.[15]

Flail Chest

A flail chest can markedly impact the mechanics of breathing. If the flail segment is small, and the paradoxical motion minimal, the patient may be able to tolerate this alteration in breathing. In those cases, the paradoxical motion of the flail segment is controlled by bulky dressings or even tape (i.e., strapping). However, a sandbag or IV bag should never be used over a flail segment as it may cause further injury.

Patients often do not breathe deeply because of the pain associated with a flail chest. In those cases, and providing the patient is hemodynamically stable, it may be desirable to provide the patient with analgesia rather than positive pressure ventilation. Positive pressure ventilation should be seen as the treatment of last resort. Underlying lung injury, particularly a pneumothorax, can be worsened with positive pressure ventilation; in the case of simple pneumothorax, positive pressure ventilation can create a tension pneumothorax.

However, if the flail segment is large, or it markedly compromises the mechanics of breathing, as seen by a heaving paradoxical motion and profound hypoxia despite administration

▷ ▷ ▷ ▷ ▷ ▷ ▷ ▷ ▷ ▷ ▷ ▷ ▷ ▷

STREET SMART

Some research and protocols suggest the use of continuous positive airway pressure (CPAP) for the treatment of flail chest. CPAP helps with oxygenation while minimizing intrathoracic pressures.

of analgesia and high-flow, high-concentration oxygen, it may be necessary to perform positive pressure ventilation. Positive pressure ventilation creates a type of **internal pneumatic splint**. The effect of the positive pressure is to stop the paradoxical motion of the flail segment while supporting the patient's ventilation.

The use of positive pressure ventilation, via either bag-mask assembly or intubation, is desirable whenever the patient has hypoxia that does not resolve with high-flow, high-concentration oxygen via nonrebreather mask or the patient requires a large amount of narcotic analgesia that subsequently depresses respiration.

CASE STUDY (CONTINUED)

The Paramedic's partner changes the patient from high-flow, high-concentration oxygen through a nonrebreather mask at 15 L/min to a bag-mask assembly. Shortly after making the change, the Paramedic notes that it is harder to ventilate the patient. His partner notes that the patient has lost a radial pulse and that the patient has become unconscious.

CRITICAL THINKING QUESTIONS

1. What are some of the predictable complications associated with simple pneumothorax?
2. What are some of the predictable complications associated with the treatments for a tension pneumothorax?

Evaluation

The Paramedic should repeat the initial and secondary assessment, time permitting. Also, she should reevaluate the patient's stability after any interventions. For example, covering an open pneumothorax with an occlusive dressing may lead to the development of a tension pneumothorax, so the Paramedic should check lung sounds, vital signs, and inspect the neck for any tracheal deviation. A simple pneumothorax, either open or closed, can quickly become a tension pneumothorax.

Tension Pneumothorax

When there is an open pneumothorax, the Paramedic should apply an occlusive dressing and secure the dressing on three sides. The occlusive dressing prevents most air from entering the communicating wound while also allowing air to escape out of the chest cavity through the unsecured fourth edge. If all four sides of the bandage are secured, the patient will be at risk for developing a tension pneumothorax since air may enter the pleural cavity through an injured lung but cannot escape through the communicating injury. If a tension pneumothorax should occur, the Paramedic should release one side of the dressing, called burping the dressing, to see if the tension pneumothorax resolves.

If the tension pneumothorax does not resolve, or the patient has a closed simple pneumothorax that has evolved—either spontaneously or with the help of positive pressure ventilation—into a tension pneumothorax, then the Paramedic will need to perform needle decompression.

A needle decompression, or **needle thoracostomy**, involves placing a needle into the pleural space in order to relieve the built up pressure that is compromising ventilation and circulation.

There are two sites to insert the needle during a needle thoracostomy (Figure 5-5). The preferred site in the prehospital setting is the anterior site. The anterior site permits easy identification of landmarks and ease of monitoring, particularly if the patient is on a long backboard.

To perform a needle decompression at the anterior site, the Paramedic identifies the second intercostal space, at the level of the angle of Louis, and at the midclavicular line. Next, the Paramedic prepares the site with an antiseptic such as iodine-based solution. With the site visualized, the Paramedic places a 14- or 16-gauge needle perpendicular to the plane of the chest and advances the needle up and over the third rib until resistance is lost and a hiss of escaping air is heard. It is important to insert the needle above the rib to avoid the intercostal arteries, part of the neurovascular bundle, that run inferior to the rib.

The alternative site is the lateral site. This site, found at the mid-axillary line (MAL) at the fifth intercostal space (5th ICS), is used when the anterior chest has trauma (obscuring landmarks) or the patient is a child.

The choice of needle is dependent on the patient's size. Males with large pectoral muscles will need longer needles, whereas children will need shorter and smaller needles.

Some Paramedics also will use a prefilled saline syringe on the needle. As the needle is advanced into

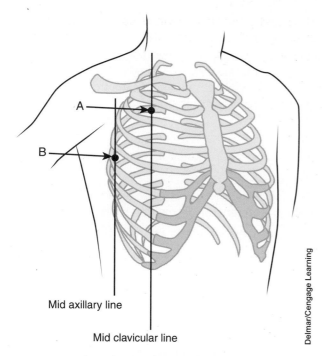

Mid axillary line

Mid clavicular line

Delmar/Cengage Learning

Figure 5-5 Needle thoracostomy sites a Paramedic can use to relieve pressure.

the chest, gentle traction on the plunger of the syringe will cause air bubbles to surface once the pleural space has been entered, which provides a visual confirmation of placement.

Immediately following the insertion of the needle, there should be an immediate relief of symptoms of the tension pneumothorax; for example, a return of radial pulses.

Some Paramedics place a flutter-type valve, in some cases created with the finger of a glove, over the needle. Others use an Ashmann's® valve, instead. These devices permit the escape of air from the chest while preventing the return of air into the chest via the needle. Many Paramedics leave the needle open to air, thereby creating an open pneumothorax from a tension pneumothorax.

It should be noted that an emergency needle decompression is not always successful initially, so it may need to be repeated (needles clog). In addition, it is only a temporary technique, preserving the patient's circulation, until a chest tube can be inserted (**Skill 5-1**).

For a step-by-step demonstration of Needle Thoracostomy, please refer to Skill 5-1 on page(s) 112–113.

CASE STUDY CONCLUSION

The Paramedics quickly examine the patient for any gross bleeding but find no blood. The Paramedics then elect to perform a more detailed assessment in the ambulance on the way to the hospital. The patient is quickly immobilized and transported to the nearest trauma center.

CRITICAL THINKING QUESTIONS

1. What is the most appropriate transport decision that will get the patient to definitive care?

2. What are the advantages of transporting a patient with chest trauma to these hospitals, even if that means bypassing other hospitals in the process?

Disposition

The location of the incident in relationship to receiving facilities will dictate where and how the patient is transported. Patients who have any of the previously listed conditions need to be taken to a trauma center. The exception to this is if the patient is in cardiac arrest. The patient may then be taken to the nearest facility. If resuscitated there, he will be transferred to a trauma center or the resuscitation will be terminated in the field. The transport goal of any trauma patient is to have the patient transported to definitive care as quickly as possible. In order to accomplish this goal, the patient may need to be transported via helicopter. Local protocol will dictate how the trauma patient should be transported.

Paramedics are commonly called upon to transfer a critically ill trauma patient from a community hospital to a

trauma center. Some of these patients have had tube thoracostomies performed, leaving a chest tube in place to drain a hemothorax. Tube thoracostomies also relieve the tension and maintain the reinflation of a lung affected by a tension pneumothorax (Figure 5-6).

During the transport of a patient who has had a tube thoracostomy placed, the Paramedic needs to continually re-evaluate the patient to ensure a tension pneumothorax does not redevelop. The Paramedic must also monitor the equipment and patient to identify and intervene early if complications develop (Table 5-1 and **Skill 5-2**).

For a step-by-step demonstration of Tube Thoracostomy Maintenance, please refer to Skill 5-2 on page 114.

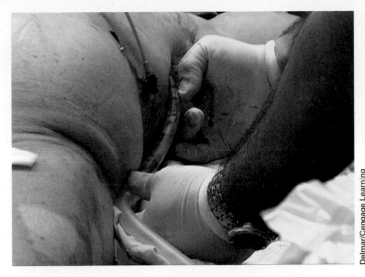

Figure 5-6 Tube thoracostomy allows continual drainage of a hemothorax and expansion of the lung in a pneumothorax.

Delmar/Cengage Learning

Table 5-1 Potential Complications during Transport with a Chest Tube

- Clot in the chest tube inside the patient
- Clot in the patient tube
- Dependent loop in the patient tube full of fluid
- Kink in the patient tube (bedrail, position)
- Partial dislodgement of the tube
- Partial disconnection of the patient tube from the chest tube connector
- Overfilled water seal
- In-line connections not secured
- Patient tube clamp closed
- Chest drain kit not upright
- Chest drain kit not sufficiently below the patient's chest
- Suction pressure below minimum operating pressure
- Disconnected suction tube

Skill 5-1 Needle Thoracostomy

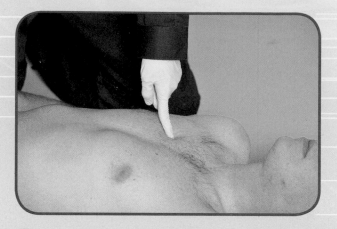

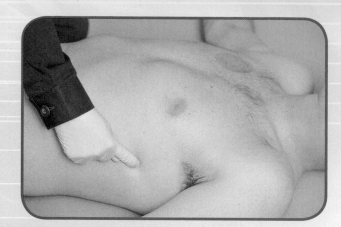

1 Identify landmarks and prep the skin.

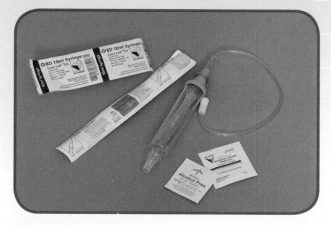

2 Assemble the kit (follow specific manufacturer's recommendations).

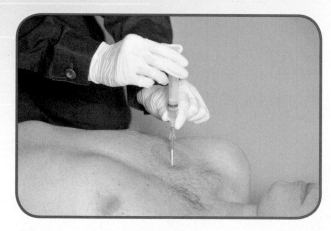

3 Insert the needle at a 90-degree angle to the chest wall until the saline in the syringe bubbles.

Delmar/Cengage Learning

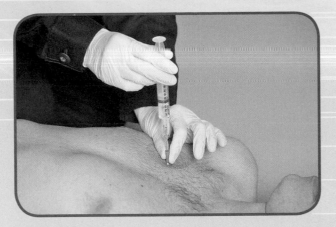

4 Advance the catheter.

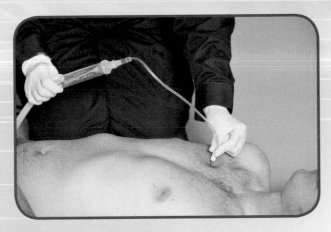

5 Attach the setup to the catheter (with or without suction).

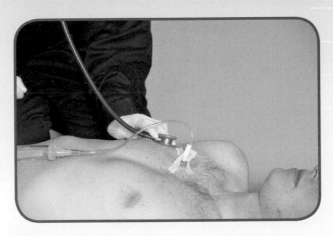

6 Secure the catheter and reassess the patient.

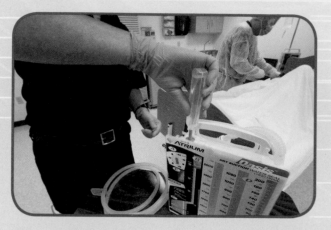

1 While the care provider places a chest tube, set up the chest drainage kit following manufacturer's recommendations.

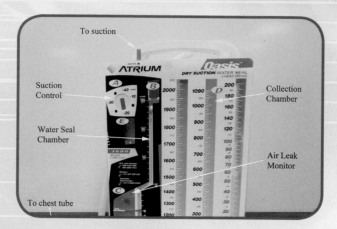

To suction

Suction Control

Water Seal Chamber

To chest tube

Collection Chamber

Air Leak Monitor

2 Anatomy of a typical chest tube drainage kit (see specific manufacturer's documentation).

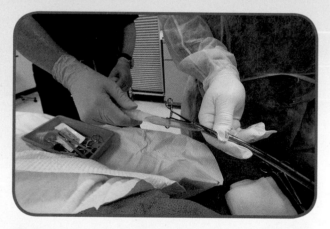

3 Connect tubes from the drain kit to the chest tube (patient tube) and to the suction source (suction tube).

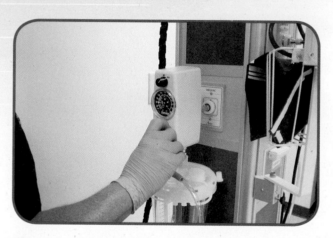

4 Turn the suction on to the appropriate setting.

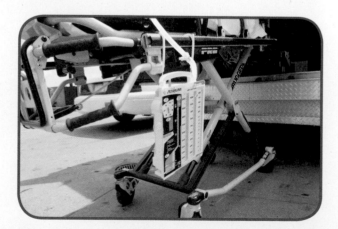

5 Maintain the chest drainage kit in an upright position below the level of the chest during transport.

CONCLUSION

Every Paramedic will have to take care of trauma patients with thoracic trauma. Trauma patients present with complex injuries. The Paramedic is required to have a detailed understanding of the mechanism of injury, kinematics, and pathophysiology. Armed with this information, the Paramedic can correctly treat the patient while en route to definitive care.

KEY POINTS:

- Thoracic trauma is a leading cause of morbidity and mortality in adults.

- Thoracic trauma is due to blunt and penetrating trauma.

- Rib fractures are common. Most concerning to Paramedics are rib fractures that create a flail segment, paradoxical motion, and altered mechanics of breathing.

- A simple pneumothorax can develop into a potentially life-threatening tension pneumothorax, especially after the application of positive pressure ventilation.

- The three cardiovascular injuries are aortic disruption, myocardial contusion, and myocardial rupture.

- Cardiac tamponade is a rapidly lethal condition where as little as 150 mL can compromise cardiac output and create hypoperfusion.

- Flail segments as evidenced by paradoxical chest wall motion should only be treated with positive pressure ventilation when there is evidence of ineffective mechanics of breathing.

- A floating sternum may indicate other potentially more life-threatening injuries to the right ventricle and trachea/bronchus.

- Myocardial contusions present with dysrhythmia in many cases and can lead to dysrhythmias and sudden cardiac death.

- Aortic disruptions are often lethal. Partial aortic disruptions present with differing blood pressures left to right and even loss of one pulse before the other.

- Bowel sounds in the chest are suggestive of diaphragmatic rupture/herniation. This injury is often accompanied by other potentially more life-threatening injuries.

- Traumatic asphyxia as evidenced by the following triad of symptoms—craniocervical cyanosis, facial edema, and subconjunctival hemorrhage—is rarely fatal.

- Treatment of a minor flail chest (i.e., one that does not compromise breathing) is treated with analgesia and bulky dressing. Major flail chest may need to be treated with positive pressure ventilation, medication-facilitated intubation, and paralysis.

- Tension pneumothorax, a simple pneumothorax plus hypotension, needs to be decompressed.

- Thoracic trauma patients need to be transported to a Level I or Level II Trauma Center.

REVIEW QUESTIONS:

1. What are the signs of a significant flail segment?
2. What are the signs and symptoms of a tension pneumothorax?
3. What is the key symptom of myocardial contusion?
4. What other potentially life-threatening injuries can accompany a diaphragmatic hernia?
5. What is the triad of symptoms associated with traumatic asphyxia?

CASE STUDY QUESTIONS:

Please refer to the Case Study in this chapter, and answer the questions below:

1. What is the predictable injury pattern based on the mechanism of injury?
2. What signs would make the Paramedic suspect that the patient has a pulmonary contusion as well?
3. What other condition would explain the paradoxical pulses, jugular venous distention, and muffled heart sounds?

REFERENCES:

1. Hubble MW, Hubble JP. *Principles of Advanced Trauma Care.* Clifton Park, NY: Delmar; 2002.
2. Karmy-Jones R, Jurkovich GJ, Shatz DV, et al. Management of traumatic lung injury: a Western Trauma Association Multicenter review. *J Trauma.* Dec 2001;51(6):1049–1053.
3. Fujiwara K, Naito Y, Komai H, et al. Right atrial rupture in blunt chest trauma. *Jpn J Thorac Cardiovasc Surg.* Jul 2001;49(7):476–478.
4. Ansari MZ, Chaudhry MA, Singal A, Joshi R. Unusual cardiac injury following blunt chest trauma. *Eur J Emerg Med.* Sep 2001;8(3):229–231.
5. Perron AD, Brady WJ, Erling BF. Commotio cordis: an underappreciated cause of sudden cardiac death in young patients: assessment and management in the ED. *Am J Emerg Med.* Sep 2001;19(5):406–409.
6. Nau T, Seitz H, Mousavi M, Vecsei V. The diagnostic dilemma of traumatic rupture of the diaphragm. *Surg Endosc.* Sep 2001;15(9):992–996.
7. Boulanger BR, Milzman DP, Rosati C, Rodriguez A. A comparison of right and left blunt traumatic diaphragmatic rupture. *J Trauma.* Aug 1993;35(2):255–260.
8. Carter BN, Giuseffi J, Felson B. Traumatic diaphragmatic hernia. *Am J Roentgenol Radium Ther Nucl Med.* Jan 1951;65(1):56–72.
9. Rizoli SB, Brenneman FD, Boulanger BR, Maggisano R. Blunt diaphragmatic and thoracic aortic rupture: an emerging injury complex. *Ann Thorac Surg.* Nov 1994;58(5):1404–1408.
10. Pryor JP, et al. Beyond the battlefield, the use of hemostatic dressings in civilian EMS. *Jnl Emerg Med Srv.* March 2008; 33(3): 102–9.
11. Dunsire MF, Field J, Valentine S. Delayed diagnosis of cardiac tamponade following isolated blunt abdominal trauma. *Br J Anaesth.* Aug 2001;87(2):309–312.
12. Rubikas R. Diaphragmatic injuries. *Eur J Cardiothorac Surg.* Jul 2001;20(1):53–57.
13. Worthy SA, et al. Diaphragmatic rupture: a frequently missed injury in blunt thoracoabdominal trauma. Available at: **http:// www.emedicine.com/emerg/topic136.htm.** Accessed on Nov. 9, 2004.
14. Lee MC, Wong SS, Chu JP, et al. Traumatic asphyxia. *Ann Thorac Surg.* Jan 1991;51(1):86–88.
15. Feliciano DV, Rozycki GS. Advances in the diagnosis and treatment of thoracic trauma. *Surg Clin North Am.* Dec 1999;79(6):1417–1429.

CHAPTER 6

ABDOMINAL AND GENITOURINARY TRAUMA

KEY CONCEPTS:

Upon completion of this chapter, it is expected that the reader will understand these following concepts:

- How injuries in solid organs tend to cause hemorrhagic shock
- The tamponade effect of subcapsular bleeding
- Referred pain associated with solid organ bleeding

ANATOMY CONCEPTS:

Prior to reading this chapter the Paramedic student should be familiar with the following anatomy and physiology concepts:

- Hollow and solid abdominal organs
- Retroperitoneal space
- Urogenital tract

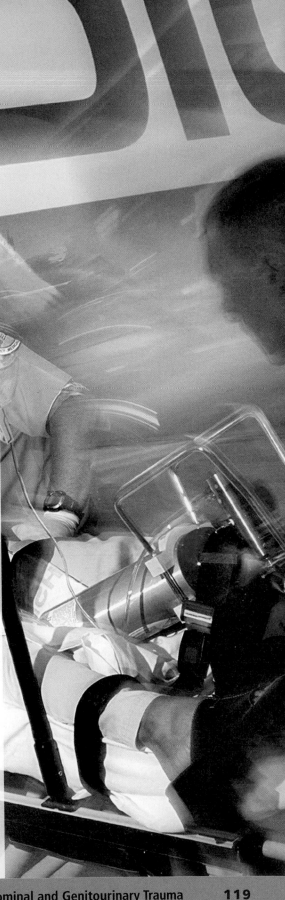

CASE STUDY:

"Gang violence is on the rise. Police presence stepped up," the supervisor says, reading the headlines of the newspaper. No sooner had the words spilt from the supervisor's lips than the tones went off. "Shots fired at the Corner of Clinton and Madison. Officers on-scene report officer down, gunshot to abdomen. Unit 624 and supervisor 6-2 respond echo response. Use caution for other responding units."

CRITICAL THINKING QUESTIONS

1. What potentially life-threatening injuries could occur from a gunshot wound to the abdomen?
2. What are the implications if the officer was wearing a soft ballistics vest?

OVERVIEW

Abdominal trauma occurs regularly both in the multitrauma patient and as isolated trauma. Due to the mobility of many of the abdominal structures and the "stretchability" of the abdomen, injuries to the abdominal contents may not be apparent immediately after the injury. For example, the peritoneal cavity can accommodate up to 3 liters of blood within the cavity without exhibiting abdominal distention.[1] When changes in sensation associated with age, head injury, and intoxication are also present, the patient with abdominal hemorrhage may not complain of pain to the same extent as someone with an intact awareness. Patients who sustain a spinal cord injury have a higher incidence of intra-abdominal injury[2] that challenges the Paramedic in the setting of a hypotensive patient with a spinal cord injury and possible intra-abdominal injury. With this in mind, Paramedics must maintain a high index of suspicion for intra-abdominal injury.

Chief Concern

Abdominal injuries may be caused by blunt trauma or penetrating trauma. Penetrating trauma is most commonly caused by knife or bullet wounds but can also be caused by shrapnel and other sharp objects that penetrate the abdominal wall. Injuries from penetrating trauma applied to the abdomen may not be limited to the abdomen, however. Depending on the object's trajectory, the object's speed and mass, and secondary collision with the bony boundaries of the abdomen, objects that penetrate the abdomen may end up in the thorax, extremities, or neck. In a similar fashion, penetrating trauma to the lower thorax may cause injury to the abdominal organs. The organs in the upper abdomen move with the diaphragm's movement during inspiration and expiration, again exposing them to the effects of penetrating trauma to the thorax.

Blunt trauma involves force over a large area that may involve the entire torso. These forces can be divided into direct forces to the body and deceleration forces within the body. Using a motor vehicle crash as an example, one crash is in actuality three separate collisions which occur within milliseconds of each other: the first between the vehicle and the object that stops it, the second between the occupant's body and the inside of the vehicle, and the third between the organs and the inner wall of the abdomen. In this third collision, the sudden deceleration applies shear forces to the organs, which are susceptible to injury at the points where they are anchored to the body. These shear forces may cause vascular injury, hollow viscus injury, or solid organ injury. Direct application of forces to the abdomen is more likely to cause solid organ injury (e.g., lacerations or hematomas). Fracture of the lower ribs from blunt thoracic trauma is another source of injury to the spleen and liver, both of which lie beneath the lower ribs.

Abdominal injuries can be generally divided into injuries to the solid organs, injuries to the hollow organs, vascular injuries, and injuries to the genitourinary system (Table 6-1). The peritoneum is a thin dual layer of tissue that serves to surround many of the abdominal organs, similar to the pleura in the thoracic cavity. The parietal peritoneum is the layer against the muscular inner abdominal wall, whereas the visceral peritoneum encapsulates the abdominal organs and forms the boundary of the peritoneal cavity. Although most organs are contained within the peritoneal cavity, some organs are considered retroperitoneal (Figure 6-1) because they are located behind the parietal peritoneum and are not located within the peritoneal cavity.

Although the retroperitoneal location of these structures helps protect them, it also makes it more difficult for the Paramedic to suspect injury. Often bleeding within the retroperitoneal space causes back pain rather than abdominal pain, which may lead the Paramedic to suspect a spinal injury rather than an intra-abdominal injury. Bleeding into the peritoneal cavity will often cause hypotension due to the large volume of the peritoneal cavity, whereas patients with retroperitoneal bleeding are less likely to be hypotensive initially. Bleeding in the retroperitoneal cavity also will tamponade due to the smaller, less distensible space, often limiting blood loss from the injury.

Solid Organ Injury

The solid organs (see Table 6-1) are highly vascular organs with a rich arterial blood supply. Injury to the solid organs, therefore, carries the potential for a significant blood loss in a short period of time. Solid organ injury is commonly responsible for hypotension secondary to intra-abdominal hemorrhage. Injuries to the solid organs include lacerations, hematomas, and vascular injury. Lacerations are an actual

Table 6-1 Abdominal Organ Classification

Solid Organs	Hollow Organs	Vascular	Geniturinary

• Liver
• Spleen
• Pancreas
• Kidneys
	• Esophagus (distal end)
	• Stomach
	• Small intestine:
	  ○ Duodenum
	  ○ Jejunum
	  ○ Ileum
	• Large intestine:
	  ○ Cecum
	  ○ Ascending colon
	  ○ Transverse colon
	  ○ Descending colon
	  ○ Sigmoid colon
	  ○ Rectum
		• Arterial
		  ○ Abdominal aorta
		  ○ Celiac artery
		  ○ Superior mesenteric artery
		  ○ Inferior mesenteric artery
		  ○ Renal arteries
		  ○ Iliac arteries
		• Venous
		  ○ Inferior vena cava
		  ○ Celiac vein
		  ○ Portal vein
		  ○ Superior mesenteric vein
		  ○ Inferior mesenteric vein
		  ○ Renal veins
		  ○ Iliac veins
			• Kidneys
			• Ureters
			• Urinary bladder
			• Urethra
			• Male:
			  ○ Testes
			  ○ Spermatochord
			  ○ Prostate
			  ○ Penis
			• Female:
			  ○ Vagina
			  ○ Cervix
			  ○ Uterus
			  ○ Fallopian tubes
			  ○ Ovaries

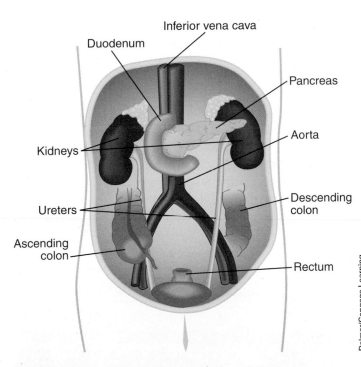

Figure 6-1 Retroperitoneal structures are located behind the parietal peritoneum rather than within the peritoneal cavity.

tear in the organ, whereas a hematoma may occur within or around the solid organ.

A thick fibrous capsule surrounds the solid organs. This capsule will sometimes contain blood loss and tamponade bleeding from a liver laceration or splenic laceration. Although this may initially limit blood loss, delayed rupture of the capsule can occur up to several days after the initial injury. Paramedics should consider the possibility of delayed rupture for patients with a history of recent trauma, especially if medical care was not sought initially for the injury. **Subcapsular hematomas** are hematomas that form between the surface of the organ and the inner face of the capsule surrounding the solid organ. Subcapsular hematomas can form from an adjacent laceration or from a leak in the vascular supply to the organ. If the capsule ruptures, the blood leaks into the peritoneal cavity, causing the appearance of free fluid on imaging that is performed at the emergency department. Significant hemorrhage and hypotension may occur with capsule rupture.

Pain from solid organ injuries can initially be misleading. Impulses of pain receptors from the organ itself travel along the autonomic nerves supplying the organ and often will cause referred pain rather than pain localized to the organ. Referred pain from the liver is appreciated in the right shoulder, whereas referred pain from the spleen is felt in the left shoulder. This referred pain is often achy in nature and is not affected by the shoulder's movement. Pain from the pancreas and kidneys, both of which are retroperitoneal organs, will often refer to the midback and flank, wrapping toward the groin, respectively. In contrast, the capsule sensory nerves come through the spinal nerves and will localize pain to the affected organ. Pain from the capsule will occur from stretching of the capsule and may improve when the capsule ruptures. Once the capsule is ruptured, however, blood leaks out and irritates the peritoneum. At that point, the pain will become diffuse across the abdomen and may be difficult to localize.

The presence of free fluid is assessed in the emergency department or aboard a medevac helicopter by performing a **Focused Abdominal Sonography in Trauma (FAST)** exam (Figure 6-2).[3] During the FAST exam, the Paramedic places an ultrasound probe against the patient's right upper quadrant and left upper quadrant to assess for peritoneal free fluid, and then places it over the pubic bone to assess for free fluid in the pelvis. The heart is also assessed for fluid in the pericardium by placing the probe under the xiphoid process. The lungs are assessed for the presence of a pneumothorax on the anterior upper chest. Free fluid, indicated by a dark black strip on the ultrasound image, is assumed to be blood in the setting of trauma (Figure 6-3).

Ultrasound technology has become small enough that some EMS systems have deployed ultrasound on ambulances[4] as well as aeromedical units.[5] Prehospital ultrasound is more common in Europe where physicians often respond as part of the EMS system.[6] Portable ultrasound units have been deployed with the military in the current combat theaters.[7] Portable ultrasound units were also successfully used during the Armenian earthquake in 1988 and Turkish earthquake in 1999 to assist with the triage of patients in those remote locations.[8] Although a more detailed discussion of the examination's technique is beyond the scope of this textbook, with increasing use in the field and improved portability, sonography may become more common in the future.

If the Paramedic suspects a solid organ injury, she should also suspect a hollow viscus injury. One study that reviewed the Pennsylvania state trauma registry noted that, in adult patients with a major or high grade solid organ injury from blunt trauma, there was a high likelihood of a hollow viscus injury.[9] This makes sense as higher grade solid organ injuries usually occur from higher blunt forces.

Liver

The liver is composed of four lobes and a total of eight segments, each with their own blood supply (Figure 6-4). The liver is attached to the diaphragm by the coronary ligament and to the anterior body wall by the falciform ligament, also called the **ligamentum teres hepatis.** This ligament also divides the liver into a right and left lobe. These ligaments can apply a shearing force to the liver during deceleration, causing lacerations. The liver sits in the lower thoracic cage

Figure 6-2 This emergency physician is performing a FAST exam in the emergency department.

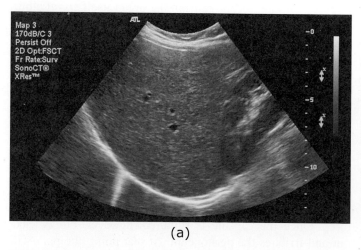
(a)

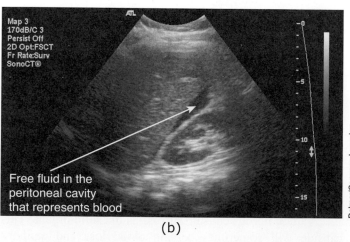
(b)

Figure 6-3 (a) A normal ultrasound image of the right upper quadrant compared with (b) an image from the right upper quadrant of a patient with free fluid indicated by the arrow.

Free fluid in the peritoneal cavity that represents blood

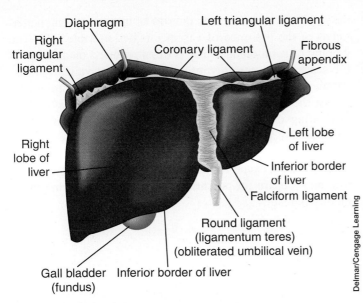

Figure 6-4 Liver anatomy. Due to the ligamentous connections, deceleration applies shear forces to the liver which may cause lacerations.

when it moves inferiorly, along with the diaphragm, during inhalation. As previously mentioned, lower rib fractures or blunt trauma to the lower thorax on the right can cause liver injury. Referred pain from the liver will develop around the right shoulder. Pain from the liver injury may worsen with breathing. The patient may also describe the pain as lower right-sided chest pain rather than abdominal pain.

Spleen

The spleen is located in the left upper quadrant, lying just inferior to the diaphragm. As one of the body's filters, the spleen has a rich blood supply. As with the liver, the spleen often sits in the lower left thorax and moves inferiorly with inspiration. Referred pain from a splenic injury can be felt in the left shoulder. Blood from a splenic rupture often travels down the splenorenal ligament toward the left flank, causing ecchymosis along the patient's left flank. Trauma to the lower left thorax can also involve the spleen. The Paramedic should suspect an underlying splenic injury when evidence exists of a lower left rib fracture and/or during a T-bone motor vehicle collision on the driver's side.

Pancreas

The pancreas is a retroperitoneal organ located posterior to the stomach and anterior to the abdominal aorta (Figure 6-1). In this position, the pancreas is somewhat protected from blunt trauma and is more commonly injured in penetrating trauma.[10] Blunt mechanisms that may injure the pancreas include handlebar and steering wheel trauma to the epigastric area. Pancreatic injury may not be apparent to the patient immediately after the trauma. Therefore, the patient may not call EMS for up to 48 hours after the injury.

Kidney

Although the kidneys are also retroperitoneal organs, they are not as well protected as the spleen. Injury may occur due to deceleration forces, direct impact against the adjacent flank, or secondarily through a posterior lower rib fracture. Penetrating trauma is also a common source of injury to the kidney and urinary system.

Injuries to the kidney can involve the collecting system, which includes the kidney itself and its connection to the ureter, or the vascular supply. Shear forces can be great enough to dislocate the kidney from its blood supply, causing significant retroperitoneal bleeding. Penetrating injury can also do the same, though more often it affects the organ itself.

The ureter is not often injured. However, penetrating trauma through the ureter can cause urine to leak into the peritoneal cavity. The ureter can be damaged by bone fragments or shear forces that occur with pelvic fractures, especially where the ureter crosses over the pelvic brim (Figure 6-5).

Patients who have sustained kidney trauma may complain of back or flank pain on the side of the injury. Back

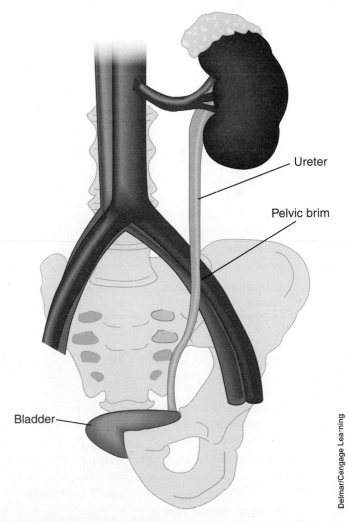

Figure 6-5 The ureter is susceptible to injury as it crosses the pelvic brim.

pain can be severe if a **retroperitoneal hematoma** (internal bleeding posterior to the peritoneum) develops. If the patient calls EMS some time after the trauma occurs, the patient may report **gross hematuria** (visible blood in the urine), urinating anything from pink-tinged urine to frank blood. Gross hematuria indicates trauma with bleeding some point along the urinary system, not necessarily only trauma to the kidney itself.

Solid Organ Injury Grading

The American Association for the Surgery of Trauma developed a grading system in the 1990s to help describe injuries to the abdominal organs.[11] The grading scheme for injuries to

the solid organs is based on the size of lacerations and hematomas or the presence of vascular injuries (Table 6-2). The grading of solid organ injury is often reported on abdominal CT scans. Although this information is not available to the Paramedic on initial assessment at the scene of a traumatic injury, the Paramedic will encounter this grading system in the setting of interfacility transfers between a community hospital and a trauma center. Familiarity with the concept of the grading system will not only allow the Paramedic to understand the extent of the patient's injuries, but also anticipate and prepare for potential decompensation during interfacility transfer.

Table 6-2 Solid Organ Injury Scaling System[11-14]

Grade	Liver	Spleen	Kidney	Pancreas
I	**Hematoma:** Subcapsular < 10% surface area	**Hematoma:** Subcapsular < 10% surface area	**Contusion:** Microscopic or gross hematuria	**Hematoma:** Minor contusion without duct injury
	Laceration: < 1 cm depth	**Laceration:** < 1 cm depth	**Hematoma:** Subcapsular without laceration	**Laceration:** Superficial without duct injury
II	**Hematoma:** Subcapsular 10% to 50% surface area Intraparenchymal < 10 cm diameter	**Hematoma:** Subcapsular 10% to 50% surface area Intraparenchymal < 5 cm diameter	**Hematoma:** Perirenal confined to retroperitoneum	**Hematoma:** Major contusion without duct injury or tissue loss
	Laceration: 1 to 3 cm depth, < 10 cm length	**Laceration:** 1 to 3 cm depth not involving a vessel	**Laceration:** < 1 cm depth without urine leak	**Laceration:** Major laceration without duct injury or tissue loss
III	**Hematoma:** Subcapsular > 50% surface area Ruptured subcapsular or parenchymal hematoma Intraparenchymal hematoma > 10 cm diameter	**Hematoma:** Subcapsular > 50% surface area Ruptured subcapsular or parenchymal hematoma Intraparenchymal hematoma > 5 cm	**Laceration:** > 1 cm depth without collecting system rupture or urine leak	**Laceration:** Distal transaction or a parenchymal injury with duct injury
	Laceration: > 3 cm parenchymal depth	**Laceration:** > 3 cm depth or involving vessels		
IV	**Laceration:** Parenchymal disruption involving 25% to 75% of hepatic lobe	**Laceration:** Laceration of segmental or hilar vessels with loss of blood flow to > 25% of spleen	**Laceration:** Extends through renal cortex, medulla, and collecting system	**Laceration:** Proximal transaction or a parenchymal injury involving the ampulla
			Vascular: Main renal artery or vein injury with contained hemorrhage	
V	**Laceration:** Parenchymal disruption involving > 75% hepatic lobe	**Laceration:** Completely shattered spleen	**Laceration:** Completely shattered kidney	**Laceration:** Massive disruption of the pancreas head
	Vascular: Venous injury	**Vascular:** Hilar vascular injury disrupting blood flow to entire spleen	**Vascular:** Avulsion of renal hilum which interrupts blood supply to the kidney	
VI	**Vascular:** Hepatic avulsion from blood supply			

Hollow Viscus and Diaphragmatic Injury

Hollow viscus injury is a generic term used to describe any number of injuries that can occur to the hollow abdominal organs (see Table 6-1). Hollow viscus injury occurs more often in the setting of penetrating trauma and is quite rare in blunt abdominal trauma.[15] It is estimated that hollow viscus injury occurs in up to 80% of patients sustaining a gun shot wound to the abdomen and up to 30% of abdominal stab wounds that penetrate into the peritoneal cavity.[15] In one large study reviewing records from almost 230,000 patients who had blunt abdominal injury mechanisms, only 1% of patients were found to have a hollow viscus injury from blunt trauma.[16]

Hollow viscus injuries are associated with solid organ injuries,[9] chance fractures of the lumbar spine,[17] penetrating injury from lower rib fractures,[18] and lower extremity fractures in pedestrians struck by automobiles.[19] Chance fractures commonly occur in patients who are improperly wearing their lap belt in motor vehicle crashes. Interestingly, the incidence of hollow viscus injury increased rapidly after seat belts were placed in automobiles, likely due to the rapid compressive forces applied on the bowel and sharp increase in pressure inside the hollow viscus, causing rupture.[20]

In rare cases, hollow viscus injury can occur from pelvic fractures[21] and in cases when airbags have deployed.[22] Rupture of the stomach is rare in blunt injury. However, when it occurs it is associated with injury that is more severe than a hollow viscus injury to other organs.[23]

As most of the hollow viscus organs are located in the peritoneum, leakage from a hollow viscus rupture spills into the peritoneal cavity. This leakage may include food particles, stomach acids, enzymes, bile, and stool. These materials should not be in the peritoneal cavity and can cause significant irritation of the peritoneum, just as blood irritates the peritoneum. Bacteria also pass into the peritoneal cavity through the rupture, contaminating the peritoneum. Infection is common and may not present until several hours to days later if the hollow viscus injury is not discovered during the initial evaluation. A patient may also have received what is believed to be minor abdominal trauma but then experiences worsening abdominal pain, fever, nausea, and vomiting, which prompts the call for assistance.

One particular injury that often presents late is that of a duodenal hematoma (Figure 6-6). The duodenum is the first part of the small intestine just downstream from the stomach. The duodenum is a retroperitoneal organ that is in close proximity to the spine. Due to its location, duodenal injury is very uncommon in blunt trauma, only occurring approximately 25% of the time in blunt abdominal injury.[24] In blunt abdominal injury, duodenal hematomas are caused by significant force applied to the epigastric area. Common mechanisms that can cause a duodenal hematoma include

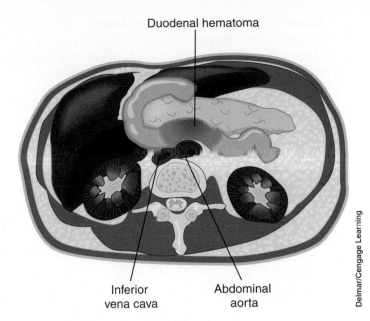

Figure 6-6 A duodenal hematoma compresses the duodenum as it expands, eventually causing a functional bowel obstruction.

striking a steering wheel, striking the end of a handlebar, or receiving a forceful kick or punch to the epigastrum.[24,25] In pediatric patients, over half of all duodenal injuries were the result of non-accidental trauma. In addition, one-third of the injuries did not show up until 48 hours after the original injury.[24] Duodenal hematomas cause a functional obstruction of the gastrointestinal tract, compressing the duodenum as the hematoma expands. Although the patient often complains of worsening epigastric pain, back pain may also occur due to the retroperitoneal location of the duodenum.

Injuries to the diaphragm can occur in both penetrating and blunt trauma. In penetrating trauma, the projectile or object passes through the diaphragm. In blunt trauma, the deceleration forces applied on the solid organs can produce tears in the diaphragm where the ligament attaches to the diaphragm. Abdominal contents, especially hollow organs, can protrude through the diaphragmatic tear. If diaphragmatic rupture occurs (Figure 6-7), the abdominal organs will cross the diaphragm and move into the thorax, displacing the lung and heart. This causes difficulty in ventilating the patient and creates other symptoms similar to a tension pneumothorax. Diaphragmatic rupture is exceedingly rare, occurring in less than 5% of blunt abdominal trauma patients.[26] Due to the liver's size and position immediately inferior to the diaphragm, diaphragmatic rupture more commonly occurs on the left side of the diaphragm.[27,28]

Vascular Injury

Abdominal vascular injury can be devastating and can potentially cause life-threatening intra-abdominal hemorrhage. Due to the size of the vessels, mortal injury can occur

Traumatic Rupture of Diaphragm with Massive
Displacement of Chest and Abdominal Organs

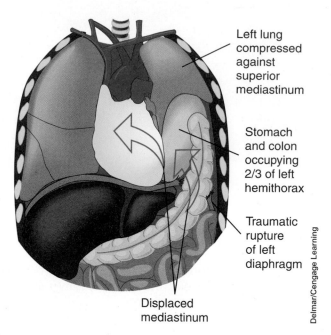

Left lung compressed against superior mediastinum

Stomach and colon occupying 2/3 of left hemithorax

Traumatic rupture of left diaphragm

Displaced mediastinum

Delmar/Cengage Learning

Figure 6-7 In a diaphragmatic rupture, the abdominal contents compress thoracic contents.

to either the arterial or venous structures in the abdomen (Figure 6-8). In penetrating injury, direct vessel damage occurs from the projectile or the penetrating object. This often produces vessel laceration and bleeding. In contrast, blunt abdominal trauma applies shear forces on the vessels where they branch, in areas where ligaments support them or they attach to the abdominal organs. Shear force can cause irregular tears in the vessel that resist the body's normal process of vessel constriction with injury.

Aortic injuries have also been associated with lumbar fractures, especially in children with improper lap belt restraints in motor vehicle crashes.[29–31] Injury to the iliac vessels and their branches may also occur from pelvic fractures with the sharp edges of the fractures lacerating the vessel.[32,33] In many of these patients, the Paramedic will notice the pelvis is unstable during physical examination. Significant pelvic hemorrhage has also been reported after fracture of the pubic ramus, also secondary to vessel laceration. In this chapter's case study, for example, the patient not only has pain in the area of both pubic rami but also has groin and abdominal swelling and bruising of the abdomen, groin, and perineum.[34] Chapter 7 presents a more detailed discussion of pelvic injuries.

Genitourinary Injury

Genitourinary injury includes injuries to the kidneys, ureters, urinary bladder, urethra, external genitalia, and reproductive organs. Penetrating trauma to any portion of the abdomen as

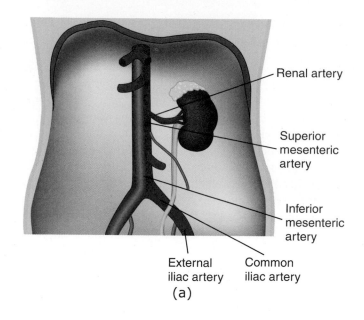

Renal artery

Superior mesenteric artery

Inferior mesenteric artery

External iliac artery

Common iliac artery

(a)

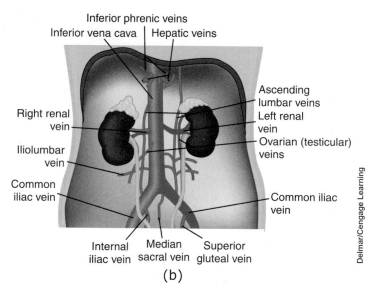

Inferior phrenic veins
Inferior vena cava   Hepatic veins

Right renal vein

Iliolumbar vein

Common iliac vein

Ascending lumbar veins
Left renal vein
Ovarian (testicular) veins

Common iliac vein

Internal iliac vein   Median sacral vein   Superior gluteal vein

(b)

Delmar/Cengage Learning

Figure 6-8 Abdominal vessels: (a) arteries and (b) veins.

well as the buttocks and upper legs can potentially involve the genitourinary system. In high-velocity penetrating trauma, injury may also occur from the shock wave as the projectile passes through the abdomen near the structures. Blunt trauma typically affects the kidneys, urinary bladder, or external genitalia due to the accessible location of these structures.

Trauma to the kidney was previously discussed in the section on solid organ injuries. Blunt trauma to the urinary bladder most often occurs from pelvic fractures.[35] In a small percentage of patients, the bladder will rupture from seat belt compression against a distended bladder. In addition to bladder injuries, pelvic fractures are also responsible for ureter, urethra, vaginal, and rectal injury, with genitourinary injury occurring in almost 5% of patients who have sustained a pelvic fracture.[36] Straddle injuries, where the blunt force targets the perineum, are responsible for male testicular, penile, and urethral injury. In female patients, straddle injury causes soft-tissue and pelvic injury.

Blunt force to the testicles can cause testicular rupture, hematoma, or dislocation. Most often, patients with isolated testicular trauma will seek medical attention up to five days after the actual injury.[37] Testicular rupture is also reported to occur after blunt trauma by a police bean bag, a nonlethal weapon used to subdue violent individuals.[38] Penile fractures occur when the tunica albuginea (Figure 6-9) ruptures when blunt force is applied to the fully erect penis, forcibly bending the penis.[39] There is immediate pain, loss of erection, and swelling of the penis, scrotum, and lower abdomen. Impotence can occur if this condition is not surgically repaired. Testicular injury can also occur during sexual intercourse.[35]

Injury to the external genitalia of either gender can also occur in the setting of self-mutilation or assault.

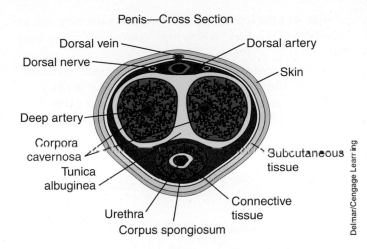

Figure 6-9 Cross-sectional anatomy of the penis. The tunica albuginea, the elastic covering of the corpus cavernosum, thins out as the corpus cavernosum fills with blood during erection.

▶ CASE STUDY (CONTINUED)

All the Paramedics can see is a wall of blue as police officers attend to their fallen comrade in addition to providing perimeter security. Shouting "Make a hole!" the curtain separates to reveal an officer on the ground, visibly shaken but smiling at the Paramedic. His first words are, "My gut hurts." His name is Zacarias, but everyone calls him Zak. Today he wore his vest. "Probably saved my life." Zak says.

CRITICAL THINKING QUESTIONS

1. What are the important elements of the history that a Paramedic should obtain?
2. Why would the use of beta blockers be problematic?

History

The Paramedic can obtain some historical information just by observing the scene during the initial impression even before contacting the patient. In the case of a motor vehicle crash, observing the damage to the vehicles can provide clues to the forces that have been applied to the patient. This observation of the mechanism of injury will allow the Paramedic to predict and assess for the likely injuries. The Paramedic should obtain as much information as possible about the mechanism that caused the injury, either directly from the patient or from bystanders. If the patient's condition permits, or if personnel are available, the scene should be surveyed in a little more detail, looking for factors such as vehicular damage, windshield deformity, steering wheel deformity, and the presence and use of safety devices (such as a helmet or seat belt). In the setting of a fall, the height of

the fall and the material the patient fell onto is also important in predicting injury patterns.

In regards to abdominal and genitourinary injury, the Paramedic should ask about abdominal pain. If the patient has abdominal pain, the Paramedic should obtain additional information on the pain, including its location, quality, radiation, relief, recurrence or exacerbating factors, severity, and time of onset. Time of onset becomes important given that some abdominal injuries may develop in a delayed fashion or be ignored by the patient during the initial injury. For patients who do not indicate recent trauma but offer a chief concern of abdominal pain, the Paramedic should always ask about recent trauma or injury as part of the history.

In some cases, the patient will recall what seemed at the time to be minor trauma but which may be significant in uncovering an underlying delayed injury. The Paramedic should also be aware of pain referral patterns, including the right and left shoulder and the back, which may indicate abdominal organ injury.

The Paramedic should try to elicit an exact mechanism, if possible. Direct force to the abdomen, as well as the type of force, may indicate potential underlying injuries. Application of a generalized force or a deceleration mechanism should cause the Paramedic to suspect vascular or hollow viscus injury in addition to solid organ injury.

A history of hematuria, or blood in the urine, in the setting of trauma indicates an injury somewhere along the urinary tract. When combined with flank or upper quadrant pain, the Paramedic should suspect a kidney injury. If lower abdominal pain is present, an injury to the urinary bladder or ureter is suspected. Finally, pain in the genitals suggests trauma to the external genitalia. Past medical, surgical, and social history; allergies and reactions; and current medications should be obtained in the usual manner if the patient's condition permits.

► CASE STUDY (CONTINUED)

The Paramedic asks another officer to secure Zak's gun. "I'll take that" says the police sargeant, reaching out with an arm that has so many hash marks on the sleeve it looks like a ladder.

Cutting Zak's shirt open, and being careful to avoid the bullet hole, the Paramedic can see one bullet in the vest at the center mass. Unstrapping the patient's vest and cutting off his undershirt, the Paramedic sees an angry looking welt proximal to the xiphoid process.

CRITICAL THINKING QUESTIONS

1. What are the elements of the physical examination of a patient with suspected abdominal trauma?
2. Why is a rapid trauma examination a critical element in this examination?

Examination

Once the Paramedic performs a rapid primary assessment and addresses any life-threatening conditions, she then moves to the head-to-toe examination. Vital signs should also be obtained and are usually delegated to another crew member.

When assessing the abdomen, the Paramedic should follow the inspection, auscultation, palpation, and percussion sequence. The Paramedic first assesses the exposed abdomen for wounds, lacerations, and ecchymotic areas that may indicate the presence of underlying injury (Figure 6-10). In the case of penetrating trauma to the chest or upper legs, the abdomen must be thoroughly inspected to detect additional wounds that may be present. Wounds that are located in the lower thorax may involve force that passed through the diaphragm and into the abdominal cavity, causing injury to the abdominal structures in the upper quadrants and epigastrium.

In the setting of multisystem trauma, auscultation of the abdomen has limited usefulness to the Paramedic given the unreliability of the finding and other higher priorities. In the setting of a delayed call for assistance or isolated abdominal trauma, the lack of bowel sounds may indicate intra-abdominal injury. Similar to patients who undergo bowel surgery, an ileus or slowing down of the normal movement of material through the gastrointestinal system may indicate an intra-abdominal injury.

Palpation should start with the quadrant furthest away from the location of pain. A distended or hard abdomen is a sign of peritonitis, which in the setting of trauma is assumed to be secondary to hemorrhage or hollow viscus perforation. Tenderness localized to the upper right quadrant or right costal margin may indicate liver injury, whereas pain localized to the left upper quadrant or left costal margin may indicate a splenic injury. Tenderness in the lower quadrants may indicate hollow viscus, genitourinary, or vascular injury. Vascular and genitourinary injury should be suspected if pelvic instability or bony tenderness is discovered on physical examination.

If a field ultrasound becomes available and the Paramedic is credentialed to perform a FAST exam, the examination may be helpful in triaging a patient who is otherwise stable to a trauma center if the FAST exam is positive for free fluid in the peritoneal cavity or the pelvis.

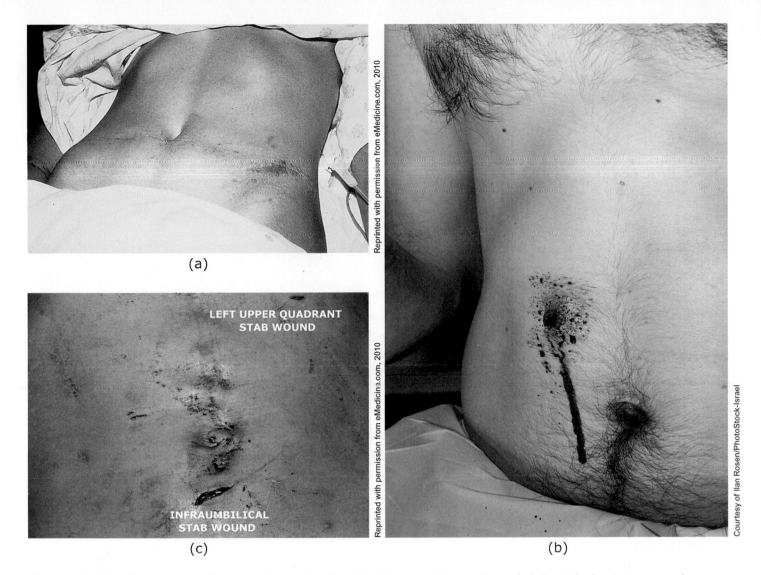

(a)

LEFT UPPER QUADRANT
STAB WOUND

INFRAUMBILICAL
STAB WOUND

(c)

(b)

Figure 6-10 Examples of traumatic abdominal findings on inspection. (a) Seat belt sign caused by a seat belt riding up over the hips. (b) Abdominal gunshot wound. (c) Abdominal stab wound.

CASE STUDY (CONTINUED)

As the Paramedic finishes her assessment, she notes the stretcher is being pulled out of the ambulance. Zak also notices the stretcher and asks, "You don't think I need to go to the hospital right now, do you doc?"

CRITICAL THINKING QUESTIONS

1. What is the significance of the location of the bullet wound?
2. What diagnosis did the Paramedic announce to the patient?

Assessment

As previously discussed, abdominal injuries may be difficult to detect for a variety of reasons. Distracting painful injuries, such as a femur fracture, may mask the pain of an intra-abdominal injury. Altered mental status, whether due to a head injury, alcohol, or illicit substances, can also blunt the sensation of pain and mask injury. In these situations, the patient may not offer a concern of abdominal pain; however, palpation during the physical examination may produce abdominal tenderness. Other physical signs discussed previously should also cause the Paramedic to have a high index of suspicion for intra-abdominal injury.

In the setting of multiple trauma, multiple studies have confirmed that intra-abdominal injury is the most common cause of hypotension in the field.[40-43] The abdominal cavity can hold up to 3 liters of blood, or one-third to one-half of the body's blood volume, before abdominal distention occurs. Although the thoracic cavity can hold between 1.5 and 2 liters of blood and can also be a source for hypotension, respiratory distress and a narrowing pulse pressure will occur in thoracic cavity hemorrhage whereas a widening pulse pressure will occur if the source is intra-abdominal.

CASE STUDY (CONTINUED)

The police sergeant answers the question before the Paramedic can respond. "You're going to the medical center. The investigators will meet you there to get your statement. Now get off my scene!" he growls. Wise words, the Paramedic thinks, but for a different reason. Although using analgesia crossed her mind, she decides to "package and transport" the patient immediately and perform all treatments en route.

CRITICAL THINKING QUESTIONS

1. What is the national standard of care of patients with suspected intra-abdominal injury?
2. What are some of the patient-specific concerns and considerations that the Paramedic should consider when applying this plan of care that is intended to treat a broad patient population presenting with intra-abdominal injury?

Treatment

The Paramedic's initial treatment priorities should center around managing life-threatening airway, breathing, and circulatory issues. Often abdominal injuries will either be the source of hypotension requiring treatment for hemorrhagic shock or will require only supportive treatment en route to the emergency department. In the setting of poor perfusion, high-flow, high-concentration oxygen should be applied to help maximize oxygen delivery.

In the stable patient, the Paramedic should consider other treatments as appropriate. She may administer analgesia to help decrease the patient's discomfort provided the patient's mental status is intact and there is a normal Glasgow Coma Scale. The Paramedic may also administer anti-nausea medications to counteract nausea and vomiting that may be present with the abdominal injury. She can also apply ice wrapped in a towel to injured external genitalia to help decrease swelling and pain.

CASE STUDY (CONTINUED)

While en route to the hospital, "on the red" and with a police escort, Zak asks for a drink of water. The Paramedic recognizes the sign and looks at the ECG monitor. Zak's heart rate is climbing. She immediately reaches for a blood pressure cuff and tells the driver to call in a "trauma alert." "What's all the fuss?" asks Zak.

CRITICAL THINKING QUESTIONS

1. What are some of the predictable complications associated with blunt force abdominal injury?
2. What are some of the predictable complications associated with the treatments for blunt force abdominal injury?

Evaluation

The vital signs of patients who have experienced abdominal trauma should be closely observed during transport to the emergency department. Patients with abdominal trauma are at risk for life-threatening internal hemorrhage, although younger and healthier patients have the ability to compensate for a long time before hypotension develops. A widening pulse pressure, especially with a lower-than-normal diastolic blood pressure, or unexplained tachycardia with a normal blood pressure should alert the Paramedic early to the onset of hemorrhagic shock. The Paramedic should be prepared to intervene, if necessary, during transport. Ecchymosis may develop gradually after the initial injury. The Paramedic should also observe the patient for truncal ecchymosis that develops during transport.

► CASE STUDY CONCLUSION

As they arrive at the hospital, the crew is immediately greeted by the emergency physician. "Let's get him inside," he says. "The press is all over the ER and looking for the story." Zak appears unconcerned about the news, or, more appropriately, Zak looks lethargic.

CRITICAL THINKING QUESTIONS

1. What is the most appropriate transport decision that will get the patient to definitive care?
2. What are the advantages of transporting a patient with suspected blunt force abdominal trauma to these hospitals, even if that means bypassing other hospitals in the process?

Disposition

Patients who have sustained abdominal trauma and are hypotensive should be transported to the closest appropriate facility. Hypotension in the setting of trauma is three times more likely to require an emergent intervention by the emergency physician or trauma surgeon than trauma without hypotension.[44,45] If significant intra-abdominal hemorrhage is suspected, the Paramedic should transport the patient to the closest appropriate trauma center. If a FAST exam performed in the field is positive for free peritoneal or pelvic fluid, the patient should be transported to the closest appropriate trauma center. Patients with isolated injury, normal vital signs that have remained stable during care, a minor mechanism, and no other apparent injuries may be suitable for transport to a community hospital. If the Paramedic has any questions on the appropriate destination for a specific patient, he should consult a physician at the closest trauma center for recommendations.

CONCLUSION

Abdominal injuries, both isolated injuries and those that are part of multisystem trauma, present a challenge to the Paramedic due to the injuries that may be hidden beneath the skin. The Paramedic must maintain a high index of suspicion for abdominal injury in order to properly assess and manage these patients.

▶ KEY POINTS:

- The abdomen contains the abdominal cavity and portions of the thoracic cavity, as well as the retroperitoneal cavity.

- Solid organ injuries include subcapsular hematomas, liver lacerations, splenic rupture, and kidney contusions.

- Solid organ injury grading helps the Paramedic anticipate decompensation during interfacility transport.

- Hollow viscus injury is very uncommon in blunt trauma and more likely to be seen in gunshot wounds.

- Aortic injury is a potentially life-threatening trauma that is often associated with lumbar fractures that can be due to improperly worn seat belts.

▶ REVIEW QUESTIONS:

1. Where do solid abdominal organs radiate their pain?
2. Why would hypotension from bleeding into the retroperitoneal space present later in the patient's clinical course?
3. A trauma patient has severe back pain at the costovertebral angle that radiates to the groin. Suddenly, the pain is gone, but the patient starts to become increasingly tachycardiac. What happened?
4. What causes liver lacerations in blunt trauma?
5. Blood is seen at the external meatus of the penis and the patient complains of flank pain. What injury should be suspected?

▶ CASE STUDY QUESTIONS:

Please refer to the Case Study in this chapter, and answer the questions below:

1. Suppose the police officer in this case was not wearing a ballistic vest. What would be the predictable injuries based on a through and through bullet wound?
2. What if the bullet had struck just below the umbilicus instead?
3. The patient starts to complain of difficulty breathing. What is a possible explanation?

REFERENCES:

1. Moore FA, Moore EE. Initial management of life threatening trauma. In: Souba WW, ed. *ACS Surgery: Principles & Practice* (6th ed.). New York: WebMD; 2008.

2. Salim A, Ottochian M, Gertz RJ, et al. Intra-abdominal injury is common in blunt trauma patients who sustain spinal cord injury. *Am Surg*. 2007;73(10):1035–1038.

3. Heller M, Jehle D. *Ultrasound in Emergency Medicine* (2nd ed.). Buffalo, NY: Center Page; 2002.

4. Smith CA. Ultra assessment tool. EMS crews begin using portable ultrasound units in the field. *JEMS*. 2003;28(7):46–54.

5. Melanson SW, McCarthy J, Stromsky CJ, et al. Aeromedical trauma sonography by flight crews with a miniature ultrasound unit. *Prehosp Emerg Care*. 2001;5(4):399–402.

6. Nelson BP, Chason K. Use of ultrasound by emergency medical services: a review. *Int J Emerg Med*. 2008;1(4):253–259.

7. Brooks AJ, Price V, Simms M. FAST on operational military deployment. *Emerg Med J*. 2005;22(4):263–265.

8. Ma OJ, Norvell JG, Subramanian S. Ultrasound applications in mass casualties and extreme environments. *Crit Care Med*. 2007;35(5 Suppl):S275–279.

9. Nance ML, Peden GW, Shapiro MB, et al. Solid viscus injury predicts major hollow viscus injury in blunt abdominal trauma. *J Trauma*. 1997;43(4):618–622.

10. Ahmed N, Vernick JJ. Pancreatic injury. *South Med J*. 2009;102(12):1253–1256.

11. American Association for the Surgery of Trauma. Injury scoring scale: a resource for trauma care professionals. Available at: **http://www.aast.org/library/traumatools/injuryscoringscales.aspx**. Accessed December 28, 2009.

12. Moore EE, Shackford SR, Pachter HL, et al. Organ injury scaling—spleen, liver, and kidney. *J Trauma*. 1989;29(12):1664–1666.

13. Moore EE, Cogbill TH, Jurkovich GJ, et al. Organ injury scaling II: pancreas, duodenum, small bowel, colon, and rectum. *J Trauma*. 1990;30(11):1427–1429.

14. Moore EE, Cogbill TH, Jurkovich MD, et al. Organ injury scaling: spleen and liver (1994 revision). *J Trauma*. 1995;38(3):323–324.

15. Hughes TMD, Elton C. Pathophysiology and management of bowel and mesenteric injuries due to blunt trauma. *Injury*. 2002;33(4):295–302.

16. Watts DD, Fakhry SM, for the EAST Multi-Institutional Hollow Viscus Injury Research Group. Incidence of hollow viscus injury in blunt trauma: an analysis from 275,557 trauma admissions from the EAST Multi-Institutional Trial. *J Trauma*. 2003;54(2):289–294.

17. Tyroch AH, McGuire EL, McLean LD, et al. The association between chance fractures and intra-abdominal injuries revisited: a multicenter review. *Am Surg*. 2005;71(5):434–488.

18. Tsaur I, Niedermeyer B. Rare complication of a dislocated rib fracture. Unusual clinical course following a motorcycle spill. *Der Unfallchirurg*. 2008;111(10):850–855.

19. Hannon M, Hadjizacharia P, Chan L, et al. Prognostic significance of lower extremity long bone fractures after automobile versus pedestrian injuries. *J Trauma*. 2009;67(6):1384–1388.

20. Cox EF. Blunt abdominal trauma: a 5 year analysis of 870 patients requiring celiotomy. *Ann Surg*. 1984;199(4):467–474.

21. Nicolau AE, Tutuianu R, Veste V, et al. Small bowel perforation caused by compound pelvic fracture found in diagnostic laparoscopy. *Chirurgia (Bucur)*. 2006;101(4):423–428.

22. Liverani A, Pezzatini M, Conte S, et al. A rare case of blunt thoracoabdominal trauma with small bowel perforation from air bags. *Il Giornale de Chirurgia*. 2009,30(5).234–236.

23. Oncel D, Malinoski D, Brown C, et al. Blunt gastric injuries. *The American Surgeon*. 2007;73(9):880–883.

24. Jurkovich GJ. Injuries to the pancreas and duodenum. In: Souba WW, ed.. *ACS Surgery: Principles & Practice* (6th ed.). New York: WebMD; 2008.

25. Thomas M, Basnu NN, Gulati MS, et al. Isolated duodenal rupture due to go-karting accidents—braking news. *Ann R Coll Surg Engl*. 2009;91(4):340–343.

26. Punyadasa AC, Tee A. Pseudopneumothorax—hold that chest tube! *Int J Emerg Med*. 2008;1(1):59–60.

27. Kishore GS, Gupta V, Doley RP, et al. Traumatic diaphragmatic hernia: tertiary centre experience. *Hernia*. Nov 12, 2009 [Epub ahead of print].

28. Peer SM, Devaraddeppa PM, Buggi S. Traumatic diaphragmatic hernia—our experience. *Int J Surg*. 2009;7(6):547–549.

29. Anderson SA, Day M, Chen MK, et al. Traumatic aortic injuries in the pediatric population. *J Pediatr Surg*. 2008;43(6):1077–1081.

30. Crawford CH, Puno RM, Campbell MJ, Carreon LY. Surgical management of severely displaced pediatric seatbelt fracture-dislocations of the lumbar spine associated with occlusion of the abdominal aorta and avulsion of the cauda equine: a report of two cases. *Spine*. 2008;33(10):E325–328.

31. Swischuk LE, Jadhav SP, Chung DH. Aortic injury with chance fracture in a child. *Emerg Radiol*. 2008;15(5):285–287.

32. Abrassart S, Stern R, Peter R. Morbidity associated with isolated iliac wing fractures. *J Trauma*. 2009;66(1):200–203.

33. Cestero RF, Plurad D, Green D, et al. Iliac artery injuries and pelvic fractures: a national trauma database analysis of associated injuries and outcomes. *J Trauma*. 2009;7(4):715–718.

34. Chiu Y, Wong TC, Yeung SH. Haemodynamic instability secondary to minimally displaced pubic rami fractures: a report of two cases. *J Orthop Surg* (Hong Kong). 2009;17(1):100–102.

35. Dandan I, Farhat W. Lower genitourinary trauma. eMedicine online emergency medicine textbook, updated April 16, 2009. Available at: **http://emedicine.medscape.com/article/828251-overview**. Accessed December 30, 2009.

36. Bjurlin MA, Fantus RJ, Mellett MM, Goble SM. Genitourinary injuries in pelvic fracture morbidity and mortality using the national trauma databank. *J Trauma*. 2009;67(5):1033–1039.

37. Mulhail JP, Gabram SG, Jacobs LM. Emergency management of blunt testicular trauma. *Acad Emerg Med*. 1995;2(7): 639–643.

38. de Brito D, Challoner KR, Sehgal A, Mallon W. The injury pattern of a new law enforcement weapon: the police bean bag. *Ann Emerg Med*. 2001;38(4):383–390.

39. Mohite PN, Shah S, Parikh A, Patel R. Fractured penis during sexual intercourse in a 38 year old male: a case report and a review of literature. *Internet J Emerg Intens Care Med*. 2008;11(1). Available at **http://www.ispub.com/.** Accessed December 30, 2009.

40. Mackersie RC, Tiwary Ad, Shackford SR, et al. Intra-abdominal injury following blunt trauma. Identifying the high-risk patient using objective risk factors. *Arch Surg*. 1989;124:809–813.

41. Chan L, Bartfield JM, Reilly KM. The significance of prehospital hypotension in blunt trauma patients. *Acad Emerg Med*. 1997;4:785–788.

42. Aranda M, Petersen SR, Hunt C, et al. An episode of prehospital hypotension in trauma patients: a marker for doom or just crying wolf? [Abstract]. *J Trauma*. 1997;42:160.

43. Shapiro NI, Kociszewski C, Harrison T, et al. Isolated prehospital hypotension after traumatic injuries: a predictor of mortality? *J Emerg Med*. 2003;25:175–179.

44. Lipsku AM, Gausche-Hill M, Henneman PL, et al. Prehospital hypotension is a predictor of the need for emergent, therapeutic operation in trauma patients with normal systolic blood pressure in the emergency department. *J Trauma*. 2006;61(5):1228–1233.

45. Lalezarzadeh F, Wisniewski P, Huynh K, et al. Evaluation of prehospital and emergency department systolic blood pressure as a predictor of in-hospital mortality. *Am Surg*. 2009;75(10): 1009–1014.

CHAPTER 7

ORTHOPAEDIC TRAUMA

KEY CONCEPTS:

Upon completion of this chapter, it is expected that the reader will understand these following concepts:

- Common mechanisms of injury for orthopaedic trauma
- The various degrees of sprains
- Four common shoulder injuries
- The various grades of ankle sprains
- The four types of tendons that most often rupture
- Classifications of open fractures
- Pediatric Salter-Harris fractures
- Common types of fractures
- Blood loss from fractures
- Common dislocation reduction methods
- Common external splints
- Compartment syndrome

ANATOMY CONCEPTS:

Prior to reading this chapter the Paramedic student should be familiar with the following anatomy and physiology concepts:

- Appendicular skeleton
- Major blood vessels in the extremities
- Major muscles
- Tendons and ligaments

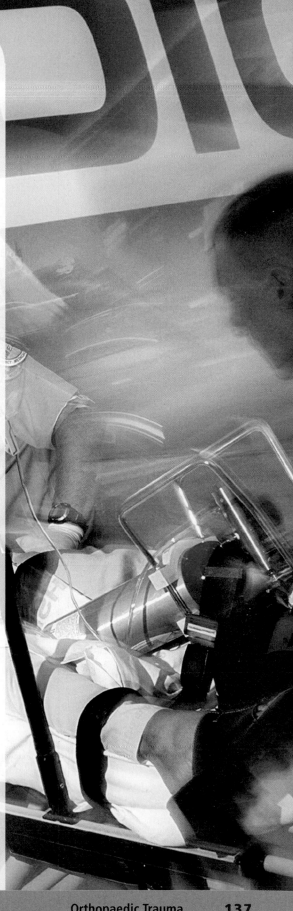

CASE STUDY:

The earthquake devastated the community. The members of the rapid response disaster medical assistance team sent to the area expect that they will encounter patients with musculoskeletal trauma. Although the Paramedics are used to treating musculoskeletal injury on a daily basis, secondary to motor vehicle collisions and athletic events, the number of injuries they are expecting to encounter is dramatic. To prepare, the team starts pouring over their manuals before arriving at the airport.

CRITICAL THINKING QUESTIONS

1. What are some of the possible musculoskeletal injuries that patients will present with at an earthquake?
2. What types of musculoskeletal injuries might the team sustain during rescue efforts?

OVERVIEW

The musculoskeletal system is very prone to injury. **Orthopaedics**, the study of those injuries, covers the universe of musculoskeletal injuries including injuries to the bones, joints, ligaments, tendons, and muscles. This chapter discusses only orthopaedic injuries of the appendicular skeleton.

Orthopaedic injury is the result of trauma, physical injury to the body caused by violent forces. In the case of blunt or penetrating trauma, an understanding of the mechanism of injury and its kinematics can lead the Paramedic to have a high index of suspicion for the patient's predictable injury pattern.

However, in the case of orthopaedic trauma, many of these forces are internal. Understanding these internal forces requires knowledge of kinesiology, the study of human movement, and biomechanics, the application of mechanical principles to the human body. Many healthcare professionals, from orthopaedic surgeons to certified athletic trainers, have extensively studied orthopaedic injuries using kinesiology and biomechanics. Studies have been done on the physics of collisions in football, physics of ball throwing, and the impact of cycling wheel design on the cycler. In fact, every sport has been studied in an effort to improve human performance while reducing injury as well. By applying knowledge of kinesiology and biomechanics, the Paramedic can also predict the injury associated with athletic and non-athletic activities.

Chief Concern

With any concerning mechanism of injury, the Paramedic must consider the possibility of sprains, strains, fractures, and dislocations. Although these injuries are all different, one constant they all share is the presence of pain. The Paramedic, either working independently or cooperatively with the EMT, generally has a comprehensive knowledge of these musculoskeletal injuries and can help bring about a better patient outcome.

Biomechanics

It is a mistake to consider the skeletal system as static and unchanging. The skeletal system is always in a process of remodeling; that is, osteoclasts absorb bone, whereas osteoblasts form new bone in order to meet current conditions. Any forces applied to the skeletal system act upon that remodeling process. **Biomechanics** is the study of the forces muscles exert upon the skeleton. Any force—tensile (pulling), compressive (pushing), shearing, bending, or torsion (twisting)—applied to the muscles or skeleton will displace tissue and thereby impact remodeling. In some cases, such as during locomotion (walking), this is advantageous. In other cases, it can lead to injury (Figure 7-1).

Whenever a force is applied against a tissue, the degree of displacement is a function of the tissue's flexibility. Initially,

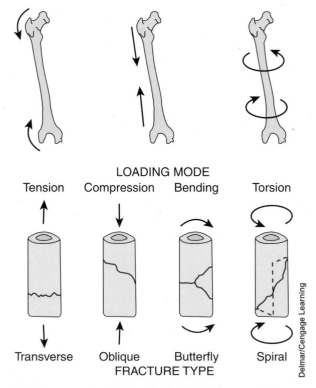

LOADING MODE

Tension Compression Bending Torsion

Transverse Oblique Butterfly Spiral
FRACTURE TYPE

Delmar/Cengage Learning

Figure 7-1 Fracture mechanisms include tensile, compressive, shearing, bending, or torsion forces.

the tissue changes shape. If the surface returns to its previous shape (i.e., elastic deformity), there is no trauma. However, if the tissue is changed or permanently deformed, called plastic deformation, an injury occurs.

In some cases, the plastic deformation is the result of continuous force (i.e., load to failure that results in the tissue reaching the "breaking point"). This occurs with bone fracture, muscle strain, and sprained ligaments. In other cases, the plastic deformation is the result of fatigue failure, the cyclical subthreshold loading that results in microscopic damage and eventually total failure. This is the case in repetitive motion disorders.

This musculoskeletal system failure can be the result of great force or, alternatively, minor repetitive motions. The common feature that predicts injury is tissue health (i.e., its elasticity). For example, the incidence of bone fractures is a function of use, disease, and aging (specifically osteoporosis). The incidence of sprains is a function of use and previous injuries, including microscopic tears. These forces, when applied to the musculoskeletal system, result in sprains, strains, dislocations, and fractures.

Sprains, Ruptures, and Dislocations

Some joints are very stable whereas others are not. However, all are prone to injury. The following sprains are not necessarily placed in order of harm. The harm of any musculoskeletal injury is in the degree of disability that results. For example, although a fracture may seem to be a devastating injury, a fracture can heal, leaving no residual disability. However, a sprain can have life-long implications.

Sprains and Strains

A tendon is connective tissue that connects muscles to bones. A **strain** is an injury to a tendon. This injury can be caused by the tearing, twisting, or pulling of muscle. A **sprain** is an injury to the ligaments that connect bone to bone. Injuries to ligaments tend to make a joint unstable.

Sprains are defined in degrees according to severity. Overstretching a ligament, such as in the case of hyperextension of the knee, can result in a minor tear, or first degree injury to the ligament. Continued stretching will result in a partial tear that is accompanied by pain, swelling, and bruising, known as a second degree tear.

If the limb's ligaments are pushed beyond their range of motion, there may be a complete tear of the ligament (a third degree sprain) and even avulsion of bone (a fourth degree sprain). When a third degree sprain occurs, the bone to which the tendon is attached cannot move (i.e., there is a loss of motion), and a tendon defect can be appreciated on palpation.

Destruction of the joint's integrity, by disruption of the bone and ligament, is considered a fifth degree sprain. Loss of the joint, a sixth degree tear, often results in amputation.

Sprained Shoulder

Due to sprains, strains, and dislocations, the shoulder may be one of the joints most likely to be injured because it has very little stability in certain positions. The sprained shoulder can lead to bursitis, tendinitis, and even a frozen shoulder. The shoulder is particularly prone to sprains, owed to the numerous ligaments and tendons that create the shoulder.

The shoulder complex (i.e., the shoulder girdle) consists of three joints—the sternoclavicular joint, the acromioclavicular joint, and the glenohumeral joint—and a pseudojoint, the scapulothoracic articulation. Numerous muscles, tendons, and ligaments make these joints functional so that the patient can experience a wide range of motion.[1]

Any number of motions can produce injury to the shoulder. Sudden traction on an outreached arm, such as occurs during a martial arts demonstration, can stretch the brachial plexus, injuring the nerves that control the shoulder. An object dropped on top of the shoulder can lead to a ligamentous tear. A blow to the anterior or posterior shoulder (e.g., as occurs during contact sports) can lead to ligamentous tears. Even an arm that is forcefully rotated and/or abducted beyond the shoulder's range of motion can result in sprains, strains, and dislocations. Such an injury can occur whenever a ball (e.g., football, baseball, tennis, volleyball, etc.) is thrown. However, the most common MOI for a shoulder injury is a simple fall on an outstretched hand, leading to a "shoulder separation."

Because the shoulder is a loose ball-in-socket joint, it depends on numerous muscles, tendons, and ligaments to maintain its position in the socket through its range of motion. Grouped together, these muscles, tendons, and ligaments can be divided into either static stabilizers or dynamic stabilizers. The static stabilizers maintain congruity in the shoulder complex, even in the face of neuromuscular pathology. The dynamic stabilizers, however, are under constant neuromuscular control (i.e., muscular tension).

These dynamic stabilizers are made up of four muscles that together are referred to as the rotator cuff. The muscles of the rotator cuff help to keep the humeral head in the glenoid. Injuries to the rotator cuff can lead to shoulder instability and a higher risk of humeral dislocation.

A sprain in these stabilizers, known as a **rotator cuff tear**, leads to destabilization of the shoulder joint and pain. The pain is anterolateral, at the deltoid insertion, with associated weakness and loss of range of motion. The Paramedic may also appreciate a crepitus in the area, and the patient may say that the shoulder is "catching," thus limiting her motion.

Another injury associated with the rotator cuff is outlet impingement, known as **shoulder impingement syndrome**. Normally, there is a narrow space between the acromion and the humeral head. Rotator cuff dysfunction (e.g., secondary to arthritis) can result in loss of that narrow space and loss of ROM. When a patient has shoulder impingement syndrome, the patient experiences severe pain whenever the humerus is internally rotated or elevated. This motion compresses the acromion against the tendons and bursa. The pain is often worst at night.

Patients with a rotator cuff injury will complain of pain, weakness in the affected limb, and a loss of range of motion (ROM). The Paramedic should take a careful history of the mechanism of injury, as sports physicians and orthopaedic surgeons can identify the likely muscle and tendon injury by comparing the MOI to their knowledge of biomechanics. The Paramedic should also inquire if the patient heard a popping sound or felt a "catch" during the motion.

Pain is often elicited over the anterolateral shoulder. The patient may complain of pain at night, usually because the patient is lying on the affected shoulder. The patient may also express apprehension with overhead motion.

Injury can occur to the sternoclavicular joint as well. The sternoclavicular joint, a freely movable synovial joint, is the only point where the shoulder is attached directly to the axial skeleton. A blow to the anterior shoulder, such as occurs during a football tackle, can roll the shoulder backward and the clavicle forward, resulting in a **sternoclavicular (SC) sprain**.

The patient immediately experiences pain proximal to the angle of Louis that worsens with any movement of the associated shoulder. If the clavicle is dislocated, then the bone will jut out of the chest wall at the angle of Louis. This emphasizes the importance of checking the entire shoulder when examining the patient. The sprained SC joint should be treated like a clavicle fracture, with a figure-eight wrap and ice.

Sprained Thumb

Force applied laterally to the thumb can injure the ulnar collateral ligament (UCL). The sprained UCL, also called "gamekeeper's thumb" (named for an injury that occurred to gamekeepers when they dispatched a rabbit) or "skier's thumb" (for injuries that occur when a skier falls while grasping the ski pole), connects to the base of the thumb and leads to instability of the metacarpophalangeal (MCP) joint.[2] Weakness in the MCP causes pain and weakness when using a pincher grasp.

Twisted Knee

The knee is a complex joint consisting of four main ligaments—the anterior cruciate, posterior cruciate, lateral collateral ligaments, and the medial collateral ligament. These ligaments help to hold the knee together and stabilize the joint. Although all of these ligaments are at risk of being injured, the anterior cruciate ligament (ACL) may be the most commonly injured.

The ACL connects the femur to the tibia. Without it, the tibia would move forward, off the femur, and create a dislocated knee, which is discussed shortly. Therefore, the ACL is critical to knee stability so that the patient's knee does not "give out."

The other commonly injured ligament is the medial collateral ligament (MCL). This ligament, found inside the knee and also running from the femur to the tibia, is responsible for keeping the knee "together." An MCL injury is divided into three grades. Grade I is an incomplete tear that is generally not debilitating. Grade II is also incomplete, but the patient with this grade complains of pain when the knee is twisted (i.e., trying to pivot). Grade II injuries require rest and rehabilitation. Grade III MCL tears are complete, requiring the use of a knee brace and perhaps even surgery.

Knee sprains often involve injuries to the ACL, MCL, and the knee's meniscus. Knee sprains occur during activities that require twisting of the knee, such as sports like basketball or football; during recreation, such as skiing; or during heavy lifting with twisting. Female athletes have a much higher incidence of sprained knees than their male counterparts.

Patients with a twisted knee may complain of sudden pain in the knee and an associated "pop" sound that is immediately followed by instability of the joint, often causing the patient to sit down and flex the knee. Swelling of the knee is immediate and can be impressive.

There is a simple test to check for ACL injuries. While the knee is flexed at approximately 90 degrees, the Paramedic grasps the tibia with both hands, thumbs proximal to the knee and parallel to the tibia, and gently pulls forward. The patient with an ACL injury will experience pain; this is called the anterior draw test. (The assumption is that a fracture has been ruled out.)

Twisted Ankle

Ankle injuries are common and typically consist of a combination of ligamentous sprain and soft-tissue injury. Swelling compounds the injury. Unfortunately, ankle injuries have a tendency to reoccur, secondary to ligament laxity following injury.[3,4]

The most common etiology for ankle sprains is sports, which account for 81% of reported ankle sprains based on one study.[5,6] Whether due to recreational activities such as ice skating, sports such as cross-country running, or trauma from falls or simply walking on icy sidewalks, the ankle is prone to injury.

The ankle is a hinged synovial joint that provides approximately 100 degrees of flexion; the other movements are owed to other joints, making forward motion possible. The ankle proper consists of the talus and fibula, which form a mortise. The joint is also strengthened by a five-way intersection of ligaments. The posterior inferior tibiofibular ligament, coupled with the anterior tibiofibular ligament, provides plantar flexion and dorsiflexion. The posterior talofibular ligament (PTFL), coupled with the anterior talofibular ligament (ATFL) that runs in front of the lateral malleolus, provides lateral stabilization. The final ligament in the ankle is the calcaneofibular ligament (CFL) that runs from the distal fibula to the calcaneous along the lateral malleolus.

Inversion, the most common injury-causing event, results in injury to the last three ligaments, particularly the anterior talofibular ligament, and lateral failure of the ankle.[7]

The patient with a twisted ankle will complain of a sudden pain upon inversion of the ankle (i.e., "rolling the ankle"). Typically, the point of maximal tenderness will be proximal to the lateral malleolus. There should not be any hard projections or crepitus in the area, as these may suggest a fracture. Squeezing the posterior calf at the midshaft should not elicit pain. If it does, then a syndesmosis injury should be suspected. The presence of swelling and ecchymosis should thus lead the Paramedic to suspect a ruptured ligament.

Ankle sprains are categorized into one of three grades. The key to a grade I sprain is that the patient is often walking on the ankle. A grade II sprain has a moderate degree

of swelling and some instability of the ankle, making walking without assistance difficult. Pain is worse when one bears weight on the ankle, and the patient should not be permitted to ambulate for fear of making a partial tear of the ligament complete. A grade III sprain is a complete tear of the ligament, leading to full instability of the ankle. Without the support of the ligaments, the ankle must be supported by splint to prevent further damage.[8]

High Ankle Sprain

Along the anterior ankle is the syndesmotic ligament that joins the tibia and fibula together. An injury to this ligament, sometimes called a high ankle sprain, is a form of inversion injury. These high ankle sprains occur when the foot is planted, as if to turn, and forcefully externally rotated. Although the ankle proper remains intact, the ligaments above the ankle are injured, and thus destabilize the ankle. Subsequently, the ankle fails.

The patient with a high ankle sprain complains of a dull ache at the shin and severe pain with rotation of the ankle. However, palpation of the structures at the ankle, and specifically the lateral malleolus, does not elicit pain. The squeeze test, mentioned earlier, may be helpful in differentiating an ankle sprain from a high ankle sprain.

Like all sprains, a syndesmosis may avulse bone from either the tibia or the fibula, or both. A high ankle sprain typically needs surgical intervention and placement of a syndesmosis screw.

Midfoot Sprain

The foot is a highly complex structure, formed by 26 bones with 57 articulations and numerous ligaments and tendons. The foot bends at the midfoot because of five tarsometatarsal (TMT) joints and the Lisfranc ligament that helps to support that movement, particularly along the axis of the heel to the great toe.

A force applied along the TMT can injure the Lisfranc ligament, resulting in a midfoot sprain and, with bone movement, a Lisfranc fracture/dislocation. These injuries can occur in equestrian sports when a rider falls with his ankle in the stirrups, among gymnasts on their dismount,[10] with a ballet dancer "en pointe," and with sprinters coming out of the blocks, to name a few mechanisms of injury.[11]

Dependent on the injury's severity (i.e., sprain, dislocation, or fracture), the patient may or may not have pain.

However, almost all patients have pain when they bear weight on the foot. The Paramedic should examine the foot's planter surface for ecchymosis and swelling. Palpation of the arch should elicit pain as well as motion of the toes.[12]

STREET SMART

A driver whose foot slips off the brake during an MVC can experience a midfoot sprain. These drivers are seen limping on-scene and complain of pain "at the bottom of the feet."

Tendon Rupture

Tendons are tough, fibrous, connective tissue that is capable of sustaining forces many times the body's weight. However, every tissue has its breaking point, and when the tendon reaches that point it ruptures. Owing to the great amount of force that is required, four tendons—each in a position of great stress—tend to rupture: the biceps, quadriceps, patellar, and Achilles tendons.

Tendons will tend to rupture if there is direct trauma, eccentric loading, muscle degeneration secondary to changes of aging, or previous steroid injection in the area due to previous injury. Also, certain fluoroquinolone antibiotics have also been implicated in tendon rupture. Medications in the "statin" family have also been associated with tendon rupture; it is thought that many statins interfere with the repair of microtears, leading to weakness and catastrophic rupture.[13]

STREET SMART

The elderly are prone to rotator cuff injury and associated biceps tendon degeneration. Coupled with muscular degeneration, a change related to aging, the elderly patient is at risk for tendon biceps rupture from seemingly minor trauma. Often these patients complain of shoulder ache more than shoulder pain.

Biceps Tendon Rupture

The biceps brachii, located in the upper arm, is often ruptured due to excessive loading with lifting (i.e., weightlifting or eccentric movements), particularly with a load in the arm. The vast majority of these ruptures are of the proximal biceps tendon, over the humeral head, and at the insertion into the scapula.

When the tendon ruptures, the patient experiences a sudden sharp pain along the anterior shoulder along with an audible pop. Inspection of the anterior shoulder may reveal a hollow space, creating the "Popeye" look (Figure 7-2).

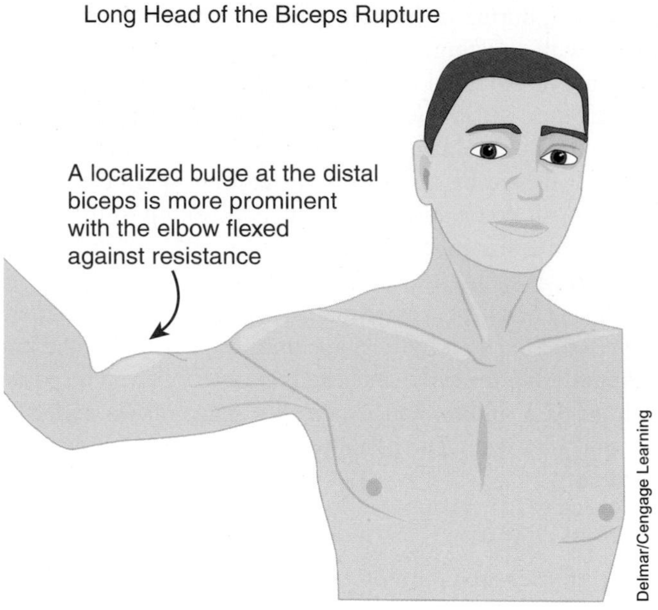
Long Head of the Biceps Rupture
A localized bulge at the distal biceps is more prominent with the elbow flexed against resistance
Delmar/Cengage Learning

Figure 7-2 Biceps tendon rupture may be indicated by a sudden pain and an audible pop.

Quadriceps Tendon Rupture

Although quadriceps tendon rupture is rare, it can be devastating. This disabling injury usually occurs during eccentric contracture in which the muscle is being forced to lengthen during contraction (such as springing up from a fall) or due to direct trauma. The incidence of quadriceps tendon rupture may be increasing due to obesity.[14] Both quadriceps tendon rupture and patellar tendon rupture tend to occur more frequently in the face of connective tissue disorders such as systemic lupus erythematosus (SLE) or steroid use/abuse.

Quadriceps tendon rupture often occurs in men (8:1) over the age of 40, secondary to degenerative changes.[15] Problems of nutrition, secondary to diabetes, and decreased blood flow have been implicated in tendon degeneration. Other conditions also implicated are chronic renal failure, hyperthyroidism, and gout.

The patient may state that the "knee gave out" following a fall. The patient may have acute pain proximal to the knee and complain of difficulty with ambulation. The Paramedic may appreciate suprapatellar swelling with defect in the painful area, so the Paramedic should compare the swollen knee with the opposite knee. The patient may be able to flex the leg but will be unable to extend it.

If the patient is ambulatory, the Paramedic may observe that the patient is walking with the hip elevated (i.e., "hitched") and the knee "locked" as the leg is "swung through." The patient in this condition will be unable to climb stairs.

Although conservative treatment (i.e., immobilization) is acceptable in minor cases of partial tendon tear, in most cases surgical repair within 48 hours is usually required (Figure 7-3).

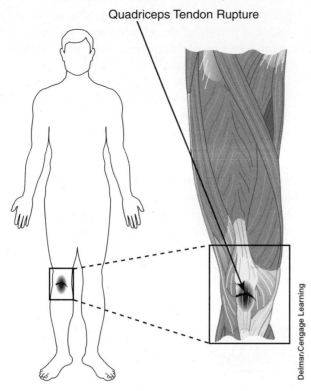

Quadriceps Tendon Rupture

Delmar/Cengage Learning

Figure 7-3 Quadriceps tendon rupture is rare, but can be devastating.

Patellar Tendon Rupture

Patellar tendon rupture is the extreme of patellar tendinopathy. Tendinopathy of the patellar tendon is thought to be due to repetitive stress on the knees. For this reason, patellar tendinopathy has earned the nickname of "jumper's knees." Any athletic endeavor, such as basketball or volleyball, in which the athlete lands with feet planted and knee flexed is a likely cause of this injury. Unlike the quadriceps tendon rupture, patellar tendon rupture tends to occur to those under the age of 40.[16]

Like those with a quadriceps tendon rupture, patients with a patellar tendon rupture complain of anterior knee pain. However, unlike the quadriceps tendon rupture, the patient cannot relate the injury to a specific event. Instead, there is a series of events (i.e., basketball game) after which the discomfort begins. And unlike the quadriceps tendon rupture, the patient generally maintains a full range of motion.

The Paramedic should be aware that there are a number of patellofemoral joint complaints, some related to patellar tendon sprain/rupture. Collectively referred to as **patellofemoral joint syndrome**, it is thought to affect as many as 25% of athletes. The patellofemoral joint syndrome is characterized by knee pain that often involves athleticism, such as sports, hiking, or even repetitive deep knee bends. In cases in which the pain is associated with trauma, the Paramedic should consider fractures: patellar fractures, distal femoral fractures, and proximal tibia fractures, which are discussed shortly.

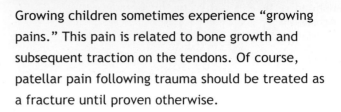
Achilles Tendon Rupture

Achilles, the ancient Greek warrior, was allegedly invulnerable, except for his heel. Like the warrior of the past, an Achilles tendon rupture can stop a weekend warrior playing recreational sports dead in his tracks, unable to push off the injured leg to walk. The Achilles tendon (i.e., tendon calcaneus), the largest tendon in the body, is found at the end of the gastrocnemius muscle in the calf and inserts into the calcaneus. This ropelike tendon is vital for running, climbing stairs, and so on.

An Achilles tendon is difficult to rupture as it can take an estimated peak load of six to eight times the person's body weight.[17] However, direct trauma, such as stepping into a hole or falling from a height, can rupture the Achilles tendon. Patients at risk for an Achilles tendon rupture may have degenerative changes of age (30 to 50) along with a sudden increase in intensity of athleticism (seen in the weekend warrior). The specific biomechanical event is usually a sudden twisting off, midline force applied during dorsiflexion, or a forced plantar flexion (i.e., push off).

Those individuals at risk for Achilles tendon rupture are those on corticosteroids and patients with diabetes that results in peripheral vascular insufficiency, specifically of the posterior tibial artery.[18] Patients will describe a sharp pain in the back of the lower leg, as if they were shot in the back of the leg, and hearing a "pop." Walking is immediately painful.

The Paramedic may note the patient has a tender, swollen, and ecchymotic calf with a depression that can be palpated about two inches above calcaneus. With the patient prone, the Paramedic squeezes the calf. Normally, there is passive plantar flexion. If the Achilles tendon is ruptured, there is not; this is called the Thompson test.

Surgery to repair the ruptured Achilles tendon is possible. Although surgery has a higher complication rate, it also has a lower re-rupture rate (Figure 7-4).[19]

Dislocations

Joints have a range of motion that is part of their functionality. If the joint is moved beyond its normal limits, injury occurs. Under the general rubric of disarticulation (the separation of a joint), there are two subcategories. A **subluxation** is a misalignment of bones in a joint that results in the joint's instability, sometimes called a partial dislocation. A luxation, or **dislocation**, is the complete movement of the bone out of

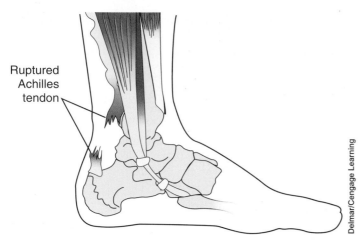

Ruptured
Achilles
tendon

Delmar/Cengage Learning

Figure 7-4 A ruptured Achilles tendon can occur from direct trauma to the area.

the joint. The resulting disarticulation of the joint results in loss of range of motion as well as concurrent tendon and ligament damage.

Dislocated Shoulder

The shoulder is a ball-and-socket joint formed by the humerus where it inserts in the glenoid fossa of the scapula. As a shallow socket, it provides for a great range of motion but at a loss of stability. As discussed in the section on shoulder sprains, static and dynamic stabilizers hold the shoulder together. This includes 15 muscles and ligaments, specifically the anteroinferior glenohumeral ligament.

Any force—be it lateral, inferior, or anterior—can lead to a dislocated shoulder. However, the most common dislocations, in some 95% to 98% of cases, are anterior dislocations. Anterior dislocations can occur as a result of a direct blow from behind, driving the shoulder forward while distracting forces pull on the limb, or from a fall on an outstretched hand. Sports implicated in shoulder dislocations include swimming and tennis. A small percentage of patients, usually older patients, have atraumatic dislocations. Their shoulders dislocate during movement in their sleep.

Patients with a shoulder dislocation tend to experience many more subsequent shoulder dislocations as a result of anterior glenohumeral instability. This occurs in as many as 70% of the cases.[20] This history is often confirmed by the patient's apprehension to placing the arm in abduction with extension and external rotation (i.e., the position of a pitcher throwing a ball).

The patient with a dislocated shoulder will be guarding the shoulder, holding it in slight abduction and externally rotated, and complaining of pain in the affected shoulder. In most cases, the patient will report a single traumatic event or a history of dislocations.

The physical examination will reveal a hollow below the acromion, flattening of the deltoid, and the prominence of the head of the humerus along the anterior aspect of the upper shoulder. The shoulder will also have a "squared off" appearance.

Some patients may describe the "dead-arm syndrome," a pain-induced paresis of the affected arm. The patient will complain of heaviness and numbness in the affected limb and an inability to hold an object.[21]

As in all cases of musculoskeletal injury, the Paramedic should assess distal pulses, bilaterally, for quality of pulse. Similarly, he should assess distal neurological function. Some 8% to 10% of patients with an anterior dislocation had axillary nerve involvement resulting in numbness over the lateral upper arm. Similarly, wrist and elbow extension, as well as paresthesia to the dorsum of the hand, should be assessed for possible radial nerve involvement.

Reduction of a shoulder dislocation, discussed shortly, should be reserved for limb-threatening emergencies. It is estimated that a compression fracture of the humeral head, called a Hill–Sachs lesion, is seen in as many as 50% of patients with an anterior dislocation, particularly in younger patients, and 88% of patients with recurrent dislocations (Figure 7-5).

STREET SMART

Recurrent anterior shoulder dislocations are often the result of an avulsion of the anteroinferior glenoid ligament (i.e., Bankart lesion). The resulting injury creates a "tear" in the rotator cuff and the labrum, which permits the humerus to dislocate more easily. A "soft-tissue repair" is the correction of a Bankart lesion.

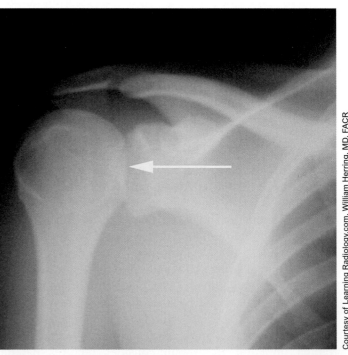

Courtesy of Learning Radiology.com, William Herring, MD, FACR

Figure 7-5 A Hill–Sachs lesion is seen in as many as 50% of patients with an anterior dislocation.

Elbow Dislocation

The elbow can dislocate from a fall on outstretched hand (FOOSH) or if the patient falls on the point of the elbow. The elbow is especially prone to dislocation when the forearm is partially flexed, driving the radius and ulna backwards. An elbow dislocation can occur during participation in sports, such as gymnastics, rollerblading, or skateboarding. In fact, some 50% of elbow dislocations occur in sports. In 90% of the cases, the dislocation is posterior. An elbow dislocation is the most common dislocation in children.[22]

Because the elbow is largely stabilized by bone, instead of ligaments, elbow dislocations are often associated with fractures. The medial epicondyle is the most common fracture, although the radial neck may also be fractured. Because of the nature of the dislocation, the Paramedic should assess an associated injury/fracture of the distal wrist. Also, as most people fall with both hands outstretched, the opposite elbow and wrist should also be examined for injury/fracture (Figure 7-6).

The patient usually complains loudly about the pain and the injury is obvious. Examination of the affected limb will show an exaggerated prominence of olecranon and a shortened forearm.

The elbow has two compartments. A posterior dislocation may damage the anterior compartment, which contains a neurovascular bundle consisting of the ulnar/median nerve and the brachial artery. Injury to the ulnar nerve, particularly if the medial epicondyle of the humerus is fractured, will result in loss of touch to the fourth and fifth digit.[23] Both the median and ulnar nerve motor function can be tested by having the patient touch the thumb, innervated by the median nerve, with the fifth finger, innervated by the ulnar nerve.

Nursemaid's Elbow

The Paramedic may be called to assess a child who "refuses to move his arm" in which the caregivers adamantly deny any trauma. This is the classic presentation of "nursemaid's elbow," a form of radial subluxation with a tear of the annular ligament.[24] The atraumatic dislocation is usually due to axial traction applied to the child's outreached arm (Figure 7-7). Typical mechanisms of injury include lifting the child by the arm over an obstacle, spinning a child around by the arms, pulling a child back when the child pulls away, and pulling a child's arm through the sleeve of a coat.

Nursemaid's elbow typically affects children between ages 1 to 4, who may be apprehensive when the Paramedic asks to examine the arm. The child will present with the forearm flexed at a 15- to 20-degree angle and slightly pronated. The Paramedic may appreciate some swelling in the elbow and note some point tenderness at the head of the radius, proximal to the elbow. The child will have difficulty bending, or refuse to bend, the elbow. As it is impossible to rule out a radial head fracture, the Paramedic should treat suspected nursemaid's elbow as though it was a radial head fracture and splint the arm in the position found. Fortunately, the immediate danger of neurovascular compromise, and therefore the need to reduce the fracture in the field, is extremely low.[25]

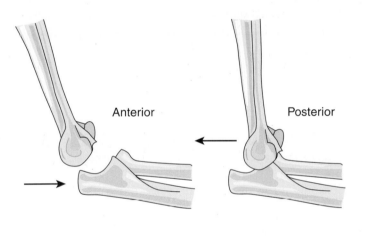

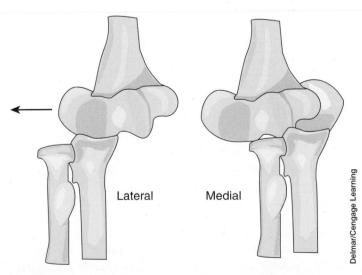

Figure 7-6 A dislocated elbow can occur from a fall on an outstretched hand or landing on the point of the elbow.

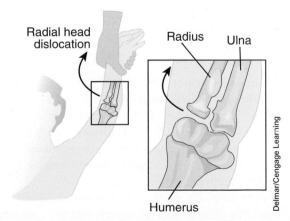

Figure 7-7 Nursemaid's elbow is a form of radial subluxation with a tear of the annular ligament.

Hip Dislocation

The femur is firmly held in place by five strong ligaments, making a hip dislocation unlikely. However, because of the high morbidity associated with a hip fracture, Paramedics need to be able to identify and treat the hip dislocation.

The etiology of most hip dislocations is either direct trauma, such as from a motor vehicle collision, or sports-related issues. In sports, about 90% of hip dislocations are posterior hip dislocations. The exception is found in skiers and snowboarders, in which case the majority of dislocations are anterior.[26]

The biomechanics of a hip dislocation in sports are a large force striking the knee, such as when it falls on the ground, while the hip is flexed, forcing the hip posterior. This mechanism of injury might be seen in a "pile on" during a scrimmage. Alternatively, anterior hip dislocations occur when the femur is abducted at such an angle that, when a force is applied to it, the hip comes out of joint. Rotational forces involved in a fall during skiing make this scenario more likely.

Traumatic hip dislocations are generally created when a force is applied along the axis of the femur. The mechanism of injury in this case can be a motor vehicle collision in which the seated occupant, with knees flexed, slides forward, striking the knee against the dashboard and transmitting the force down the axis of the femur. Alternatively, the driver could be "standing on the brake," locking the knees. When the foot strikes the floorboard, the forces are transmitted along the axis of the femur, creating a posterior hip dislocation.

STREET SMART

The use of seat belts and development of airbags has markedly decreased the incidence of hip dislocations in motor vehicle collisions. However, when a hip dislocation does occur, the patient will be unable to get out of the car on his or her own power. Extrication of the patient often requires heavy rescue to cut the car away from the patient.

Focused injury along the axis of the femur can cause an isolated hip dislocation. Because of the large amount of force needed to dislocate a hip, associated injuries, such as pelvic fractures, often accompany a hip dislocation. A hip dislocation is a surgical emergency. Studies have shown more morbidity when there is an increased time between the injury and reduction of the hip.[27]

The Paramedic's suspicion of a hip dislocation is first based on the mechanism of injury and an understanding of kinematics and biomechanics. When approaching the patient, the Paramedic may appreciate that the patient is immobile (a dislocated hip prevents the patient from rising). The patient often complains loudly of pain in the pelvis and the lower back, particularly if it is a posterior dislocation. After assessing for life-threatening injuries, the Paramedic can focus on the patient's hip. With a posterior hip dislocation, the leg will be flexed, adducted, and internally rotated. The Paramedic should expose the entire hip to examine for a hematoma, a sign of vascular injury, even though vascular injuries generally only occur with anterior hip dislocations. Next, the Paramedic should examine any evidence of sciatic nerve involvement, such as loss of sensation to the posterior leg. Simple dorsiflexion may also reveal injury to the sciatic nerve.

Potential complications of posterior hip dislocations include sciatic nerve involvement. Studies have suggested up to 20% of posterior hip dislocations are complicated by sciatic nerve injury. Open traumatic hip dislocations have high infection rates with 50% mortality. Other complications include deep vein thrombus, secondary to prolonged immobilization, and avascular necrosis (AVN) of the femoral head. The time to reduction is critical in reducing the risk of AVN of the femoral head. The development of AVN can lead to long-term disability secondary to post-traumatic osteoarthritis. Over one-half of patients with a hip dislocation will have chronic pain due to post-traumatic osteoarthritis and/or limited use of the hip following a hip dislocation.

STREET SMART

Some infants are born with a developmental dislocation of the hip (DDH). Breech birth is thought to account for some 25% to 45% of cases. With the hips and knees at 90 degrees, the hip is brought through a passive range of motion. A click sound is heard when the hip is replaced. A Pavlik harness is used to treat DDH or, postoperatively, a short leg spica cast may be used.

Patellar Dislocation

The patella, the largest sesamoid bone in the body, is the bony prominence noted on the distal anterior thigh. The patella is actually part of an elaborate network of ligaments, the quadriceps muscle, and other soft tissue. The patella, acting as a pulley and a lever, is key to a kinetic energy chain that permits forward locomotion. Disruptions of that kinetic energy chain can be devastating to the patient's ability to walk.

The patella has both dynamic and static stabilizers that hold the patella in place. When these ligaments are injured, the patella becomes unstable and prone to dislocation. Patellar dislocations can be either acute, as the result of trauma, or chronic, as a result of patellofemoral syndrome. In acute patellar dislocations, traumatic forces—direct trauma or sudden change in direction—cause sprains of these ligaments as well as soft-tissue damage. Acute patellar dislocations occur in almost all sports, such as with weightlifters, distance runners, and swimmers.[28]

Patellar injuries are common, as 35% of all knee injuries involve the patella.[29] With an acute patellar dislocation, the patient feels a sudden pain, as the femur rotates over the tibia, and the "knee gives out." Subsequently, there is rapid swelling, tightness of hamstrings and quadriceps, and pain with flexion.

Upon inspection, the Paramedic will note the laterally displaced patella (Figure 7-8). The patella is normally kept midline, in part, by the MCL, which prevents lateral movement. When the MCL is disrupted, the patella can become displaced. Among patellar dislocations, 97% are lateral. Patients with recurrent patella dislocations may attempt reduction by moving the leg from flexion to extension. The patella can then be observed to move in a J track back into the patellar groove.

Generalized complaints of knee pain, in the absence of trauma, are suggestive of patellofemoral joint syndromes. Patients with patellofemoral joint syndrome may complain of pain from the hips to the shins, a joint pain line that represents the place of the patella in the kinetic energy chain.

Patients with patellofemoral joint syndrome will variously describe the pain as ranging from dull and achy to sharp and shooting. The pain tends to focus around the knee and the patella and the leg feels like it is about to "give out." The key differences between acute dislocation and patellofemoral joint syndrome is the lack of localized swelling and a midline patella.

Knee Dislocation

Unlike the kneecap dislocation (patellar dislocation), the knee dislocation is a surgical emergency. A knee dislocation occurs with the displacement of the tibia and femur, during which all three major ligaments are disrupted. With an unstable knee, the neurovascular bundle in the popliteal space is at risk. As a result of lacerations of the popliteal artery (a limb-threatening event), the lower leg becomes ischemic, sometimes resulting in amputation. Complicating matters, a dislocated knee is often associated with multitrauma and other life-threatening injuries. Fortunately, it is estimated that 50% of knee dislocations spontaneously reduce before the patient's arrival at the trauma center, allowing the Paramedic to tend to life-threatening emergencies.[30]

A knee dislocation can occur as a result of large forces applied in any of five directions (i.e., anterior, posterior, lateral, medial, or rotational). Examples of mechanisms of injury include striking the tibia on the dashboard in an MVC (posterior) or hyperextension of the knee during a fall (anterior). The result is sprains of both the cruciate ligaments as well as one or both collateral ligaments.

The patient with a knee dislocation will present with severe leg pain and an obvious "step off" that shows the femur is not aligned with the tibia and fibula (Figure 7-9). The Paramedic's focus should be to assess distal neurovascular function. It is estimated that as many as 80% of knee

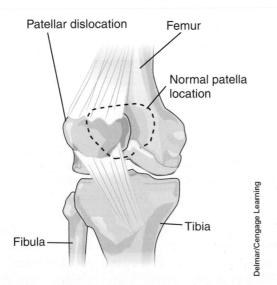

Figure 7-8 Almost all patellar dislocations are lateral.

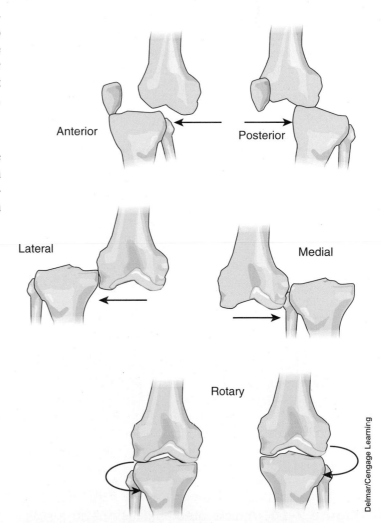

Figure 7-9 Knee dislocation can occur as a result of large forces applied in any of five directions.

dislocations will have vascular compromise, typically involving the popliteal artery, and as many as 40% of patients will have nerve injury, typically involving the peroneal nerve. If the popliteal artery is damaged, the Paramedic may note a stocking-like distal cyanosis, absent pedal pulses, and a cool extremity.[31] If the peroneal nerve, a branch of the sciatic nerve, is damaged, the patient will experience pain along the shin, dorsal foot, and foot–drop.

Ankle Dislocation

An ankle dislocation is not a dislocation of just one joint but any one of 57 articulations. An ankle dislocation is more often than not associated with multiple bone fractures as well.

An ankle can dislocate in any of the four axes: posterior, superior, anterior, and lateral. A lateral ankle dislocation is the result of a forced eversion/inversion. In a major MVC, the driver can sustain a lateral ankle dislocation when the foot slips off the brake. An anterior ankle dislocation occurs when the foot is fixed, as when someone steps into a hole, and a posterior force is applied to the tibia (i.e., when the body falls backwards). The ankle can also dislocate superiorly, when a force drives the talus upward, such as what would occur in a fall. However, the most common ankle dislocation is a posterior dislocation, when the talus is forced backward and is often accompanied with a fracture at the lateral malleolus.[32]

In every example, the dislocated ankle will be deformed and the Paramedic may note significant edema (Figure 7-10).

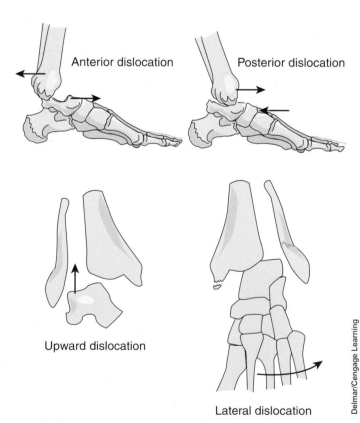

Anterior dislocation

Posterior dislocation

Upward dislocation

Lateral dislocation

Delmar/Cengage Learning

Figure 7-10 A dislocated ankle is not a dislocation of just one joint but any one of 57 articulations.

The patient will complain of pain and point tenderness at the ankle. Therefore, the Paramedic should closely examine the ankle for broken skin, which suggests an open fracture. The skin in the ankle is relatively thin and is easily interrupted. Malleoli tenting, raised skin in the area of the dislocation, helps to confirm ankle dislocation. The distal foot should be examined for evidence of neurovascular compromise.[33] Specifically, the posterior tibial artery, posterior to the medial malleolus, should be identified as well as the anterior tibial artery, which becomes the dorsalis pedis artery. Nerves at risk include the deep peroneal, which is proximal to the dorsalis pedis and innervates the great toe, and the tibial nerve, which enters the foot next to the posterior tibia and becomes the sural nerve innervating the lateral foot and little toe.

Fractures

Classification of Fractures

Although a **fracture** is simply a broken bone, there is nothing simple about a fracture. Fractures can occur because of either direct force or an indirect force. Furthermore, a direct force can either be applied to a local area or applied over a large area. Examples of a focused direct force are a small force applied to a localized area, such as a nightstick fracture of the ulna, or a distributed direct force, such as a crushing injury of the femur during a building collapse. Direct force can result in a simple fracture (i.e., a single break) or comminuted fractures, where there are multiple breaks.

An indirect force is a result of the application of a tensile force, which is a shearing, bending, compressive, or torsion force to the bone along or across its axis. A tensile force typically produces a transverse fracture in which the bone is literally distracted into two halves. The opposite force, a compressive force, often results in either a simple fracture or a comminuted fracture. Torsional forces create a simple fracture called a spiral fracture, whereas bending creates a simple fracture that is either transverse or an oblique fracture.

The energy involved in the trauma also impacts the degree and type of fracture. A high-energy mechanism tends to result in fragmentation of the bone (i.e., a comminuted fracture) and a large amount of soft-tissue injury, whereas low-energy mechanisms tend to cause a displaced fracture. Displaced fractures heal faster, with quicker callus formation and stabilization of the fracture and union/remodeling of the bone.

Fractures are also classified as closed, meaning the bones remain within the limb, or open, meaning that the skin has been breeched. That breech can be internal, from bone ends, or external, such as from a gunshot wound (GSW).

The amount of soft-tissue damage has implications for the patient. A classification system called the **Gustilo–Anderson system**, based on the amount of soft-tissue injury, is used for prognosis of fracture healing, risk of infection, and probability of amputation.

A type I open fracture consists of a wound that is less than 1 cm in length, has minimal soft-tissue damage, and is considered a clean wound. A type I open fracture is usually the result of a simple transverse or short oblique fracture and has a good prognosis for healing with little chance of infection or probability of amputation.

A type II open fracture consists of a wound that is greater than 1 cm in length and moderate soft-tissue damage. Often, the mechanism of injury is not the bone from within but a penetrating projectile, such as a gunshot wound. The result is necrotic tissue in the vicinity of the fracture that impairs fracture healing.

A type III open fracture involves extensive devitalization of the surrounding muscles and widespread wounds that may require a skin flap. These wounds are seen in mass casualty incidents, such as tornados, farm injuries (power-takeoff trauma, in particular), and high-velocity gunshot wounds, or short range shotgun blasts. These wounds often have associated neuromuscular trauma as well as vascular injury. In many cases, limb salvage is not possible and life-saving amputation is the only option.[34]

Fractures may be classified as complete or incomplete. Both comminuted fractures and all of the variations of a displaced fracture (i.e., oblique, transverse, and spiral) can be complete fractures. An example of an incomplete fracture is a greenstick fracture. Pediatric bones, being more elastic, tend not to break but rather splinter, hence the name "greenstick fracture." However, any type of fracture can be incomplete. Careful management of the injury prevents the incomplete fracture from becoming a complete fracture (Figure 7-11).

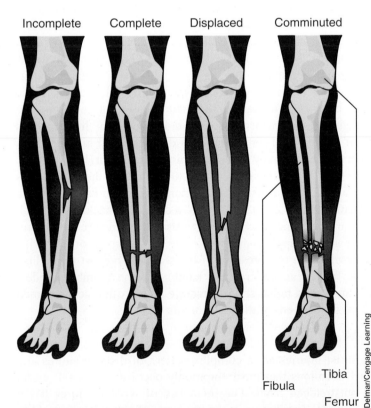

Incomplete   Complete   Displaced   Comminuted

Tibia
Fibula
Femur

Figure 7-11 Types of fractures include incomplete, complete, displaced, and comminuted.

Osteoporosis

Bone health and bone density are due, in part, to adequate amounts of calcium, the presence of vitamin D, and parathyroid hormones. Deficiencies of any of these three can lead to osteoporosis, a condition in which the bone mineral density is diminished and the bone is therefore weaker. Osteoporosis is a common cause, or contributing factor, in fractures—especially atraumatic fractures, sometimes called fragility fractures. A fragility fracture occurs with a trauma that will not normally cause a fracture (e.g., a fracture from a standing position onto the floor).

Osteoporosis can be divided into two classifications. Type I, post-menopausal osteoporosis, is the result of loss of estrogen, which accelerates bone loss. Type II, called senile osteoporosis, is a function of an aging skeleton and conditions of aging such as decreased kidney function, hypoparathyroidism, and digestive tract malabsorption.

The Paramedic should suspect osteoporosis if the patient is elderly (i.e., over 70 years of age), has kyphosis (Dowager's hump), and is slight of build, suggestive of the wasting of aging.

Osteoporosis has been implicated in atraumatic hip fractures. The risk of death within one year following a hip fracture increases by 10% to 20%. Only one-third of patients will return to their normal level of activity, and as many as 50% of these patients will be rehabilitated in a nursing home.[35]

Pediatric Fractures

Paramedics should be concerned about a special type of fracture that is specific to the pediatric population: a fracture of the growth plate. The growth plate, found at the interface of the metaphysis and the epiphysis, is where bone growth occurs. It is also the bone's anatomic weak point. A fracture of that growth plate, called a physeal fracture, disrupts bone growth.

Physeal fractures, or **Salter–Harris fractures**, are divided into five classifications according to the fracture's location. A type I Salter–Harris fracture is a transverse fracture between the metaphysis and epiphysis, the growth plate zone. A type II Salter–Harris fracture includes a type I fracture as well as a fracture of the metaphysis, whereas a type III fracture includes a type I fracture and a fracture of the epiphysis. A Salter–Harris type IV fracture includes types I, II, and III (i.e., complete separation of the metaphysis from the epiphysis) and fractures of both the metaphysis and epiphysis of the bone. Although a type III fracture can lead to permanent disability and a type IV fracture can lead to permanent bone deformity, a Salter–Harris type V is actually a compression fracture of the growth plate secondary to axial loading (Figure 7-12).[36]

Fractures of the Upper Extremities

The upper extremities include those bones in the appendicular skeleton found in the shoulder girdle. Because of the close approximation of these bones, any substantial energy applied

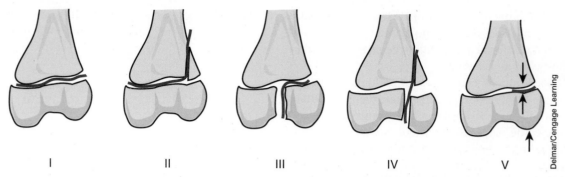

I II III IV V

Delmar/Cengage Learning

Figure 7-12 Salter–Harris fractures are divided into five classifications according to the fracture's location.

to one tends to be transmitted to all. Therefore, whenever a fracture is found, secondary to direct trauma, the Paramedic should suspect another fracture from indirect trauma.

Humeral Fractures

The humerus, found in the upper arm, is prone to fracture from direct trauma, such as a blow to the arm, or indirect trauma, such as a fall on an outstretched arm and subsequent axial loading. However, the humerus is a strong and pliable bone that resists fracture; in fact, 80% of proximal humerus fractures are simple transverse or oblique fractures.[37] The "classic" midshaft fracture (i.e., diaphyseal fracture) is more common in adults, whereas proximal humerus fractures are more common in the elderly.

Patients with a diaphyseal fracture may have deformity of the upper arm. Because of the proximity of the radial nerve to the humerus, those with a gross deformity of the humerus may concurrently develop radial nerve palsy. Wrist extension and abduction/extension of the thumb helps the Paramedic assess the motor function of the radial nerve.

Patients with proximal humeral fractures, particularly the elderly, may complain of shoulder pain and examination findings, swelling, and ecchymosis. These symptoms might lead the Paramedic to suspect a dislocated shoulder. For this reason, all dislocations should be treated as fractures.

Ulna Fracture

Three-quarters of ulnar fractures are distal fractures proximal to the wrist. In some cases, the ulnar fracture is associated with a dislocation of the radioulnar joint, called a **Monteggia's fracture**. This dislocation is owed to the close association of the radius and ulna; they even share a common interosseous membrane. Therefore, the Paramedic should suspect a "forearm" fracture even if the obvious deformity is to the ulna. This fracture/dislocation is seen in cases in which the patient falls forward onto a pronated outstretched hand (Figure 7-13).

Radial Fractures

Radial fractures can be divided into distal, mid-forearm, and proximal fractures. A radial head fracture is often the result of a fall onto an elbow. This occurs in 20% of elbow trauma. A suspected radial head fracture deserves a careful

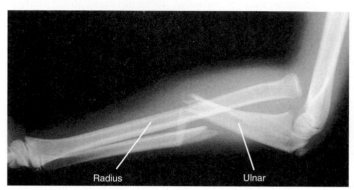

Radius   Ulnar

Image reprinted with permission from eMedicine.com, 2010

Figure 7-13 Nearly 75% of ulnar fractures are distal fractures proximal to the wrist.

neurovascular examination as all three major nerves of the forearm pass through the elbow and near the radial head. Because of this, radial nerve function is of particular concern.

A particular type of radial fracture, a midshaft radial fracture, is called Galeazzi's fracture. **Galeazzi's fracture** is the counterpart to Monteggia's fracture. Whereas Monteggia's fracture features an ulna fracture with dislocation of the radioulnar joint, Galeazzi's fracture features a fracture of the radius with a dislocation of the radioulnar joint. In both kinds of fracture, the forearm axis is disturbed and biomechanics are altered, thereby preventing pronosupination (Figure 7-14).

A classic distal radial fracture is called the Chauffeur's fracture. This fracture got its name from the days when the hand crank used to "kick over" a car would backfire and kick back, breaking the chauffeur's wrist.[38] The fracture is the result of a force applied directly to the radial aspect of the wrist, resulting in compression of the scaphoid against the radius. A fall on an outstretched hand, with the thumb extended, causes this radial styloid fracture and is often accompanied by dislocations of the metacarpals.

Wrist Fractures

Wrist injuries are a complex pattern of distal fractures and dislocations that most commonly occur due to a fall on an outstretched hand. The incidence of wrist fractures has a bimodal distribution at the extremes of age and a reversal in frequency by sex (i.e., youthful boys and elderly women are most susceptible).[39]

Conversely, if the patient falls onto a flexed hand, a "reverse Colles" or **Smith fracture** will occur. With volar displacement of the hand, there is an obvious intra-articular "step off" at the wrist.

Typically, either a Colles or Smith fracture can be treated nonsurgically with simple splinting.[40] However, the fracture can be complicated by interruption of the neurovascular bundle. Although all three of the nerves that innervate the hand pass through the wrist, the median nerve is most commonly injured. An injury to the median nerve is like an acute attack of carpel tunnel syndrome with sensory disturbance from the thumb to the index finger.

Carpal Fractures

The cuboidal-shaped carpel bones lie in two rows with eight bones each. The proximal row contains the scaphoid bone, known as the navicular bone, which is the most commonly fractured carpal bone. Although all of the carpal bones are prone to fracture, the scaphoid bone is most problematic. Unlike other carpal bones, the scaphoid bone has only one blood supply. Any complete fracture risks both nonunion, thereby making the wrist unstable, but also avascular necrosis in some 10% to 15% of cases (Figure 7-16).

The scaphoid bone tends to fracture when the patient falls on an outstretched hand (i.e., hyperextension). The patient with a scaphoid fracture will complain of pain in the wrist, proximal to the thumb. Palpation of the anatomic sniff box, the void proximal to the wrist at the base of the thumb, will elicit point tenderness in most cases. Any attempts at forced dorsiflexion will also elicit pain.

In some cases, the fracture is not apparent on the original radiograph, or is obscured by swelling. The patient later complains of loss of range of motion, an ache in the wrist, and pain in the hand whenever lifting or gripping an object.

Hamate Fracture

The hamate, a triangular carpal bone found in the wrist, is important for grasping clubs, racquets, and bats. The hamate

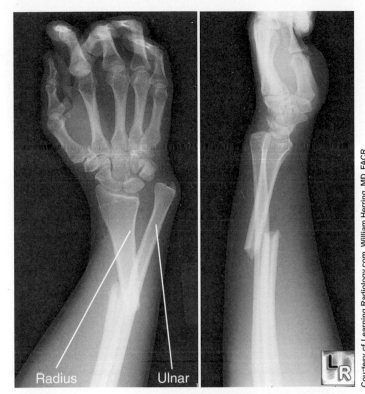

Figure 7-14 Radial fractures can be divided into distal, mid-forearm, and proximal fractures.

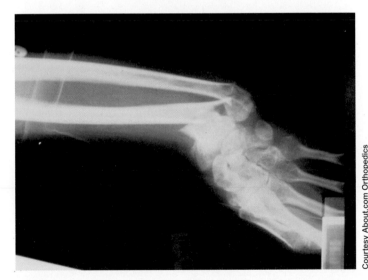

Figure 7-15 A Colles fracture is a distal radial fracture that produces a characteristic "silver fork" deformity.

In 1814, an Irish surgeon described a fracture of the wrist that was to later bear his name, the Colles fracture. A **Colles fracture** is a distal radial fracture that follows a fall on an outstretched hand, or an MVC in which the driver grabs the steering wheel. The resultant fracture produces a characteristic "silver fork" deformity (i.e., dorsal displacement of the hand above the plane of the forearm) (Figure 7-15). Some 50% of Colles fractures have associated ulnar fractures as well.

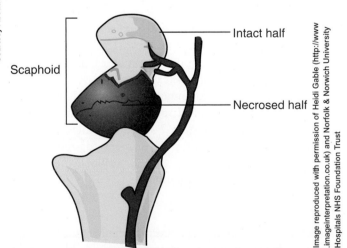

Figure 7-16 Avascular necrosis can occur with the scaphoid bone.

can be injured through repetitive swinging motions during sports using these implements (the circular projection called the hook is at particular risk).

The patient may complain of pain in the palm of his hand, often when gripping an object, but has no pain in his thumb. Although not a medical emergency, a patient may call EMS when tingling or numbness of the digits is experienced, secondary to ulnar nerve involvement.

Hand Injury

Fractures and dislocations of the fifth and/or fourth metacarpals are generally the result of a direct blow to the ulnar border of the hand, such as may happen when striking a solid object, like a wall, with a closed fist. Interestingly, although a fracture of the fifth metacarpal is dubbed a "boxer's fracture," modern boxers who wear boxing gloves seldom have this fracture.

The patient with a suspected boxer's fracture will have a painful, swollen hand with a loss of motion of the fifth finger. If the fracture has an associated dislocation, and many do, there may be a palpable "step off" as well. Classically, the patient will be unable to flex the finger toward the thumb, which indicates a loss of range of motion.

Generally, the hand should be immobilized in the position of function, with 20 to 30 degrees of extension at the wrist and 90 degrees of flexion at the finger. The splint should immobilize the entire forearm, with the volar aspect of the splint ending at the palmar crease.

Thumb Injury

The "opposable" thumb is critical to allow humans pinch and grasp. Injury to the thumb's joints, or the two phalanges therein, can impair the patient's ability to perform work or the activities of daily living. An injury to the thumb's carpometacarpal joint (CMC), also called a **Bennett's fracture**, can occur as a result of direct trauma or a fall on an outstretched hand with the thumb slightly flexed.

The patient with a thumb injury will complain of acute pain and loss of range of motion. It is not uncommon for the patient to guard the hand and to display apprehension when the Paramedic examines the thumb, as even the slightest stress on the thumb can produce pain and halt the patient's voluntary cooperation with the examination.

The Paramedic should immobilize the thumb in the position found, preferably with a spica-like splint that includes a gutter for the thumb (Figure 7-17). The patient should be transported to the emergency department for radiographic examination and consultation with an orthopaedic surgeon who may elect to "pin" the thumb.

Mallet Fracture

A common distal phalangeal injury is the mallet fracture. A **mallet fracture** occurs when something, like a baseball or basketball, strikes the end of the patient's finger, the distal finger is pushed beyond its normal range of motion

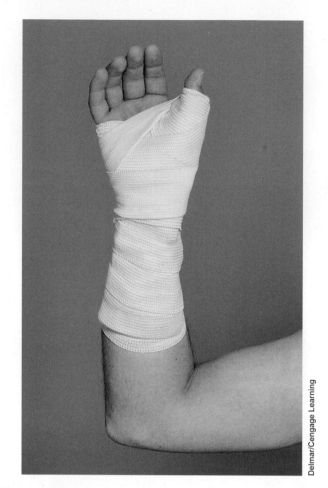

Figure 7-17 A spica-like splint includes a gutter for the thumb.

Delmar/Cengage Learning

(hyperflexed), and the extensor tendon is damaged. The "jammed finger" can be a minor injury (sprained finger) or so severe that the tendon avulses a piece of bone. The Paramedic should inspect under the nail bed, since blood under the nail bed, or a detached nail, is suggestive of an open fracture. In most cases, the finger is splinted with a dorsal aluminum splint or a commercially available plastic splint. The Paramedic should apply ice to the wound to reduce swelling.

Fractures of the Lower Extremities

Like the shoulder girdle, the bones of the lower extremities communicate through the pelvic girdle. Also like the shoulder girdle, direct trauma in one extremity can be transmitted to the entire girdle and create indirect trauma. Generally speaking, it takes a great deal more force to fracture bones in the pelvic girdle than the shoulder girdle. For this reason, there may be more soft-tissue damage and hemorrhage associated with a lower extremity fracture.

Pelvic Fracture

The pelvis (pelvic ring, consisting of three bones) is held together at the sacroiliac (SI) joints posteriorly and the pubis symphysis anteriorly by ligaments. Within this ring are many

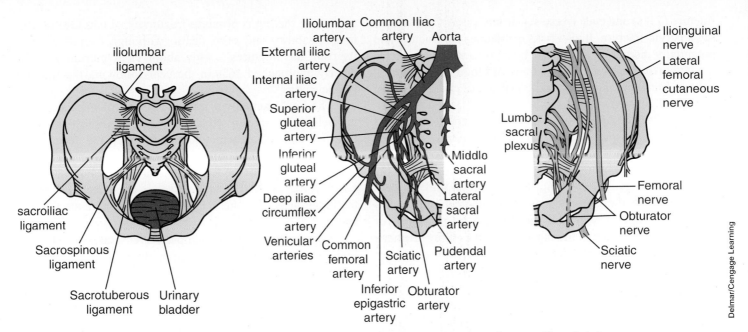

Figure 7-18 Structures of the pelvic girdle include the pelvic ring and sacroiliac joints.

major blood vessels such as the common iliac artery that gives rise to the internal and external iliac arteries, as well as the sciatic nerve. Also housed within the pelvis are the organs of the genitourinary system (Figure 7-18).

Pelvic fractures can be divided into stable fractures (fracture of one of two arches with or without associated fractures of the femurs) and unstable fractures (involves both arches and is the result of great force). About two-thirds of pelvic fractures are stable fractures. Often osteoporotic patients have a stable hip fracture. Pelvic fractures that are the result of great force fall into three categories: force applied across the pelvis (i.e., laterally), force on top of the pelvis (i.e., antero-posterior (AP) compression), or force by vertical shear. The majority of hip fractures occur in MVCs and the remainder occur primarily in car versus pedestrian collisions, motorcycle crashes, falls, and crush injuries, in that order.[41]

The first category, lateral compression, may occur in a "T-bone" MVC, for example. During moderate lateral compression, the pelvic ring is compressed, reducing the volume of the pelvis. This pelvic fracture, called a closed book pelvic fracture, is relatively stable, though bladder rupture is a potential complication. During a severe lateral impact with rotation, such as when the patient is run over by a car, lateral crushing forces tend to cause a "windswept pelvis." With a windswept pelvis, most of the pelvic ligaments are disrupted, resulting in a very unstable hip. While the patient is supine, the pelvis appears asymmetric with abduction of one hip and adduction of the contralateral hip.

AP compression is seen in frontal, or "head-on," MVCs as well as motorcycle collisions, pedestrians struck by a motor vehicle, or crush injuries from a collapsed structure, such as a cave-in. These forces, when applied to the AP aspect of the pelvis, tend to cause dislocation of the pubic symphysis anteriorly and the sacroiliac joint posteriorly. Severe forces

applied to the pelvis can result in an "open book fracture," so named because the posterior ligaments remain intact and act as a hinge whereas the anterior ligaments are completely disrupted."[42]

If all of the ligaments—anterior and posterior—are disrupted, the pelvis is extremely unstable and has a high number of associated neurovascular injuries. Because there is no internal stability, the pelvis must be lifted as a unit, preferably with a pelvic binder in place. Pelvic binders will be discussed shortly.

The last mechanism of injury is vertical shear. Vertical shear occurs when a force is applied from the direction of the feet toward the head, such as what occurs in a fall from a height when the patient lands on one foot first. Also referred to as a **Malgaigne fracture**, this pelvic fracture typically involves one-half of the pelvis. The affected hemipelvis has an upward shift and may have associated lumbar fractures, avulsion of the ischial spine, and stretching of the sacral nerves.

Immediately upon inspection of the pelvis, the Paramedic should make a determination of whether the patient has an open versus closed pelvic fracture. An **open pelvic fracture** is associated with significant musculoskeletal and genitourinary trauma and has a 55% mortality rate.[43] An open pelvic fracture can be hidden, occurring inside the vagina or rectum. Therefore, if a Paramedic sees gross hemorrhage from the vagina or rectum, she should suspect an open fracture.

Although palpation along the pelvis, assessing for crepitus, is appropriate, the application of pressure over the pubis and iliac crests is not appropriate. The Paramedic should avoid "rocking" the pelvis or "springing" the pelvis (i.e., applying alternating compressing force and distracting force to the iliac crest). First, this application of force to a potentially fractured pelvis has poor specificity for the presence of fracture (71%) and even worse sensitivity (59%)[44] for detecting a pelvic fracture. It also risks displacing the fracture and potentially disrupting any pelvic hematoma that has stopped the hemorrhage. As much as 4 liters of blood can be lost by venous bleeding into retroperitoneal space from a pelvic fracture.

The Paramedic should assess the patient's genitals (scrotum/labia), and the inguinal area in general, for bleeding and ecchymosis. Gross hematuria, or blood at the external urethral meatus, suggests urethral disruption, as does perineal/genital swelling. Scrotal/labial and perineal hematomas in these areas may indicate deeper intrapelvic hemorrhage. The flanks should also be assessed for ecchymosis. Bruising in the flanks, known as Grey–Turner's sign, is suggestive of bleeding into the retroperitoneal space from the pelvis.

The presence of incontinence, both bowel and bladder, may be related to injury of the spinal nerves in the lower lumbar/sacrum. The patient may also complain of perineal numbness. The perineal numbness and saddle paresthesia are symptoms associated with a neurological disorder called **cauda equina syndrome**, which is the result of associated lower lumbar fractures and nerve compression.[45]

The three most common complications associated with a pelvic fracture are a femur fracture (in 48% of cases according to one study), thoracic injury, and peripheral nerve damage.[41] Therefore, it is imperative that the Paramedic assess the entire lower extremity from the costal margin of the thoracic cage to the toes.

STREET SMART

The patient with a suspected pelvic fracture should not be log-rolled. Log-rolling these patients may lead to the creation of an open book fracture. Rather, these patients should be lifted onto the backboard, either manually or by orthopaedic/scoop stretcher.[46]

A straddle injury can also be associated with a pelvic injury. A straddle injury is an injury of the superior and inferior pubic rami as a result of an acute deceleration and contact to the perineal area. This might occur with a fall onto a fence, crossbar of a bike, or a gymnastics bar. Although obvious soft-tissue trauma to the external genitalia may be more worrisome, the internal damage to the urinary tract, specifically urethral disruption and pelvic fractures, may be more problematic. Fortunately, these injuries seldom affect pelvic stability.

Hip Fracture

The words "I've fallen and cannot get up" signal the need for many EMS calls. Invariably, they are spoken because of a hip fracture. From osteoporosis to malignant tumors

to trauma, the hip is prone to fractures that can lead to lifelong disability and even death. Although overall mortality from hip fractures is only about 15%, mortality in the elderly approached 36% in the year following the fracture in one study.[47]

The hip is actually a joint consisting of the femur and the pelvis. The site in which the femur fits into the pelvis, in a ball-and-socket arrangement, is called the acetabulum (sometimes called the vinegar cup). The neck of the femur connects the head of the femur with its shaft at approximately a 130-degree angle. This angle places a great deal of stress on the femur neck, and shearing forces can fracture the femoral neck.

A hip fracture can be an impacted femoral head, a broken femoral neck, a fractured trochanter, or all of these. Fractures of the femoral head, either simple or comminuted, are rare. They are usually the result of a force along the axis of the femur, such as striking the underside of the dashboard with the knee and having the force transmitted to the femoral head. Often these fractures are associated with hip dislocations and other femur fractures.

The most common femoral fracture is the femoral neck fracture, which is usually referred to as a hip fracture. These fractures occur in the elderly, especially patients with osteoporosis, from seemingly minor trauma. In some cases, simply turning the hip leads to rotational forces that can break the femur's neck. Although incomplete stress fractures may heal with rest, complete fractures can lead to compromised blood flow to the head of the femur, avascular necrosis, and/or nonunion.

Trochanter fractures can be further divided into three classifications. The greater trochanter fracture is often an avulsion fracture caused by forceful contraction of the iliopsoas muscle. The avulsion fracture is the result of grade III sprain and is seen in gymnasts and dancers.

Intertrochanteric fractures, between the greater and lesser trochanter, are often the result of osteoporosis. These "hip" fractures can be either stable or unstable. In the past, these fractures were treated with prolonged bedrest. However, the hazards of immobility (i.e., bedsores, deep vein thrombus, muscular atrophy, malformation, etc.) have led to an increasing number of surgical interventions such as open reduction and internal fixture (ORIF).

Subtrochanteric fractures are actually fractures of the proximal shaft of the femur but are still considered hip fractures. Although indistinguishable in the field, these fractures tend to occur as a result of high-energy trauma, such as MVC and skiing accidents.

Pathologic Hip Fractures

The pathologic hip fracture is an atraumatic hip fracture. Pathologic hip fractures can occur because of hyperparathyroidism and renal failure, which affect calcium levels, as well as metastatic cancer and Paget's disease.

Paget's disease is a chronic and progressive disease that is more common in patients over age 50 and increases in frequency with the patient's age. Its medical name, osteitis deformans, speaks to a major effect of Paget's disease: deformity of the bones. Paget's disease affects about 3% to 4% of the population over the age of 40.

Metastatic disease from multiple varieties of cancer (such as breast, renal prostatic, lung, multiple myeloma) can metastasize to bone. Alternatively, the cancer can be a primary bone cancer, called an osteosarcoma. In every case, the cancer erodes the bone and compromises the structural integrity.

The kidneys are responsible for minerals such as calcium and phosphate within the body. With renal failure, mineral levels can fall and lead to bone demineralization and osteoporosis, a syndrome called renal osteodystrophy. Demineralized bones are brittle and prone to pathologic fractures.

The body needs vitamin D to utilize calcium. In the past, an absence of vitamin D led to a condition called rickets. That condition has largely been eliminated since vitamin D is now added to many foodstuffs including milk. However, some medications, such as heparin, lasix, and certain anticonvulsants, can decrease vitamin D levels, leading to bone demineralization and pathologic fractures.

Finally, the overproduction of the parathyroid hormone can lead to serum hypercalcemia and bone demineralization. Commonly due to a parathyroid adenoma, it affects patients over 50 years old and women more than men. It is estimated that hyperparathyroidism is a primary or contributing cause of 10% of hip fractures, specifically fractures of the femoral neck.

Femur Fractures

It takes a tremendous amount of force to break the femur, the largest and strongest bone in the body. However, when a break does occur it can be catastrophic. Beyond the immediate loss of mobility, a fractured femur can lose over a liter of blood into the thigh, leading to hypotension and shock.

Strictly speaking, a femur fracture involves a bone break from the condylar, the rounded end of the bone at the knee, to the shaft. Fractures of the proximal femur, subtrochanteric to the femoral head, are considered hip fractures.

Femur fractures can occur from major trauma (e.g., from a motor vehicle collision) or from minor trauma (e.g., fractures occurring from osteoporosis). Femur fractures from seemingly minor trauma, such as a fall from a standing position, are suspicious. In these cases, the Paramedic should consider the possibility of a pathologic fracture secondary to chronic diseases or metastatic cancer.

All long-bone fractures, including fractures of the femur shaft, can be spiral/transverse, comminuted, or open. Upon inspection, the Paramedic should expose the entire length of the thigh from knee to pelvis. The Paramedic may note gross deformity, with or without laceration; bony crepitus with muscle spasm; and shortening of the leg. The thigh may appear swollen and feel tense secondary to formation of a hematoma in the muscle. The Paramedic should immediately proceed to assess for the presence or absence of peripheral pulses. Absence of a peripheral pulse may indicate impending compartment syndrome or shock and represents a medical emergency.

Although the Paramedic should also assess distal neurological function, the femur fracture may be a distracting injury, making the patient an unreliable reporter. Fortunately, nerve damage secondary to a midshaft femur fracture is rare.

Although the traction splint can relieve a great deal of the patient's pain, the Paramedic should consider the use of muscle relaxants, such as benzodiazepines, as well as analgesia.

The Paramedic should irrigate open femur fractures to remove gross contaminates and then place a moist sterile dressing, secured with a bandage, over the open fracture. This dressing should be regularly monitored. If the bandage is too tight, it may act like a constricting band and increase the risks of compartment syndrome.

Supracondylar femur fractures occur when an axial load is applied to the bent knee. Fractures can also occur proximal to prosthetic knee replacements. As the distal femur is funnel shaped, it tends to fracture proximal to the interface of the diaphyseal bone and the metaphyseal bone adjacent to the epiphyseal plate (Figure 7-19). Due to the supracondylar fracture's proximity to the knee, concurrent injury to the ligaments of the knee, particularly the ACL, is common.

Patients with a supracondylar fracture will present with the classic signs of a fracture: pain, deformity, and weakness. Because of the proximity of major nerves, the Paramedic should not be distracted by the injury but focus instead on verifying distal neurological function.

As femur fractures can bleed heavily into the thigh, the Paramedic should assess for the signs of compartment syndrome, which will be discussed shortly, as this is a potentially more devastating consequence of the fracture. Most supracondylar fractures will require stabilization via open reduction and internal fixation. External bracing is not generally viable because it is impossible to immobilize the joint above and below. Treatment of the femur fracture is described shortly.

Knee Fracture

The knee is a joint that consists of the patella (anterior), the femur (superior), and the tibia (inferior). Knee fractures include distal femur fractures, patellar fractures, and proximal tibial fractures.

Most patellar fractures occur as the result of direct trauma, a fall onto a flexed knee, or striking the dashboard in a MVC. Tibial fractures can occur as a result of axial loading and indirect trauma. Approximately 30% of knee fractures, particularly those involving the tibial plateau, will have associated injury of the ligaments.

The quadriceps is attached to the superior pole of the patella. Forceful contraction of the quadriceps can avulse portions of the articular surface. Fractures involving the cartilage in a joint are called osteochondral fractures and sometimes result in "free bodies," fragments of bone and cartilage, floating in the knee.[48]

The patient with a suspected knee fracture will present with diffuse pain over the knee and associated swelling of the knee. In cases of a patellar fracture, it is possible to elicit point tenderness over the patella and palpate the bony fragments.

Stress Fractures

One form of fracture, called a **stress fracture**, is the result of repetitive loading of the musculoskeletal interface, which is an overuse injury. A stress fracture (i.e., jogger's fracture) was originally described by Breithaupt to explain foot pain in marching military recruits in 1855. It starts as an incomplete fracture that, if untreated, can evolve into a complete fracture. A combination of poor conditioning, short adaptation time for bone remodeling to stress, and general poor bone health, secondary to insufficient diet, can lead to stress fractures.

The patient with a stress fracture will present with point tenderness, swelling, and pain upon beginning a stress-invoking activity. The key to accurately determining a stress fracture is persistent pain following cessation of the activity.

A minor condition that can lead to a stress fracture is shin splints. **Shin splints**, also known as medial tibial stress syndrome, are a result of inflammation of the peroneal tendon that creates pain over the lower half of the anterior shin. A cause of shin splints is pes planus (flat feet), which cause the posterior tibialis to become overstretched and inflamed. This also puts stress on the tibia.

Ankle Fracture

Whereas ankle sprains are very common, the likelihood of an ankle fracture is remote. In fact, they make up less than 15% of all ankle injuries. This is owed, in part, to the

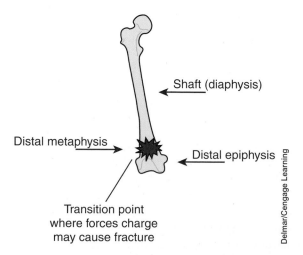

Figure 7-19 Distal femur fractures tend to occur proximal to the interface of the diaphyseal bone and the metaphyseal bone adjacent to the epiphyseal plate.

Shaft (diaphysis)

Distal metaphysis

Distal epiphysis

Transition point where forces charge may cause fracture

Delmar/Cengage Learning

large number of tendons and ligaments in the ankle that help protect it. An ankle fracture is a fracture of any of the bones that make up the ankle: the tibia, fibula, talus, and calcaneus. The first three bones allow for dorsiflexion and plantar flexion, whereas the calcaneus allows inversion and eversion. Excessive movement in any of these four directions can lead to a sprain or fracture; in some cases, the fracture is an avulsion fracture that is part of a third degree sprain.

Ankle fractures are classified as unimalleolar, bimalleolar, and trimalleolar, because of the dominant nature of the tibia in the ankle. A lateral malleolus fracture is a fracture of the fibula, whereas a medial malleolus fracture is a fracture of the tibia. A unimalleolar, or first degree, ankle fracture is generally stable, whereas a bimalleolar fracture (second degree) is unstable. It is usually found along the mediolateral axis. Often the patient is unable to ambulate with a bimalleolar fracture. A trimalleolar fracture (Cotton fracture) involves the medial, lateral, and posterior malleoli of the tibia. It is unstable in both mediolateral and anteroposterior axes. Both the trimalleolar and the bimalleolar fractures usually require an open reduction and internal fixture.

A Paramedic should suspect an ankle fracture when gross deformity, swelling, and ecchymosis is observed with the affected ankle. Palpation generally will elicit extreme point tenderness and crepitus over the affected ankle.

Calcaneus Fracture

The calcaneus, as the lever arm of the gastrocsoleus complex, is critical to walking. Although rare (less than 2% of all fractures), fracture of the calcaneus (heel fracture) can have life-long implications to a person's gait and standing.

A calcaneus fracture can be the result of a heel strike during a fall or other high-energy axial loading. These fractures—a compression fracture with impacted bony fragments—are painful and primarily felt on the outer side of the ankle or heel pad. Examination of the heel may reveal ecchymosis along the heel and sole of the foot, known as Mondor signs. Gentle compression of the heel will elicit pain when there is a calcaneus fracture present. The Paramedic should examine both feet, even if the patient only complains of pain in one heel, as bilateral calcaneus fractures are not uncommon. That suspicion should be based on the mechanism of injury.

CASE STUDY (CONTINUED)

Two Paramedics are assigned by the operations chief to the urban search and rescue (USAR) team. After one of the scent dogs went on "alert," the team started digging the patient out. The Paramedics are waiting at the bottom of the rubble pile as the patient is brought down to them in a rigid frame basket.

The patient appears to be a roughly 50-year-old male. At first glance, the patient looks awake and alert. However, a closer look reveals some obvious deformities of the extremities. With the basket on the ground, the Paramedics introduce themselves and start their assessment.

CRITICAL THINKING QUESTIONS

1. What are the important elements of the history that a Paramedic should obtain?
2. Why would the patient's past medical history be important?

History

The Paramedic's first step in assessing a traumatized patient is to assess the mechanism of injury, the kinematics involved, and the biomechanics of the body in relation to that mechanism of injury (or the biomechanics if athleticism is involved). Specifically, the Paramedic should be concerned with the lines of force.

The Paramedic must consider if the force was linear, such as a blow to a limb, and if so, whether it was point specific (such as gunshot wounds) or diffuse (such as a crush injury from a collapsed wall). The path of energy with a linear line of force, both point specific and diffuse, allows for easier prediction of the injury patterns.

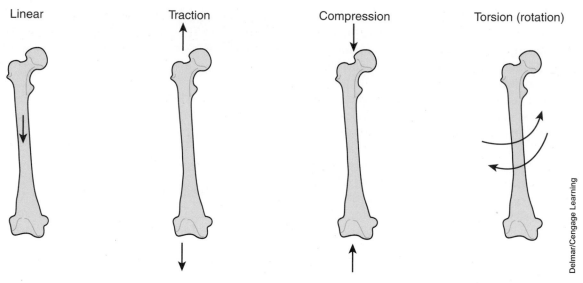

| Linear | Traction | Compression | Torsion (rotation) |

Delmar/Cengage Learning

Figure 7-20 Lines of force include traction, compression, and torsion.

Other lines of force include traction (resulting in distraction of joints and ligaments), compression (resulting in impaction), and torsion (resulting in shearing injury). These lines of force tend to create more indirect trauma; that is, injury at a point other than the point of impact or force. There are numerous examples of indirect trauma, such as greenstick fractures, Colles fractures, impacted hip fractures, and so on (Figure 7-20).

Naturally, if the injury is sports related, the Paramedic should document the nature of the sport. This description should include the position the patient played (for example, was the patient a flanker versus a hooker in rugby) and the nature of participation (for example, was the athletic event intramural, amateur, semi-pro, collegiate, and so on). In some cases, a certified athletic trainer (ATC) may be present and should be consulted. An ATC can be a valuable source of information and has extensive knowledge of sports-related injuries.

In addition to a standard OPQRST (**O**nset, **P**rovokes, **Q**uality, **R**adiates, **S**everity, **T**ime) history of the pain, the Paramedic should ascertain if the pain was immediate, which is suggestive of rupture or fracture, or delayed, which is suggestive of the pain of inflammation. Also, the Paramedic should ask the patient if he heard any sounds, such as snapping or popping, just before the pain. Although the Paramedic should not encourage weightbearing, he should ask the patient if there was any weightbearing on the affected limb prior to EMS arrival.

The Paramedic should also question the patient about the presence of associated symptoms such as loss of range of motion in the affected joint, weakness of the extremity, and paresthesia. Again, the Paramedic should not ask the patient to perform range of motion activities.

Past Medical History

The Paramedic should obtain a careful past medical history, starting with allergies and ending with events preceding the injury using SAMPLE. For example, in the course of treatment lidocaine is injected as a local anesthetic, radiographic dye is injected for medical imaging, and cortisone is injected as an anti-inflammatory. Many people have allergies to one or more of these substances.

Medications that affect the musculoskeletal system include anticoagulants, such as heparin, and nonsteroidal anti-inflammatory drugs (NSAIDs). Chronic use of NSAIDs is suggestive of recurrent injury. Furthermore, use of NSAIDs during the acute phase of a musculoskeletal injury may change clotting times, impacting hematoma formation.

The Paramedic should obtain a standard past medical history, focusing on those diseases that impact bone health. This includes diabetes, which affects healing; renal disease, in that chronic kidney disease can lead to mineral and bone disorders; parathyroid disease, which affects calcium levels; and gastrointestinal disorders that affect mineral and vitamin absorption. Other comorbidities that increase the risk of fractures are Paget's disease and osteoporosis, which were both discussed previously.

The saying goes "sprains beget sprains." Therefore, the Paramedic should ask if the patient has a history of previous injury and, if so, when was the last time this "joint" was injured. A history of previous fractures, particularly fractures from minor trauma or atraumatic fractures, suggests osteoporosis.

The Paramedic should take a careful history of the events that preceded the injury. In some cases, a patient can pass out from pain during the event (some postulate this is vasovagal syncope). Others pass out before the event, leading to the fall, fracture, and pain. Pre-event syncope is suggestive of a cardiac event, a potentially life-threatening dysrhythmia, and should be investigated.

Fracture Risk

Suppose an elderly person falls from a standing position onto a carpeted floor. The patient denies neck or back pain, but the Paramedic sees a notable kyphosis. Should this patient be immobilized on a backboard, a procedure that will likely create back pain for this patient, or is the mechanism of injury insufficient to warrant spinal immobilization?

One of the difficulties Paramedics face when assessing the elderly following a fall is determining the risk of fracture. Osteoporosis, as discussed earlier, is a function of aging and, to some degree, affects greater than one-half of Americans over 50 years of age.[49] Osteoporosis has been implicated as a contributing factor in the over one-quarter million hip fractures; as a result, one-half of this population will never walk without assistance and a quarter of them will need long-term care.

The key determination in assessing fracture risk is the degree of osteoporosis. Part of that risk analysis for osteoporosis is **bone mineral density (BMD)**, which is used to diagnose osteoporosis and is useful in predicting risk of fracture. A BMD, reported as a "T-score," of $(-)1.0$ or greater is normal, translated as a low risk of fracture. A score of $(-)2.4$ to $(-)1.0$ is considered osteopenia, or a moderate risk of fracture. Any T-score less than $(-)2.5$ is osteoporosis and poses a greater risk of fracture. Many patients, particularly women, can tell you their "bone health," especially if they have been diagnosed with osteopenia or osteoporosis.

An indirect indicator of bone health is the medications prescribed. Some medications, such as Os-Cal®, are calcium replacement therapies for patients with osteopenia and osteoporosis. Even TUMS® has been prescribed as a mineral replacement therapy. One somewhat controversial treatment is estrogen therapy, used either as estrogen replacement or as a selective estrogen receptor modulator (SERM). Examples of estrogen replacement medications are Premarin® and Estrace®, and an example of a SERM medication is Evista®. However, there is a risk of certain types of breast cancer with the use of these medications.

The biphosphates, such as Fosamax®, Boniva®, Actonel®, and the injectable biphosphate Zometa®, have shown promise in preventing and treating osteoporosis by slowing bone turnover and increasing bone formation. These medications are often coupled with vitamin D and calcium. The last group of medication, calcitonin, the hormone responsible for calcium levels in the body, is used following a fracture attributed, in part, to osteoporosis. The presence of these medications should alert the Paramedic to an increased risk of fracture due to pre-existing osteoporosis.

Finally, the best indicators of fracture risk are age and a history of previous fractures. People of advanced age, more than 75 years, carry a great risk of fracture from minor trauma. An indicator of bone health is the presence or absence of kyphosis. Kyphosis, an extreme curvature of the upper back, known as hunchback or dowager's hump, is indicative of osteoporosis (Figure 7-21).

As in all paramedicine, the first rule is "do no harm." If the Paramedic has a high index of suspicion that a fracture is possible, then she must take appropriate measures to protect the patient from further injury.

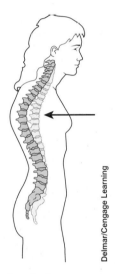

Delmar/Cengage Learning

Figure 7-21 Kyphosis is an extreme curvature of the upper back.

CASE STUDY (CONTINUED)

After completing their primary assessment, the Paramedics start to methodically assess the patient's entire body, starting at the head and working to the toes. The Paramedics carefully expose, then assess, the patient's shoulder girdle and the pelvic girdle.

CRITICAL THINKING QUESTIONS

1. What are the elements of the physical examination of a patient with suspected multiple musculoskeletal trauma?

2. Why is a neurovascular examination a critical element in this examination?

Examination

The Paramedic's examination of the patient with orthopaedic trauma starts with an assessment from "the doorway." The Paramedic starts with a global impression of the patient, looking for signs of distress or pain. Pained facial expressions, diaphoresis, and pallor are signs the patient is injured and that the sympathetic nervous system is responding. Next, the Paramedic notes the patient's stance. For example, the classic sign of an upper extremity injury, particularly of the shoulder, is when the patient stands, guarding the affected arm with the other uninjured arm and even tilting the head toward the affected side.

Next, the Paramedic turns her attention to the affected limb. A gross inspection should tell the Paramedic if the limb is positioned correctly from an anatomic perspective. The Paramedic considers if the limb is valgus (has an abnormal displacement of the limb away from the midline) or varus (an abnormal twist or bend in the limb inward toward the midline).

The Paramedic inspects the entire limb, from the joint above to the joint below. Failure to expose the entire limb may leave proximal fractures from indirect trauma hidden. With the limb completely exposed, the Paramedic examines the limb for breaks in the skin. Any breaks in the skin proximal to the injury can reasonably be assumed to be the result of an open fracture, even if bone is not observed. A sign of imminent open fracture is tenting of the skin. If tenting is observed, then the limb should immediately be realigned into its natural anatomical position.

It is often helpful to compare limbs. Asymmetry, secondary to muscle atrophy or swelling, becomes more apparent through this technique. Discoloration, secondary to vascular insufficiency or hematoma formation, is also more apparent.

The classic triad for a fracture is a painful, swollen deformity, so if these conditions exist the Paramedic should suspect a fracture. However, the Paramedic still must perform a more thorough examination.

The primary concern for most patients is pain, which should be addressed. However, the primary concern for Paramedics is neurovascular compromise. The Paramedic should perform a careful assessment for distal neurovascular function, utilizing knowledge of innervations and circulation. Some Paramedics use Doppler stethoscopes to obtain distal pulses. These "D-scopes" are remarkably sensitive and useful in noisy environments, such as the back of a moving ambulance. Once the pulse is obtained, the site is marked for ease of reassessment later. Pulse oximetry can also be used to assess distal circulation.

Palpation of the affected limb should assess for minor deformity and defects. A "**step off**" is an indication of either dislocation or displaced fracture and its location should be carefully noted using anatomical terms before swelling obscures the defect. Gentle palpation should also uncover point tenderness, another sign of fracture. In some cases, the Paramedic may appreciate crepitus, a grating sensation felt under the skin that is suggestive of a fracture.

CASE STUDY (CONTINUED)

After completing their examination, the Paramedics suspect the patient has a midshaft femur fracture as well as a grade III open fracture of the ankle, on the Gustilo-Anderson scale. The Paramedics are concerned with loss of life, secondary to hemorrhagic blood loss into the thigh, as well as loss of limb, from the ankle fracture. The Paramedics immediately call for a casualty evacuation (CaseVac) and alert the surgical team at the field hospital.

CRITICAL THINKING QUESTIONS

1. Why does the patient need immediate care?
2. What diagnosis did the Paramedic announce to the patient?

Assessment

Following a careful injury history and physical examination, the Paramedic may come to suspect a sprain, dislocation, or fracture. In most cases, the Paramedic assumes the worst case, a fracture, and treats accordingly.

The three disorders that a Paramedic must address are pain, distal neurovascular compromise, and blood loss from soft-tissue damage. The last disorder, blood loss from soft-tissue and vascular damage, can be substantial. It is estimated that as much as a pint of blood, or 500 cc, can be lost from a humerus fracture, that one to two units (or pints) of blood can be lost in a lower leg fracture (tibia/fibula), and as much as 1,000 to 1,500 cc of blood can be lost into the femur. However, the greatest blood loss occurs in a pelvic fracture, up to 4 liters, with most of this bleeding being occult, into the retroperitoneal space. In addition, up to 40% of patients with a pelvic fracture have intra-abdominal bleeding. Limiting the pelvic space and creating venous tamponade can control life-threatening bleeding, which is discussed further in the "Treatment" section. Therefore, the Paramedic must continuously monitor for signs of hypoperfusion and treat accordingly (see Chapter 11 on trauma resuscitation).

CASE STUDY (CONTINUED)

The Paramedics prepare to "package" the patient on a flexible litter, as the USAR team needs the hard framed basket. Before the patient is transferred to the flexible stretcher, his limbs need to be immobilized. The "busted" ankle presents a problem with using the traction splint (i.e., there is no purchase point for the hitch). Since they packed light, the Paramedics only have some flexible aluminum splints, soft dressings, and cravats. Some imagination is needed to solve this dilemma.

CRITICAL THINKING QUESTIONS

1. What is the standard of care of patients with suspected midshaft femur fracture?
2. What are some of the patient-specific concerns and considerations that the Paramedic should consider when applying this plan of care?

Treatment

The clinical objectives of fracture management are threefold: pain management, prevention of further injury, and control of hemorrhage. The maxim in EMS has been that any musculoskeletal injury should be assumed to be a fracture until proven otherwise. Therefore, discussions of sprain versus strain versus fracture, in the field, are somewhat academic and the diagnosis is left to the emergency physician.

In the case of the long-bone fracture, these three objectives can be best met by returning the bone to its neutral anatomic position and a natural alignment. However, the reduction of joints—a complex apparatus of ligaments, tendons, bones, and a neurovascular bundle—is generally reserved to those special situations where there is a loss of distal circulation, which is a limb-threatening condition. The reduction of various joints is discussed in the following paragraphs. Otherwise, the Paramedic is well-advised to splint the injured joint in the position found and let the emergency physician reduce the joint.

Reduction

Before any reduction is attempted, the Paramedic obtains immediate manual stabilization of the injury, preventing movement of the joints above and below. This single act may provide the patient with the greatest relief from pain. In a sense, the Paramedic is providing a temporary external splint that prevents further bone damage until a more permanent splint can be applied.

With the limb immobilized, the Paramedic assesses distal neurovascular function. Understanding innervation, the Paramedic assesses the different nerve pathways for loss of motor function (paralysis) or loss of sensation (paresthesia). For example, the median nerve innervates the thumb, forefinger, middle finger, and one-half of the ring finger; the superficial branch of the radial nerve innervates the dorsum of the hand; and the ulnar nerve innervates the other half of the ring finger and the little finger (Figure 7-22).

Next, the Paramedic should consider analgesia. Fentanyl citrate may be the drug of choice (DOC), administered intranasally, because of its short onset of action (within 5 to 10 minutes), ease of administration, and analgesia that is equivalent to intravenous morphine.[50]

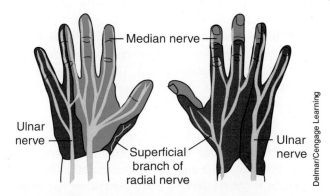

Figure 7-22 The nerves of the hand are the median, the radial, and the ulnar nerves.

If the Paramedic notes involuntary muscle spasm by the presence of muscle terseness in the fracture's vicinity, he should consider administering a benzodiazepine, such as midazolam. The twofold advantage of benzodiazepines is relief of smooth muscle spasm and amnesia.

The reduction of the long-bone fracture is straightforward. The Paramedic grasps distal from the injury site, along the long axis of the bone, and applies gentle traction. This traction should correct rotational, lateral misalignment (valgus), and medial misalignment (varus) deformities.

Reduction of a dislocation or fracture while in the field is generally not recommended. Field reduction risks neurovascular injury and is done only when there is a loss of pulses and/or paralysis and a risk of loss of limb or limb function. An infrequently performed skill, field reduction should only be done after performing a risk–benefit analysis. The Paramedic must weigh the time to transport and arrival to definitive care against the risk of loss of limb or function, and the increased difficulty in reducing a joint after a lengthy period of time, which may imply surgical reduction. Field reduction should only be done after consultation with medical control, if possible.

All attempts at reduction should be preceded with analgesia (provided the patient is hemodynamically stable) and use of muscle relaxants, such as the benzodiazepines. However, caution is advised when using these two agents together as conscious sedation may occur. Although anxiolysis is desirable, a drug-induced depression of consciousness (procedural sedation) may make it difficult for the patient to cooperate and risks the need for airway control.

Shoulder Reduction

In general, there are two techniques for reduction of the shoulder: one using traction and one using leverage.[51] The original method of shoulder reduction, the **Hippocratic method**, uses a form of countertraction. With the patient supine, the Paramedic grasps the wrist of the extended arm, then places a foot into the axilla and applies steady countertraction. Although effective, this method risks axillary nerve injury, humeral shaft fracture, and glenoid capsule damage.

In 1980, Manes presented a new technique, intended for use in the elderly. With the **Manes method**, the patient is seated. The Paramedic stands behind the patient and inserts her flexed forearm into the axilla of the patient's affected arm. Then, the Paramedic places her other hand on the patient's forearm and applies gentle traction. This technique is effective for those with little muscle mass (i.e., elderly, children, and some women) (Figure 7-23).

In the hanging arm technique (i.e., the **Stimson method**), the patient lies prone on a stretcher, with a sandbag (or similar weight) placed under the clavicle. With the hanging arm in forward flexion, a 10-pound counterweight pulls traction. This method is most effective when the patient has received analgesia (Figure 7-24). It requires that the patient's shoulder eventually tires and reduction is achieved. This relatively

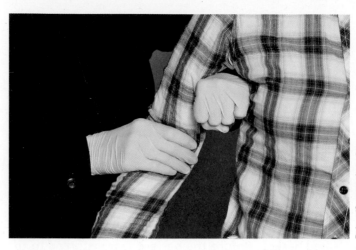

Figure 7-23 The Manes method is effective for those with little muscle mass.

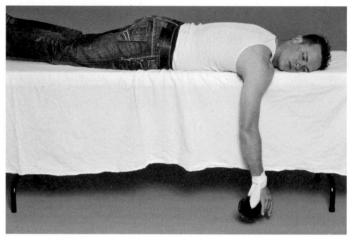

Figure 7-24 The Stimson method of shoulder reduction reduces risks of neurovascular injury.

passive method of shoulder reduction reduces risks of neurovascular injury.

The alternative to traction is the use of leverage. The oldest leverage technique may be **Kocher's method**, first described in 1870. With the arm adducted, and stabilizing the elbow in the palm of the hand, the Paramedic grasps the wrist, forms a 90-degree bend at the elbow, and rotates the arm externally until resistance is felt. Then, lifting the limb until the shoulder is reduced, the Paramedic ends by rolling the forearm into the body to a splintable position. Although effective, this method should be used with caution in the elderly or osteoporotic patient as it risks causing a humeral fracture (Figure 7-25).

The newest leverage techniques use scapular manipulation. Scapular manipulation focuses on repositioning the glenoid fossa rather than manipulation of the humerus.[52] The scapular manipulation technique (SMT), first described by Bosely and Miles in 1979, creates less anxiety and requires less sedatives or analgesics.[53] With the patient prone or seated and the arm hanging, similar to the Stimson method, and

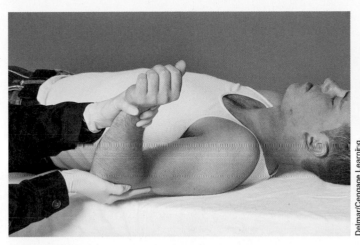

Figure 7-25 Kocher's method should be used with caution in the elderly or osteoporotic patient.

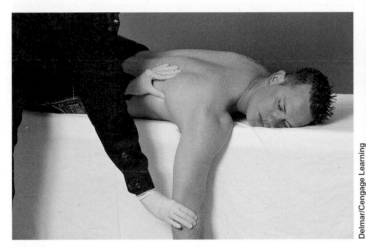

Figure 7-26 Scapular manipulation creates less anxiety and requires less sedatives or analgesics than other leverage methods.

allowing time for relaxation, the Paramedic applies traction to the arm held in 90 degrees of forward flexion. Then the inferior tip of the scapula is moved medially and dorsally with the Paramedic's thumbs (Figure 7-26).

Elbow Reduction

The elbow is a complex union of the ulnar nerve, median nerve, and brachial artery. Any reduction of the elbow, particularly if bony fragments exist, risks damage to this neurovascular complex.

One reduction method, the Parvin method, has the patient lying prone with the entirety of the humerus on the bed and the forearm perpendicular to the humerus (Figure 7-27a). The Paramedic grasps the humerus with one hand, with the thumb on the olecranon. Grasping the wrist, the Paramedic applies 5 to 10 pounds of downward traction while simultaneously pushing the olecranon forward. Alternatively, the patient can be lying supine (e.g., on a stretcher). This technique takes two providers but may be easier to perform in the back of an ambulance (Figure 7-27b).

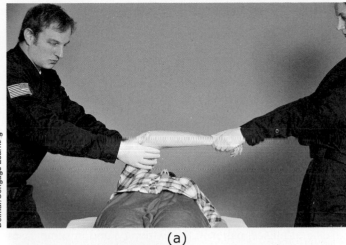

(a)

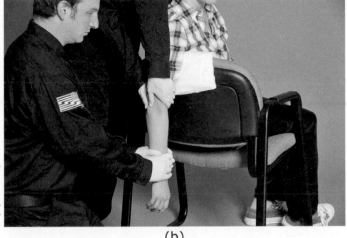

(b)

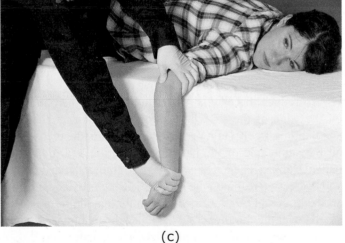

(c)

Figure 7-27 Reduction of the elbow. (a) Parvin method. (b) Supine on stretcher. (c) Traction.

An alternative method also requires two providers but may be procedurally easier to perform. The patient's affected limb can be draped over the back of a chair, with a pillow in the axilla (Figure 7-27c). With traction steadily applied to the wrist, the Paramedic applies forward force at the olecranon until the elbow is reduced.

Finger Reduction

Dislocations of the fingers are relatively common; however, the risk of neurovascular injury is minimal. Many patients apply traction along the axis and self-reduce the injury. If the patient has done this, the Paramedic should buddy splint the finger, apply ice, and transport the patient for medical attention as needed.

Knee Reduction

The primary concern with a dislocated knee is neurovascular injury, particularly of the popliteal artery. Up to 64% of dislocated knees involve interruption of the popliteal artery.[30] The indications for reduction of the knee include absence of peripheral pulses, pallor in the extremity, and in some cases a palpable thrill behind the knee in the popliteal fossa can be appreciated, suggesting compression of the popliteal artery.[31] Some 25% to 35% of knee dislocations also damage the peroneal nerve, as evidenced by impaired dorsiflexion and decreased sensation behind the great toe.[31]

If reduction of the posterior knee dislocation is indicated, one Paramedic stabilizes the distal femur of the supine patient while longitudinal traction is applied to the lower leg until the entire leg is in alignment. After reduction, the Paramedic should splint the knee in slight flexion, approximately 15 degrees, and apply a compression bandage with recurrent wraps to reduce swelling.

Patella Reduction

A dislocated patella is painful. Swelling from the dislocation occurs almost immediately, making reduction more difficult over time, thus favoring early reduction. The most common patellar dislocation is lateral displacement of the patella. As there are no neurovascular structures proximal to the patella, the risk of injury is minimal. Loss of distal circulation with a patellar dislocation suggests concurrent injury of the femur and/or tibia, and a complicated knee dislocation.

To reduce the patella, the Paramedic has the patient sit on the edge of the stretcher, with the leg bent at the knee and hanging freely (Figure 7-28). The Paramedic then stands on the same side of the patellar dislocation and grasps the patient's ankle. The leg is gently raised to flex the quadriceps and decrease tension on the patella. The leg is extended while applying gentle traction medially to the patella to assist the patella over the femoral condyle. Once the patella is reduced, the entire leg should be immobilized in full extension.[54]

Hip Reduction

Although a hip dislocation is an orthopaedic emergency, the determination of hip dislocation versus hip fracture is almost impossible to make in the field. A hip reduction in the field should only be attempted if there is a loss of distal neurovascular function, or the time to reduction may be greater than six hours. Even then, the Paramedic should consult with medical control.

A common technique used for closed reduction of the hip is the **Bigelow method** (Figure 7-29). With the patient supine,

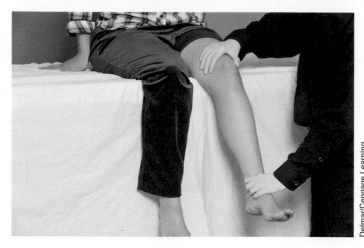

Figure 7-28 Patella reduction can be done with the patient sitting on the edge of the stretcher.

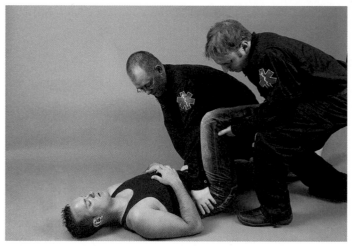

Figure 7-29 Hip reduction can be achieved with the Bigelow method and Stimson maneuver.

one Paramedic provides posterior traction along the anterior superior iliac, in effect pinning the hips to the stretcher and stabilizing the hips. Another Paramedic grasps the lower leg at the bent knee and applies steady longitudinal traction, levering the femur into the acetabulum by abduction and external rotation. As the quadriceps are powerful and may be in spasm, the Paramedic may need to grasp the ankle with one hand and place the crook of the elbow of the other arm under the knee to obtain sufficient force to overcome the quadriceps.

An alternative to the Bigelow method is the **Stimson maneuver**. The Stimson maneuver is the reverse of the Bigelow method. With the patient prone instead of supine, the leg hangs over the edge of the stretcher. The Paramedic applies downward pressure to the pelvis to stabilize the hip and downward traction on the back of the knee. Rotation of the ankle reduces the hip.

Splinting

Movement of bone ends in a fractured bone displaces clots, risks further neurovascular injury, and creates a great deal of pain. Splinting long-bone fractures prevents pain as well as further injury.

There are some basic principles of splinting for all injuries. First, the bone ends above and below the suspected fracture/dislocation should be manually stabilized. Next, the Paramedic should assess distal neurovascular function.

Before splinting, the Paramedic should consider analgesia. Before applying a splint to a long bone, the Paramedic moves the long bone to its natural anatomic position, if possible. If the injury involves a joint and distal neurovascular function is intact, then the Paramedic should splint the joint in the position found. If distal neurovascular function is compromised, then the Paramedic should reduce the joint as described earlier and splint the affected limb.

One mnemonic useful for pre- and post-splinting is FACTS: **F**unction, **A**rterial pulses, **C**apillary refill, **T**emperature, and **S**ensation (Table 7-1). The Paramedic should check the "FACTS" before and after splinting and every 5 to 10 minutes thereafter.

A large number of splints are available on the market. A splint should be easy to apply, provide a rigid "external skeleton," and permit access to the distal extremity for assessment of neurovascular function. The splint should also control the joints above and below the injury site. Following splinting, the Paramedic should provide supportive care. The mnemonic RICE is used to summarize supportive care: **R**est, **I**ce, **C**ompression, and **E**levation of the affected limb above the heart.

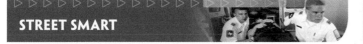

STREET SMART

It is important to observe and describe the condition of the injury site before the splint is applied.

Dressings, bandages, and splints obscure the injury.

Upper Extremity Splints

The upper extremity, the shoulder girdle, presents some interesting challenges for splinting. This is owed, in part, to the flexibility of the joints and to the importance that the hands and arms have for activities of daily living.

Fractures of the midclavicle can be treated with a figure-eight splint (Figure 7-30). While the patient is standing upright, the Paramedic instructs him to place his hands on the hips, rolling the shoulders backward as much as tolerated. Using cravats or stockinette draped across each shoulder and under the contralateral axilla, the splint is tied off.

Fractures of the upper humerus, or dislocations of the shoulder, are typically splinted with a sling and swathe. With

a pad in the axilla for comfort, the Paramedic applies the sling to hold the arm at a 90-degree inclination perpendicular to the body. Then an elastic compressive bandage, often a six-inch Ace® wrap, is used to immobilize the arm to the chest and minimize movement of the injured limb (Figure 7-31).

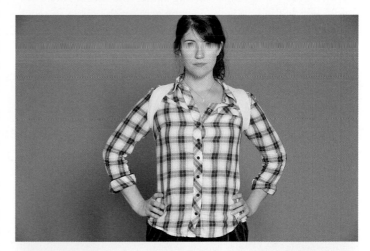

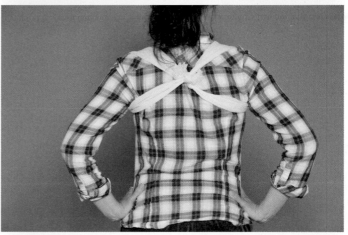

Delmar/Cengage Learning

Figure 7-30 A figure-eight splint can be used to treat fractures of the midclavicle.

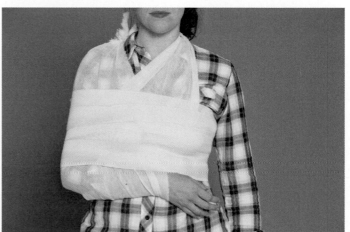

Delmar/Cengage Learning

Figure 7-31 A sling and swathe are typically used for fractures of the upper humerus, or dislocations of the shoulder.

Table 7-1 FACTS

F	Function: distal motor function
A	Arterial pulses
C	Capillary refill
T	Temperature, skin
S	Sensation

The use of the **Velpeau bandage** is an alternative to the sling and swathe and is sometimes preferred by patients with a dislocated shoulder as it allows the arm's weight to be supported. The Paramedic places the injured hand on the uninjured shoulder and the arm across the chest. Using a six-inch Ace® wrap and starting under the axilla, the Paramedic winds the bandage over the arm on the chest in recurrent wraps, leaving the elbow exposed, until secure. Then the wrap direction is changed and the wrap goes over the injured shoulder and under the elbow. This last wrap supports the upper arm. Finally, the wrap is tied around the entire torso and secured with fasteners or tape. It is advisable to back up fasteners with tape (Figure 7-32).

For fractures of the humerus, or the elbow, the **sugar tong splint** and a sling and swathe are effective in immobilizing the humerus as well as the joints above and below the suspected fracture. Forming malleable splinting material into a tong shape, measured from the axilla to the elbow and the elbow to the acromion process, the upper arm is immobilized laterally and medially. Using a recurrent bandage, starting at the axilla and wrapping to the elbow, the splint is held in place. Then the sling and swathe, described earlier, is applied (Figure 7-33).

For midshaft radial or ulnar fractures, the Paramedic can use either a posterior gutter splint (Figure 7-34) or a double sugar tong splint (Figure 7-35). For a **posterior gutter splint**, also known as an ulnar gutter splint, the Paramedic measures a malleable splinting material for a length from the distal palmar crease to the midshaft humerus, ensuring joints above and below the fracture are immobilized. The splinting material is then formed into a gutter and held in place with an Ace® wrap.

An alternative splint is the double sugar tong splint. The **double sugar tong splint** is more effective than the posterior gutter splint as it prevents both pronation as well as supination. To start, two "sugar tongs" are preformed from malleable splint material. With the elbow flexed, the first "sugar tong" is applied along both the anterior and posterior aspects of the forearm and held in place with an Ace® wrap. Note the approximate 20-degree flexion of the wrist. The second "sugar tong" is applied along the medial and lateral aspects of the upper arm, overlying the first splint. This splint is then held in place with another bandage.

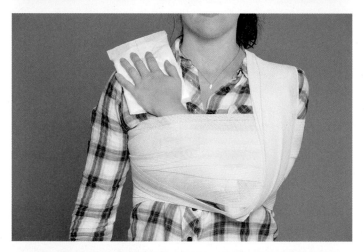

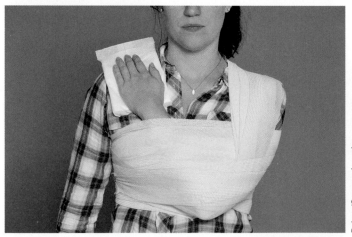

Delmar/Cengage Learning

Figure 7-32 The Velpeau bandage is an alternative to the sling and swathe that allows the arm's weight to be supported.

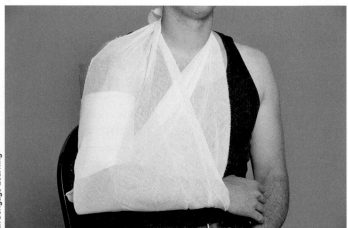

Delmar/Cengage Learning

Figure 7-33 The sugar tong splint with sling and swathe are effective in immobilizing the humerus as well as the joints above and below the suspected fracture.

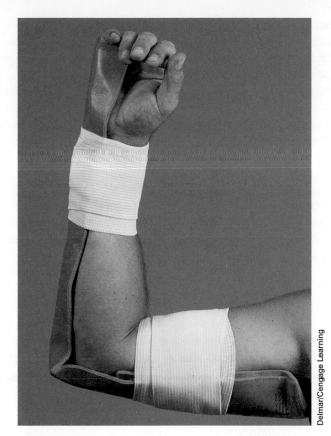

Figure 7-34 A posterior gutter splint is also known as an ulnar gutter splint.

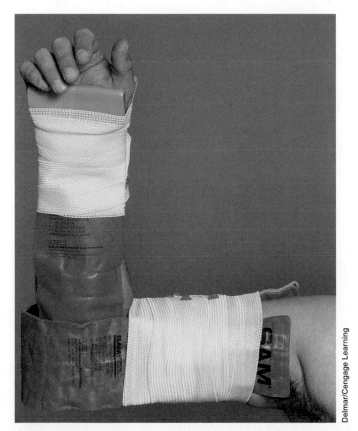

Figure 7-35 The double sugar tong splint prevents both pronation as well as supination.

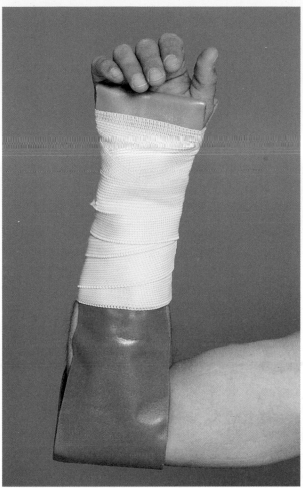

Figure 7-36 The short arm volar splint is useful for distal fractures of the radius or ulna, as well as the wrist.

For distal fractures of the radius or ulna, as well as the wrist, the **short arm volar splint** is useful (volar means palmar surface). Again, the malleable splinting material is made into a sugar tong splint. The Paramedic should note the position of the hand. To preserve the "position of function," some Paramedics have the patient grasp a roller bandage. The splint is then held in place with a bandage (Figure 7-36).

Fractures of the hand and wrist can also be immobilized with a volar splint that extends to the distal interphalangeal joint, called a **Colles splint**. This splint is also useful for immobilizing a Colles fracture. Using malleable splinting material, a splint should be formed that keeps the wrist in 15 to 20 degrees of flexion and the metacarpal joint at a 90-degree angle, with the phalanges fully extended (Figure 7-37).

Gutter splints can be modified to immobilize the fourth and fifth metacarpals, called a **boxer's splint**. Although the splint immobilizes both the wrist and the fourth and fifth digits, it is not recommended for distal forearm fractures as it permits supination/pronation of the hand.

Similarly, a volar splint can be modified into a radial gutter splint immobilizing the lateral hand and digits. Extending from the proximal forearm to the distal interphalangeal joint,

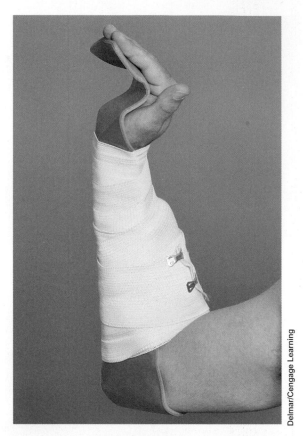

Figure 7-37 A Colles splint is a volar splint that extends to the distal interphalangeal joint.

thereby immobilizing the index finger and middle finger, the radial gutter splint surrounds the anterior wrist. The curvature of the palmar surface should keep the metacarpophalangeal (MCP) joint at 70 degrees, the proximal interphalangeal (PIP) joint at 30 degrees of flexion, and the distal interphalangeal (DIP) joint at 5 to 10 degrees of flexion. This position is called the wine glass position and helps to maintain the hand in the position of function. It is important that the thumb be permitted to extend through an opening in the splint. There are many commercial models of the radial gutter splint available (Figure 7-38).

The **thumb spica splint** is used for suspected gamekeeper's thumb/skier's thumb or suspected scaphoid fractures. Like the radial gutter splint, the thumb spica splint starts at the mid-forearm and wraps the thumb to the distal interphalangeal (DIP) joint. Like the radial gutter splint, the thumb spica splint keeps the hand in the wine glass position (Figure 7-39).

Simple fractures of the distal phalanges, or dislocation of the interphalangeal joints, are immobilized by either buddy taping or finger splints. **Buddy taping** is simply taping the injured finger to the next finger. To add rigidity to the assembly, the Paramedic can insert a tongue depressor between the fingers. The patient will appreciate it if you wrap the splint in gauze dressing.

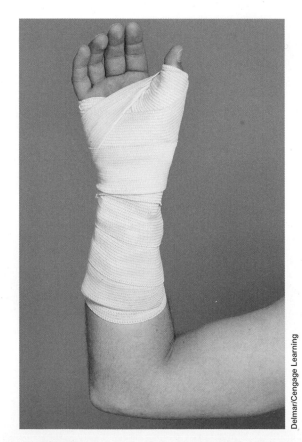

Figure 7-39 The thumb spica splint is used for suspected gamekeeper's thumb/skier's thumb or suspected scaphoid fractures.

Figure 7-38 Radial gutter splint.

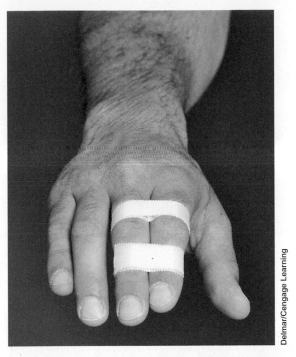

Figure 7-40 Buddy taping and finger splint help immobilize simple fractures.

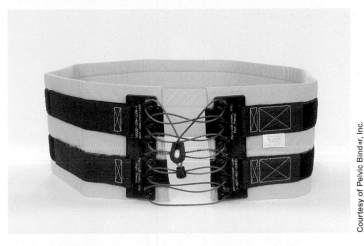

Figure 7-41 A pelvic binder helps reduce the pelvic volume.

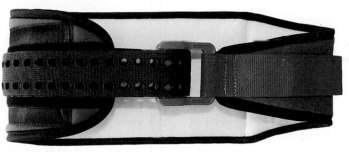

Figure 7-42 The pelvic sling allows access to the anterior pelvis for central venous cannulation and urinary catheterization.

The **finger splint** should maintain the proximal interphalangeal (PIP) joint at an approximate 15 to 20 degrees of flexion (Figure 7-40).

Lower Extremity Splint

Splinting the pelvic girdle can be a challenge. Associated structures often receive collateral damage, leaving more than one bone or ligament to immobilize. The importance of stabilizing a pelvic fracture to prevent an open book fracture cannot be overemphasized.[55] The blood loss into the pelvis from a fracture can be life-threatening, so the Paramedic's first priority is to "reduce the pelvic volume" (the space within the pelvis). By reducing the pelvic volume, there is less space for blood to accumulate and more opportunity for clot formation and venous tamponade.

In the past, Paramedics used sheets to create a form of **pelvic binder**. Using a draw sheet folded approximately 20 cm wide, the Paramedic slid the sheet under the small of the patient's back and moved down over the anterior superior iliac spine (ASIA) and over the ischial tuberosity. Then the Paramedic creates a square knot, places a dowel in the middle, and turns like a corkscrew to tighten the sheet, creating a form of Spanish windlass.

Another adaptation of a current technology is the updated pelvic binder. These pelvic binders use a corset-type device that is laced up the middle and tightens with a pulley system that then locks in place (Figure 7-41).

Similar to a pelvic binder is the pelvic sling. The **pelvic sling** has an approximately 20-cm circumferential belt with an anterior ratchet device. The pelvic sling allows access to

the anterior pelvis for central venous cannulation and urinary catheterization, permits use of the traction splint, and has a self-limiting locking device to prevent overtightening of the pelvic sling (Figure 7-42).

Another effective device is the pneumatic anti-shock garment (PASG)/military anti-shock trousers (MAST). The PASG/MAST uses inflatable chambers to create a circumferential pressure around the pelvis. Applied in one of several ways (e.g., slid up the legs and pelvis like a pair of pants), the PASG/MAST are effective in reducing the pelvic volume and may have the added benefit of increasing the blood volume to the core organs. PASG/MAST should not be used if the patient has pulmonary edema or penetrating chest trauma (Figure 7-43).

In 1860, John Hilton developed the first traction splint, which was later modified by Dr. H. O. Thomas. Many soldiers' lives were saved due to use of the Thomas splint during World War I. It remained the standard of care for femur fractures through the beginnings of volunteer rescue squads in the 1930s, and eventually was placed on the original "essential equipment" list for ambulances proposed by the American College of Surgeons Committee on Trauma.[56]

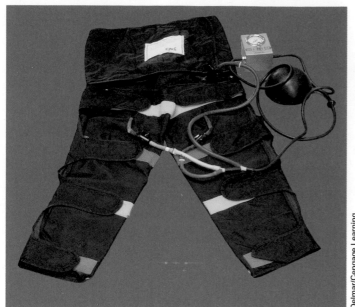

Figure 7-43 The PASG/MAST uses inflatable chambers to create a circumferential pressure around the pelvis.

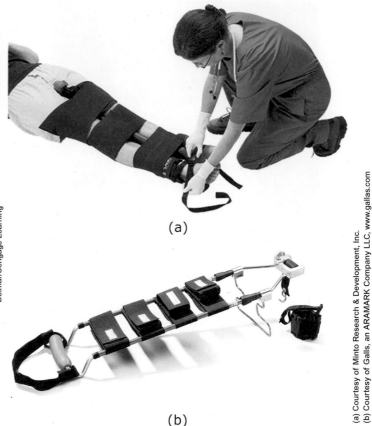

(a)

(b)

Figure 7-44 (a) Unipolar and (b) bipolar traction splints are improved versions of the Thomas splint.

(a) Courtesy of Minto Research & Development, Inc.
(b) Courtesy of Galls, an ARAMARK Company LLC, www.galls.com

In essence, the Thomas splint provides an external metal skeleton to replace the fractured femur. It provides stability and, using a Spanish windlass, applies traction to the femur. This traction helps stabilize the limb ends and permits clot formation. The traction may be responsible for controlling hemorrhage, as a femur fracture can lose between two and four units of blood.

However, these splints are not intended to treat pelvic fractures. In fact, the splint depends on the integrity of the pelvis upon which it rests as a foundation for the traction. Similarly, these splints cannot be used if the knee is fractured/dislocated due to a risk of injury to the peroneal nerve. They also cannot be used if the patient's ankle is amputated or avulsed, as this is a point of fixation for traction.

More recently, there have been improvements on the Thomas splint including the addition of a cranking device to pull steady traction. These variations can be broken down into two classifications: unipolar traction splint and bipolar traction splint (Figure 7-44).

Another traditional splint is the Robert Jones bandage, also known as the Jones compression dressing. The **Robert Jones bandage** is a bulky compression bandage used for knee injuries. Starting with a shell of bulky dressing, such as cotton wool or foam, around the knee from midshaft femur to mid-calf, the Paramedic winds a layer of recurrent bandage around the entire length of the dressing. To add stability, the Paramedic can add wooden slats or a malleable splinting material once the basement wrapping is in place. Another wrap is then added to hold the rigid splint in place.

The advantage of a Robert Jones bandage is that it provides compression, thereby preventing edema, while maintaining stability of the affected joint (Figure 7-45).

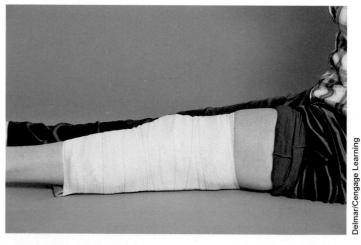

Figure 7-45 A Robert Jones bandage (i.e., "Bulky Jones Bandage") provides compression while maintaining stability of the affected joint.

Distal leg and ankle injuries can be stabilized using a **posterior leg splint**. Using a malleable splinting material, the Paramedic measures from the head of the metatarsal to the mid-calf and forms a gutter splint. Before the gutter splint is put in place, the Paramedic places padding behind the ankle, proximal to the fibular neck, to avoid

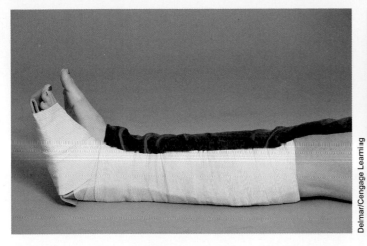

Figure 7-46 A posterior leg splint can be used to stabilize distal leg and ankle injuries.

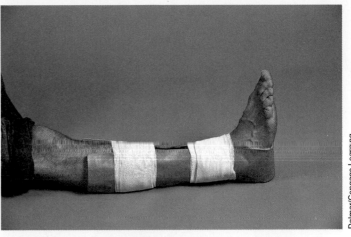

Figure 7-47 A stirrup splint provides lateral and medial support to prevent eversion/inversion of the ankle.

compression of the peroneal nerve. With the splint in place, the Paramedic uses a bandage to wrap in a recurrent fashion (Figure 7-46).

If an ankle fracture/dislocation is suspected, then the Paramedic should consider a stirrup splint. The **stirrup splint** provides lateral and medial support to prevent eversion/ inversion of the ankle. The stirrup splint is similar to the sugar tong splint, but is applied to the ankle. Once the malleable splinting material has been preformed and placed in a supportive position, it is held in place by a recurrent bandage, allowing the patient's toes to be exposed for neurovascular assessment (Figure 7-47).

CASE STUDY (CONTINUED)

During the course of the patient's care, the patient's limb begins to become pale. At first, the Paramedics do not realize it until they slightly move the patient's limb to apply a bandage and the patient lets out a blood-curdling scream. That causes the Paramedics to sit back and reconsider the situation.

CRITICAL THINKING QUESTIONS

1. What are some of the predictable complications associated with prolonged entrapment?
2. What are some of the predictable complications associated with the treatments for conditions related to prolonged entrapment?

Evaluation

When evaluating an extremity injury, the Paramedic should be concerned about a complication often associated with extremity injury: compartment syndrome. **Compartment syndrome**, one of the reperfusion injuries, shares some characteristics and complications with the other reperfusion injury, crush syndrome.

Almost all organs in the body are surrounded by connective tissue membranes: the lungs (the pleura), the heart (the pericardium), and the brain (the meninges). Muscles are no different. Groups of muscles are surrounded by a tough sheet of fibrous connective tissue called fascia. Muscles within these fascia are called compartments.

The muscles in the forearm have three compartments. The volar compartment contains flexor and pronator muscles and, within it, the median nerve, the deep branch of the radial nerve, and the major blood vessels. The dorsal compartment contacts the wrist and finger extensors. The third compartment is the mobile wad compartment, which contains the radial forearm muscles responsible for flexing the forearm and extending/abducting the hand.

The muscles in the lower legs are divided into four main compartments: anterior, lateral, deep posterior, and superficial posterior. The anterior compartment lateral to the tibia contains muscles that dorsiflex the ankle and extend the toes and the anterior tibial artery as well. The lateral compartment,

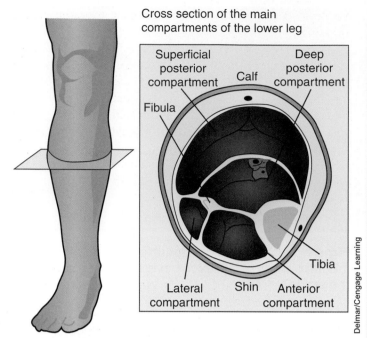

Cross section of the main compartments of the lower leg

Figure 7-48 Compartments of the lower leg: anterior, lateral, deep posterior, and superficial posterior.

lateral to the fibula, contains muscles that permit eversion of the foot and the superficial peroneal nerve that permits feeling on the top of the foot. The deep posterior compartment contains muscles that flex the great toe and phalanges, as well as provide inversion and plantar flexion of the foot. It also contains the posterior tibial nerve that permits feeling on the sole of the foot. The superficial posterior compartment contains muscles such as the gastrocnemius, which is responsible for plantar flexion of the foot, and the soleus, which inserts into the calcaneus through the Achilles tendon. This compartment also contains the sural nerve that allows sensation to the lateral foot and distal calf. In addition, there are 10 compartments in the hands and nine in the foot as well (Figure 7-48).

Pathophysiology of Compartment Syndrome

Whenever pressure builds up inside a compartment, either as a result of compressive external forces or obstruction to venous outflow, these forces decrease tissue perfusion, which leads to cellular hypoxia and ischemia (Table 7-2). Tissue perfusion is the result of capillary perfusion pressure. The normal rate is about 25 mmHg—minus the interstitial fluid pressure, which is normally about 5 mmHg—within the compartment. As the interstitial fluid pressure increases, it overcomes the capillary perfusion pressure until tissue perfusion equals zero and ischemia occurs. In other words, when the pressure within the compartment reaches 25 to 30 mmHg, perfusion stops. When perfusion stops, vasoactive substances (histamine and serotonin) are released, increasing capillary permeability. Acid increases due to anaerobic metabolism and muscles undergo necrosis, releasing potassium and myoglobin.

Table 7-2 Causes of Compartment Syndrome

- Obstruction to outflow, leading to increased compartment pressure
  - Fractures
  - Gunshot and stab wounds
  - Snake bite
  - Overuse/weightlifting
  - Minor trauma and hemorrhage with anticoagulants
  - Hemophilia
- Compressive external forces leading to a smaller compartment
  - Splints and dressings
  - Circumferential burns
  - MAST/PASG
  - Crush injury
    - Coma
    - Narcotics overdose
    - Stroke

STREET SMART

Unrecognized infiltration of intravenous fluids can cause compartment syndrome, particularly in the hand. The Paramedic should regularly monitor IV sites for signs of infiltration (i.e., swelling and tenderness) and document the site's condition.

A compartment syndrome of the forearm, such as might occur from lying on the forearm while in a coma from a heroin overdose, can lead to **Volkmann's contracture**.[57] Volkmann first described compartment syndrome in 1872 as the result of a too tight bandage on an elbow fracture. The forearm appears tense from overpressurization and the patient experiences paralysis and paresthesia from compression of the median nerve and severe pain from passive extension of the fingers.

Tibial fractures are responsible for approximately 45% of the cases of compartment syndrome. Tibial compartment syndromes, like all compartment syndromes, present with the classic 5 "P's" of the compartment syndrome: pain, paresthesia, pallor in the extremity, pulselessness (a late sign), and poikilothermia, a cold distal extremity. Pain and paresthesia are the most predictive features.[58]

Pain, out of proportion to the injury, is characteristic of compartment syndrome. The pain is a crescendo pain described as deep, aching, and made worse with movement, even passive stretching of the limb. Pain is often coupled with paresthesia, a stocking-like numbness that progresses as the nerves are compressed. In the anterior compartment syndrome, paresthesia is seen in the great toe, due to compression of the peroneal nerve, for example.

To confirm pulselessness in an extremity, the Paramedic should apply the pulse oximeter probe to the distal toe or finger, then occlude the arterial pulses one at a time. This will confirm the absence of one of the arterial pulses.

The complications of compartment syndrome are twofold: immediate and delayed. The immediate problem is muscle loss from hypoperfusion. The first action is to remove the compressive force, if that is the problem (e.g., removing the bandage from a splint, cutting a cast lengthwise, or performing an escharotomy of a circumferential burn). In most instances, Paramedics need to consider immediate transport to the closest appropriate facility. In as little as three hours muscle damage can be irreversible, and in six hours nerve damage is permanent. During transport, it is appropriate to apply ice. However, the limb should not be elevated as this action lowers the mean arterial perfusion pressure.

In some cases, the compartment syndrome is so advanced (or, in the case of interrupted arterial perfusion, is so rapid) that immediate fasciotomy may be indicated. **Fasciotomy**, a surgical procedure where the fascia is cut to relieve tension, is considered an advanced Paramedic skill and must be performed only under special conditions and after training. In the field, fasciotomy, so-called "dirty fasciotomy," has been advocated under a limited set of circumstances; for example, prolonged evacuation from a wilderness setting and tactical situations with delayed evacuation.

An alternative to field fasciotomy may be use of mannitol. Mannitol, a hyperosmotic diuretic, draws fluid out of the compartment, reducing the intercompartmental pressure. It has been shown to be effective, thus eliminating the need for a fasciotomy.[59]

Prolonged compartment syndrome can lead to crush syndrome. If reperfusion is established, a washout of potassium and myoglobin puts the patient at risk for dysrhythmia (including sudden cardiac death) and rhabdomyolysis (leading to acute renal failure). Crush syndrome treatment is discussed in Chapter 8.

CASE STUDY CONCLUSION

Once the Paramedics have immoblized the patient's limb and administered a healthy dose of opiates, the patient is moved to the litter and carried by hand down to a predesignated evacuation point. A medevac helicopter is standing by to airlift the patient to the trauma center.

CRITICAL THINKING QUESTIONS

1. What is the most appropriate transport decision that will get the patient to definitive care?
2. What are the advantages of transporting a patient with suspected acute alcohol withdrawal to these hospitals, even if that means bypassing other hospitals in the process?

Disposition

Most orthopaedic injuries can be transported to community hospitals where treatment—and perhaps more importantly, rehabilitation—can be arranged. If the patient is a multitrauma victim, the patient should be transported to a trauma center where life-threatening injuries can be treated first. In every case, the Paramedic should document the patient's history and physical condition, particularly when reassessing the injured extremity.

CONCLUSION

Although orthopaedic injuries are an everyday occurrence, all of these injuries have the potential to cause life-long disability. Proper assessment and treatment in the field can be the first step toward a full recovery with possible return of all function.

KEY POINTS:

- The musculoskeletal system is in a constant state of change.

- Sprains occur in degrees, from a mild first degree sprain to loss of the joint in a sixth degree tear.

- Injuries to the shoulder include shoulder separation, rotator cuff tears, shoulder impingement syndrome, and sternoclavicular sprains.

- Sprained knees are graded I, II, and III.

- One of the most common orthopaedic injuries is a twisted ankle, which is graded like the ankle sprain as I, II, and III.

- Four tendons tend to rupture: biceps, quadriceps, patellar, and Achilles.

- Dislocation is a complete luxation, or separation, of a joint, whereas a subluxation is a partial separation of a joint.

- The shoulder is the most common dislocation, and the anterior shoulder dislocation is the most common shoulder dislocation.

- A patellar dislocation is not a knee dislocation.

- Open fractures are graded on the Gustilo-Anderson system, which is graded type I to III.

- Fractures are either complete or incomplete, and either open or closed.

- Pediatric fractures of the growth plates are classified as Salter-Harris fractures: I-V.

- Midshaft or diaphyseal humerus fractures are common in adults, whereas fractures of the humeral head (proximal fractures) are more common in the elderly.

- A fracture/dislocation of the ulna, or Monteggia's fracture, is common in the wrist; its counterpart is Galeazzi's fracture, a midshaft radial fracture.

- Classic wrist fractures are the Colles fracture and the reverse Colles, or Smith, fracture.

- The scaphoid (i.e., navicular) bone is the most common carpal fracture and is prone to avascular necrosis.

- A fall on an outstretched thumb can cause a Bennett's fracture.

- Pelvic fractures are either open or closed; closed pelvic fractures are associated with higher mortality rates.

- Impacted femoral head, broken femoral neck, and fractured trochanter are all types of hip fractures.

- Paget's disease is a chronic and progressive disease of the bones.

- Dislocated knees are a medical emergency.

- Ankle fractures are unimalleolar, bimalleolar, and trimalleolar.

- Osteoporosis risk is measured by bone mineral density, or T-score.

- Blood loss from fractures can be significant: 500 cc in the humerus, 1,000 to 1,500 cc in the femur, and over 1,500 cc in the pelvis.

- Manual stabilization is the first step of every limb reduction/fixation.

- The Hippocratic method, the Manes method, the Stimson method, Kocher's method, and scapular manipulation are all techniques for shoulder reduction.

- Reductions in the field are only performed if there is vascular compromise.

- The Bigelow and Stimson maneuvers are used to reduce hip dislocations.

- The mnemonic FACTS is useful for assessing fractures/dislocations: function, arterial pulses, capillary refill, temperature, and sensation. The mnemonic RICE is useful for remembering the treatment of fractures/dislocations: rest, ice, compression, and elevation.

- Common external splints are the sugar tong, the gutter splint, the spica splint, and the volar splint.

- Open book pelvic fractures are life-threatening conditions and are treated with pelvic binders.

- A complication of fractures and fracture management is compartment syndrome.

- The five P's are characteristic of compartment syndrome: pain, paresthesia, pulselessness, poikilothermia, and pallor.

REVIEW QUESTIONS:

1. What is "biomechanics?"
2. What are the six degrees of sprain?
3. What are the three types of open fractures using the Gustilo–Anderson system?
4. What are the four lines of force responsible for fractures?

CASE STUDY QUESTIONS:

Please refer to the Case Study in this chapter, and answer the questions below:

1. Suppose in this case the patient's shoulder had been dislocated in the process of extrication and the patient subsequently lost pulses. What are the methods of reducing a shoulder?

2. After reducing the shoulder, the Paramedics note that the only splinting material they have left is a bandage. How can they bandage this shoulder post-reduction?

3. If CasEvac is delayed, what treatments can the Paramedics start in the field to treat the compartment syndrome?

REFERENCES:

1. Tzannes A, Murrell GA. Clinical examination of the unstable shoulder. *Sports Med*. 2002;32(7):447–457.
2. Peterson JJ, Bancroft LW. Injuries of the fingers and thumb in the athlete. *Clin Sports Med*. Jul 2006;25(3):527–542, vii–viii.
3. van Rijn RM, van Os AG, Bernsen RM, Luijsterburg PA, Koes BW, Bierma-Zeinstra SM. What is the clinical course of acute ankle sprains? A systematic literature review. *Am J Med*. Apr 2008;121(4):324–331.e6.
4. McKeon PO, Mattacola CG. Interventions for the prevention of first time and recurrent ankle sprains. *Clin Sports Med*. Jul 2008;27(3):371–382, viii.
5. Fong DT, Man CY, Yung PS, Cheung SY, Chan KM. Sport-related ankle injuries attending an accident and emergency department. *Injury*. Oct 2008;39(10):1222–1227.
6. Ivins D. Acute ankle sprain: an update. *Am Fam Physician*. Nov 15 2006;74(10):1714–1720.
7. Wexler RK. The injured ankle. *Am Fam Physician*. Feb 1 1998;57(3):474–480.
8. Gross MT, Liu HY. The role of ankle bracing for prevention of ankle sprain injuries. *J Orthop Sports Phys Ther*. Oct 2003;33(10):572–577.
9. Lohrer H, Alt W, Gollhofer A. Neuromuscular properties and functional aspects of taped ankles. *Am J Sports Med*. Jan–Feb 1999;27(1):69–75.
10. Chilvers M, Donahue M, Nassar L, et al. Foot and ankle injuries in elite female gymnasts. *Foot Ankle Int*. Feb 2007;28(2):214–218.
11. Desmond EA, Chou LB. Current concepts review: Lisfranc injuries. *Foot Ankle Int*. Aug 2006;27(8):653–660.

12. Nunley JA, Vertullo CJ. Classification, investigation, and management of midfoot sprains: Lisfranc injuries in the athlete. *Am J Sports Med*. Nov–Dec 2002;30(6):871–878.

13. Pullat RC, Gadaria MR, Karas RH, et al. Tendon rupture associated with simvastatin/ezetimibe therapy. *Am J Cardiol*. July 1, 2007;100(1):152–153.

14. Kelly BM, Rao N, Louis SS. Bilateral, simultaneous, spontaneous rupture of quadriceps tendons without trauma in an obese patient: a case report. *Arch Phys Med Rehabil*. Mar 2001;82(3):415–418.

15. Kannus P, Józsa L. Histopathological changes preceding spontaneous rupture of a tendon. A controlled study of 891 patients. *J Bone Joint Surg Am*. Dec 1991;73(10):1507–1525.

16. Lian Ø, Refsnes PE, Engebretsen L, Bahr R. Performance characteristics of volleyball players with patellar tendinopathy. *Am J Sports Med*. May–Jun 2003;31(3):408–413.

17. Kader D, Saxena A, Movin T, Maffulli N. Achilles tendinopathy: some aspects of basic science and clinical management. *Br J Sports Med*. Aug 2002;36(4):239–249.

18. Schepsis AA, Jones H, Haas AL. Achilles tendon disorders in athletes. *Am J Sports Med*. Mar–Apr 2002;30(2):287–305.

19. Khan RJ, Fick D, Keogh A, et al. Treatment of acute Achilles tendon ruptures. A meta-analysis of randomized, controlled trials. *J Bone Joint Surg Am*. Oct 2005;87(10):2202–2210.

20. Dodson CC, Cordasco FA. Anterior glenohumeral joint dislocations. *Orthop Clin North Am*. Oct 2008;39(4):507–518, vii.

21. Seroyer ST, et al. Shoulder pain in the overhead throwing athlete. *Sports Health*. March/April 2009;1(2):108–120.

22. Lattanza LL, Keese G. Elbow instability in children. *Hand Clin*. Feb 2008;24(1):139–152.

23. Shin R, Ring D. The ulnar nerve in elbow trauma. *J Bone Joint Surg*. May 2007;89(5):1108–1116.

24. Shabet S, Folman Y, Mann G, Kots Y, Fredman B, Banian M, et al. The role of sonography in detecting radial head subluxation in a child. Case Report. *J Clinical Ultrasound*. May 2005;33(4):187–189.

25. Toupin P, Osmond MH, Correll R, Plint A. Radial head subluxation: how long do children wait in the emergency department before reduction?. *CJEM*. Sep 2007;9(5):333–337.

26. Matsumoto K, Sumi H, Sumi Y, Shimizu K. An analysis of hip dislocations among snowboarders and skiers: a 10-year prospective study from 1992 to 2002. *J Trauma*. Nov 2003;55(5):946–948.

27. Yang EC, Cornwall R. Initial treatment of traumatic hip dislocations in the adult. *Clin Orthop Relat Res*. Aug 2000;(377):24–31.

28. Thijs Y, De Clercq D, Roosen P, Witvrouw E. Gait-related intrinsic risk factors for patellofemoral pain in novice recreational runners. *Br J Sports Med*. Jun 2008;42(6):466–471.

29. Mehta VM, Inoue M, Nomura E, Fithian DC. An algorithm guiding the evaluation and treatment of acute primary patellar dislocations. *Sports Med Arthrosc*. Jun 2007;15(2):78–81.

30. Seroyer ST, Musahl V, Harner CD. Management of the acute knee dislocation: the Pittsburgh experience. *Injury*. Jul 2008;39(7):710–718.

31. Zoys GN. Knee dislocations. *Orthopedics*. Mar 2001;24(3):294–299; quiz 300–301.

32. Crawford AH, Al-Sayyad MJ. Fractures and dislocations of the foot and ankle. In: Green NE, Swiontkowski MF, eds. *Skeletal Trauma in Children* (3rd ed.). Philadelphia: WB Saunders Company; 2003:516–537.

33. Ufberg J, McNamara R. Management of common dislocations. In: Roberts JR, Hedges JR, eds. *Clinical Procedures in Emergency Medicine* (4th ed.). Philadelphia: WB Saunders Company; 2004:984–986.

34. Fernández-Valencia JA. *Orthopaedia—Collaborative Orthopaedic Knowledgebase*. Available at: **http://www .orthopaedia.com/x/r4EqAQ**. Accessed December 13, 2009.

35. Vestergaard P, Rejnmark L, Mosekilde L. Increased mortality in patients with a hip fracture-effect of pre-morbid conditions and post-fracture complications. *Osteoporos Int*. Dec 2007;18(12):1583–1593.

36. Mubarak SJ, Kim JR, Edmonds EW, Pring ME, Bastrom TP. Classification of proximal tibial fractures in children. *J Child Orthop*. Mar 17 2009.

37. Kontakis G, Koutras C, Tosounidis T, Giannoudis P. Early management of proximal humeral fractures with hemiarthroplasty: a systematic review. *J Bone Joint Surg Br*. Nov 2008;90(11):1407–1413.

38. Greenspan, A. *Orthopaedic Imaging: A Practical Approach* (4th ed). Philadelphia, PA: Lippincott Williams and Wilkins; 2004:170.

39. Armstrong PF, Joughlin VE, Clarke HM. Pediatric fractures of the forearm, wrist, and hand. In: Green NE, Swiontkowski MF. *Skeletal Trauma in Children* (2nd ed.). Philadelphia, PA: WB Saunders; 1998:161–196.

40. Földhazy Z, Törnkvist H, Elmstedt E, Andersson G, Hagsten B, Ahrengart L. Long-term outcome of nonsurgically treated distal radius fractures. *J Hand Surg [Am]*. Nov 2007;32(9):1374–1384.

41. Scalea TM, Burgess AR. (2004). Pelvic fractures. In: Moore EE, Feliciano DV, Mattox KL, eds. *Trauma* (5th ed.). New York: McGraw-Hill; 2004: 779–805.

42. Frakes M, Evans T. Major pelvic fractures. *Crit Care Nurse*. 2004;23:18–30.

43. Heetveld MJ, Harris I, Schlaphoff G, Sugrue M. Guidelines for the management of haemodynamically unstable pelvic fracture patients. *ANZ J Surg*. 2004;74:520–529.

44. Grant PT. The diagnosis of pelvic fractures by "springing." *Arch Emerg Med*. 1990;7(3):178–182.

45. Small SA, Perron AD, Brady WJ. Orthopedic pitfalls: cauda equina syndrome. *Am J Emerg Med*. Mar 2005;23(2):159–163.

46. Lee C, Porter K. The prehospital management of pelvic fractures. *J Emerg Med*. 2007;24(2):130–133.

47. Radcliff TA, Henderson WG, Stoner TJ, Khuri SF, Dohm M, Hutt E. Patient risk factors, operative care, and outcomes among

older community-dwelling male veterans with hip fracture. *J Bone Joint Surg Am*. Jan 2008;90(1):34–42.

48. Bharam S, Vrahas MS, Fu FH. Knee fractures in the athlete. *Orthop Clin North Am*. Jul 2002;33(3):565–574.

49. National Osteoporosis Foundation. *America's Bone Health: The State of Osteoporosis and Low Bone Mass in Our Nation*. Washington, DC: National Osteoporosis Foundation; 2002.

50. Wolfe, T. Intranasal fentanyl for acute pain: techniques to enhance efficacy. *Ann Emerg Med*. 2007;49(5):721–722.

51. Mattick A, Wyatt JP. From Hippocrates to the Eskimo—a history of techniques used to reduce anterior dislocation of the shoulder. *J.R. Coll. Surg. Edinb*. Oct 2000;45:312–316.

52. Doyle W, Ragar T. Use of the scapular manipulation method to reduce an anterior shoulder dislocation in the supine position. *Ann Emerg Med*. 1996;27(1):92–94.

53. Baykal B, Sener S, Turkan H. Scapular manipulation technique for reduction for traumatic anterior shoulder dislocations: experiences of an academic emergency department. *J Emerg Med*. 2005;22(5):336–338.

54. Kling MP. Patellar dislocation reduction. In: Reichman EF, Simon RR, eds. *Emergency Medicine Procedures*. New York: McGraw-Hill Professional; 2003:640.

55. Coppola PT, Coppola M. Orthopaedic emergencies. Emergency department evaluation and treatment of pelvic fractures. *Emerg Med Clin North Am*. 2000;18(1):1.

56. Bledson B, Barnes D. Traction splint. An EMS relic? *Jnl Emer Med Svc*. August 2004:65–67.

57. Owen CA, Mubarak SJ, Hargens AR, et al. Intramuscular pressures with limb compression clarification of the pathogenesis of the drug-induced muscle-compartment syndrome. *N Engl J Med*. May 24 1979;300(21):1169–1172.

58. Ulmer T. The clinical diagnosis of compartment syndrome of the lower leg: are clinical findings predictive of the disorder? *J Orthop Trauma*. Sep 2002;16(8):572–577.

59. Daniels M, Reichman J, Brezis M. Mannitol treatment for acute compartment syndrome. *Nephron*. Aug 1998;79(4):492–493.

CHAPTER 8

SOFT-TISSUE INJURY

KEY CONCEPTS:

Upon completion of this chapter, it is expected that the reader will understand these following concepts:

- Types of soft-tissue injuries
- Healing process
- Wound closure
- Assessment and treatment of crush injury
- Hemostatic agents to aid hemostasis
- Dressings and bandages

ANATOMY CONCEPTS:

Prior to reading this chapter the Paramedic student should be familiar with the following anatomy and physiology concepts:

- Integumentary system
- Coagulation
- Inflammation

Following the frigid cold of winter, everyone welcomed the warm, sunny, spring day. However, for one man, that warmth gave way to the alarms and sirens of emergency response teams. Apparently, the man had taken advantage of the warm weather to work on his car in the driveway and was now pinned beneath it after the jack collapsed. The caller doesn't know how long the patient has been under the car.

CRITICAL THINKING QUESTIONS

1. What are some of the possible soft-tissue injuries that the Paramedic might suspect based on the mechanism of injury?

2. Are any of these soft-tissue injuries potentially life-threatening conditions?

OVERVIEW

Traumatic wounds can result from a number of sources and often involve shearing and tearing forces. In one study of 1,000 wounds, the distribution of traumatic wounds was 42% secondary to blunt trauma; 34% due to sharp, nonglass objects; 13% due to glass; and the remainder dues to bites and other minor injuries.[1] Regardless of the etiology, soft-tissue injuries can be potentially life-threatening issues, although in most cases the damage is more psychological than physiological.

Chief Concern

Soft-tissue injuries can range from the minor skin abrasion to the life-threatening crush injury. Soft-tissue injuries can affect the superficial epithelial layers or impact deeper muscle and nervous tissues. Soft-tissue injuries can be a minor annoyance, as in the case of a bruise or abrasion, or can be the source of significant pain and suffering, as in the case of burns, which will be discussed in Chapter 9. Although soft-tissue injury to the skin is visible and apparent, injury to deeper soft tissues—such as tendons, ligaments, and muscles—is not so apparent. This chapter will focus on soft-tissue injuries of the skin, exclusive of burns. Sprains, strains, and muscular injuries were discussed in Chapter 7 on musculoskeletal injuries.

Similar to burns, soft-tissue injuries can be looked at as superficial, partial thickness, or full thickness. It helps to think about soft-tissue injuries in this way because it is based on anatomy and is consistent with the terminology for burns and frostbite.

Abrasions

An **abrasion**, by definition, is a wound that does not go below the epidermis. Therefore, abrasions, also known as scrapes, are superficial soft-tissue wounds. Bleeding from an abrasion is minor and capillary in nature. Although an abrasion is typically not life-threatening, it can be the source of an infection and a cause of pain. For these reasons, abrasions should be cleaned and decontaminated, then dressed with a sterile dressing. The Paramedic should offer analgesia to the patient in severe cases.

Lacerations

A traumatic force that tears, cuts, or rends the flesh, leaving a jagged wound, creates a **laceration**. A laceration can be superficial or full thickness. The laceration that extends past the dermis will reach a layer of loose connective tissue called the **superficial fascia**. This superficial fascia constitutes the subcutaneous layer of skin and can be recognized in a laceration. The superficial fascia encloses the fatty tissues that insulate and cushion the skin. This fatty layer can be debrided without significant harm. Often it is debrided because devitalized fat (fat without perfusion) serves as a medium for infection. The resulting dead space tends to refill naturally. In extreme cases, tissue expanders can be used to fill the void.

Since nerves travel within the superficial fascia, superficial lacerations tend to be painful. Injection of anesthetics, such as lidocaine, dissipates along this connective tissue plane and results in localized pain relief.

Full thickness lacerations penetrate past the superficial fascia and into the deep fascia that encloses muscles (Figure 8-1). This thick and fibrous layer is visible to the naked eye and appears like off-white colored cellophane wrap. Deep fascia provides the muscles with another layer of protection from infection. Interruption of both the skin and the deep fascia permits the introduction of infection into the muscle. In almost every case, a deep laceration requires wound exploration for contaminants, irrigation, and closure with sutures.

Punctures

As the name implies, a **puncture wound** penetrates through the skin and, like the laceration, can be either be superficial or full thickness. The Paramedic is normally unable to visualize the depth of the puncture wound. This is a notable difference between a laceration and a puncture wound. Therefore, the Paramedic is unable to ascertain if the puncture wound is superficial or full thickness in the field. The Paramedic should not probe the wound to determine its depth.

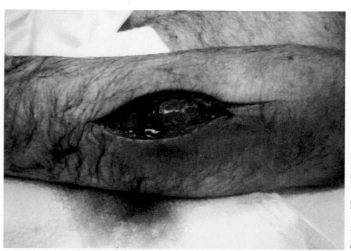

Courtesy of Brecht Palombo

Figure 8-1 Full thickness lacerations penetrate past the superficial fascia and into the deep fascia that encloses muscles.

A more significant concern to the Paramedic is what underlying organs may have been injured when the puncture wound occurred. There are a number of causes of puncture wounds, including gunshot wounds (GSW), knife wounds, and so on. If a GSW is suspected, the Paramedic should inspect the patient's body for an exit wound and plot a suspected course of trajectory. In some cases, there is no exit wound and the trajectory is thus not apparent. In that case, the Paramedic cannot determine which organs are injured. Alternatively, there may be multiple exit wounds, depending if the bullet shattered bone and fragmented. Whenever possible, the Paramedic should try to determine the caliber and type of weapon used.

Although there is less velocity in a knife wound than a bullet wound, the knife's damage, as seen in a cone, can be extensive. Again, the Paramedic should try to determine the length of the knife and whether there is a single knife wound or multiple knife wounds.

A puncture wound created by a needle or splinter sometimes creates a felon into a distal fingertip. A **felon** is a purulent infection that results when bacteria-laden foreign material is injected into the pulp of the finger, most commonly the thumb or index finger. These infections are very painful and require careful incision and drainage by a physician in most cases.

Starting as a small abscess following a puncture wound from a nail or needle, **necrotizing fasciitis** can become a life-threatening soft-tissue infection (Figure 8-2). Once beta-hemolytic streptococci is "seeded" under the skin, it flourishes in the dark moist space between the dermis and the subcutaneous layer, spreading along the fascia. During its spread, the enzymes from the infection literally liquefy the fascia as it spreads. Often the spread of necrotizing fasciitis extends well beyond the visible surface manifestations. In some cases, amputation is required to halt its progression.[2]

Avulsions and Amputations

There are over 30,000 traumatic amputations annually in the United States and 65% involve the upper limb, from fingers to elbow to shoulder. The majority of amputations (80%)

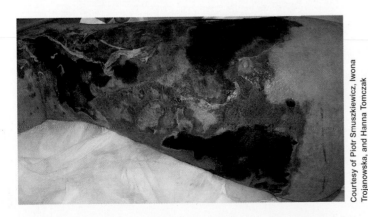

Courtesy of Piotr Smuszkiewicz, Iwona Trojanowska, and Hanna Tomczak

Figure 8-2 Necrotizing fasciitis can become a life-threatening soft-tissue infection.

Table 8-1 Partial List of Mechanisms of Injury That Can Cause Amputation

- Conveyers
- Printing press
- Snow blower
- Lawnmower
- Circular saw
- Band saw
- Drill presses
- Roll presses
- Food slicer
- Meat grinder
- Tractor power takeoff
- Augers

occur in working males, and the patient's typical age at the time of an amputation is 15 to 40. Most amputations occur while the patient is working on a machine. The fingers are the most common amputation.

The mechanism of injury helps to determine whether the separation of a body part from the body is an amputation or an avulsion (Table 8-1). An **amputation** is the separation of a limb or digit by a shearing force. Any focused energy on a specific point can cause a shearing force. Amputations usually have a clean line of demarcation where the force impacted the body. Alternatively, an **avulsion** is usually caused by a tearing force. These forces rend the limb from the body, often leaving a jagged or tattered stump behind. Both amputations and avulsions can be either partial or complete. A common partial avulsion is an ear that is torn off the head during combat.

Avulsions tend to bleed, as torn blood vessels are unable to retract as easily as the transected blood vessels in an amputation. In addition, avulsions have less of a chance of reimplantation than an amputation. The sharp guillotine force involved in an amputation minimizes local tissue trauma whereas the tearing forces of an avulsion crush and mangle a larger area, creating more tissue damage.

STREET SMART

One study showed that most traumatic amputations from a blast injury were actually found midshaft, and not at joints as might be suspected. This is thought to be due to axial force being applied to the limb.[3]

Wound Healing

The skin, although only 1 to 2 mm thick, is a remarkable organ with many functions. As the largest organ in the body, the skin protects the body from infection, provides thermal control, serves as a sensory organ, and maintains the body's aesthetics. When the skin is injured, it can adversely impact the patient's quality of life. In the case of burns, injuries to the skin can be life-threatening.

Whenever the skin is wounded, the body immediately starts wound healing. Wound healing can be divided into three phases: hemostasis, proliferative, and remodeling.

During the **hemostasis stage**, as the name suggests, bleeding is controlled. At first, the tissue retracts, leading to the compression of arterioles and venules. This reflexive vasoconstriction can last for 10 minutes, permitting the clot to form. Leaking tissue-clotting factors from injured cells initiates the clotting cascade. Thrombin and fibrin form fibrinogen, which helps with platelet plug formation. These platelet plugs are the start of clot formation and hemorrhage control.

Almost simultaneously, the characteristic signs of a wound develop. The area starts to become reddened, swollen, warm, and painful as the body's immune system starts to attack invading microbes. As neutrophils start to clear debris, via phagocytosis, the body starts the next phase, the proliferative phase.

During the **proliferative phase**, which starts on about day two and may last three weeks, fibroblasts start to form a bed of collagen and rudimentary tissue. This formation, called **granulation**, replaces the fibrin clot. Granulation starts on the inside and pushes the scab up and out, a process called **wound contraction**. During this process, new blood vessels are formed, a process called **angiogenesis**, to provide the growing tissue with nutrients. The development of new blood vessels to provide nutrients to the growing skin, called **neovascularization**, is critical to wound healing. Evidence of neovascularization is seen in the bright red appearance of the young scar. The loops of capillaries, surrounded by fibroblasts, give the scar its characteristic grainy appearance and announce the granulation stage of healing. This granulation is most pronounced in wounds that heal by secondary intention.

Primary wound healing, healing by first intention, occurs within hours of an incision. These wounds, which are usually clean wounds, heal well. That is, they heal with good cosmetic result and little scar formation, because of the close approximation of the wound edges.

If the wound is contaminated, preventing close approximation of the wound edges, a lengthy process of wound healing, called **delayed primary wound healing**, occurs as macrophages must wall off foreign material. Wound decontamination by Paramedics in the field can help to shorten this delayed wound healing. In most cases where there has been contamination, the wound will have to be sutured in order to bring the wound edges into closer approximation. If a wound is not properly decontaminated, and/or the wound is not sutured, then chronic inflammation can result and lead to prominent scarring.

In some cases of wounds with gross contamination, the Paramedic purposely leaves the wound open to start the inflammatory response. The wound is then closed a day or so later with sutures to promote primary wound healing.

Healing by secondary intention, or secondary wound healing, occurs when the wound is purposefully left open to air and the body is allowed to close the wound itself via granulation. Healing by secondary intention involves a more intense inflammatory response and is seen as more useful in grossly contaminated wounds.

In all cases, the body is trying to seal the wound to prevent further contamination, infection, and hemorrhage. It is the Paramedic's responsibility to assist the body with this function by artificially creating sterile barriers and promoting clot formation via bandaging.

During the final phase, called the **remodeling phase**, the body starts to return the skin to a more normal condition. Within six weeks, the new skin covering the wound (scar) will have 80% to 90% of its wound "bursting" strength. Within 6 to 12 months, the wound will change its texture, color, and thickness to match the surrounding skin (Figure 8-3).

Chronic Wounds

However, scar formation is not uniform in all wounds or all patients. Some wounds become chronic wounds. Examples of chronic wounds include venous ulcers, diabetic ulcers, and pressure sores. Paramedics can have an impact on some of the causes of chronic wounds, as dressings and bandages help to prevent repeated trauma to the wound. In addition, irrigation for decontamination can reduce foreign bodies and subsequent inflammation and infection. Systemic support can help to prevent hypoxia and ischemia induced by hypoperfusion.

These chronic wounds can also be the result of poor circulation (i.e., venous stasis), or a result of pressure necrosis. Patients with diabetes are particularly prone to venous stasis

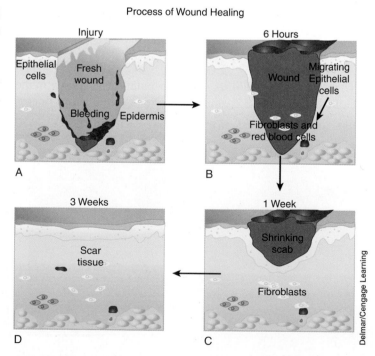

Process of Wound Healing

Figure 8-3 Wound healing occurs in several phases.

and chronic wounds, particularly in the feet. A pressure sore (bedsore) is a classic example of a chronic wound that results from pressure necrosis. Immobility, often coupled with fecal contamination, makes these pressure sores particularly problematic to heal.

Pressure sores are an ulceration of the skin that occurs because of prolonged pressure along prominences of the body such as the sacrum, elbows, knees, and ankles. The combination of compression of the skin, preventing perfusion, and shear forces that are created as the skin slides against the deep fascia in opposing directions, plus the friction created by the bedding against the skin, culminate to create a pressure sore. Wound formation is further accelerated whenever there is moisture (from sweat, feces, or urine) that macerates the skin.

Other factors that accelerate the development of pressure sores include advanced age, with accompanying decreased healing capacity; poor nutrition; smoking that causes peripheral vasoconstriction; and diabetes mellitus that causes poor circulation.

Pressure sores are very problematic in the nursing home and extended care populations. To help identify and quantify risk factors, in order that appropriate treatment plans may be initiated, the **Braden risk assessment scale** was created and is used extensively in the long-term care industry (Figure 8-4). This scale includes evaluations of sensory perception, moisture, activity, mobility, nutrition, and friction/shear.

Pressure sores can be divided into four stages using the National Pressure Ulcer Advisory Panel's staging system. These stages are analogous to the various types of burns discussed in the next chapter: superficial, partial thickness, full thickness, and affecting bone and muscle.

Stage one pressure sores are superficial injuries to the skin that are characterized by nonblanchable reddened areas. Like a superficial burn, these wounds heal when the stimulus is removed (pressure) and left open to air.

A stage two pressure sore is a partial thickness wound that affects the epidermis but does not extend into the dermis layer. The interface between the dermis and the epidermis is not visible to the human eye; however, the dermis layer is

Progression of a Pressure Sore

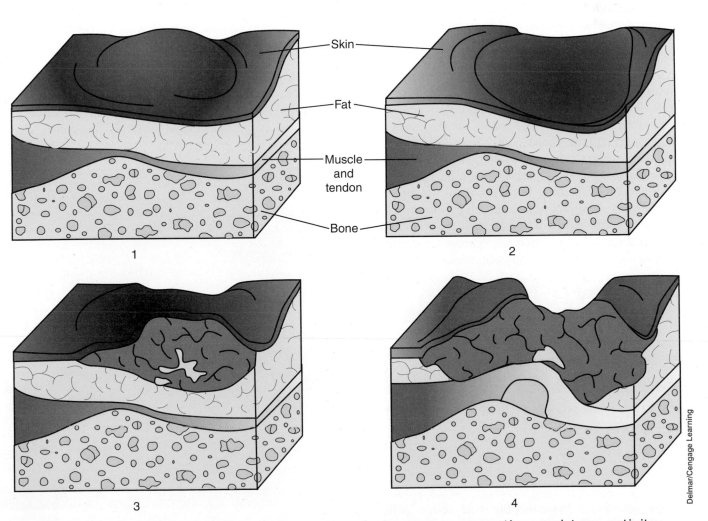

Figure 8-4 The Braden stages of pressure sores evaluate sensory perception, moisture, activity, mobility, nutrition, and friction/shear.

the "living" layer that continuously reproduces the epidermis. Therefore, a partial thickness wound is capable of healing itself. Stage two pressure wounds can develop blisters like a partial thickness burn. Examples of stage two injuries include abrasions, skin tears, and skin burns from tape.

A stage three pressure sore is a full thickness wound that cannot heal without interventions such as tissue grafting and special biodressings. The appearance of a stage three pressure sore can be deceiving. Like an iceberg, the majority of the damage from this wound is hidden under the skin. Only the presence of an open wound on the surface alerts the Paramedic to deeper damage. This phenomenon is consistent with the inside out theory of pressure sore formation that suggests pressure sores start deep at the interface of the fascia and dermis. Stage three wounds are particularly difficult to heal for this reason and are very prone to infections.

The last pressure sore, sometimes called a stage four pressure sore, extends into the deeper muscles and even into the bones. These wounds are often found on the patient's dorsum, where the wound has been hidden from sight in a bedridden patient. Patients—such as stroke patients, comatose patients, or patients with altered sensory perception—lying supine or decubitus for prolonged periods of time develop these wounds, sometimes referred to as **decubitus ulcers**. A stage four decubitus ulcer can lead to osteomyelitis, necrotizing tissue fasciitis, and muscle necrosis.

There are multiple methods of wound repair including autolytic debridement using moist dressings, mechanical debridement using soaked packed dressings, and surgical debridement. One of the newer wound healing technologies is the V.A.C. therapy system. With the V.A.C. system, the Paramedic places foam dressing into the wound, connects a tube to the dressing and applies suction to the tube, which pulls exudate and infectious debris from the wound, collecting it in a canister.[4]

Although Paramedics may encounter treatments in progress when caring for a patient with a pressure sore, the Paramedic's focus should be on treating the whole patient. Assessment for sepsis and systemic support for oxygenation and perfusion are the Paramedic's priorities.

STREET SMART

Poor nutrition is a major contributor to poor wound healing and chronic wounds. Through social service referrals by Paramedics, patients in need can obtain help in providing proper nutrition through services such as Meals on Wheels.

Scar Formation

In some patients, a **hypertrophic scar** results following wound healing. Although these raised prominent scars tend to fade over time as the wound regresses, that process may take years. Hypertrophic scars more often occur with healing by secondary intention, in cases where there is hematoma formation, or when local inflammation competes with systemic inflammation, such as occurs following trauma, sepsis, and burns.

Abnormal wound healing sometimes results in keloid formation (Figure 8-5). **Keloids**, lesions that can develop up to one year after an injury and are thought to be due to genetic influences, are the result of an overgrowth of scar tissue. Keloids are different than hypertrophic scars because the keloid formation extends past the confines of the original scar and they tend to be more permanent. Keloids are not cancerous.

The formation of scars is impacted by skin tension, which may be either static or dynamic. As skin hangs on the skeleton, like a curtain from a rod, there is always some constant **static tension**. And like a curtain's pleats, the skin has folds, or static tension lines called **Langer's lines**. In between these lines there is also tension.

When the skin is interrupted (e.g., by a laceration), the amount of tension between these folds helps to predict how much the wound will gap. Therefore, the greater the gap in the wound, due to static tension, the greater the size of the scar. Areas of great tension include the anterior tibia, for example. Areas of little tension include a horizontal laceration of the eyelid.

Static tension has its greatest impact when a ragged wound is revised into a straight line but unequal pressures are exerted across that line. An increased scar will occur.

Dynamic tension lines, also called **Kraissl's line**, exist along planes of movement and the underlying muscle creates

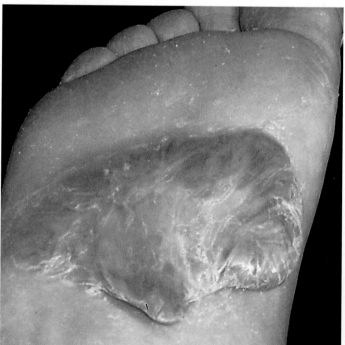

Figure 8-5 Keloid scars are the result of an overgrowth of scar tissue.

the tension. An example of dynamic tension lines is when wrinkles appear on a person's forehead during a frown. Any laceration, particularly a deep laceration that impacts muscle, which crosses these lines will heal with clearly visible scars, regardless of the technique of wound closure employed. The type of skin tension, static or dynamic, impacts on the method of wound[5] closure chosen.

Wound Closure

To support primary wound healing, there are three primary methods of wound closure: sutures, staples, and adhesives. The classic method of wound closure is sutures.

Essentially there are two types of sutures: running sutures and interrupted sutures. Running sutures consist of continuous sutures that rapidly close a wound. This method is appropriate when rapid hemorrhage control is needed or a large wound is present. Interrupted sutures are more time-consuming to complete but provide for better approximation of the wound edge, leading to decreased scar formation. Interrupted sutures also have the advantage that if a suture is broken or an infection develops, the repair of the entire wound isn't necessarily compromised as some sutures may be left to maintain the position of the wound edges.

Surgical sutures are available in nonabsorbable materials such as stainless steel and synthetic fibers (such as polyesters or polypropylene) or absorbable sutures made of either collagen or synthetic polymers. The classic collagen suture, called cat gut, is obtained from the intestines of animals.

Skin staples are actually an ancient means of wound closure, as they appeared in ancient Hindu medicine. The skin staple, using metal staples, is fast and relatively painless. With a rotating head, skin staplers allow the provider to visualize the wound, ensure close approximation of the wound edges with skin forceps, and quickly close the wound. Steel skin staples also have a lower infection rate than do sutures.

The last wound closure method involves a special class of adhesives called cyanoacrylate tissue adhesives. These "skin glues" are used both internally and externally to close wounds. They allow for rapid closure and tight tissue union, with the resulting tight wound edge approximation minimizing scar formation. Skin glues are also useful in pediatrics, as they are not painful, and in cases where the patient may not return for suture removal. As a bonus, many of these skin glues exert an antimicrobial action. Finally, skin glues are flexible and water resistant, making them ideal for closing wounds on hands and across stress lines in the skin.

It should be noted that wound tape, including nylon-reinforced strips such as Steri–strips®, can be used to close percutaneous wounds. These tapes are generally used for more superficial wounds or as an adjunct to deep sutures. One advantage of adhesive tapes over sutures is the lack of residual cross marks left by sutures, thereby making wound tapes more attractive for certain applications.

Under certain circumstances, a formerly closed wound will reopen, or **dehiscence**. Risk factors for dehiscence of a closed wound, such as that from a recent surgery, include age (particularly in patients over age 70), comorbidities such as diabetes, and a poor nutritional status. As a result of decreased granulation, delayed epithelialization, and poor neovascularization, the tissues become "friable" and fragile. Friable tissue easily disintegrates. Wound healing is particularly impaired following transplant surgeries when the patient is placed on immunosuppressant medications and steroids. This population is at special risk. Obesity and smoking are other recognized risk factors for dehiscence.

Special Case of Crush Injury

A devastating and potentially life-threatening soft-tissue injury is crush injury. As the name implies, **crush injury** is the result of a large force being distributed over a large area of the body, such as an extremity. A crush injury can cause crush syndrome or compartment syndrome.

In crush injury, the massive forces compress the limb, causing extensive damage to muscle cells, leading to a condition called **crush syndrome**. In a study of the earthquake in Tangshan Province, China, where 164,851 people were crushed, 2% to 5% of survivors of collapsed buildings developed crush syndrome. If left untreated, approximately 50% of patients with crush syndrome will go into acute renal failure, and 50% of those patients will require renal dialysis.

In three-quarters of cases of crush syndrome, the lower limbs are affected. In another 10% of cases, the upper limbs are affected. Hands and feet are excluded in the definition of crush injuries because they lack sufficient muscle mass to cause crush syndrome.

Crush syndrome may initially have been described by Dr. Bywaters when he documented the injuries from building collapse, then called Bywater's syndrome, during the London blitz of World War II. Etiologies of crush syndrome, in addition to building collapse, include earthquake, trench or mine cave-in, landslide, train derailment with entrapment, and avalanche.

Crush syndrome is the result of the physical breakdown of muscle tissue from compressive forces that leads to **traumatic rhabdomyolysis** (rapid breakdown of skeletal muscle). The immediate physical destruction of muscle cells releases myoglobin, amino acids, purines, and potassium into the surrounding tissues. Subsequent ischemia from hypoperfusion of the limb creates lactate acid, from converted purines, and an increasing acid load during the first hour of entrapment.

The three factors that are taken into account when considering crush syndrome are the muscle mass involved (the larger the mass, the greater the chance), the length of time elapsed during compression (can begin at one hour but typically occurs at four to six hours), and distal circulation (loss of pulses). However, there is no correlation between the severity of injury or length of entrapment and the levels of myoglobin and other toxins. Therefore, crush syndrome should be considered in every case of entrapment.

Crush syndrome is a **reperfusion injury** that occurs when the limb is released and blood flow is restored to the limb. As the blood flow returns, the potassium-laden, acidotic blood trapped within the limb is released into the general circulation. The combination of a sudden increase in the systemic acid load and the hyperkalemia can serve as the catalyst for ventricular fibrillation and sudden cardiac death.

Traumatic rhabdomyolysis is a secondary syndrome that sometimes occurs with crush injury. As the myoglobin is released into the bloodstream, it coagulates in the acidic blood (as a protein, it coagulates in acid). This insoluble coagulant enters into the kidney, blocking the collecting tubules in the nephron and forming renal plugs (casts of the tubule). As the kidney fails and acute tubular necrosis occurs, acid is not excreted and the acid load in the bloodstream climbs. This acidemia helps to perpetuate the impact of the initial rhabdomyolysis. If left untreated, the patient eventually dies from hyperkalemia-induced dysrhythmia and/or massive vasodilation from acidosis.

CASE STUDY (CONTINUED)

The patient, a 58-year-old male, is still awake and alert as the fire rescue crew arrives. The extrication team quickly stabilizes the vehicle with step blocks, and the Paramedic then gets down to the patient's level to explain what is going to happen. Then he starts getting the history of the event. The man explains that he feels like he is going to pass out. He is not sure how long he has been under the car; it felt like hours, but he started to work at 8 a.m. and his wife found him when she came out to get him for lunch.

The patient has an extensive past medical history including hypertension, diabetes, and coronary artery disease. He is on several medications for his medical conditions, including Plavix®.

CRITICAL THINKING QUESTIONS

1. What are the important elements of the history that a Paramedic should obtain?
2. What are the confounding factors for wound healing?

History

The history, and particularly the mechanism of injury (MOI), should lead the Paramedic to have a high index of suspicion about the presence of soft-tissue injuries. One of the most common soft-tissue injuries is injury to the face, often caused by motor vehicle collision (MVC). Other causes include assaults and animal bites.

Perhaps no other injury has as dramatic a psychological impact as does a facial injury. A person's self-image and self-esteem are attached to his facial appearance. It has been estimated that some three million patients seek emergency medical care for facial injuries. Although these are generally not life-threatening situations, these patients want immediate medical attention so that the best possible cosmetic result can be achieved. The rest of the medical history may identify potential problems with wound healing.

Medications, by classification, that can impair wound healing include corticosteroids, anticoagulants, antineoplastic (chemotherapy), and nonsteroidal anti-inflammatory drugs such as aspirin or ibuprofen. Note that the last classification of medications includes many over-the-counter drugs that patients may not consider as "medications" even though they take them daily.

Some medications are taken intermittently yet exert a long-term influence on healing. For example, patients with asthma may be placed on steroid therapy during acute exacerbations of their disease. These corticosteroids impair wound healing.

All forms of chronic disease that impact oxygen transport, as shown in the Fick principle (oxygenation, ventilation, respiration, circulation, and cellular respiration), will adversely impact wound healing. The past medical history can be helpful in revealing wounds that may not heal well and therefore require more immediate medical attention.

Immunosuppression from human acquired immunodeficiency virus (HIV), acquired immune deficiency due to chemotherapy for cancer, and diabetes mellitus impact healing.

Diabetes has long been recognized as a confounder of wound healing, particularly for peripheral injuries. The combination of poor peripheral circulation and distal neuropathy makes serious wounds more likely. Annually 86,000 amputations, ranging from a toe to a leg, are the result of diabetes. The risk is greatest if gangrene has set in. Some providers, including Paramedics, always have the patient with diabetes remove her shoes and socks and then examine the feet for reddened areas (i.e., hot spots) and blisters that signal early ulcer formation.

Tobacco smoke, with its many toxins, retards healing. The nicotine, a potent vasoconstrictor, slows blood flow to the skin. Carbon monoxide in the smoke diminishes the oxygen transport to the wound. These are just a few of the many negative effects that smoking has on wound healing. As a part of the history, the Paramedic should obtain the patient's smoking history and relay that information to the physician.

Radiation therapy dramatically impacts skin for the patient's lifetime. If the patient has a history of cancer, the Paramedic should inquire if the patient had radiation therapy and, if so, what parts of the body were exposed to radiation.

When inquiring about the last meal, what the Paramedic is really trying to elicit is a nutritional status. Poor nutrition, even in the face of adequate caloric intake, can compromise wound healing. For example, a deficiency in vitamin C (ascorbic acid), found in vegetables and fruit, can lead to a disease called scurvy. Vitamin C is a critical cofactor for collagen synthesis and is important for wound healing.[6] Other critical nutrients include vitamin A and zinc.

Malnutrition can be the result of social barriers such as poverty. Other barriers include psychological barriers such as depression and dementia and physical barriers such as blindness and stroke. Medical conditions such as malabsorption syndromes and congestive heart failure can also lead to malnutrition.

▶ CASE STUDY (CONTINUED)

The Paramedic manages to get intravenous access via the external jugular vein, and medical control orders a sodium bicarbonate bolus and infusion "just in case." As soon as the vehicle is lifted by airbags, the patient is extricated to a backboard via a long axis drag.

Following the primary assessment, which reveals no immediate life-threatening injury, the Paramedic starts a head-to-toe assessment while the gurney is being prepared. The patient has multiple abrasions; a deep laceration to the left thigh, possibly from something on the undercarriage; and a massive bruise across a protuberant abdomen. Although most of the bleeding has stopped, some of the wounds are still weeping. The Paramedic directs the EMT to dress the wounds while they are en route to the hospital.

CRITICAL THINKING QUESTIONS

1. What are the elements of the physical examination for soft-tissue injury?
2. What are the descriptions of wound drainage?

Examination

Due to the traumatic nature of these calls, a robust effort at initial assessment and resuscitation should precede a detailed physical examination of the patient. In cases of severe life-threatening hemorrhage, the Paramedic may reverse the traditional ABC approach to trauma assessment (CAB), and

apply a tourniquet. Tourniquet application is discussed in the "Treatment" section.

When proceeding with the examination, it is important for the Paramedic to first expose the area to be inspected. The saying goes, "You can't treat what you don't see." The Paramedic should cut or tear clothing to expose underlying injury as necessary. The entire area should be exposed if an injury is suspected but not apparent in order to ensure complete examination of the wound. Penetrating objects found in the wound should be left in place and stabilized with bulky dressing as needed. The Paramedic should look for both entry and exit wounds for all suspected GSW.

The mnemonic DCAP BTLS serves well as a reminder for the elements of the detailed physical exam. Starting at the top of the head, at the scalp, the Paramedic should proceed in a systematic fashion from head to toe looking for deformities, contusions, abrasions, punctures, burns, tenderness, lacerations, and swelling. These signs indicate soft-tissue injury.

The scalp is commonly lacerated. Because of the highly vascular nature of the scalp, scalp wounds often bleed copiously. However, the Paramedic should not allow the bleeding scalp wound to divert attention away from the more life-threatening underlying head injury. The Paramedic should carefully palpate the laceration with a gloved hand while feeling and looking for deformities that may indicate a fracture, such as a step off, or an open cranium. To improve visualization, it may be necessary to irrigate the area with copious amounts of sterile solution. In some cases, the patient's hair may need to be cut, using a pair of shears. Only rarely is a razor needed.

When performing a scalp examination, the Paramedic should examine the entire cranium. Minor to moderate lacerations, such as from flying glass, may be clotted with matted hair that overlies the laceration and obscures its visualization. If the Paramedic finds glass fragments, they should be carefully removed, using tweezers if possible, to prevent further injury from sharp edges.

While examining the scalp, the Paramedic should also examine the earlobe. Avulsions, partial or complete, are one of the more common soft-tissue ear injuries. If the earlobe is still attached. it can be simply taped in place until sutured. As the earlobes are highly vascular, even reattached ears tend to heal well. For this reason, the avulsed earlobe should be found and transported to the emergency department like any amputated limb (this process is discussed shortly).

Like scalp wounds, eyebrow lacerations may indicate a fracture of the underlying supraorbital rim or the frontal sinus. Because eyebrows are a different type of hair than what is on the scalp, and does not grow back over a scar, the eyebrows should not be clipped or shaved to improve visualization.

One of the most disconcerting injuries can be an eyelid laceration. The eyelid's purpose, to protect the eye, mandates that the Paramedic perform a careful examination of the eye for any associated injury such as a hyphema, or lens displacement, as well as foreign bodies. An orbital floor fracture (blowout fracture) may be evidenced by **enophthalmos** (receded eyeball) or **exophthalmos** (bulging eyeball).

A "black eye" is the result of a contusion of the soft tissues and the collection of blood under the eye. However, the presence of a black eye should alert the Paramedic to the possibility of more serious injuries. For example, bilateral periorbital ecchymosis (i.e., raccoon eyes) leads the Paramedic to

suspect a basilar skull fracture. A unilateral periorbital ecchymosis may indicate an orbital floor fracture. If the patient complains of diplopia (double vision) or has enophthalmos, then the Paramedic should palpate the entire orbital rim for signs of fracture. Whenever the Paramedic notes a black eye, a complete ocular evaluation is appropriate.

Soft-tissue injuries to the nose, like those to the scalp and eyebrow, suggest underlying fractures of the nasal bones or cartilage, such as a deviated septum. It may be necessary for the Paramedic to apply nasal packing to control epistaxis, since this is often associated with soft-tissue injuries to the nose, as discussed in Chapter 3.

The ducts of the eyes—the parotid and the lacrimal glands—are occasionally involved with injuries to the eyes. The parotid gland located proximal to the eye and superficially within the cheek can be injured with facial wounds. The presence of clear liquid flowing from a cheek wound, as well as a sagging upper lip, is suggestive of a parotid gland/duct injury.

Injuries to the nose may involve the lacrimal glands. The lacrimal glands, proximal to the nose, will leak tears if the gland/duct is injured. Both of these glands are important to vision and to the eye's health.

The lips are particularly vascular, so soft-tissue injuries to the lips often result in bleeding. Most injuries are minor, such as the "split lip," and the injury goes up to but does not pass the vermilion border (border of the lip and skin). Minor lip lacerations and contusions can occur as a result of a blunt force, such as being thrown against the steering wheel, which crushes the flesh of the lip against the hard teeth behind the lip. On occasion, a protruding tooth can also cause a lip laceration. Lip lacerations that extend past the vermilion border indicate a significant tearing force was applied to the lip. This type of injury may have injured the underlying orbicularis oris muscle; in addition, the facial bones should be carefully examined.

STREET SMART

Properly worn mouth guards not only help protect teeth but can also reduce the incidence of a split lip. If a lip laceration is noted, the Paramedic should suspect that the patient was momentarily rendered unconscious, before the blow was landed, and that the mouth guard fell out.

Tongue injuries can occur as a result of a fall or a blow to the face, as would happen if someone is punched. Although most of these injuries are benign, avulsions of the tongue, gaping wounds (> 1 cm), and actively bleeding lacerations may require medical intervention that includes suturing. One-third or greater partial avulsions and complete avulsions will need a special procedure, referred to as the flap procedure, which is performed by a specialist. These specialists are generally available in a trauma center.

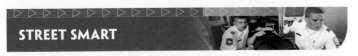
As often occurs with any soft-tissue injury, there is often associated nerve injury. The two nerves that are of particular concern are the facial nerve and the trigeminal nerve. The facial nerve (i.e., the seventh cranial nerve) controls facial expressions such as frowning via the temporal or frontal branch, as well as innervations of the lacrimal gland. To test the facial nerve, the Paramedic should ask the patient to frown, smile while showing teeth, or close the eyes and prevent them from being opened.

The trigeminal nerve (i.e., the fifth cranial nerve) has, as the name suggests, three branches: the ophthalmic, the maxillary, and the mandibular branches. The ophthalmic branch is the sensory nerve for the forehead, the maxillary branch is the sensory nerve for the cheek, and the mandibular branch is the sensory nerve for the chin. However, only the mandibular branch of the trigeminal nerve has motor nerves. These motor nerves control the jaw's movement during mastication and are tested by asking the patient to smile.

The trigeminal nerve is a major facial nerve and injury to it can lead to an excruciatingly painful condition called trigeminal neuralgia. For this reason, it is important to document suspected trigeminal nerve damage as evidenced by lack of facial sensation at the forehead, cheek, and chin, or the inability to smile. In this manner, the origins of the trigeminal neuralgia can be associated with the trauma.

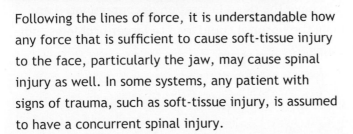
Straddle Injuries

A **straddle injury** is a special type of soft-tissue injury that involves the perineum. A straddle injury occurs when the genitals (in particular) and the perineum (in general) strike an object. This may result from trauma, a kick to the groin, falling off a bicycle and striking the crossbar, or being ejected from a motorcycle and striking the instrument cluster. All straddle injuries should be assumed to be serious, as injuries to either the genitals or the urinary tract can have life-long implications.

Wound Examination

Following the head-to-toe examination and identification of all soft-tissue injuries, the Paramedic should make a focused wound assessment of each injury. When examining a wound, the Paramedic should observe and document the size, depth, exudate type, and amount of exudate, as well as associated peripheral edema. When estimating (or, better yet, using a small ruler), the Paramedic should describe the wound in centimeters. The description should include the depth of the wound. Abrasions are superficial, whereas lacerations are full thickness. What differentiates a laceration from an incision are the edges. With an incision, the edges are clean, whereas with a laceration the edges are jagged and more difficult to approximate for closure with sutures. A laceration can be thought of as a jagged incision. If supporting structures such as tendons or fascia are visible, that should also be documented. The tendon and/or fascia suggest injury to deeper structures, and the wound may need to be reopened and explored. In some instances, the tendon and/or fascia retract into the wound, making the Paramedic the only witness.

Wounds initially weep fluids called **exudates**. If the fluid is bright red, or a clot is present, then the Paramedic should document that blood as present in the wound. Blood-tinged liquid drainage is called serosanguineous, whereas clear fluid is just serous.

If the fluid is opaque, tan, or yellow, the exudate is considered **purulent**. If the exudate has an offensive odor, suggestive of infection, then it is called foul purulent. All purulent or foul purulent exudate should be called to the physician's attention (Table 8-2).

Directly measuring the exudate is nearly impossible in the field. Rather than measure the amount, Paramedics

Table 8-2 Wound Drainage Classification

- *Serous.* Clear or yellow-tinged color which is watery plasma.
- *Sanguineous.* Red color which is bloody from fresh bleeding.
- *Serosanguineous.* Pink color which is a mixture of plasma and red blood cells.
- *Purulent.* White (pus), yellow, green, or brown color with a thick consistency that is a mixture of white blood cells and living or dead organisms.

generally describe the amount of exudate present in terms of wound appearance and/or amount of dressing soaked.

If the wound is dry or moist in appearance, but not enough to be absorbed through a thickness of gauze dressing, then the amount is listed as **scant**. If the dressing is saturated through, and involves approximately 25% of the dressing, then the amount is listed as small. If more than 25%, but not all of the dressing, is saturated, then the exudate amount is described as moderate. If greater than three-quarters of the dressing is soaked, the drainage is considered large.

The Paramedic should also document the condition of surrounding tissue. For example, localized edema may indicate cellulitis, and a red band or streak from a wound may indicate **lymphangitis**, an infection that has taken a tract through the lymphatic system.

Special Case of Bites

Bite injuries can be broken down into human bites and animal bites. Both have a high incidence of infection and both can transmit diseases, including rabies and hepatitis B and C. Human bites can occur as a result of a clenched fist injury or an occlusive bite. In the first case, the dorsal knuckles of the attacker are split by the patient's teeth and leave a laceration or "bite." Bacteria introduced under the skin can penetrate the joints and tendons.

The more classic bite injury is the occlusive bite. Although not as common as dog and cat bites, a true estimate of occlusive bite injury is difficult to obtain due to underreporting. For example, it is not uncommon for toddlers to bite one another. However, these superficial bites rarely become infected. Generally, thorough cleansing with soap and water is all that is needed. More problematic is when one person bites another person's fingers, either completely or partially amputating the finger.

As both clenched fist injury and occlusive bites can occur during a criminal act, it is important that the Paramedic examine and document the wound(s) for location, size, and shape, as well as whether there are deeper punctures, superficial lacerations, or avulsions. Hand injuries should be examined for associated fractures and tendon injury. The American Board of Forensic Odontology suggests that photographic evidence be taken of the injury for use in criminal prosecutions later. Although it is not the Paramedic's responsibility to take these pictures, law enforcement officers may want to take photographs before the wound is dressed and before soft-tissue swelling obscures the injury.[8]

The majority of animal bites (approximately 90%) are from dogs. However, other animals—from ferrets to snapping turtles—can also bite. Animal bites, particularly cat and dog bites, are more problematic. First, the sharp pointed teeth of these animals tend to puncture the skin and inoculate bacteria deep into the tissues. Some 64 different pathogens have been identified in the saliva of dogs and cats.[9] Therefore, it is imperative that a physician examines all animal bites so that prophylactic antibiotics can be started.

The second problem with animal bites is that large animals, such as dogs, can exert tremendous pressure—between 200 to as much as 450 pounds per square inch—between their molars. These bone-crushing molars can produce extreme pressures and can lead to crushing injury to bones, nerves, and muscles. Therefore, the Paramedic should suspect a fracture for any circumferential occlusive animal bite.

Most animal bites occur in the upper extremities and the face. Depending on the area of the attack, the Paramedic will have to focus the examination. Part of every examination of an animal bite should include not only a description and location of the soft-tissue injury, but also the distal motor and sensory function.

STREET SMART

Rabies has to be suspected whenever any mammal—such as foxes, raccoons, or skunks—bites a human. Therefore, the Paramedic should document the type of animal, particularly noting its observed behaviors before the attack.

CASE STUDY (CONTINUED)

The patient keeps repeating he is fine and does not want to go to the hospital. At this point, the Paramedic explains to the patient that he needs to go to the hospital to have the deep laceration decontaminated and sutured, as well as to check for tetanus prophylaxis. Avoiding the hospital could lead to larger problems, not necessarily today but tomorrow, in terms of his wound healing.

CRITICAL THINKING QUESTIONS

1. What is the importance of making a determination about the type of wound?
2. What is the prognostic implication?

Assessment

Generally, wounds can be classified as bleeding or non-bleeding and either clean or dirty. A wound is considered dirty if it contains devitalized (necrotic) tissue or foreign bodies (including bullets), or has been contaminated with debris, soil, and so on. The utility of these designations is twofold. Bleeding must be controlled in bleeding wounds and dirty wounds should be decontaminated as soon as possible.

CASE STUDY (CONTINUED)

The patient reluctantly agrees to go to the hospital provided the lights and sirens are not used. He is already embarrassed and doesn't want any more attention. He also wants his wife to accompany him. While waiting for his wife to get her purse and his "cards," the Paramedic starts his treatment. His first priorities, after the ABCs, are to control the patient's hemorrhaging and decontaminate his wounds where he can before dressing them.

CRITICAL THINKING QUESTIONS

1. What is the national standard of care of patients with soft-tissue injuries?
2. What are some of the patient-specific concerns that the Paramedic should consider when applying this plan of care that is intended to treat a broad patient population presenting with soft-tissue injuries?

Treatment

As bleeding can be a life-threatening situation if not controlled, the first priority of treatment for soft-tissue injuries is bleeding control. The next priority is gross wound decontamination and then wound dressing.

Minor Bleeding

Bleeding in the clear majority of minor abrasions and superficial lacerations is self-controlled. The wounds only need to have gross contamination, such as grass or glass, removed and the area irrigated with copious amounts of sterile solution. Many of these minor soft-tissue injuries can be left open to air, and the body's natural clotting mechanisms will achieve satisfactory hemostasis.

The traditional wound dressing for a minor laceration or abrasion is the adhesive bandage (e.g., Band-Aids®). In some cases, such as large-spread abrasions, the wounds can be painful. In these cases, a clear semiocclusive biodressing, such as Tagaderm®, may be applied. These clear adhesive bandages generally do not stick to the wound and are easily removed later.

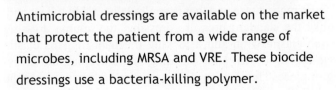

STREET SMART

Antimicrobial dressings are available on the market that protect the patient from a wide range of microbes, including MRSA and VRE. These biocide dressings use a bacteria-killing polymer.

Moderate Bleeding

Most moderate bleeding is venous bleeding. Under normal circumstances, field dressings (described shortly) will initially provide hemostasis and protect the wound from further trauma. If the venous bleeding is more robust, and cannot be controlled by simple field dressings, then the Paramedic may consider use of a hemostatic agent. A **hemostatic agent** facilitates the coagulation of blood to stop hemorrhage by collecting clotting factors.

Perhaps the first of the modern hemostatic agents is zeolite. A granular mineral composed of silicon oxide, aluminum oxide, and other elements, zeolite acts to absorb water, thereby congealing the blood faster. This process is an exothermic reaction (produces heat) that can result in burns. A newer formulation does not produce the heat that the earlier formulation did and its advantage offsets its hazard. Zeolite has been used to stop severe arterial bleeding and, because it is a powder, it can be applied on wounds that are not suitable for either tourniquet or compression dressings. Another key advantage of zeolite hemostat is that it is relatively inexpensive.

One hemostatic agent in use in the field is Poly–N–acetyl glucosamine (P-NAG), also called chitin (when acetylated) or chitosan (when not acetylated). This naturally occurring biodegradable complex polysaccharide is thought to work by attracting circulating cells, scavenging nitric oxide (helps vasospasm), and adhering to tissues. It has been used for brisk bleeding control and is US FDA approved. An advantage of this dressing is that it does not require special storage.

One of the earliest hemostatic agents was human fibrin dressings, which were used as early as 1915. Because of

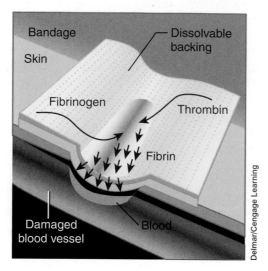

Figure 8-6 Dried fibrin dressing is easy to apply.

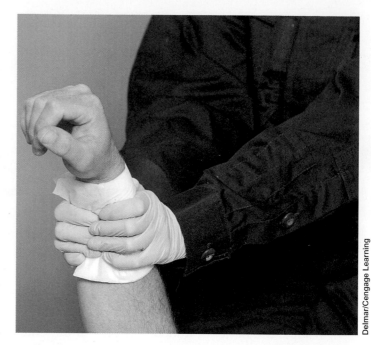

Figure 8-7 Direct pressure is often all that is needed to control bleeding.

concerns about hepatitis transmission, its use diminished. However, new blood testing technologies have renewed interest in this agent. Dried human fibrin—containing fibrinogen, thrombin, factor XIII, and calcium—has no special storage requirements and is easy to apply (Figure 8-6). Dried human fibrin has been shown to be effective in stopping hemorrhage from GSW, penetrating liver injuries, and even aortic puncture.[10]

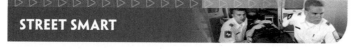

STREET SMART

Bleeding from a scalp wound must be controlled. However, unlike other wounds, the application of direct pressure to the wound to control bleeding may be contraindicated if the laceration overlies an open cranial vault fracture. Therefore, it is imperative that the Paramedic closely examine the wound prior to dressing it to stop the bleeding.

Severe Bleeding

In the past, the mantra for bleeding control was "direct pressure, elevate, and pressure point." Recent research has called into question some of these practices. For example, it is unclear if limb elevation and pressure points actually have any impact on severe bleeding, leading some Paramedics to abandon these practices. Instead, severe bleeding is dealt with by direct pressure, pressure dressings, and tourniquets (not necessarily in that order).

Ordinarily bleeding, even severe bleeding, can be controlled with direct pressure. If the bleeding is venous in nature, then application of a sterile dressing over the wound with a gloved hand is usually all that is needed to stop the

bleeding. If the bleeding is arterial, however, it may be necessary for the Paramedic to stick the tips of her fingers into the wound and press the artery up against the adjunct bone (Figure 8-7). remembering that most major arteries are proximal and adjacent to a bone. This direct pressure should immediately stop the bleeding. If it does not, then the Paramedic should consider using a tourniquet instead.

With arterial bleeding under control by direct pressure, the Paramedic may note some venous back bleeding occurring in the wound, particularly in the upper extremities. The forearm has two arterial sources, and compression of one artery still allows blood flow to the extremity and out the venous outflow tract.

Pressure dressings have existed for decades as a proven and effective method of bleeding control. Their use does not present the risk of limb ischemia like the tourniquet. The single largest detriment to pressure dressings is the time required for application and the need for additional personnel to properly apply them.

The **standard pressure dressing** (i.e., battle dressing) used for decades consisted of a pad of gauze attached to a cotton cravat. It was sometimes split to make a four-tail dressing.

The newest version of the pressure dressing is the **Israeli trauma bandage**, sometimes simply called a trauma bandage (Figure 8-8). Like the standard pressure dressing, it has a sterile inner gauze pad that is applied directly to the wound. Unlike the standard pressure dressing, the trauma dressing has an elastic wrap and a locking mechanism. This elastic wrap serves to help slow bleeding while keeping the dressing in place. The locking device, a tension bar, prevents the bandage from slipping.

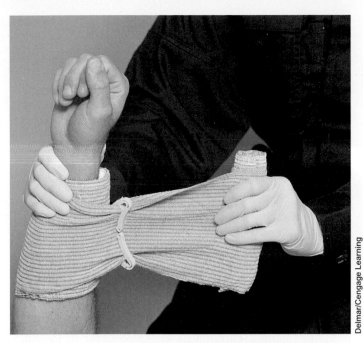

Figure 8-8 The Israeli trauma bandage is the newest version of the pressure dressing.

Tourniquets

In some cases, arterial hemorrhage cannot be controlled by direct pressure or it may be obvious that the hemorrhage is severe and the patient will bleed to death. In those cases, the Paramedic should consider using a tourniquet. Indications for use of the tourniquet include penetrating trauma to an extremity, "care under fire," amputation, and whenever bleeding is not controlled with direct pressure.

Although in the past the tourniquet was considered the tool of last resort, recent evidence has reversed that position.[11] In cases of obvious extreme hemorrhage, a tourniquet should be the first device employed to stop bleeding. Although concerns about complications from tourniquet application (discussed shortly) may be valid, the loss of blood can ultimately cost the patient her life. Essentially, tourniquets place life before limb.

Early Romans used tourniquets to stop bleeding before amputation, although the physician Galen argued against it. The first true tourniquet to stop hemorrhage may have been created by Jean Louis Petit. Petit developed a screw-like tourniquet and named it the tourniquet (French *tourner*–to turn). In the 1800s, Johann Frederick August von Esmarch developed a flat rubber bandage, called the Esmarch bandage, that was used to **exsanguinate** (drain blood; Latin: *sanguis*: blood) from limbs before surgery. Amputations were common at that time. In fact, Civil War soldiers carried a tourniquet on their person for immediate application if struck by a Minnie ball. In 1904 Harvey Cushing (the surgeon who noted Cushing's triad in head-injured patients) developed a **pneumatic tourniquet** for orthopaedic surgery that is similar to the present day blood pressure cuff. These surgical tourniquets are still in use today and provide the basis for much that is known about tourniquet complications.[12]

Tourniquets have been made from belts, triangle bandages, shirt ties, rubber tubing, and every imaginable material that can be placed circumferentially around a limb. However, not all of these tourniquets are effective. To be effective, a tourniquet should use the lowest possible tourniquet inflation pressure to achieve arterial occlusion. This is done in order to minimize the risk of nerve and muscle damage.

The optimal tourniquet should have a width of material that is at least 1 inch. This helps to ensure distribution of pressure across the tourniquet and prevents tissue damage. It is preferable if the tourniquet's compression can be augmented by a mechanical device such as a windlass, ratchet, or cam that can be operated with one hand. Although a tourniquet can be made from belts and other articles in the field, these tourniquets often apply inadequate pressure to the limb, which may produce more bleeding. The Paramedic should ideally use a commercially available device that is designed to be used as a tourniquet.

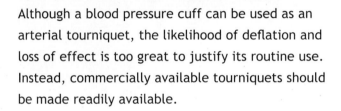

STREET SMART

Although a blood pressure cuff can be used as an arterial tourniquet, the likelihood of deflation and loss of effect is too great to justify its routine use. Instead, commercially available tourniquets should be made readily available.

The tourniquet is applied several inches above the wound, between the wound and the heart (life before limb), if possible. The Paramedic applies continuous pressure until the bleeding stops. After application of the tourniquet, the Paramedic will observe for cessation of bleeding.

The simplest tourniquet may be the "Russian tourniquet." The Russian tourniquet is simply a length of cotton cloth wrapped around the arm and tied off with a square knot. A stick is then placed in the knot. Turning the stick applies pressure to the arm. The stick is tied off to the limb with another length of cotton cloth or cravat.

A tourniquet can also be made with a long (> 200 cm) elastic (rubber) band (Figure 8-9). The elastic is laid lengthwise down the limb and then crossed over the limb. The Paramedic applies pressure and ties the tail off.

The Combat Application Tourniquet® (CAT) (Figure 8-10) is effective, as is the Emergency and Military Tourniquet® (EMT) (Figure 8-11).[13] Some Paramedics place the letter "T" on the patient's forehead to alert others that a tourniquet is in place. Leave the limb uncovered if possible so that others can see.

Local effects of tourniquet application include nerve injury, muscle injury, arterial injury, and skin damage. Nerve injury usually manifests as a **neuropraxia** (nerve not

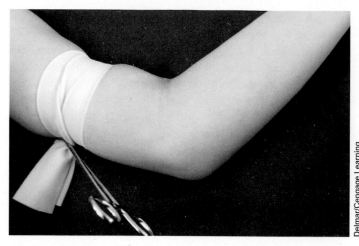

Figure 8-9 Use of an elastic tourniquet requires a long elastic band.

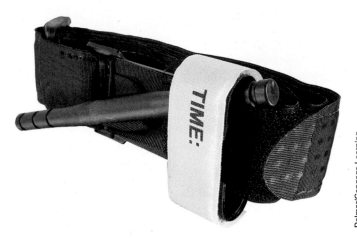

Figure 8-10 The Combat Application Tourniquet is an effective means to stop bleeding.

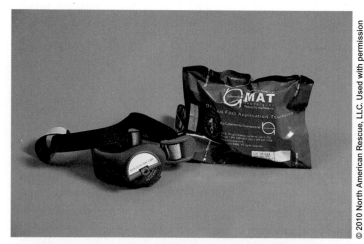

Figure 8-11 The Emergency and Military Tourniquet is another effective means to stop bleeding.

transmitting impulses after an injury) and can range from mild paresthesia to full paralysis. This neuropraxia is most likely to occur in the radial nerve in the arm and the sciatic nerve in the leg. Fortunately, permanent damage is rare. If it does occur, it is generally because the tourniquet has been on for more than two to four hours and is related to overpressure.

Tourniquets have also been implicated in muscle injury. The intracellular environment stays at baseline for the first 15 minutes after the tourniquet is placed. After that, the environment becomes steadily more acidotic. On average, muscle can withstand ischemia for up to four hours without permanent damage from the ischemia. After that point, the intracellular environment is severely acidotic, energy stores are depleted, and there is a marked increase in CO_2 and lactate production. Microvascular congestion also occurs within the muscle at about this time, which can worsen ischemia.

Although direct arterial injury is rare, there is the risk of plaque rupture in vessels that are atheromatous (plaques prone to rupture). Thrombosis may also occur in the limb, further blocking the microcirculation and decreasing the likelihood of reperfusion.

Finally, the tourniquet can produce direct trauma to the skin, including pressure necrosis and friction burns. The edges of the tourniquet should be rounded to avoid digging into the skin underneath the tourniquet.

"[The tourniquet is] to be regarded with respect because of the damage it may cause, and with reverence because of the lives it undoubtedly saves. It is not to be used lightly in every case of a bleeding wound, but applied courageously when life is in danger."

—Hamilton Bailey, *Surgery of Modern Warfare*, 1941[14]

▷ ▷ ▷ ▷ ▷ ▷ ▷ ▷ ▷ ▷ ▷ ▷ ▷

STREET SMART

Tourniquet pain may occur 45 minutes to an hour after application of the tourniquet. It generally starts with a dull ache and progresses to severe pain. In anticipation of this inevitable event, the Paramedic should consider early administration of appropriate opiate analgesia, if not contraindicated by hypotension.

Amputated Limbs

The therapeutic goal of treating an amputation is reimplantation. Recent strides in microsurgery and technology have made it possible to reimplant almost any limb provided the limb is properly preserved.

Amputations are either complete or partial. As in any fracture, the Paramedic should immediately stabilize any partial amputation and perform a check of the distal circulation, sensation, and motor function. A partial amputation should then be splinted in the position of function, if possible. Some Paramedics will place a saline-moistened sterile dressing around the entire limb to prevent further contamination or trauma. A pulse oximeter may be used to continuously monitor distal circulation.

If the limb is missing, then the Paramedic's first priority is to determine if it is the result of an amputation or a complete avulsion. The mechanism of injury will help the Paramedic with that determination. Amputated limbs tend not to bleed, whereas avulsed limbs can bleed profusely. If the limb is steadily bleeding, then the first priority is hemorrhage control. It may be necessary to use a tourniquet, particularly if the patient has a complete avulsion.

Once the bleeding is controlled, the Paramedic must protect the stump. A field dressing placed over the stump is usually sufficient; again, some Paramedics use saline-moistened sterile dressing to protect the stump. If the stump has visible contamination, the Paramedic may use sterile saline in a syringe to gently irrigate the stump. No other solution, including antiseptic solutions, should be used.

Naturally, the Paramedic will want to find the missing limb. However, efforts to find the severed limb should not delay the patient's transportation to the hospital (preferably one with a transplant specialist) if the patient is hemodynamically unstable. If and when the limb is recovered, it should be treated with the same care as was the stump.

Again, the objective of field care for an amputation is reimplantation. Local keys to limb salvage include the absence of devitalized (necrotic) tissue and bacterial contamination, as well as distal perfusion. However, the first priority in patient care is the patient (remember, life before limb). Aggressive resuscitation of the trauma patient makes the patient a better candidate for a successful reimplantation.

Field Amputation

Amputation has been an accepted medical procedure since ancient times; its use was even described by Hippocrates. Amputation may have reached its peak during the Civil War when 40,000 amputations were performed in the Union Army alone. A good surgeon could remove a limb in 10 minutes. As was true then, so it is now. Amputation in the field is reserved for true "life or limb" situations. Like early Civil War surgeons, the Paramedic may hesitate to consider amputation. Nonetheless, amputation is still a viable option under a very limited number of circumstances.

A survey of emergency physicians in almost 200 major U.S. cities revealed 18 physicians (53% by surgeons, 36% emergency physicians) who performed a total of 26 field amputations in the past five years, the majority of them for patients in motor vehicle collisions.[15] This illustrates that field amputation is rare. With the reintroduction of tourniquets to the field, the number of field amputations may fall even further.

The decision whether to amputate or not can be supported by the use of the Mangled Extremity Severity Score (MESS) (Table 8-3).[16] This score takes into account the amount of soft-tissue damage, limb ischemia, hypotension, and the patient's age. MESS scores of less than 7 suggest that the limb is salvageable, whereas scores greater than 7 indicate amputation. If the limb has been entrapped for more than six hours, the score is doubled.

A field amputation is outside of the scope of practice of most Paramedics. However, a number of emergency physicians have been trained in this procedure and may be available to respond to the scene. In those cases where the physician has been called to the scene, the Paramedic may be called upon to assist. The first priority of patient care is controlling hemorrhage. This is best accomplished by applying a tourniquet before the procedure. The next priority is anesthesia, if available, and analgesia as tolerated. Depending on the resources available, the Paramedic and physician may elect to perform rapid sequence intubation to control the airway and provide deep sedation during the procedure. During the actual procedure, the Paramedic will need to assist. The soft tissues are cut by a scalpel and the bone(s) cut with a saw as distal as possible. The stump is then bandaged and the patient transported to a trauma center for revision of the stump. If the entrapped limb can be freed, it should be properly preserved and transported to the trauma center in the event reimplantation is possible or tissue can be used for the revision.

Table 8-3 Mangled Extremity Severity Score (MESS)

Skeletal/soft-tissue injury	Low energy (stab, simple fracture, pistol gunshot wound)	1
	Medium energy (open or multiple fractures, dislocation)	2
	High energy (high speed MVC or rifle GSW)	3
	Very high energy (high speed trauma + gross contamination)	4
Limb ischemia	Pulse reduced or absent but perfusion normal (double score if > 6 hours)	1
	Pulseless, paresthesias, diminished capillary refill	2
	Cool, paralyzed, insensate, numb	3
Shock	Systolic BP always > 90 mmHg	0
	Transient hypotension	1
	Persistent hypotension	2
Age (years)	< 30 years old	0
	30 to 50 years old	1
	> 50 years old	2

Wound Care: Irrigation

Owing to the special nature of a laceration or incision, specifically how deeper tissues are penetrated by the object, it is important that the Paramedic perform a thorough irrigation. Before proceeding with a wound irrigation, the Paramedic may want to consider providing the patient with analgesia. Traditionally morphine has been used prior to wound care; however, other medications such as fentanyl are also being used. Fentanyl, which is 100 times more potent than morphine, has a short duration of action and a safer hemodynamic profile.

Some Paramedics will take a 19-gauge blunt needle or a catheter from a 16-gauge angiocatheter and a large saline-filled syringe and copiously irrigate the area. This irrigation is important to prevent wound infection. When irrigating a wound, the Paramedic should wear eye protection to prevent potentially infectious microfine spray from getting into the eyes, thereby infecting the Paramedic. The solution in the wound should be allowed to run out freely and not collect within the wound.

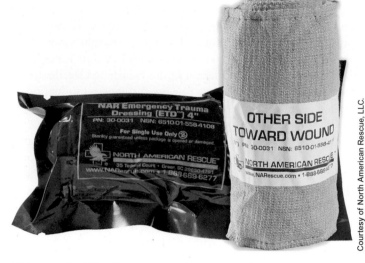

Figure 8-12 Emergency trauma dressing protects the wound from contamination and further trauma.

STREET SMART

Although rare, cases of gas gangrene still do occur when the barnyard contaminates wounds. It is important that even minor wounds be properly cleaned and medical attention sought for wounds that occur on the farm.

Wound Dressing

A dressing's purpose is to protect the wound from microbes and further trauma while supporting the healing process. Dressings are therefore sterile and must be applied with, minimally, clean technique and, preferably, with sterile technique. A bandage supports many dressings; in some cases, the bandage and dressing are combined, such as is the case with a **field dressing** (Figure 8-12). A bandage is clean, but not necessarily sterile, and is intended to hold a dressing in place. Hypothetically, a bandage can be reused once it is cleaned. A dressing, in contrast, cannot be reused.

The traditional dressing is the gauze dressing with which most Paramedics are familiar. Although the gauze dressing is inexpensive and relatively easy to apply, it has several disadvantages. First, it does not protect the wound from bacteria, particularly if the dressing is moist with exudate. One study showed that bacteria was able to pass through 64 layers of moist gauze.[17] Second, when the gauze dressing is changed it often lifts the clot off the wound, causing rebleeding and a delay in healing. Third, a gauze dressing, even the new elastic gauze dressing, is difficult to apply to the body's contours.

Finally, gauze dressings applied to an older wound will often lift any newly formed epithelium.

The choice of which dressing to use is decided, in part, on the wound's characteristics. For example, for wounds such as abrasions, and those with scant drainage or exudate, it may be permissible to use a film dressing.

A **film dressing** is a thin, transparent, semipermeable membrane that permits moisture to escape and oxygen to enter. Because these dressings "breathe," they prevent the maceration (a softening of the dermis as seen when skin is submersed in water for a long time) that is associated with more traditional first aid strips. These dressings permit direct observation of the wound while protecting the wound from trauma (i.e., friction and infection). Film dressings are used for minor abrasions, scalds, and as a dressing over intravenous sites. Most of these dressings have a layer of acrylic adhesive that makes applying the dressing easy. A dressing should be chosen that is larger than the wound. The wound's borders should be clean and free of oils that would undermine the dressing.

Film dressings may also be used as a bandage to hold foams, discussed shortly, in place. Film dressings come in all sizes and go by the names of OpSite®, Tagaderm®, and Bioclusive® (Figure 8-13).

To properly release a film dressing, in order to prevent damage, the Paramedic should apply light pressure to the center of the dressing while the edges are carefully lifted. Once the dressing is free, and because of the moisture from the wound, the dressing should be able to be lifted off in one piece.

Foam dressings absorb exudate while protecting the skin. Foam dressings have high absorbency, conform to all body shapes, and provide protection from further trauma by cushion. Foam dressings can also be used under compression

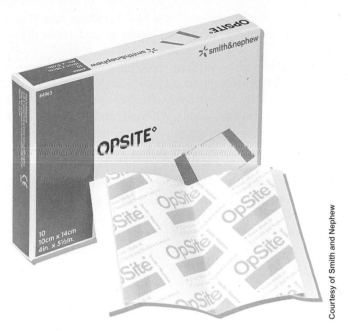

Figure 8-13 Film dressings come in a variety of sizes.

bandages so that the bandage both absorbs moderate exudate as well as prevents edema formation.[18] Some dressings even contain activated charcoal to adsorb odors.

Hydrogels are an interesting crossover between film dressings and foam dressings. Hydrogels are transparent membrane dressings, like the film dressing, that are also absorbent, like the foam dressings. These dressings also absorb heat, making them ideal for use as a burn dressing (superficial and partial thickness burns). Finally, these dressings can be cooled by refrigeration so that when applied to a strain or sprain they serve in the place of ice.

Topical Antibiotics

Although Paramedics traditionally do not consider the use of topical antibiotics, **silver dressings** provide some antimicrobial action in addition to wound coverage. Silver is particularly well known for its antimicrobial properties, particularly against methicillin-resistant Staphylococcus aureus (MRSA) and vancomycin-resistant enterococci (VRE). Previously used in burn care, in the form of silver sulfadiazine cream, silver is broad spectrum and inactivates all bacteria. The use of silver nitrate dressings in burn patients during the 1960s reduced death from sepsis from 60% to 28%.[19] Silver dressings are particularly useful for burns and wide area abrasions such as those that occur in motorcycle crashes (Figure 8-14).

Another topical antibiotic is iodine. Used since the mid-1800s as an antimicrobial, iodine is found in the form of a decontaminant wash, as a skin prep for intravenous access, and as a hand scrub. When used as skin prep, it is a 10% concentration. When it is used in a wound, it is diluted to 1% and allowed to dry for five minutes before a dry sterile dressing (DSD) is applied over the wound.

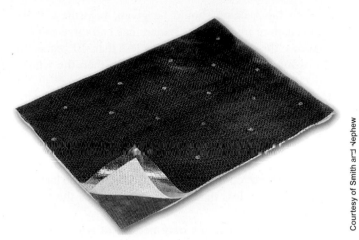

Figure 8-14 The construction of a typical silver dressing.

Bandages

A **bandage** is any material used to support a dressing. Triangular bandages, also called cravats, have long been used by Paramedics. Another bandage that is particularly useful in the upper extremities is the tubular bandage. Made from an open weave or stockinette, this bandage is slid over the axis of the extremity to hold the dressing in place.

All sorts of tape have been used to hold bandages in place. Paramedics have even used duct tape or a strong, waterproof tape to secure bandages in the wilderness. However, most Paramedics prefer to use softer cloth variety surgical tape.

A number of newer adhesive bandages, in all shapes and sizes, are also available. These bandages have been created for odd shapes, such as the fingertip or knuckle. Many of these bandages have an antibiotic impregnated dressing as well.

STREET SMART

The use of tape to hold a dressing in place can cause trauma itself. Skin stripping and tension blisters can be caused by the adhesive on the tape. This is particularly true in the case of the elderly. In those cases, using paper tape and carefully removing tape can prevent further trauma.

Tetanus Prophylaxis

Tetanus prophylaxis, techniques to prevent the painful disease caused from neurotoxins in clostridium tetani, is more a function of the number of previous doses for tetanus immunization than the length of time that has elapsed from previous vaccinations. If the patient has less than three (3) doses of tetanus vaccination, or is uncertain of his tetanus vaccination status, then the vaccine should be given, regardless if the wound is clean or minor. If the patient has had three or more vaccinations, the last vaccination was less than 10 years ago, and the wound is either minor or is clean, then the tetanus vaccine is not needed.

If the patient has had three or more vaccinations for tetanus and the wound is "dirty" (i.e., contaminated with soil, saliva, or feces), and the last tetanus was received less than five years ago, then the tetanus vaccine is not needed. Similarly, if the wound is penetrating, crushing, or a soft-tissue wound from heat or cold (burns or frostbite), and the last tetanus shot was given less than five years ago, then the tetanus vaccine is not needed.

These recommendations only pertain to adults and not to children (< than 8 years of age) or the elderly (> 64 years of age). The tetanus vaccine of 250 units—often tetanus, reduced diphtheria, and pertussis (TdP) or only tetanus and reduced diphtheria (TD)—should be given intramuscularly (IM) using a small one-inch 23- to 25-gauge needle.[20]

Futures in Wound Care

With the increase in the number of patients with diabetes, and the subsequent increase in the number of cases of chronic wounds, coupled with an aging population, the need for new means of treating wounds has become clear. These technologies could conceivably be used in the field by Paramedics— particularly in austere conditions, such as occur during disasters—as a temporary treatment.

One promising new therapy to improve wound healing in those cases is negative wound therapy. As a topical treatment, negative wound therapy applies a negative pressure to the wound, extracting exudate in the process, and maintaining moisture within the wound, which is critical to wound healing. This negative pressure device is a disposable, open cell antimicrobial gauze dressing with either a foam base or nonadherent contact layer, all of which is covered with a semipermeable film dressing. An evacuation tube in the dressing is attached to some suction apparatus that maintains a negative pressure. The benefits of this apparatus are numerous, such as increased local blood flow, increased epithelial cell migration, decreased swelling, and fewer dressing changes.

One of the more difficult problems that a surgeon is faced with is replacing large areas of skin that have been lost to trauma or infection. Although the burn patient is the first patient population that comes to mind, and is discussed in the next chapter, another group—those patients with Ehlers–Danlos syndrome—is representative of this problem. Patients with **Ehlers–Danlos syndrome** are born with a congenital abnormality of collagen formation. This leads to fragile skin prone to injury with seemingly minor trauma and poor wound healing that invariably leads to extensive scarring.

Recently these patients have been treated with **bioengineered skin equivalent (BSE)**, a human skin substitute that consists of dermal cells seeded into a bovine collagen matrix and grown in the laboratory. In the future, BSE may be used to treat difficult skin defects that are the result of trauma.

Another medical procedure under evaluation is the use of artificial dermal regeneration templates. An artificial dermal regeneration template provides the body with the scaffolding for dermal regeneration using a bilayer matrix made of bovine collagen and other chemicals.

Wound Care: Wound Closure

Many Paramedics are asked if a wound needs to be sutured. In general, all wounds need medical attention, particularly if the laceration overlies a stress line, or involves the hand, feet, or face. However, some physicians feel that a minor laceration (i.e., less than 2 cm), without complications such as gross contamination, if left open to the air, may actually heal better (i.e., leave less scarring) than if sutured.

It is generally optimal to close a wound, by either sutures or staples, within six to eight hours. However, concomitant trauma may require wound closure to wait for up to 24 hours. Of particular concern are wounds to the hands and feet, as they have obvious implications relating to function and long-term disability. These wounds should be seen and sutured within eight hours. Alternatively, an uncomplicated facial wound can wait for as long as 24 hours before wound closure.

Wounds that generally are closed and allowed to heal by primary intention include clean (i.e., decontaminated and/or debrided) wounds that are bleeding slightly and appear fresh.

Wounds such as ulcerations, pressure sores, punctures, and partial thickness abrasions are usually left open to air and allowed to heal by secondary intention and granulation. In those cases, the wound is closely monitored for secondary infection that will impair healing.

Contaminated wounds (wounds that contain saliva, soil, or feces) or gunshot wounds are left for delayed primary closure. Leaving the wound open allows the body to rid itself of infection, after extensive decontamination and/or debridement. The wound is then closed four to five days later.

While en route to the hospital, a 40-minute transport time, the patient starts to become tachycardic, then hypotensive. The Paramedic attributes the initial tachycardia on-scene to "nerves" and pain. However, the hypotension is troubling, and the tachycardia is not impressive. At that moment, the Paramedic remembers that the patient was on a beta blocker. Opening the first IV "wide open," the Paramedic starts to look for a second venous access.

CRITICAL THINKING QUESTIONS

1. What are some of the predictable complications associated with crush syndrome?
2. What are some of the predictable complications associated with the treatments for crush syndrome?

Evaluation

The evaluation of the multitrauma patient with soft-tissue injury should be ongoing and focused on complications that can reasonably be foreseen. These complications include "hidden hemorrhage," or injury to underlying organs. In some cases, the soft-tissue injury is so impressive that more subtle underlying injury is ignored. In other cases, the soft-tissue injury is accompanied by crush injury, a potentially life-threatening complication.

Crush Injury

Crush injury delivers its fatal blow in a one-two punch in the field. The first effect of crush injury is the massive hypovolemia that occurs as a result of three events that occur at the moment of release. As a reperfusion injury, a quantity of blood volume is sequestered in the entrapped limb(s). As much as 12 liters of fluid can be trapped in the crushed limb in the space of 48 hours[21]. This volume of fluid is lost to the third space, interstitial space, over time. This loss alone can be sufficient to be fatal in some cases. Then, upon release of the entrapped limb(s), a rush of blood enters the limb, further depleting the blood volume. Finally, acid trapped in the limb is released to the systemic circulation, which causes vasodilation and a worsening hypovolemia.

Next, in the moments immediately following the limb's release, acidotic and hyperkalemic blood rushes into the systemic circulation. Acidotic and hyperkalemic blood can stun the heart, sending it into a fatal dysrhythmia (ventricular tachycardia or ventricular fibrillation).

Fortunately, Paramedics have a number of viable field treatments that can be used to pretreat the patient. Therefore, it is imperative that Paramedic care be initiated before the extrication. Even if the establishment of intravenous access may be time-consuming, it is important that the Paramedic delay the extrication until the patient has been properly prepared.

The order of treatment can be thought of as ABCDE: Airway, Breathing, Circulation, Drugs, and ECG preceding extrication. Establishing and maintaining an airway is important, not only to prevent hypoxia and acidosis from anaerobic respiration (which adds to the acid load), but to ensure adequate ventilation. Ventilation (breathing) is a critical component of the total treatment plan, which is discussed shortly.

After ensuring a patent airway, the Paramedic should consider establishing intravenous access. Some medical authorities suggest using a 2- to 3-liter bolus to overcome the immediate loss of intravascular volume and then 1.5 liters per hour. The therapeutic goal of intravenous fluid resuscitation is twofold. The first reason is to replace lost fluid volume that occurred secondary to third spacing. The second reason is to dilute the acidosis and hyperkalemia. Lactated Ringer's, a potassium-containing solution, should be avoided in favor of normal saline solutions (0.9% sodium chloride in sterile water).

Fluid resuscitation in the elderly, children under 12 years of age, and those with pre-existing renal failure should be closely monitored to prevent fluid overload. Approximately 10 cc/kg is suggested in most cases. Although 20 cc/kg is the norm in most cases, these particularly sensitive patient populations should probably receive smaller boluses serially while monitoring for signs of fluid overload. Signs of fluid overload include pulmonary edema, jugular venous distention, and a third heart sound (i.e., a ventricular gallop). These signs should be assessed after every 500 cc of infusion.

In some cases, it is not possible to gain access to the patient so that an intravenous line can be established. If so, some medical authorities advocate placing a tourniquet on the affected limb. This tourniquet can help prevent the immediate impact of reperfusion injury upon extrication and allow treatment to be instituted before the tourniquet's release. A tourniquet may remain in place for up to four hours, although no maximum safe duration has been established.

With intravenous access established, the Paramedic should administer sodium bicarbonate, as this reverses acidosis. The reversal of acidosis is dependent upon adequate ventilation to drive the bicarbonate–acid formula toward neutrality (Table 8-4).

To indirectly monitor blood acid, Paramedics may use end-tidal carbon dioxide ($EtCO_2$) levels. $EtCO_2$ levels are

Table 8-4 Acid–Base Reaction

$$(HCl^+) + (NaHCO_3) \longrightarrow/\longleftarrow (NaCl) + (H_2CO_3) \longrightarrow/\longleftarrow (H_2O) + (CO_2)$$

Acid + Bicarbonate Sodium Chloride + Carbonic Acid Water +Carbon Dioxide

best measured by monitoring the exhalation of an intubated patient but can be measured by sidestream capnography in a non-intubated patient. If medication-facilitated intubation is indicated, the use of etimodate can be considered to facilitate the intubation. Etimodate is an ultra-short acting hypnotic, less than five minutes, which has a safe hemodynamic profile (less likely to cause hypotension).

Second, the sodium in the sodium bicarbonate acts as a competitive electrolyte against the hyperkalemia. Hyperkalemia is a serious risk to the patient's life; therefore, it should be treated aggressively and prophylactically.

Finally, the Paramedic should place the patient on the ECG monitor. The ECG monitor can help provide an indirect measurement of the patient's **hyperkalemia** (elevated levels of electrolyte potassium). A normal potassium level is between 3.5 and 4.5 mEq/L. Potassium is mildly elevated when the level is between 5.5 and 6.5 mEq/L, and is demonstrated on the ECG monitor as a peaked T wave. A moderate hyperkalemia, between 6.5 and 7.5 mEq/L, is shown on the ECG with prolonged PR interval and depressed or elevated ST segments. If a 12-lead ECG is obtained, these changes will be global (in all 12 leads).

Severe and potentially life-threatening potassium levels between 7.5 and 8.5 widen the QRS. With potassium levels above 8.5, which is a life-threatening condition, there is a loss of P waves and a widening of the QRS into a sine wave (sinusoid pattern). A progression of ECG changes accompany increasing potassium levels (Figure 8-15).

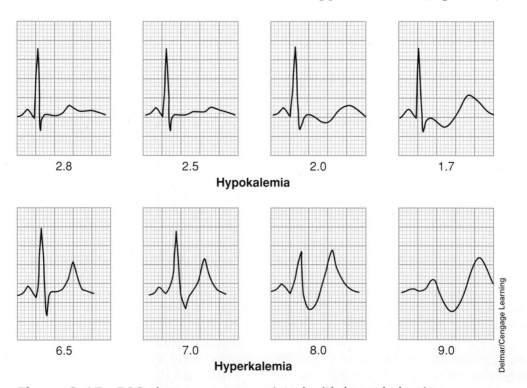

| 2.8 | 2.5 | 2.0 | 1.7 |

Hypokalemia

| 6.5 | 7.0 | 8.0 | 9.0 |

Hyperkalemia

Delmar/Cengage Learning

Figure 8-15 ECG changes are associated with hyperkalemia.

As an alternative to sodium bicarbonate, when IV access cannot be obtained, or in conjunction with sodium bicarbonate, the Paramedic can administer albuterol via small volume nebulizer. Albuterol drives potassium into cells and is highly effective as a short-term treatment![22]

Traumatic Rhabdomyolysis

Following the patient's release from entrapment, it is common for the Paramedic to administer one or two ampoules of sodium bicarbonate, in doses of 50 mEq to a total of 300 mEq, in 24 hours to reverse acidosis and prevent traumatic rhabdomyolysis. The therapeutic goal of bicarbonate therapy is to alkalinize the urine to a pH of 6.5. Urine pH can be checked in the field using simple litmus paper or urine dip sticks.

Keeping the urine alkaline helps to ensure that myoglobin remains soluble in solution and does not form renal casts that occlude the filtration system in the kidneys and cause acute tubular necrosis. To help keep the kidneys functioning, some systems have Paramedics administer mannitol. This **forced diuresis** (increase in urination through administration of fluids and/or diuretics) is caused by the hyperosmolar qualities of mannitol. The usual dose is 0.25 g/kg of 20% solution mannitol over 10 to 30 minutes to a maximum dose of 2 g/kg/24 hours. Diuresis should start to occur in 15 to 30 minutes. However, mannitol should be administered cautiously, if at all, to patients with congestive heart failure.

Elderly patients may need dopamine to support the heart during fluid loading. In these cases, dopamine is not for hypotension but for inotropic support.

The Paramedic should have a high index of suspicion that a lethal dysrhythmia may occur upon disentanglement if the ECG monitor shows the wide ECG and/or runs of ventricular tachycardia. A cardiac arrest of this nature is due to the hyperkalemia. Defibrillation is often unsuccessful without treatment of the underlying problem. In this case, the Paramedic may choose to deviate from standard advanced cardiac life support guidelines and administer sodium bicarbonate and calcium first rather than epinephrine.

Although medical authorities differ over which treatment to initiate first, the two treatments are sodium bicarbonate and calcium. To treat the hyperkalemia with sodium bicarbonate, the Paramedic should administer 1 mEq/kg slow IV push. Alternatively, the Paramedic can use either 10% calcium gluconate in 10 cc intravenously over two minutes or 10% calcium chloride in 5 cc over two minutes.

If sodium bicarbonate and calcium chloride are used in the treatment of cardiac arrest, then each medication should be followed by a large fluid bolus. When combined, calcium chloride and sodium bicarbonate form the precipitate calcium bicarbonate (chalk) and sodium chloride (table salt).

CASE STUDY CONCLUSION

The patient is transported expeditiously to the trauma center, where the Paramedic has already alerted the trauma team. Although the patient appears to be stabilizing, the Paramedic knows that traumatic rhabdomyolysis may have occurred and kidney dialysis may be in the patient's future. En route, the Paramedic keeps an eye on the patient's respiratory rate, end-tidal carbon dioxide levels, as well as ECG. Although the monitor shows "spikey" T waves, there has not been any runs of ventricular tachycardia, or worse. If any appear, the Paramedic has calcium chloride ready to use.

CRITICAL THINKING QUESTIONS

1. What is the most appropriate transport decision that will get the patient to definitive care?
2. What are the advantages of transporting a patient with suspected crush injury to these hospitals, even if that means bypassing other hospitals in the process?

Disposition

Patients with significant soft-tissue damage should be transported to a trauma center for medical evaluation and follow-up. The Paramedic should document all wounds, including notes on the type, location, and depth of wound as well as drainage, and what type of dressing was used. The method of bleeding control should also be documented (i.e., dry sterile dressing, direct pressure, or pressure dressing). If a tourniquet was used, the Paramedic should make its presence well known and, if possible, stand by the patient until the emergency staff has been notified.

The patient with reperfusion injury (crush injury) has the potential for traumatic rhabdomyolysis. Even with aggressive resuscitation with intravenous fluids and sodium bicarbonate therapy > 30%, the patient may go on to develop acute renal failure (ARF).[23] The International Society of Nephrology has established a renal disaster relief task force to provide emergency dialysis in cases of disaster. However, a large number of cases of traumatic rhabdomyolysis can be prevented by Paramedic care in the field.

CONCLUSION

In the course of a lifetime everyone experiences some soft-tissue injury. The clear majority are minor but some are life-threatening and require the attention of a Paramedic. Although many soft-tissue injuries are merely an annoyance, some are painful and require the careful administration of analgesia.

KEY POINTS:

- Soft-tissue injuries include abrasions, lacerations, punctures, avulsions, and amputations.

- Wound healing starts with hemostasis and proceeds through proliferative and remodeling stages.

- During the hemostasis stage, there is vasoconstriction, fibrinogen collection, platelet plugging, and clot formation.

- During the proliferative phase, fibroblasts start granulation, wound contraction occurs, and there is angiogenesis and neovascularization.

- Wounds heal by primary or secondary intention.

- Pressure sores, chronic wounds measured on the Braden risk assessment scale, occur in four stages.

- Keloids are a form of hypertrophic scar.

- Scar formation is affected by static and dynamic tension lines in the skin.

- Wounds may be closed with sutures, staples, bioglues, or special tapes.

- Crush injury, a reperfusion injury, can lead to crush syndrome with traumatic rhabdomyolysis and other reperfusion injury.

- Enophthalmos or exophthalmos may represent soft-tissue injury around the eye.

- Wounds drain serous, sanguineous, serosanguineous, and purulent drainage.

- Treatment involves bleeding control, wound decontamination, and wound dressing.

- Hemostatic agents include minerals, complex polysaccharides, and fibrin.

- Tourniquets are used to control massive arterial bleeding.

- Dressings are sterile covers placed over a wound to help coagulate blood and protect the wound from contamination, whereas bandages hold a dressing in place.

- Three special dressings are the film dressing, the foam dressing, and the hydrogels.

- Silver and iodine are antibiotics used with dressings.

- Tetanus prophylaxis is an important consideration in wound treatment.

- Ehlers-Danlos syndrome is a congenital skin disease that appears like a burn.

- Crush injury creates massive hypovolemia, followed by traumatic rhabdomyolysis.

- Sodium bicarbonate is the drug of choice when treating crush injury.

REVIEW QUESTIONS:

1. What is necrotizing fasciitis?
2. What are the differences between an avulsion and an amputation?
3. What are the four stages of pressure sores?
4. What are the four classifications of wound drainage?
5. What are the three methods of controlling severe bleeding?

CASE STUDY QUESTIONS:

Please refer to the Case Study in this chapter, and answer the questions below:

1. In this case, suppose the patient had his leg severed and was bleeding heavily. What would have been the Paramedic's initial response?

2. Using the ECG as a rough gauge of hyperkalemia, what would be the patient's suspected potassium level if there is a loss of P waves and a widening of the QRS during the course of care?

3. If the patient in the scenario had gone into cardiac arrest, what would be the initial drug of choice (DOC)?

REFERENCES:

1. Hollander JE, Singer AJ, Valentine S, Henry MC. Wound registry: development and validation. *Ann Emerg Med.* 1995;25:675–685.

2. Beasley R. *Beasley's Surgery of the Hand.* New York: Thieme Medical Publishers; 2003.

3. Hull JB, Cooper GJ. Pattern and mechanism of traumatic amputation by explosive blast. *J Trauma: Injury, Infect, Crit Care.* March 1996;40(3S):198–205.

4. Banwell PE. Topical negative therapy in wound care. *J Wound Care.* 1999;8(22):79–82.

5. Trott A. *Wounds and Lacerations.* Atlanta GA: Elsevier Health; 2005.

6. Raugi GJ. Adult scurvy. *J Am Acad Dermatol.* 1999;41(6): 895–906.

7. Benbadis SR, et al. Value of tongue biting in the diagnosis of seizures. *Arch. Intern Med.* Nov 27, 1995;155(21):2346–2349.

8. Freeman AJ, Senn DR, Arendt DM. Seven hundred seventy eight bite marks: analysis by anatomic location, victim and biter demographics, type of crime, and legal disposition. *J Forensic Sci.* Nov 2005;50(6):1436–1443.

9. Talan DA, Citron DM, Abrahamian FM, et al. Bacteriologic analysis of infected dog and cat bites. *N Engl J Med.* Jan 14, 1999;340(2):85–92.

10. Alam, H.B., et al. Hemorrhage control in the battlefield: role of new hemostatic agents. *Mil Med.* Jan 2005.

11. Lakstein D, Blumenfeld A, Sokolov T, Lin G. Bssorai R; Lynn M, Abraham RB. Tourniquets for hemorrhage control on the battlefield: a 4-Year accumulated experience. *J Trauma: Injury, Infect, Crit Care.* May 2003;54(5):S221–S225.

12. Wakai A, Winter DC, Street JT, et al. Pneumatic tourniquets in extremity surgery. *J Am Acad Orthop Surg.* 2001;9(5):345–351.

13. Kragh JF Jr, Walters TJ, Baer DG, et al. Practical use of emergency tourniquets to stop bleeding in major limb trauma. *J Trauma.* 2008;64(2):S38–50.

14. Bailey H. *Surgery of Modern Warfare.* Edinburgh: E&S Livingston; 1941.

15. Kampen KE, Krobner JR, Jones JS, Dougherty JM, Bonness RK. In-field extremity amputation: prevalence and protocols in Emergency Medical Services. *Prehosp Disaster Med.* 1996;11(1):63–66.

16. Johansen K, et al. Objective criteria accurately predict amputation following lower extremity trauma. *J Trauma.* 1990;30:568.

17. Mertz PM, Marshall DA, Eaglestein WH. Occlusive dressings to prevent bacterial invasion and wound infection. *J Am Acad Dermatol.* 1985;12:662–668.

18. Bates–Jenson B, Sussman C. *Wound Care* (3rd ed.). Philadelphia PA: Lippincott Williams & Wilkins; 2006.

19. Fraser JF, Bodman J, Sturgess R, Faoagali J, Kimble RM. An in-vitro study of the antimicrobial efficacy of a 1% silver sulphadiazine and 0.2% chlorhexidine digluconate cream, 1% silver sulfadiazine cream and a silver coated dressing. *Burns.* 2004;30(1):35–41.

20. CDC. Preventing tetanus, diphtheria, and pertussis among adults: use of tetanus toxoid, reduced diphtheria toxoid and acellular pertussis vaccines. Recommendations of the Advisory Committee on Immunization Practices (ACIP). MMWR Recomm. Rep. 2006;55 (RR-17);1–33.

21. Centers for Disease Control and Prevention Available at: **http://www.bt.cdc.gov/masscasualties/blastinjury-crush.asp.** Accessed July 2009.

22. Better OS. Rescue and salvage of casualties suffering from the crush syndrome after mass disasters. *Mil Med.* 1999;164(5): 366–369.

23. Smith J, Greaves I. Crush injury and crush syndrome: a review. *J Trauma.* 2003;54:S226–S230.

CHAPTER 9

BURN TRAUMA

KEY CONCEPTS:

Upon completion of this chapter, it is expected that the reader will understand these following concepts:

- Incidence of burn trauma
- Types of burn trauma
- Pathophysiology of burn trauma
- Burn assessment
- Burn treatment

ANATOMY CONCEPTS:

Prior to reading this chapter the Paramedic student should be familiar with the following anatomy and physiology concepts:

- Anatomy of the skin

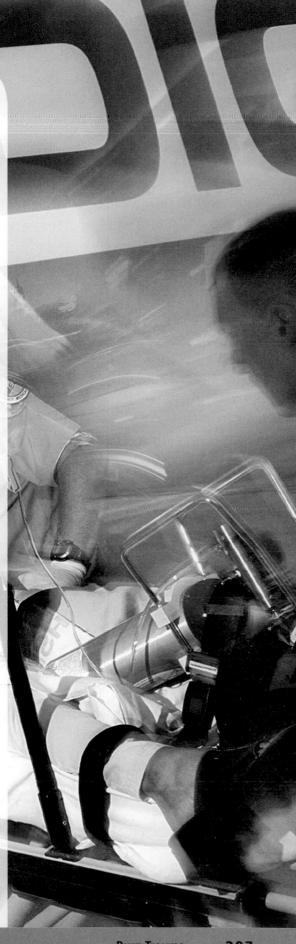

CASE STUDY:

The initial dispatch only mentioned an explosion with fire at the old paper mill. However, dispatch quickly came back to revise the report. "Man with burns, EMS requested to the west gate to meet engine 7."

As the Paramedic puts the ambulance in gear and wheels out of the garage, his mind races with possibilities. "Man with burns" he ponders. "Could the burns be thermal burns, chemical burns, or electrical burns?" Since the paper mill is a veritable kindling box of combustible paper products, thermal burns seem most likely.

After safely crossing the intersection choked with fire apparatus, the Paramedic and his partner enter the west gate to meet the engine company. As the Paramedic dismounts, he thinks to himself, "Explosion, an explosion requires a spark. Maybe these burns are electrical burns from a short circuit or something." One firefighter emerges from the huddle of firefighters around the patient and frantically motions them to come over to the patient.

CRITICAL THINKING QUESTIONS

1. What are some of the possible causes of burn trauma in this case?
2. Which type of burn trauma may be most lethal on-scene?

OVERVIEW

Approximately one-and-a-quarter-million people are burned in the United States annually. Of those, approximately 50,000 require hospitalization. Approximately 1 in 10 hospitalized burn patients will die as a result of their burns.[1] Among the deaths that occur as a result of burns, the majority are due to burns from fire. The remaining deaths are due to motor vehicle fires, plane crashes, electrical and chemical burns, and so on.[2]

Death from burns is the third leading cause of unintentional death in children ages 1 to 4, surpassed only by motor vehicle collisions and falls. Although there has been a decline in pediatric mortality from burns—largely due to flame-retardant bed clothing, self-extinguishing cigarettes, and other safety enhancements—burns from fire and hot liquid scalds still scar many children.

However, the number of deaths from burn trauma alone is relatively low. Modern resuscitation techniques and burn care has drastically improved survival. Most deaths from burn trauma actually are a result of carbon monoxide poisoning, cyanide poisoning, and asphyxiation.

Although it is difficult to separate death from fire and death from smoke inhalation, it is known that 50% of burn deaths will occur in the first 10 days following the incident, with a large percentage of those deaths occurring during the first 24 hours. During this period of time, Paramedics can have the greatest impact on these patients' long-term survival.

Chief Concern

Burns originate from several sources: chemical, electrical, and thermal sources. Regardless of the etiology, burns have one constant: pain. Part of the Paramedic's mission is to relieve the patient's pain and suffering.

However, pain is only part of the problem. Patients with burns can suffer from a number of life-threatening complications—some that threaten to suffocate them, and others that put organs like the heart and kidneys in danger. Some of these complications can occur on-scene, whereas others (such as burn–shock) can occur later. The Paramedic's early assessment and intervention in the complex burn patient's care can reduce the patient's mortality and morbidity.

Thermal Burns

Thermal burns can be the result of exposure to flames, steam, molten liquids, or contact with a hot object. Although contact with molten liquids (such as cooking grease) or with hot objects (such as frying pans and other cooking utensils) can cause burns, open flame is more frequently thought of as a cause of thermal burns. Yet exposure to extremes of cold can also cause burns. The pathophysiology of these two thermal injuries is very similar.

Pathophysiology of Burns

Temperature and pH, two essential physical conditions, must remain relatively constant within the body in order for the normal biochemical processes, such as enzymatic actions, to occur at the cellular level. Extremes of temperature, either heat (in the form of flame or steam) or cold (secondary to cold water drowning), can disrupt these biochemical processes and result in cellular injury or death.

At temperatures above 48°C (118°F), biochemical reactions within the cells start to malfunction. Upon exposure to very high temperatures, or to prolonged high temperatures, proteins can start to denature, a process called coagulation. These cells and tissues are not salvageable, and eventually necrosis (Greek for death) occurs. This necrotic tissue can generally be identified by either its semisolid white curd-like appearance or by the blackened hard eschar.

The tissue surrounding necrotic tissue sends out chemical mediators that initiate the inflammatory response, a protective systemic reaction that includes histamine, serotonin, and bradykinins. Locally, these chemical mediators cause increased capillary permeability and subsequent shifts of fluids from various other adjoining compartments (intravascular, interstitial, and intracellular) to the injured tissue.

Eventually, these compartmental shifts of fluid create a relative hypovolemia secondary to the formation of burn edema. Key to this concept of burn edema is the realization that total body fluid may not decrease but instead may be misplaced. The development of hypovolemia secondary to the sequestered fluids is a process that takes hours to days to develop. It does not occur immediately while the patient is in the field.

A more important consideration for Paramedics is the systemic effects of burn trauma upon the body. The body responds to the stress of a physical insult of this magnitude by secreting epinephrine, norepinephrine, and vasopressin. The ensuing vasoconstriction creates an increased systemic vascular resistance, thereby increasing the heart's oxygen demand (mVO_2) as well as diminishing blood flow to core organs such as the kidneys.

Classic signs of stress (i.e., tachycardia, tachypnea, and hypertension) should alert the Paramedic to the possibility of collateral damage to the core organs. For example, a patient with a history of coronary disease may be prone to angina following a burn. Yet the typical signs of acute coronary syndrome such as chest pain may be masked by the burn pain, which is a distracting injury.[3]

Chemical Burns

Between 2% and 6.5% of admissions to burn centers are for chemical burns. The American Association of Poison Control Centers (AAPCC) reports approximately 25,000 cases of exposure to acid and nearly twice as many exposures to alkaline substances. However, there are as many bleach exposures reported as acid and alkaline exposures combined.[4]

Chemicals are a part of everyday life and can be found in any industrial, agricultural, and even domestic setting. Drain cleaner is an example of a household chemical that can cause a burn. However, a discussion of every chemical manufactured, which would number in the thousands, is beyond the scope of this textbook. Therefore, it is more helpful to discuss general classes of chemical burns and to divide chemicals into three major classifications: alkalis, acids, and biochemical agents.

Alkaline chemicals (those with pH greater than 7 and which turn litmus paper blue, also known as bases) are possibly the most problematic of the chemicals. Examples of alkali include lime, potassium hydroxide, and sodium hydroxide. Alkalis dissolve fats (a process called **saponification**), bind with proteins, and extract water from cells (a process called **dessication**). These three processes culminate in an injury called liquefaction necrosis. **Liquefaction necrosis**, which can be imagined as a hot knife running through butter, literally melts the skin as it proceeds and allows for deeper penetration of the alkali into the deeper tissue. The extent of these **caustic burns** (a burn that destroys organic tissue through a chemical process) is not as obvious upon gross examination for this reason. Acids are considered corrosive, whereas bases are considered caustic.

Some common alkali include sodium hydroxide and potassium hydroxide, which are both used in drain cleaners and oven cleaners. Calcium hydroxide and calcium oxide are a part of cement. Sodium hypochlorite, or common household bleach, are common ammonia solutions.

Acids, in contrast, physically **denature** (break down) proteins through a process of hydrolysis that changes proteins into their base amino acids, thereby destroying them in the process. This process is called **coagulation necrosis**. Coagulation necrosis causes acid burns to be self-limiting. As the acid burns the skin, it creates a layer of **eschar** (Greek for scab). The scab consists of blackened necrotic tissue that prevents deeper penetration of the acid into the skin and thus limits the depth of the burn.

Examples of commonly encountered acids include sulfuric acid (used in toilet bowl cleaners and automobile batteries), nitric acid (used in fertilizer manufacture), and hydrofluoric acid (used in rust removers and tire cleaners). Hydrochloric acid used in swimming pool cleaners, phosphoric acid used in disinfectants, acetic acid used in cooking (vinegar), and formic acid used in airplane glue are other common acids.

Another mechanism for a burn is biochemical agents, such as desiccants, oxidizers, and protoplasmic poisons. These biochemical agents react chemically with tissues and cause injury. Protoplasmic poisons, such as hydrofluoric acid, chemically bind with cellular proteins and form salts. Desiccants dry out the cells in the skin. Boric acid applied to a carpet, for example, is a weak desiccant that dries out flea eggs and dehydrates flea larvae, killing them in the process. Oxidizers inappropriately accelerate some chemical reactions, leading to the formation of unusable intermediate substrates.

Exposure to a chemical agent should be thought of as a poisoning or toxicological emergency. Any burn injury should be regarded as secondary to the larger problem of poisoning. Regardless of the mechanism of injury, any chemical exposure can lead to cell death and serious burn injury.

Common Chemical Exposures

The most common chemical exposures that a Paramedic will encounter in the civilian world will be from acids and alkalis. Chemical exposures to oxidants, such as white phosphorus, are more likely to occur during warfare or training for warfare. Likewise, exposures to vesicants, such as mustard gas, are more likely to occur as a result of a terrorist attack.

Phenol

Phenol has many names (hydroxybenzene, benzenol, phenyl alcohol, and phenic acid), but is perhaps best known by its old name: carbolic acid. Phenols are weak organic acids created from coal tar, through a process called fractional distillation. It is used in the manufacture of many products including explosives and fertilizers, and is mixed with slaked lime for use in sewage treatment. Phenols are also used in medicine as chemical facial peels, antipruritics (e.g., Campho-Phenique®), and even throat lozenges (e.g., Chloraseptic®).

Phenol is an aromatic hydrocarbon. Aromatics emit (off-gas) gasses. Its sickeningly sweet acrid odor can be detected even at low concentrations (i.e., less than 0.05 parts per million). A colorless gas at room temperature, it is heavier than air. Therefore, patients found unconscious on the ground are at greater risk of exposure.

Its mechanism of injury is corrosive, denaturing proteins and poisoning the protoplasma. At concentrations greater than 250 ppm, it is immediately dangerous to life. Even one hour's exposure to 50 ppm can cause debilitating and permanent injury.

On contact with the skin, phenol forms a white covering (precipitated proteins), but the gas from phenol can penetrate deep into the dermis and enter the body. Systemically, phenol binds with albumin, an abundant blood protein, and also causes red blood cells to lyse. These systemic effects can rapidly lead to global hypoxia due to the red blood cell lysis as well as dramatic fluid shifts within internal fluid compartments from altered colloidal osmotic pressure.

Hydrofluoric Acid

Hydrofluoric acid is commonly used in the manufacture of fertilizers, pesticides, solvents, and high-octane fuels. It is particularly useful for dissolving silica. Silica is used to clean stone and marble and to polish glass and metal casings.

Hydrofluoric acid, in its anhydrous form (i.e., without water), is colorless and a strong acid. Burns involving hydrofluoric acid that are greater than 160 square cm (approximately 25 square inches) can cause systemic toxicity. Chemical burns of even 2% total body surface area can be fatal.

However, for every rule there is an exception. Acid burns are typically self-limiting, due to coagulation necrosis. However, this is not the case with hydrofluoric acid. Hydrofluoric acid in its aqueous form is a weaker acid. However, aqueous hydrofluoric acid is lipophilic, meaning it is attracted to fat, particularly fats or lipids in the cell wall.

Systemically, fluoride ions in the hydrofluoric acid penetrate into deeper tissues and bind with calcium and magnesium. This causes severe injuries, including decalcification of the bone, a secondary injury.

For patients with hydrofluoric acid exposure, it is problematic that symptoms are sometimes delayed. If the patient's total body surface exposure area is greater than 50%, then the patient will experience immediate pain and tissue destruction. However, if the total body surface area exposed to aqueous hydrofluoric acid is less than 50%, then the patient may be asymptomatic for up to eight hours. If the exposure area is less than 20% of the total body surface area, then symptoms can be delayed for up to 24 hours.

Anhydrous Ammonia

Anhydrous ammonia is a colorless gas with a pungent smell that is recognized by most as a cleaning product for drains and as an oven cleaner at concentrations as low as three parts per million (ppm). Ammonia can also be released as a product of partial combustion of wood and nylon and may therefore be dangerous to firefighters. A more notorious use of anhydrous ammonia is in the illicit production of methamphetamines.

More problematic, however, is the common use of anhydrous ammonia both as a fertilizer on the farm (farmers use one-third of the commercially available ammonia) and as a pressurized coolant for industrial refrigeration. A small amount of anhydrous ammonia gas escaping from a commercial cooler, such as is used in a grocery store warehouse, can put civilians living downwind at great risk of potentially toxic exposures.

As an alkali, anhydrous ammonia becomes a vapor under normal atmospheric conditions and is readily absorbed into skin and deeper tissues. In cases of direct exposure with liquid anhydrous ammonia, and compounding the insult, are the cutanous tissue burns created (i.e., freezer burns). The presence of freezer burns is a function of the duration of contact and the concentration of the anhydrous ammonia.

On the surface, the burn will have a soft-appearing gray-yellow tinge, masking the systemic effects that are occurring in the deeper tissues. Anhydrous ammonia mixed with water becomes a strongly alkaline solution called ammonium hydroxide. Ammonium hydroxide breaks tissue down (liquefaction necrosis) and liberates water in the process. The liberated water in turn perpetuates the conversion of anhydrous ammonia into more ammonium hydroxide until the hydroxyl ions are exhausted.

In its gaseous form, anhydrous ammonia is inhaled into the lungs and reacts with water to form ammonium hydroxide. This chemical reaction is exothermic (heat producing), and the subsequent heat can cause thermal burns to the respiratory tract, leading to the patient's characteristic cough and wheeze secondary to bronchial swelling. At 1,000 ppm, the ammonia becomes caustic to the airway; at higher concentrations, it can result in laryngospasm.

STREET SMART

One method of producing the illicit substance methamphetamine, the so-called "Nazi method," uses anhydrous ammonia, often obtained illegally from farms. The danger of exposure to ammonia is so great that many jurisdictions consider the mere presence of children in the "meth lab" to be de facto evidence of child abuse.

Calcium Oxide

Calcium oxide, more commonly referred to as lime, is a caustic alkali. One of its more common applications is being mixed in cement in a two-thirds lime concentration. The dry cement will have a pH of 12.5. Calcium oxide is also used as a binding material in the production of pulp for the paper industry.

Although the skin provides a substantial barrier to prevent direct tissue contact with lime, the body's ingestion, inhalation, or internal exposure to lime results in a chemical reaction with the cells, which leads to emulsification of cell walls (liquefactive necrosis). Heat is the by-product of this chemical reaction, resulting in thermal damage to the endothelial walls of the capillaries and subsequent thrombosis formation.

Electrical Burns

Electrical injuries, which can range from mild shocks to severe trauma, account for more than 20,000 emergency visits annually and over 1,000 deaths. Most electrical injuries, approximately 60%, occur from contact with typical household electricity.

Physics for Paramedics

Household electricity is a form of technical electricity (manmade electricity), as opposed to environmental electricity or lightning. It is the result of the flow of negatively charged atomic particles, called electrons, toward a positive pole or a ground. The flow of electrons, called current, is an effort to attain an electrical balance of charged particles, or neutrality.

A common unit of measurement which measures the difference between the two electrical poles in this electrical pathway or circuit, as well as the strength of the current, is called the **voltage (V)**, named after the Italian physicist Volta. The amount of that electrical current is called the **amperage**. As an example, the amount of current flowing through a lighted 100-watt bulb is approximately 1 ampere.

An analogy can be made with water. Although a high mountain stream flowing downhill may have a great deal of speed (voltage), it does not have the volume, measured in gallons per minute (analogously amperage), that the mighty Mississippi River has. Therefore, it does not have the Mississippi River's destructive power. In terms of the mechanism of injury, the more amperage that an electrical current has, the greater the potential damage it can create.

A single electron going through a copper wire may actually only travel 1 millimeter per second, or in a vacuum at about one-tenth the speed of light. However, the electrical signal travels at nearly the speed of light because of the production of electromagnetic waves, alternating fluctuations of magnetic and then electrical fields. These electrical fields, radiating from an electrical source, can pass through any object in the vicinity, including the Paramedic, in an effort to find a **ground**, or zero potential.

All substances allow the passage of electrical current to some degree. If electricity flows freely through the object, the object is called a **conductor**. If the object opposes the passage of an electrical current, it is called a **resistor**. This electrical resistance is measured in **ohms**.

The amount of current that passes into the body is a function of the electrical voltage and the resistance, known as Ohm's law: Current (I) = Voltage (E) / Resistance (R).

Skin, being inert, does not allow the passage of electricity into the body easily and is thus a resistor (normal skin resistance is about 25,000 ohms), depending on its moisture content, thickness, and contamination. However, when the skin is wet it readily allows the passage of electricity because water is an excellent conductor of electricity. In this case, as little as 1,500 ohms are required to pass through the skin and into the body. Conversely, an electrician's dry, calloused hands may resist 1,000,000 ohms of electricity before the electrician senses the electrical current.

All resistance to electrical flow creates heat as a by-product to some degree. The greater the resistance, the greater the ohms, and therefore the greater the heat produced. For example, the energy needed to overcome the resistance found in the palm of a hand may generate heat in excess of 1,000°C.

An important aspect of an electrical burn is the length of the patient's contact. For example, as little as 50 volts over 10 seconds can lead to partial thickness burns. The resulting blisters markedly diminish the skin's resistance, allowing for further burn trauma.

This intense heat, which is the mechanism of injury for an electrical burn, can lead to near-instant mummification of the tissue. This mummification creates a clearly defined char wound.

Secondary injury from an electrical burn can occur as a result of injury to the muscle. The resulting muscle damage is similar to a crush injury, discussed in Chapter 8, and can result in rhabdomyolysis.

An electric **arc**, a high voltage light flash, can produce temperatures as high as 4,000°C. These pale blue-violet flashes are formed when electricity goes between two objects of greatly different electrical potentials, such as a high power line and a person. The resulting arc actually creates a plasma trail that can vaporize skin and bone.

Pathophysiology of Electrical Burns

Combining these factors—type of electrical current (AC/DC), the amount of current (volts), the duration of contact with the patient, and the area of contact (in terms of the thickness of the skin)—determines the extent of burn trauma. For example, a 1-second contact with 1 milliampere (mA) is just at the threshold of human perception, creating a sense of tingling in the hands; however, a 1-second contact with 100 mA can lead to respiratory paralysis and ventricular fibrillation. At approximately 5 mA, the sensation is more like warmth than tingling, owed to the buildup of heat from the skin's resistance to the flow of electrical current.

As he approaches the patient, the Paramedic considers the idea that the patient may have a chemical burn. During paper-making, black liquor—a mixture of alkaline chemicals—is used to break down wood into pulp for paper. White lightning, another caustic substance, is also used in paper processing. Both chemical mixtures are heated to high temperatures, making them a double threat to workers. The Paramedic recalls some nasty chemical burns he's seen from patients exposed to black liquor.

Even before he kneels down, he calls out to the plant foreman, "Get me those MSDS sheets!" Almost before the words left his mouth, like an echo, the foreman replies, "They are already on their way."

After one look at the man, the Paramedic knows the patient is facing double trouble. The patient not only has been exposed to a large volume of the chemicals, but the chemicals are still on him, increasing the duration of contact. The Paramedic's first order of business is to get those clothes off him and get him decontaminated.

CRITICAL THINKING QUESTIONS

1. What are the important elements of the history that a Paramedic should obtain?
2. What is the importance of the MSDS sheets?

History

Heat is generally transferred by either direct contact or radiation. Therefore, it is important for the Paramedic to ascertain if the burn is secondary to exposure to fire or secondary to contact with a burning material. If the burn is a contact burn, then the next question is whether the object was solid (such as a stove top) or liquid (such as scalding hot water).

STREET SMART

Although burns can obviously be deadly, the poisons contained in the smoke can be lethal as well. Critical questions must be asked whenever a patient has a burn. These questions include: "What type of fire?" (i.e., open flame or a smoldering smoky fire) and "Was the patient in a confined space?"

Exposure to the products of partial combustion, such as carbon monoxide and/or cyanide, which are found in smoke from a smoldering fire can poison a patient, compounding the severity of the injuries. Entrapment in a confined space, voluntary or otherwise, can increase the duration of exposure to these toxic gasses.

If the material was liquid, the next question is, "How thick was the liquid?" A property of all liquids is viscosity; the more viscous (thicker) a liquid, then the greater the likelihood of a deeper burn over even a short amount of exposure time. Some of the most severe burns are secondary to hot oils, molten grease, or coal tar. Molten metals, perhaps the thickest liquid known, almost instantly produce a full thickness burn.

The duration of contact is also important to understanding the severity of burns. In the case of a thermal burn, even an almost instantaneous flash, such as occurs in an arc burn, can produce a burn. However, prolonged contact with an open flame is more likely to produce trauma.

History for a Patient with Chemical Burns

Key to obtaining a patient's history when dealing with a chemical burn is to ascertain the offending chemical agent. The Paramedic must take care to ensure the correct chemical is identified, as many chemicals have similar sounding names and comparable spellings. Routinely confounding the situation is the presence of multiple chemicals, each with individual characteristics. Many of these interact with one another to create a third and greater potential of harm.

Once the chemicals have been identified, it is important for the Paramedic to determine their physical form (i.e., liquid, solid, or gas). Although physical contamination may be apparent, like a thermal burn, the injury on the outside may be less important than the injury on the inside.

Such is the case with chemical exposure, which likely involves an inhalation injury.

The next order of business is to determine the volume of the exposure. Many chemicals can be toxic at very small volumes and even smaller concentrations. Atmospheric gas detectors are available for some chemicals. These gas detectors can either register present or not present, or the concentration of the gas in the air in parts per million (ppm).

The final determination is the total time of exposure. In some cases, a prolonged exposure to a dilute chemical can be more injurious than a short exposure to a concentrated chemical.

Prior to EMS arrival, some patients may attempt self-care and decontamination. Instructions for decontamination and simple first aid are found on the material safety data sheet (MSDS) available at the work site.

To complete the history, using the SAMPLE tool, the Paramedic should determine if there are any coexisting injuries and/or comorbidities that could complicate the patient's care.

History for a Patient with Electrical Burns

After establishing scene safety, the Paramedic should identify the mechanism of injury. After turning off the power source, the Paramedic must assess the electricity source. Common household electric circuits have been "stepped down" to about 110V from 440V through the use of transformers, which reside on the power poles from which electricity is distributed to the residence. These distribution lines receive electricity from higher-powered transmission lines that can carry 1,000V. Any transmission line that carries more than 1,000V is called a high tension line.

Toddlers, for example, may be likely to chew through common household electrical cords and suffer burns to the lips. Adventuresome adolescents may climb power poles, or even power towers, and come in contact with transmission lines.

After establishing the source of the electricity (distribution versus transmission), the Paramedic should try to establish the current's pathway. The most common lethal pathway is from hand to hand, crossing the chest. However, the most commonly occurring pathway is from hand to foot, as the electricity tries to find ground. However, if the patient or the Paramedic steps into an electrical field, then it is possible for the electricity to pass from foot to foot as the circuit is created.

A key factor to technical electrical injuries is the duration of contact. Technical electricity is an alternating electrical current (AC). Alternating current electricity cyclically reverses the electrical current, usually at 60 **hertz (Hz)** or cycles per second, adding efficiency to the transmission of electricity.

When a patient comes in contact with any electricity, the stimulus may cause a muscular contraction. In the case of direct current (DC), such as found in a battery, this contact leads to one massive muscular spasm. Muscular contraction from a direct current surge often throws a patient clear from the danger. In contrast, when a patient comes in contact with alternating current at approximately 15 to 150 Hz, the muscles spasm in a repetitive and rhythmic fashion (i.e., clonus), preventing the muscles from relaxing long enough to release the patient's grasp of the power line. This is called the "let-go" current. The resultant phenomenon may cause persistent paralysis of the diaphragm, among other muscles, resulting in asphyxia.

▶ CASE STUDY (CONTINUED)

Following a gross decontamination, the Paramedic, attired in proper PPE, starts the primary assessment, focusing on the patient's airway and breathing. The patient seems able to maintain his own airway when the Paramedic lifts the oxygen mask to look into his mouth. Next, the Paramedic focuses on the patient's breathing. Although he has a pulse oximeter available, he knows it will not yield much information. What the Paramedic really wants is the carbon monoxide detector, but that is back in the ambulance.

The Paramedic isn't concerned about hypoxia, since the patient is awake and his mentation is good. However, the near circumferential burns across the patient's chest do give the Paramedic a reason for concern. He knows the patient is going to have trouble breathing against the eschar that is about to form.

CRITICAL THINKING QUESTIONS

1. What are the elements of the physical examination of a patient with a burn?
2. Why are the near circumferential chest burns a concern to the Paramedic?

Examination

Upon arrival at the patient's side, the Paramedic performs an initial assessment. He starts with a consideration of the mechanism of injury, followed by the possibility of spinal trauma and the need for manual stabilization, and then proceeds with a routine initial assessment.

While performing the initial assessment, the Paramedic should observe for signs of serious burn trauma. Confusion and combativeness, for example, may be due to hypoxia secondary to pulmonary burns from inhalation of superheated gasses or poisoning by products of partial combustion, such as carbon monoxide or cyanide. Other evidence of hypoxia includes open mouth breathing, gasping breaths derived from air hunger, and/or nasal flaring.

While assessing the airway, the Paramedic may also note singed nasal hairs, grossly swollen lips, or a soot-blackened tongue, as well as a reddened mucous membrane in the oropharynx. These are signs the patient may have inhaled smoke and/or superheated air. A persistent productive cough of black sooty phlegm, or bronchorrhea, is a significant sign of inhalation burns.

The Paramedic should also evaluate the patient for the presence of **stridor**, an abnormal high-pitched musical sound, in the throat. Auscultation of the throat, while generally not part of an initial assessment, may be necessary in order to determine the presence of stridor. Audible stridor, heard without a stethoscope, should immediately alert the Paramedic to the possibility of complete airway closure and the need for immediate definitive control of the airway, possibly by endotracheal intubation.

Further signs of hypoxia, suggestive of pulmonary involvement, include the presence of cyanosis in the lips, sclera, or nail beds. The use of pulse oximetry at this point is of questionable value.

Carbon monoxide, found in smoke, competes with oxygen. Carbon monoxide favorably binds with hemoglobin, with an affinity 250 times greater than oxygen, forming carboxyhemoglobin. It also blocks oxygen from the receptor sites, creating hypoxia. Unfortunately, pulse oximetry cannot distinguish between oxyhemoglobin and carboxyhemoglobin, so it may give a falsely high reading for oxygen saturation.

Yet, these pulse oximeters continue to register a pulse rate as well as oxygen saturation. One of the earliest signs of hypoxia is an elevated pulse rate. The Paramedic can use a pulse oximeter as a pulse register for purposes of assessing the patient's response to oxygen therapy.

Handheld carbon monoxide detectors, whose operation is similar to a pulse oximeter, are available. Although specific operation of each machine varies from manufacturer to manufacturer, light is generally passed through an accessible capillary bed and returned to a sensor.

A more problematic issue for the patient's respiration than carbon monoxide poisoning is a circumferential burn of the patient's thoracic. Charred inflexible skin, or eschar, acts as a constricting band around the patient's chest, preventing it from expanding. Without the ability to expand the chest wall, the patient cannot inhale, resulting in suffocation. Under emergency conditions, and with specific medical direction, some Paramedics may perform a field escharotomy (superficial incisions to release the underlying pressure).

Sources of hypoperfusion, evidenced by signs such as absent radial pulses, should be quickly established and aggressively treated. The source of the hypoperfusion cannot be burn edema, as that takes about 8 to 12 hours to develop. However, hypoperfusion can be the result of hemorrhage from occult trauma that is masked by the burn trauma.

In the same perspective, burn patients can suffer secondary injuries from falls or explosions that preceded the fire. These injuries may be overlooked during the Paramedic's disability assessment because of the presence of the burns. A head injury is potentially a more lethal condition, in the prehospital phase, than a burn.

Finally, the Paramedic should expose the patient to check for other life- or limb-threatening injuries as well as to assess the extent of the burn. Any jewelry the patient is wearing should be removed and secured as soon as possible. Rings, earrings, and body jewelry can retain heat, further burning the patient. These items can also have a tourniquet-like effect as the burn edema occurs, leading to distal digital ischemia.

Examination of the Patient with Chemical Burns

Hydrofluoric Acid

Initially, a hydrofluoric acid exposure will create redness, localized edema, and possible blistering. External signs of contact with more concentrated hydrofluoric acid can include small white burns, secondary to protein coagulation, and/or blisters or a classic silvery-gray scale. These benign-appearing lesions are deceptive, as the larger problem occurs under the skin where the hydrofluoric acid has been absorbed and causes serious systemic effects.

Binding with free calcium in the bloodstream, the systemic effects of hydrofluoric acid exposure include abdominal pain, muscle pain, paresis, hypotension, dysrhythmias and convulsions. Nausea and vomiting early in the course of care should alert the Paramedic to the possibility of systemic absorption.

Phenol

Although phenol burns initially appear gruesome, and tend to become the focus of immediate care, the systemic effects are more deadly. Although treatment of the external burn is important, the Paramedic should focus her attention on the assessment and treatment of the systemic effects of the exposure.[5]

Outwardly, the cutaneous manifestations of a phenol exposure will manifest a painless white covering made of precipitated proteins. Phenol, an anesthetic, often numbs the injured tissue, leading patients to dismiss the importance of the burn. If there is an area of greater than 60 square inches of affected skin, there is a substantial risk of immediate death from the exposure.

The Paramedic's initial assessment of the patient exposed to phenol should focus on systemic signs of poisoning (such as nausea and vomiting) as well as signs of sympathetic stimulation (i.e., tachycardia and diaphoresis). If left untreated, or at a later stage in the evolution of the phenol exposure, pulmonary edema and hypotension may occur. Initial sympathetic stimulation later gives way to central nervous system depression as manifested by hypotension, convulsions, and coma.

Anhydrous Ammonia

As a corrosive, ammonia is immediately irritating, causing a burning sensation in the oropharynx and nasopharynx as well as fits of coughing. Initial life-threatening symptoms will focus on the respiratory system, where ammonia will interact with the moist mucous membranes to form ammonium hydroxide. This chemical reaction is also exothermic, producing heat in the process, and leads to more cellular injury.

Contact with the respiratory tract, through inhalation, can cause immediate edema of both the bronchioles and the alveolus as a result of the cellular breakdown of the cell walls (liquefaction necrosis) through saponification. Deep penetration of the lung fields is possible with inhalation of ammonia.

Calcium Oxide

Exposure to cement dust (64% calcium oxide) is one mechanism of exposure to calcium oxide, otherwise known as Quick Lime. With a pH of 12.5, calcium oxide acts like the alkaline ammonia, causing liquefaction necrosis. The lower limbs, in proximity to the dust, are most often exposed, representing about 86% of injuries. There is a gradual progression of symptoms from 12 to 48 hours post-exposure.

Inhalation of aerosolized calcium oxide is more problematic. The corrosive effects upon the respiratory tract cause the typical triad of a burning throat, persistent cough, and complaints of shortness of breath. Inhaled lime damages the squamous epithelial cells lining the respiratory tract, producing subsequent edema and bronchoconstriction and/or bronchospasm. During most exposures, the most commonly exposed organs are the pharynx and the esophagus.[6]

Examination of the Patient with Electrical Burns

Electricity has to overcome the skin's resistance at the point of contact before coursing through the body toward the ground. As energy builds to overcome the skin's natural resistance, heat is produced. This amassed heat causes a burn at the point of entry.

Once the electricity reaches ground, it must once again amass sufficient energy to overcome the skin's resistance before exiting the body. The resultant discharge can be dramatic, with the electricity literally exploding from the body. The exit wound, called a blowout wound, can be impressive, whereas the entry wound can be small and hard to detect.

Variables such as the part of the body affected, the surface area of the contact point, and so on, make it difficult to accurately distinguish entrance wounds from exit wounds. The point of contact with the electrical source, a piece of information that Paramedics are most often able to obtain while on-scene, is more helpful than anything else in distinguishing the entrance wound from the exit wound.

Electricity has been known to cause muscular contractions strong enough to fracture bones and dislocate shoulders. There are even reports of bilateral scapular fractures in cases where the electricity traveled across the chest from one arm to the other arm.

STREET SMART

When confronted with an electrical burn patient whose clothes seem to have ignited, the Paramedic should consider the possibility of an arc burn. Flashes from an arc are hot enough to ignite clothing.

CASE STUDY (CONTINUED)

"Stick to the discipline," the Paramedic urges himself, knowing that injury hidden under the burn is more likely to kill the patient on-scene than the burns themselves. Several leading diagnoses come to mind, including hypoxia secondary to toxic inhalation, respiratory failure secondary to restrictive lung disorder, and traumatic brain injury secondary to blast.

While attending to the primary assessment, the Paramedic calls to his partner to request "the bird" so they can fly the patient to the burn center. She yells back, "The dispatcher wants to know what kind of burns he has and his burn percentage."

CRITICAL THINKING QUESTIONS

1. What is the significance of the burn type and percentage?
2. Why was air medical services requested early into this patient's care?

Assessment

The Paramedic's first step when assessing a burn's severity is to decide the burn's depth. Burns are grossly categorized into superficial, partial thickness, and full thickness burns.

Superficial burns, as the name implies, involve the outermost layer of the skin, the epidermis (Figure 9-1). The epidermis is essentially a layer of dead cells, the corny layer, with a basement of germinal cells that continually replace any cells that are lost through abrasion or other everyday rubbing. A superficial burn generally appears reddened and may be slightly edematous over time. A key finding that differentiates superficial burns is that superficial burns blanch under pressure.

Partial thickness burns extend into the dermis, a reticular layer of specialized cells and blood vessels below the epidermis, which is also referred to as the true skin (Figure 9-2). Since pain receptors are located in the dermis, partial thickness burns are often painful for this reason.

A partial thickness burn's appearance can range from bright red to mottled, and the emergence of fluid is a significant finding. Visible moisture, either on the surface or sequestered in a blister, indicates that the epidermis has been breached.

Blisters are thin-walled sacks of clear fluid that develop on the skin. Large blisters are called bulla. Some concern has been raised that the fluid in these blisters, specifically vasoactive substances that decrease circulation to the wound, may be deleterious to wound healing.

However, in the prehospital setting, Paramedics should attempt to leave these blisters, or bulla, intact. Paramedics must exercise special caution to avoid breaking blisters on the hands, palms, or fingers, as these blisters can be particularly painful for the patient. If a blister or bulla should break, the Paramedic should apply a sterile dressing over the wound, leaving the intact flap to act as a biological dressing.

A **full thickness burn**, as the name suggests, extends past the skin's protective barrier and exposes the body to infection and insults from the environment (Figure 9-3). A full thickness burn can even extend into muscle, impairing motion and mobility in the process.

The appearance of a full thickness burn can range from a white, waxy look to a black, leathery surface consistent with charred flesh. More importantly, full thickness burns are insensate, and the absence of pain in the burn wound is pathognomic (i.e., specifically diagnostic) for a full thickness burn. The identification of a full thickness burn is further supported by the absence of bleeding, as a combination of cautery and microthrombii seal capillaries.

Some emergency medical experts group partial and full thickness burns together as **deep burns**. This classification may be useful in the prehospital setting. Since burns, and burn edema, develop over time, final determination of the extent of a burn is often withheld for 24 hours until the burn fully develops. This process is where the burn "declares" itself.

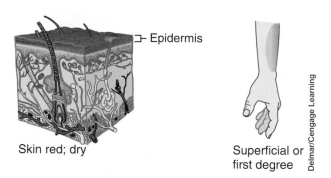

Skin red; dry — Superficial or first degree

Epidermis

Figure 9-1 Superficial burns involve the outermost layer of the skin, the epidermis.

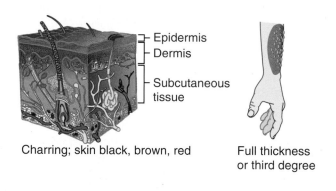

Epidermis — Dermis — Subcutaneous tissue

Charring; skin black, brown, red — Full thickness or third degree

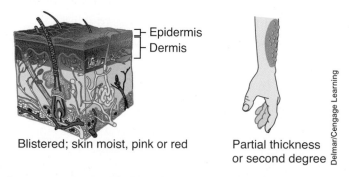

Epidermis — Dermis

Blistered; skin moist, pink or red — Partial thickness or second degree

Figure 9-2 Partial thickness burns extend into the dermis, a reticular layer of specialized cells and blood vessels below the epidermis.

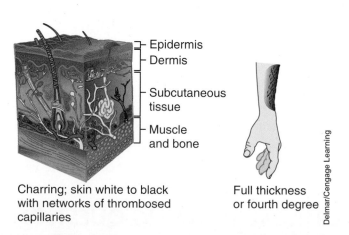

Epidermis — Dermis — Subcutaneous tissue — Muscle and bone

Charring; skin white to black with networks of thrombosed capillaries — Full thickness or fourth degree

Figure 9-3 Full thickness burns extend past the skin's protective barrier and expose the body to infection and insults from the environment.

Some laypersons and medical providers still use the terms first, second, and third degree burns. These older designations imply an increasing importance and gravity with each degree of burn. However, even a superficial, or first degree burn, can be life-threatening, especially if certain suntan-enhancing agents of the Psoralen family (P-UVA) are used, though this use has been largely discontinued. P-UVA is used for the treatment of psoriasis and dermatitis.

It is uncommon to have only a full thickness wound unless there is a specific point of contact with a hot object. Flames, for example, create an irregular concentric injury on the portion of the body closest to the source. Each area of such a burn has variations, explained by **Jackson's thermal burn theory and zones of injury**.

The outermost ring of a burn is generally superficial and is called the zone of hyperemia. **Hyperemia**, which is secondary to inflammatory mediators such as histamine and prostaglandins, results in dilation of capillary beds and is manifest by reddened skin (superficial burn).

Within the zone of hyperemia is the zone of **stasis**, where edema and blisters form because of microvascular injury. Subsequent edema and infection decrease oxygenation and nutrition to the tissue within the wound and can result in necrosis. This is why some experts group partial and full thickness wounds together.

In the center of the burn wound is the zone of **coagulation**, the area of direct tissue destruction. Outwardly, there is a visible layer of eschar and necrosis.[7]

The physical location of the burn trauma on the body has some implications regarding the extent of injury. For example, the skin on the back is thickest, perhaps 0.20 to 0.24 inches, whereas the skin on the eyelids is the thinnest, approximately 0.02 inches thick.

Burn Estimates

After identification of the burn trauma, the Paramedic estimates the total body surface area (TBSA) involved, which assists in determining the burn's severity. This has implications for patient disposition as well as fluid resuscitation.

Some systems simplify the determination of burn area by performing serial halves: for example, the front of the body is one half, the upper portion of the front of the body is one half of one half, and therefore 25%, and so on. However, most Paramedics rely on Wallace's rule of nines.

Wallace's rule of nines divides the body into 11 quadrants, each equivalent to 9% of the total body surface area. Although the rule of nines is quick and may be useful for determining large burn areas, it is notoriously inaccurate as it results in overestimating burn area.

The Lund–Browder chart, the preferred method of burn estimation, assigns body surface estimations according to the specific area involved (Figure 9-4). The Lund–Browder chart is actually five charts, each representing people in a different age range: 1 to 4 years of age, 5 to 9 years of age, 10 to 14 years of age, 15 to 18 years of age, and 19 or greater years of age.

Another method, the palmar method, is useful for small burns as well as irregularly shaped burns, such as a hot water scalding. In an adult, the palm of the hands is approximately 1% of the total body surface area. In a child, the palm of the hands represents one-half of 1% of the TBSA, whereas the entire palmar surface of the hand is more approximate of the TBSA. Regardless of the method of burn estimation used, only the deep burns (i.e., partial and full thickness burns) are used to estimate the TBSA involved.[8]

PROFESSIONAL PARAMEDIC

Paramedics, as patient advocates, must always be alert to the possibility of child abuse. Pediatric burns, a common everyday occurrence, are of special concern. In a moment of rage, parents can injure a child, resulting in a burn. Specific burns, with characteristic stocking and donut burn patterns, immediately raise questions of child abuse. The question that should be foremost in every Paramedic's mind is, "Does the injury match the mechanism of injury and the developmental age of the child or is there a potential for child abuse?"

Assessment of Electrical Burns

Pulmonary complications from electric shock in the field are generally limited to involvement of the phrenic nerve and diaphragm paralysis. Pleural effusions, which are occasionally seen in these cases, occur later in the patient's history.

Cardiac complications of electrical injury can range from sustained sinus tachycardia with global, nonspecific ST segment changes that persist for weeks to atrial fibrillation and heart blocks to ventricular fibrillation and cardiac arrest.

A more problematic issue may be the vascular damage that occurs with electrical injury. The inflammatory response that occurs following the passage of electricity through the body leads to diffuse mural thrombus formation, arterial occlusion, and ischemia of muscles.

Electric shock can cause a number of abdominal complications including stress ulcers (called **Curling's ulcer**), hypodynamic ileus, and localized abdominal muscle injury. Nausea and vomiting are common complaints, occurring in 25% of patients who suffer from an electric shock.[9]

Trying to estimate the extent of injury from an electrical burn is like trying to estimate the size of an iceberg, where 70% of the iceberg is underwater and not visible. Electrical injuries may have only a limited external burn yet have an extensive internal injury.

Once electricity has entered the body, it tends to follow blood vessels and nerves. As the electricity travels along the

Lund and Browder's Burn Estimate Diagram

AREA	Inf.	1-4	5-9	10-14	15	Adult
HEAD	19	17	13	11	9	7
NECK	2	2	2	2	2	2
ANT. TRUNK	13	13	13	13	13	13
POST. TRUNK	13	13	13	13	13	13
R. BUTTOCK	2.5	2.5	2.5	2.5	2.5	2.5
L. BUTTOCK	2.5	2.5	2.5	2.5	2.5	2.5
GENITALIA	1	1	1	1	1	1
R.U. ARM	4	4	4	4	4	4
L.U. ARM	4	4	4	4	4	4
R.L. ARM	3	3	3	3	3	3
L.L. ARM	3	3	3	3	3	3
R. HAND	2.5	2.5	2.5	2.5	2.5	2.5
L. HAND	2.5	2.5	2.5	2.5	2.5	2.5
R. THIGH	5.5	6.5	8	8.5	9	9.5
L. THIGH	5.5	6.5	8	8.5	9	9.5
R. LEG	5	5	5.5	6	6.5	7
L. LEG	5	5	5.5	6	6.5	7
R. FOOT	3.5	3.5	3.5	3.5	3.5	3.5
L. FOOT	3.5	3.5	3.5	3.5	3.5	3.5

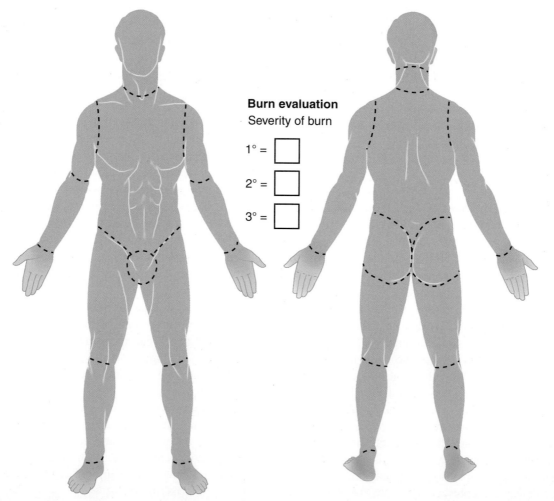

Burn evaluation
Severity of burn

1° = ☐

2° = ☐

3° = ☐

Delmar/Cengage Learning

Figure 9-4 The Lund–Browder chart assigns body surface estimations according to the specific area involved.

blood vessels, resistance creates thermal energy. The heat produced injures the internal lining, the tunica intima, and an inflammatory response ensues. In some cases, a thrombus may form, occluding the vessel, resulting in loss of blood flow downstream and subsequent pain secondary to ischemia.

As the electricity travels along peripheral nerves, it can interrupt nerve function, causing numbness, paresis, or paralysis. Depending on the affected nerve, the paresis can be patchy along the axis of the extremity.

Many major veins, arteries, and nerves travel in proximity to a bone. Due to this close approximation, bones can also be heated, thereby heating the cells within the marrow of the bone. This increased heat affects the production of red blood cells.

CASE STUDY (CONTINUED)

Focusing on the impending airway and ventilation problems, the Paramedic elects to use medication-facilitated intubation immediately and starts the premedication regime as the helicopter lands. With the assistance of the flight crew, the patient is electively intubated and put on a transport ventilator. Without a concern about respiratory depression, the flight crew immediately administers a large dose of morphine for analgesia.

CRITICAL THINKING QUESTIONS

1. What is the national standard of care of patients with burn trauma?
2. What are some of the patient-specific concerns and considerations that the Paramedic should consider when applying this plan of care that is intended to treat a broad patient population presenting with burn trauma?

Treatment

The Paramedic's first priority of patient care is personal protection, including standard precautions. Because of the large amount of bodily fluids that Paramedics often encounter in burn trauma, they should use adequate personal protective equipment that shields them from potentially infectious bodily fluids before treating the patient.

The universal treatment for all burns begins with removing the patient from the source of the burn. This should be accomplished in a safe and expeditious manner, so as to minimize dangers to the Paramedic by mitigating hazards. For example, the Paramedic can use fire service turnout gear. The next task is to remove the source of the burn from the patient.

With the patient clear of the danger, the Paramedic should extinguish any burning materials that remain on the patient, such as smoldering leather. Use of tepid to cool tap water is effective in many cases, or sterile water (if available). However, the use of cold water and/or ice may cause further damage and is therefore not recommended. Sterile saline should also be avoided.

As a rule, the Paramedic should remove any burning materials from the patient. The exception to this rule is tar. Tar should not be removed from the skin as it will damage viable tissue under the tar in the process. Tar should first be cooled with clean water until it is cool to touch.

The Paramedic should perform an initial assessment to determine the patient's further treatment needs. Although a burn may appear appalling, death in the prehospital setting is more likely to come from suffocation. Thus, the Paramedic's top priority is maintaining a patent airway or preventing other fatal complications of trauma rather than focusing on the burn itself.

Evidence of airway swelling, such as audible stridor or a hoarse voice, should be investigated and remedied immediately. Aggressive airway control, including endotracheal intubation, should be considered. Although some paralytics would not be considered later in a burn patient's care for fear of developing hyperkalemia, in the prehospital setting (first hour following the burn) it is acceptable to use medication-facilitated intubation to ensure and secure an airway.

Following intubation, the Paramedic should use a commercial device to secure the endotracheal tube in place. Frequently, tape does not adhere well to burnt skin. Swelling in the area may also undermine the tape, leading to failure and potential misplacement of the endotracheal tube.

Circumferential burns of the thoracic area can be the most deadly burns of all. The formation of hard, nonyielding eschar literally leads to suffocation of the patient. Unable to expand the chest, the patient is unable to breathe and the only hope of survival lies in an emergency escharotomy.

An **escharotomy** is a surgical incision into the depth of the burnt tissue. The opening, generally in parallel lines along the mid-axillary line and horizontally along the plane of the diaphragm, allows for expansion and movement. Typically, the procedure is performed using a portable electrical cauterizing tool and the incisions are made into the necrotic tissue. Generally, analgesia is not needed because the incisions are made into the insensate full depth burn.

Since audible stridor and circumferential burns are observable, the Paramedic can immediately realize and rectify the danger. More insidious, and just as lethal, is the presence of poisonous gasses.

The majority of burn center fatalities are attributable to smoke inhalation, since smoke contains poisonous gasses such as carbon monoxide and cyanide. Carbon monoxide and cyanide are by-products of incomplete combustion, creating the invisible gasses found in visible smoke.

Smoke Inhalation

Smoke inhalation, not burns, causes the majority of fire-related deaths in the United States. For example, the mortality rate for a person with 40% TBSA burns, about 3%, increases to 27% when complicated by smoke inhalation. Smoke inhalation kills via three major mechanisms: asphyxiation, carbon monoxide poisoning, and cyanide poisoning.

An oxygen-poor environment, created by the presence of fire, may be the first cause of asphyxiation. As fire consumes oxygen to support combustion, oxygen concentrations can fall below 10%, leading to asphyxiation.

The next cause of asphyxiation is loss of the upper airway secondary to burns and swelling. Often these upper airway burns are accompanied by facial burns. Evidence of facial burns that may involve smoke inhalation include burnt eyebrows and eyelashes, **carbonaceous sputum** (combination of secretions, mucosal slough, and smoke residue), and **singed vibrissae** (stiff nasal hairs).

However, not all facial burns are accompanied by upper airway burns. Likewise, not all upper airway burns have accompanying facial burns. Therefore, the Paramedic must remain vigilant to the possibility of upper airway burns in every burn trauma case.

Evidence of upper airway burns can include stridor (sometimes audible only by stethoscope), hoarseness, and respiratory distress manifested by tachypnea, retractions, and carbonaceous sputum. Because of the risk of asphyxiation secondary to airway closure, the Paramedic should consider intubation for patients with this symptom pattern.

The final cause of asphyxiation is lower airway burns. Inhalation of superheated gasses, such as steam, can cause burns to the lower airway. This is more likely to occur in a confined space.

Signs of lower airway burns include wheezing, frank crackles, and a persistent nonproductive cough. As physiologic changes occur due to inflammation (i.e., capillary edema and atelectasis), there will be worsened ventilation-perfusion (V-Q) match and a worsening of the patient's

Table 9-1 Inhalation Gasses	
Sulfur dioxide	Petroleum products (oil, fuel), coal
Nitrogen dioxide	Diesel, lacquers, and wallpaper
Carbon monoxide	Petroleum products
Hydrogen cyanide	Polyurethane and nitrocellulose
Hydrogen sulfide	Coal

condition regardless of the administration of high-flow, high-concentration oxygen and positive pressure ventilation.[10] Inhalation of superheated gasses can also cause pneumothorax.[11]

Smoke inhalation can also kill patients through inhalation of the toxins carbon monoxide and cyanide. These systemic poisons, absorbed via the pulmonary tree, cause profound hypoxia. Among the common gasses found in inhalation poisonings, the most dangerous may be cyanide (Table 9-1).

STREET SMART

Inhalation of microparticles of combustion can be seen in the carbonaceous sputum that firefighters bring up hours and even days after a fire, sometimes referred to as "fire boogers." These particles often contain known carcinogens. Good pulmonary toilet (coughing, expectoration, and suctioning) is needed to clear these potential carcinogens, and medical follow-up may be in order.

Carbon monoxide has approximately 200% more affinity for hemoglobin than oxygen, thereby preventing respiration and the inevitable cascade of hypoxia and acidosis. Carbon monoxide binds with hemoglobin and creates carboxyhemoglobin ($HbCO_2$). Elevated $HbCO_2$ levels greater than 40% to 60% can lead to an immediate loss of consciousness (Table 9-2). If left untreated, the patient exposed to carbon monoxide will develop a large acid load, secondary to anaerobic respiration, which in turn leads to massive vasodilation. The patient will then succumb to shock. Therefore, the suspicion of carbon monoxide poisoning is based, in part, upon the symptom complex associated with the shock syndrome. The presence or absence of the classic cherry red skin used by many to describe carbon monoxide poisoning is not reliable or consistent from patient to patient. It is a late sign and should be used as only one sign of many that leads the Paramedic to suspect carbon monoxide poisoning.

Management of carbon monoxide poisoning revolves around administration of high-flow, high-concentration oxygen. As carbon monoxide does not affect the amount of dissolved oxygen in the blood, an attempt to increase dissolved oxygen in the blood is made using high-flow, high-concentration oxygen; continuous positive airway pressure;

Table 9-2 Carbon Monoxide Poisoning

%HbCO$_2$	
< 20%	Headache, confusion, loss of concentration
20% to 40%	Nausea, vomiting, visual disturbances, and fatigue
40% to 60%	Combativeness, frank shock, and cardiac dysrhythmia
> 60%	Decompensated shock and cardiac arrest

and positive pressure ventilation to increase the amount of oxygen in the blood that is not bound to hemoglobin. High-flow, high-concentration oxygen can reduce the half-life of carbon monoxide from four hours to one hour.[12] The rapid transportation of a patient to a hyperbaric chamber has come under discussion, due to its limited availability and unproven efficacy. The decision to transport someone to a hyperbaric chamber should be based on local protocols.[13]

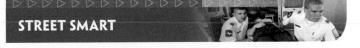

STREET SMART

If signs of global ischemia appear on a burn patient's 12-lead ECG, the Paramedic should suspect hypoxemia. This in turn should lead to an aggressive search for the cause of the hypoxemia.

The frequency of cyanide poisoning has increased as a result of changes in materials used in houses and furnishings. When burned, certain materials—such as wool, polyurethane, and silk—produce noxious fumes that include cyanide. The concentration of these toxins is increased in confined spaces. The Paramedic must consider cyanide poisoning in patients with an altered mental status who do not respond to high-flow, high-concentration oxygen.

Cyanide causes hypoxia by inhibition of cytochrome oxidase, an enzyme needed in the electron transport chain for aerobic metabolism. One therapeutic approach is to provide an alternate binding site for the cyanide. These "kits," such as the Lilly kit or the Pasadena kit, consist of amyl nitrite ampules, sodium nitrite, and sodium thiosulfate. The typical administration calls for 10 mL of sodium nitrite (3%) intravenously over two to four minutes along with inhalation of amyl nitrite, which is often given while the intravenous access is established. The administration of sodium thiosulfate follows the administration of the nitrites: 12.5 g intravenously over 10 minutes. The nitrites create a methemoglobin within the blood that, when coupled with carbon monoxide poisoning, makes use of these kits potentially lethal.

The newest treatment is the use of hydroxocobalamin. Hydroxocobalamin is the chemical precursor to vitamin B12 and contains cobalt. Cyanide is attracted to metals, such as ferric ion found in hemoglobin and cobalt found in hydroxocobalamin. Therefore, the hydroxocobalamin works competitively with the hemoglobin for the cyanide. The typical dose is 50 mg/kg administered intravenously over 30 minutes, and administered more rapidly in cardiac arrest. Once the cyanide attaches to the hydroxocobalamin, it is harmlessly excreted in the urine. The only major side effects appear to be red urine (chromaturia) and reddened skin.[14,15] Many laboratory values are altered for up to 48 hours after administration, therefore the Paramedic should attempt to obtain blood tubes for the hospital.

Burns and Hypoperfusion

Burns release inflammatory chemical mediators, such as prostaglandins, kinins, histamines, and cytokines, that create edema. This burn edema may take as long as 8 to 12 hours, and sometimes 48 hours, to fully manifest and create the hypotension associated with hospital burn care (i.e., burn shock).

In the prehospital setting, signs of hypoperfusion, including tachycardia and hypotension, must be attributed to other potentially more life-threatening traumatic injuries. The Paramedic must be diligent in identifying and treating those traumatic injuries, such as by staunching the loss of blood with direct pressure. Barring identification of a visible source of the shock, the patient must be expeditiously transported to a trauma center for more thorough and invasive examination.

Although unstable patients need immediate transportation to definitive care, many burn patients are relatively stable, physiologically speaking. These patients may benefit from considered care: venous access, analgesia, and protective dressings.

Fluid Resuscitation

Dr. Frank Underhill, based on his understanding of the relationship of increasing hematocrit to fluid loss (plasma volume deficit), advocated the aggressive use of intravenous solutions during burn resuscitation back in 1897. Despite this understanding, hypovolemia remained a leading cause of burn death as late as the 1940s up until the advent of modern intravenous techniques.

Burn shock, secondary to burn edema, typically occurs in deep burns that involve one-third or more of the total body surface area. Fluid resuscitation initiated after the formation of burn edema can be ineffective in preventing or reversing burn shock. Despite advances in intravenous therapy, inadequate fluid resuscitation remains a source of mortality for burn patients.

In contrast, overly aggressive fluid administration (over-resuscitation) can lead to increased burn edema formation, abdominal compartment syndrome, and acute respiratory distress syndrome as a result of a phenomenon called **fluid creep**.[16] What is needed is a balanced approach to fluid resuscitation that takes into account the TBSA of the burn and also maintains perfusion to the patient's vital organs: the heart, lungs, and brain.

The leading measure of sufficient fluid administration in the hospital setting is urine output. However, this measure has limited usefulness in the prehospital setting. Without this measure, some burn experts question the utility of aggressive prehospital fluid resuscitation, particularly if the patient's transportation to a burn center is less than 60 minutes.

Other burn experts suggest that prehospital resuscitation helps to generate a more positive fluid balance for the patient and that this may improve the patient's long-term survival. The initial fluid of choice is debatable, with some leaning toward normal saline, whereas others prefer lactated Ringer's, and still others tend toward compound sodium lactate solution (Hartmann's solution). Yet most agree that dextrose-containing solutions should be avoided at the outset or at least until the patient's energy demands can be calculated.

A similar argument involves the dispute about the volume needed for resuscitation. Some EMS systems maintain that in the prehospital setting 1 liter per hour for adults, 500 mL per hour for adolescents (ages 10 to 15), and 250 mL for children (> 5 years of age) is adequate, whereas others depend on the Parkland formula.

The Parkland formula (Table 9-3), developed in the burn center at Parkland Hospital, Dallas, Texas, was intended as a guideline for the first 24 hours of fluid resuscitation. Adult patients with serious deep burns receive the first half of this calculated fluid volume over the first eight hours following the burn trauma and the remainder over the next 16 hours.

The goal of EMS fluid resuscitation is to help support the patient during the first 24 hours. During this period of time, burn edema forms and the burn declares itself.

Pain Management

For many people, the thought of a burn immediately conjures ideas of excruciating pain. The source of that burn pain is stimulation of exposed skin nociceptors (the pain-sensing nerve endings within the skin), which occurs primarily in partial thickness burns. Full thickness burns are insensate, secondary to physical destruction of the nociceptors.

Inflammatory chemical mediators, released by the body during the burn trauma, further sensitize nociceptors, making the burn hypersensitive to any mechanical force, such as rubbing or contact.

Therefore, the first—and often most effective—treatment of burn pain is to encase the burn with impervious dressing that, in essence, acts as a temporary skin covering. This prevents contact with the burn until a more lasting covering, such as skin grafts, can replace the dressing.

Even with adequate burn dressings in place, the patient will still experience pain from the burn. Burn pain that occurs while at rest, called **background pain**, is a constant in the

patient's experience and will remain until the inflammatory response subsides. Pain occurring while procedures are being performed (**procedural pain**) is the result of mechanical manipulation and pressure, such as occurs during the application or reinforcement of dressings.

The goal of prehospital pain management, or **analgesia**, should be zero background pain and tolerable procedural pain. The importance of adequate pain management cannot be overemphasized. The patient's first experience with analgesia will be during the first dressing. Appropriate analgesia establishes patient confidence in the healthcare team and, perhaps more importantly, begins to have a positive impact on the psychological trauma that accompanies burn trauma.

In the prehospital setting, the drug of choice for analgesia at this time remains morphine sulfate. Before proceeding with analgesia, and before applying the burn dressing, the Paramedic must make an assessment of the patient's pain. Traditional models for assessment of pain intensity, such as the verbal numeric pain scale, are satisfactory for the task at hand, establishing a baseline of the background pain.

The Paramedic should then administer pharmacological analgesia, typically in a dose of 0.01 mg/kg of morphine sulfate. Morphine is an excellent analgesic because it can be administered in small incremental doses until comfort is reached. Unfortunately, the onset of action of intravenous morphine can take as long as 10 minutes. Morphine should not be given intramuscularly or subcutaneously in burn patients because of shifting fluids and erratic uptake.

For this reason, some EMS systems prefer the shorter-acting opioid fentanyl. Intravenously, fentanyl is rapid acting with a typical onset of action within one minute. It also has a short duration of action (i.e., a mean half-life of 90 minutes). This combination of characteristics makes fentanyl ideal for the prehospital setting. The typical starting dose is usually about 1 mcg per kg, which can be repeated until analgesia is achieved.

Some Paramedics complement opioid analgesics with sedatives such as diazepam or midazolam. Supplementation with these anxiolytics helps to decrease the patient's anticipation of pain. However, the power of verbal analgesia should not be underestimated. Words of reassurance comfort the patient, lessen anxiety, and improve analgesic effectiveness.

If the opioid analgesic is supplemented with an anxiolytic, such as diazepam, many Paramedics decrease the opioid dose by approximately 25% in an attempt to eliminate the risk of respiratory depression and/or apnea.

It should be noted that some EMS systems use inhaled nitrous oxide (N_2O) for analgesia. Nitrous oxide has been used successfully for analgesia since its first use by Humphrey Davy in 1799 for a toothache.

The administration of nitrous oxide, with oxygen, via a face mask or oxygen-powered ventilation device and its short duration of action makes nitrous oxide ideal for prehospital use. Rapidly absorbed via the lungs, it provides satisfactory, patient-controlled analgesia within minutes, with little or no risk of overdose. Because nitrous oxide is a gas, it expands

Table 9-3 Parkland Formula

Total volume infused in first 24 hours = 4 mL/kg × %TBSA (partial & full thickness) burns.
Infuse the first half in the first 8 hours, then the second half over the next 16 hours.

in the body; therefore, it should not be used if there is a suspicion that an air-filled organ may rupture, as might occur during an explosion.

Field Dressings

With adequate analgesia administered, the Paramedic applies the field dressing. Burn dressings are grossly categorized as either interactive or noninteractive.

Interactive dressings include those dressings that work directly with the body to heal the skin. These interactive dressings include clotting factors, collagen fiber mesh, and/or a synthetic epidermal layer that replaces the patient's skin until either new skin develops or the patient receives an autograft or cultured skin. At present, these interactive dressings are not available in the out-of-hospital environment.

Noninteractive dressings are temporary dressings that must be changed. They include low adherence dressings such as roller gauze dressings and transparent semipermeable membrane dressings.

For centuries, well-intentioned people have applied wet dressings to burns, hoping to stop the burning and pain associated with a burn. Recently, iatrogenic problems of hypothermia (hypothermia caused by the treatment) and wound contamination have caused some Paramedics to question the utility of wet dressings. For this reason, some Paramedics restrict the use of wet dressings on burns that are reddened, blanch under pressure, and are sensate (i.e., partial thickness burns). Conversely, all blackened and painless burns (full thickness burns) are dressed with dry sterile dressings.

Regrettably, most deep burns are a combination of both partial and full thickness burns and the size of the wound varies. Thus, another approach is necessary. Based upon the TBSA affected, some Paramedics dress burns that are less than 10% with a wet dressing, whereas burns greater than 10% are covered by dry sterile dressing.

Although referred to as a wet dressing, the dressing is actually damp; that is, no moisture can be squeezed out of the dressing. One method of obtaining a moist, but not wet, dressing is to pour water into the packaging, which is generally impervious, and then squeeze the gauze dressing inside the package until no water drips out.

In the past, lay rescuers have applied a variety of creams and salves, including butter and grease. Many of these "home remedies" are of dubious benefit, and some are definitely harmful. Barring any medical advances, Paramedics do not apply ointments to burns in the field.[17]

Decontamination of Chemical Burns

Treatment begins with the universal algorithm for all burns: remove the patient from the source of the burn, then remove the source of the burn from the patient. The first leg of the algorithm involves patient rescue, the disentanglement and extrication of the patient from the mechanism of injury while being ever mindful of personal safety.

With the patient in a safe place, the Paramedic removes the source of the burn from the patient. When the source of the burn is a chemical, this process is called decontamination.

Decontamination begins by removing all of the patient's clothing. Clothing can be permeated with chemicals, allowing the burning process to continue. Furthermore, certain chemicals are volatile and may "off-gas" (produce a dangerous vapor).

The patient's jewelry also should be removed. Chemicals trapped under or around rings, watches, and so on, may not only continue to cause burns from the continuous contact, but the metals in the jewelry may interact with the chemicals to produce new and possibly more toxic chemical compounds.

Water is the universal solvent and effectively neutralizes a large number of chemicals. Therefore, copious amounts of water are generally used to decontaminate most chemical exposures. Because large volumes of water are needed to properly decontaminate the patient, the use of tap water is acceptable in most cases. The use of simple litmus paper can help the Paramedic qualitatively measure the decontamination's progress.

The importance of irrigation of chemical burns with copious amounts of water cannot be understated. Patients who receive irrigation within 10 minutes of the chemical exposure have a fivefold decrease in full thickness injury and a twofold decrease in their hospital stay.[18] However, care should be taken to try to avoid contaminating noncontaminated skin with contaminated water from the irrigation flush.

However, not all burn wounds should be irrigated. Water applied to elemental metals—sodium, potassium, lithium, and magnesium—can cause an exothermic reaction that worsens the burn. Those burns should be covered with mineral oil and visible fragments manually removed with tweezers or forceps. The Paramedic should then place a mineral oil-soaked gauze dressing over the wound.

Anhydrous Ammonia

Anhydrous ammonia requires water immediately, within seconds of exposure. Immediate decontamination is so important that farmers, frequent users of anhydrous ammonia, are encouraged to carry water bottles on their person just in case of accidental exposure. It is noteworthy that anhydrous ammonia can also be used to make the illicit drug methamphetamine and may be found on-site at a "meth" lab.

Hydroflouric Acid

Immediate prehospital treatment of hydrofluoric acid is potentially life-saving. It is also relevant to the patient's long-term disability. Exposures to hydrofluoric acid can be problematic. Even when the exposed area has been thoroughly rinsed and the patient's pain has stopped, internal damage can continue. The key to proper management of the hydrofluoric acid exposure is to prevent the hydrofluoric acid from binding with calcium in the body, thereby causing hypocalcemia.

Minimally, proper decontamination for hydrofluoric acid includes flushing the affected skin. Flushing should begin even before all the patient's clothing is removed, and should continue for about five minutes. However, flushing for greater than five minutes will delay treatment with the proper antidote as well as potentially complicate patient care by inducing hypothermia in the patient.

Flushing should be followed by application of calcium gluconate gel (2.5%) onto the wound. The Paramedic should wear gloves while applying calcium gluconate and massage it into the wound until the pain stops and/or the redness disappears. By wearing gloves, the Paramedic prevents secondary exposures. The calcium gluconate bonds with the fluoride in the hydrofluoric acid to form the insoluble chemical calcium fluoride.

In some EMS systems, the application of 0.13% benzalkonium chloride (Zephrian®) solution-soaked compresses is advocated instead of 2.5% calcium gluconate gel. The Paramedic should replace the compresses every two to four minutes. It should be noted that it is not acceptable to use benzalkonium chloride for burns to the eyes as it is an eye irritant.

At concentrations of less than 50%, hydrofluoric acid may not immediately cause burns. Nevertheless, absorption of the chemical into the body may cause considerable internal injury, including destruction of bone. Therefore, the decision to apply the antidote gel calcium gluconate should be based on exposure, not on evidence of burn trauma.

Special care should be applied to patients with chemical exposure under the fingernails and to the hands. The Paramedic can place calcium gluconate gel inside a nonlatex examination glove to ensure continuous moist contact with the calcium gluconate on the affected area.

If the pain becomes unbearable, it is possible to inject calcium gluconate 5% solution into the periphery using a 27-gauge or smaller needle and subcutaneously injecting approximately 0.5 mL per square centimeter. Calcium gluconate comes in standard 10% solutions as a prefilled syringe and therefore must be diluted in equal parts or 50/50. A word of caution: Calcium gluconate is not the same as calcium chloride for injection. Calcium chloride for injection can be corrosive and create further injury.

A new antidote, hexafluorine, has been tested experimentally for decontamination of hydrofluoric acid splashes. It has shown some success and may come into routine EMS use in the future.

The use of local anesthetics should be avoided. Pain is an important clinical indicator of the treatment's effectiveness, and any efforts to mask the pain will diminish the treatment's effectiveness.

If the patient inadvertently inhaled hydrofluoric acid, it creates a pungent smell. The Paramedic must then be concerned about the risks of airway swelling and obstruction. To help prevent this potentially fatal outcome (hydrofluoric acid can be lethal with as little as a 50 ppm concentration), 3 mL of 2.5% calcium gluconate may also be nebulized.

If the patient ingested the hydrofluoric acid, then any calcium-containing antacid, such as Mylanta®, Maalox®, Tums™, and so on, may be an effective antidote. Patients who have ingested hydrofluoric acid are likely to have systemic manifestations of poisoning yet may be unaware of their exposure secondary to the pain of burns (distracting injuries). Therefore, the Paramedic must maintain a high index of suspicion for ingestion whenever burns to the face have occurred.

Phenol

Patients who are contaminated with phenol put Paramedics at risk for secondary contamination via either direct contact or through vapors that off-gas from heavily contaminated clothing. Paramedics should wear butyl rubber gloves and aprons to protect against accidental secondary exposure.

Like hydrofluoric acid, the systemic effects of phenol exposure can be more problematic than the actual burn. Immediate decontamination can greatly improve the odds of patient survival and decrease morbidity, for there is no known antidote for phenol poisoning.

Phenol is poorly soluble in water and is therefore resistant to irrigation during decontamination. Although irrigation with water is the first-line treatment, it is important to only irrigate when large quantities of water are available. Irrigation with small quantities of water may serve to only expand the area of exposure and hasten absorption. Irrigation should continue until there is no detectable odor of phenol present.

Some EMS systems use a topical application of 50% polyethylene glycol (PEG) diluted 50/50 for easier application. If PEG is not available, then glycerin solutions or even vegetable oil can be used to dissolve the phenol. For small exposures, isopropyl alcohol can be used to dissolve the phenol. However, the Paramedic must use caution to avoid letting the mucous membranes absorb the isopropyl alcohol, leading to isopropyl alcohol toxicity.

Calcium Oxide

Calcium oxide, common lime found in cement, can cause serious burns. Because of this, the patient's first instinct may be to wash it off. However, the most effective first aid is to brush away the calcium oxide, taking precautions to prevent the powder from spreading. After removing all contaminated clothing (especially boots where the dust tends to collect, leaving a cuff burn), gross contamination should be brushed off, then the remainder gently blotted.

Following gross decontamination, the Paramedic should irrigate the affected area with large quantities of water, while on-scene and prior to transportation, until the chemical is removed.

Ocular Burns

Chemical exposure, such as industrial strength ammonia cleaners, on the eyes can lead to permanent blindness. What is more problematic is that the effects of such an exposure may be mild, or even subclinical, initially and may not fully manifest for several weeks.

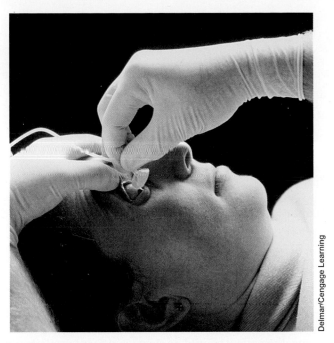

Figure 9-5 Application of the Morgan lens provides a mechanism for controlled irrigation of the eye.

All cases of chemical exposure to the eyes should be treated as a chemical burn. A chemical burn to the eyes mandates immediate irrigation with copious amounts of water in an effort to neutralize and/or dilute the chemicals' contact with the eye's surface.

A frequently used device for eye irrigation is the Morgan lens®. The Morgan lens provides a mechanism for controlled irrigation of the eye, called lavage, until better conditions than irrigation by hand are available.

The process of using a Morgan lens begins by applying a topical ocular anesthetic, such as lidocaine. However, a topical anesthetic is not always necessary. The relief obtained from the ocular lavage is typically sufficient to gain patient cooperation.

With the Morgan lens properly attached to an intravenous solution of lactated Ringer's, as per manufacturer's recommendations, the Paramedic initiates a flow of irrigating solution. With fluids flowing, the Morgan lens is gently placed under the upper lid and then the lower lid, while the Morgan lens floats above the eye's surface on a cushion of solution (Figure 9-5).

With the lens in place, the Paramedic should use a free flow of approximately 2,000 mL initially, followed by a continuous irrigation at approximately 50 to 60 mL an hour or until arrival at definitive care. Once the irrigation is initiated, it is important that the irrigation is continuously maintained and the lens is not allowed to run dry.

Treatment of Electrical Burns

The most pressing complication of electrical shock may be cardiac dysrhythmia. Ventricular fibrillation, a common sequela, is potentially lethal, and three times more likely to be lethal if the current passes from arm to arm. Artificial ventilations, external cardiac compressions, and direct current countershock (defibrillation) are critical life-saving procedures. Premature ventricular contractions, premature atrial contractions, and tachycardia are generally benign and self-resolving.

Barring cardiac arrest, the Paramedic should focus on the initial assessment and attend to immediate life threats. If the electric shock was with low voltage, such as household current, and the patient has no obvious residual effects, the value of intravenous access is questionable. However, if the patient came in contact with a high tension line, the risk of internal injury is greater.

Like in a thermal burn, the Parkland formula is useful for estimating initial fluid resuscitation volumes for a patient who has come in contact with a high tension line. Alternatively, some EMS medical directors advocate an initial 20 cc/kg bolus until further medical evaluation can help to more accurately estimate the internal burn injury. Some EMS systems use lactated Ringer's instead of normal saline solution (NSS), 0.9% sodium chloride in sterile water, fearing that large volumes of NSS can induce hyperchloremia.

If the Paramedic establishes intravenous access, she should draw routine laboratory bloods. Creatine kinase (CK) levels, obtained from blood samples, can be helpful in determining the extent of the patient's injury. For example, it can assist in determining the damage to muscle.

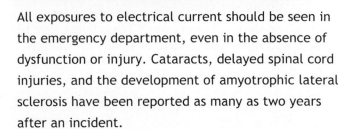

STREET SMART

Toddlers often explore their world with their mouth. This includes sucking on extension cord sockets and biting electrical wires. The resulting low-voltage electric burn of the lips and mouth leaves a grayish white area that is depressed, whereas the surrounding area becomes raised, due to swelling.

STREET SMART

All exposures to electrical current should be seen in the emergency department, even in the absence of dysfunction or injury. Cataracts, delayed spinal cord injuries, and the development of amyotrophic lateral sclerosis have been reported as many as two years after an incident.

CASE STUDY (CONTINUED)

The flight crew is interested in the volume of fluids that were administered and are relieved to hear that the Paramedic elected to limit the infusion to a maintenance drip. With the patient packaged, airway controlled, respiratory monitoring indicating that the patient's respiratory gasses were within normal perimeters, intravenous access secured, plenty of opiates on-board, and vital signs stable, the Paramedic turns the patient over to the flight crew, confident that everything that can be done has been done.

CRITICAL THINKING QUESTIONS

1. What is the implication of hypotension in a burn trauma patient in the field?
2. What is the typical fluid resuscitation for a burn patient?

Evaluation

Although the guidelines for burn resuscitation, such as the Parkland formula, are based on a 24-hour time period, the associated third spacing of fluids does not take place in the first few hours immediately following a burn. If hypotension occurs during the first few hours following the burn trauma, the patient should be suspected of internal bleeding.

CASE STUDY CONCLUSION

The Paramedics watch as the "chopper" lifts off and makes its slow turn south. They know that the patient will be in the burn unit within the hour, and receiving the best care possible. However, the day is far from over. The radio squawks, directing them to report to "rehab" immediately.

CRITICAL THINKING QUESTIONS

1. What is the preferred destination for the patient with burn trauma?
2. What are the exceptions in those cases?

Disposition

The first few hours of care are critical for the burn patient whether the burns are chemical, electrical, or thermal.

There are approximately 125 specialized "burn centers" in the United States. However, the majority of burns are managed in trauma centers or local hospitals. If needed, patients are transferred to a burn center at a later time.

If the patient has concurrent trauma along with the burns, the patient should be transported to a trauma center for initial stabilization before transfer to the burn center.

Certain burns are considered high-risk burns (Table 9-4). In these cases, the Paramedic should consider transportation, by ground or air, to a burn center.[19] These burns have been shown to be a significant cause of morbidity or mortality.

Table 9-4 American Burn Association Criteria for Burn Center Admission

- Full thickness (third degree) burns over 5% TBSA
- Partial thickness (second degree) burns over 10% TBSA
- Any full thickness or partial thickness burn involving critical areas (e.g., face, hands, feet, genitals, perineum, skin over any major joint), as these have significant risk for functional and cosmetic problems
- Circumferential burns of the thorax or extremities
- Significant chemical injury, electrical burns, lightning injury, coexisting major trauma, or presence of significant preexisting medical conditions
- Presence of inhalation injury
- Greater than 15% TBSA in adults
- Greater than 10% TBSA in children
- Hand and foot burns that can lead to significant morbidity if not treated properly; therefore, most are treated with aggressive therapy. However, if there is careful follow-up, the patient may be monitored on an outpatient basis.

CONCLUSION

As burns are one of the leading causes of death in adults and children, it is important that the Paramedic know how to assess and treat all burns regardless of their etiology. However, there is one constant in all types of burns, whether thermal, electrical, or chemical: pain. The burn's outward appearance, whether minor or severe, can distract the Paramedic from the burn's deeper and potentially more lethal complications.

▶ KEY POINTS:

- Death from burns does not occur as often as death from carbon monoxide, cyanide, and asphyxiation.

- Chemical mediators—histamine, serotonin, and bradykinins—lead to increased capillary permeability and third spacing hours and days after the burn.

- Chemical burns from alkalis (i.e., caustic burns) lead to saponification and dessication and culminate in liquefaction necrosis.

- Chemical burns from acids (i.e., corrosive burns) lead to protein denaturing, coagulation, and hydrolysis, and culminate in coagulation necrosis that forms an eschar.

- Common chemical exposures are phenols, hydrofluoric acid, anhydrous ammonia, and calcium oxide (i.e., lime).

- Units of electrical measurement include voltage (strength) and amperage (volume) to determine current.

- Current is a function of voltage over resistance (ohms).

- Materials are either conductors or resistors.

- Key to the history of a chemical burn is identification of the offending agent and determination of the volume and duration of exposure.

- Key to the history of an electrical burn is identification of the current pathway, identification of the type of electricity (AC/DC), and the determination of the volume and duration of contact.

- Examination of the thermal burn patient focuses on airway compromise, inhalation of toxic gasses, and other traumatic injury.

- Examination of the chemical burn patient focuses on decontamination and symptomatic relief.

- Examination of the electrical burn patient focuses on rendering the patient safe and providing routine trauma care.

- Burns have been reclassified according to the depth of skin involvement: superficial, partial thickness, and full thickness.

- Burns have zones of injury according to Jackson's thermal burn theory: hyperemia, stasis, and coagulation.

- Three methods are used to determine the extent of burns: Wallace's rule of nines, the Lund-Browder chart, and the palmar method.

- The first priority in all chemical, electrical, and thermal burns is Paramedic safety.

- Priorities of patient care are airway control and ventilation.

- Smoke inhalation is a major cause of morbidity and mortality secondary to carbon monoxide and cyanide poisoning.

- Carbon monoxide causes anaerobic respiration, acidosis, shock, and death.

- Cyanide poisoning has the same pathway as carbon monoxide.

- The therapeutic goal of analgesia for burn patients is zero pain; however, tolerable pain is often all that can be accomplished due to the complexities of burn care.

- Although controversy exists over burn dressings, it is still the standard of care to use wet dressings for burns that cover less than 10% of TBSA.

- Decontamination of anhydrous ammonia requires copious amounts of water.

- Decontamination of hydrofluoric acid involves a flush as well as application of calcium gluconate.

- If phenols off-gas, the risk of accidental secondary exposure is high. The Paramedic should wear respiratory protection as well as butyl rubber gloves and an apron.

- Decontamination of phenol includes irrigation with copious amounts of water as well as 50% polyethylene glycol (PEG), vegetable oil, or isopropyl alcohol.

- Decontamination of calcium oxide starts with brushing off dry chemicals, taking respiratory precautions, and then irrigating with copious amounts of water.

- Ocular burns are treated with a Morgan lens.

- Fluid resuscitation in the field should be conservative, 1 L/hr for adults, 500 mL/hr for adolescents, and 250 mL/hr for children, to avoid "fluid creep."

- Hypotension in the field is due to trauma, not burns.

- The saying goes, "trauma trumps burns." Burn patients with major trauma, as defined by the federal triage guidelines, should go to a trauma center.

- Although burn care provided in a burn center is optimal, many burns are treated at a trauma center or even a local hospital.

REVIEW QUESTIONS:

1. How do chemical burns from acids differ from chemical burns from alkali?
2. Why are AC electricity-induced burns more dangerous than DC electricity-induced burns?
3. What is Jackson's thermal burn theory?
4. The clinical pathways for carbon monoxide and cyanide are similar. How can they be differentiated?
5. Besides water, what else is used to decontaminate a chemical burn?

CASE STUDY QUESTIONS:

Please refer to the Case Study in this chapter, and answer the questions below:

1. What is potentially the most life-threatening injury on-scene?
2. What is the theory behind conservative fluid resuscitation in the field for burn patients?
3. If in this case the patient had a "significant" chemical injury, but was also suffering from hypotension and a secondary hemorrhage from an unknown etiology, what would be the appropriate transportation decision? Remember, the helicopter is on the ground and time is not an issue.

REFERENCES:

1. Centers for Disease Control and Prevention. Available at: **http://www.cdc.gov/homeandrecreationalsafety/fire-prevention/fires-factsheet.html.** Accessed February 2005.

2. American Burn Association. *Advanced Burn Life Support Provider Manual.* Chicago, IL: American Burn Association; 2005.

3. Williams J, et al. Carbon monoxide poisoning and myocardial ischemia in patients with burns. *J Burn Care Rehabil.* 1992;13:210–213.

4. Lai MW, Klein-Schwartz W, Rodgers GC, Abrams JY, Haber DA, Bronstein AC. 2005 Annual Report of the American Association of Poison Control Centers' national poisoning and exposure database. *Clin Toxicol (Phila).* 2006;44(6-7):803–932.

5. Lin TM, Lee SS, Lai CS, Lin SD. Phenol burn. *Burns.* Jun 2006;32(4):517–521.

6. Salzman M, O'Malley RN. Updates on the evaluation and management of caustic exposures. *Emerg Med Clin North Am.* May 2007;25(2):459–476.

7. Hettiaratchy S, Dziewulski P. ABC of burns: pathophysiology and types of burns. *BMJ.* Jun 2004;328:1427–1429.

8. DeSanti L. Pathophysiology and current management of burns. *Adv Wound Care.* July-August 2005;18:323–332.

9. Wright HR, Drake DB, Gear AJL, Wheeler JC, Edlich RF. Industrial high-voltage electrical burn of the skull, a preventable injury. *J Emerg Med.* 1997;15(3):345–349.

10. Herndon D. Total burn care. *Elsevierl.* 2007:265–270.

11. Serinken M, et al. Bilateral pneumothorax following acute inhalation injury. *Clin Tox.* 2009;47(6):595–597.

12. Weaver LK, et al. Carboxyhemoglobin half life in carbon monoxide poisoned patients treated with 100% oxygen at atmospheric pressure. *Chest.* 2000;117:801–808.

13. Juurlink DN, et al. Hyperbaric oxygen for carbon monoxide poisoning (review). *The Cochrane Database of Systemic Reviews.* 2005;1.

14. Borron SW, Baud FJ, Megarbane B, et al. Hydroxocobalamin for severe acute cyanide poisoning by ingestion or inhalation. *Am J Emerg Med.* Jun 2007;25(5):551–558.

15. Erdman AR. Is hydroxocobalamin safe and effective for smoke inhalation? Searching for guidance in the haze. *Ann Emerg Med.* Jun 2007;49(6):814–816.

16. Saffle JI. The phenomenon of fluid creep in acute burn resuscitation. *J Burn Care Res.* 2007;28(5):770–772.

17. 12th Annual San Antonio Trauma Symposium, September 19-21, 2006, Henry B. Gonzalez Convention Center San Antonio, Texas. Emerging advances in burn resuscitation. *Journal of Trauma-Injury Infection & Critical Care.* June 2007;62(6)Supplement:S71–S72.

18. Leonard LG, Scheulen JJ, Munster AM. Chemical burns: effect of prompt first aid. *J Trauma.* May 1982;22(5):420–423.

19. American College of Surgeons Committee on Trauma. *Burns in Advanced Trauma Life Support.* Chicago, IL: American College of Surgeons; 2002:155.

CHAPTER 10

PEDIATRIC TRAUMA CONSIDERATIONS

KEY CONCEPTS:

Upon completion of this chapter, it is expected that the reader will understand these following concepts:

- Suspected injury patterns based on mechanism of injury and kinematics
- Pediatric head injury
- Unique pediatric spinal cord injury
- Unique pediatric thoracic injury

ANATOMY CONCEPTS:

Prior to reading this chapter the Paramedic student should be familiar with the following anatomy and physiology concepts:

- Differences in adult and pediatric anatomy
- Lifespan development

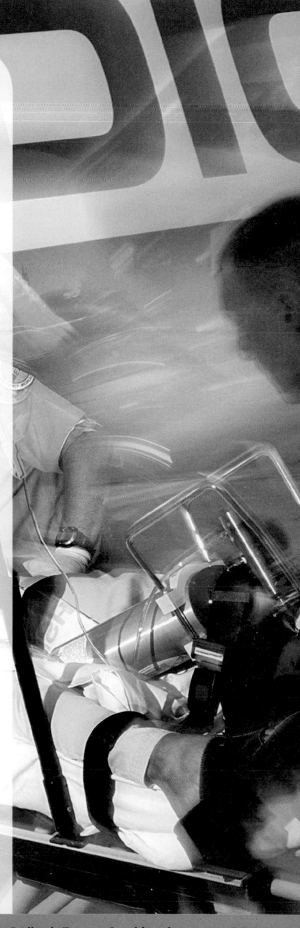

CASE STUDY:

With siren screaming and lights flashing, the ambulance pulls out of the bay on a car versus pedestrian call. The report from police on-scene is that a child crossed the road in front of a stopped school bus only to be hit by a motor vehicle coming from the opposite direction.

By the time the ambulance pulls onto the scene it is dusk. All the crew can see is a crumpled body on the ground that appears to be a school-aged child and several adults standing around. One of the adults appears to be kneeling next to the child, holding head stabilization. Standing next to the four-door sedan is a middle-aged woman and a police officer. She is visibly distraught. The Paramedic turns his attention to the child on the ground.

CRITICAL THINKING QUESTIONS

1. What is the predictable injury pattern that would be suspected based on the mechanism of injury?
2. Are any of these injuries potentially life-threatening conditions?

OVERVIEW

Unintentional injury is the leading cause of death for people ages 1 through 44.[1] Among the 15- to 24-year-old age group, homicide is the second leading cause of death. For the pediatric age groups, injury is likely the most common reason for accessing EMS. Injury in the pediatric population is responsible for over six million visits to the emergency department per year.

Although there are similarities in the pathophysiology of injury between adults and children, there are also many differences in the types of injuries sustained by children as compared with adults. Additionally, the types of injuries may vary based on the child's age as a result of normal growth and development. This chapter will explore the pathophysiology and treatment of traumatic injury in pediatric patients.

Chief Concern

Just as adults may sustain multiple trauma, children may be part of one as well. Using the information presented in the preceding chapters and reviewing the many different types of injuries present by body system, this section will highlight the differences based on the pathophysiology of children.

Injury Patterns

The source of trauma varies by age group, with certain mechanisms more prevalent in certain age groups than in others (Table 10-1). In the non-ambulatory age group, many injuries are due to non-accidental trauma or falls, whereas in the older age group, homicide and suicide become more prevalent.

Similar mechanisms of injury will also cause different injury patterns based upon the child's age (Table 10-2). For example, although the intent of restraint systems in motor vehicles is to be protective, a young child who is not restrained—or improperly restrained—in a car seat may develop significant neck, intra-abdominal, or spinal injuries from seat belts, whereas a teenager will tend to develop injuries in a pattern similar to adults.

Waddell's triad is a set of three injuries that occur as a combination when the pediatric patient is struck by a vehicle. However, the validity of Waddell's triad has been called into question in recent studies.[2] Toddlers who are struck by an automobile also may have significant crush injuries to the extremities, torso, and head as a result after becoming pinned underneath an automobile tire. A younger child struck by an automobile is more apt to sustain head, cervical spine, or chest injuries from direct impact with the bumper, whereas an older child will more often suffer lower extremity, abdominal, or pelvic injuries from impact with the bumper.

One major difference between children and adults is the way children respond to severe injury. Provided the child remains well oxygenated, children possess an excellent physiologic reserve and can maintain a reasonable blood pressure even after a significant blood loss. This is partly due to the responsiveness of the child's sympathetic nervous system to

Table 10-1 Common Sources of Pediatric Trauma by Age Group

Age	Sources of Injury
0–1	• Child abuse
	• Burns
	• Falls
	• Drowning
1–4	• Motor vehicle crashes
	• Drowning
	• Falls
	• Pedestrian events
5–9	• Motor vehicle crashes
	• Pedestrian crashes
	• Bicycle injuries
	• Drowning
	• Burns
	• Falls
	• Sports and recreational injuries
10–14	• Motor vehicle crashes
	• Bicycle crashes
	• Drowning
	• Sports and recreational injuries
	• Gunshot wounds
	• Suicide
	• Burns
15–19	• Motor vehicle crashes
	• Pedestrian injuries
	• Drowning
	• Gunshot wounds
	• Homicide
	• Suicide
	• Sports and recreational injuries

Table 10-2 Common Injuries by Mechanism

Mechanism	Injuries
Motor vehicle crashes	• Blunt thoracoabdominal trauma • Head injury
Pedestrian trauma	• Head injury • Chest injury • Femur fractures • Tibia/fibula fractures
Near drowning	• Hypoxia • Coma • Brain damage
Falls	• Head injury • Spinal & extremity fractures • Internal chest & abdominal injuries
Bicycle-motor vehicle collision or falling forward over the handlebars	• Head and neck trauma • Extremity fractures • Abrasions • Lacerations
Poisoning	• Coma • Kidney failure • Hepatic failure
Gunshot wounds & stabbings	• Injury to organs and tissues in the direct path of the sharp object or projectile • Pneumothorax • Hemothorax • Tension pneumothorax • Cardiac tamponade

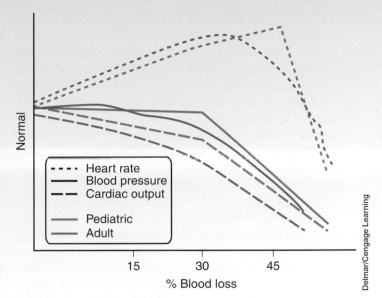

Figure 10-1 Pediatric vital sign response to blood loss is partly due to the responsiveness of the child's sympathetic nervous system.

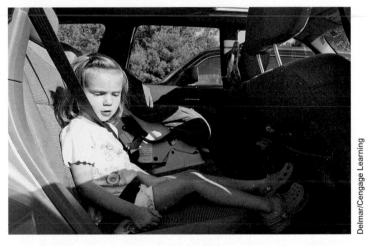

Figure 10-2 Cervical spine and neck soft-tissue injuries can result when younger children are improperly restrained.

clamp down the vasculature and stimulate the heart rate and force of contraction to maintain an adequate blood pressure. Although these features help maintain the child's blood pressure significantly longer than an adult with a similar proportional blood loss, when the child decompensates, she does so rapidly (Figure 10-1).

As the child becomes a young adult, the reserve is still present although it is not as robust as in the younger age group. In contrast, adults tend to require proportionally less blood loss in order to cause vital sign alterations. Children also often appear less sick than adults given similar injuries. This can lure the Paramedic into a false sense of assurance that the child is well.

In motor vehicle crashes, properly restrained children rarely sustain injury when vehicle speeds are under 15 miles per hour. In addition, properly restrained infants have survived unscathed in crashes with greater speeds because of the protection of the car seat. Unrestrained children are at risk for head and high cervical spine injuries due to their relatively immature spinal joints and heavier head. If the child is improperly restrained (Figure 10-2), such as not using a booster seat, the lower cervical spine, neck vessels, and airway can be injured due to the deceleration force applied on the neck where the seat belt crosses the lower neck.

Some children may find the shoulder harness portion of the seat belt uncomfortable because they are not sized properly for the restraint. Deceleration injuries to the hollow viscus, abdominal aorta, inferior vena cava, and lumbar spine may occur as the unrestrained upper body folds over the seat belt, focusing all of the deceleration forces to the narrow area of the abdomen under the strap. This also occurs, as in adults, when the lap portion of the belt is worn above the iliac crests.

As with adults, height is a major factor in the injury patterns that occur with falls. Generally, a fall from three times the child's height or greater is considered a significant fall and the child is thus at risk for severe injury. Due to their proportionately larger and heavier head, younger children tend to fall head first, thus injuring their brain and upper cervical spine. The surface struck also factors into the severity of the injuries. Softer materials tend to dissipate energy prior to impact, thus lessening the force applied to the internal structures. Deceleration injuries to the blood vessels and solid organs of the torso may also occur upon impact.

Bicycle injuries tend to follow a pattern similar to that of pedestrian–auto collisions, especially for younger children riding smaller bicycles. Injuries to the lower extremities occur more often than those to the upper extremities due to the lower extremity's contact area with the bumper or automobile. Head and neck injuries occur most often from secondary collision with the windshield, hood, roof, or ground, but may also occur from primary collision, especially in younger children. One injury that tends to be specific to bicycles is handlebar injuries. Sudden stops may cause the child to launch over the handlebars. In addition to the expected head, cervical spine, and upper extremity injuries, the child is also susceptible for abdominal solid organ injury or hollow viscus injury if the upper abdomen struck the handlebars during the incident. Lower extremity injury from handlebars is not as common in children as in adults.

Trauma Injuries

Head Injury

Head injuries are the leading cause of traumatic death in children. Serious head injuries are also five times more common than intra-abdominal injuries in the pediatric population. The pediatric brain is more susceptible to secondary injury from hypoxia than the adult brain. This is due to the rapid growth of the brain that occurs in the first several years of life and the markedly increased blood flow required to support that growth. The cerebral blood flow of a child peaks at age 5 at a flow rate twice an adult's cerebral blood flow.

Prior to skull fusion, the fontanels can accommodate some increase in pressure due to the elasticity of the skin and soft tissue. Although this is a benefit in decreasing secondary injury due to increased intracranial pressure, it also means that a small infant may lose almost her entire blood volume into the cranial vault and thus develop severe hemorrhagic shock. The usual signs of a closed head injury develop much later, if at all.

After the first year, the pediatric brain fills the skull much more tightly than the adult brain. With age, brain tissue atrophies, pulling away from the inner table of the skull. This places some tension on the veins that bridge across the dura mater as the brain atrophies. In the adult, due to the increased potential movement of the brain within the skull, subdural hematomas are more likely to develop in blunt head injury mechanisms. In children, because the brain does not

have as much room to move, brain injuries tend to be more diffuse.

Although most injuries are diffuse brain injuries, both subdural hematomas and epidural hematomas do occur in pediatric patients. Epidural hematomas are far less common than subdural hematomas and in general are associated with temporal bone skull fractures and injuries to the middle meningeal artery. Subdural hematomas in 75% of patients are bilateral, exhibiting the classic coup-contrecoup injury pattern. As with adults, subdural hematomas result from tears in the bridging veins across the dura. This more often occurs from deceleration injury rather than direct injury.

Increased intracranial pressure due to cerebral edema develops in the pediatric brain more quickly than in the adult. The signs and symptoms associated with mass effect also occur earlier in children than in adults due to the smaller potential space in the skull. As long as pediatric patients remain well oxygenated, however, they tend to fare much better with less residual deficit from the injury than an adult with a similar injury.

In pediatric patients, skull fractures are often linear and nondisplaced, meaning depression or elevation of a fragment does not occur. These fractures typically heal well without surgery. However, surgical intervention is required for epidural and subdural hematomas and displaced skull fractures.

In adults, decerebrate posturing is a grave sign indicating severe brain injury that involves the brainstem. Significant deficit is usually present in adult survivors. In children, however, decerebrate posturing does not mean the brainstem was involved in the injury. Decerebrate posturing usually occurs secondary to increased intracranial pressure from cerebral edema rather than from herniation as in adults. As with most other injuries, children have a better prognosis than adults with similar injuries.

Altered mental status after a head injury makes the Paramedic suspicious that the patient has either a cerebral hemorrhage or a concussion. One objective measure that can be used to gauge the severity of a child's head injury is the **Modified Glasgow Coma Score for Children** (Table 10-3). As with the Glasgow Coma Score, the individual areas are assessed in an age-appropriate manner and the score totaled. The range is between 3 for a fully comatose child up to 15 for a neurologically intact child.

Seizures may occur after a head injury and are more common in children than in adults. These seizures are called **post-concussive seizures** and generally resolve on their own within a few minutes. Patients with a prior seizure disorder may seize after a head injury depending upon the level of control of the baseline seizure disorder. It is also possible that the patient sustained a head injury because he had a seizure. If the seizure lasts more than five minutes, then it should be treated.

Scalp lacerations can cause significant hemorrhage due to the scalp's vascularity. Since the child's normal blood volume is significantly less than an adult's normal blood volume, vigorous bleeding from a scalp laceration is sufficient

Table 10-3 Modified Glasgow Coma Score for Children

Activity	Score	> 1 Year Age	< 1 Year Age
Eye opening	4	Spontaneously	Spontaneously
	3	To verbal command	To shout
	2	To pain	To pain
	1	No response	No response
Motor response	6	Obeys commands	Spontaneously
	5	Localizes pain	Localizes pain
	4	Withdraws to pain	Withdraws to pain
	3	Abnormal flexion (decorticate)	Abnormal flexion (decorticate)
	2	Abnormal extension (decerebrate)	Abnormal extension (decerebrate)
	1	No response	No response
Verbal response	5	Appropriate words & phrases	Smiles, coos, babbles
	4	Disoriented, inappropriate words	Cries but is consolable
	3	Persistent cries and screams	Persistent cries, screams
	2	Grunts, meaningless sounds	Grunts, agitated, restless
	1	No response	No response
Total 3–15			

to cause significant hemorrhagic shock. Inattention to heavily oozing scalp wounds may cause the Paramedic to miss an easily treatable source of hemorrhage.

Neck and Facial Injury

The mechanisms that cause neck and facial injuries in children were discussed earlier in the chapter. Facial bone fractures are relatively uncommon in pediatric patients and are exceedingly rare in patients under 6 years old.[3] The low frequency of facial bone fractures in younger children is believed to be due to the relative proportions between the cranial vault and the face, with the infant's high cranium-to-face ratio decreasing significantly by age 5 and then dropping down to the usual adult proportion by adolescence. The high cranium-to-facial bone ratio effectively protects the facial bones from injury as the forces are more likely applied to the cranium rather than directly to the facial bones. With the increased flexibility of the pediatric bone structure, the facial bones will bend more than break, which may ultimately cause more functional problems as the face heals.

Neck soft-tissue injuries occur in a fashion similar to adults who sustain soft-tissue injuries. As previously discussed, seat belt injuries are common in the pediatric population due to the sizing and placement of restraints.

Spinal Trauma

In children, the spinal column is still transitioning from softer cartilage to bone during the first several years of life. The flexibility of the spine and supporting ligaments in children makes spinal fracture much less common in children than adults. As a result, serious injury to the cervical spine is rare in children under 15 years old.[4]

The location of cervical spine injury in children will vary by age. In children under 12 years old, the upper cervical spine is injured more often than the lower cervical spine. In these children, cervical spine injuries most commonly occur at the level of the occiput, C1 or C2. This is due to the proportionately larger and heavier head. In children above the age of 12 years old, the body proportion is more similar to that of an adult, and the spinal injury focus shifts toward the lower cervical spine. This, combined with more activities that apply a fulcrum to the lower cervical spine, make this area more likely to be injured.

The type of injury also differs between children and adults. In children, especially the younger children, the cervical musculature is weaker than in the adult. The ligaments that bind together the vertebrae are also more elastic and more easily stretched. The vertebrae themselves are softer and more cartilaginous than those in the adult. These factors all make subluxation (Figure 10-3), or sliding of one vertebrae on another, more common than cervical spine fracture. Subluxation of the cervical vertebrae will more often cause an incomplete spinal cord injury or a nerve root injury. Complete transection of the spinal cord from a subluxation is rare.

Two types of spinal cord injury that are more common in the pediatric patient than the adult patient are spinal cord injury without obvious radiographic abnormality (SCIWORA) and stingers.[4] Both occur more often in pediatric patients due to the flexibility of the cervical spine as just described.

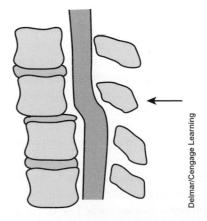

Delmar/Cengage Learning

Figure 10-3 With a subluxation injury, one vertebrae slides in relation to the one below it, compressing and damaging the spinal cord.

In a **spinal cord injury without obvious radiographic abnormality (SCIWORA)**, the patient exhibits signs and symptoms that are typical of a spinal cord injury although X-rays or CT scans performed in the emergency department are normal. However, when an MRI is performed later, it will show damage to the spinal cord. Almost half of the patients who have a neurologic complaint or sign at the time of injury will have a delayed onset of paralysis up to four days after the injury. This may be due to edema surrounding the injury. Fortunately, if the patient is alert and oriented, there were no neurologic complaints (i.e., paralysis, weakness, paresthesia, or anesthesias) at any time, and no abnormalities are noted on physical examination, then it is very unlikely that a patient has a SCIWORA.

A **stinger** results from the stretching of nerves. It is a transient neurologic symptom that has occurred at the time of injury and resolves after a short period of time, often before the patient's arrival at the emergency department. A stinger can be as simple as tingling in a specific dermatome or may involve weakness that resolves. Some stingers are described as a sharp pain followed by a feeling of flowing warmth in the area. Stingers are more common in the adolescent and teen population, especially in those who participate in contact sports. Even if the stinger has resolved prior to the Paramedic's contact with the patient, the patient should be treated as if he is having a potential spinal cord injury.

Chest Trauma

The function of the bony thorax (ribs, sternum, thoracic vertebrae) is to protect the underlying important organs in the chest and upper abdomen. Children have a significant amount of flexibility in the bony thorax, and thus are more prone to internal injury without signs of external injury. Rib fractures are rare due to the flexibility of the bony thorax. Therefore, if a rib fracture is clinically present, the Paramedic must suspect a severe internal injury is present. Pulmonary contusions are the most common type of chest injury in children, occurring more frequently than rib fractures and pneumothoraces. Pulmonary contusions may be difficult to detect clinically because there is often no overlying injury. Impaired gas exchange occurs due to the blood leaking into the interstitial space between the alveoli and pulmonary capillaries. This makes oxygenation of the patient difficult. Paradoxically, it is often not difficult to bag-ventilate the patient. This is in stark contrast to a tension pneumothorax in which the patient becomes more and more difficult to bag-ventilate as the tension pneumothorax worsens.

In children, tension pneumothorax is the most commonly missed life-threatening injury. Tracheal deviation, a late sign that is difficult to detect in adults, is almost impossible to detect in younger children. Therefore, the Paramedic must maintain a high degree of suspicion for the developing tension pneumothorax. Hemothorax can occur in children and may cause life-threatening hemorrhage.

Blunt injury to the chest is more likely to cause great vessel injury or disrupt the pulmonary tree in children as compared with adults. The flexibility of the bony thorax in children allows transmission of more energy from the blunt force to the underlying organs than in adults. In adults, the fracture of a rib or the sternum dissipates a large portion of the blunt force energy, reducing the amount that reaches the thoracic organs. Pericardial tamponade is rare in children.

Commotio cordis is one condition more prevalent in pediatrics that has received a lot of attention among those involved with pediatric sports. In commotio cordis, a blunt force localized to the midsternal area causes sudden cardiac arrest. It is now known that this force, when applied to the sternum and transmitted to the heart, may in some cases cause the equivalent of an R on T phenomenon, sending the child into ventricular tachycardia, ventricular fibrillation, or torsades de pointes. Although many children have been successfully resuscitated by the use of nearby automated external defibrillators, many have not. Modifications to protective gear worn by children in sports prone to commotio cordis should help in the prevention of the condition.

Abdominal and Genitourinary Trauma

The abdomen in children is much more compact than in adults. Children also tend to have less abdominal fat, thus offering less protection from blunt force. The child's abdominal muscles are also weaker than in adults and are less protective. The spleen and liver spend more time in the thoracic cavity than in adults, making them prone to injury in patients with thoracic trauma.

The spleen is the most commonly injured abdominal organ in the child.[4] The capsule is much thicker than in the adult, and ruptures less often. However, the vast majority of the child's spleen injuries do not require surgery to remove the spleen (splenectomy). If a splenectomy is required in order to control hemorrhage, the child is at a significant risk of sepsis due to the loss of the spleen's immune system function. Pediatric patients who undergo a splenectomy, as in adult patients, will require life-long antibiotics as a prophylaxis for sepsis from relatively minor infections. The liver is the second most commonly injured abdominal organ. As with splenic injuries, liver injuries in children are treated much less often with surgery than in adults.

Hollow viscus injuries from blunt trauma are less common in children than in adults. Children, due to the smaller area, will commonly have injuries to the spleen and hollow viscus when the pancreas is injured. The pancreas is somewhat protected, as it is nestled up against the spine. Therefore, it requires significant blunt force to cause an injury.

Genitourinary injuries occur in 10% to 15% of pediatric patients who have an abdominal injury. Kidney injuries are the most common part of the genitourinary system to be injured. As with adults, a fracture in the anterior portion of the pelvis can injure the child's bladder or urethra. However, urethral injury is rare in children. Testicular injury is also very uncommon in children. Zipper injuries to the penis are more common in the toddler who is toilet training, but may occur in older children as well.

Although the FAST exam is commonplace in the adult emergency department, its use in pediatric trauma has only recently been explored. Several studies looking at the use of FAST in children have concluded it is a feasible tool to use in pediatric trauma patients. The Paramedic may be exposed to the FAST exam in the emergency department or in disaster situations, just as with adult patients.

Orthopaedic Trauma

The skeleton is much more flexible in the younger child, than in adults. Because of this flexibility, bone injury in the pediatric population may be a more incomplete injury rather than a complete fracture as in adults. **Greenstick fractures** occur when the force applied to the bone causes one side of the cortex to break while the other side bends or deforms (Figure 10-4). Greenstick fractures get their name from the injury that occurs when a fresh twig in spring is bent.

Buckle fractures also occur in children and not in adults (Figure 10-5). **Buckle fractures** typically occur in younger children when force has been applied as an axial load to the extremity. This causes a deformity in the softer bone similar to what occurs when a stick of butter is dropped on end from the dinner table onto the floor. This elasticity, similar to that of the bony thorax, means that significant force is required to cause a pelvic fracture in younger children. Both pelvic and

femur fractures can cause life-threatening hemorrhage due to vascular injury in the pelvis and due to the femur's significant blood supply.

Another type of orthopaedic injury that is specific to pediatric patients involves injury to the epiphysis, or the growth plate (Figure 10-6). The growth plate is an area of cartilage at one end of the long bone and is responsible for the formation of new bone. This softer bone is easily damaged. If the epiphysis is damaged and not treated properly, that damage threatens the growth of the extremity.[5] The Salter–Harris classification (Figure 10-7) is used to describe the types of injuries that involve the growth plates and helps guide definitive treatment by the orthopaedist. In one study, the higher Salter–Harris classification, the higher rate of growth disturbance when looking at the femur. Over 60% of patients with a Salter–Harris category 4 demonstrated growth plate disturbance.[5]

Burns

Thermal injury to children occurs in both accidental trauma and in non-accidental trauma. Sources of injury in accidental trauma include flame, objects heated to a high temperature, and scalding water or grease. In non-accidental trauma, scalding water, lit cigarette butts, and lighters are common sources. As with any injury to a child, injuries that are suspicious or

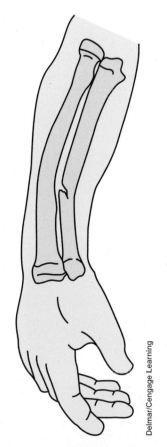

Delmar/Cengage Learning

Figure 10-4 Greenstick fractures are incomplete fractures that occur in children due to the flexibility of the skeleton.

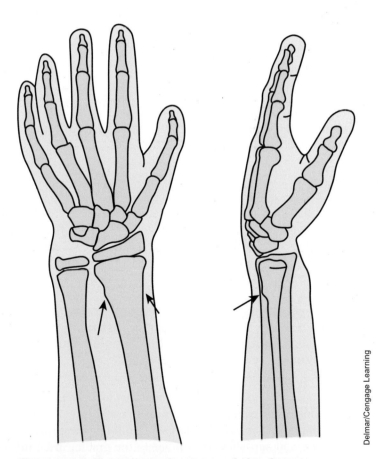

Delmar/Cengage Learning

Figure 10-5 Buckle fracture of the forearm. Note the deformity of the bone that occurs without a break in the bone's cortex.

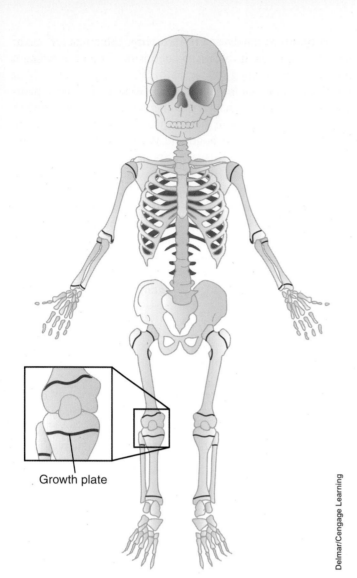

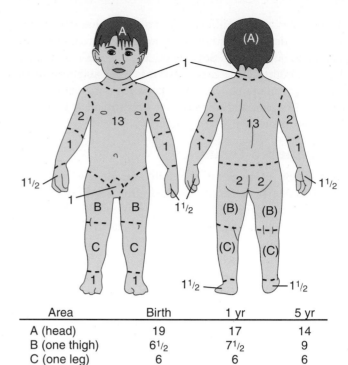

Area	Birth	1 yr	5 yr
A (head)	19	17	14
B (one thigh)	6½	7½	9
C (one leg)	6	6	6

Figure 10-6 Pediatric bony anatomy is unique due to the presence of growth plates.

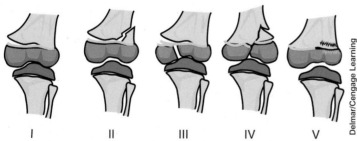

Figure 10-7 The Salter–Harris classification of epiphyseal injury describes the types of injuries that involve the growth plates.

do not match the history should be reported to the appropriate authorities for investigation.

Although the grading of burns into full thickness, partial thickness, and superficial is similar to the grading used for adults, the rule of nines has been modified for use in pediatric patients (Figure 10-8). The rule of nines is based on adult body surface area proportions and is used to estimate

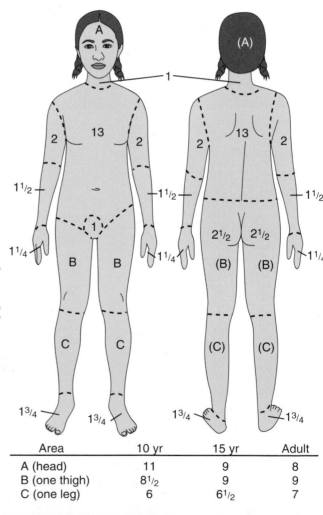

Area	10 yr	15 yr	Adult
A (head)	11	9	8
B (one thigh)	8½	9	9
C (one leg)	6	6½	7

Figure 10-8 Modifications made to the rule of nines based on pediatric body proportions by age.

Delmar/Cengage Learning

the body surface area affected by the burn. Since the physical proportion is different based upon the child's age, several different modifications have been made based upon these changing proportions. The Paramedic should use the one that best approximates the patient's physical proportions in estimating body surface area affected by a burn.

Psychological Considerations

The Paramedic must also be keenly aware of the psychosocial aspects of caring for critically injured pediatric patients. Not only must the child be calmed and treated, but caregivers, friends, or other children on-scene may require reassurance and direction.

The psychological effects of severe trauma can continue well past the injury and treatment. Often children who have been severely injured demonstrate regressive behavior immediately after the injury, affecting the Paramedic's approach in obtaining the history and performing a physical examination on the child. In the short term, after hospitalization, emotional instability may occur with regressive behavior in the face of perceived threats or likelihood of injury. This may present a challenge if a Paramedic is called to assess a child after a minor injury and the assessment causes flashbacks to the major injury in the distant past. It is estimated that 60% of children who sustain multisystem injury will have personality changes one year after the injury. Half of those patients will also have residual deficits that are cognitive, physical, and affective. These deficits will also impair learning.

The best approach when caring for an injured child is to remain calm, soothing, and reassuring to both the child and the child's caregivers. Calming and reassuring the caregivers often helps calm and reassure the child.

▶ CASE STUDY (CONTINUED)

While the crew is attending to the injured child, the Paramedic takes a quick moment to look over the car. "Hmm . . ." he murmurs as he observes a dent and some handprints on the hood. That suggests the child most likely turned toward the car, as would be predicted, striking his head on the hood, leaving a dent. Next he would have been thrown backward, creating a classic coup-contrecoup injury.

While the Paramedic is reviewing the mechanism of injury, the bus driver yells out, "I have the school nurse on the phone! Anybody want to talk to her?" Turning to an EMT, the Paramedic says, "Go and try to get as much past medical information as possible while we package the patient."

CRITICAL THINKING QUESTIONS

1. What are the important elements of the history that a Paramedic should obtain?
2. What special considerations are there for obtaining a pediatric history?

History

As with adult patients who have sustained an injury, the Paramedic can obtain a lot of information through observation prior to and during initial patient contact. Clues from the scene and bystanders will help the Paramedic determine the mechanism of injury and therefore the forces applied to the child. From this, the Paramedic can predict the likelihood of the presence of certain types of injuries. The timing of the injury is also important as some of the previously discussed injuries are frequently not apparent at the time of the obvious injury. For this reason, the Paramedic is prudent to ask about the potential for injury, no matter how insignificant it was to the caregivers, in nearly all pediatric patients the Paramedic encounters.

Once the mechanism is ascertained in the conscious pediatric patient, it is often helpful to start with the location of pain. This may further refine the Paramedic's paramedical diagnosis of likely injuries. Following the OPQRST mnemonic, the Paramedic should elicit the other associated factors in the child's concern. A past medical and surgical history, list of medications, and allergies can be obtained from the caregivers.

The Paramedic should view any history of a loss of consciousness or change from the patient's baseline mental status or activity as a potential intracranial hemorrhage until proven otherwise. The Paramedic should also note symptoms of a spinal cord injury or stinger. In addition, the Paramedic should view dyspnea as a potential sign for serious intrathoracic injury even in the setting of a lack of external signs. Vomiting occurring many hours or days after the injury may indicate the presence of a head injury or a hollow viscus injury, depending upon the mechanism.

The Paramedic should also elicit information regarding the use of restraint and safety gear from the patient, bystanders, or caregivers. The Paramedic should note whether the safety devices or restraint were used properly. This information allows the Paramedic to predict injury patterns based upon proper or improper use of the protective devices.

The crew works at a feverish pace to stabilize the child's cervical spine and to maintain the unconscious child's airway. The child, whose name is Zack, has an irregular breathing pattern, so the Paramedic decides to assist his breathing with a bag-mask assembly. Vital signs are in progress when the Paramedic calls for the child to be moved to the backboard and off-scene. "What about the leg?" asks one of the EMTs. The left leg has an obvious angulated open femur fracture. "Splint it with the rest of the body on the backboard," the Paramedic replies. The EMT winces at the idea of straightening an obviously open femur fracture, but the Paramedic reminds him that time is of the essence.

CRITICAL THINKING QUESTIONS

1. What are the elements of the physical examination for pediatric multitrauma patients?
2. What special age–specific considerations must be taken during the physical examination of the pediatric patient?

Examination

As with adult trauma patients, the Paramedic should focus her initial pediatric patient examination on the airway, breathing, and circulation. Conditions that endanger the patency of the airway, impair oxygenation and ventilation, or disrupt circulation require the Paramedic's immediate attention. The Paramedic must remember that tension pneumothorax is the most commonly missed life-threatening pediatric injury. Therefore, she must carefully examine the chest during both the primary and secondary examinations. The Paramedic must also remember that the pediatric patient's ability to overcompensate for hemorrhage and shock is challenging as compared with the adult patient. These compensatory mechanisms may make the child appear well initially, with a rapid decompensation occurring later during EMS contact time.

Once the patient's life-threatening conditions are improved, the Paramedic can then proceed to the thorough head-to-toe examination. The Paramedic may need to modify her approach based upon the child's emotional age at the time of the injury. Younger children may be uncomfortable with a head-to-toe approach and may be more cooperative and less anxious with a toe-to-head approach. Older children may feel more at ease if allowed to assist with the examination or play with the Paramedic's examination tools. Regardless of the exact order of the examination, the Paramedic should perform a thorough examination of the patient, exposing the patient as appropriate for environmental conditions.

As the patient is loaded into the ambulance, the Paramedic asks the sheriff on-scene if he will call the trauma center and tell them they are inbound with a pediatric trauma patient and to emphasize that they suspect a head injury.

"What about the leg?" the Sheriff asks. "Sure, tell them everything, but emphasize the suspected head injury and that we will be there in less than 20 minutes."

CRITICAL THINKING QUESTIONS

1. What is the importance of making a determination of suspected injuries?
2. What is the prognostic implication?

Assessment

The key to treating critically injured patients is to identify shock early and intervene aggressively to prevent decompensation. If the Paramedic waits until the systolic blood pressure begins to drop before treating the injured child, the Paramedic will lag behind the progression of shock and have a more difficult time in stabilizing the child.

Somnolence, altered mental status, or inappropriate responsiveness can signal the presence of a head injury in a pediatric patient. However, these signs may also be an early indication of hypoxia. As the critically injured child may have poor peripheral perfusion, a pulse oximeter finger probe may not pick up an adequate waveform to determine the patient's oxygenation. If available, the Paramedic may use a forehead probe or earlobe probe to pick up circulation sufficiently to provide a reading. Regardless, with any significant trauma, the Paramedic should administer supplemental oxygen to the pediatric patient to help improve oxygen delivery.

As previously mentioned, pediatric patients have the ability to compensate well for their injuries and then rapidly decompensate. This is largely due to the increased sensitivity of the pediatric blood vessels to circulating catecholamines (e.g., natural epinephrine). These circulating catecholamines cause vasoconstriction and tachycardia that can support a normal or near normal blood pressure for a significant period of time (Figure 10-1). Depending on the degree of vasoconstriction, the pediatric patient can be in early shock and maintain a normal heart rate. In late shock, the pediatric patient will experience bradycardia, typically from depletion of the catecholamine stores, hypothermia, and hypoxia. A seriously injured child who becomes bradycardic is near death and requires aggressive intervention by the Paramedic. Capillary refill time is an early indicator of shock in the pediatric patient due to the significant vasoconstriction. A pediatric patient with a delayed capillary refill is in shock and requires aggressive intervention regardless of the blood pressure.

One tool used to gauge the severity of injury in the pediatric patient is the **Pediatric Trauma Score** (Table 10-4), which is computed by adding the scores for the individual categories and may range from +12 to −6. A Pediatric Trauma Score less than 8 indicates severe injury. The initial studies with this tool demonstrated good correlation with injury severity in children.[6] The Pediatric Trauma Score may be useful in some settings to determine if triage to a trauma center is needed or to alert trauma team activation at the trauma center.[7] Its use is usually dependent on local or regional practice.

Table 10-4 The Pediatric Trauma Score

Category	+2	+1	−1
Weight	> 20 kg	10–20 kg	< 10 kg
Airway	Normal	Maintained	Invasive (intubated or supraglottic airway)
Systolic BP	> 90 mmHg	50–90 mmHg	< 50 mmHg
Central nervous system	Awake	Obtunded	Coma
Open wound	None	Minor	Major
Skeletal trauma	None	Closed fracture	Open fracture or multiple fractures

CASE STUDY (CONTINUED)

After performing spinal immobilization, the EMT concentrates on maintaining an airway and ventilating Zack. The Paramedic knows that Zack's irregular respirations and unconsciousness are due to a head injury. In the ambulance, he asks that the head of the stretcher be elevated approximately 20 degrees. He reasons that this will help "drain the brain" and thereby decrease intracranial pressure as well as decrease the chances of aspiration in the unprotected airway.

CRITICAL THINKING QUESTIONS

1. What is the national standard of care of pediatric patients with suspected head injury?

2. What are some of the patient-specific concerns that the Paramedic should consider when applying this plan of care that is intended to treat a broad patient population presenting with head injury?

Treatment

As with adults, the treatment of a critically injured child begins with ensuring the child has a patent airway, that the child has adequate oxygenation and ventilation, and that the child has adequate perfusion. Any life-threatening issues found during the primary survey require immediate treatment by the Paramedic.

In managing the airway of children, the younger child may require support with a folded towel or small blanket under the shoulders to maintain a neutral position of the cervical spine, improve visualization, and prevent kinking of the softer, more pliable airway of the child. The debate over pediatric intubation is not limited to medical causes of respiratory failure. In some cases, it may be appropriate to utilize effective bag-mask ventilation to ensure adequate oxygenation and ventilation. In other cases, especially when encountering facial bleeding, vomit, or other foreign material in the airway, it may be more appropriate to endotracheally intubate the child.

An appropriately sized single-lumen, blind supraglottic airway may also be used. Although placement of the single-lumen, blind supraglottic airway is typically easier, it may not provide the same level of protection from foreign material as endotracheal intubation. The Paramedic should also remember that if a surgical airway becomes necessary, needle cricothyrotomy is the only surgical procedure appropriate in children under 12 years old.

One common impediment to ventilation is the tension pneumothorax. As previously discussed, tension pneumothorax may not be easily appreciated in children. The needle chest decompression procedure for pediatric patients is similar to that of adults. However, the needle length and caliber should be shorter for smaller children. In adults, the chest wall is typically rather thick. However, in children there is typically less muscle and fat in the chest wall, so a longer needle length is not needed to enter the pleural cavity. In smaller children, a smaller gauge needle, such as a 1-inch, 20-gauge intravenous catheter, may also be acceptable.

To support circulation, the Paramedic may administer normal saline boluses at 20 mL/kg after obtaining intravenous or intraosseous access. For smaller children, the use of a large volume syringe (for example, 30 or 60 mL) attached to a three-way stopcock is an effective way of delivering the bolus rapidly while at the same time preventing fluid overload. In older children, intravenous fluids may be administered through a burette. To use this method, the volume to be administered is placed in the burette, then the roller clamp between the IV fluid bag and the burette is clamped and the roller clamp between the burette and the patient is opened, allowing the bolus to flow freely. This fluid bolus is administered up to three times in the unstable patient before the Paramedic considers blood products, which should be administered in a volume of 10 mL/kg boluses.

If the Paramedic suspects head injury, the head of the stretcher or the head of the backboard can be elevated approximately 20 degrees to prevent the physiologic increase in intracranial pressure that occurs when the patient lies supine. Post-concussive seizures that last longer than five minutes should be treated with a benzodiazepine. The patient's oxygenation and ventilation status must be closely watched in patients with a suspected injury who have received a benzodiazepine. The Paramedic should consider aggressive airway management if any indication for hypoxia or hypoventilation occurs.

Table 10-5 Assessment and Critical Interventions in the Pediatric Trauma Patient

Assessment	Critical Actions
Airway Summary	
Airway obstruction	• Open airway
	• Jaw thrust
	• Needle cricothyrotomy
Breathing Summary	
Apnea	• BVM
	• Endotracheal intubation
	• Gastric decompression
Tension pneumothorax	• Needle decompression
Open pneumothorax	• Occlusive dressing
	• Needle thoracostomy if tension develops
Hypoxia	• Oxygen therapy
	• Endotracheal intubation
Circulation Summary	
Hypotension/hypoperfusion	• Normal saline 20 mL/kg boluses
	• Blood products 10 mL/kg boluses
Disability Summary	
Head injury	• Elevate head of backboard 20 degrees
Post-concussive seizure	• Administer benzodiazepine if seizure lasts > 5 minutes
SCIWORA/stinger	• Immobilization

Pediatric patients who have any neurologic complaints during their history or neurologic deficits on examination should be fully immobilized on a long spine board with a cervical collar (Table 10-5). For younger children, other immobilization devices exist that are more appropriate for a smaller sized patient. The patient should be immobilized even if the neurologic sign or symptom was transient and is resolved at the time of the examination.

CASE STUDY (CONTINUED)

While deciding whether to intubate the child, the EMT is doing an acceptable job of ventilating the child. However, Zack starts to seize. "No worries," the Paramedic announces, "he has a post-concussive seizure." Nevertheless, the Paramedic knows that this is a sign of increasing intracranial pressure and he is prepared to give diazepam if the seizures don't break. The Paramedic also considers administering lidocaine as part of the preinduction portion of the intubation.

CRITICAL THINKING QUESTIONS

1. What are some of the predictable complications associated with head injury?
2. What are some of the predictable complications associated with the treatments for head injuries?

Evaluation

The injured pediatric patient must be carefully monitored and reassessed for the development of a tension pneumothorax and shock during transport. Tension pneumothorax can be difficult to detect in the injured child. Pediatric patients also compensate well for shock for a prolonged period of time. Early detection and aggressive intervention are the keys to caring for a critically injured child.

CASE STUDY CONCLUSION

The ambulance pulls into the hospital parking lot. Shutting down the lights and siren as they pull into the bay, there is an eerie silence until the back doors swing open. "Welcome to Children's Hospital," exclaims the resident. "What have we got?"

While unloading Zack, the Paramedic starts to give the report. As Zack enters into the trauma bay, a crush of people descend upon him, literally pushing the Paramedic out of the way. That is alright with the Paramedic. He got the patient there alive, now it's their turn to help Zack.

CRITICAL THINKING QUESTIONS

1. What is the most appropriate destination for a pediatric multitrauma patient?
2. Why is it acceptable to bypass other hospitals to get the patient to these facilities?

Disposition

Pediatric patients who have sustained significant injury should be transported to the closest appropriate pediatric-capable trauma center (Table 10-6).[8] Hospitals designated as pediatric trauma centers have a wide range of services available to expertly care for the child who has sustained multiple injuries. Children who have an isolated single system injury (e.g., isolated single long-bone fracture) may be transported to a nonpediatric trauma facility depending upon the capabilities in the Paramedic's system. As these capabilities may change, the Paramedic will need to be knowledgeable as to the capabilities at the hospitals within her region.

Table 10-6 Criteria for Transport Directly to the Closest Appropriate Pediatric Trauma Center[8]

Physiologic Criteria

- GCS < 14
- Systolic blood pressure < 90 or (70 + 2 × age)
- Respiratory rate either < 10 or > 29 in children older than 1 year; < 20 in infant younger than 1 year old

Anatomic Criteria

- Penetrating injury to head, neck, torso
- Flail chest
- Two or more proximal long-bone fractures
- Crushed, degloved, or mangled extremity
- Amputation proximal to the wrist or ankle
- Pelvic fractures
- Open or depressed skull fracture
- Spinal cord injury

Mechanism Criteria

- Fall greater than 10 feet or two to three times the child's height
- High-risk auto crash
  - Passenger compartment intrusion > 12 inches at occupant site or > 18 inches any site
  - Ejection from automobile
  - Death in same passenger compartment
  - Vehicle telemetry data consistent with high risk of injury
- Auto vs. pedestrian/bicycle > 20 mph impact, thrown, or run over
- Motorcycle crash > 20 mph
- Burns with other trauma should triage to trauma center

CONCLUSION

The critically injured child can present unique challenges to the Paramedic that are different than those presented by adult patients. Not only does the child's physiology provide distinct differences that require close attention, but the psychosocial issues that occur, especially with younger children, can test the Paramedic's capabilities. By being thorough and remembering to ensure the patient is well oxygenated and well perfused, the Paramedic will be able to expertly manage even the most challenging injured child.

KEY POINTS:

- Trauma (i.e., unintentional injury as compared to homicide) remains the leading cause of death in children and young adults.

- There are similarities and differences between pediatric and adult trauma.

- Children compensate in shock well, then decompensate rapidly.

- Children tend to fall head first, leading to traumatic brain injury.

- Head injury is the leading cause of trauma death in children.

- Subdural hematomas occur in infants but not as often in children.

- Children have a better prognosis following increased intracranial pressure.

- A modified Glasgow Coma Scale is used in pediatrics.

- Pediatric trauma patients may experience spinal cord injury without obvious radiographic abnormality.

- Children are prone to solid abdominal organ injury in trauma.

- Psychological care is as important as physical care in some instances.

- As in adults, pediatric trauma starts with an assessment of the mechanism of injury, as well as an application of knowledge of kinematics, to ascertain a predictable injury pattern.

- Somnolence is a sign of traumatic brain injury in a child.

- Bradycardia is a premorbid sign.

- Standard adult trauma care is appropriate when the patient's size is taken into consideration.

REVIEW QUESTIONS:

1. Differentiate posturing in children and adults.
2. Why are high cervical injuries more likely to occur in children?
3. Describe the unique pediatric spinal cord injury.
4. What is unique about pediatric thoracic injury?
5. What unique cardiac event occurs in children while playing sports?

CASE STUDY QUESTIONS:

Please refer to the Case Study in this chapter, and answer the questions below:

1. Based on the mechanism of injury, what is the predictable injury pattern?
2. What are the potential life threats from these injuries?
3. Which is more problematic?

REFERENCES:

1. Centers for Disease Control. Ten leading causes of death by age group, United States–2006. Available at: **http://www.cdc.gov/injury/Images/LC-Charts/10lc%20-%20 By%20Age%20Group%202006-7_6_09-a.pdf.** Accessed January 15, 2010.

2. Orsborn R, Haley K, Hammond S, Falcone RE. Pediatric pedestrian verses motor vehicle patterns of injury: debunking the myth. Air Medical Journal 1999;18(3):107–110.

3. Meier JD, Tollefson TT. Pediatric facial trauma. *Curr Opin Otolaryngol Head Neck Surg.* 2008;16(6):555–561.

4. Clark JR, Hubble JP. Pediatric trauma. In: Hubble MW, Hubble JP. *Principles of Advanced Trauma Care.* Clifton Park, NY. Delmar Cengage Learning; 2002:599–620.

5. Basener CJ, Mehlman CT, DiPasquale TG. Growth disturbance after distal femoral growth plate fractures in children: a meta analysis. *J Orthop Trauma.* 2009;23(9):663–667.

6. Tepas JJ, Mollitt DL, Talbert JL, Bryant M. The pediatric trauma score as a predictor of injury severity in the injured child. *J Pediat Surg.* 1987;22(1):14–18.

7. Simon B, Gabor R, Letourneau P. Secondary triage of the injured pediatric patient within the trauma center: support for a selective resource-sparing two-stage system. *Pediatr Emerg Care.* 2004;20(1):5–11.

8. Sasser SM, Hunt RC, Sullivent EE, et al. Guidelines for field triage of injured patients: recommendations of the national expert panel on field triage. Morbidity and Mortality Weekly Report January 23, 2009;58(RR-1):1-35. May be accessed from: **http://www.cdc.gov/mmwr/PDF/rr/rr5801.pdf.**

CHAPTER 11

TRAUMA RESUSCITATION

KEY CONCEPTS:

Upon completion of this chapter, it is expected that the reader will understand these following concepts:

- Shock versus hypoperfusion
- Goal-directed therapy in shock–trauma
- Permissive hypotension
- Hemorrhage control

ANATOMY CONCEPTS:

Prior to reading this chapter the Paramedic student should be familiar with the following anatomy and physiology concepts:

- Systemic response to hypoperfusion
- Sympathetic nervous system
- Coagulation cascade
- Mechanics of ventilation

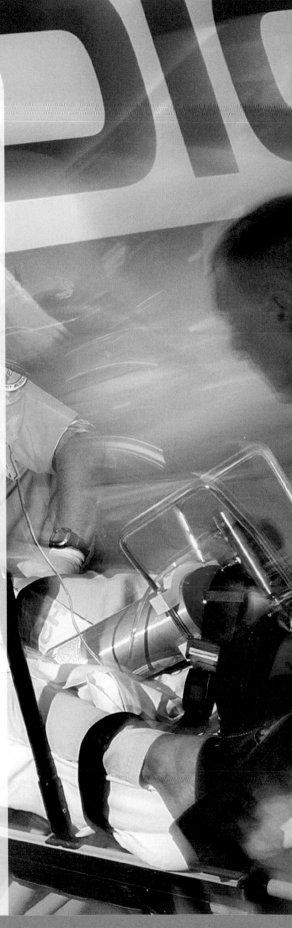

"Patient with shotgun wound, Police on-scene, scene secure, perpetrators in custody and police request that EMS expedite," comes the message over the radio. Turning onto the boulevard, and turning on the lights and siren, the Paramedic training officer turns to the young Paramedic beside her and says, "These calls tend to get messy. Be sure to have your PPE. Now, based on the mechanism of injury, what are some predictable injury patterns? Let's start with a wound to the head."

This is the Paramedic's first shooting. As an intern, he had seen cardiac arrests and even a childbirth, but he had never been to a shooting. Now, as a rookie, his training officer is putting him through his paces. He understands that she is just preparing him for the onslaught of sensations and emotions he is about to feel. "Now, keep the discipline, what do you start with?" asks the training officer.

CRITICAL THINKING QUESTIONS

1. What are some of the possible life-threatening injuries that would be suspected based on the mechanism of injury?

2. What are the special scene dynamics with an officer involved shooting?

OVERVIEW

The preceding chapters detailed the breadth of trauma care, from the pathophysiology to injury patterns to treatment. When faced with a critically ill patient with multiple injuries, the Paramedic needs to adopt an approach that prioritizes treatment and prevents the Paramedic from becoming focused on one problem while ignoring others. As with the critical medically ill patient, the critically injured patient requires a holistic approach to care in order to improve the patient's outcome.

Chief Concern

Shock is defined as inadequate oxygenation of the end organs and tissues and is independent of the patient's blood pressure and other physiologic parameters. With this in mind, the Paramedic's overarching goal in treating the critically ill trauma patient with multiple injuries is to enhance the delivery of oxygen to the tissues. In contrast to the shock seen in critically ill medical patients, hemorrhagic shock is the most common type of shock in injured patients. Neurogenic shock occasionally occurs in the setting of spinal cord injury or significant brain or brainstem injury, but is a far less common cause of shock in the critically injured patient. The Paramedic must also keep in mind other causes of shock, such as medical causes, as a medical event may have preceded the traumatic event.

Oxygen Delivery to the Tissues

The delivery of oxygen to the tissues is dependent upon four components: a clear and unobstructed airway, adequate oxygenation, adequate ventilation, and adequate circulation (Table 11-1).

In the setting of multi-organ trauma, there are many things that can interfere with the airway. In addition to oral secretions and vomit, other considerations in managing the airway are blood, teeth, and bony fragments in the airway. Unstable facial fractures may also interfere with mask seal, airway adjunct placement and function, and supraglottic airway placement and function. Neck hematomas may displace the trachea and therefore the intubating landmarks. Direct injury to the neck may also disrupt the trachea or distort the airway anatomy, increasing the difficulty of intubation and potentially affecting the placement and balloon seal of a supraglottic airway.

As with the critically ill medical patient, critically injured trauma patients often benefit from supplemental high-flow, high-concentration oxygen. Administering high-flow, high-concentration supplemental oxygen to the patient quickly saturates all available hemoglobin molecules and increases the amount of dissolved oxygen in the blood. Replacement of nitrogen with oxygen provides an oxygen reservoir to provide a time buffer during airway management procedures.

Table 11-1 Four Components Required for Adequate Delivery of Oxygen to the Tissues and Conditions that Interfere with these Components

- Clear and unobstructed airway
  - Foreign matter
  - Facial fractures
  - Neck hematoma
  - Upper airway injury
- Adequate oxygenation
  - Impaired ventilation
  - Impaired oxygen diffusion
  - Decreased circulating volume/hemoglobin
- Adequate ventilation
  - Rib fractures
  - Thoracic vertebrae fractures
  - Chest wall contusions
  - Flail chest
  - Pneumothorax
  - Hemothorax
  - Pulmonary contusion
- Adequate circulation
  - Massive hemorrhage
    - Chest
    - Abdomen
    - Pelvis
    - Femur
  - Mechanical
    - Pericardial tamponade
    - Tension pneumothorax/hemothorax
    - Blunt myocardial injury
      - Dysrhythmias
      - Impaired contractility

Ventilation, the movement of air in and out of the lungs, is integral to the introduction of oxygen into the body and the removal of carbon dioxide. Ventilation is affected by several conditions that can occur in trauma. A pneumothorax or hemothorax reduces the volume of lung space that is ventilated and can participate in gas exchange. In a spontaneously breathing patient, injuries to the chest wall may impair respiratory mechanics that create the negative intrathoracic pressure required for ventilation. Rib fractures and thoracic vertebrae fractures produce significant pain which worsens with deep inspiration, limiting the patient's ability to take a sufficiently deep breath. Chest wall contusions may also be painful enough to impair chest excursion. A flail segment will decrease the negative intrathoracic pressure generated, thus decreasing lung expansion.

Pulmonary contusions impair ventilation by not allowing that section of the lung to expand and contract normally. Pulmonary contusions also affect the diffusion of oxygen and carbon dioxide across the membrane between the alveoli and the pulmonary capillaries in that section of lung affected by the pulmonary contusion. As with a pneumothorax, patients who develop a large pulmonary contusion may become difficult to ventilate as the lung stiffens from the edema and blood in the interstitial space between the alveoli and the pulmonary capillaries. Massive abdominal hemorrhage can apply pressure on the underside of the diaphragm and impair lung expansion. Finally, a diaphragmatic hernia may be large enough to allow abdominal contents to pass into the thoracic cavity, also decreasing the ability of the lung on the affected side to expand to provide sufficient ventilation.

In hemorrhagic shock, the circulation and perfusion is most often affected by blood loss. In significant hemorrhage, both plasma and hemoglobin are lost early on, rapidly decreasing the blood's oxygen-carrying capacity. Significant blood loss can occur with abdominal hemorrhage, as the abdomen may accommodate over half of a patient's circulating blood volume. Up to 25% to 30% of the patient's circulating blood volume can be lost in the thorax, and pelvic and femur fractures may produce blood loss of over 1 liter. Blood loss from any of these conditions can easily produce moderate to severe hemorrhagic shock.

In addition to blood loss, circulation can be affected by mechanical factors that impede blood circulation. Traumatic pericardial tamponade mechanically reduces ventricular filling and impedes cardiac output. A tension pneumothorax, massive hemothorax, or hemopneumothorax can also impair ventricular filling. Blunt myocardial injury can produce dysrhythmias that decrease cardiac output by decreasing the number of systolic beats producing forward blood flow. In more severe cases, a blunt myocardial injury may affect the contractility of the right ventricle (the anterior-most portion of the heart in the chest), decreasing preload and thus decreasing afterload.

Finally, in a small number of patients with a spinal cord injury or with a massive head injury, shock may actually be secondary to loss of vascular tone, similar to septic or anaphylactic shock. In these cases, hypotension and shock can occur even in the absence of significant hemorrhage. Volume replacement may help improve hypotension and shock. However, with massive fluid administration in a patient without blood loss, fluid overload is a real complication even in patients with normal cardiac function. Vasopressors may be required in order to decrease vascular volume and support the blood pressure, similar to the treatment for septic shock.

Pathophysiology of Hemorrhagic Shock

In critically injured patients, the most likely cause of shock is hemorrhagic shock. In treating hemorrhagic shock, it is helpful to understand the pathophysiology of hemorrhagic shock and the mechanisms the body uses to compensate for acute blood loss.

Acute Blood Loss

The pathway to shock begins with hemorrhage that the body cannot rapidly stop and which overcomes the initial stages of the coagulation system (Figure 11-1). After a sufficient amount of blood loss, circulating volume decreases. This causes a drop in preload in that less blood is available to return to the heart for oxygenation. Decreasing preload, or chamber filling pressures, affects the force of contraction based upon the Frank-Starling mechanism, in which the heart uses some of its stretch in filling to generate a higher force of contraction up to a point (Figure 11-2). When the preload decreases, the amount of blood in the left ventricle is decreased, thus decreasing the pressure in the left ventricle at the end of diastole and ultimately decreasing the stroke volume.

As the cardiac output is directly affected by the stroke volume (Figure 11-3), when the stroke volume decreases, the cardiac output also decreases. The mean arterial blood pressure is dependent on the cardiac output and the central venous

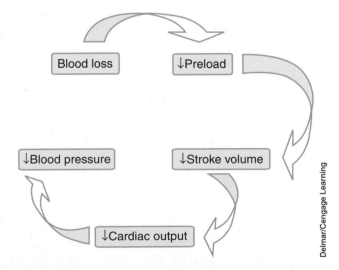

Figure 11-1 The genesis of hemorrhagic shock begins with hemorrhage that the body cannot rapidly stop.

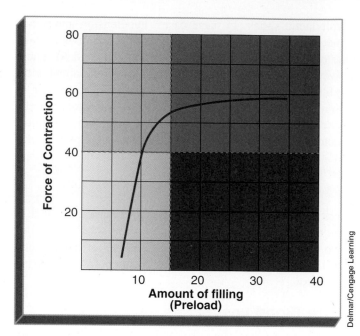

Figure 11-2 The Frank-Starling mechanism in which force of contraction, and thus stroke volume, is dependent on the volume of blood, and thus the pressure at the end of diastole, in the ventricle.

Computing cardiac output:

CO = HR × SV

where CO = cardiac output
HR = heart rate
SV = stroke volume

Figure 11-3 Computations used for cardiac output.

Computing the mean arterial blood pressure:

MAP = (CO × SVR) + CVP

where MAP = mean arterial pressure
CO = cardiac output
SVR = systemic vascular resistance
CVP = central venous pressure

Figure 11-4 Computations used for the mean arterial blood pressure.

---

pressure (Figure 11-4), both of which are affected in hemorrhagic shock. The central venous pressure is the pressure in the central venous system during diastole, which is essentially the preload, or pressure that allows the heart to fill. As previously mentioned, the central venous pressure (preload) will fall in hemorrhagic shock. The cardiac output decreases in hemorrhagic shock due to the drop in stroke volume. The systemic vascular resistance is dependent on the diameter of the vessels in the vascular system.

In distributive shock states, such as spinal cord injury or severe brain injury, the loss of vascular tone significantly decreases the systemic vascular resistance, thus decreasing the mean arterial pressure without contribution of the changes in cardiac output and central venous pressure from hemorrhage.

Compensatory Mechanisms

The body has several different mechanisms available to compensate for hemodynamically significant hemorrhage. The end result of most of the compensatory mechanisms is to stimulate the sympathetic nervous system to help increase the blood pressure and improve perfusion to the core organs. These mechanisms shunt blood away from the gut, skeletal muscle, and skin, and preferentially circulate it toward the coronary, cerebral, and renal circulation. The shunting of blood increases central venous return, increasing the preload and in turn increasing cardiac output. As shock progresses, blood will be shunted from the kidneys last.

Baroreceptors located in the carotid bodies and aortic arch sense the blood pressure in the central arterial vessels by sensing the stretch in the arterial wall at these locations. Stimuli from baroreceptors are fed into the medulla oblongata and are used to adjust the tone of the sympathetic nervous system. For example, if the baroreceptors detect an increase in stretch in the arterial vessels corresponding to an increase in blood pressure, the medulla oblongata will decrease sympathetic nervous system tone. This allows the vessel diameter to increase slightly and heart rate to slow until the baroreceptors' stimulus returns to the normal level. If the signal from the baroreceptors indicates less stretch than usual, which is indicative of a decrease in arterial blood pressure, the opposite occurs with vessel diameter decreasing and heart rate increasing. This short-term regulation of blood pressure allows the body to respond to changes in position, altitude, and circulating volume, maintaining the systolic blood pressure within a relatively steady range that is normal for that person. Some medical conditions and medications decrease the body's ability to rapidly compensate for changes in blood pressure. This mechanism does not compensate for conditions that cause chronic hypertension.

In a patient undergoing severe hemorrhage, the baroreceptors sense a significant change in the stretch of the walls of the central arteries. This is turn stimulates the sympathetic nervous system to decrease vascular system diameter, thereby increasing systemic vascular resistance and increasing central venous pressure. The sympathetic nervous system also increases the patient's heart rate, which in turn increases cardiac output. The end result is to maintain the mean arterial pressure.

When the sympathetic nervous system is stimulated, it also causes epinephrine to be secreted from the adrenal gland. The circulating epinephrine helps augment the sympathetic nervous system by directly stimulating the body's adrenergic receptors. This also helps increase vascular tone and heart rate.

The decrease in blood pressure also acts at the capillary level. Capillary blood flow is dependent on the central venous pressure. When the central venous pressure falls, the pressure within the capillaries also drops. In hemorrhage sufficient enough to produce hypotension, this drop in pressure causes a fluid shift out of the cells and from the interstitial space into the capillaries in an effort to increase circulating plasma. Although this does not create additional oxygen-carrying capacity, it works with the other compensatory mechanisms to improve the patient's blood pressure by increasing circulating volume.

The drop in blood pressure also triggers the release of antidiuretic hormone (vasopressin) from the posterior pituitary of the brain into the circulation. Antidiuretic hormone signals the kidneys to conserve water by retaining sodium. This mechanism is used to temporarily increase circulating volume. The thirst mechanism is also activated, encouraging the patient to ingest fluids as another way of temporarily increasing circulating volume.

Chemoreceptors located in the medulla oblongata, carotid, and aorta sense pH, carbon dioxide, and, to a lesser extent, oxygen content in the blood and cerebrospinal fluid. Chemoreceptors in the medulla oblongata detect the pH of the cerebrospinal fluid, and will increase respiratory rate in response to a decrease in cerebrospinal fluid pH. Chemoreceptors in the aorta detect both pH and carbon dioxide levels in the central circulation. In addition to pH and carbon dioxide, chemoreceptors in the carotid detect oxygen. The chemoreceptors in the aortic arch and the carotid produce less of a change in respiratory rate than the central chemoreceptors in the medulla oblongata. In addition to directly increasing the respiratory rate by stimulating the respiratory center, the heart rate and vascular tone are affected by impulses sent to stimulate the sympathetic nervous system. Chemoreceptors are most often activated when the mean arterial pressure drops below 60 mmHg. However, they may be activated at a higher blood pressure if the patient is hypoxemic or acidotic.

As a last ditch effort to improve blood pressure and cerebral perfusion, when the mean arterial pressure drops below 40 to 60 mmHg, an intense cerebral discharge develops. This discharge is meant to provide intense sympathetic stimulation to keep the vascular system constricted in an effort to maintain the blood pressure.

If the patient survives this episode of hemorrhagic shock, the **hematopoietic system** increases production of red blood cells, gradually replacing red blood cells lost during hemorrhage. Although this is an important part of homeostasis, this process can take several weeks at an increased level of production to return the blood's hemoglobin content to a normal level. This is not useful in combating the acute loss of the blood's oxygen-carrying capability in hemodynamically significant hemorrhage.

Decompensation

At some point, the body cannot compensate further for acute blood loss. When this happens, the supply of epinephrine has been exhausted; this usually occurs after the intense sympathetic discharge caused by cerebral ischemia and hypoxia. In addition, increased acidemia impairs epinephrine's effectiveness at producing vasoconstriction and tachycardia. The patient's blood pressure falls as the vascular system relaxes when sympathetic stimulation and circulating epinephrine are insufficient to maintain vasoconstriction. Hypotension decreases blood supply to the kidneys, brain, and heart. Decreased cerebral blood flow causes ischemia and edema, which can worsen intracranial pressure, especially in patients with intracranial hemorrhage. Myocardial ischemia is caused by decreased coronary artery blood flow. Capillary beds in the ischemic organs begin to leak, allowing fluid to move from the vascular space to the interstitial space, increasing swelling.

The end effect of decompensation is a rapid drop in blood pressure and blood flow, ultimately leading to cardiac arrest. If the Paramedic can aggressively intervene before decompensation occurs, the patient's outcome is generally improved. Once the patient decompensates, it is often difficult to reverse the downward spiral.

Initial Patient Contact: Sick versus Not Sick

During the initial contact with an injured patient, experienced Paramedics can often identify those patients who are critically ill just by looking at them. Although not an inclusive list, several factors comprise the global assessment on contact that allows the seasoned Paramedic to determine at a glance who needs immediate transport (Table 11-2). Patients who have one or more of these observable conditions should be rapidly extricated from the scene and transported to the nearest appropriate trauma center. All these observations tie into the four components required to ensure adequate delivery of oxygen to the tissues.

Clear and Unobstructed Airway

The Paramedic's first key component in achieving the goal of oxygen delivery is ensuring the patient has a clear and unobstructed airway. This initial pathway from the atmosphere to the lungs is one place where the delivery of oxygen to the tissues can become disrupted.

Table 11-2 Observations Indicating the Need for Immediate Transport of a Critically Injured Patient

- Decreased level of consciousness
- Noisy respirations
- Pale, gray, mottled, or cyanotic skin
- Abnormal respiratory pattern
- Abnormal chest wall movement
- Uncontrolled external hemorrhage in combination with any of the above

Assessment

Airway assessment begins during the Paramedic's initial encounter with an injured patient. A patient who is speaking fluently, clearly, and engages properly in conversation is likely well oxygenated at that time. However, a patient with altered mental status may have altered mental status secondary to hypoxia, hypotension, intoxicants, or head injury. Patients who have altered mental status also may have difficulty in maintaining a patent airway. Critically injured patients will generally be transported to the emergency department in a supine position. Relaxation of airway musculature can impede the airflow through the upper airway enough to impair oxygenation.

Audible gurgling or snoring with respirations indicates to the Paramedic that the patient's airway is partially obstructed. Inspection may reveal the source of the partial obstruction. Often in the patient with a decreased level of consciousness, extra tissue in the upper airway partially obstructs the airway when the airway musculature relaxes. Saliva, blood, and vomit are also common causes of partial airway obstruction. Bleeding may come from the nose or nasopharynx, intraoral bleeding, or externally from the face.

Severe facial injury may either make airway management more difficult or may make it more straightforward. Unstable facial bones not only can cause copious amounts of bleeding but can also make it difficult to maintain an adequate mask seal when performing bag-mask ventilation. In situations in which the face has been completely destroyed (Figure 11-5), the usual landmarks that assist in performing airway management techniques are not present to help guide the Paramedic. In select cases, tissue loss from the mandible may actually make the middle airway landmarks easier to see.

Trauma to the neck can potentially produce an airway obstruction. In some cases, it is obvious to the Paramedic that neck trauma is producing a partial or complete airway obstruction. Observing any wounds or asymmetry in the neck, palpating the neck for masses, noting the tone of the patient's voice, and asking if it is normal all provide the Paramedic with valuable information regarding the patency of the airway. Hematomas may expand rapidly, making it necessary for the Paramedic to frequently reassess the airway.

Management Plan

Airway management should be undertaken aggressively in patients with potential compromise of the airway. Traditionally, patients with a Glasgow Coma Scale below 8 should be intubated, although the Paramedic may consider using a supraglottic airway when performing a rapid sequence intubation in patients with a difficult airway. Nasotracheal intubation may be a viable option in patients with issues in mandible mobility. Nasotracheal intubation, however, is contraindicated in patients who have a suspected basilar skull fracture due to concerns of passing the tip of the nasotracheal tube through the cribiform plate and into the brain.

It should be noted that, in one study, patients who sustained a head injury and underwent rapid sequence intubation had a poorer outcome than those that received either supplemental oxygen only or bag-mask ventilation at the trauma center.[1] When the pulse oximeter readings were reviewed, it was clear that the patients that underwent rapid sequence intubation were more likely to have episodes of hypoxemia. One episode of hypoxemia in a patient with a traumatic brain injury significantly increases that patient's morbidity and mortality.[2] These studies illustrate the need for adequate preoxygenation of the patient prior to performing airway management techniques, including rapid sequence intubation.

Repeated intubation attempts also decrease the likelihood of intubation success. In one study of flight providers, the success rate dropped dramatically after the second attempt at intubation.[3,4] This focus on airway management also detracts the Paramedic from treating the entire patient.[3] There is a good chance that if an injured patient is critical enough to require airway management, then that patient also has a litany of other injuries that require treatment. While the Paramedic is distracted by struggling with the airway, the patient can easily slip into worsening shock or cardiac arrest.

Based upon this information, Paramedics should ensure that the patient is adequately preoxygenated prior to initiating airway management techniques. The Paramedic should also limit the total number of attempts at intubation to two before switching to another means of airway management. In some patients, a more rapid approach to airway management in the critically injured patient may be to perform a rapid sequence intubation, placing a supraglottic airway after induction and paralysis.

In a small percentage of patients, it may be appropriate for the Paramedic to use a surgical airway technique as the initial approach at airway management. In patients with deformity of the airway anatomy, massive mandible injury, or unrecognizable facial landmarks, it may be prudent to move

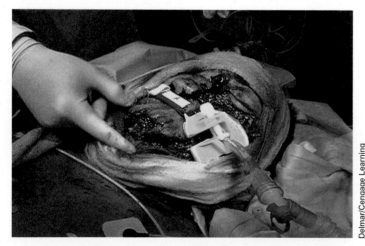

Figure 11-5 The facial trauma caused by a shotgun blast to the face significantly increased the level of difficulty in performing airway management techniques on this patient.

Delmar/Cengage Learning

directly to a surgical airway if placing one is more likely to be successful than performing intubation or a supraglottic airway. It is difficult to protocolize this type of decision as it is largely based on the Paramedic's experience and comfort level with the airway management techniques available to him.

Adequate Oxygenation

The second key factor needed to adequately deliver oxygen to tissues involves ensuring adequate oxygenation of the patient. In order to transport oxygen to the tissues, it must first travel into the bloodstream so it can be distributed throughout the body.

Assessment

Altered mental status is often the first objective sign of hypoxemia. This can include a wide range of responses from confusion to somnolence to combativeness. The mucous membranes of the lips and tongue are often the first areas to become cyanotic. Pallor may be secondary to hypoxemia or may be from circulatory collapse. Pulse oximetry may provide an objective measure of hypoxemia; however, it is often difficult for the finger probe to detect an adequate plethysmograph, or oximetry waveform due to shunting of blood from the skin. In some cases, a forehead pediatric probe may detect enough capillary blood flow to determine a reading.

Management Plan

All critically injured trauma patients should receive high-flow, high-concentration oxygen via nonrebreather mask, bag-mask ventilation, endotracheal intubation, or a supraglottic airway. Many conditions that accompany the critically injured patient, namely acidosis and increased carbon dioxide, decrease oxygen's affinity for hemoglobin. Supplemental oxygen is often essential in these situations in order to help boost oxygen saturation up to 100% by increasing the partial pressure of oxygen seen by hemoglobin, thus encouraging the binding of oxygen. After several vital capacity breaths or approximately two to five minutes on a nonrebreather mask at 15 liters per minute of oxygen, the nitrogen in the dead space of the lungs is washed out, replaced by the oxygen, thus creating a natural reservoir of oxygen. This reservoir may help extend apnea time during airway management techniques or help maintain oxygenation in a patient who is supine on a long spine board for a prolonged period of time.

In the setting of the critically injured multisystem trauma patient, there are few consequences of administering supplemental oxygen to the patient.

Adequate Ventilation

The Paramedic's third key factor in providing adequate oxygen delivery to the tissues is ensuring adequate ventilation of the patient. Without adequate movement of air in and out of the lungs, oxygen diffusion into the pulmonary capillaries and carbon dioxide diffusion into the alveolar space will not occur.

Assessment

Ventilation is primarily assessed by observing the patient's chest for symmetric rise and fall and auscultating the breath sounds. Any asymmetry may indicate the presence of rib fractures, a flail chest, or a pneumothorax. Auscultation of breath sounds will provide the Paramedic with an appreciation of the equality of breath sounds as well as how well air moves in and out of the lungs.

The Paramedic can also observe the patient for signs of an increased work of breathing. This includes observing for the use of accessory muscles, pursed lip breathing, sternal retractions, and intercostal retractions. Obvious trauma to the chest, including wounds, impaled objects, or areas of ecchymosis, may indicate the need for a closer examination of the area. Wounds may in fact be an open pneumothorax if the wound penetrates the pleural space.

Palpation can detect instability in the chest wall and provide the Paramedic with another means for assessing chest excursion. The trachea can be palpated just above the sternal notch to assess if it is in a midline position. However, tracheal deviation is a late sign of intrathoracic injury, whereas other collections of signs and symptoms are more likely to indicate a tension pneumothorax (Table 11-3).

Management Plan

Once the Paramedic determines that a patient is not ventilating adequately, he must ensure the patient's respirations are assisted with bag-mask ventilation while he prepares for more definitive airway management. Ventilations should be timed with the patient's inhalation and allow sufficient time for chest recoil to occur before the next breath. The volume of the assisted ventilation should provide adequate chest rise when combined with the patient's natural breath.

If a tension pneumothorax is suspected, the Paramedic should proceed with a needle thoracostomy, placing a large bore needle that is at least 5 cm long in the second intercostal

Table 11-3 Signs and Symptom Complexes Suggestive of a Tension Pneumothorax (Not All Need to Be Present)

- Severe dyspnea
- Decreased pulse oximetry on high-flow, high-concentration supplemental oxygen
- Hypotension
- Elevated jugular venous pressure
- Absence of breath sounds on the affected side
- Hyperresonant percussion note on the affected side
- Penetrating trauma to the wound over the affected side

space at the midclavicular line. For the vast majority of adults, a regular venous catheter normally used for intravenous access has insufficient length to penetrate the thoracic cavity.[5] Ideally, a kit that contains a sufficiently long large bore needle, a flutter valve or Heimlich valve, tubing, and a means to secure the catheter should be used. The **Heimlich valve** may be attached to portable suction to allow complete re-expansion of the lung during transport.

Open pneumothorax should be treated with an occlusive dressing. Alternatively, a regular dressing can be used if secured in a manner that leaves one side or one corner open to act as a **flutter valve** (a one-way valve used to prevent air from returning into the thoracic cavity). The Paramedic must constantly reassess the patient to ensure the open pneumothorax has not progressed to a tension pneumothorax. If a flail segment is present, it should be stabilized with a bulky dressing secured in place to help splint that segment and restore near normal chest wall motion.

Adequate Circulation

The Paramedic's final key factor in providing adequate oxygen delivery to the tissues lies in ensuring adequate circulation. In the setting of the critically injured patient, this may be challenging for two main reasons. The first reason is that, in the setting of uncontrolled hemorrhage, liberal fluid administration (a mainstay in the treatment of most other classifications of shock) can produce several consequences that may ultimately worsen the patient's outcome. The second reason lies in the identification of shock other than hemorrhagic shock as the underlying cause of the patient's poor perfusion. It is easy for the Paramedic to overlook an underlying medical condition that may have preceded the traumatic event by becoming focused on the injury itself.

Assessment

Skin color and capillary refill are early indicators that a patient has poor perfusion and is in shock, even with a relatively normal blood pressure and heart rate. In younger patients without underlying medical conditions, the previously discussed compensatory mechanisms may work well enough to maintain vital signs within a normal range while the patient demonstrates poor peripheral perfusion. In these healthy patients, the sympathetic nervous system activation from blood loss may raise the pulse rate from 60 beats per minute to 90 beats per minute, markedly improving the cardiac output while the pulse is still considered within the normal range. Yet, that sympathetic nervous system activation will cause enough peripheral vasoconstriction for the patient to demonstrate pallor and decreased capillary refill.

The blood pressure may also provide an early indication of shock in the injured patient. Sympathetic nervous system activation has a greater effect on the more muscular arterial system and less of an effect on the venous system. When auscultating the blood pressure of a patient who is in early compensated shock, the Paramedic will observe the systolic pressure at near normal or at the lower end of normal, whereas the diastolic blood pressure will be low. This widened pulse pressure is indicative of hemodynamically significant blood loss, further supported by a high normal or low tachycardiac heart rate.

Uncontrolled hemorrhage should always be assumed to cause hemodynamic instability. For example, scalp injuries can easily seep through loose bandages and dressings over time, resulting in significant blood loss and shock due to poor bleeding control.

Although hemorrhagic shock is by far the most common cause of shock in the critically injured patient, neurogenic shock is another likely cause. It may be difficult to determine the difference between the two in the patient who is unconscious and not responsive. For example, a conscious patient can indicate deficits in sensation that cannot be appreciated in a patient who cannot speak. Likewise, a patient who has an altered mental status may not be able to follow commands when the Paramedic is performing a physical exam, making it difficult to appreciate extremity weakness or cranial nerve injury. In this situation, the Paramedic needs to utilize his observation skills to pay attention to any voluntary movement of the extremities. Palpation of the extremities may also provide the Paramedic with a sense of muscle tone, which will be flaccid immediately after the spinal cord injury. Although spinal cord injuries are traditionally thought of as having a discrete level below which there is no sensation or motor function, in reality most spinal cord injuries are either incomplete or secondary to cord contusions that may not present in a classic pattern. This, combined with injuries to the nerve plexuses in the axilla and the pelvis, may produce conflicting information on the neurologic examination.

The sympathetic nervous system pathways utilize the spinal cord as the means for distributing the sympathetic nerves through the body. Because of this, a spinal cord injury will disrupt the sympathetic nervous system below the injury, causing the vessels supplied by the sympathetic nerves to relax and return to their normal size. This allows blood to pool in the skin below the injury, while the baroreceptors in the aortic arch and the carotid bodies detect a drop in blood pressure from the redistribution of blood. The sympathetic nervous system is activated and constricts the vessels supplied by nerves above the level of injury. Clinically, when the Paramedic examines the patient, he will see warm, pink skin below the level of the injury and cool, clammy, pale skin above the level of the injury. This is one recognizable sign in an obtunded patient that hypotension is likely due to a spinal cord injury.

Management Plan

In the setting of hemorrhagic shock, two main treatments help stabilize and resuscitate the critically injured patient. These two interventions involve stopping any external bleeding and providing fluid resuscitation using either crystalloid fluids (normal saline or lactated Ringer's) or blood products.

Hemorrhage Control

Control of bleeding is an integral step in resuscitation. If external bleeding is not controlled, further fluid resuscitation will only worsen blood loss. Heavy venous bleeding can, in a short period of time, add up to hemodynamically significant blood loss. Scalp wounds are notorious for profuse bleeding. Therefore, the Paramedic should take care to provide sufficient bandaging to scalp wounds to minimize blood loss. This may include pressure on wounds on the upper scalp that are at risk for developing large hematomas under the scalp. Because the head is also a large area responsible for heat loss, large bleeding scalp wounds can contribute to hypothermia, which can impair coagulation.

Tourniquets, once relegated to last resort situations, have become more important in hemorrhage control of the extremities. Much of the data that led to this paradigm shift comes from military research; however, the issue of uncontrolled extremity hemorrhage from penetrating trauma is also an issue in civilian medicine.[6] Data from the Iraqi and Afghanistan conflicts demonstrated improved survival when tourniquets were used for extremity hemorrhage.[7] In one study, survival was significantly improved if the tourniquet was applied before the patient became hypotensive. These studies also demonstrated that the complications often cited as the reason for deferring tourniquet use until last resort—including unintended loss of limb, long-term neurologic deficits, renal failure, and muscle damage—were no higher in the group that had tourniquets applied than the group that didn't.[8]

In combat situations, the Tactical Combat Casualty Care Course recommends applying a tourniquet first for any extremity bleeding except for minor bleeding.[9] Once the casualty is evacuated to a safe location, the need for a tourniquet can be reassessed. This recommendation recognizes that, during care under fire, it can be hazardous to both the combat medic and the casualty to follow the traditional direct pressure, elevation, and pressure point recommendations for hemorrhage control. In fact, one research study examining participants' abilities to completely occlude the femoral artery at the femoral pressure point found the average length of time a participant needed to apply enough pressure to stop blood flow as measured by a Doppler stethoscope on the pedal pulse was 20 seconds.[10] This study places in question the true feasibility of using pressure points as a means of hemorrhage control.

These studies led to the development of recommendations for civilian use of tourniquets (Figure 11-6).[11,12] These recommendations take into consideration the type of incident and estimated transport time. Recommendations for reassessment and removal are also included. In long transport situations, it is reasonable to reassess the limb for continued bleeding as it normally takes a clot approximately a half hour to stabilize. Once that clot has stabilized,

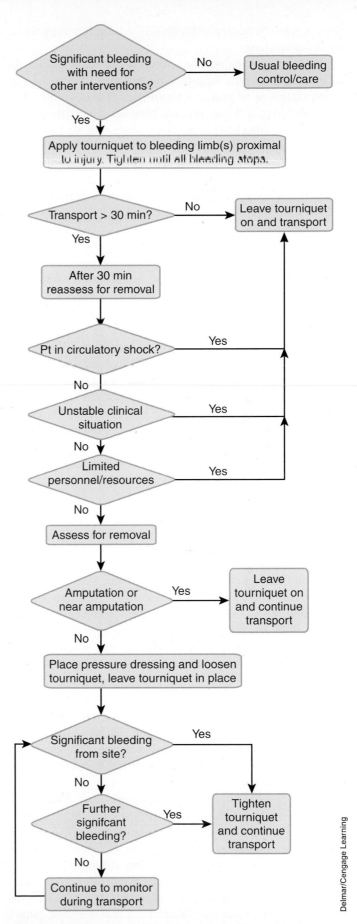

Figure 11-6 Algorithm for tourniquet use by civilian EMS.

bleeding may be controlled without the tourniquet, minimizing complications.

In essence, this algorithm suggests that, if the Paramedic is faced with a vigorously flowing extremity bleed, the recommendation is to utilize a tourniquet first to gain control of the bleeding, and then provide bandaging and other bleeding control methods. If a commercially available tourniquet is not available, a blood pressure cuff inflated 20 to 30 mmHg above the patient's systolic blood pressure can be used to gain control. Most blood pressure cuffs, however, are not able to maintain a constant pressure for an extended period of time and will likely need to be reinflated.

Fluid Resuscitation

The second main treatment to support the critically injured patient's circulatory system is fluid resuscitation. Herein lies two decades of debate that has gravitated toward a minimal fluid resuscitation strategy in the setting of uncontrolled hemorrhage.

It was recognized in both World War I[13] and World War II,[14] at least in young, fit soldiers, that hypotension could be tolerated for prolonged periods of time while the soldier was awaiting surgery for presumed intra-abdominal bleeding. In fact, hypotension was thought to be protective, effectively slowing down bleeding and allowing the coagulation cascade to work.

Resuscitation research focusing on hemorrhagic shock in the 1950s used a model that was not reflective of the typical timeline that occurs when a patient sustains an injury with intra-abdominal or intrathoracic bleeding. The model used involved inducing bleeding in the subject animal (e.g., pig, dog, rat), and then allowing the animal to bleed to lose a pre-determined volume of blood—typically enough to put the animal in class III or class IV shock. Once that volume was reached, bleeding was stopped and fluid resuscitation began.[15] Using this model, animals had better outcomes with high volume fluid resuscitation. This high volume fluid resuscitation strategy formed the basis for the traditional administration of 2 liters of crystalloid fluid into critically injured patients, which the U.S. military used during the Vietnam conflict. Interestingly, during the Vietnam conflict, while soldiers were surviving to the intensive care unit, many were developing what was called at the time "Da Nang Lung." This was eventually recognized as adult respiratory distress syndrome (ARDS), and many deaths occurred later in the course of trauma treatment because of it.[16]

There are two camps in the debate over fluid resuscitation. The traditional camp follows the high volume resuscitation recommended by animal research from the 1950s that was carried out during the Vietnam conflict. In contrast, the **permissive hypotension** camp subscribes to more controlled fluid resuscitation using physiologic measures to determine the need for administration of additional fluid. The crux of the traditional fluid resuscitation camp's argument is to maintain a near normal blood pressure to maintain organ perfusion, recognizing that prolonged ischemia can have devastating consequences, especially to the intestines and kidneys. The permissive hypotension camp argues that hypotension is protective, as it lowers the blood pressure enough to allow the coagulation system to work at stabilizing any clots that have formed. This action may temporarily stop internal bleeding until the bleed can be surgically corrected. This debate centers only on patients with uncontrolled hemorrhage. Patients whose hemorrhage is controlled (e.g., injuries on an extremity) may benefit from more aggressive fluid resuscitation.

Animal research on fluid resuscitation in hemorrhagic shock that began in the 1980s used a different model than the previous research in the 1950s. The predominant model used induces bleeding in the animal, allows the animal to bleed for a certain period of time, initiates fluid resuscitation, and then controls bleeding.[15] The timing used in these experiments better reflects the typical prehospital and hospital phase of treatment. In one well-conducted study in which bleeding was initiated with a tear in the pig's aorta, the researchers captured the blood volume and measured a bleeding rate. As the pig became hypotensive, the bleeding rate decreased until it was minimal and the pig's blood pressure stabilized. As fluid resuscitation began, once the systolic blood pressure climbed to about 80 mmHg, 76% of the pigs started bleeding again.[17] Multiple studies consistently demonstrated significant rebleeding rates once the systolic blood pressure was greater than 80 to 90 mmHg or the mean arterial pressure rose above 60 mmHg. Regardless of the type of fluid used, the rise in blood pressure was felt to disrupt the newly formed clot that had essentially reduced bleeding and stabilized the patient.

There are other consequences to high volume fluid administration. Administration of as little as 750 mL of intravenous fluid will dilute clotting factors remaining within the circulatory system, impairing the body's ability to continue to form and stabilize clots. Not only are clotting factors diluted, but the red blood cells in the blood are diluted, further decreasing oxygen-carrying capacity. Combine diluted clotting factors and hemoglobin with an increased blood pressure that disrupts clots that are in the process of stabilizing and the stage is set for the cyclic resuscitation of additional bleeding, hypotension, fluid administration, normalization of blood pressure, and additional bleeding.

High volume intravenous fluid administration also activates the cytokine system and inflammatory system response. Some cytokines attach to coagulation factors, further impeding the coagulation cascade's function and increasing bleeding time. The inflammatory processes serve to increase the permeability of capillary vessel walls, allowing plasma to leak out of the circulatory system and into the interstitial space. This capillary leak is most profound in the kidneys, lung, and intestines. In the lung, the capillary leak causes fluid to move into the interstitial space between the alveoli and the pulmonary capillaries, impeding oxygen and carbon dioxide exchange at a microscopic level and at a macroscopic level, making the lungs more difficult to ventilate. In the kidneys, the fluid leaking into the interstitial space impairs the kidneys' ability to filter the blood and produce urine, sending the patient into acute renal failure. Capillary leak in the intestines allows enough fluid to move into the abdominal cavity that the pressure within the abdominal cavity elevates to the point where the pressure causes ischemia of the bowel. The capillary leak also provides a pathway for bacteria to move from inside the intestines, where bacteria normally exist, into the peritoneal cavity, placing the patient at risk for an infection. Once this inflammatory process begins, it cannot be stopped. With aggressive supportive care, some patients will recover; however, the mortality rate is very high.[18]

One clinical trial studying hypotensive patients who sustained penetrating trauma to the torso, undertaken in Houston and published in 1994, is the only controlled trial addressing the issue of fluid resuscitation. Hypotensive patients who were picked up by Paramedics on even days underwent traditional fluid resuscitation including two large bore intravenous lines and rapid administration of up to 2 liters of lactated Ringer's. On odd days, patients did not receive any intravenous fluids from Paramedics or from the emergency department, with fluid resuscitation beginning once the surgeon had controlled the internal bleeding. The patients in the second group had a higher survival-to-discharge rate, fewer complications, and a shorter hospital course than the patients who were in the traditional fluid resuscitation group.[19]

One group of patients of special concern are those who have a traumatic brain injury and are hypotensive. Even one episode of hypotension increases the morbidity of patients who have a traumatic brain injury. In this situation, the mean arterial pressure is insufficient to overcome intracranial pressure and provide adequate cerebral blood flow. When the brain becomes ischemic, as occurs from the global decrease in cerebral blood flow, the brain swells. Because the skull is rigid, this swelling further elevates intracranial pressure and decreases cerebral blood flow. In these patients, the Paramedic will need to keep the systolic blood pressure at approximately 100 mmHg, rather than the 80 to 90 mmHg target range normally used in hypotensive patients (Table 11-4).

During the Iraqi and Afghanistan conflicts, military physicians have utilized various massive transfusion treatment pathways. They recognize that in some critically injured soldiers, blood loss is so extensive that multiple transfusions are required within a short period of time in order to replace blood loss. Although a unit of packed red blood cells replaces the oxygen-carrying capacity of blood, it is usually devoid of clotting factors, platelets, and other blood proteins. If clotting factors are not replaced, the patient's

Table 11-4 Recommended Endpoints when Following Limited Fluid Resuscitation (Permissive Hypotension)

Administer small boluses of intravenous crystalloid (25 to 250 mL) until reaching one of the following endpoints:
- Palpable radial pulse
- Appropriate mentation in a non-head-injured patient
- Mean arterial pressure of 40 to 60 mmHg or a systolic blood pressure of 80 to 90 mmHg (MAP > 60 mmHg in patients with suspected traumatic brain injury)

clotting factors eventually are depleted and massive hemorrhage recurs. In a 2009 article, the authors noted that many studies recommend replacing blood, fresh frozen plasma, and platelets unit for unit in order to replace clotting factors and platelets in addition to red blood cells.[20] The Paramedic may encounter this treatment pathway when transferring a critically injured patient from a community hospital to a trauma center.

Neurogenic Shock

Neurogenic shock, a form of distributive shock, generally responds poorly to intravenous fluid administration. Depending upon the location of the spinal injury and in the absence of additional bleeding, many of these patients will have a systolic blood pressure that remains in the 90 to 100 mmHg range and is able to perfuse the brain. If the spinal cord injury is higher or the neurogenic shock is caused by hemorrhage in the brain, then vasopressor medications may be required in order to raise the blood pressure to an adequate level. In these situations, the vasopressor of choice in neurogenic shock is either norepinephrine or phenylephrine. These vasopressors act purely on the alpha-adrenergic receptors that produce vasoconstriction and generally do not significantly elevate the heart rate as can happen with dopamine or dobutamine. If neither of those vasopressors is available, then dopamine is a reasonable choice until the others become available.

Adrenal Insufficiency

Patients with a history of adrenal insufficiency may not be able to mount an appropriate stress response when faced with critical injuries. These patients often carry a medical alert bracelet or card advising the Paramedic of this condition. Many patients carry a kit with injectable steroids they can self-administer in the event of a crisis. If there is an indication that the critically injured patient has adrenal insufficiency, then the Paramedic should consider administering intravenous hydrocortisone 100 mg or methylprednisolone (Solumedrol®) 125 mg in addition to the treatments discussed previously.

"Rookie, you did good!" the trainer says as she pats the Paramedic on the back. "Let's review the call, shall we?" she says as she begins to wash her hands. The patient's gunshot wound is to the chest. The patient, an apparent victim of his own weapon turned against him by would-be robbers, is conscious on arrival, but just barely. His airway is currently patent, although several pellets to the patient's throat made the rookie Paramedic nervous. The brunt of the blast is located to the anterior chest on the right side. Breath sounds are diminished, but the patient has a strong, albeit rapid, radial pulse.

The first change that alerted the rookie Paramedic to the developing tension pneumothorax is the weakening radial pulse, which he re-checked often. In addition, the patient's oxygen saturations were dropping despite the administration of high-flow, high-concentration oxygen via nonbreather mask. After consultation with his field training officer, the Paramedic performed a needle thoracostomy. The patient's relief is almost immediate.

CRITICAL THINKING QUESTIONS

1. What other injuries are predictable for a close proximity shotgun blast?
2. What is the most appropriate transport decision that will get the patient to definitive care?

CONCLUSION

This chapter presented a holistic approach to the critically injured patient. The key to effectively managing a critically injured patient who has sustained multiple system trauma is to ensure the patient has a patent airway, is well oxygenated, is well ventilated, and has adequate circulation to perfuse the brain. Following these basic factors will help the Paramedic effectively manage these critical patients.

KEY POINTS:

- Shock is the body's inability to get oxygen to the cells.

- Oxygenation, ventilation, and respiration are part of shock.

- Neurogenic shock is the result of vasodilation.

- Hemorrhage leads to loss of preload, stroke volume, and cardiac output.

- Baroreceptors sense the loss in blood pressure.

- Circulating epinephrine is secreted to augment the sympathetic nervous system.

- The hematopoietic system replaces lost blood volume.

- Decompensation is the result of acidemia.

- The primary assessment details the order of assessment and treatment.

- Tension pneumothorax is a treatable life threat.

- Profound extremity hemorrhage is best controlled by tourniquet.

- Titrated fluid resuscitation and permissive hypotension have become the standard of care.

- Hypotension must be treated aggressively in the traumatically brain-injured patient.

- Neurogenic shock is a form of distributive shock.

- Norepinephrine, phenylephrine or dopamine, not fluid resuscitation, is the treatment for neurogenic shock.

- Patients with adrenal insufficiency will need additional support during the treatment of shock including injectable steroids.

REVIEW QUESTIONS:

1. What assessments "made from the doorway" suggest the need for immediate transport of the critically ill patient?
2. What are the signs of a tension pneumothorax?
3. Explain the paradigm shift that suggests tourniquets are superior to previous methods of bleeding control.
4. Explain the concept of permissive hypotension.
5. What are the clinical endpoints for the administration of fluids during resuscitation of the shock–trauma patient?

CASE STUDY QUESTIONS:

Please refer to the Case Study in this chapter, and answer the questions below:

1. Assuming the shotgun wound is to the head, what is the predictable injury pattern based on the mechanism of injury?
2. Assuming the shotgun wound is to the chest, what is the predictable injury pattern based on the mechanism of injury?
3. Assuming the shotgun wound is to the abdomen, what is the predictable injury pattern based on the mechanism of injury?

REFERENCES:

1. Davis DP, Hoyt DB, Ochs M, et al. The effect of Paramedic rapid-sequence intubation on outcome in patients with severe traumatic brain injury. *J Trauma*. 2003;54:444–453.

2. Robertson C. Desaturation episodes after severe head injury: influence on outcome. *Acta Neurochirurgica Supplementum*. 1993;59:98–101.

3. Wang H. Out of hospital endotracheal intubation—where are we now? *An Emer Med*. 2006;47(6):532–541.

4. Stephens SW, Brown T, Cofield SS. Value of multiple prehospital intubation attempts. *Prehosp Emerg Care*. 2007;11(1):123.

5. Ball CG, Wyrzykowski AD, Kirkpatrick AW, et al. Thoracic needle decompression for tension pneumothorax: clinical correlation with catheter length. Canadian Journal of Surgery 2010 53(3):184-188.

6. Dorlac WC, DeBakey ME, Holcomb JB, et al. Mortality from isolated civilian penetrating extremity injury. *J Trauma*. 2005;59(1):217–222.

7. Kragh JF, Walters TJ, Baer DG, et al. Survival with emergency tourniquet use to stop bleeding in major limb trauma. Annals of Surgery 2009;249(1):1–7.

8. Kragh JF, Walters TJ, Baer DG, et al. Practical use of emergency tourniquets to stop bleeding in major limb trauma. *J Trauma*. 2008;64(2 Supplement):S38–S50.

9. National Association of EMTs. Tactical Combat Casualty Care Course. Available at: **http://www.naemt.org/education/ PHTLS/TCCC.**aspx. Accessed February 10, 2010.

10. Swan KG, Wright DS, Barbagiovanni SS, et al. Tourniquets revisited. *J Trauma*. 2009;66(3):672–675.

11. Doyle GS, Taillac PP. Tourniquets: a review of current use with proposals for expanded prehospital use. *Prehosp Emerg Care*. 2008;12(2):241–256.

12. Lee C, Porter KM, Hodgetts TJ. Tourniquet use in the civilian prehospital setting. *Emerg Med J*. 2008;24(8):584–587.

13. Cannon WB, Fraser J, Cowell EB. The preventative treatment of wound shock. *JAMA*. 1918;70(9):618–621.

14. Beecher HK. *Resuscitation and Anesthesia for Wounded Men: the Management of Traumatic Shock*. Springfield, IL. Charles Thomas; 1949.

15. Stern SA. Low volume fluid resuscitation for presumed hemorrhagic shock: helpful or harmful? *Curr Opin Crit Care*. 2001;7(6):422–430.

16. Rhee P, Koustova E, Alam HB. Searching for the optimal resuscitation method: recommendations for the initial fluid resuscitation of combat casualties. *J Trauma*. 2003;54 (5 Supplement):S52–S62.

17. Dondeen JL, Coppes BS, Holcomb JB. Blood pressure at which rebleeding occurs after resuscitation in swine with aortic injury. *J Trauma*. 2003;54(5 Supplement):S110–S117.

18. Lenz A, Franklin GA, Cheadle WG. Systemic inflammation after trauma. *Injury*. 2007;38(12):1336–1345.

19. Bicknell WH, Wall MJ, Pepe PE, et al. Immediate versus delayed fluid resuscitation for hypotensive patients with penetrating torso injuries. *NEJM*. 1994;331(17):1105–1109.

20. Sihler KC, Napolitano LM. Massive transfusion: new insights. *Chest*. 2009;136(6):1654–1667.

SECTION 11

ENVIRONMENTAL MEDICINE

This section on environmental medicine discusses conditions requiring outdoor care, such as heat and cold emergencies, mountain medicine, water emergencies, and poisonous envenomations.

CHAPTER 12

HEAT EMERGENCIES

KEY CONCEPTS:

Upon completion of this chapter, it is expected that the reader will understand these following concepts:

- Spectrum of heat illnesses
- Pathophysiology of heat illness
- Two types of heat exhaustion
- Two types of heatstroke
- Field treatment of heatstroke
- Complications associated with heatstroke

ANATOMY CONCEPTS:

Prior to reading this chapter the Paramedic student should be familiar with the following anatomy and physiology concepts:

- Thermoregulation
- Oxyhemoglobin curve
- Oxidative phosphorylation

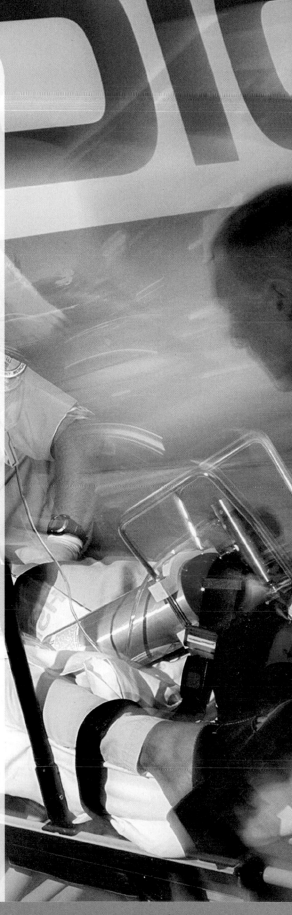

CASE STUDY:

Sean has always been interested in running. His passion for the sport started seven years ago when he joined his high school's cross-country team. He always placed high in the shorter events, but his endurance and stamina were issues in events over 5 kilometers. After graduation, Sean began endurance training to push his body and allow it to withstand extended stress. As an adult, and now in medical school, he has set his sights on competing in the New York City Marathon. But 26.2 miles through city streets is a daunting task; he knows he will have to condition his body to continue even after the brain is screaming to stop! Fortunately, most marathons are held during the fall, so heat is not much of a factor.

CRITICAL THINKING QUESTIONS

1. What are some possible causes of heat illness for a marathoner?
2. What type of heat illness would be most lethal on-scene?

OVERVIEW

Migrant field workers in southern California, steel workers in Pittsburgh, and a roofer in Montana all have one thing in common: a risk of heat illness. Heat illness claims more lives than all other weather-related emergencies combined.[1] In addition, heat illnesses are the second most common cause of death among high school athletes. Predominantly a summertime emergency, deaths from heat illness more commonly occur during a **heat wave** (two days of high heat [>90°F] and high humidity [>80% relative humidity]).

If left untreated, heat illnesses have a very high mortality. However, early recognition and prompt intervention by the Paramedic in the field can dramatically lower the mortality rate. To treat heat illnesses, the Paramedic must understand how the body adjusts to high temperatures, how the body can decompensate, and how the Paramedic can support the body in its efforts to regain homeostasis.

Chief Concern

High temperatures, high humidity, and dehydration cumulatively can create heat stress on the body. Unabated heat stress leads to a spectrum of heat illnesses ranging from heat exhaustion to deadly heatstroke. However, without some heat the body cannot function. A review of human physiology explains how the body maintains the warmth it needs in order to function.

Physiology Review

The body's regulatory systems attempt to maintain the body within a temperature range that averages around 98.6°F (37°C). The external environment (i.e., the ambient temperature and humidity surrounding the body) sometimes challenges the body with extra heat and/or interferes with the body's ability to dissipate heat. These challenges, collectively known as heat stress, are constantly monitored by the body's regulatory mechanisms. When heat stress is high, the body's regulatory mechanisms activate systems within the body to help maintain a near constant internal milieu or homeostasis.

The hypothalamus plays a major role in helping maintain homeostasis. The hypothalamus, located in the portion of the midbrain known as the diencephalon, senses temperature changes and sends chemical signals to the body, particularly the integumentary system, to respond to an increased internal core temperature.

The integumentary system is the largest organ system in the body. When stimulated by the hypothalamus, it has the ability to help maintain normal internal body temperature through heat generation or to increase heat loss through vasodilation and subsequent radiation (evaporation of sweat). To accomplish this, the anterior hypothalamus stimulates the parasympathetic nervous system to stimulate muscarinic receptors (one of the two cholinergic receptors). The muscarinic receptors in turn stimulate blood vessels in the skin and the eccrine glands (also known as sudoriferous glands)

located in the dermal layer of the skin to produce sweat. The creation of sweat lowers the body's core temperature, as evaporation of sweat lowers surface temperature and, along with radiation, cools the body. As the body cools and the internal core temperature drops, the anterior hypothalamus stops sending signals to the parasympathetic receptors in the skin and the person stops sweating (Figure 12-1). This process is known as a feedback loop that continues as long as the brain senses it needs to lose heat (positive feedback).

Evaporative Heat Loss

Sweat is comprised primarily of water. The transport ion that is responsible for getting water to the skin's surface is sodium. The body uses this natural "attraction" to excrete water to

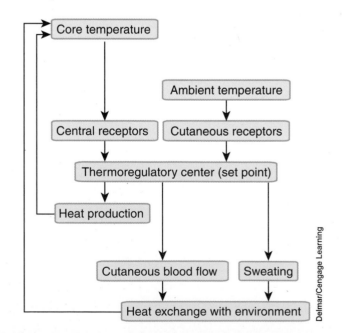

Figure 12-1 A relationship exists between the body's ambient temperature and core temperature.

the skin surface. The ionic concentration of sweat is normally sodium 0.9 g/L, potassium 0.2 g/L, calcium 0.015 g/L, and magnesium 0.0013 g/L.[2]

As sweat reaches the skin surface, it evaporates into the atmosphere, taking heat with it. During this process, called **thermolysis**, the dissipated heat lowers the body's internal core temperature. The movement of sodium and water out of the body lowers the core body temperature, but it also begins the process of dehydration. Sodium is vital for muscle contraction, both cardiac and skeletal, and loss of these electrolytes can have physiological consequences as well.

Heat Index

The key to body cooling is evaporation, which works best in low humidity and low temperatures. When temperature and humidity climb, there is a point where evaporation stops. When evaporation stops, the person retains the heat and is at risk for heat illness.

The **heat index**, sometimes called the misery index, is a function of ambient temperature and humidity (Figure 12-2). Combining these factors creates a "perceived" temperature. For example, although the temperature may only be 86°F (30°C), if the humidity is 90% then it will feel like it is 105°F (40.6°C). Anytime the perceived temperature is over

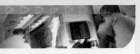
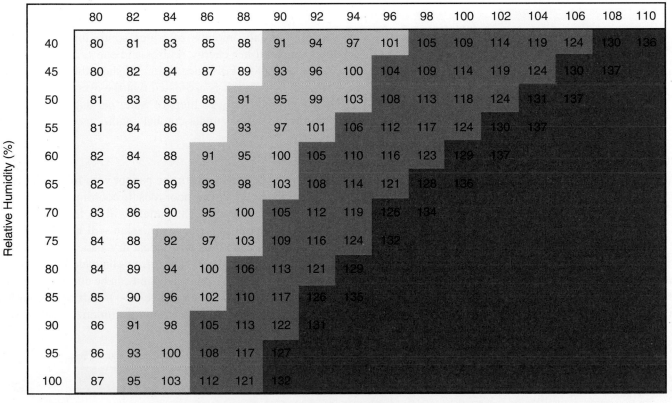

Temperature (°F)

Relative Humidity (%)	80	82	84	86	88	90	92	94	96	98	100	102	104	106	108	110
40	80	81	83	85	88	91	94	97	101	105	109	114	119	124	130	136
45	80	82	84	87	89	93	96	100	104	109	114	119	124	130	137	
50	81	83	85	88	91	95	99	103	108	113	118	124	131	137		
55	81	84	86	89	93	97	101	106	112	117	124	130	137			
60	82	84	88	91	95	100	105	110	116	123	129	137				
65	82	85	89	93	98	103	108	114	121	128	136					
70	83	86	90	95	100	105	112	119	126	134						
75	84	88	92	97	103	109	116	124	132							
80	84	89	94	100	106	113	121	129								
85	85	90	96	102	110	117	126	135								
90	86	91	98	105	113	122	131									
95	86	93	100	108	117	127										
100	87	95	103	112	121	132										

Likelihood of Heat Disorders with Prolonged Exposure or Strenuous Activity

☐ Caution   ☐ Extreme Caution   ■ Danger   ■ Extreme Danger

Delmar/Cengage Learning

Figure 12-2 The National Oceanic and Atmospheric Administration (NOAA) heat index is a function of ambient temperature and humidity.

105°F (40.6°C), the patient is at risk for heat illness. When the heat index climbs to 130°F (54.5°C), the patient is at risk for heatstroke.

Pathophysiology of Hyperthermia

Hyperthermia interferes with cellular metabolism, specifically the sodium–potassium pump. Most chemical reactions in the body are pH dependent, and the body tries to maintain the pH within a very narrow range of 7.35 to 7.45. Normally, the sodium pump moves sodium out of the cell. Increased heat, and subsequent cell shrinkage, causes the cells to lose sodium and elevate sodium levels in the blood. As a result, any sodium-dependent action potentials (such as nerve conduction and muscle contraction) are affected and the person loses strength, has diminished reflexes, and has an altered sensorium overall.

Increased heat leads to loss of intracellular water. The subsequent cell shrinkage directly affects the cell's structure, with formation of blebs on the cell wall, swelling of mitochondria, and collapse of the cytoskeleton, all of which lead to cell destruction.

The effect of hyperthermia is particularly problematic for red blood cells. When exposed to heat, red blood cells change shape from a disc to a sphere. This spherical shape is much less efficient in carrying oxygen. Coupled with a shift in the oxyhemoglobin curve, the patient suffers hypoxia and experiences anxiety and agitation.[4]

STREET SMART

Heat stress can induce a sickle cell crisis in a patient with sickle cell disease. As the cell volume decreases, the hemoglobin starts to sickle. Sickling collapse has been listed as a contributing cause in the deaths of 10 college football players. These athletes often collapse in the first few minutes of exertion, remain conscious, but succumb later.[5]

Heat Illness

When heat stressors overtake the body's ability to compensate, a heat illness occurs. Heat illness can occur as a result of increased external heat stressors (high temperature and/or high humidity), increased internal heat production, or decreased capacity to dissipate heat.

The obvious cause of heat illness is extremes of heat. However, an individual's response to heat stress is varied and may be attributed to pre-existing dehydration, salt depletion, and pathologic hyperventilation. Certain medical conditions and medications can excerbate heat illness as well (discussed further in the "History" section).

Heat illnesses are not separate entities with unique pathologies, but rather artificial delineations along a continuum of heat illnesses that serve to help the Paramedic decide treatment priorities (Figure 12-3). Therefore, heat illness should be seen as a continuum that starts with heat fatigue, proceeds to heat exhaustion, and ends with heatstroke. An analogy can be made comparing heat illness to shock, which can be categorized as compensated, decompensated, and irreversible.

Heat Fatigue

The onset of heat illness can be insidious, starting with **heat fatigue**. The patient may notice a decline in coordination and difficulty with task performance. However, it is also possible that the only symptom the patient may experience is weakness. These behaviors are warning signs of impending heat exhaustion.

To prevent heat exhaustion, and treat heat fatigue, the patient should stop working, get out of the sun, and drink small amounts of water. The patient should be encouraged to drink small amounts of water approximately every 15 minutes until her energy returns and she is able to perform complex motor skills once again. To show the importance of staying hydrated, it is estimated that the average soldier will need approximately 16 liters of water per day during routine summer operations under combat conditions.

Heat Exhaustion

The classic presentation for the patient with **heat exhaustion** is generalized weakness, poor muscle coordination, and alterations in mental status. The patient will be tachycardic and tachypneic but normotensive. The skin will have poor turgor and mucous membranes will appear dry. Patients with accompanying dehydration will have furrows on their tongue as well.

The etiology of heat exhaustion can be due to either water depletion or salt depletion (Table 12-1). **Salt depletion heat exhaustion** usually occurs in non-acclimatized patients and

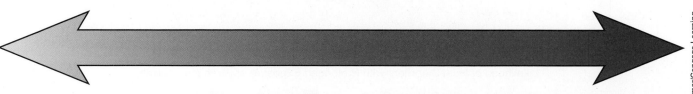

Heat fatigue–Heat exhaustion–Heat syncope–Heat cramps–Heatstroke–Anhydrosis–Exertional rhabdomyolysis

Delmar/Cengage Learning

Figure 12-3 The continuum of heat illnesses serves to help the Paramedic decide treatment priorities.

Table 12-1 Symptom Pattern Heat Exhaustion: Salt Depletion versus Water Depletion

Signs and Symptoms	Salt Depletion	Water Depletion
Acclimatized	No	Yes
Thirst	No	Yes
Nausea	Yes	Yes
Vomiting	Yes	No

can also occur during prolonged periods of strenuous exercise in even temperate temperatures. The salinity of the sweat secreted is high, leading to systemic hyponatremia.

Patients with salt depletion heat exhaustion often do not complain of thirst and have nausea with vomiting. Muscle cramps accompany the majority of cases of salt depletion heat exhaustion.

Conversely, **water depletion heat exhaustion** occurs when the person fails, either voluntarily or involuntarily, to replace fluid losses. These patients often complain of thirst and may be nauseous but generally do not vomit. These patients present as hyperthermic, tachycardic, and hyperventilating.

A key finding that may differentiate heat fatigue from heat exhaustion is orthostatic hypotension. Although true orthostatic hypotension is the result of autonomic failure, secondary orthostatic hypotension may occur if the patient has heat exhaustion, especially if the patient is dehydrated as well.

Heat syncope can be a warning sign of heat exhaustion. As much as eight (8) pints (3.8 liters) of blood can be shunted to the skin to radiate heat. To prevent systemic hypotension and subsequent syncope, the blood flow to the spleen and muscles is shut down, thus explaining the lethargy that accompanies heat exhaustion. Simultaneously, the heart rate increases as well as the stroke volume, leading to greater cardiac output. If the patient was previously dehydrated, has impaired hemodynamic regulation vis-á-vis cardiac disease, or takes medications such as diuretics or beta blockers, these compensatory mechanisms may be insufficient. The result is heat-related syncope.[4]

The treatment of heat exhaustion focuses on whether the heat exhaustion is due to salt depletion or water depletion. Those with salt depletion heat exhaustion are treated with electrolyte replenishment. Patients with water depletion heat exhaustion are treated with fluid replacement.

For patients suspected to have water depletion heat exhaustion, judicious administration of 1 to 2 liters of normal saline over a period of hours is routine. However, caution should be exercised. Too rapid administration of intravenous fluid can lead to dilutional hyponatremia and cerebral edema with an increase in intracranial pressure and a possiblity of seizures.

Heat Cramps

Heat cramps (muscle spasms due to loss of water or sodium) often accompany heat exhaustion (in as many as 60% of cases). Three antecedent conditions must be met before heat cramps occur: (1) The patient must work at a sustained pace for several hours, (2) the patient must sweat profusely, and (3) the patient must drink large volumes of water. The resultant cramps of the skeletal muscles are painful and localized, and can occur in several large muscle groups including the thighs and the abdomen.

Heat cramps occur after exposure to heat (e.g., in the evening), and often occur when the muscles are cooled in the shower. Although not a prehospital emergency, in most cases Paramedics should be familiar with heat cramps in case they encounter them during extended operations. Typically the treatment of heat cramps is 0.1% saline solution orally (PO) or two crushed salt tablets in 1 liter of water) or intravenous administration of normal saline at a volume of 10 mL/kg.

Heatstroke

At the extreme of the continuum of heat illness is heatstroke (sunstroke). Heatstroke is a potentially lethal condition that can be broken down into two varieties: exertional and classic heatstroke (Table 12-2).

Exertional heatstroke (EHS) is, as the name suggests, the result of strenuous physical activity. The normal basilar rate of heat production is about 100 kcal/hr. However, during periods of exertion, the rate can reach 1,000 kcal/hr. If this activity occurs outdoors and in the sun, an additional 150 kcal/hr can be added. Through evaporation of sweat, the human body can dissipate up to 600 kcal/hr, assuming a relative humidity less than 75%.[6] The cumulative impact of the endogenous heat and the environmental heat overwhelms the body's capacity for thermolysis through evaporation and radiation. As a result, the patient develops heatstroke.[7]

Persons at risk for EHS are athletes at summer session, new military recruits in boot camp, rookie firefighter/police recruits in academy, and other unacclimatized and unconditioned individuals. Factors that place these populations at

Table 12-2 Classic versus Exertional Heatstroke

	Classic	Exertional
Presentation		
Age	Elderly	Adult male
Health	Chronic illness	Fit
MOI	Dyshomeostasis	Exogenous heat
Symptom		
Sweating	Anhydrosis	Diaphoresis
Medications		
	Diuretics, antipsychotics, antihypertensives	None
Complications		
Renal failure	< 5%	25% to 30%
Rhabdomyolysis*	Rare	Common

Note: *Discussed later in the chapter.

greater risk include obesity, dehydration, lack of sleep, and use of sympathomimetics.

Nonexertional heatstroke (classic heatstroke) is usually seen in elderly patients who, because of medical conditions or age, are unable to compensate for a change in temperature and/or humidity. Patients at risk are the infirmed who are unable to control their environment, those with cardiovascular disease who lack reserve, and those on certain medications, which are discussed shortly. The symptom triad for classic heatstroke is hyperthermia, altered mental status, and **anhydrosis** (a lack of sweat).

Special Case of Malignant Hyperthermia

Certain medications can cause a malignant hyperthermia. For example, certain individuals with a genetic predisposition can have an episode of life-threatening hyperthermia triggered by certain anesthetics. Of concern for Paramedics are the depolarizing agents, such as succinylcholine.

Untreated malignant hyperthermia is a medical emergency that has been associated with a 70% mortality rate. The Paramedic might suspect malignant hyperthermia when the patient demonstrates muscle rigidity following administration of succinylcholine, a state not expected with a paralytic. Masseter muscle spasm may also occur and is associated with malignant hyperthermia. The third indicator of malignant hyperthermia is a marked increase in end-tidal CO_2 (i.e., an increase that is two to three times normal). Treatment for malignant hyperthermia begins with stopping the succinylcholine, inducing hyperventilation with the goal to return end-tidal carbon dioxide to within a normal range, and transporting the patient. Hospitals with an operating room will have the medication dantrolene available to treat malignant hyperthermia, although dantrolene is ineffective in treating routine heatstroke.[8]

CASE STUDY (CONTINUED)

"Man down on the route" blares dispatch through the radio. The two Paramedics from Unit 9 were the first on the scene where a runner had collapsed next to the checkpoint. The runner, Sean, is lying on the road. Witnesses say he collapsed but they do not think he passed out. The first action the Paramedics do is remove Sean from the hot pavement. They know that pavement is a heat sink and will radiate heat, increasing the ambient temperature and worsening the heat illness.

Although slow to react, Sean is able to answer some questions. As a medical student, Sean understands the importance of history in the care of a patient, so he does his best to answer every question. Yes, he thought he had adequately hydrated. No, he did not drink any water while on the course. Yes, he had prepared for the race. Yes, he is nauseous but he has not vomited.

Sean is insistent that he is alright and just wants to finish the race. However, when he tries to stand up he passes out. The Paramedics know what they have to do. One calls for a "bus" to the checkpoint to transport the patient while the other starts her assessment.

CRITICAL THINKING QUESTIONS

1. What are the important elements of the history that a Paramedic should obtain for a patient experiencing a heat emergency?
2. What is the importance of the history?

History

Often the first step in ascertaining if a heat illness exists is determining if the patient is one of the populations at risk. Populations at highest risk for heat illness are those in construction (roofers, highway workers), agriculture (farmers), and restaurant work (kitchen workers). Others at risk include foundry workers, plant operators, bakers, and laundry workers.[3] Public safety workers, and especially firefighters, are also at risk for heat illness. The turnout gear of a firefighter, with NFPA 1971 vapor barriers, can increase the endogenous heat load by 500% in some cases.

Exertional heatstroke is preceded by exercise, and the largest percentage of patients with heat illness are laborers.[9] Exertional heatstroke is typically seen in younger males and in greater numbers among African Americans.

In one OSHA study, almost one-half of the heat illnesses occurred on the first day on the job, and 80% occurred within the first four days on the job.[10] This may have been due to a lack of acclimatization. Over time, workers become used to the heat (acclimatization). This is a function of the body's adaptation. The kidneys retain more salt and water, the body sweats faster, and the sweat contains less salt. The process of acclimatization takes one to two weeks to occur. In the interim, the person is at increased risk for heat illness. In 1986, the National Institute for Occupational Safety and Health (NIOSH) suggested progressively longer periods of work in hot conditions, a program of acclimatization.[11]

STREET SMART

It takes an overweight person 50% longer to acclimatize than a fit person. Therefore, obese patients are at greater risk of heat illness during a heat wave than the average person.

Classic heatstroke occurs during summertime heat waves. The incidence of heatstroke during a heat wave in cities is about 20 cases per 100,000 population.[12] Particularly vulnerable to classic heatstroke during a heat wave are the elderly and the infirmed. These patients are often found in nursing homes and extended care facilities. Heatstroke occurs in the elderly so often during a heat wave that many states have enacted laws that require air conditioning in nursing homes.

In some cases, the Paramedic receives the call for a "sick person" with fever and weakness and finds a delirious patient. The patient sometimes experiences a convulsion, leading the Paramedic to suspect meningitis. A high temperature could be the result of infection-induced **hyperpyrexia** or hyperthermia. It is difficult to distinguish advanced sepsis from heatstroke in many cases because they share common signs and symptoms.[8]

Key to a suspicion of heatstroke is syncope. The Paramedic should inquire if there was any loss of consciousness (fainting). Seizures can also accompany these episodes of syncope. Seizures are particularly problematic as they increase the heat load at a time when the body can least afford it.

Medications, particularly sympathomimetics, psychotropics, and cardiovascular medications, can increase the patient's risk for heatstroke (Table 12-3). These medications either generate more heat or decrease the body's ability to respond to heat stress.

Ingestion of stimulants such as sympathomimetics can lead to a hypermetabolic state. Common sympathomimetics include cocaine, methamphetamines, and MDMA (ecstasy). Sympathomimetics increase the endogenous heat produced by the body. The use of recreational drugs is particularly problematic if the individual is outdoors, adding another heat stress to the body.

Certain drugs (e.g., the anticholinergics) can also cause the sweat glands to malfunction. Acetylcholine is responsible for sweating. Anticholinergics inhibit sweating, thus defeating the body's ability to dissipate heat. Medications with

Table 12-3 Medications Implicated in Heat Illness

- Alpha adrenergics
- Anticholinergics
- Benzodiazepines
- Beta blockers
- Calcium channel blockers
- Diuretics
- Psychotropics
- Phenothiazines
- Thyroid medications
- Tricyclic antidepressants

anticholinergic properties include antihistamines (diphenhydramine) and antipsychotic medications, specifically the neuroleptics. Commonly prescribed neuroleptics include the phenothiazines (chlorpromazine, promethazine, and prochlorperazine), the thioxanthenes (thiothixene and zuclopenthixol), and butyrophenones (haloperidol and droperidol).

A number of medications prescribed for cardiovascular conditions can cause problems. Patients taking beta blockers, such as atenolol or metoprolol, are unable to mount a compensatory tachycardia and are more likely to experience heat syncope as well as heatstroke. Patients taking diuretics, such as hydrochlorothiazide, which can worsen dehydration, are more prone to heat illnesses.[13]

Commonly prescribed antihypertensives, such as calcium channel blockers, predispose the patient to heatstroke. Even laxatives taken for constipation can lead to diarrhea and dehydration, leaving the patient at risk for heat illness.

Heatstroke can also be a manifestation of a disease. The thyroid gland is responsible for producing hormones that control metabolism. Graves' disease (hyperthyroidism) produces abnormally high levels of thyroid hormone. During a thyroid storm (thyrotoxic crisis), excessive thyroid hormones create a hypermetabolic state that includes hyperthermia. Untreated, thyrotoxic crisis can lead to malignant hyperthermia, heatstroke, and death.

Another hormone-related cause of hyperthermia is pheochromocytoma. Although rare, a pheochromocytoma is an epinephrine-secreting tumor of the adrenal gland. The result, like a thyrotoxic crisis, is a hypermetabolic state. In some cases, patients with pheochromocytoma develop hyperthermia and heatstroke.

Hyperthermia can also occur as a result of hypothalamic hemorrhage. Hypothalamic hemorrhage is associated with subarachnoid hemorrhage and traumatic brain injuries. The hypothalamus is responsible for temperature regulation; therefore, any injury to the hypothalamus can lead to hyperpyrexia and heat illness.

Heat illness can also be the result of the body's inability to sweat. Medical conditions that prevent a patient from sweating include burns, psoriasis, and cystic fibrosis. In the case of burns, there are no sweat glands; in the case of cystic fibrosis and psoriasis, the sweat glands malfunction.[14]

The Paramedic should also inquire about the patient's last oral intake. Hydration is critical to the prevention of heat illness. It has been reported that potable water was available in the majority of cases of exertional heatstroke and yet laboratory reports showed that these patients were dehydrated.

One of the historic elements that can help distinguish exertional heatstroke from classic heatstroke is time to onset of symptoms. Exertional heatstroke can happen within hours of exposure to heat, whereas classic heatstroke tends to take days to develop. The onset of classic heatstroke is more insidious.[15]

Heatstroke and the Homeless

Poor and socially isolated individuals lack access to water, shelter from the heat, and, particularly in the northern states, air conditioning. Some of these individuals purposely limit their intake of water because of a lack of bathroom facilities, which leaves them dehydrated.

These vulnerable homeless are at risk for heatstroke. This risk occurs from a combination of environmental exposure, impaired mobility, dehydration, use of alcohol, and even a lack of available sunblock. An additional compounding factor can be psychotropic medications, which are commonly prescribed to patients in this population.

To earn a subsistence wage, the homeless may work in "labor pools." These temporary employment situations require long hours of strenuous work, and the people who work them are often outdoors and exposed to the heat. These jobs leave the person at risk for heatstroke.

To mitigate the hazard of heatstroke, some cities open public pools and "cooling stations"—such as churches, museums, and community centers—during heat waves.[16] These community cooling centers are part of a public health response to limit fatalities during heat waves, particularly among the homeless.[17]

Patients in alcohol withdrawal are also at risk for heatstroke. Detoxification may be voluntary or involuntary (such as might occur while incarcerated). Detoxification is particularly stressful to the body, yet less than 28% of jails reported detoxification services in the Arrestee Drug Abuse Monitoring (ADAM) program and only 1% of inmates received detoxification in jail.[18]

STREET SMART

Meningitis/encephalitis can present with high fever (hyperpyrexia or hyperthermia), confusion, and even coma, which are symptoms similar to heatstroke. The Paramedic should look for petechiae and purpura, evidence of a systemic infection. However, a patient in the late stage of heatstroke can present with petechiae/purpura, secondary to disseminated intravascular coagulation. When in doubt, the Paramedic should take respiratory precautions against meningitis.

CASE STUDY (CONTINUED)

The Paramedic's initial exam shows that Sean has a patent airway with no need to suction. His breathing is rapid and shallow, and his lungs are clear bilaterally. There are no signs of trauma to the chest. His radial pulses are thin and thready, and his skin is hot and dry. As her partner arrives with the stretcher, the Paramedic performs a rapid assessment of the head, eyes, ears, nose, and throat (HEENT) which reveals dilated, reactive pupils with a pale conjunctiva. Sean's mouth has a dry mucosa. The rest of the exam is unremarkable except the blistering noted to both feet and an abrasion to the left knee. After placing Sean on the stretcher, the Paramedics place him into the ambulance. The Paramedic takes a quick set of vital signs: blood pressure of 110/96; pulse of 150 and regular; respiratory rate of 28 and regular; oxygen saturation of 97%; capnography of 50 Torr; Glasgow Coma Score of 12 (eyes open spontaneously, incomprehensible sounds, & withdraws from pain). They decide to begin transporting out of Central Park and to New York Hospital. As her partner begins driving and notifying dispatch, the Paramedic starts her treatment.

CRITICAL THINKING QUESTIONS

1. What are the elements of the physical examination of a patient with suspected heat illness?
2. Why is a Glasgow Coma Scale a critical element in this examination?

Examination

The patient with heatstroke will present with various stages (Table 12-4). One of them is the sudden onset of altered mental state in approximately 80% of cases. This combination of delirium, hallucinations, confusion, and even coma are the result of central nervous system dysfunction and rising intracranial pressure secondary to cerebral edema.

Most notable in the physical exam is the elevated temperature of over 106°F (41°C). These patients are "hot to the touch" and described as having hot, dry skin. Recently there has been a de-emphasis on anhydrosis as a sign of heatstroke, as many patients with exertional heatstroke are still sweating. Anhydrosis is a late finding in classic heatstroke.[19]

The patient may exhibit a sustained tachycardia, often greater than 130 beats per minute. In general, the body does not sustain a tachycardia without underlying pathology. However, the blood pressure may be near normal initially, secondary to the body's compensatory mechanisms, and with a widened pulse pressure. Hypotension is a late sign that may be due to hypovolemia, a consequence of dehydration and/or myocardial dysfunction.

The body's attempts at compensation can be seen, and the patient's condition determined, by observing a few physical signs. As a core temperature (needed for a true diagnosis of hyperthermia) is difficult to obtain in the field, use of these physical signs of hyperthermia can be very helpful.

Initially, peripheral vasodilation leads to high central venous pressures, as manifest in jugular venous distention (JVD). As thermal injury occurs, there is production of thromboxanes (coagulation cascade), leukotrienes (inflammation), oxygen-free radicals, and nitric oxide. The last product, nitric oxide, leads to widespread vasodilation, increased vascular permeability with third spacing of fluids, and reduced venous return to the heart.

The loss of central venous pressure, as seen by a widening pulse pressure,[20] leads to reduced cardiac output and resulting hypoperfusion and shock syndrome. Subsequent cerebral hypoperfusion can lead to altered mental states, seizures, and coma. Seizures are problematic as muscular activity raises the body's core temperature further and hastens the patient's decline.

As the hypothalamus becomes dysfunctional, homeostatic mechanisms, such as vasodilation and diaphoresis, stop. When this happens, anhydrosis may be observed. The cumulative effect of generalized hypoxemia, organ ischemia, electrolyte imbalance, and loss of the potassium–sodium pump's efficiency is depressed myocardial function. A 12-lead ECG may demonstrate diffuse ST–T elevation, nonspecific patterns of ischemia, or indications of generalized ischemia.[21,22] These changes are not indicative of myocardial ischemia secondary to coronary artery disease but rather global ischemia secondary to extracardiac conditions.

The Paramedic may also note that the patient's respiratory rate was initially increased but, as the patient decompensates, there is a fall in respiration, further worsening the hypoxemia.

Table 12-4 Stages of Heatstroke*

Signs	Early Stage	Late Stage
Mental status	Confused	Seizures/coma
Heart rate	Elevated	Elevated
Respirations	Elevated	Decline
Blood pressure	Normal	Hypotensive
Skin	Diaphoresis	Anhydrosis
Pulse pressure	Normal	Widened
JVD	Marked	Absent
ECG	Normal	ST-T wave elevations

Note: *These are generalized stages. Patients can and will present with mixed presentations.

STREET SMART

Patients with heatstroke will present with dilated, normal, or pinpoint pupils. Several studies have suggested a correlation between high core temperature, pinpoint pupils, and higher mortality. However, drugs implicated in heatstroke (i.e., anticholinergics and sympathomimetics) cause pupillary dilation (mydriasis).[23] Therefore, pupillary reaction is undependable in the differential diagnosis of heatstroke.[24]

CASE STUDY (CONTINUED)

The combination of confusion and the hyperdynamic vital signs make the Paramedic think that Sean is experiencing the early stages of heatstroke. She applies the electrodes for an ECG, looking for ST segment and T wave changes. Sean is still too diaphoretic.

CRITICAL THINKING QUESTIONS

1. What is the significance of the altered mental status?
2. What diagnosis did the Paramedic announce to the emergency department?

Assessment

The preceding signs and symptoms would suggest a field diagnosis of hyperthermia to the Paramedic,[25] or possibly suspected heatstroke. However, there are other etiologies for hyperthermia other than heatstroke: malignant hyperthermia, some endocrine disorders such as thyroid storm, and pheochromocytoma, as well as serotonin syndrome from selective serotonin reuptake inhibitor toxicity.

Fortunately, a careful history can often provide the true origins of the hyperthermia in those cases. A more difficult case is the septic patient. The septic patient will present as hyperdynamic with an elevated temperature at first and then may rapidly decline. Although the temperature is useful in this differential, as fevers seldom reach 105.8°F (41°C), temperatures are difficult to obtain in the field and may have a poor correlation to core temperature.

Late stage heatstroke will also present with the signs of increased intracranial pressure (i.e., Cushing's triad) and posturing, secondary to cerebral edema. Increased intracranial pressure should be treated in the same manner as traumatic brain injury.

From a field perspective, the key clinical feature that distinguishes heat exhaustion from heatstroke is an altered mental status. Any alteration in mental status is a medical emergency.

CASE STUDY (CONTINUED)

The Paramedic jumps in the patient compartment, turns up the air conditioner, and starts to put icepacks in Sean's axilla and groin. Instead of using chemical ice packs, the Paramedics elect to put ice cubes into plastic one-quart bags and store them in a cooler along with some sopping wet towels that absorb the melt water. They also have several small battery operated fans strategically placed in the ambulance to start a current of wind over Sean's body.

The Paramedic's partner yells back, "Is that necessary? We are only 15 minutes from the hospital." The Paramedic replies, "Even a little bit helps!" as she returns to her patient care duties.

CRITICAL THINKING QUESTIONS

1. What is the national standard of care of patients with heatstroke?
2. What are some of the patient-specific concerns and considerations that the Paramedic should consider when applying this plan of care that is intended to treat a broad patient population presenting with heatstroke?

Treatment

A core temperature of 107.6°F (42°C) exceeds the thermal maximum that cells can endure without damage. At this temperature, cells start to die from protein denaturing. Organs then start to fail within 45 minutes.[26] Therefore, it is imperative that the Paramedic start treatment as soon as possible. Delays in treatment are associated with a mortality rate as high as 80%, whereas early aggressive cooling can lower the mortality rate to 10%. Patients with temperatures as high as 114°F (46°C) have survived heatstroke with early and aggressive intervention.

After removing the patient with heatstroke from the environment and disrobing him as needed, the first treatment priority remains the ABCs. The airway needs to be aggressively managed if the patient cannot maintain it on his own. If the patient is obtunded but still has intact airway reflexes, the Paramedic may have to consider medication-facilitated intubation.

Following airway is breathing. Heatstroke has a triple impact on oxygenation. First, increased temperatures have a dramatic effect on the oxyhemoglobin curve, causing a rightward shift. Coupled with a change in red blood cell morphology, red blood cells become spherical at high temperatures, and hypoxia ensues. A higher partial pressure of oxygen—via high-flow, high-concentration oxygen—is needed to treat the hypoxemia.

In many cases, high-flow, high-concentration oxygen will not be enough. During heatstroke, marked acidosis occurs secondary to cellular dysfunction and further shifts the oxy-hemoglobin curve to the right. This metabolic acidosis is evidenced by a marked increase in end-tidal carbon dioxide.[27] A positive correlation has been shown between correction of acid levels and neurological outcome in one series.[28] Therefore, the Paramedic should consider ventilation as well as oxygenation.

The Paramedic should perform basic life support measures such as bag-valve-mask ventilation with oral or nasal airway insertion to keep the oxygen saturation above 90%. If saturation drops below 90%, or visible chest rise cannot be achieved, or if the patient is obtunded, intubation is the next step. If laryngoscopy cannot be performed, a supraglottic airway should be used to secure the airway.

The therapeutic goal of ventilation/oxygenation is to obtain an end-tidal carbon dioxide ($EtCO_2$) level within the normal range, 35 to 45 mmHg, while maintaining a minimal oxygen saturation (SpO_2) of greater than 90%.

Vascular access is imperative for fluid and sodium replenishment, especially when the patient's mental status cannot tolerate PO intake. In addition to peripheral vein access, adult interosseous devices are effective.

However, the Paramedic must be cautious with the amount of fluid administered. Paramedics need to remember that the patient may have higher plasma osmolarity that is causing cerebral swelling and altered mental status. As a result, antidiuretic hormone (ADH) may have been secreted to combat the initial dehydration. This hormone has a very long half-life, causing it to remain active for a long period of time. Kidneys may not be able to diurese additional fluids until the effects of the ADH are diminished. Prehospital treatment is the start of the patient's recovery, although overly aggressive fluid resuscitation can produce adverse reactions.[29] Maldistribution of fluids due to third spacing is generally correctable with cooling. However, fluid resuscitation should be limited except in special circumstances (i.e., those patients with hypoperfusion). The treatment for patients with heat exhaustion focuses on fluid replacement, whereas treatment for heatstroke focuses on rapid cooling rather than fluid replacement. The therapuetic goal of cooling is to lower the temperature about 0.4°F per minute.

Hypoglycemia is commonly encountered in the patient with heatstroke, particularly in exertional heatstroke. The Paramedic should obtain a blood glucose and consider intravenous administration of 25 grams of dextrose 50% in water.

It is imperative that cooling be started in the field and that the cooling be effective, but not overly effective. If the patient is cooled too quickly (overshoot), then the patient will start to shiver and rebound hyperthermia will occur. The most effective field treatments use **evaporative techniques**. In one technique, the Paramedic gently sprays a cool mist over the patient. The water should be cooler than tepid or lukewarm water (i.e., at about 60°F [15°C]). The mist should moisten the skin but not be allowed to drip, as heat loss is greatest with evaporation. To speed evaporation, the Paramedic can use a high-powered fan to circulate air over the patient (Figure 12-4).[30]

An alternative technique is **strategic ice packing**. Ice packs are placed strategically at pulse points (places where deep arteries rise to the surface). Strategic ice packing is convenient in the ambulance, although not as effective as evaporative techniques.[31]

Some experts feel that **ice water immersion** (placing the body in very cold water) is the gold standard for treatment of heatstroke. Ice water immersion can reduce core temperature in 20 to 40 minutes.[20] However, overshoot, induced hypothermia, and shivering frequently occur with this technique. Although benzodiazepines can be used to stop shivering and prevent rebound hyperthermia, ice water immersion is not practical in the field.[32,33]

Another technique that can be used in conjunction with evaporative cooling and/or strategic ice packs is **iced gastric lavage/gavage**. A lavage/gavage system, using an orogastric tube, can lower the core body temperature 0.3° F (0.15°C)/min. The techniques use 10 cc/kg ice water instilled into the stomach for one minute, then suctioned out of the stomach for one minute.[34]

Other methods of rapid cooling such as gastric lavage, rectal enema, cold humidified oxygen, and even cooling blankets have not proven superior to either cold water immersion or evaporative techniques at cooling the body. Once the patient's core temperature reaches 100.4°F (38°C), efforts at cooling the body should stop. However, at a steady decline of 0.4°F (0.2°C) per minute, it would take 15 to 30 minutes to lower the patient's temperature to 100.4°F (38°C) in most cases.

Many athletic trainers at football camps keep a tub of ice water available during practice in the event that a player experiences heatstroke. (Between 1995 and 2009, 33 football players died from heatstroke.) First, the patient is suspended over the tub on a stretcher while ice water towels are draped over the patient. If that is ineffective, the patient is placed in the tub.

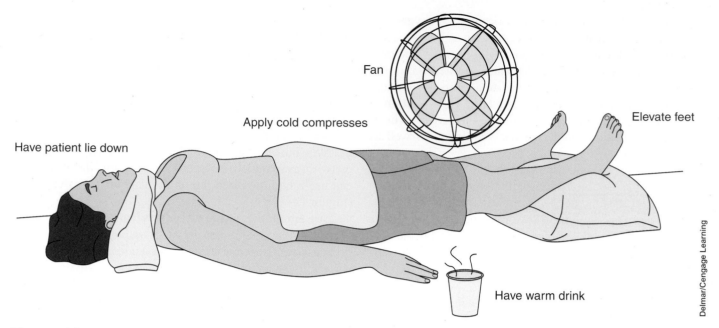

Figure 12-4 Evaporative cooling is the most effective field treatment for heatstroke.

Fan

Apply cold compresses

Elevate feet

Have patient lie down

Have warm drink

Delmar/Cengage Learning

Special Case of Exertional Rhabdomyolysis

It is estimated that up to 25% of patients with exertional heatstroke will develop **rhabdomyolysis**. Rhabdomyolysis occurs as a result of vigorous exercise that injures skeletal muscle. The risk of exertional rhabdomyolysis (muscle meltdown) is greater for novel overexertion (e.g., that exertion experienced by recruits during academy or rookies in summer football camps).

Treatment for exertional rhabdomyolysis is the same as for crush injury: an infusion of intravenous fluids, in some cases as much as 10 liters during the course of treatment, and sodium bicarbonate. The patient should be immediately transported for possible kidney dialysis, critical care, and hemodynamic monitoring.

CASE STUDY (CONTINUED)

As the Paramedic suspected, Sean suddenly appears unconscious. As she uses painful stimulus to arouse him he starts to posture. The Paramedic yells to her partner, "He is out of it," to which her partner responds by turning the lights and siren on.

With venous access already established, the Paramedic starts to prepare a bolus when Sean seizes. "This is bad," the Paramedic murmurs. "This guy needs Valium before this seizure kills him." As she prepares the Valium, she wonders, "Hmm, maybe this guy was not so dry as we thought. When he said he was adequately hydrated, did he overhydrate?"

CRITICAL THINKING QUESTIONS

1. What is the implication of a seizure in a patient with heatstroke?
2. What is the typical fluid resuscitation for a patient with heatstroke?

Evaluation

Seizures are particularly devastating to the patient with heatstroke. Seizures create a tenfold increase in heat production at a time when the body can ill afford an additional heat load.[35] These seizures may be the result of hypoxia, hypoperfusion, and hypoglycemia, three factors that should be dealt with during the primary assessment. After ruling these factors out, seizures may be the result of hyponatremia.[36]

Sweat carries sodium with it, so excessive sweating increases sodium loss. Sodium is important to the body's ability to maintain hemostasis and is the most prevalent extracellular electrolyte. The passage of sodium into muscle and nerve cells through ion channels increases the polarity or electrical charge and causes muscle cells to depolarize, or contract. When there is a lack of sodium in the blood, or **hyponatremia**, there can be decreased depolarization.[37]

During the process of dehydration and sodium loss, the body attempts to conserve fluid by secreting the antidiuretic hormone (ADH). Release of this hormone instructs the kidneys to retain as much fluid as possible through reabsorption.

There are two mechanisms that can cause hyponatremia: excessive loss of sodium (described under exertional heatstroke) and excessive water intake. Excessive water intake results in a condition known as water intoxication or hyperhydration and can lead to **dilutional hyponatremia**. The increase in fluid alone will not stop the secretion of ADH, which has a long half-life and remains active for a long time, but instead will increase water in the plasma. This increase causes a shift in water concentration in brain cells, leading to cerebral swelling. This results in confusion and, in extreme cases, seizures and coma.[38]

Hyponatremia occurs because of inappropriate replacement of fluid losses with hypotonic fluids. For example, during endurance events, as well as military training camps, patients unwittingly drink water in the mistaken belief that they will prevent heat illness.

Multiple medications can also cause hyponatremia. These medications couple with classic heatstroke to produce hyponatremia-induced seizures. These medications include thiazide diuretics and angiotensin-converting enzyme inhibitors (commonly prescribed for hypertension and heart failure), loop diuretics, and psychotropic medications including selective serotonin reuptake inhibitors.

Early signs of hyponatremia include increased thirst, muscle cramps, lethargy, and skeletal muscle spasms. The most common symptoms, in one study, were mental status changes, emesis, and nausea—all symptoms consistent with exertional heatstroke. Subsequently, the patients experienced seizures.[39]

The first priority of hyponatremia-induced seizures in the heatstroke patient is control of the seizure activity. Typically, benzodiazepines are used to control seizure activity. However, hyponatremia-induced seizures are often refractory to benzodiazepines and the seizure progresses to status epilepticus. If that is the case, then the Paramedic may need to resort to the use of paralytics. Although these paralytics do not stop the underlying seizure activity in the brain, they do stop the muscle contractions that contribute endogenous heat to increase the core temperature and worsen the heatstroke.

Usually sodium replacement using intravenous therapy is the gold standard for the treatment of hyponatremia. However, it is difficult to establish in the field without monitoring blood serum levels. Normal saline (0.9% sodium chloride in sterile water) should be infused starting with a "keep vein open" (KVO) rate of 15 gtts/minute and increased according to medical control instructions.[40]

Although the etiology of the seizure activity may be hyponatremia, cerebral edema with its attendant increased intracranial pressure is also present. After controlling the seizure, the Paramedic must take steps to control the increasing intracranial pressure. Intubation with carefully titrated hyperventilation to maintain an end-tidal carbon dioxide level between 32 and 35 mmHg will help to slow the raising intracranial pressure. Hyperventilation should be instituted if the patient presents with decorticate or decerebrate posturing, fixed and dilated pupils, or Cushing's triad.

STREET SMART

"Ravers," participants in all night parties, may take MDMA (esctasy), drink large amounts of fluids, and exercise vigorously while dancing. These activities can lead to hyperthermia and hyponatremia-induced seizures.[41]

CASE STUDY (CONCLUSION)

As the ambulance is pulling in, the Paramedic quickly rechecks her interventions. Although Sean is not responding as quickly as she had hoped, the Paramedic knows the priority is rapid delivery to the hospital. She feels that her interventions en route will have a positive effect on his outcome. A quick physical exam reveals the following:

His airway is still patent and controlled by the patient, his breathing is 24 breaths per minute, and his oxygen saturation is 99%. Although his skin has cooled to a normal temperature, his Glasgow Coma Score is only 12 (eyes open, incomprehensible sounds, and flexion to pain).

CRITICAL THINKING QUESTIONS

1. What is the preferred destination for the patient with heatstroke?
2. What are the exceptions in those cases?

Disposition

Although many cases of heat fatigue and heat exhaustion are treated and released in the field, heatstroke is a medical emergency that requires rapid transportation to the closest facility capable of providing cooling. Although the emergency department can institute techniques of internal cooling, such as gastric and bladder irrigation with cold water and even peritoneal lavage, none has been shown to be as advantageous as the external cooling that is started in the field.

In severe cases of heatstroke that are refractory to these standard treatments, the emergency physician may consider cardiopulmonary bypass or extracorporeal membrane oxygenation (ECMO). Even some studies of the use of hyperbaric oxygen (HBO) have shown promise. However, at the present time external cooling using evaporative techniques or immersion therapy are the standard of care.[42]

CONCLUSION

The body is constantly challenged by many different stressors, each one activating a process of compensatory mechanisms designed to provide metabolic balance and achieve homeostasis. These mechanisms are only a short-acting and temporary measure. They will allow the body to combat the stressor until the stressor can be removed. In the case of heat, this involves removing oneself from the environment. However, some situations may prevent the body from leaving the environment. The most important treatment that EMS can perform is removing the patient from the stressful environment. In cases of extreme heat, Paramedics must assist the body by providing the needed balance to resume normal metabolism. Once achieved, the body will then be able to care for itself and function normally.

KEY POINTS:

- Heat illness has a higher mortality rate than all other weather-related issues—tornados, hurricanes, lightning, floods, and blizzards—combined.

- Survival from heatstroke depends, in large part, to the actions the Paramedic takes in the field.

- Evaporative loss accounts for the majority of the body's ability to dissipate heat.

- When evaporative loss stops, heat illness ensues. The heat index accounts for humidity in an estimate of perceived temperature.

- Heat has a dramatic impact on oxygenation, both at the level of the red blood cell and on the oxyhemoglobin curve.

- Heat negatively impacts on sodium-dependent processes such as nerve conduction and muscle contraction, leading to weakness, slowed reflexes, and altered mental status.

- Heat illness is on a continuum from heat fatigue to heat exhaustion to heatstroke.

- Heat exhaustion can be the result of salt depletion or water depletion.

- Patients with salt depletion-induced heat exhaustion are not acclimatized, do not complain of thirst, and often vomit.

- Treatment of salt depletion-induced heat exhaustion focuses on electrolyte replacement.

- Heat cramps often accompany heat exhaustion.

- Heatstroke is a life-threatening medical emergency caused by increased external heat stressors, increased internal heat production, a decreased ability to dissipate heat, or a combination thereof.

- Heatstroke is either classified as exertional heatstroke or classic heatstroke.

- Classic heatstroke has a triad of symptoms: hyperthermia, altered mental status, and anhydrosis.

- Classic heatstroke is difficult to differentiate from sepsis in the elderly.

- Many drugs can quicken the onset of heatstroke, including sympathomimetics, cardiovascular medications, and psychotropics.

- Exertional heatstroke most commonly occurs in outdoor workers.

- Heatstroke is often preceded by heat syncope.

- Heatstroke can also be a symptom of an underlying disease such as Graves' disease, pheochromocytoma, and hypothalamic stroke.

- Exertional heatstroke (EHS) takes hours to develop, whereas classic heatstroke takes days to develop in many cases.

- Besides hyperthermia, the patient with heatstroke will have sustained tachycardia, be normotensive, and have jugular venous distention (JVD).

- Anhydrosis is a late finding in classic heatstroke and is often not seen in exertional heatstroke.

- As ECG changes are observed, the patient may also experience seizures/coma, anhydrosis, and a widening pulse pressure.

- Although the definition of heatstroke is a temperature of 105.8°F (41°C), a core temperature is difficult to obtain in the field. Therefore, the Paramedic must resort to the symptom pattern for a diagnosis.

- Airway and ventilation, to increase oxygenation and reverse acidosis, remain a priority in the care of the patient with heatstroke.

- Rapid cooling using evaporative techniques, with cooling mist and fans, or conductive techniques, using ice packs and ice baths, is instrumental in reversing heatstroke in the field.

- Rhabdomyolysis is a common complication of exertional heatstroke.

- Hyponatremia-induced seizures are the result of increased intracranial pressure and can be caused by hyperhydration.

REVIEW QUESTIONS:

1. What is the heat index and what is its implication regarding the rate of heat illness?
2. What is the pathophysiology behind heat syncope?
3. Differentiate exertional heatstroke and classic heatstroke.
4. What medication that a Paramedic might administer would induce malignant hyperthermia and what would be some signs of impending malignant hyperthermia?
5. What is part of the differential for heatstroke?

CASE STUDY QUESTIONS:

Please refer to the Case Study in this chapter, and answer the questions below:

1. What type of heat exhaustion did the Paramedic suspect that Sean had and how was that substantiated by the patient's presentation?
2. What are the three impacts of heatstroke on oxygenation?
3. In a resource-rich environment like New York City, what alternative destinations could Sean been taken to if he did not respond to basic cooling methods?

REFERENCES:

1. Centers for Disease Control and Prevention. Heatwaves. Available at: **http://www.cdc.gov/climatechange/effects/heat.htm.** Accessed July 2009.
2. Montain SJ, Cheuvront SN, Lukaski HC. Sweat mineral-element responses during 7 h of exercise-heat stress. *Int J Sport Nutr Exerc Metab.* 2007;17(6):574–582.
3. Perron A. et al. Association of heat index and patient volume at a mass gathering event. *Preh. Emer Care.* 2005;9(1):49–52.
4. Auerbach PS, ed. *Wilderness Medicine: Management of Wilderness and Environmental Emergencies.* St. Louis, MO: Mosby; 1995:167–212.
5. Hoffman EK, Dunham PB. Membrane mechanisms and intracellular signalling in cell volume regulation. *Int Rev Cytol.* 1995;161:173–262.
6. Buono MJ, Sjoholm NT. Effect of physical training on peripheral sweat production. *J Appl Physiol.* 1988;65:811–814.

7. Chou, H.L. et al. Exertional heatstroke: a care report and review of articles. *J Emerg Crit Care Med*. 2009;20(1):33–38.

8. Bouchama A, Knochel JP. Heatstroke. *N Engl J Med*. 2002;346;1978–1988.

9. Adelakun A, Schwartz E, Blais L. Occupational heat exposure. *Appl Occup Environ Hyg*. 1999;14:153–154.

10. Memorandum to Welsh, Len. Investigation of 25 heat related emergencies in summer 2005. California OSHA. February 17, 2006.

11. NIOSH publication 86-112: *Working in Hot Environments*.

12. Heat-related illnesses and deaths—United States, 1994–1995. *MMWR Morb Mortal Wkly Rep*. 1995;44:465–468.

13. Wexler RK. Evaluation and treatment of heat-related illness. *Am Fam Physician*. 2002;65:2307–2314.

14. Shuster S, Johnson C. The abnormality of sweat duct function in psoriasis. *Br Jnl Derm*. 2006;81(11):846–850.

15. Glazer J. Management of heatstroke and heat exhaustion. *Am Fam Physician*. 2005;71(11):2133–2140.

16. Kellerman AL, Todd KH. Killing heat. *N Engl J Med*. 1996;335:126–127.

17. Rampulla, J. Hyperthermia & heatstroke: heat-related conditions. The healthcare of homeless persons. Boston Healthcare for Homeless Program. Available at: **www.nhchc.org/hyperthermia.pdf.** Accessed December 31, 2009.

18. Fiscella K, et al. Alcohol and opiate withdrawal in US jails. *Am J Public Health*. 2004;94(9):1522–1524.

19. Hubbard R. Novel approaches to the pathophysiology of heatstroke: the energy depletion model. *Ann Emerg Med*. 1997;16(9):1066–1075.

20. Casa DJ, McDermott BP, Lee EC, Yeargin SW, Armstrong LE, Maresh CM. Cold water immersion: the gold standard for exertional heatstroke treatment. *Exerc Sport Sci Rev*. Jul 2007;35(3):141–149.

21. Muniz A. Ischemic electrocardiographic changes from severe heatstroke. *South Med J*. 2004;97(10):S10–S11.

22. Wakino S, et al. A case of severe heatstroke with abnormal cardiac findings. *Inter Hrt Jnl*. 2005:46(3):543–550.

23. McGurire GG, Scott RA, Tong TG, et al. Pupil size in heatstroke. *West J Med*.1975;122:255.

24. Martinez M. Drug associated heatstroke. *South Med J*. 2002;95(8):799–803.

25. McGugan EA. Hyperpyrexia in the emergency department. *Emerg Med*. 2001;13(1):116–120.

26. Bynum GD, Pandolf KB, Schuette WH, Goldman RF, Lees DE, Whang-Peng J, et al. Induced hyperthermia in sedated humans and the concept of critical thermal maximum. *Am J Physiol*. 1978;235:R228–2236.

27. Bouchama A, De Vol EB. Acid-base alterations in heatstroke. *Intensive Care Med*. 2001;27:680–685.

28. Hart GR, Anderson RJ, Crumpler CP, Shulkin A, Reed G, Knochel JP. Epidemic classic heatstroke: clinical characteristics and course of 28 patients. *Medicine*. 1982;61:189–197.

29. Sterns RH. Severe symptomatic hyponatremia treatment and outcome. *Ann Intern Med*. 1987;107:656–664.

30. Hadad E, Rav-Acha M, Heled Y, Epstein Y, Moran DS. Heatstroke: a review of cooling methods. *Sports Med*. 2004;34:501–511.

31. Gaffin SL, Gardner JW, Flinn DS. Cooling method for exertional heatstroke. *Ann Intern Med*. 2000;132:678.

32. Bouchama A, Dehbi M, Chaves-Carballo E. Cooling and hemodynamic management in heatstroke: practical recommendations. *Crit Care*. 2007 [serial online];11(3):1–17.

33. McDermott BP, Casa DJ, Ganio MS, Lopez RM, Yeargin SW, Armstrong LE, et al. Acute whole-body cooling for exercise-induced hyperthermia: a systematic review. *J Athl Train*. Jan-Feb 2009;44(1):84–93.

34. Erickson TB, Prendergast HM. Procedures pertaining to hyperthermia. In: Roberts JR, Hedges JR, Chanmugan AS, et al. *Clinical Procedures in Emergency Medicine* (4th ed.). Philadelphia, PA: WB Saunders; 2004:1358–1370.

35. Dematte JE, O'Mara K, Bueschr J, Whitney CG, Forsythe S, McNamee T, et al. Near-fatal heatstroke during the 1995 heat wave in Chicago. *Ann Intern Med*. 1998;129:173–181.

36. Backer HD, Shopes E, Collins SL, Barkan H. Exertional heat illness and hyponatremia in hikers. *Am J Emerg Med*. Oct 1999;17(6):532–539.

37. Upadhyay A, Jaber BL, Madias NE. Incidence and prevalence of hyponatremia. *Am J Med*. Jul 2006;119(7 Suppl 1):S30–S35.

38. Ayus JC, Krothapalli RF, Arieff AI. Treatment of symptomatic hyponatremia and its relation to brain damage. *N Engl J Med*. 1987;317:1190–1195.

39. O'Brien KK. et al. Hyponatremia associated with overhydration in U.S. Army trainees. *Mil Med*. 2001;166(95):405–410.

40. Montain SJ, Sawka MN, Wegner CB. Hyponatremia associated with exercise: risk factors and pathogenesis. *Exer Sports Sci Rev*. 2001;29(3):113–117.

41. Holmes SB, Banerjee AK, Alexander WD. Hyponatraemia and seizures after ecstasy use. *Postgrad Med J*. Jan 1999;75(879):32–33.

42. Niu KC, et al. A hyperbaric oxygen therapy approach to heatstroke in multiple organ dysfunction. *Chin J Physiol*. 2009;52(3):169–172.

COLD EMERGENCIES

KEY CONCEPTS:

Upon completion of this chapter, it is expected that the reader will understand these following concepts:

- Pathophysiology of hypothermia
- Hypothermia as a disorder
- Assessment of the hypothermic patient
- Treatment of the hypothermic patient

ANATOMY CONCEPTS:

Prior to reading this chapter the Paramedic student should be familiar with the following anatomy and physiology concepts:

- Homeostasis
- Thermogenesis
- Integumentary system
- Changes of aging

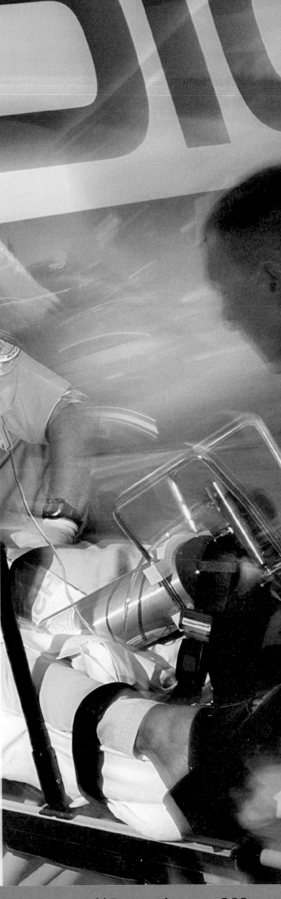

CASE STUDY:

"Check the welfare," the radio squawked. A routine call, the Paramedic pulled the ambulance away from the post. Again the radio squawks, "Elderly woman down, possible broken hip, found on the kitchen floor by police." It seems the neighbors have a system to check on each other. Every morning Mrs. Maud lifts her shades in the kitchen. The neighbors called the police when they noticed she did not lift her shade or pick up her morning paper. The police had forced the door and found her on the floor. When the Paramedics arrive, she is barely conscious with shallow breathing and she is "ice cold" to the touch.

CRITICAL THINKING QUESTIONS

1. What are some of the possible causes of the patient's altered mental status?
2. How is altered level of consciousness related to the "ice cold" skin?

OVERVIEW

Winter inevitably brings about cold emergencies. With an incidence of cold emergencies of 1 per 100,000 populations, most EMS systems can anticipate seeing at least one cold-related illness annually.[1] According to one study conducted over a five-year period, cold illness accounts for an average of 647 deaths annually, with over 50% of these occurring in elderly patients.[2,3] Hypothermia occurs everywhere: It is as likely to affect people in the city as it is in the country, and it affects people from both the deserts of Arizona and the North Dakota hills. Regardless of their geographic location in the United States, Paramedics will treat patients with cold emergencies.

Chief Concern

All mammals, including humans, are warm-blooded and must produce warmth in order to survive. A **thermoneutral** body temperature is between 97.7°F and 99.5°F (36.5°C and 37.5°C). When the internal, or core, body temperature is within this range, the body's metabolic reactions can best occur. However, extremes of temperature—either above or below this range—interfere with the body's enzymatic reactions or retard the body's metabolic processes. The spectrum of cold illness ranges from mild to moderate to severe hypothermia. In extreme cases, hypothermia can lead to serious injury and death.

At odds with the body's "need" to maintain an internal core temperature of approximately 99°F (37.2°C) are the forces of evaporation, conduction, convection, and radiation (Figure 13-1). On average, about 65% of the body's heat is lost through simple radiation of heat to the atmosphere. Wearing a layer of clothing helps to decrease this loss. Another 15% is lost through conduction (contact with colder objects, such as wind and water).

Exposure to wind can rapidly induce hypothermia. In 1945, Passel and Siple created the wind chill temperature

(WCT) index. Passel and Siple postulated that the combination of temperature and wind could lower the temperature the skin experiences. In 2001, the National Weather Service (NWS) updated the wind chill temperature index. This revised version is based on a human face model and does not include the effects of heat from the sun, which may increase the temperature on the skin by 10°F to 20°F (Figure 13-2).

Heat loss via conduction in cold water is particularly problematic. Cold water has 30 times the conductive heat capacity of air. Therefore, heat is rapidly lost in those patients who are immersed in cold water.

Typically, the remainder of the body's heat loss occurs through evaporative losses contained within the moisture of the patient's expired air or sweat. The latent heat of evaporation, the heat contained in the moisture from each warmed expired breath, is about 0.54 kcal (kilos per calorie) per gram of water. This rate is affected by humidity and respiratory rate.

The body has many complex thermoregulatory mechanisms to help ensure that the body's **core temperature**, the temperature in the vital organs (heart, lungs, and brain) and core organs (liver, kidneys, and spleen), remains within this narrow range.

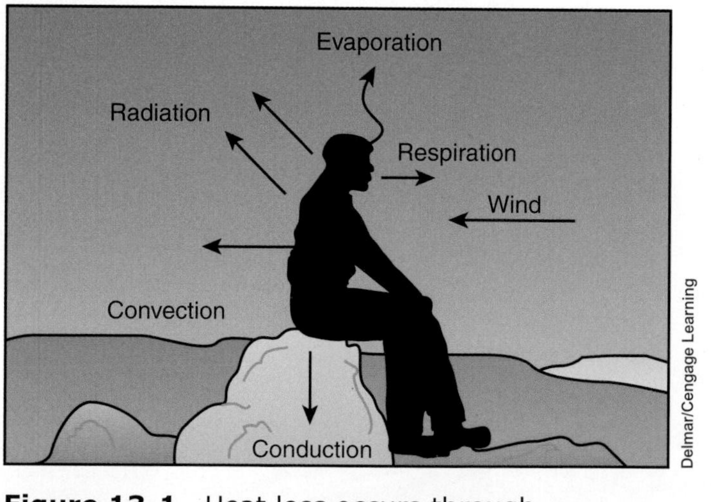

Thermoregulation

The body's temperature is largely controlled by the hypothalamus, an area situated in the center of the brain. This small pea-sized nucleus of neurons serves as the link between the nervous system and the endocrine system and monitors many life functions, including core temperature. Acting like a thermostat, the hypothalamus regulates heat production. Through its connection with the nervous system, particularly the sensory nerves in skin that transmit signals via the spinothalamic tract, the hypothalamus can "sense" changes in core temperature and effect changes in the body to produce, retain, or dissipate heat. The body has several means to produce heat as a part of the process called **thermogenesis**.

For example, if the hypothalamus senses a drop in core body temperature, it can increase muscle tone. This state of muscular contraction or tension requires the use of energy. Producing energy to contract the muscle releases heat as

Figure 13-1 Heat loss occurs through evaporation, conduction, convection, and radiation.

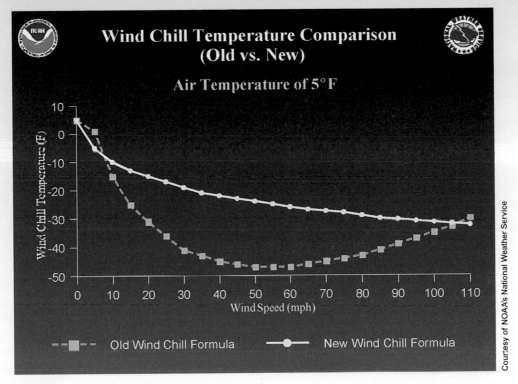

Figure 13-2 The National Weather Service updated the wind chill index in 2001.

its by-product. This is most dramatically demonstrated by **shivering**, the rhythmic contraction of muscle at a rate of 10 to 20 contractions per second. The human body can normally produce 40 to 60 kcal per square meter of body surface area. Shivering can increase heat production by two to five times that amount.

The body also has other non-shivering mechanisms for thermogenesis, and epinephrine plays a key role in them. The hypothalamus mediates between the nervous system and the endocrine system and activates the adrenal glands to secrete epinephrine. Epinephrine's effects are several-fold. First, epinephrine controls peripheral blood flow through its stimulation of the alpha-receptors, closing precapillary sphincters within the skin's capillary beds, and through vaso-constriction. This effectively shunts blood away from the skin and redirects the warm blood to the core. Epinephrine can

reduce blood flow in the skin from a normal 2,500 mL per minute to as little as 500 mL per minute. This reduction in blood flow is evidenced by cool and pale skin.

These peripheral tissues essentially go into a state of reduced metabolism (anaerobic metabolism) while maintaining minimal function. This fact should be significant for the Paramedic. Later, when warmth returns, blood flow through the area will pick up the by-products of this anaerobic metabolism, such as lactic acid.

Epinephrine can also increase glycogen metabolism. The average body holds about 2,000 kcal of heat-producing glycogen. Initially, heat is produced in the liver and muscles by the anaerobic reduction of glycogen by epinephrine (epinephrine promotes glycolysis) into its primary substrate, glucose. This glucose now serves a second purpose by supplying energy for shivering. When the muscles use all of their glycogen stores, creating a condition called **glycogen debt**, the patient experiences extreme fatigue, cessation of shivering, and rapid decline into severe hypothermia.[4]

Hypothermia Defined

Hypothermia is a suboptimal body temperature, one that—if allowed to persist—is incompatible with life. The disorder hypothermia does not occur in degrees. Rather, hypothermia should be thought of as occurring along a continuum, one that is punctuated with events that can be used as artificial boundaries to describe levels of hypothermia. Like the patient in compensated shock who cannot be thought of as being stable, the patient with mild hypothermia is in transition to moderate and then severe hypothermia unless the Paramedic intervenes.

Mild hypothermia occurs when the body's core temperature drops between 89.6°F and 95°F (32°C and 35°C). Moderate hypothermia occurs between 82.4°F and 89.6°F (28°C and 32°C). Prolonged core temperatures below 82.4°F (28°C) are not compatible with life.

As it is difficult to obtain a core body temperature in the field, the Paramedic must rely on physical findings to make a determination of the level of hypothermia. It should be stressed that physical findings can vary tremendously from patient to patient. Therefore, the determination of the level of hypothermia, without a core temperature, is somewhat hypothetical.

Etiology of Hypothermia

Most hypothermia is unintentional. When hearing the term "hypothermia," most Paramedics think of a patient with a prolonged exposure to cold while outdoors, perhaps while ice fishing or snowshoeing. Although many cases of unintentional hypothermia do occur while people engage in winter recreation, there are other situations in which hypothermia may occur.

Hypothermia may be a risk in cases of prolonged entrapment, such as a motor vehicle collision or a building collapse. Hypothermia may also occur due to prolonged exposure to tepid water. Any condition that leads to unconsciousness and/or immobility—such as stroke, opiate overdose, or intoxication—is a predisposing factor to hypothermia.

However, there are a significant number of cases of urban hypothermia, such as the one described in this chapter's case study. To understand how urban hypothermia can occur, it is necessary to understand how the body retains heat and the forces that drain heat from the body.

As a by-product of metabolism, the body creates heat. Although this heat is necessary to continue further biochemical reactions, excessive heat can actually interfere with these metabolic processes. Therefore, the body takes measures to help control the internal body temperature. The thermoregulatory center within the hypothalamus is responsible for maintaining optimal body temperature within the proper range. This control is accomplished primarily through evaporation of sweat and radiation of heat from capillary beds at the surface of the skin.

When the body is exposed to cold, the hypothalamus directs sweat glands to stop producing sweat and, perhaps more importantly, directs capillary beds to shut down and shunt blood away from the skin toward the core. This is described in more detail shortly.

Extent of the Problem

In the course of their lives, many people have experienced mild hypothermia. It is thought by authorities that most of these cases go unreported. These cases of mild hypothermia are generally well tolerated and do not result in significant problems of morbidity or mortality.

At issue are the cases of life-threatening hypothermia. A key difference in the morbidity and mortality seems to exist between patients with moderate hypothermia (21% mortality) and those with severe hypothermia (> 40% mortality). Therefore, it is imperative that the Paramedic recognizes severe hypothermia and responds appropriately to the threat.

Pathophysiology of Hypothermia

Hypothermia has profound effects on both the cardiovascular system and the pulmonary system. The pulmonary system is impacted at a macro level as well as a micro level. At the macro level, the cold causes vasoconstriction of the pulmonary vasculature. This vasoconstriction results in increased resistance to blood flow and pulmonary hypertension. The effect of hypothermia is to create a right-to-left shunt. Blood does not come into contact with the air and gas exchange is diminished at the alveolar level.

The second effect of cold occurs upon the oxyhemoglobin dissociation curve (ODC). Cold shifts the ODC to the left, making oxygen bind more tightly to the hemoglobin. As a result, although the patient's pulse oximetry may read an SpO_2 of near 100%, the oxygen is not off-loading at the cellular level. This results in tissue hypoxia and may be one of the causes of cardiac irritability.

Cold can also compromise the cardiovascular system, as the muscles of the heart become stiffer and less able to pump effectively. This diminished stroke volume is normally compensated for by an increase in heart rate: cardiac output equals stroke volume times heart rate (CO = SV × HR). However, the heart's pacemakers also are slowed. During severe hypothermia, the heart rate can drop into the twenties. In the case of the young person, the heart may simply go into asystole. This diminished cardiac capacity occurs at a time when a greater volume of blood is returning to the heart as a result of peripheral vasoconstriction. Since the heart cannot handle the increased work, backwards heart failure occurs and noncardiogenic pulmonary edema develops.

When the onset of hypothermia is gradual, the patient may also experience **cold diuresis** (excessive urination due to decreased temperatures).[5] As blood is shunted to the core, the kidneys become engorged with blood. As the core temperature drops, renal cell dysfunction sets in. Coupled with lower levels of ADH, the kidneys start to excrete large volumes of dilute urine. Along with movement of fluids into the interstitial space, the patient suffers from hypovolemia. Treatment for this condition is discussed later.[6]

Local Cold Injuries

A survey of cold injuries is not complete without a discussion of local cold injuries, even though the treatment of local cold injuries is basic. **Frostbite**, a freezing of tissue, is an example of a localized cold injury. Frostbite can occur because of prolonged exposure to cold temperatures, such as might occur with cross-country skiing, or a sudden exposure to a cold-producing agent such as anhydrous ammonia found on a farm.

Frostbite can be classified, like a burn, as either superficial frostbite or deep (full thickness) frostbite. Like a superficial burn, superficial frostbite, also known as **frostnip**, involves just the epidermal layers of the skin. And like a superficial burn, superficial frostbite is initially reddened and may develop some blanched areas. Often there is diminished sensation in the area as well.

Generally, frostnip resolves spontaneously when the patient is rewarmed. The key to treating this superficial frostbite is to ensure that it does not evolve into deep frostbite. In the past, some practitioners advocated rubbing the frostbitten area with snow to increase circulation. However, by rubbing snow on the frozen area, ice crystals within the affected tissue damage more cells, thereby worsening the injury. The therapeutic goal is to not allow the injury to worsen. This is best accomplished by getting the patient out of the cold environment and removed to someplace warm.

Deep frostbite occurs when the freezing extends past the epidermal layer and moves into the subcutaneous tissues. Patients with deep frostbite have an area of the body that is generally hard on palpation, has a white appearance, and lacks sensation.

As frostbite frequently involves the periphery—such as toes, nose, fingers, and ears, all of which are important appendages—it is important to get treatment as soon as possible. As with all cold injuries, the first priority is to get the patient out of the environment, remove wet and especially constrictive clothing, and then apply a dry dressing to the wound.

If available, the treatment of extremity injuries is immersion. The affected extremity is gradually immersed into tepid water (no warmer than 104°F). Most patients complain of severe pain with reperfusion of the affected extremity. Therefore, liberal use of analgesics, to the extent the patient can tolerate, is advised.

If immersion rewarming is not available, then the Paramedic should splint the extremity and transport the patient immediately. The affected limb should not be rewarmed by use of chemical hot packs or other means (the use of hot packs and rewarming is discussed later in the chapter). Under no circumstances should the extremity be rewarmed if there is a chance of it refreezing.

Trench foot (immersion foot) is a special case of cold injury that was first described in World War I. Appearing similar to frostbite, trench foot occurs at temperatures above freezing, often in tropical jungles. **Trench foot** is localized tissue damage that occurs from prolonged exposure to moisture that is below body temperature. The tissue is initially reddened, then becomes pale or mottled and finally purple or blue. Eventually, the tissues die. Untreated toes can be lost within six hours and the entire foot within 24 hours. Because the damage is more superficial, walking on the affected limb can worsen the injury. Therefore, the patient should be evacuated by litter and not allowed to walk.

The treatment of trench foot, like other cold injuries, consists of removing the affected extremity from the environment, removing wet socks, drying the area, and padding the injury with a dry dressing.[7]

STREET SMART

Frostbite is not only a function of temperature. It can also occur above sub-zero temperatures, especially with a wind chill.

Mrs. Maud is 78 years old and is a wisp of a woman, barely weighing 50 kgs. Although she is independent, her simple surroundings suggest she is living at a subsistence level. Like a lot of elderly patients, she has a list of medical conditions, such as osteoporosis, hypothyroidism, hypertension, and a previous stroke. She broke her hip once before. Her medications include a beta blocker. All this information is on the "vial of life" left on the refrigerator door.

CRITICAL THINKING QUESTIONS

1. What are the important elements of the history that a Paramedic should obtain?
2. What is the implication of taking certain medications to hypothermia?

History

Like all trauma, the first step in assessing the patient is determining the mechanism of injury. Although the obvious mechanism of injury in a cold emergency may be prolonged exposure to cold during outdoor recreation, there are others. For example, persons trapped in a mudslide following a summer thunderstorm may experience hypothermia. Cold injury secondary to cold-water immersion is a constant threat for commercial fishermen and water sport enthusiasts. Anytime the body is subjected to sustained temperatures below 98.6°F (37°C), in the right conditions the patient may become hypothermic.

Certain pediatric patient populations are at increased risk for cold injuries and hypothermia. Infants, for example, have immature nervous systems and may be unable to control body temperature. Children with non-environmental hypothermia should be evaluated for possible sepsis, endocrine disorders, and toxic ingestion.[8] The higher risk for hypothermia among children is a function of a larger body surface area to mass coupled with poor judgment.

The elderly are also more at risk for cold injuries and hypothermia. Several changes of aging predispose the elderly to hypothermia, such as diminished subcutaneous fat for insulation. Diminished physiologic capacities serve to undermine the elderly patient's ability to withstand cold stress, which may cause him to succumb to the cold. For example, shivering is the mainstay of thermogenesis during hypothermia. However, the elderly patient's decreased muscle mass decreases his ability to shiver. In addition, shivering requires energy. Malnutrition or undernutrition, secondary to altered gastrointestinal function, reduces the amount of energy available to shiver. Shivering also requires oxygen. Diminished respiratory reserves and functional lung capacity reduce the amount of oxygen available. Finally, medications commonly prescribed to the elderly, such as beta blockers, may diminish the elderly patient's ability to respond to cold stress.[9]

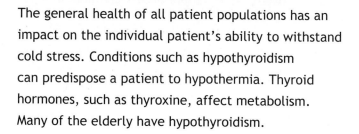

STREET SMART

The general health of all patient populations has an impact on the individual patient's ability to withstand cold stress. Conditions such as hypothyroidism can predispose a patient to hypothermia. Thyroid hormones, such as thyroxine, affect metabolism. Many of the elderly have hypothyroidism.

Some drugs can induce hypothermia (Table 13-1). For example, patients taking antipsychotic medications may have an adverse drug reaction that can lead to hypothermia. This, in turn, diminishes the patient's ability to respond to cold stress and can be a significant contributing cause of hypothermia. Many medications can impact the nervous system.

Certain diseases and conditions can also make a person more prone to hypothermia. As the skin plays a major role in the body's warmth, persons with skin disorders such as burns and psoriasis are prone to hypothermia. Likewise, since the

Table 13-1 Medications Associated with Hypothermia

- Sedatives
- Alcohol
- Opiates
- Barbiturates
- Anticonvulsants
- Antihistamines
- Antipsychotics
- Antidepressants
- Antipyretics

endocrine system, and particularly thyroxine and epinephrine, plays a major role in heat production, certain endocrine disorders make a patient more prone to hypothermia (e.g., hypothyroidism [myxedema] and primary adrenal insufficiency [Addison disease]).

Finally, the central nervous system, through its sensory pathways and the hypothalamus, controls heat production. Drugs such as opiates and narcotics, as well as certain antipsychotic medications such as tricyclics, can depress the central nervous system and make the patient more prone to hypothermia. In fact, any neurological condition that can leave a patient insensate to heat loss, such as stroke or spinal cord injury (spinothalamic tract), can render a person prone to hypothermia.

CASE STUDY (CONTINUED)

The Paramedic kneels next to Mrs. Maud and explains she is going to examine her. Mrs. Maud moans a barely audible and incomprehensible sound. Resting a hand on Mrs. Maud's shoulder, the Paramedic is taken aback by how cold her skin feels. "That is odd," she thinks, "It only went down to 50 last night and it's warm here in the sun. Why isn't Mrs. Maud shivering if she is that cold?" Looking down the length of the patient, she notes the incontinence—possibly due to a pelvic fracture or cold diuresis—that seems to have hastened the hypothermia.

CRITICAL THINKING QUESTIONS

1. What is the significance of the lack of shivering?
2. What impact does hypothermia have on mental status?

Examination

Optimally, measurement of the patient's core temperature is used to determine the level of hypothermia. Unfortunately, most standard thermometers depend on peripheral locations (i.e., oral, rectal, or axillary), and then adjust these measurements to correspond with the core temperature. These peripheral locations are often the first ones affected by vasoconstriction. Standard thermometers also have a lower limit of 93.2°F (34°C), making them impractical for measuring hypothermia. However, special low core thermometers are available. Newer tympanic membrane thermometers also hold promise. Studies have shown that tympanic thermometers are comparable to esophageal thermometers at measuring core temperatures and are simple and fast.[10] The most accurate means of obtaining a core temperature in the field is with the use of rectal thermometers. However, due to the difficulty of obtaining rectal temperatures in the field, Paramedics must depend on physical findings to help make the diagnosis of hypothermia.

The most notable physical finding for the patient with mild hypothermia is shivering. The presence of shivering helps the Paramedic to distinguish between mild and moderate hypothermia and has implications for the urgency of care.

Mortality is rare in cases of mild hypothermia. Shivering can continue for several hours provided the patient has adequate energy supplies and substances like drugs or alcohol do not inhibit the patient's shivering.

The patient with mild hypothermia will generally be hyperdynamic as well, as tachypnea, tachycardia, and hypertension will be present. This is a result of epinephrine's effects. The patient's skin should be cool and pale, for example.

Mild hypothermia will initially result in loss of fine motor coordination, and will progress to impairment of gross motor function, including stumbling and falling. The latter may significantly impair the patient's ability for self-help or self-rescue.

Patients with mild hypothermia may also present with altered judgment. Mildly hypothermic patients may have an uncharacteristic irritability to suggestion or may not be cooperative with care. This altered judgment is sometimes seen in a phenomenon called **paradoxical undressing**, in which patients with hypothermia often state they have an overwhelming feeling of warmth and take off their clothes just before losing consciousness.[11] Another peculiar behavior is **terminal burrowing**, wherein the patient enters into a confined space. Theories suggest that terminal vasodilation or a malfunction of the hypothalamus is responsible for these behaviors. Their consequences are obvious.

One means of remembering the signs and symptoms of mild hypothermia is to remember the "umbles": stumbles, mumbles, fumbles, and grumbles. Along with shivering, the "umbles" are seen in mild hypothermia.

Special Case of Intoxication

The Paramedic should exercise caution when treating a suspected hypothermic patient if the patient may also be intoxicated. Alcohol has a threefold impact on the hypothermic patient. First, alcohol is a vasodilator, leading to the temporary sensation of warmth. However, it ultimately increases the loss of heat over the long term. Next, alcohol depresses the shivering reflex, which is a vital compensatory mechanism. Again, this hastens the onset of moderate to severe hypothermia. Finally, alcohol impairs judgment. The altered judgment may occur from alcohol intoxication or may be the result of hypothermia. When given the choice, the Paramedic and the patient are better served to err on the side of mild hypothermia and to treat the patient

accordingly, rather than return later to treat the severely hypothermic patient.

As the body temperature approaches 82°F (32°C), the compensatory mechanisms start to fail. Shivering stops and consciousness starts to wane. At approximately 86°F (30°C), the patient may lose consciousness. At 86°F (30°C), the pulse also starts to slow and cardiac output is diminished. This results in loss of peripheral pulses. It is important that the Paramedic take a full minute to obtain an accurate pulse in the hypothermic patient.

The most dramatic manifestation of altered cardiac physiology is spontaneous dysrhythmia, such as atrial fibrillation. However, atrial fibrillation may be difficult to distinguish from sinus bradycardia with muscle tremor-induced artifact.[12] Many of the intervals—such as PR, QRS, and QT intervals—lengthen in response to slowed conduction secondary to hypothermia. The appearance of the pathomimetic J wave, also called an **Osborne wave** (Figure 13-3),

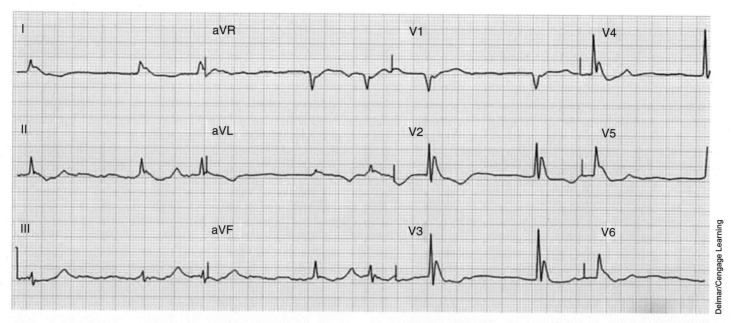

Figure 13-3 A J wave that is pathomimetic for hypothermia may be seen on an ECG.

Delmar/Cengage Learning

may also be seen. The J wave, although pathognomonic to hypothermia, is present in only about one-third of patients.

During moderate hypothermia, the pupils become sluggish, then dilated, and then fixed, as occurs during the progression of papillary response in a severe brain injury. These findings highlight the impact that hypothermia has upon the central nervous system. Like the pupils, the patient's mental status will change from apathetic and lethargic to stuporous and onto coma.

The patient with severe hypothermia (< 82.4°F [28°C]) may appear dead. Unresponsiveness (coma), severe hypotension, and loss of pulses—secondary to myocardial depression, hypoventilation to the point of apnea, and fixed dilated pupils—may lead to a diagnosis of death. However,

Table 13-2 Levels of Hypothermia

Level	Core Temperature	Clinical Signs	Rewarming
Mild	90°F–95°F (32°C–35°C)	• Shivering • Fine motor impairment • Judgment impaired • Hyperdynamic	Passive external
Moderate	82°F–90°F (28°C–32°C)	• Shivering stops • Altered mental status • Hypodynamic	Active external
Severe	< 82°F (< 28°C)	• Unconscious • Absent pulses	Active internal

all of these conditions are potentially reversible. The saying goes, "The patient is not dead until he is warm and dead."

Different levels of hypothermia have corresponding clinical signs and unique rewarming techniques (Table 13-2). However, these signs and techniques are intended to serve only as a guide. As every patient is an individual, some may not fit the guideline criteria.

▶ CASE STUDY (CONTINUED)

"Let's be careful with Mrs. Maud," says the Paramedic. "I know this is a medical emergency, but let's handle her carefully or we will be getting a whole lot busier, if you know what I mean."

The absence of a radial pulse, coupled with the profound bradycardia on the ECG monitor, suggests to the Paramedic that Mrs. Maud has severe hypothermia. Initially, the ECG monitor startles everyone. Mrs. Maud is in asystole; however, the Paramedic reminds everyone that she is still talking, even if it is not understandable. Moving the electrodes to the center of mass and changing the lead to MCL1 improves the picture.

CRITICAL THINKING QUESTIONS

1. What are the degrees of hypothermia?
2. How does the Paramedic determine compensated versus decompensated hypothermia?

Assessment

Hypothermia, like hypoxia, is a disorder. Traditionally, the diagnosis of hypothermia has been divided into three levels—mild or minor, moderate, and severe—and treatments are assigned accordingly. However, another way to look at hypothermia is with the same model used to describe hypotension: compensated versus decompensated. This model recognizes the importance of supporting the body's own mechanisms and also emphasizes the importance of intervention when the body is unable to compensate. This approach to the treatment of hypothermia is supported by the incidence of morbidity and mortality associated with compensated (mild) hypothermia and decompensated (moderate to severe) hypothermia.

The first order of business is to get Mrs. Maud off the floor. While the first responders head to the ambulance to get the "scoop" stretcher, the Paramedic starts to cut off the patient's wet clothes and examine Mrs. Maud. Although her leg is shorted and rotated, that is not her biggest problem.

Placing a dry blanket over Mrs. Maud, the Paramedic asks the first responders to create a thermal wrap while she establishes intravenous access, which is no small task as the vasoconstriction has left no visible external veins. Probing blindly in the antecubital fossa, the Paramedic eventually gets a flash. After ensuring that it is not arterial, she starts a low drip of saline at room temperature. The Paramedic remembers a guideline from her lessons: "If it took hours to cause hypothermia, then it should take hours to treat it."

Suddenly, a first responder walks into the room and announces, "Look what I found in the bathroom next to her medicines." He is holding a hot water bottle. Excellent thought, the Paramedic agrees, as the Paramedic directs the first responder to fill it with tepid tap water and put it on the patient's pelvis.

CRITICAL THINKING QUESTIONS

1. What is the national standard of care of patients with hypothermia?
2. Why is there the concern for "after drop?"

Treatment

The first order of business in all cases of hypothermia, regardless of the level or degree of hypothermia, is to try to stabilize the patient's current temperature. The issue of rewarming is secondary. To help the patient stabilize his temperature, the Paramedic should remove the patient's wet clothing, as the patient can lose 30 times more heat through thermal conductivity with the wet clothing.

Next, the Paramedic should cover the patient, as hypothermia is further aggravated by heat loss from radiation. Remember that radiation is one of the body's primary mechanisms to naturally dissipate heat. The goal is to help the body retain whatever heat is being created, no matter how little the amount.

Finally, the Paramedic should remove the patient from the environment, especially from exposure to wind. This will help to reduce convective heat loss. A simple blanket is typically sufficient. There are plasticized polymer blankets that are coated in reflective films, in many cases aluminum foil, that can reflect body heat back to the patient. In some cases, a hypothermia wrap is created. These wraps consist of a layer of polypropylene—which wicks moisture away from the body, keeping it dry—and layers of insulating materials. Wool is particularly well suited as an insulation material, as it maintains its heat-retaining capacity even when wet. Then, the entire package, including the patient, is wrapped in plastic or similar impervious material to prevent moisture from the environment from wicking away heat (Figure 13-4).

These techniques are all considered **passive rewarming**, wherein the patient's own body heat is used to rewarm the patient. Thermogenesis for passive rewarming is dependent, in large part, upon muscular activity, such as shivering. The body's ability to shiver is premised on having adequate supplies of oxygen and glucose to maintain aerobic metabolism. High-flow, high-concentration oxygen is often in order, as is the administration of glucose-containing solutions. Glucose may be administered orally if the patient can maintain an independent airway. Otherwise, intravenous administration may be necessary.[13]

If the patient is capable of maintaining an airway, it may be wise to provide the patient with some food. The saying goes, "Eat for heat." Simple carbohydrates, those energy foods that provide for a quick release of sugar, should be provided to the patient to support shivering. If the patient can tolerate simple carbohydrates, then the Paramedic can provide foods containing proteins and fats. These foods sustain the patient for a longer period of time. The analogy can be made to stoking a fire: using kindling (i.e., simple sugars) to start the fire, then adding increasingly larger branches (i.e., complex foodstuffs, such as carbohydrates and proteins), then finally logs (i.e., fats).

STREET SMART

Although having the patient self-assist with rescue may seem like a good idea, the muscular activity actually pushes cold blood from the extremities into the core. For this reason, the patient with moderate to severe hypothermia (i.e., non-shivering) should not be encouraged to walk.

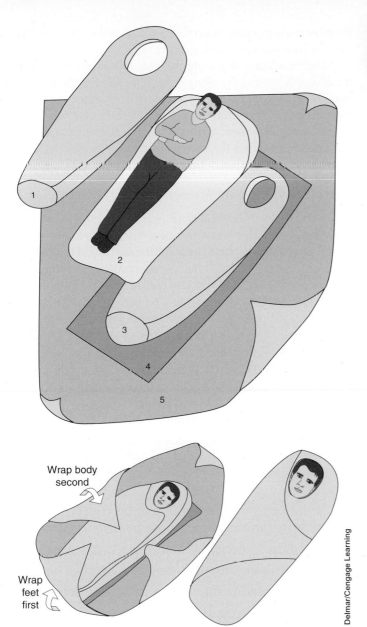

Figure 13-4 A hypothermia wrap prevents moisture from the environment from wicking away the patient's heat.

Wrap body second

Wrap feet first

Delmar/Cengage Learning

Alcohol, a vasodilator, increases heat loss through peripheral vasodilation and therefore should be avoided. Since caffeine is a diuretic, causes increased water loss, and leads to further dehydration, it should also be avoided.

In some cases, the patient is incapable of producing sufficient heat to rewarm himself. This is the key difference between mild hypothermia and moderate to severe hypothermia. In these cases, the Paramedic may need to provide the patient with heat through **active rewarming** (taking steps to add heat to the body). Although active rewarming may appear to be desirable, it is fraught with potentially lethal complications. In many cases, patient survival is best served by patiently waiting for the patient to rewarm passively, if at all possible.[14]

STREET SMART

Epinephrine can be very effective in shunting blood away from the skin. Paramedics who have dressed a wound outdoors in the frigid cold have seen "bleed through" of their dressings once the patient is in the warm ambulance and peripheral blood flow returns.

Active Rewarming

The Paramedic must carefully consider active rewarming. A malignant hypothermia syndrome—represented by the triad of severe hypotension, dysrhythmia, and hyperkalemia—can lead to death. In most cases, if the patient was cooled slowly—that is, if hypothermia developed slowly, (for example, "terrestrial" hypothermia occurs over hours to days)—then the patient should be warmed slowly, using passive rewarming (i.e., endogenous heat production and minimization of external heat loss). However, the physical health of some patients will not permit slow passive rewarming. Such is the case in severe hypothermia and cardiac arrest.

Thermoregulation and the body's ability to warm itself ceases below 86°F (30°C). This is a key factor when the Paramedic decides whether to allow the patient to passively rewarm or to perform active rewarming procedures. If the patient's temperature is at or below 86°F (30°C), the patient will continue to deteriorate unless further active intervention is taken.

Once the decision is made to actively rewarm the patient, the Paramedic must decide whether to use active external rewarming or active internal rewarming. The simplest form of active rewarming, and the most quickly executed method, is external active rewarming.[15]

Active External Rewarming

Once the conditions for passive rewarming have been achieved, the Paramedic can proceed with active external rewarming. The traditional method of active external rewarming uses chemical hot packs applied to areas where major veins rise to the surface of the skin. As major arteries tend to run alongside major veins, these points will be recognized as pulse points. Any source of external heat, such as hot water bottles and heated blankets, is acceptable.

Hot packs, which are easily accessed, are applied to the carotid pulse point (proximal to the larynx) and the femoral pulse point (proximal to the groin). The Paramedic should exercise caution when using chemical hot packs. These hot packs tend to warm up very fast, reaching temperatures of 160°F (71.1°C), then cool down. Special chemical heat packs, such as the *Heat Wave*™, can produce a more steady heat at 100°F (37.8°C) and sustain that temperature for up to 10 hours. The temperatures of standard chemical hot packs can burn vulnerable skin that is already compromised. Therefore, the hot pack should be covered initially to protect the skin from burn trauma.[16]

The Paramedic should also ensure that the heat pack is intact. Often chemical heat packs are inserted under clothing or wrapped in towels, for example, and placed out of sight. These packs often contain calcium chloride, or magnesium sulfate, which can be corrosive to the skin.

Other methods of passive external rewarming include the use of radiant heat lamps (some ambulances have these built into the head liner in the patient compartment) and electric-powered heat guns.

The Paramedic should also exercise caution when warming the body's core. Rapid rewarming of the extremities can lead to the after drop phenomenon. Perhaps first described by Baron Dominick Jean Larrey, who is attributed with invention of the "flying ambulance," **after drop phenomenon** occurs when cold extremities are warmed. The subsequent vasodilation sends cold, acidotic, and hyperkalemic blood surging to the core. The result is an actual drop in body core temperature (after drop) which—combined with the acidotic, hyperkalemic blood—can lead to ventricular fibrillation and sudden cardiac death. This phenomenon is not universally agreed upon. Some experts assert that there are insufficient volumes of blood in the periphery to cause a drop in the core temperature following rewarming of the extremities, particularly if the onset of hypothermia was gradual.

Active Internal Rewarming

If available, the Paramedic may consider the initiation of warm, humidified oxygen. The oxygen, at approximately 104°F to 113°F (40°C to 45°C), can be administered via either mask or, preferably, endotracheal tube. Not only does warmed humidified oxygen increase the patient's rewarming by 1.8°F to 3.6°F (1°C to 2°C), it also stems the loss of heat from the respirations.

A number of compact and portable oxygen-warming devices are available, from the "mechanical nose" that uses the patient's own latent heat of respiration, to battery operated non-invasive core rewarming systems.

The Paramedic should not hesitate to intubate the patient if needed to control the airway and/or to administer warmed, humidified oxygen to the patient's core. In the past, there was a concern that intubation could induce ventricular fibrillation in the patient. However, a prospective multicenter study demonstrated that was not the case, as zero episodes of ventricular fibrillation resulted from intubation of hypothermic patients.[17]

Special Case of Rewarming Shock

When the onset of hypothermia is gradual, the patient may experience cold diuresis, which was described earlier. While in the hypothermic state, the contracted blood volume is sufficient for the patient who is vasoconstricted. When the body is rewarmed, however, vasoconstriction is reversed and a normal vascular space returns. The patient, who is volume contracted, will develop hypoperfusion that can even lead to cardiac arrest. To prevent **rewarming shock**, the Paramedic should infuse 1 to 2 liters of normal saline (0.9% NaCl), heated to 113°F (45°C) if possible, prophylactically (20 cc per kg for children) in anticipation of rewarming shock. The Paramedic should avoid lactated Ringer's, as the hypothermic liver is incapable of metabolizing the lactate.

STREET SMART

In severe hypothermia, the medulla and the respiratory centers become unresponsive to increasing carbon dioxide levels. The body resorts to hypoxia drive and in rare situations the administration of oxygen may lead to respiratory arrest. The prepared Paramedic understands this phenomenon and is prepared to ventilate the patient.

CASE STUDY (CONTINUED)

Despite the utmost care during handling, Mrs. Maud appears to have gone into cardiac arrest. With no peripheral or central pulses, an absence of heart sounds, and asystole on the ECG monitor, the Paramedic orders compressions while she prepares for intubation.

Local medical protocols advise only one shock for ventricular fibrillation, no medications (including atropine and epinephrine), and no pacing even though this is a witnessed asystole. "OK, let's make this CPR count," the Paramedic says as the patient is packaged for transport.

CRITICAL THINKING QUESTIONS

1. What are some of the predictable complications associated with hypothermia?
2. What are some of the predictable complications associated with the treatments for hypothermia?

Evaluation

The Paramedic should withhold CPR if there is any sign of a rhythm, regardless of the absence of peripheral pulses. Bradycardia is frequently witnessed at rates as low as 20 bpm. The body is in a "metabolic icebox" and this heart rate is all that may be necessary. The chilled heart is often refractory to the Paramedic's efforts at transcutaneous pacing or the use of atropine.

Hypothermic patients are prone to ventricular fibrillation, particularly if handled roughly. Therefore, extra efforts should be taken to ensure that the patient is truly in cardiac arrest. Because the patient's skin is cold, the ECG electrodes may register asystole despite the presence of electrical activity. Electrode gel needs to heat to melt and form a conductive "bridge" with the body core. Similarly, shivering may be mistaken for ventricular fibrillation. For these reasons, the Paramedic typically takes the carotid pulse for a minute to ensure true cardiac arrest.

If the patient is truly in ventricular fibrillation, then CPR should be commenced and a single attempt at defibrillation may be in order.[18] Note that, since the chilled heart will most likely not respond to defibrillation, further attempts at defibrillation should be withheld until the patient is rewarmed. This is consistent with the American Heart Association recommendations in its advanced cardiac life support.[19]

In most cases, the administration of anti-arrhythmic medication is also inappropriate. Common anti-arrhythmic medications such as lidocaine and procainamide, for example, are inactivated in cold temperatures.

Unless the patient has an obviously lethal wound, such as a frozen chest, then CPR should be continued until the patient is delivered to the hospital or the rescuer is fatigued. The Alaska protocol calls for the EMT to perform CPR for 60 minutes if the patient is in ventricular fibrillation.

▶ CASE STUDY CONCLUSION

The ambulance starts to the trauma center, where extracorporeal core rewarming is available. After giving the radio alert, the Paramedic reflects, "Is it possible she bled out in her hip or pelvis?"

CRITICAL THINKING QUESTIONS

1. What is the most appropriate transport decision that will get the patient to definitive care?
2. If the patient was in cardiac arrest would that alter the transportation decision?

Disposition

Transportation to a hospital capable of extracorporeal core rewarming (ECR) is preferable when the patient has hypothermia. Although heated lavage of the bladder (via catheter) and the gastrointestinal tract (via orogastric tube) is possible at a community hospital, the transfer of heat is minimal and therefore of limited benefit. However, warmed saline irrigations of the lungs via bilateral thoracostomy tubes may be effective. In cases of multiple patients, options may be limited. Cases of mild to moderate hypothermia may be transferred to the community hospital as a function of triage. Cases of severe hypothermia, in contrast, should be transported to hospitals capable of ECR.

Hemodialysis, as well as venovenous, arteriovenous, and cardiopulmonary bypass, are four methods of extracorporeal rewarming. The availability of these services, and the needed specialists to perform them, should be evaluated on a community-by-community basis and factored into the decision on the patient's destination.[20]

CONCLUSION

All patients with suspected hypothermia should be transported for medical evaluation. Complications of hypothermia include aspiration pneumonia, pulmonary edema, coagulopathies, pancreatitis, and electrolyte disorders. If treated appropriately, starting in the field, hypothermia and its attendant complications are survivable with minimal sequela. However, ignored or mistreated hypothermia can be deadly.

▶ KEY POINTS:

- Cold emergencies occur in all climates and locations.

- An internal core temperature around 99°F (37°C) must be maintained for homeostasis.

- Approximately 65% of the body's heat is lost through radiation. Wind increases that loss. Passel and Siple's wind chill chart accounts for the increased heat loss attributed to wind's convection.

- Thermogenesis is limited and augmented by shivering in an emergency.

- Shunting of blood keeps core organs warm.

- Shivering is supported by muscular glycogen but creates a glycogen debt.

- Hypothermia is divided into mild (89.6°F to 95°F [32°C to 35°C]), moderate (82.4°F to 89.6°F [28°C to 32°C]), and severe (< 82.4°F [28°C]) categories.

- Hypothermia affects oxygenation by vasoconstriction of the pulmonary vasculature, creating a pulmonary shunt, and shifting the oxyhemoglobin curve to the left, allowing oxygen onto red blood cells but not releasing it at the cellular level.

- Hypothermia affects the cardiovascular system by slowing the heart when there is increased venous return, due to peripheral vasoconstriction, leading to backwards heart failure and noncardiogenic pulmonary edema.

- Hypothermia can lead to hypovolemia because of cold diuresis.

- Frostnip, and the more severe frostbite, are examples of localized cold injuries.

- The J wave, or Osborne wave, on the ECG is pathognomonic for hypothermia.

- Spontaneous dysrhythmias, such as atrial fibrillation, are common with hypothermia.

- Altered mental status is a constant in all three levels of hypothermia; however, absence of shivering can be used to distinguish mild from moderate hypothermia.

- Stabilization begins with removing the patient from the environment, stripping the patient of wet clothes, and then covering the patient with a blanket. Further treatment is dependent on the degree of hypothermia.

- Techniques for rewarming are passive warming, active external rewarming, and active internal rewarming.

- Active external rewarming consists of the use of hot packs or warming blankets, whereas active internal rewarming consists of the use of warmed humidified oxygen, mechanical noses, and warmed intravenous solutions.

- Aggressive external rewarming can flood the core with cold, acidotic blood that actually worsens the patient's hypothermia, called the after drop phenomenon.

- If any pulse is detected, the Paramedic should withhold CPR (see local protocols) and medications if the patient goes into arrest.

- Hospitals are capable of performing extracorporeal core rewarming with dramatic results. Therefore, patients with hypothermia who are dead should be treated until they are warm and dead.

REVIEW QUESTIONS:

1. Describe the process of cold diuresis.
2. What factors make the elderly more prone to hypothermia than others?
3. How does intoxication affect hypothermia?
4. How can a profoundly hypothermic patient be mistaken as dead?
5. What is the utility of looking at hypothermia as either compensated or decompensated?

CASE STUDY QUESTIONS:

Please refer to the Case Study in this chapter, and answer the questions below:

1. What implication would shivering have in this case?
2. Why is a beta blocker problematic in this patient?
3. What would be the significance if the back door had been left open?

REFERENCES:

1. Centers for Disease Control and Prevention (CDC). Hypothermia-related deaths—United States, 2003–2004. *MMWR Morb Mortal Wkly Rep*. Feb 25 2005;54(7):173–175.
2. Baumgartner, E.A. Hypothermia and other cold-related morbidity emergency department visits: United States, 1995–2004. *Wilderness Environ Med*. 2008;19;233–237.
3. Hypothermia-related deaths—United States, 1999–2002 and 2005. *MMWR Morb Mortal Wkly Rep*. March 2006;55(10): 282–284.
4. Sessler DI. Thermoregulatory defense mechanisms. *Crit Care Med*. Jul 2009;37(7 Suppl):S203–S210.
5. Giesbrecht G, Wilderson J. *Hypothermia, Frostbite and Other Cold Injuries* (2nd ed.). Seattle: The Mountaineers Books; 2006.
6. Polderman KH. Mechanisms of action, physiological effects, and complications of hypothermia. *Crit Care Med*. Jul 2009;37 (7 Suppl):S186–202.
7. Long WB, Edlich RF, Winters KL, Britt LD. Cold injuries. *J Long Term Eff Med Implants*. 2005;15(1):67–78.
8. Greenberg RA, Rittichier KK. Pediatric nonenvironmental hypothermia presenting to the emergency department. *Pediatric Emergency Care*. February 2003;19(1):32–34.
9. Merck Manual of Geriatrics Section 8 Metabolic and Endocrine Disorders. Chapter 67 Hyperthermia and Hypothermia. Last updated February 2006. Available at: **http://www.merck.com/**. Accessed August 2009.
10. Walpoth BP, et al. Assessment of hypothermia with new "tympanic" thermometer. *J Clin Monit Comput*. March 1994;10(2):91–96. Danzl D. Accidental hypothermia. In: *Wilderness Medicine: Management of Wilderness and Environmental Emergencies* (4th ed.). St. Louis, MO: Mosby; 2002:135–217.
11. Wedin B, Vanggaard L, Hirvonen J. "Paradoxical undressing" in fatal hypothermia." *J. Forensic Sci*. July 1979;24(3):543–553.
12. Adams DC, Heyer EJ, Simon AE, et al. Incidence of atrial fibrillation after mild or moderate hypothermie cardiopulmonary bypass. *Crit Care Med*. Feb 2000;28:309–311.
13. Biem J, Koehncke N, Classen D, Dosman J. Out of the cold: management of hypothermia and frostbite. *CMAJ*. Feb 4 2003;168(3):305–311.
14. Bernard SA, Gray TW, Buist MD, et al. Treatment of comatose survivors of out-of-hospital cardiac arrest with induced hypothermia. *N Engl J Med*. Feb 21 2002;346(8):557–563.
15. McCullough L, Arora S. Diagnosis and treatment of hypothermia. *Am Fam Physician*. Dec 15 2004;70(12): 2325–2332.
16. Feldman KW, Morray JP, Schaller RT. Thermal injury caused by hot pack application in hypothermic children. *Am J Emerg Med*. Jan 1985;3(1):38–41.
17. American Heart Association. Part 10.4: hypothermia. Circulation 2005; 112(Suppl 24):IV-133-IV-135.
18. Cummins RO, ed. Hypothermia. In: *ACLS for Experienced Providers*. Dallas, TX: American Heart Association, 2003: 83–95.
19. 2005 American Heart Association Guidelines for Cardiopulmonary Resuscitation and Emergency Cardiovascular Care. *Circulation*. Nov 2005;112(24 Suppl):IV–136–IV–138.
20. Casas F, Alam H, Reeves A, Chen Z, Smith WA. A portable cardiopulmonary bypass/extracorporeal membrane oxygenation system for the induction and reversal of profound hypothermia: feasibility study in a swine model of lethal injuries. *Artif Organs*. Jul 2005;29(7):557–563.

CHAPTER 14

MOUNTAIN MEDICINE

KEY CONCEPTS:

Upon completion of this chapter, it is expected that the reader will understand these following concepts:

- Altitude sickness syndromes
  - Acute mountain sickness
  - High altitude cerebral edema
  - High altitude pulmonary edema
- Minor disorders of altitude
  - Ultraviolet keratitis
  - High altitude retinal hemorrhage
  - Khumbu cough
- Role of acclimatization in preventing mountain syndromes
- Assessment and diagnosis of altitude sickness syndromes
- Treatment of altitude sickness syndromes

ANATOMY CONCEPTS:

Prior to reading this chapter the Paramedic student should be familiar with the following anatomy and physiology concepts:

- Pulmonary physiology
- Pathophysiology of increased intracranial pressure

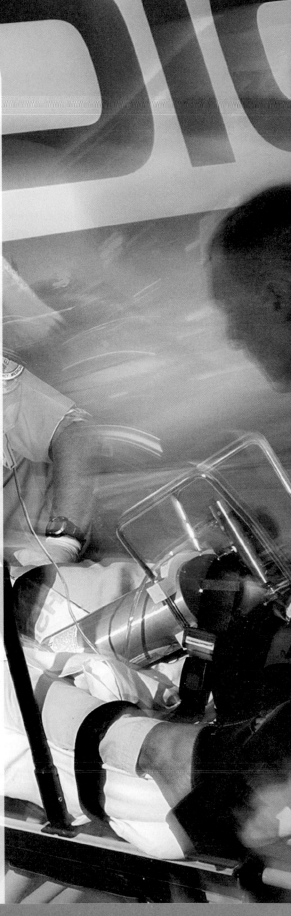

CASE STUDY:

At 10:30 a.m. three climbers from the East leave the parking area at Lupine Meadows (altitude 6,700 feet) in Grand Teton National Park bound for a two-day climb of the Glacier Route on the Middle Teton at 12,804 feet above sea level. Two of the climbers have significant rock climbing experience, and one was in the Tetons the previous season.

After about three hours of steady uphill climbing, they reach the snowline at Garnet Meadow where they rest, hydrate, and eat. One of the climbers, the most inexperienced of the group, is already starting to tire and states he isn't feeling very well today. However, after the brief break they resume their ascent to their proposed campsite at 10,800 feet.

CRITICAL THINKING QUESTIONS

1. What are some of the possible altitude sickness syndromes that may be suspected based on the mechanism of injury?

2. Are any of these altitude sickness syndromes potentially life-threatening conditions?

OVERVIEW

Travelers to mountainous areas of the United States and abroad can encounter several altitude-induced problems. The ease of travel around the world makes altitude illness a real possibility for people setting out on everything from a simple ski vacation in the Rockies to participating in outdoor sport venues such as mountain climbing and adventure racing. The universe of mountain medicine includes bites and stings, heat and cold illness, and even anaphylaxis. This chapter will focus on altitude sickness.

Chief Concern

Three common problems are generally encountered during a person's ascent to altitude: acute mountain sickness (AMS), high altitude pulmonary edema (HAPE), and high altitude cerebral edema (HACE). Before discussing these disorders, it is important to look at the levels of altitude.

A **moderate altitude** is considered to be any elevation between 8,000 and 12,000 feet; therefore, anything below 8,000 feet is considered low altitude. Recreationalists of all types easily reach this altitude. Many ski areas in the United States fall into this range. Snowmobiling, hiking, mountain climbing, adventure racing, and general tourism can and do also occur at these moderate altitudes. Anecdotal reports from physicians at popular resort areas such as Park City, Utah, for example, suggest that AMS is prominent as people fly in from more modest elevations in the United States for a week of skiing.

High altitude starts at 12,000 feet and extends to 18,000 feet. Many mountains in the United States—including the ranges in Alaska—as well as the Canadian Rockies reach these heights. There are human populations in Asia that live as high as 17,500 feet. Trekking, which has become very popular with people around the globe and generally takes place in Nepal, Tibet, and Pakistan, reaches these heights and beyond, up to about 20,000 feet. Many participants in trekking "expeditions" become sick, with some becoming incapacitated and ultimately evacuated. Trekking companies generally employ a medical professional (usually a physician or a Paramedic schooled in wilderness medicine and altitude-related illness) to accompany the group.

Any elevation above 18,000 feet is considered **extreme altitude**. There are many mountains in Asia (Himalaya), Russia (Pamirs), South America (Andes), and Africa that reach above 18,000 feet. These altitudes are generally visited by teams of climbers who attempt the high peaks of the world. Most people who spend weeks or months at an elevation of 18,000 feet or above are experienced in technical climbing. They are also well educated regarding travel at altitude, and accustomed to extreme weather conditions. However, in recent years there has been a significant increase of "guided" climbs of the world's tallest peaks like Mt. Everest. Some of the clients who are guided up peaks of this magnitude are poorly prepared for the physical and mental rigors of these expeditions. Consequently, many of them fall victim to the full range of altitude disorders as well as exposure to extreme elements.

Acclimatization

Inspired air contains 20.93% (21%) oxygen. As a person ascends in altitude, the barometric pressure decreases. Although the amount of oxygen remains the same, because the barometric pressure of the atmosphere decreases as one ascends, there are fewer oxygen molecules available in the inspired air. Dalton's law of partial pressures explains this. Dalton's law states the pressure of a mixed gas is equal to the sum of the pressures of the individual gasses it contains. At sea level, the barometric pressure is 760 mmHg, and 21% oxygen has a partial pressure of oxygen of 159.6 mmHg. The arterial oxygen is maintained at about 90 mmHg. At 15,000 feet, the barometric pressure is 429 mmHg and the air still contains 21% oxygen. However, at that elevation the partial pressure of oxygen drops to 90 mmHg. As a result, the arterial oxygen is only 44 mmHg (hypoxia is defined as arterial oxygen below 60 to 70 mmHg), and the hemoglobin saturation is 80%. The drop in the partial pressure of oxygen (pO_2) results in hypoxia. At 18,000 feet the atmospheric pressure and the pressure of oxygen in the air, is approximately half that at sea level.[1]

As pO_2 falls at altitudes above 9,000 to 10,000 feet, chemoreceptors create a hypoxic stimulus, increasing ventilation. Over time and with controlled ascent, the human body can compensate somewhat for the reduction in available oxygen molecules through a process commonly known as **acclimatization**.

Anybody who is traveling to altitude is at risk of acute mountain sickness, regardless of age, level of physical fitness, prior medical history, or previous experience from altitude sickness without acclimatization. Although physical fitness would seem to be protective, research has shown that this is not entirely true.[2] Many other factors need to be included to determine who gets sick at altitude. Among these are rate of ascent, maximum altitude reached, nutrition, hydration, past history of altitude illness, and prophylactic use of certain drugs known to be beneficial to acclimatization (which are discussed later).

Additionally, frequent travelers to mountainous areas who have never had anything more than a temporary mild headache should not adopt a cavalier altitude about travel to altitude. More severe forms of altitude illness can and do strike even the most experienced mountaineers.

Normal Response to Altitude

The body's normal response to an increase in altitude (Figure 14-1) includes faster, deeper breathing (i.e., Kussmaul-like hyperventilation); some shortness of breath during exertion, but not at rest; periodic breathing similar to Cheyne–Stokes breathing at night with frequent awakening; and increased urination. Additional physiological responses include increased cardiac output, higher pulmonary arterial pressure, a relative increase in red blood cells, and fluid shifting from the blood to the tissues.[1]

Polycythemia, increased red blood cell production, begins after a few days to weeks at altitude. The hypoxia stimulates the kidneys to release a hormone called erythropoietin, which travels to the bone marrow. This hormone stimulates the production of additional red blood cells. With more red blood cells, the blood can carry more oxygen. However, this process can take days to weeks to fully develop.[3] Chronic polycythemia is seen in those who live at higher altitudes and is sometimes called chronic mountain sickness (CMS). The problem is characterized by an excess of red blood cell production in people living permanently above an altitude of 8,000 feet (2,500 meters). The symptoms of this very incapacitating disease include headaches, chronic weakness and fatigue, digestive troubles, and sleep disturbances. Pulmonary and systemic hypertension are also commonly found. This condition is common in the Andean populations in South America as well as the high mountain villages in Nepal, Pakistan, and Tibet.

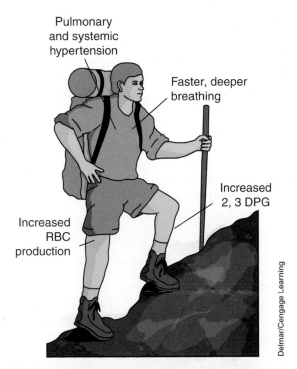

Pulmonary and systemic hypertension

Faster, deeper breathing

Increased 2, 3 DPG

Increased RBC production

Delmar/Cengage Learning

Figure 14-1 The normal physiological response to altitude includes changes in breathing and urination.

As the atmospheric pressure drops, the body also manufactures an enzyme called 2,3-diphosphoglycerate or 2,3-DPG. This enzyme lessens the affinity of oxygen to remain bound to hemoglobin and helps release more oxygen to tissues at lower pressure. As altitude increases and pressure drops, the body produces more 2,3-DPG, which keeps the oxygen transfer going.

As breathing becomes faster and deeper, CO_2 levels in the blood fall. Because a healthy individual runs on hypoxic drive (i.e., increased blood CO_2 levels), as CO_2 levels fall so does the inducement to breathe. The climber then becomes hypoxic, a headache often ensues, and the climber's secondary drive to breathe (the hypoxic drive) stimulates the climber to breathe.

If an individual is awake, this is easy to control. As hypoxia occurs secondary to hypoventilation, the climber takes a breath. Some climbers make a conscious effort to control their breathing to prevent the onset of hypoxia-induced headaches. However, when the climber is sleeping there is no conscious control of breath. As a result, a periodic Cheyne–Stokes-like breathing pattern develops due to the competition between the two respiratory triggers.[4]

If an individual is given an appropriate amount of time for the body to adjust to the altitude increase, these symptoms remain mild. If one continues to ascend to higher altitude too fast, however, symptoms become more frank and can cause increased distress and more serious conditions (which are discussed later in this chapter).

Hypoxia produces changes in the brain and lungs that lead to overperfusion of capillary beds with increased pressure, fluid leakage from the capillaries, and edema formation.[5] Acclimatization can be helped by the prophylactic use of acetazolamide (Diamox®). **Acetazolamide**, a carbonic anhydrase inhibitor, works by stimulating respirations and enhancing excretion of bicarbonate in the kidneys, thus acidifying the blood and balancing the respiratory alkalosis effect of the altitude-induced hyperventilation.

Acetazolamide has also been found to reduce pulmonary arterial pressures in animals, thus reducing fluid shift from pulmonary capillary beds into the alveoli and reducing the incidence of pulmonary edema.[6] The standard dosing is 125 mg twice daily beginning a day before the ascent and continuing for two to five days after arrival.[1] Acetazolamide also helps reduce episodes of periodic breathing at night by increasing the blood acid content through the increase in bicarbonate excretion, which engages the hypoxic drive and stimulates breathing. Recommended dosage for treatment of periodic breathing is 125 mg by mouth before bed.

As with any pharmacological treatment, there are side effects of acetazolamide. These include numbness and tingling in the extremities and around the mouth, as well as increased diuresis. This increase in urine output can exacerbate the chronic fluid loss common at altitude that is caused by exertion (perspiration) and water loss through the respiratory system. Because acetazolamide is a sulfa-based drug, it is contraindicated for those with sulfa allergies.

Ginkgo biloba has been studied in recent years as a prophylactic treatment for altitude illness. Although the studies are limited at this point, they do show promise. The recommended dose is 120 mg by mouth, twice a day, starting five days prior to ascent and continuing at altitude.[7] Possible side effects of Ginkgo are increased bleeding and, on occasion, hemorrhagic stroke.

Many diseases can mimic the effects of high altitude illness. Although poor health while at altitude is most likely caused by the altitude, ruling out other causes of illness is prudent.

Major Disorders of Altitude

Acute Mountain Sickness

When arriving at altitude, some people develop a transient illness called **acute mountain sickness (AMS)** that begins 6 to 24 hours after arrival, although symptoms can develop sooner. Although the exact cause of the illness is not completely known, there is evidence that the pathological effects are a result of cerebral edema. Lower PaO_2 levels at altitude cause vasodilatation. If not mediated, this causes leakage of fluid from the blood into brain tissue, causing the edema. This is directly related to the oxyhemoglobin dissociation curve. The **oxyhemoglobin dissociation curve** describes the relationship between available oxygen and oxygen carried by hemoglobin.

At a pO_2 of 80 mmHg, the SpO_2 is about 95%, which is expected in a healthy patient at sea level. A fall in pO_2 to 40 mmHg, which represents the oxygen pressure at 18,000 feet, results in a precipitous drop in SaO_2 to approximately 72%. At the summit of Mt. Everest, the highest point on Earth at 29,035 feet (8,850 meters), the pO_2 is only one-third that found at sea level.

Altitudes above 26,247 feet (8,000 meters) are considered the "death zone." Death zone is an appropriate name because above 26,247 feet (8,000 meters) life cannot be sustained for very long. Metabolism requires two things: oxygen and fuel. With reduced oxygen available, fuel can't be burned. At altitude, fuel (food) consumption declines and what does get eaten is less effective because of slowing digestion. Soon the body starts to consume itself in an effort to produce the necessary metabolic rate to maintain body temperature. At these altitudes, cells do not reproduce, and small things like a cut to the hand or cracked skin due to the harsh environment will not heal. However, pO_2 is not the only factor determining oxygen saturation. The amount of hemoglobin in the blood can greatly affect the SaO_2, even if the pO_2 is low.

People with increased diuresis at altitude are also less likely to develop AMS.[8] The diuresis may aid acclimatization through the excretion of excess base (i.e., sodium bicarbonate in the urine), as well as increasing dehydration that increases intravascular oncotic response and hypovolemia decreasing hydrostatic pressures.[9]

High Altitude Cerebral Edema (HACE)

High altitude cerebral edema (HACE) is a life-threatening condition caused by increased intracranial pressure (ICP) due to reduced pO_2 at altitude and the resulting leakage of fluid that compresses brain tissue. Although a different mechanism, HACE causes many of the same signs and symptoms as those found in a traumatic brain injury, resulting in increased ICP.

Fortunately, HACE has a low incidence, although the exact numbers are not known. The usual onset is 24 to 36 hours after arrival at altitudes over 10,000 feet (3,000 meters). There are several common risk factors for the development of HACE, including rapid ascent, past history of altitude illness, pulmonary abnormalities, and exertion. As in AMS, it's thought that there may be a genetic predisposition to development of HACE in certain individuals; however, this has not been well studied. The hallmarks of HACE—ataxia and altered level of consciousness—have a couple of theoretical causes. One theory suggests that HACE is actually caused by vasogenic edema or a disruption in the blood–brain barrier.[5] Whether this disruption of the blood–brain barrier is caused by mechanical means (increased capillary pressures) or is chemically mediated is still being investigated.

High Altitude Pulmonary Edema (HAPE)

Most deaths from altitude illness occur from **high altitude pulmonary edema (HAPE)**.[5] HAPE is a noncardiogenic edema caused by increased pressure in the pulmonary capillaries. HAPE usually occurs on the second night at a new altitude and rarely occurs after four days at a given altitude. This condition is caused by fluid shift into the alveoli from the pulmonary capillaries. As the alveoli fill with fluid, less oxygen is able to diffuse into the blood, which causes pO_2 in the blood to fall. This lack of oxygen becomes apparent in reduced brain function, reducing a person's ability to think clearly, which is a dangerous situation in an extreme environment.

HAPE is most often preceded by HACE. When this sequence occurs, the outcome is usually poor and there is a high likelihood of death unless treated quickly and aggressively.[1] HAPE has much of the same etiology as the other altitude disorders that have been discussed: too rapid an ascent, causing a lack of proper acclimatization, and heavy exertion, with both leading to an increase in pulmonary arterial pressures.

A cold environment may also play a role by increasing pulmonary capillary pressures. Normally, small pulmonary arterioles constrict to protect the capillaries, which prevents overpressuring and fluid leakage. In people who develop HAPE, this constriction is not uniform, causing capillary leakage in some areas of the lungs but not others.

Minor Disorders of Altitude

The following minor disorders may be seen either independently or in combination with the major mountain syndromes. Awareness of these disorders, and prevention of these disorders, is superior to treating the aftermath.

Ultraviolet Keratitis—Snow Blindness

Snow blindness (i.e., ultraviolet keratitis) is a very painful eye condition caused by exposure to extreme solar ultraviolet radiation. This typically occurs from wearing no protection or inadequate eye protection in high glare conditions.

When increased ultraviolet light on snow and ice at altitude burns the underprotected cornea of the eye, it causes this painful and debilitating condition. Symptoms of snow blindness include a gritty feeling in the eyes, redness and tearing, pain on movement of the eyes, and headache. Treatment is supportive, giving the eyes a chance to recover from the "sunburn." The Paramedic should remove the person from sunlight, blindfold both eyes, and cover them with cool, wet bandages. The patient should then seek medical attention after evacuation. Recovery from snow blindness may take two to three days. Prevention requires wearing appropriate protection for altitude (Table 14-1).

High Altitude Retinal Hemorrhage

High altitude retinal hemorrhages occur frequently at altitudes above 14,000 feet and are caused by a lack of oxygen to the retina. There is little evidence that these occur because of, or in conjunction with, other altitude disorders. However,

Table 14-1 Guidelines for the Proper Selection of Eyewear for Altitude

- 99% to 100% UV absorption (UVA, UVB, UVC)
- Polycarbonate or CR-39 lens (lighter, more comfortable than glass)
- 5% to 10% visible light transmittance
- Large lenses that fit close to the face
- Wrap around or side shielded to prevent incidental light exposure

some researchers believe that retinal hemorrhages are a sign of poor acclimatization.

This painless condition rarely affects vision unless the hemorrhage is large. In that case, a part of the visual field in the affected eye may be blurry. There is no treatment for high altitude retinal hemorrhage because the blood is usually reabsorbed in one to two weeks.

CASE STUDY (CONTINUED)

During the ascent from the meadow to the campsite, the climber who was feeling poorly earlier, a 24-year-old male, is noticeably struggling with the increased altitude, slowing his pace relative to his partners, and complaining of nausea and a headache. On arrival at the campsite, the 24-year-old male is exhausted with an increased headache and severe nausea, causing him to vomit. It is now about 3:30 p.m., so the group decides to pitch their three-man tent and rest, cook dinner, and prepare for an early morning start for the 12,804-foot summit.

The ill climber has a fitful night sleep. It is later reported by one of his tent mates that the ill climber seemed to stop breathing at times during the night, sometimes for several seconds at a time. At 6 a.m., he is in more distress with labored breathing and mild confusion. Although complaining of having to urinate, he is unable to unzip his sleeping bag to exit the tent. At this point, the two other climbers are alarmed at their friend's deteriorated condition, and it becomes obvious that he needs medical attention. Fortunately, one of them has a cell phone and is able to make a 9-1-1 call at 6:15 a.m., which is transferred to the Jenny Lake Ranger Station in the park.

After receiving the cell phone report on the ill climber's general condition, the rangers decide to dispatch two rangers to the site by helicopter. At 6:50 a.m., a park helicopter with the two park rangers/medics lifts off from the Rescue Cache at Lupine Meadows for the short flight to the area where the climbers are camped at 10,800 feet.

The history of the incident gained from the other climbers is that they had arrived from New York yesterday and were only going to be in the area for four days. They left their hotel in Jackson and drove to the trailhead the previous morning when they started their climb. The patient denies any past medical history, medications, or allergies, and considers himself a fit individual who regularly competes in triathlons back home.

CRITICAL THINKING QUESTIONS

1. What are the important elements of the history that a Paramedic should obtain?
2. What is the importance of the climbers arriving from New York?

History

Patients with acute mountain sickness may complain of dizziness, headache, nausea, fatigue, insomnia, and anorexia. Headache is almost universally common in people who travel above 6,000 feet (2,000 meters) and is a key indicator of AMS. The headache's severity can range from mild (described as a "hangover") to debilitating. The headache is described as either being in the back of the head or the temples. Straining (for example, to lift a pack) or bending over (for example, to retrieve something from a pack) often makes the headache worse.

Many climbers—particularly those climbers/trekkers or mountaineers who are at moderate elevations in the mountains for sport, recreation, or competition—will use alcohol, sleep aids, and narcotics for pain management. These three drugs all can induce respiratory depression, worsening AMS. AMS, in turn, can progress to HACE.

HAPE often occurs on the second night of a climb and can occur regardless of the individual's fitness level. The hallmarks of HAPE are complaints of extreme fatigue, restlessness at night, and shortness of breath with mild exertion (or, more seriously, shortness of breath while at rest). The patient with HAPE feels extreme fatigue gauged by comparison with companions or others at the same altitude.

The initial symptom of HACE is often the headache of AMS, as HACE is the more extreme form of AMS. Patients with HACE may present with neurologic symptoms including confusion and changes in behavior (some irrational), as well as hallucinations. The progression of symptoms from confused to coma can occur in just a few hours.

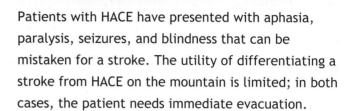

STREET SMART

Patients with HACE have presented with aphasia, paralysis, seizures, and blindness that can be mistaken for a stroke. The utility of differentiating a stroke from HACE on the mountain is limited; in both cases, the patient needs immediate evacuation.

CASE STUDY (CONTINUED)

On arrival at the site, a quick patient assessment reveals the patient is alert to voice, mildly confused with pale skin, and shows signs of cyanosis around the lips. Vital signs are pulse 114 and regular; respirations 30, labored and noisy; blood pressure 148/92. Lung sounds reveal crackles in scattered fields, becoming coarse in dependent areas of the lungs.

CRITICAL THINKING QUESTIONS

1. What are the elements of the physical examination of a patient with suspected spinal cord syndrome?
2. Why is a dermatome-focused neurological examination a critical element in this examination?

Examination

All climbers, trekkers, and mountaineers will experience some hyperventilation and dyspnea on exertion (DOE) at altitude. Some may even experience changes in respiratory pattern (i.e., Cheyne–Stokes respirations) with breath-holding episodes lasting up to 15 seconds. These are all normal physiologic adaptations to elevation.

What differentiates these adaptations from acute mountain sickness is loss of appetite, fatigue, and dizziness, to the point of near syncope or, perhaps more dramatically, nausea with vomiting.

HACE can be differentiated from acute mountain sickness by a simple "gait test," a modified Romberg test. The affected individual is instructed to walk heel-toe for several steps, and then asked to turn around and walk back. If the person has difficulty (i.e., ataxia), the Paramedic can assume he has some degree of HACE.

Altered mental status is also a sign of HACE. Often, the person exhibits lassitude and confusion, which can progress to unconsciousness—and ultimately death—if not recognized as HACE and treated early. Some patients may exhibit signs similar to a stroke (CVA) and be incapacitated, unable to assist in their treatment and evacuation.

A physical exam of a person with HAPE will show pale cool skin, peripheral cyanosis, tachycardia and tachypnea at rest, patchy crackles on lung auscultation (areas of no pulmonary arteriole constriction), and, in later stages, frothy pink sputum.

A dry, persistent, and sometimes debilitating cough, called the **Khumbu cough**, can be the precursor to HAPE and should not be discounted. It is thought to be, at least in part, due to the low humidity in the mountain air. The cough is so vigorous that many climbers have been known to break ribs while coughing. Attributed to bronchoconstriction secondary to breathing in cold frigid air (frigid mountain air can be nearly devoid of humidity), the high altitude cough can also occur independently of HAPE. Khumbu cough is differentiated from HAPE by the absence of shortness of breath and fatigue and adequate oxygen saturation on room air.

CASE STUDY (CONTINUED)

The working diagnosis offered by these Paramedics is acute mountain sickness that has progressed to high altitude pulmonary edema and/or high altitude cerebral edema.

CRITICAL THINKING QUESTIONS

1. What is the significance of the diagnosis?
2. Why might the patient resist the diagnosis the Paramedic announced?

Assessment

An international hypoxia symposium held in Alberta, Canada, at Lake Louise in 1991 produced the "Lake Louise Criteria," which lists the diagnostic criteria needed to make a diagnosis of altitude sickness (Table 14-2).

The clinical diagnosis of AMS is defined as a headache accompanied by one of the listed criterion. Likened to a bad hangover, untreated AMS is seen as a precursor to the more serious, and potentially life-threatening, HACE.

Table 14-2 Lake Louise Criteria

- Acute mountain sickness
  - Anorexia, nausea, vomiting
  - Fatigue or weakness
  - Dizziness or lightheadedness
  - Difficulty sleeping
- High altitude cerebral edema
  - Mental status changes
  - Ataxia
- High altitude pulmonary edema
  - Dyspnea at rest
  - Cough
  - Weakness
  - Chest tightness or congestion
  - Crackles or wheezing
  - Central cyanosis
  - Tachypnea
  - Tachycardia

To help differentiate a simple headache from AMS/HACE, the patient should drink a liter of water and take an NSAID. If the headache resolves, it was probably secondary to dehydration, a common problem in the arid mountain air. If it does not resolve, the Paramedic should assume AMS/HACE.

Hypothermia, which is a common problem at altitude, may also manifest in ataxia. Therefore, all signs and symptoms must be considered to come to a differential diagnosis of AMS/HACE.

The clinical diagnosis of HACE is defined as the onset of ataxia, altered mental status, or both in a person who has AMS or HAPE (discussed in this chapter). "Clinically and pathologically high altitude cerebral edema is the end-stage of acute mountain sickness."[5]

Evaluating the signs and symptoms in combination with a history of AMS, rapid ascent, and high exertion can lead the Paramedic to a diagnosis of HAPE. In fact, 50% of people with AMS will also have HAPE, and 14% will also have HACE.[10]

STREET SMART

A headache at 10,000 feet is not "normal." By denying the early manifestation of AMS, the patient may jeopardize herself and her teammates. Failure to acknowledge this headache may potentially lead to a life-threatening condition.

The Paramedics apply 15 liters of oxygen by a nonrebreather mask. Since the patient is not able to provide much assistance initially, he is wrapped in a hypothermia blanket, secured in a litter, and carried to the awaiting helicopter by the rangers and the other two climbers.

CRITICAL THINKING QUESTIONS

1. What is the national standard of care of patients with suspected altitude sickness?
2. What are some of the patient-specific concerns and considerations that the Paramedic should consider when applying this plan of care that is intended to treat a broad patient population presenting with altitude sickness?

Treatment

Acute mountain sickness symptoms will typically resolve with rest, fluids, and general over-the-counter analgesia. Acetazolamide may also be used at 125 mg by mouth, every 12 hours. However, someone with AMS should not proceed any higher until 100% symptom free. If symptoms do not resolve within 24 hours, descent to a lower altitude is recommended.

AMS affects people of every age, physical condition, gender, and level of mountaineering experience. Whether or not a person will develop AMS and how severely depends heavily on the patient's rate of ascent and personal physiology. Although one can't control genetic makeup, one can have control over the rate of ascent.

As a general rule, the easiest way to avoid or reduce the symptoms of AMS is to ascend slowly to allow enough time for acclimatization. This means when ascending, acclimatize for two to three nights at 8,000 to 10,000 feet (2,500 to 3,000 meters). After reaching 10,000 feet (3,000 meters), one should keep sleeping altitude gain between about 1,000 feet (300 meters) per day. For every 3,333 feet (1,000 meters) gained, an individual should stay at the same altitude for one extra night. Remember the climber's adage: climb higher during the day, sleep lower during the night.

Treatment for High Altitude Cerebral Edema

Dr. Peter Hackett, one of the world's foremost researchers in high altitude physiology and pathophysiology, says there are three treatments for HACE: descent, descent, and descent! Individuals diagnosed with HACE should be treated with oxygen, **dexamethasone (Decadron®)**, and rapid descent.

The Paramedic should administer oxygen at 4 to 6 lpm by nasal cannula or by appropriate high altitude oxygen apparatus. Dexamethasone is a glucocorticosteroid hormone and acts as an anti-inflammatory. The drug decreases brain swelling and other edema without reducing blood flow to the brain. This action reverses the effects of HACE. However, dexamethasone treats the symptoms, not the etiology, of HACE. Rapid descent of 2,000 or more feet is essential. Descent is

often made difficult by the ataxia and altered level of consciousness. However, a person suffering from HACE should be evacuated to the last "asymptomatic" altitude, or lower.

Mountaineering literature is full of stories of climbers being lowered or "short roped" by companions or guides because they are unable to descend under their own power. This is a difficult and dangerous process and demonstrates the need to recognize HACE early. Better still, an individual with unresolved signs and symptoms of AMS should not proceed higher until asymptomatic. There are no documented cases of HACE in individuals using acetazolamide.

Treatment for High Altitude Pulmonary Edema

As in other serious forms of altitude illness, HAPE requires rapid descent. Many times this individual may not be ambulatory and may have to be carried or evacuated by air, if possible. Descent should be a minimum of 2,000 to 3,000 feet lower than where symptoms first occurred. Of course, application of supplementary oxygen is critical. The combination of supplemental oxygen and descent effectively raises the pO_2 and rapidly reduces symptoms.

The therapeutic goal of pharmacological intervention is to lower pulmonary hypertension. The drugs of choice are dexamethasone, albuterol, and nifedipine. Nifedipine, a calcium channel blocker, acts to reduce pulmonary arterial pressures. Lasix (furosemide) is not effective because its mechanism of action is related to reducing left ventricular pressure, which is not the cause of fluid in the lungs in a patient with HAPE. Persons with HAPE who were otherwise ambulatory and given Lasix have later become non-ambulatory and required litter carry descent.[1] Pulse oximeters are very helpful in determining and documenting an improvement in a patient's condition.

In recent years, the development of portable hyperbaric chambers has dramatically improved the care of people stricken with HAPE in remote areas. Popular climbing and trekking areas in Asia and elsewhere have access to these devices. The best known and popular of these is the **Gamow bag** (Figure 14-2), which is essentially a sleeping bag-like

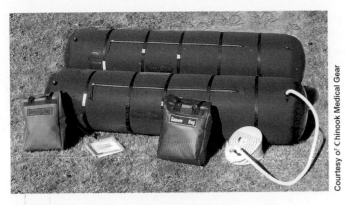

Figure 14-2 A Gamow bag is a portable hyperbaric chamber that has dramatically improved the care of people stricken with HAPE in remote areas.

Courtesy of Chinook Medical Gear

device with a foot pump that can be inflated to mimic pressures at altitudes approximately 2,000 feet lower than where the patient actually is located. This device effectively raises the pO_2 and, over time, allows the patient to recover sufficiently to descend on his or her own. People with ready access to medical care, such as at ski resorts in the United States and Europe, may recover easily in one to three days with supplemental oxygen and rest.[11]

Treatment of Khumbu Cough

To prevent and treat Khumbu cough, the patient needs to "rebreath" his own humidity. Although a simple balaclava will work, a special ski mask developed for the Finnish Olympic ski team may be more functional. A metallic net with cloth shell, the mask maintains its shape under extreme conditions.

▶ CASE STUDY (CONTINUED)

As the patient is loaded aboard the helicopter, one of the climbers mentions to the Paramedic that the patient's "drill holes"—climber jargon for urine in the snow—were dark orange and another one looked like crankcase oil.

CRITICAL THINKING QUESTIONS

1. What are some of the predictable complications associated with altitude sickness?
2. What are some of the predictable complications associated with the treatments for acute altitude sickness?

Evaluation

Several other less common disorders are found in travelers to altitude that the Paramedic should consider. For example, cerebrovascular accidents do happen, including transient ischemic attacks. As noted earlier, these can be confused with other more common altitude conditions such as HACE. A good history taking and physical exam can aid the Paramedic in differentiating between these two.

Deterioration at high altitude caused by prolonged stays at heights above 20,000 feet can occur. People on expeditions to high mountains can be trapped at 20,000 feet or above by severe weather conditions for days at a time, thereby causing significant health deterioration and jeopardizing the lives of those trapped. The dehydration of travel at altitude can contribute to pulmonary embolism or thrombophlebitis. Both of these serious conditions can result in death.

Chronic conditions that affect the heart, lungs, and blood vessels, which can be well managed at sea level, become a liability with travel to altitude. Individuals with common diseases such as diabetes and asthma should seek medical advice from a physician versed in the effects of altitude before taking part in trips that can take them over 8,000 feet in elevation. This includes many North American ski areas.

▶ CASE STUDY CONCLUSION

Nearly 15 minutes later, the helicopter lands back at Lupine Meadows where the patient is transferred to a waiting ambulance and transported to St. John's Medical Center in Jackson, WY, for further treatment.

CRITICAL THINKING QUESTIONS

1. What is the most appropriate transport decision that will get the patient to definitive care?
2. What are the advantages of transporting a patient with suspected altitude sickness to these hospitals, even if that means bypassing other hospitals in the process?

Disposition

Patients with either HACE or HAPE need to be transported to facilities familiar with these uncommon conditions. This transportation is often performed by helicopter, as time is of the essence in these cases. Often special "very high altitude" helicopters designed to fly in the rarified mountain air are used. A helicopter has even been designed that can land on the top of Mt. Everest. However, the average helicopter's ceiling is 26,247 feet (8,000 meters), and helicopters flying over 23,000 feet (7,000 meters) may have to deal with jet streams, with winds up to 300 km/hr.

There are a number of potentially serious side effects of travel to altitude. Although physical fitness alone is not necessarily protective, it is helpful in combination with other strategies for staying healthy at altitude. Some of these strategies are controlled rate of ascent, the use of pharmacologic agents such as acetazolamide (Diamox®) for both acclimatization (prophylactically) and treatment of nighttime period breathing, and use of NSAIDs such as ibuprofen and acetaminophen for mitigation of mild symptoms of AMS. The Paramedic should pay close attention to the patient's nutrition and hydration. Research has shown that a diet with liberal amounts of carbohydrates produces higher amounts of CO_2 in the body and thereby increases ventilation.[12]

Regions of moderate to high altitude present the Paramedic with unusual physiologic responses in potential patients they may treat. A solid background in the common types of problems, their signs and symptoms, as well as treatment options is essential to providing optimal care. Climbers should also be familiar with the potential signs of altitude illness (Table 14-3).

Table 14-3 Golden Rules of Climbing

The International Society for Mountain Medicine (ISMM) has published the "Golden Rules" for altitude travel:

- If you feel unwell at altitude, it's altitude illness unless proven otherwise.
- Never ascend with signs or symptoms of altitude illness.
- If your symptoms are getting worse (or if you have HAPE or HACE), descend at once!

CONCLUSION

Altitude-related ailments are a constant threat to world travelers, trekkers, and adventurers alike. Early recognition and treatment of acute mountain sickness, and its various major and minor syndromes, can decrease associated morbidity and mortality.

KEY POINTS:

- The three major altitude sicknesses are acute mountain sickness, high altitude cerebral edema, and high altitude pulmonary edema.

- The three standard elevations are moderate, high, and extreme.

- Elevation decreases partial pressure of oxygen, leading to hypoxia.

- Acclimatization consists of polycythemia, increased 2,3-DPG, and renal compensation.

- Acetazolamide, a carbonic anhydrase inhibitor, acidifies blood, offsetting altitude-induced respiratory alkalosis.

- Acetazolamide can worsen dehydration secondary to fluid loss during hyperventilation of arid mountain air.

- Acute mountain sickness can occur secondary to a drop in partial pressure of oxygen in blood.

- HACE pathology revolves around increased intracranial pressure.

- High altitude pulmonary edema (HAPE) is a noncardiogenic pulmonary edema.

- HACE and HAPE are often seen together.

- Minor mountain syndromes include ultraviolet keratitis, or snow blindness; high altitude retinal hemorrhage; and Khumbu cough.

- Alcohol, sleep aids, and narcotics induce respiratory depression and worsening AMS.

- The primary symptom of HACE is a headache.

- HACE and AMS can be differentiated by a gait test.

- Khumbu cough—a persistent, dry, hacking cough—can be differentiated from HAPE by the absence of shortness of breath between coughing fits and an acceptable room air pulse oximeter reading.

- AMS is treated with rest, fluids, and over-the-counter analgesia.

- HACE is treated with dexamethasone, oxygen, and descent.

- HAPE is treated with nifedipine, oxygen, and albuterol, as well as descent.

- Portable hyperbaric chambers, like a Gamow bag, are useful for treating HACE/HAPE.

REVIEW QUESTIONS:

1. Explain Dalton's law of partial pressures and high altitude sickness.
2. How does the body acclimatize?
3. Compare and differentiate AMS from HACE.
4. How does nifedipine help to treat HAPE?
5. What is a Gamow bag?

CASE STUDY QUESTIONS:

Please refer to the Case Study in this chapter, and answer the questions below:

1. What is the likely diagnosis for this ill-fated climber?
2. What additional physical findings would have helped to establish the diagnosis of HAPE?
3. What additional physical findings would have helped to establish the diagnosis of HACE?

REFERENCES:

1. Wilkerson J. Disorders caused by altitude. In: *Medicine for Mountaineering.* Seattle, WA: The Mountaineers; 2001:220.

2. Bircher H, Eichenberger U, Maggiorini M, Olex O, Bartch P. Relationship of mountain sickness to physical fitness and exercise intensity during ascent. *J Wilderness Med.* 1994;5: 302–311.

3. Kamler K. High altitude. In: *Surviving the Extremes* (p. 194). New York: Penguin Books; 2005:194.

4. Dietz, T. Altitude tutorial. International Society for Mountain Medicine; 2001. Available at: **www.ISMMed.org.** Accessed January 10, 2010.

5. Hackett P, Roach R. High altitude illness. *New Engl J Med.* 2001;345(2):108.

6. DeAngelis, CD. Fontanarosa PB. Eds. Clinician's Corner, JAMA 2002;287;104.

7. Dietz T. Altitude illness clinical guide for physicians. 2000. Available at: **www.high-altitude-medicine.com/AMS-medical .html.** Accessed January 10, 2010.

8. Ganoong W. Respiratory adjustments in health and disease. In: *Review of Medical Physiology* (22nd ed.). Lange Medical Publications, New York. McGraw-Hill Publishing Companies; 2005:684. Accessed: October 2008.

9. Shah M, Braude D, Crandall C, Kwack H, Rabiniwitz L, Cumbo T, Basnyat B, Bhasyal G. Changes in metabolic and hematologic laboratory values with ascent to altitude and the development of acute mountain sickness in Nepalese pilgrims. *Wilderness Environ Med.* 2006;17:171–177.

10. Hultgren H, *High Altitude Pulmonary Edema: Current Concepts.* 1996:267–284.

11. Hultgren H, Honigman B, Reves N. High altitude pulmonary edema at a ski resort, *West J Med.* 1997;164: 222–227.

12. Golja P, Flander P, Klemenc M, Maver J, Princi T. Carbohydrate ingestion improves oxygen delivery in acute hypoxia. *High Alt Med Biol.* 2008;9:53–62.

CHAPTER 15

WATER EMERGENCIES

KEY CONCEPTS:

Upon completion of this chapter, it is expected that the reader will understand these following concepts:

- Epidemiology of drowning
- Pathophysiology of drowning
- Disorders of dysbarism
- Decompression illness
- Treatment of the drowning patient

ANATOMY CONCEPTS:

Prior to reading this chapter the Paramedic student should be familiar with the following anatomy and physiology concepts:

- Airway anatomy
- Airway reflexes
- Thoracic physiology

"Cowabunga!" yells 16-year-old Brian as the rope swing arcs over the water in the quarry pit. Even though it is summer, it is still early and the water is freezing. Everyone is laughing as they wait for Brian to surface. "Hope all the beer you drank works like antifreeze!" one fellow yells. Eventually Brian does surface and everyone turns back to the fire and the beer. Only Jen continues to watch, waiting for Brian to swim to the shore so she can help him out of the water. But something is wrong. Brian seems to be moving toward shore when he quietly slips under the water's surface. Jen knows that Brian saw her watching him and wonders if he's just "playing" with her. However, when seconds turn into a minute, she becomes concerned. After a minute she yells, "Hey everybody, I think Brian is in trouble!"

CRITICAL THINKING QUESTIONS

1. What is the pathophysiology behind drowning?
2. How does the patient's age or sex impact the incidence of drowning?

OVERVIEW

When someone mentions drowning, one imagines fear-producing images of panic and suffocation. Understanding the pathophysiology of drowning and its treatment can help Paramedics hold that fear in check while they calmly and deliberately treat the patient.

What is drowning? Over 20 definitions of drowning exist, including near drowning, wet drowning, dry drowning, active drowning, passive drowning, and silent drowning. To help clear up confusion, the World Congress on Drowning developed a standard definition of drowning, in part to facilitate reporting and research on drowning. Drowning is defined as any submersion that results in primary respiratory impairment in a liquid medium.[1]

In 2005, the Centers for Disease Control and Prevention (CDC) estimated that 3,582 deaths occurred from unintentional/accidental drowning; one in four of these were children 14 years of age or less.[2] Pediatric drowning is a serious public health emergency. One survey of 9,420 children in South Carolina found that one-tenth of these children had a " serious threat" of drowning. The survey also determined that residential swimming pools were the greatest danger.[3]

Each water-emergency patient has some physical changes common to all other water-emergency patients. The Hollywood picture of a screaming child is not very accurate. The body's instinctive fight to keep the airway dry and head above water does not allow much yelling, as most of the patient's energy is directed to keeping the head up and the arms out.

Chief Concern

Whenever a water emergency occurs, the Paramedic's first thought should be, "Is there a drowning?" Drowning is a complex topic that includes fresh- versus saltwater drowning, swimming emergencies versus diving emergencies, and includes the attendant complication of cardiac arrest.

Drowning

According to the CDC, the definition of drowning is the process of "experiencing respiratory impairment from submersion/immersion in liquid." Anytime someone submerges there are physiological reactions that occur, and from these reactions the body may inhale large or small amounts of the liquid. Although the World Congress on Drowning and the CDC use a single definition of drowning, there is a utility to addressing each drowning as either a wet or a dry drowning, as it relates to the amount of liquid the patient has inhaled.

Wet Drowning

In a **wet drowning**, the patient's lungs contain at least some liquid. Wet drowning accounts for approximately 80% to 90% of recorded drowning. Most drowning starts out with the airway being protected automatically by the body through a process called laryngospasm. Eventually, asphyxia-induced hypoxia will override the protective airway reflex, the airway relaxes, and the patient inhales an agonal breath.

The patient's blood chemistry, having already been changed with the lack of oxygen, changes even more so with the inspiration of water. The patient will likely become **negatively buoyant**, a condition in which an object sinks. Upon drawing in fluid instead of air, buoyancy provided by the normally air-filled lungs is lost from the person's lungs. This occurs when about 4 mL/kg of water is aspirated, or a volume of 280 mL for the average person (by comparison, a can of soda equals 350 mL).

This fact plays a major role in determining the patient's location. Submerged patients will almost always be found within a certain distance of where they went underwater.

Dry Drowning

The other 10% to 20% of drownings are thought to be **dry drownings**, a condition in which the patient asphyxiates but the lungs stay dry. According to research from the *American Journal of Forensic Medicine and Pathology*, this percentage could be even lower, around 2%.[4]

A laryngospasm is the body's attempt to seal off the airway when water is sensed in the throat. This action can be so forceful that the patient actually suffocates. The urge to breathe cannot overpower the laryngospasm, and death occurs by suffocation.

A patient of dry drowning may be **positively buoyant**, or floating, as air remains in the lungs. This can be an easy recovery in still waters as watercraft or surface swimmers can easily recover the patient. However, it can be a challenging, long-distance search if the water is flowing and there is little to snag the body.

Fresh Water versus Salt Water

Following a drowning with aspiration (wet drowning), it is reasonable to assume that an electrolyte imbalance may complicate the clinical picture. Osmosis may cause water to enter the bloodstream, thus leading to dilution of electrolytes. However, studies have shown that typically less than 4 mL/kg of water is found in the lungs following a drowning. This small amount of aspiration of either salt or fresh water rarely leads to serious electrolyte imbalances. The exception is children who have both ingested and aspirated fresh water. In those cases, hyponatremia (low serum sodium levels) is of concern. However, hyponatremia is seldom an immediate problem in the prehospital setting.

Risk Factors for Drowning

Youth may be the greatest risk factor for drowning; in fact, one in four drowning patients is a child under 15 years of age. It is estimated that for every fatal drowning, four more pediatric drownings occur. In 2005, almost 30% of pediatric deaths from age 1 to 4 years old was from drowning. Fatal pediatric drowning (1 to 14 years) remains the second leading cause of unintentional injury-related death according to the CDC.[2]

Location plays a factor in pediatric deaths. For infants (children under 1 year of age), bathtubs, five-gallon buckets, and even toilets can be locations where a drowning will occur.[3] For preschool children (children ages 1 to 4), pools are dangerous. In general, pools are a common location for drowning. Interestingly, in many cases either one or both parents are at home at the time of the drowning and the child is out of sight for less than five minutes, thus suggesting a lack of parental supervision.[5]

As the child's age increases, the likely location of drowning changes to natural water settings, such as lakes, ponds, rivers, and the ocean. This shift is coupled with use of recreational watercraft.[6] The U.S. Coast Guard reports that the majority of boating fatalities were caused by drowning and that 9 out of 10 of those who drowned were not wearing life preservers at the time. Similar to motor vehicle collisions, alcohol is a contributing factor in half of all boating accidents and one in five reported boating fatalities.[7]

Complication of Hypothermia

Hypothermia is a common complication of drowning. For the human body to stay in water for a prolonged period of time, the water must be warmer than 91°F (33°C), referred to as thermally neutral water. The majority of fresh water in the United States is usually less than 77°F (25°C) year round and therefore below the thermally neutral water temperature.

Once a person enters the cold water, which wicks body heat away 25 times faster than air, the body temperature will start to drop (Table 15-1). Typically, life-threatening

Table 15-1 Hypothermia Chart

Stage	Core Temperature	Signs & Symptoms
Mild hypothermia	99°F–97°F°	Normal, shivering can begin
	97°F–95°F	Cold sensation, goose bumps, unable to perform complex tasks with hands, shiver can be mild to severe, hands numb
Moderate hypothermia	95°F–93°F	Shivering intense, decreased muscle coordination becomes apparent, movements slow and labored, stumbling pace, mild confusion, may appear alert
	93°F–90°F	Violent shivering persists, difficulty speaking, sluggish thinking, amnesia starts to appear, gross muscle movements sluggish, unable to use hands, difficulty speaking, signs of depression
Severe hypothermia	90°F–86°F	Shivering stops, exposed skin blue or puffy, muscle coordination very poor, confusion, incoherent/irrational behavior, but may be able to maintain posture and appearance of awareness
	86°F–82°F	Muscle rigidity, semiconscious, stupor, loss of awareness of others, pulse and respiration rate decrease, possible heart fibrillation
	82°F–78°F	Unconscious, heartbeat and respiration erratic, pulse may not be palpable
	78°F–75°F	Pulmonary edema, cardiac and respiratory failure, death may occur before this temperature is reached

hypothermia starts to set in within 30 to 60 minutes.[9] Therefore, even the most skilled swimmer will start to become fatigued and have hypothermia-induced loss of motor skills. Furthermore, the hypothermic person in cold water may not even be fully aware of rescue efforts, let alone able to assist in them.

Cold Water Reflex

There are, however, cases of patients surviving prolonged submersion in cold water. One theory postulates the physiological result of hypothermia termed **cold water reflex (Mammalian dive reflex)**. According to this theory, when the human body is suddenly exposed to cold water, the body's defense is to immediately shut down all but the vital organs. Several changes then occur. First, there is a reflexive inhibition of the respiratory center leading to hypoventilation, vagal stimulation leading to bradycardia, and a generalized shunting of peripheral blood to the core and vital organs (heart, lungs, and brain).

These changes, coupled with slowed metabolism, shut down the body's systems. This shutdown is thought to be responsible for the successful rescue and recovery of people that have been submerged for over 60 minutes. This reflex is thought to be more pronounced in children. In addition, the colder the water, the more pronounced the reflex may be. Studies are underway in which researchers are intentionally inducing hypothermia in the field in order to increase cardiac arrest survival rates after spontaneous return of circulation.[10] These studies seem to lend credence to the concept that hypothermia may improve cerebral survival in the drowning patient who is successfully resuscitated.

Dive Drowning

People have been diving for a number of reasons for centuries. Modern divers dive for sport or as part of a commercial venture, such as bridge repair. Diving without any apparatus, using breath holding, is called a free dive. Some free dives have been recorded to over 700 feet.[11] However, deeper free dives can occur when divers with self-contained underwater breathing apparatus (SCUBA) lose their air supply or during a submarine escape.

Diving drowning is a special subset of water emergencies. Although the number of actual diving deaths is low (three to nine deaths per 100,000 dives) and only 60% of those deaths are from drowning, drownings do occur. Dive drowning is usually secondary to equipment failure (i.e., problems with the air supply) or medical emergencies (such as seizures or sudden cardiac death while underwater).[12]

Some people pass out while free diving and snorkeling, a condition called **shallow water blackout (SWB)**. This condition is due to hyperventilation and subsequent hypocapnia prior to swimming. The majority of dive emergencies occur due to SCUBA diving emergencies during descent or ascent. These emergencies are part of a clinical condition owed to dysbarism.

Many pool drownings may be secondary to shallow water blackouts. Breath-holding contests or competitive swimming, without exhalation, may lead to SWB and subsequent drowning.

Dysbarism

Dysbarism refers to disorders that result from changes in pressure. They could occur from high altitudes, or, as in the case study from this chapter, from ascending and descending under the water. Dysbarism consists of decompression sickness, arterial gas embolism, and barotraumas. To understand disorders due to dysbarism, the Paramedic must understand four basic gas laws.

The lungs contain compressible gasses. Those lungs are encased within the body, which is primarily made up of non-compressible water. The internalized gas is subject to pressure changes that occur outside of the body.

When a gas is placed under pressure, assuming a constant temperature, the volume of gas will change inverse to the change in pressure; the greater the pressure, the smaller the volume. **Boyle's law** explains this phenomenon. When a diver goes to a depth of 33 feet, without exhaling, the pressure on the body increases by 1 atmosphere and the lung volume decreases by one-half. The lung volume at 66 feet (2 atmosphere) is one-third (Figure 15-1).

The problem occurs when the diver takes a breath from a SCUBA tank underwater and then ascends without exhaling. As the pressure on the lungs drops, the lungs expand proportionately. Since the lungs have a limited ability to expand, they tend to rupture. **Barotrauma** occurs from changing pressures, after which a pneumothorax can develop. Most divers are trained to manage their ascents and to avoid breath holding, usually by talking during the ascent.

The greater problem, especially for SCUBA divers, is the gasses that are dissolved in the blood. When under pressure, gasses can be forced to dissolve into water. Nitrogen is the primary gas in the air (78%), with the rest being oxygen (21%) and other minor gasses.

Dalton's law states that if pressure is exerted on a mixture of gasses, the individual gasses will all compress the same and the proportion of the pressures will all remain constant (Figure 15-2). This means that partial pressures of mixed gasses increase proportionally as the pressure increases. At some point, however, the gas is forced into solution in the blood.

As the technical/commercial diver reaches approximately 300 feet, even the oxygen in room air (21%) can create oxygen toxicity. Oxygen toxicity can impair surfactant function, leading to alveolar collapse, pulmonary edema, and

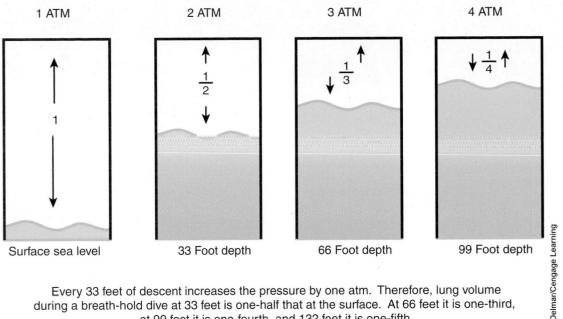

Every 33 feet of descent increases the pressure by one atm. Therefore, lung volume during a breath-hold dive at 33 feet is one-half that at the surface. At 66 feet it is one-third, at 99 feet it is one-fourth, and 132 feet it is one-fifth.

Figure 15-1 Boyle's law states that the pressure and volume of a gas are inversely proportional to each other when that gas is at the same temperature.

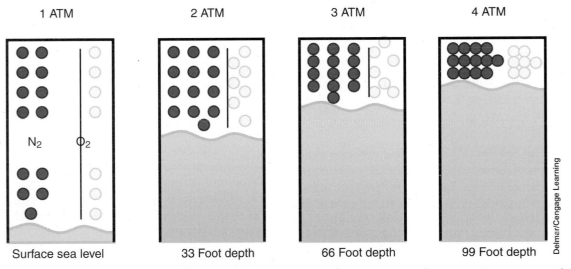

Figure 15-2 Dalton's Law states that as the pressure on the mixture of gasses increases, the partial pressures on those individual gasses increase proportionately.

central nervous system complications, including seizures. Seizures are particularly problematic when they occur during a deep-sea dive. To prevent this, most deep-sea divers inhale a mixture of helium and oxygen.

The greater problem may be the increased nitrogen that is also dissolved in the blood. Nitrogen alters the electrical properties of nervous tissues, creating an anesthetic effect. Nitrous oxide has long been known to create this effect. The resulting disorder is referred to as **nitrogen narcosis,** or "rapture of the deep." It has been suggested that every 50 feet

in a dive creates a cerebral impact equivalent to drinking one alcoholic beverage. As the diver descends deeper, reasoning is lost, the memory is foggy, the vision is narrowed, and confusion sets in.[13] Nitrogen narcosis can be particularly dangerous for divers as higher-level functions are compromised (i.e., planning, abstract thinking, initiating appropriate actions, sensory discrimination). These are critical cognitive functions for the diver.

Henry's law simply states that the amount of gas dissolved into blood and tissues is proportional to the partial

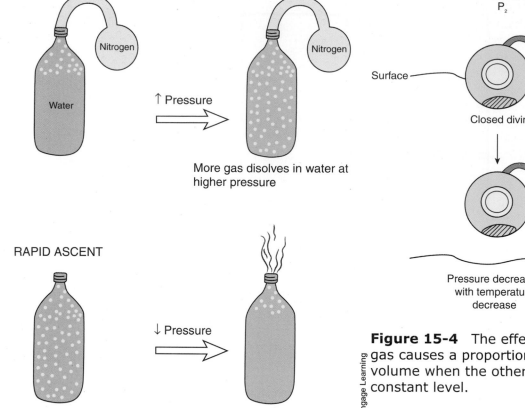

DESCENT

Nitrogen

Water

↑ Pressure

More gas disolves in water at higher pressure

RAPID ASCENT

↓ Pressure

Gas rapidly comes out of solution and into the tissues before it can be removed by the lungs

Figure 15-3 The effect of Henry's law is the reason nitrogen bubbles form in the blood during rapid ascent to the water's surface.

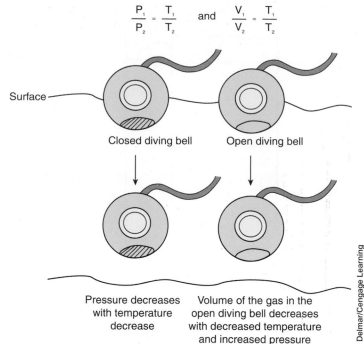

$$\frac{P_1}{P_2} = \frac{T_1}{T_2} \quad \text{and} \quad \frac{V_1}{V_2} = \frac{T_1}{T_2}$$

Surface

Closed diving bell   Open diving bell

Pressure decreases with temperature decrease

Volume of the gas in the open diving bell decreases with decreased temperature and increased pressure

Figure 15-4 The effects of temperature on a gas causes a proportionate change in pressure or volume when the other variable is maintained at a constant level.

pressure of that gas (Figure 15-3). Gas will continue to diffuse across the gas/blood interface until the partial pressures are equal on either side of the interface. As seen in Dalton's law, that increase in partial pressure can be substantial and a significant amount of nitrogen gas can be dissolved into the blood. The greater problem may occur when the diver ascends. Gasses dissolved in the blood and into the lipid tissue are now under less pressure. As a result, the gasses start to come out of solution and form bubbles within the blood. These nitrogen bubbles are the source of decompression sickness, which is discussed shortly.

The final gas law, **Charles' law**, deals with changes in temperature (Figure 15-4). If the volume is held constant (e.g., in a closed diving bell that cannot change shape), the pressure will decrease proportionate to the decrease in temperature. If the pressure is held constant, the volume will decrease with a decrease in temperature. It is common during a deep dive for divers to experience differing temperatures through layers of water called thermals. In general, the water temperature decreases the further one gets from the surface. The colder the water gets, the more pressure decreases. However, the volume decreases as well, compounding the problem created by Boyle's law.

Decompression Illness

Diving emergencies are problems related to the pressure changes that occur with changes in depth. Air-filled spaces like the lungs and the intestines create a host of symptoms that are covered under the broad umbrella term of **decompression illness (DCI)**.

It is estimated that over 1,000 SCUBA divers are affected by decompression illness every year. These illnesses can be divided into decompression sickness or arterial gas embolism. Decompression sickness involves issues within the local tissues, whereas arterial gas embolism is more systematic and a more lethal condition.

Decompression Sickness

Decompression sickness is sometimes called Caisson's disease. During the construction of the Brooklyn Bridge in the late 1800s, large watertight containers called caissons were sunk into the riverbed so that workers could make the piers and foundations for the bridge. As the workers went "top side," the nitrogen would come out of solution in their blood and they would become symptomatic: the time of onset ranged from 15 minutes to 12 hours. The name "the bends" came about because the nitrogen coming out of solution caused such severe abdominal pain that the workers would be bent over in pain. Many workers realized that relief came from going back down into the caisson.

The U.S. Navy has divided decompression sickness into two categories, although there is symptom crossover in both. The first category, decompression sickness I (DCS I), involves the skin and musculoskeletal system. This includes the more traditional symptoms of decompression sickness, such as joint and muscle pain and pain in the gut.

Over 60% of cases of decompression sickness involve DCS I. Starting with the skin, the Paramedic may note subcutaneous emphysema that is not proximal to the chest wall. Along with the lumps from the subcutaneous emphysema, a rash may form on the patient's skin. In severe cases, the skin takes on a marbled appearance called **cutis marmorata**. This nitrogen under the skin makes the skin "feel" as if it is crawling. Called **formication**, it is associated with a variable paresthesia as well as itch (pruritus).

The most common symptom reported is arthritic joint pain. This minor joint pain in the large joints (hip, shoulder) often dissipates spontaneously. It is described variously, ranges from tingling to a dull ache, and is often dismissed as overexertion. However, persistent pain left untreated can lead to osteonecrosis (death of the bone), secondary to interruption of blood to the joint. A key symptom is fatigue that lingers. This fatigue is inconsistent with the patient's athleticism and does not resolve with rest.

DCS II includes neurological involvement and thus has more ominous implications. The most common presentation of DCS II is a headache or visual disturbances, such as spots in the eyes (scotoma) or double vision (diplopia).

Ataxia may be appreciated if the patient has spinal cord involvement. Other complaints associated with spinal cord involvement include lower back pain, ascending weakness (in some cases with associated paralysis), and bladder dysfunction.

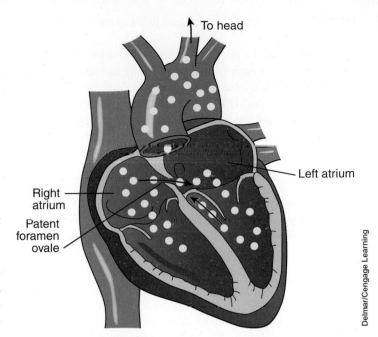

Figure 15-5 A patent foramen ovale allows venous gas bubbles to enter the systemic circulation.

The difficulty arises when a diver ascends and nitrogen bubbles form in the venous circulation. Normally these nitrogen bubbles are "filtered" out in the lungs. However, in the case of the patient with patent foramen ovale, the venous bubbles bypass the lungs by moving from the right side of the heart to the left side of the heart through the patent foramen ovale, and on to the body and brain (Figure 15-5). This leads to neurological symptoms such as weakness and dizziness.[14]

Chokes

Although **pulmonary decompression sickness** (i.e., the "chokes") is rare, its symptoms indicate the need for EMS and could signal a potentially life-threatening condition. Pulmonary decompression sickness occurs when multiple pulmonary gas emboli form. In the worst-case scenario, these gas emboli block the alveoli capillaries, leading to a rapid oxygen desaturation, right-sided heart failure, and cardiovascular collapse. Even mild cases of pulmonary decompression sickness can cause pleuritic-like chest pain that worsens with deep breathing and often is accompanied by paroxysms of dry hacking cough (hence the name the "chokes").

Immersion Pulmonary Edema

One form of dive-related pulmonary illness is not considered pulmonary decompression sickness and is thought to be due to immersion in cold water. The effect is twofold.

When the body is immersed in cold water, peripheral blood is redistributed to the core. This peripheral vasoconstriction increases peripheral vascular resistance, increasing the heart's workload and, in some cases, inducing a myocardial infarction. The effect of this increased peripheral vascular resistance upon the heart can be worsened in those patients

Nitrogen is five times more soluble in fat than muscle. Therefore, women and obese patients are at greater risk for decompression sickness.

Patent Foramen Ovale

Recent dive research has been exploring the relationship between a patent foramen ovale (PFO) and decompression sickness (DCS). During gestation, the lungs are nonfunctional and blood bypasses the lungs through an opening in the heart's septal wall called the foramen ovale (Latin for oval hole). Upon birth, this opening typically closes; if it does not, it is called an atrial septal defect and sometimes requires surgery to close.

However, in a small percentage of patients the opening closes but does not close completely, often giving rise to an "innocent" murmur. Patients with this condition, a **patent foramen ovale**, may be completely unaware of its presence. In fact, it is estimated that 10% to 20% of the population have a patent foramen ovale.

with pre-existing hypertension and leads to backwards failure more quickly.

Secondarily, the peripheral vasoconstriction also leads to increased venous return, further stressing the heart and leading to backwards failure. The complex etiology of **immersion pulmonary edema (IPE)** is poorly understood. Some young people, including special forces combat swimmers, develop IPE despite being in excellent physical condition. There is some speculation about pre-existing abnormalities of the myocardium, such as ventricular hypertrophy, or defective heart valves.[15]

Patients with IPE will feel short of breath, present with fulminate pulmonary edema as manifest by pink frothy sputum, and may be confused secondary to hypoxia. Often the symptoms of IPE occur after a shallow dive, helping to differentiate it from pulmonary decompression sickness (Table 15-2).[15,16]

It is important to get high-flow, high-concentration oxygen to the patient as soon as possible. The oxygen displaces the nitrogen in the lungs, called "nitrogen wash out," and allows the nitrogen in the blood to "off-gas" more quickly. When possible, it is better to use a flow-restricted oxygen-powered ventilation device (FROPVD) as an alternative nonrebreather mask (NRB); however, divers are more likely to be compliant with the familiar regulator of a FROPVD (Figure 15-6).[17] High-flow, high-concentration oxygen should be given to patients even if they are expected to receive hyperbaric oxygen (HBO). Patients who received high-flow, high-concentration oxygen did better than those who did not following an HBO decompression "dive."[18] Studies have shown that oxygen administration has been delayed, on average, four hours after surfacing and 2.2 hours after DCS symptoms appeared. Timely administration of oxygen is so

Table 15-2 Symptom Pattern of Decompression Sickness

- The bends
  - Pain in joints
  - Itching
  - Formication
- The staggers
  - Vertigo
  - Hearing loss
  - Loss of balance
- The tingles
  - Ascending paralysis
  - Incontinence
  - Bladder dysfunction
- The chokes
  - Shortness of breath
  - Burning chest pain
  - Dry cough

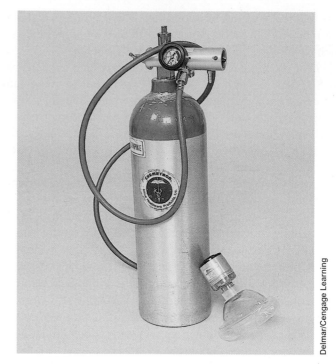

Delmar/Cengage Learning

Figure 15-6 A flow-restricted oxygen-powered ventilation device is an ideal way to get high-flow, high-concentration oxygen to the patient.

important that the Divers Alert Network (DAN) has been working to place oxygen at dive locations (remote emergency medical oxygen, or REMO).[19]

Central Arterial Gas Embolism

The most serious form of decompression illness may be cerebral arterial gas embolism. **Cerebral arterial gas embolism (CAGE)** occurs when a patient attempts a too-rapid ascent (i.e., panic ascent) without exhalation. A nitrogen gas bubble is created and passes into arterial circulation. Since arterial blood distribution goes first to the brain, cerebral blood flow is interrupted, similar to what happens in an embolic stroke. In less severe cases, there is a neurological dysfunction (e.g., seizures or difficulty thinking without confusion).[20] In many cases, the outcome is more severe and manifests almost immediately following the dive. The diver typically becomes unconscious within 10 minutes of surfacing.

▷ ▷ ▷ ▷ ▷ ▷ ▷ ▷ ▷ ▷ ▷ ▷

STREET SMART

In the past, patients with suspected DCS were placed in the Trendelenburg position. The idea was to prevent cerebral gas emboli from reaching the brain. This practice has been abandoned, however, as the Trendelenburg position has been found to increase intracranial pressure (ICP).

The time to treatment, particularly to a decompression chamber or hyperbaric oxygen chamber, is important. Administration of high-flow, high-concentration oxygen should be instituted immediately.

Pulmonary Barotrauma

Lung volume decreases during descent secondary to compression. Ferreras–Rodriquez, free diver, performed a record–breaking dive to 417 feet and his 50-inch chest was compressed to a 20-inch circumference. During a rapid ascent, such as during an emergency ascent, the rapid re-expansion of the lung can lead to damage from the rapid pressure change, called **pulmonary barotrauma**.[21]

As the diver ascends, lung expansion is limited by the rib cage. As a result of subsequent increased intrathoracic pressures and pulmonary overinflation, a pneumothorax occurs[22] and/or the pulmonary vein ruptures, which leads to arterial gas embolism.[22] Patients with a history of COPD, spontaneous pneumothorax associated with blebs, history of pulmonary cysts, or tumors secondary to lung cancer is prone to barotrauma and pneumothorax.

Pulmonary barotraumas are best treated by prevention. SCUBA divers are trained to ascend 10 meters per minute with three- to five-minute stops at 6 meters. Deeper dives require more frequent stops.[23] Frequent stops allow divers to off-load nitrogen and empty their lungs to prevent pulmonary barotrauma and decompression.

STREET SMART

Patients with a history of asthma are at risk for pulmonary complications. These patients have a limited forced vital capacity and their forced expiratory volume is decreased. This leads to air trapping and therefore an increased risk of barotrauma.

Minor Dive Syndromes

Ear squeeze, a feeling of fullness in the ear, may be the most common dysbarism disorder. In one study of ears, nose, and sinus complaints following diving, 64.6% of patients noted symptoms of ear squeeze.[24] The problem of ear squeeze is a problem of the middle ear. The Eustachian tubes equalize the middle ear with the external environment. During a diver's ascent, there is increased pressure on the tympanic membrane that can be equalized by the Eustachian tubes. One-quarter of divers complained of ringing in the ear (tinnitus)[25] as well as nausea and loss of hearing. The risk of ear squeeze increases if the patient has a pre-existing infection or inflammation of the ear.

Divers often complain of pressure within the sinuses, called **sinus squeeze**, which can lead to headaches. Sinus squeeze is worsened by an infection or pre-existing polyps. Some divers use pseudoephedrine to dry up the mucous membranes in the sinuses and prevent sinus pressure buildup. In some cases, the patient may develop an epistaxis secondary to ruptured blood vessels.

The last of the ear, nose, and throat syndromes is **tooth squeeze**. In this syndrome, air under a tooth's filling, especially older or temporary fillings, leads to pressure-induced toothache or barodontalgia. Those prone to barodontalgia include those with periodontal abscesses and multiple carious teeth.

STREET SMART

Since 1993, the **Divers Alert Network (DAN)** has been working on recommendations for how long to wait to fly in an airplane after diving. At present, DAN recommends a minimum 12-hour surface interval time (SIT) for a nondecompression dive before flying. Even with pressurized cabins in modern airplanes, a six-year study of 802 patients showed 40 cases of DCS, ranging from mild to severe.[26]

▶ CASE STUDY (CONTINUED)

The sheriff's dive team arrives and starts to set up and survey the scene. Although the teenagers all know that they were trespassing, the immediate concern is Brian. Therefore, they cannot answer the deputy's questions fast enough. Though it is fresh water, it is also stagnant water. The sheriff, who is crossed-trained as a Paramedic, knows that if the kid survived he might be in for secondary drowning down the line.

CRITICAL THINKING QUESTIONS

1. What are the important elements of the history that a Paramedic should obtain?
2. What is secondary drowning?

History

The Paramedic's first task is to survey the scene and determine the type of water (fresh versus salt), the depth of the water, and the temperature of the water. If the water is flowing, the Paramedic should be aware of low head dams and other obstacles that may cause spinal cord injury and complicate patient care.

The water temperature plays a large role in the success of resuscitation. There is a recorded case of a 2½-year-old child who was submerged for 66 minutes in 66.2°F (19°C) water and was resuscitated with a good neurologic outcome.[27] Many pools have a thermometer in the water poolside, and public pools often regularly take and record temperature readings.

Water contamination is a concern in most drownings. If possible, the Paramedic should obtain a water sample and transport it with the patient for laboratory analysis later. As antibiotic treatment is likely, any history of allergies to medications should be obtained as well.

Alcohol intoxication and substance abuse are common factors in over one-half of drownings and can complicate the physical assessment. Furthermore, alcohol intoxication can induce hypoglycemia. The Paramedic should obtain as complete an accounting as possible of activities before the accident.

Witnesses typically describe the patient as having his head above the water, struggling to stay afloat, and then quietly slipping under the water. Rarely is it reported that the patient was thrashing his arms over his head as shown in the movies, as thrashing does not help keep the patient afloat. If thrashing is observed, the patient may have had a seizure. Patients with neuromuscular disorders or seizures have an increased of risk of drowning.[28]

The Paramedic should also obtain the patient's cardiac history. Cold-water immersion has been known to cause dysrhythmias, particularly if the patient has a history of congenital prolonged QT syndrome.[29]

The Paramedic should try to ascertain the events that immediately preceded the drowning. For example, a thrashing patient suggests the patient had a seizure while in the water. If the patient was diving, such as from rock above the shoreline or from a rope swing into a quarry, then the patient might have gone in head first, with the potential of spine injury, paralysis, and then drowning.

Finally, while the drowning patient is being recovered (for more details on water rescue, refer to Chapter 28) or as soon as practical thereafter, the Paramedic should ascertain the submersion time. This time is usually calculated from the time the patient is last seen to the time of rescue.

► CASE STUDY (CONTINUED)

Driving a stake into the shore at the point Brian was last seen, the deputy ties a rope to the stake and to himself. With a flare in his hand, he swims straight out. The bright light of the flare gets dimmer and dimmer, then suddenly it becomes bright. In seconds, it is above the water. "I got him!" the deputy yells out. While the deputy swims to shore, the first responders start to wade a backboard into the water. Sliding the backboard long axis under Brian's body, the team lifts the teenager's limp body above the water and carry him to shore.

Off in the distance, more patrol cars are seen winding down the quarry road. The deputy thinks to himself, "I wonder which one has the kid's parents?"

CRITICAL THINKING QUESTIONS

1. What are the elements of the physical examination of a patient with suspected drowning?
2. Why is a rapid head-to-toe secondary examination a critical element in this examination?

Examination

For every pediatric drowning death, the American Academy of Pediatrics estimates that there are four nonfatal submersion incidents. Therefore, the Paramedic should start the patient examination expecting that the patient is "resuscitable."

The examination of the drowning patient focuses on the patient's level of consciousness. If the patient is unconscious, then the examination focuses on life signs. If the patient is in cardiac arrest, the Paramedic initiates basic life support immediately. More treatment options are described under the "Treatment" section.

If the patient is unconscious but has pulses, the examination focuses on the airway. The patient's ability to maintain and protect the airway is of primary importance, so the Paramedic should take efforts to preserve the airway.

If the patient is conscious and able to maintain the airway, the Paramedic should auscultate the lungs for adventitious breath sounds. Stridor at the trachea may indicate partial airway obstruction and the need to prophylactically intubate the patient to protect the airway, with consideration of a medication-facilitated intubation. Wheezing may be appreciated proximal to the angle of Louis where the trachea bifurcates, suggesting aspiration and the need for deep endotracheal suctioning.

An altered mental status may be suggestive of hypoxia, hypoglycemia, or head injury. For these reasons, the Paramedic should use a pulse oximetry, make a blood glucose determination, and obtain a set of vital signs to rule out Cushing's triad.

A head-to-toe physical examination, when time permits, can help the Paramedic eliminate concurrent injuries—such as fractures, soft-tissue injuries, and head injuries—that could complicate the patient's recovery.

STREET SMART

The Paramedic should have a strong index of suspicion for possible spinal injuries, particularly in unknown situations. A person can easily sustain a spinal injury diving into any body of water.

CASE STUDY (CONTINUED)

Brian is unresponsive but appears to be having agonal breathing. He is cold to the touch and probably hypothermic. This condition might help him survive his drowning.

CRITICAL THINKING QUESTIONS

1. What is the significance of the hypothermia?
2. What is the significance of agonal breathing?

Assessment

Paramedics are sometimes called to the scene where a body is found and drowning is suspected. In some instances, the patient may have been deceased for some time. Generally, unless air is trapped in the clothing, a body will sink to the bottom of a body of water, head down, until decomposition leads to the formation of gas with subsequent bloating, causing the body to float to the surface.

The typical evidence of death is rigor mortis (stiffened muscles), livor mortis (blood pooling), and algor mortis (cooling of the body). However, these signs can be misleading in the drowned patient. For example, the stiff muscles of rigor mortis can relax, absorption of water changes the color of livor mortis from blue–red to pink, and the patient's body may have cooled from the cold water.

Maceration of the skin may be a better indicator. The white wrinkled skin of maceration starts peripherally at the toes and fingers, in about two to four hours. Early decomposition is recognizable by the skin's green discoloration, and the fact that the body is found floating, usually belly up, suggests decomposition.[30]

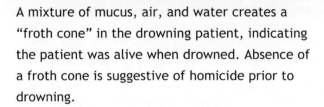

STREET SMART

A mixture of mucus, air, and water creates a "froth cone" in the drowning patient, indicating the patient was alive when drowned. Absence of a froth cone is suggestive of homicide prior to drowning.

Brian seems to have an ECG rhythm, best seen in MCL1, but the complexes are very small and the EMT on-scene cannot find a carotid pulse. "Start compressions!" the deputy yells as he quickly strips off his diving gear, "and let's blow some air into that boy's lungs!" As he yells over the din of the chaotic scene, he looks up and sees two figures, holding each other. "Must be the parents," he murmurs.

Someone yelling "Suction!" interrupts that thought, and the deputy turns back to Brian. Since air seems to be going in for now, intubation will wait until they are in the back of the ambulance.

CRITICAL THINKING QUESTIONS

1. What is the treatment of patients with suspected drowning?
2. What are some of the patient-specific concerns and considerations that the Paramedic should consider when applying this plan of care that is intended to treat a broad patient population presenting with drowning?

Treatment

Treatment starts in the water during the rescue, if possible. Basic life support, initiated early, is critical to the patient's survival. If cervical spine injury is suspected, either because of an unwitnessed drowning or a mechanism of injury that suggests the possibility of a spinal injury, then spinal precautions should be taken. However, the priority is to begin rescue breathing as soon as possible, even in the water. One study suggested that without a mechanism of injury, routine cervical spine immobilization may not be warranted.[31]

Once the patient is removed, and is found in cardiac arrest, the Paramedic should initiate chest compressions. Chest compressions in the water are of questionable effectiveness.

Over one-half of drowning patients in cardiac arrest are found in asystole, whereas approximately another 30% are in a ventricular fibrillation/tachycardia. The remainder have a bradycardia/pulseless electrical activity (PEA). These rhythms are thought to be secondary to profound acidosis and hypoxia. Although the Paramedic should institute standard advanced cardiac life support, treatment should also focus on reversing acidosis, through ventilation, and correcting hypoxia.

STREET SMART

Profound hypothermia can mimic death: cold skin, dilated and unresponsive pupils, pulselessness, profound pallor, and asystole on the monitor (ECG electrodes need warmth to work). The saying goes, "No one is dead until he is warm and dead." All hypothermic drowning patients should be resuscitated until normothermic.

If the patient is not in cardiac arrest but is unconscious, the Paramedic should immediately clear the airway to remove obvious debris as necessary. Ventilation with a bag-mask assembly or a flow-restricted, oxygen-powered ventilation device should begin immediately. Caution is advised with ventilation, carefully watching for chest rise, as higher airway resistance may be met and/or problems of barotrauma can be exacerbated with aggressive overventilation. Optimally, the patient should be ventilated with a volume of 6 mL/kg based on the patient's ideal body weight.

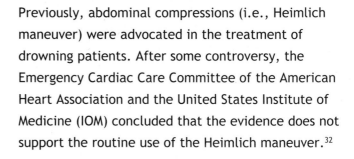

STREET SMART

Previously, abdominal compressions (i.e., Heimlich maneuver) were advocated in the treatment of drowning patients. After some controversy, the Emergency Cardiac Care Committee of the American Heart Association and the United States Institute of Medicine (IOM) concluded that the evidence does not support the routine use of the Heimlich maneuver.[32]

If the patient is conscious, the Paramedic should administer high-flow, high-concentration oxygen, particularly if the patient's SpO2 is 90% or less. The Paramedic should pay careful attention to the patient's work of breathing. A decrease in respiratory rate may be less of an indication of improvement as it is an indication of exhaustion. In those instances, the patient may need to be assisted with ventilation. Aspiration of cold water can lead to bronchorrhea and bronchospasm. When wheezes are appreciated on auscultation, then administration of albuterol (an inhaled beta agonist), small volume nebulizer, or metered dose inhaler may be indicated.

The drowned patient's intravascular volume should be optimized in order to dilute acidosis and improve circulatory status for adequate cerebral perfusion. Fluid resuscitation of 20 mL/cc may be indicated as well as inotropic support, with dopamine, as needed to maintain a normotensive state. The combination of dilution, ventilation, and oxygenation should help reverse acidosis.

The Paramedic should consider passive external rewarming through the removal of wet garments. Active rewarming has been debated for the drowning patient as therapeutic hypothermia as been shown to be helpful.[33]

A great deal more attention has been paid to cerebral resuscitation. Controlled hyperventilation, moderate hypothermia, and neuromuscular paralysis are thought to confer some neuroprotection for the patient. These procedures can be instituted in the field by Paramedics, with medical control, and continued in-hospital for four to five days. Hyperbaric oxygen therapy (HBO) may also be considered for dive-related drownings.

▶ **CASE STUDY (CONTINUED)**

"Good news," the deputy thinks. "Air is moving, and oxygen saturations are climbing despite the coarse crackles in the upper chest. Let's put a PEEP valve on that bag." A first responder palpates a pulse. Leaning down, the Deputy carefully put his fingers into the carotid groove and closes his eyes. The scene is so quiet the crew can hear a pin drop when he triumphantly announces, "Yep, continue CPR."

CRITICAL THINKING QUESTIONS

1. What are some of the predictable complications associated with cold water drowning?
2. What are some of the predictable complications associated with the treatments for cold water drowning?

Evaluation

With the accumulation of fluid in the lung as evidenced by coarse crackles, as well as dilution of surfactant leading to atelectasis, the use of continuous positive airway pressure (CPAP) has been advocated by some. Indications for CPAP include persistent hypoxia, as evidenced by SpO_2 of less than 95% in the face of high-flow, high-concentration oxygen; accessory muscle use; and auscultation of adventitious breath sounds.[34]

If endotracheal intubation is indicated, for better control of ventilation through monitoring of end-tidal carbon dioxide ($EtCO_2$), then the use of positive end-expiratory pressure (PEEP) is also indicated. Both PEEP and CPAP provide for better ventilation by recruiting atelectatic alveoli and increasing the surface area of available alveoli for diffusion.

Gastric distention is a common complication of resuscitation. It interferes with ventilation, especially of children, and represents a risk for aspiration upon regurgitation. To prevent these harms, the Paramedic should place an oro/nasogastric tube to decompress the stomach.

▶ **CASE STUDY CONCLUSION**

The thump-thump of the helicopter's rotors are heard in the distance. Someone has called for LifeStar and the fire department first responders have already set up a landing zone. Time is of the essence. If this kid is going to survive, he needs to go to the trauma center.

CRITICAL THINKING QUESTIONS

1. What is the preferred destination for the drowning patient?
2. What are the exceptions in those cases?

Disposition

The destination decision is based, in part, on level of consciousness. For the unconscious, hypothermic drowning patient who has not been responsive to standard therapy in the field, extracorporeal membrane oxygenation (ECMO) has shown some promising results.[35] ECMO is similar to a heart–lung bypass machine used in the operating room that provides oxygen to the blood outside of the body (i.e., extracorporeal). ECMO is indicated when there is a potentially reversible cause of cardiopulmonary failure; drowning patients typically do not have pre-existing organic disease that caused the cardiopulmonary failure. There are multiple reports of drowning patients who have a full neurological recovery following the use of ECMO.

Survival of all drowning patients is somewhat unpredictable. However, the Orlowski score is commonly used as a prognostic indicator of survival. A point is added for each of the following: age 3 or greater, submersion for greater than five minutes, resuscitation started after 10 minutes, and the patient being in coma on arrival to the emergency department or having an initial arterial blood gas pH of less than 7.1. If the patient has a score of 1 or 2, the patient has a 90% chance of recovery, whereas a score of 3 or more indicates that the chance of survival drops to 5%.

CONCLUSION

The risk of drowning is an unfortunate fact of life for parents in that it is the most common cause of accidental death for children from ages 1 to 14.[36] The key to preventing a child from becoming a statistic is prevention. As drowning appears to have a bimodal distribution, drownings most often occur with toddlers who are less than 4 years old and adolescents 15 to 19 years of age. Supervision of children in these age groups is important when they are around water. A four-foot tall fence, with a latched and self-closing gate, can help. The pool gates are open in 70% of pool drownings.

▶ KEY POINTS:

- Drownings can be either wet drownings (i.e., water in the lungs) or dry drownings.

- Wet drownings result in negative buoyancy, whereas dry drownings result in positive buoyancy.

- Electrolyte disturbances are rare in either freshwater or saltwater drowning.

- Pediatrics remains the major patient population affected by drowning.

- Hypothermia can cause drowning, but it also can improve survival in drowning due to the cold water reflex.

- Dive drowning is a subset of drowning.

- Hyperventilation during snorkeling can lead to shallow water blackout.

- Dysbarism is any disorder that results from changes in pressure.

- Boyle's law, Dalton's law, Henry's law and Charles' law are the gas laws.

- Boyle's law explains changes in pressure during a dive, and the resulting barotrauma on ascent.

- Dalton's law explains partial pressures, hypoxia at depth, and underwater seizures.

- Nitrogen narcosis, or rapture of the deep, is the result of the anesthetic qualities of nitrogen at depth.

- Henry's law explains how nitrogen comes out of solution during ascent.

- Charles' law explains how thermals affect pressure.

- Decompression illness is the broad title for a number of compression–decompression emergencies.

- Decompression sickness is divided into two categories: DCS I, involving the skin and musculoskeletal system, and DCS II, involving the central nervous system.

- Pulmonary decompression sickness, or the chokes, is the result of pulmonary embolisms.

- Immersion pulmonary edema is a form of noncardiogenic pulmonary edema thought to be due to cold water.

- Minor dive syndromes include ear squeeze, sinus squeeze, and tooth squeeze.

- Cerebral arterial gas embolism may be the most serious form of decompression illness.

- Hypoxia, hypoglycemia, and head injury should be ruled out in any diving emergency where the patient displays an altered mental status.

- Hyperbaric oxygen treatment is still the preferred treatment for treating suspected decompression sickness.

REVIEW QUESTIONS:

1. Describe the difference between wet and dry drownings.
2. What is the theory behind the protective effects of cold water drowning?
3. What is decompression sickness (i.e., Caisson's disease)?
4. What is the symptom pattern for the bends, the staggers, the tingles, and the chokes?
5. What patients are at risk for pulmonary barotrauma?

CASE STUDY QUESTIONS:

Please refer to the Case Study in this chapter, and answer the questions below:

1. What is the significance of fresh water in this case? Stagnant water?
2. Is there significance to the location?
3. Could Brian have drowned from a shallow water blackout?

REFERENCES:

1. van Beeck EF, Branche CM, Szpilman D, Modell JH, Bierens JJ. A new definition of drowning: towards documentation and prevention of a global public health problem. *Bull World Health Organ*. Nov 2005;83(11):853–856.
2. Centers for Disease Control and Prevention, National Center for Injury Prevention and Control. Web-based injury statistics query and reporting system (WISQARS). Available at: **http://www.cdc.gov/injury/wisqars/index.html.** Accessed March 23, 2008.
3. Brenner RA, Trumble AC, Smith GS, Kessler EP, Overpeck MD. Where children drown, United States, 1995. *Pediatrics*. Jul 2001;108(1):85–89.
4. Lunette P, Modell JH, Sajantila A. What is the incidence and significance of "dry-lungs" in bodies found in water? *American Journal of Forensic Medicine and Pathology* 2004;25(4): 291–301.
5. Present P. *Child Drowning Study. A Report on the Epidemiology of Drowning in Residential Pools to Children under Age Five.* Washington (DC): Consumer Product Safety Commission (US); 1987.
6. Gilchrist J, Gotsch K, Ryan GW. Nonfatal and fatal drownings in recreational water settings—United States, 2001 and 2002. *MMWR*. 2004;53(21):447–452.
7. Howland J, Mangione T, Hingson R, Smith G, Bell N. Alcohol as a risk factor for drowning and other aquatic injuries. In: Watson RR, ed. *Alcohol and Accidents. Drug and Alcohol Abuse Reviews. Volume 7.* Totowa, NJ: Humana Press, Inc.; 1995.
8. Quan L, Bennett E, Branche C. Interventions to prevent drowning. In: Doll L, Bonzo S, Mercy J, Sleet D (eds.). *Handbook of Injury and Violence Prevention.* New York: Springer, 2007.
9. Giesbrecht GG, Pretorius T. Survey of public knowledge and responses to educational slogans regarding cold-water immersion. *Wilderness Environ Med*. Winter 2008;19(4): 261–266.
10. Samuelson H, Nekludov M, Levander M. Neuropsychological outcome following near-drowning in ice water: two adult case studies. *J Int Neuropsychol Soc*. Jul 2008;14(4):660–666.
11. Bennett PB et al. Pippin makes record breaking breath hold dive. *Scuba Times*. July/Aug 1995.
12. Denoble PJ, Caruso JL, Dear Gde L, Pieper CF, Vann RD. Common causes of open-circuit recreational diving fatalities. *Undersea Hyperb Med*. Nov–Dec 2008;35(6):393–406.
13. Bennett P, Rostain JC. Inert gas narcosis. In: Brubakk AO, Neuman TS. *Bennett and Elliott's Physiology and Medicine of Diving* (5th ed.). United States: Saunders Ltd; 2003:304.
14. Saary MJ, Gray GW. A review of the relationship between patent foramen ovale and type II decompression sickness. *Aviat Space Environ Med*. Dec 2001;72(12):1113–1120.
15. Mahon RT, Kerr S, Amundson D, Parrish JS. Immersion pulmonary edema in special forces combat swimmers. *Chest*. July 2002;122(1):383–384.
16. Slade JB, et al. Pulmonary edema associated with scuba diving. *Chest*. November 2001;120(5):1686–1694.
17. Clendenen B. Alert diver—January/February 1996. Available at: **Diversalertnetwork.org.** Accessed November 22, 2009.
18. Longphre JM, Denoble PJ, Moon RE, Vann RD, Freiberger JJ. First aid normobaric oxygen for the treatment of recreational diving injuries. *Undersea Hyperb Med*. Jan–Feb 2007;34(1): 43–49.
19. Pollock NW. REMO2—an oxygen rebreather for emergency medical applications. *Alert Diver*. July/Aug 2004:50–55.

20. Thalmann ED. Decompression illness: what is it and what is the treatment? Divers Alert Network. Available at **Diversalertnetwork.org.** Accessed November 22, 2009.

21. Rozali A, Sulaiman A, Zin BM, Khairuddin H, Abd-Halim M, Sherina MS. Pulmonary overinflation syndrome in an underwater logger. *Med J Malaysia.* Oct 2006;61(4):496–498.

22. Mihos P, Potaris K, Gakidis I, Mazaris E, Sarras E, Kontos Z. Sports-related spontaneous pneumomediastinum. *Ann Thorac Surg.* Sep 2004;78(3):983–986.

23. Marroni A, Bennett PB, Cronje FJ, Balestra C, Cali-Corleo R, Germonpre P, Pieri M, Bonucelli C. A deep stop during decompression from 82 fsw (25m) significantly reduces bubbles and fast tissue gas. *Undersea and Hyperb Med.* 2004;31(2): 233–243.

24. Roydhouse N. 1001 disorders of the ear, nose and sinuses in scuba divers. *Can J Appl Sport Sci.* Jun 1985;10(2):99–103.

25. Zulkaflay AR, Saim L, Said H, Mukari SZ, Esa R. Hearing loss in diving—a study amongst Navy divers. *Med J Malaysia.* Mar 1996;51(1):103–108.

26. Vann RD, Wachholz CJ, Nord D, Denoble PJ, Macris G. Can divers with mild symptoms of DCI fly on commercial airliners? In: Mitchell SJ, Doolette DJ, Wachholz CJ, Vann RD. *Management of Mild or Marginal Decompression Illness.* Durham, NC: Divers Alert Network; 2005:90–99.

27. Zuckerbraun NS, Saladino RA. Pediatric Drowning: Current Management Strategies for Immediate Care. *Clinical Pediatric Emergency Medicine.* Mar 2005; 6(1):49–56.

28. Bell GS, Gaitatzis A, Bell CL, Johnson AL, Sander JW. Drowning in people with epilepsy: how great is the risk? *Neurology.* Aug 19 2008;71(8):578–582.

29. Choi G, Kopplin LJ, Tester DJ, et al. Spectrum and frequency of cardiac channel defects in swimming-triggered arrhythmia syndromes. *Circulation.* 2004;110:2119–2124.

30. Geberth V, ed. *Practical Homicide Investigation* (4th ed.). CRC Press. 2006.

31. Watson S, et al. Cervical spine injuries among submersion victims. *Jnl Trauma.* Oct. 2001;51(4):658–662.

32. Rosen P, Stoto M, Harley J. The use of the Heimlich maneuver in near drowning: Institute of Medicine report. *J Emerg Med.* May–Jun 1995;13(3):397–405.

33. Varon J, Acosta P. Therapeutic hypothermia: past, present, and future. *Chest.* May 2008;133(5):1267–1274.

34. Dottorini M, Eslami A, Baglioni S, Fiorenzano G, Todisco T. Nasal-continuous positive airway pressure in the treatment of near-drowning in freshwater. *Chest.* Oct 1996;110(4): 1122–1124.

35. Bolte RG, Black PG, Bowers RS, Thorne JK, Corneli HM. The use of extracorporeal rewarming in a child submerged for 66 minutes. *JAMA.* Jul 15 1988;260(3):377–379.

36. Centers for Disease Control and Prevention. National Center for Injury Prevention and Control. Wisqars details of leading causes of death. National Center for Health Statistics (NCHS), National Vital Statistics System. Available at: **http://webappa.cdc.gov/sasweb/ncipc/leadcaus10.html.** Accessed June 2009.

CHAPTER 16

ENVENOMATION

KEY CONCEPTS:

Upon completion of this chapter, it is expected that the reader will understand these following concepts:

- Envenomations of the following:
  - Hymenoptera
    - Apis (bees), vespids (wasps, yellow jackets, hornets), Formicidae (ants)
  - Crotalinae
    - Rattlesnake, cottonmouth, copperhead, coral snakes
  - Arachnoids
    - Black widow spider, brown recluse spider
  - Scorpions
  - Cnidaria
    - Jellyfish, corals, sea anemones
  - Mollusca
    - Cone snail, octopus
  - Spiny fish
    - Stingray, lionfish
- Assessment and treatment of envenomations

ANATOMY CONCEPTS:

Prior to reading this chapter the Paramedic student should be familiar with the following anatomy and physiology concepts:

- Central nervous system function
- Coagulation cascade

Medic 11 is dispatched to Colonial Park, at the base of the hiking trail, for a report of snakebite to a hiker. There is no other information available except that the patient has leg pain. Two Paramedics are en route to the scene.

CRITICAL THINKING QUESTIONS

1. What are some possible snakes that the hiker may have encountered?

2. Which snakes are venomous?

OVERVIEW

The management of the envenomed patient can be challenging for the Paramedic. Although some situations (such as a bee sting) are relatively common, others (such as a rattlesnake bite) are rare. These cases can test the Paramedic's knowledge as well as provoke anxiety in the patient. Familiarity with these situations can help the Paramedic to appropriately evaluate and treat the envenomed patient.

Chief Concern

Although Hymenoptera stings cause more deaths in the United States than any other envenomation, most go unreported to U.S. poison centers as they are often managed at the site of envenomation. Hymenoptera envenomation can cause a range of reactions from minimal pain and swelling to rapid loss of airway from anaphylaxis. Death is generally from allergic reaction, although there can be significant sequela from the direct action of the venom. Often EMS becomes involved if the patient has an allergic reaction to the envenomation or if the patient experiences a significant envenomation, such as occurs when encountering a swarm.

Hymenoptera Stings

The order **Hymenoptera** includes the Apis species (bees), vespids (wasps, yellow jackets, hornets), and Formicidae (ants). The vespids cause the most adverse reactions. In 1990, the Africanized honeybee (Apis *mellifera scutellata*) was introduced to the United States. Its offspring, which is a hybrid of the Africanized and European honeybees, display an exaggerated group defense behavior. Although the venom is not significantly different from the native bee population, because of its aggression and propensity to swarm, they have been called "killer bees."

Hymenoptera tend to sting in defense of their colony, nest, or hive and are often instigated to sting with the patient unknowingly close to their domain. Smells (such as perfumes), bright color, or loud noises may also initiate a sting. After stinging with their hollow stinger, bees inject their venom. They then leave the barbed venom apparatus in place as they pull away, which kills the bee. Specialized musculature around the venom sac can cause continued envenomation until the stinger is removed. The smooth, unbarbed stinger of vespids allow them to sting more than once.

Ants are ubiquitous and account for half of all insects on Earth. Although many U.S. ant species can envenomate, the imported Brazilian fire ant (*Solenopsis invicta*) is the most aggressive. Believed to have been accidentally introduced into the United States aboard cargo, these insects attack en masse and can inflict thousands of bites over a short period of time. Envenomation usually occurs after a patient inadvertently steps on their mound. These ants have flourished in the warmer areas of the United States as they have few natural predators.

The Harvester ants (*Pogonomyrmex barbatus*) can also cause toxicity to humans. However, their numbers have been declining because of competition with the imported fire ants.

Pathophysiology

The venom of Hymenoptera is a complex collection of proteins and peptides. Not only does it cause direct toxicity, it also avidly activates the immune system, resulting in an allergic reaction. The large peptide molecule, as well as the presence of protein, makes the venom very antigenic. Some of the toxic components can also cause clinical effects similar to those of allergic reaction. Significant anaphylactoid reactions can occur with the first envenomation, or after the patient had prior exposure, sensitizing them to the venom. Although death without anaphylactic reaction is uncommon, multiple stings (such as 30 to 40 wasp stings or 200 to 300 honeybee stings) can be fatal.

Some species, like Harvester ants, will bite as a means to gain access to the target and spray formic acid into the wound. Their venom also contains **hemolysin**, which can cause breakdown of red blood cells. Fire ants, in contrast, only bite to get a grip and then sting (from the abdomen), injecting a toxic alkaloid called solenopsin. This venom can also cause a significant reaction in sensitized individuals.

Snakebite

In 2007, more than 3,000 bites from poisonous snakes were reported to U.S. poison centers.[1] Countless more go unreported, both from venomous and non-venomous snakes. Although data is limited, mortality from snakebite in the United States is low, with two deaths reported to U.S. poison centers in 2007. Morbidity, however, can be high, with significant and sometimes persistent lymphatic and muscle abnormality.

Venomous snakes are indigenous to all of the United States except for Maine, Alaska, and Hawaii. Snakes hibernate in the winter, and most bites occur in the United States between the months of May to October. Snakebites can occur at any time of the day, with late afternoon being most common. Although most bites occur to the extremities as a result of the patient walking or reaching, the handling of snakes can also result in bites to the torso and face. The handling of snakes accounts for a large percentage of envenomations. Alcohol intoxication, male gender, and being in one's second decade of life are other risk factors for envenomation.

Venomous Snakes in the United Snakes

There are approximately 30 species of venomous snakes in the United States (Table 16-1). Most envenomations come from the family **Viperidae**, subfamily Crotalinae. This group includes rattlesnakes (Crotalus and Sistrurus), cottonmouths (also called water moccasins), and copperheads (Agkistrodon). Family **Elapidae**, the other family of venomous snakes in the United States, includes coral snakes (Micrurus and Micruroides) mostly found in the southeastern United States. Family Colubridae consists of the non-venomous snakes in the United States.

Venomous Snakes versus Non-Venomous Snakes

Venomous snakes bite by means of fangs (described shortly). Non-venomous snakes, in contrast, have teeth but do not have fangs. Venomous snake species can also be distinguished from non venomous snake species by the presence of a single row of scales, or plates, on its belly. Non-venomous snakes have a double row of scales (Figure 16-1).

Pathophysiology

Venom is a complex mixture of proteins, peptides, lipids, carbohydrates, and enzymes. Many of the different components in venom remain unidentified. The venom is very stable

Table 16-1 North American Venomous Snakes

- Diamondback rattlesnake (Eastern and Western)
- Timber rattler
- Prairie rattler
- Sidewinder (Mojave and Sonoran Desert)
- Massasauga (Desert and Western)
- Caroline pigmy
- Copperhead (Southern and Broadbanded)
- Cottonmouth (Northern, Eastern, Western, and Florida)
- Coral snakes (Eastern, Texas, and Sonoran)

and is not sensitive to heat. Even within the same species of snake, the venom composition can differ depending on factors such as the snake's last meal, the time of year, and the last time venom was used by the snake. Crotaline envenomation can cause abnormalities in three areas as a direct effect of the venom: local tissue injury, coagulation abnormality, and systemic effects.

Death rarely occurs and is typically noted in those patients with anaphylaxis to venom or its components or in those that did not receive adequate treatment in a timely manner.[2] Crotaline venom does not have significant neurotoxicity except in the Mojave and Eastern Diamondback rattlesnake, which differentiates them from most other Crotaline species.[3]

Coral snake venom is primarily neurotoxic and does not contain the venom components that cause local injury such as with Crotalinae. Death in these patients can be from respiratory failure, although envenomations are rare.

Anaphylaxis to Venom

Patients can have an allergic reaction to either the components of the venom or even the saliva mixed with the venom. This can occur with prior exposure to venom, or in those patients without prior venom exposure. These reactions can appear similar to anaphylaxis from any cause and can include rapid onset of airway edema, rash, and hypotension. It is important to recognize that these effects can be in addition to, or mutually exclusive of, the primary venom effects.

Pit Vipers

Crotalinae are also known as pit vipers because of the presence of a heat-sensing pit located between the eye and the nostril on either side of its head. Vipers have triangular heads and vertically aligned elliptical pupils. Pit vipers are known for their fangs. **Rattlesnakes** have the longest fangs of the pit vipers, with some reaching 3 to 4 cm in length. These needle-like structures are able to retract into the snake's mouth on a hinge-like mechanism and then extend to bite and inject venom. Although most pit vipers commonly have two fangs, some have multiple fangs. In others, a fang can be absent. For this reason, the lack of the distinctive "two fang" bite mark does not rule out an envenomation.

A startled rattlesnake can strike without warning, and may be able to strike up to half its body length. Unlike in movies, people rarely report hearing a rattle prior to the strike. Rattles may also not be present in younger snakes. Copperheads and water moccasin snakes do not have rattles.

Copperheads have rust and copper color bands on the body with a prominent copper-colored head. **Water moccasins** have a white mouth which gives rise to another of its common names, the cottonmouth. These snakes are known to be somewhat more aggressive than other pit vipers and can bite underwater.

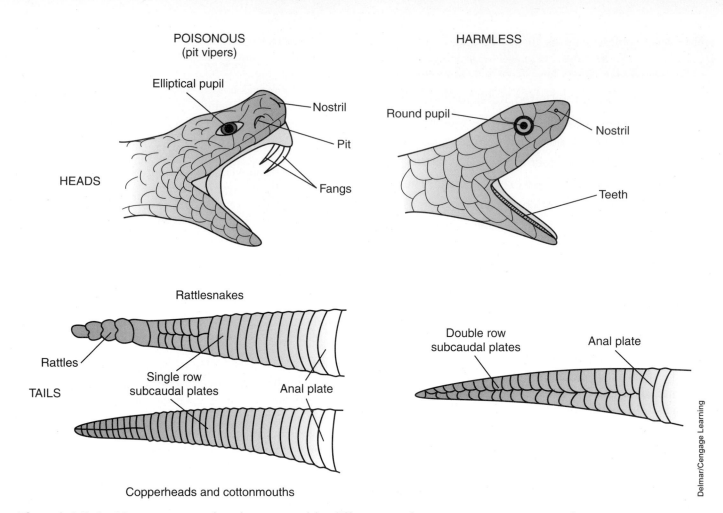

POISONOUS
(pit vipers)

HARMLESS

HEADS

Elliptical pupil

Nostril

Pit

Fangs

Round pupil

Nostril

Teeth

TAILS

Rattlesnakes

Rattles

Single row
subcaudal plates

Anal plate

Copperheads and cottonmouths

Double row
subcaudal plates

Anal plate

Delmar/Cengage Learning

Figure 16-1 Venomous snakes have notable differences from non-venomous snakes.

Elapids

The brightly colored **coral snake** is found in southern, temperate areas of the United States. They are identified by the red, yellow, and black banding that runs along their body, and are sometimes confused with the similarly colored, nonvenomous Milk or King snakes. Some people use the rhyme "Red on yellow, kill a fellow; red on black, friend of Jack," referring to the stripe pattern of the coral snake, to differentiate the snakes (Figure 16-2). This pattern recognition only refers to coral snakes within the United States. The coral snake also has a black snout, which further differentiates it from the red snout of the Milk and King snakes.

The fangs of the coral snake are smaller than those of the pit viper. Coral snakes will sometimes bite and hold on to the bite site, or "chew," leaving a bite pattern that can sometimes differentiate it from the bite of a pit viper. These snakes are elusive and will often spend time under brush. Envenomation usually occurs with handling the snake or while gardening or performing similar landscaping tasks.

Spiders

Spiders are carnivorous arthropods that are found throughout the United States. Although different species of spiders are found in various geographic regions, less than 20% of

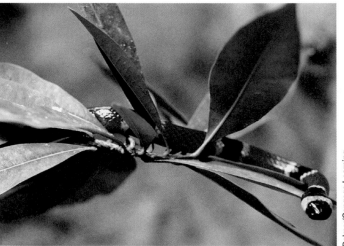

Delmar/Cengage Learning

Figure 16-2 The coral snake is quite venomous.

spiders found in the United States are of medical importance. Although most encounters with spiders are benign, there are spiders with envenomation syndromes that may result in the need for prehospital intervention.

Over the years, many different species of spiders have been implicated in medical emergencies. Information as to the ability of different spiders to cause toxicity has been ambiguous. Spiders such as the Hobo spider (originally located in the Pacific Northwest and now moving eastward) and the yellow sac spider have been intermittently implicated in the formation of necrotic lesions, similar to the brown recluse spider. The literature as to these spiders' ability to cause this lesion has been quite ambiguous. Based on this lack of data, the focus will be on two arachnoids with known medical importance: the black widow and brown recluse.

Black Widow

Although the **black widow spider** is the most well-known spider, there are five species of widow spiders in the United States: the black widow (*Latrodectus mactans*); Western black widow (*Latrodectus hesperus*); the Northern black widow, found along the East Coast, and west to eastern Texas, Kansas, and Oklahoma (*Latrodectus variolus*); the brown widow of the South (*Latrodectus bishopi*); and the brown button spider or brown widow (*Latrodectus geometricus*).

L. mactans females are approximately 8 to 10 mm, generally shiny, and jet black with a rounded abdomen. The red-hourglass markings on their ventral surface are species specific (i.e., it is noted only on *L. mactans* and not on the other four species [Figure 16-3]).

The females are significantly larger, with fangs capable of puncturing human skin. Although the male can envenomate, it is significantly smaller, and its much smaller fangs are unable to puncture human skin. The black widow is so-called because of her propensity to trap, kill, and eat the male spider after mating. Black widow females usually create complex, low-lying webs often found in areas such as garages, barns, sheds, and low-lying foliage. Black widows are not aggressive creatures and generally bite after inadvertent contact, such as after ending up in boots or sleeping bags.

In 2007, more than 2,500 widow spider bites were reported to U.S. poison centers. Although these numbers are likely underreported, there were no deaths attributed to black widow spider bites in that year.

Pathophysiology

The venom of the black widow is very potent, more so than that of a pit viper on a volume-to-volume basis. As can be expected by their size, significantly smaller amounts of venom are injected than when a patient is envenomed by a pit viper. Although there are multiple components to the venom, the primary agent responsible for most of the clinical effects is alpha latrotoxin. Alpha-latrotoxin is a neurotoxin that causes release of neurotransmitters from presynaptic nerve endings, specifically calcium. The large amount of neurotransmitters causes significant stimulation at the motor endplate of the neuromuscular junction with resultant physical findings.

Brown Recluse

The **brown recluse spider** (*Loxosceles reclusa*) is also called the fiddleback spider or violin spider. Although there are other species of Loxosceles, the recluse is the one most commonly found and is most predominant geographically.

These spiders are so named because of the brown violin-shaped marking on the dorsum of its body. They are approximately 6 to 15 mm long, and have significantly longer legs than their body (Figure 16-4). Their body color is brown to orange but can also be gray. Unlike most spiders that have four sets of eyes, Loxosceles have three sets of eyes. Although they are found in the southeast (although west of the east coast) and the southwest, the other species are found in variable locations in the United States. They are nocturnal hunters, and prefer to live in dark spaces such as garages, outhouses, under rocks, or in woodpiles. Although they are not particularly aggressive, they will bite when surprised or threatened. Similar to the black widow spider, the females are more dangerous than the males.

In 2007, more than 1,700 brown recluse bites were reported to U.S. poison centers. Although in general poison center numbers are likely underreported, there have been

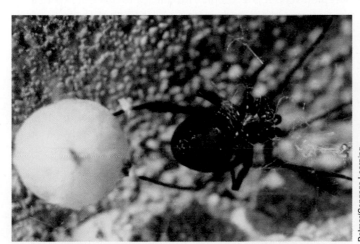

Figure 16-3 The black widow spider is one of five widow species in the United States.

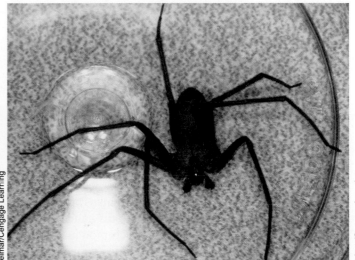

Figure 16-4 The brown recluse spider is often found in the southern and western United States.

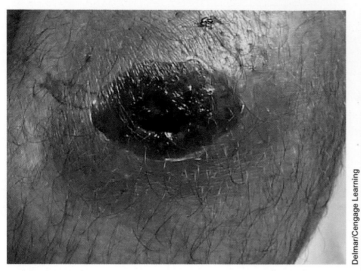

Figure 16-5 This spider bite is from a brown recluse spider.

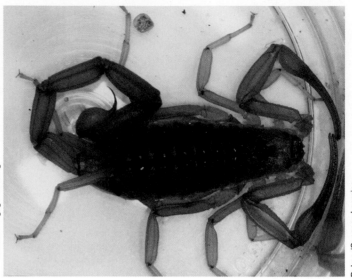

Figure 16-6 A scorpion does not bite, but spreads its venom through a sting.

studies that show that the number of reported *L. reclusa* bites outnumbers the actual identification of brown recluse spiders outside endemic areas. This discrepancy is likely from other spider bites that have been attributed to the brown recluse spider.

Pathophysiology

The reclusa injects a very small amount of venom. Similar to other spiders, the venom of the *L. reclusa* is primarily cytotoxic. Although there are many components, the two most important are hyaluronidase, which helps the venom move through tissue, and sphingomyelinase, which is the venom component responsible for the breakdown of the tissues from cell death (Figure 16-5).

STREET SMART

Although tarantulas are part of the funnel web spider family, the most deadly spiders in the world, the tarantula is not poisonous. Tarantulas sometimes catch a ride on imported bananas or are purchased as exotic pets.

Scorpions

Scorpions are arthropods that envenom humans not by biting, but by stinging with a specialized apparatus called a telson. Of the approximately 1,000 species of scorpion in the world, 20 are of medical importance (i.e., requiring medical treatment beyond first aid), and all species of these invertebrates belong to the Family Buthidae. In the United States, the only scorpion of medical importance is in the genus Centruroides,

C. exilicauda, also called *C. sculpturatus*. The bark scorpion, as it is called, is found in the southwestern United States, primarily in Arizona and isolated areas of New Mexico, Utah, and Nevada (Figure 16-6).

In 2007, although more than 1,600 scorpion exposures were reported to U.S. poison centers, no deaths were reported.[1] Death is exceedingly rare from scorpion envenomation. In fact, there was only one reported death after a Centruroides envenomation, which was likely an anaphylactic reaction to the venom.

Although painful, scorpion stings rarely cause more than a local reaction, and can be treated conservatively without lasting effects. Children are at higher risk for venom effects and have far more systemic effects from envenomation than adults.[4]

Pathophysiology

Scorpion venom is a complex mixture of toxins that is primarily neurotoxic. *C. exilicauda* toxins are active on the voltage-gated ion channels at the neuromuscular junction, which primarily affect sodium channels. This causes the repetitive firing of both sympathetic and parasympathetic nerves, allowing for the release of acetylcholine and catecholamines. The release of these substances is responsible for most of the end-organ effects. This results in sensory effects (pain), hypersecretion from parasympathetic stimulation, tachycardia and hypertension from sympathetic stimulation, and neuromotor hyperactivity. The venom's potency varies with the species of scorpion.

Marine Envenomation

Marine envenomation is not an uncommon occurrence; however, it is difficult to gauge its true incidence as many cases of marine envenomation go unreported to poison centers. In the United States, severe or fatal encounters are rare.

Cnidaria

The Phylum **Cnidaria**, which includes jellyfish, corals, and sea anemones, number over 9,000 species, although only approximately 100 cause toxicity to humans. These invertebrates are distributed throughout the world, and their toxicity can range from a painful sting without other signs or symptoms to death within a short time after exposure.

There are four classes within the phylum, all of which have members with potential toxicity to humans. They are Hydrozoa (Portuguese Man-O-War, fire coral), Cubozoa (box jellyfish), Anthozoa (sea anemone), and Scyphozoa (true jellyfish). These classes and species are distributed throughout the world, and different species from the same class can be found in many different geographic regions (Table 16-2).[5]

Although Cnidaria envenomations do occur in the United States, they are much more prevalent in countries such as Australia, the Philippines, and Malaysia. There have been fatalities documented in the United States, most of which were attributed to Portuguese Man–O–War (*P. Physalis*) (Figure 16-7).

Pathophysiology

The stinging apparatus of Cnidarians is called a **nematocyst**. They are microscopic structures found on the tentacles and around the mouth of most Cnidaria. Each nematocyst contains

Table 16-2 Venomous Marine Animals

Common	Habitat
Hawaiian box jellyfish	Hawaii
Sea wasp*	Gulf of Mexico
Portuguese Man–O–War*	Eastern U.S. coast, Gulf of Mexico
Fire coral	Caribbean
Sea nettle	Chesapeake Bay
Lion's mane or hair jelly	Northwest U.S. coast
Cabbage head	Gulf of Mexico, Caribbean
Thimble jelly	Florida, Caribbean

*Indicates documented fatalities from envenomations

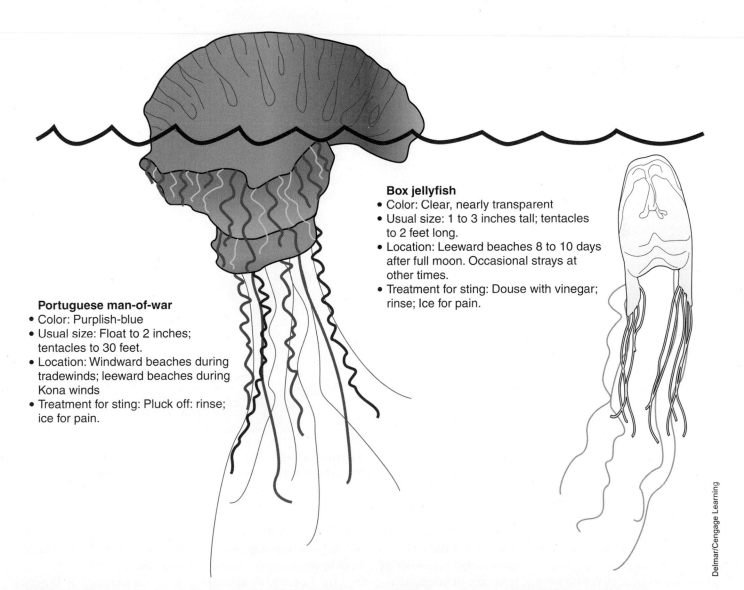

Box jellyfish
- Color: Clear, nearly transparent
- Usual size: 1 to 3 inches tall; tentacles to 2 feet long.
- Location: Leeward beaches 8 to 10 days after full moon. Occasional strays at other times.
- Treatment for sting: Douse with vinegar; rinse; Ice for pain.

Portuguese man-of-war
- Color: Purplish-blue
- Usual size: Float to 2 inches; tentacles to 30 feet.
- Location: Windward beaches during tradewinds; leeward beaches during Kona winds
- Treatment for sting: Pluck off: rinse; ice for pain.

Delmar/Cengage Learning

Figure 16-7   The Portuguese Man–O–War and box jellyfish are part of the Phylum Cnidaria.

a coiled threaded tube-like structure that contains venom. If these are disturbed, or if the creature feels threatened or is hunting prey, the tubule uncoils and fires. Specialized cells on the tubules called denticles allow for the tube to inject venom within the target. Other structures allow for the threaded tube to "hold on" to the target organism. The nematocyst fires within a microsecond, and some Cnidaria have the ability to fire threads up to 1 meter.

Cnidaria venom is very complex and is made up of multiple components, many of which are still unidentified. Although different between species, the venom is a complex mix of polypeptides and proteins. Depending on which species produced it, the venom can be dermonecrotic, cardiotoxic, or hemolytic.[6]

Other Marine Envenomation

Other minor marine animals are also capable of producing pain and rashes from bites and stings. Specifically, the Phylum Mollusca and the spiny fish will be addressed.

Mollusca

The Phylum Mollusca include the Gastropoda (cone snail) and Cephalopoda (octopus). Although neither of these is indigenous to the United States, there have been cases of captive marine creatures, as part of an exotic fish display, causing envenomation.

The cone snail is a carnivore that feeds by injecting its toxin using detachable, dart-like, radicular teeth. It is indigenous to the warm Indo-Pacific waters, and envenomation generally occurs with handling or breaking the shell. Envenomation is rare, and the syndrome can range from pain similar to that of a bee, to a progressive paralysis, coma, and cardiotoxicity caused by the multicomponent toxin. There is no specific antivenin, or antitoxin, for this toxin.

The blue-ringed octopus (*Hapalochlaena maculosa*) is a small, yellow-brown creature that can become iridescent when threatened. They are found only in the temperate waters of southern Australia, from southern Western Australia to eastern Victoria. It is a non-aggressive creature; envenomation generally occurs only when the creature is threatened. When the octopus' jaws inject its neurotoxin, tetrodotoxin, a syndrome is caused that can range from minimal skin findings to progressive paralysis and death despite resuscitation. As with the cone snail, there is no available antidote.

Spiny Fish

The stingray is a cartilaginous fish related to the shark (Figure 16-8). They are common in coastal tropical and subtropical marine waters throughout the world. Although envenomations are not uncommon in the United States, fatalities are very uncommon. Most envenomations occur when the stingray is inadvertently stepped on. The stingray tail has serrated spines covered with an integumentary layer and tapered barb. Venom glands run along the tail. Venom effects include pain out of proportion to the injury, with nausea, vomiting, diarrhea, weakness, headache, hypotension, and cardiac rhythm disturbances.

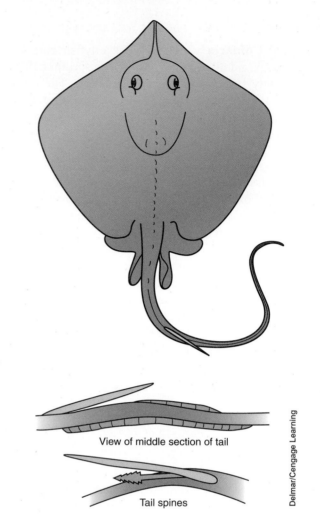

View of middle section of tail

Tail spines

Delmar/Cengage Learning

Figure 16-8 The Atlantic stingray is a cartilaginous fish related to the shark.

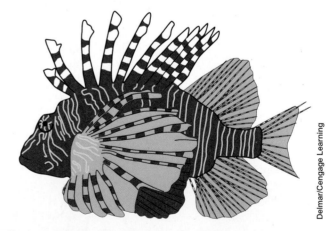

Delmar/Cengage Learning

Figure 16-9 The lionfish is characterized by its brightly colored, striped body and radiating, venomous spines.

Although no deaths have been confirmed from direct venom effects from the stingray, there are cases of confirmed death from traumatic injury from the barbed tail.

The lionfish, another spiny fish, is a member of Family Scorpaenidae (Figure 16-9). They are characterized by their brightly colored, striped bodies and radiating, venomous spines. Native to the Western Indo-Pacific, various species of lionfish can be found in warm waters virtually worldwide and have recently been observed in the Atlantic Ocean off the east coast of the United States. Toxicity is manifest by severe pain to the affected area, usually a limb, with extension up the limb. Systemic symptoms also include nausea, vomiting, diaphoresis, and syncope.

► CASE STUDY (CONTINUED)

When the Paramedics arrive on-scene, they find a 26-year-old male sitting on the ground in obvious distress. He is holding a rag to his leg. "Sir, we're here to help," the Paramedic greets. "What happened today?"

"Well, I was hiking up on Willis Pass and thought I heard something . . . the next thing I knew I felt a sharp pain to my leg. When I looked down, there was a snake on the side of the trail," explains the patient, Scott Bansky.

Mr. Bansky goes on to explain that he woke up early to get some hiking in before his afternoon shift as a DJ at a local radio station. He wasn't that far from the base of the trail and called 9-1-1 as he walked to the trailhead to await the ambulance. He guesses it occurred about 15 to 20 minutes ago. He did not get a good look at the snake but thinks it was "brown."

Mr. Bansky denies any weakness, shortness of breath, numbness, tingling, or any other injury. He has never been bitten by a snake (or anything for that matter) before and has never required antivenin. He had pain immediately after the bite and thinks it may be slightly worse now.

CRITICAL THINKING QUESTIONS

1. What are the important elements of the history that a Paramedic should obtain?
2. Is it important to identify the offending snake?

History

When the Paramedic first arrives on the scene of an envenomation, scene safety is of the utmost importance. It is not safe to attempt to capture the snake or creature (spiders and scorpions are rarely found, and only sometimes seen) to bring it to the emergency department. Identification can be helpful, but not at the risk of the prehospital providers or others on-scene. Although cases exist in which the knowledge of the specific snake changed a clinical course or direct care, if it is an indigenous snake, there is only one antivenin utilized in the United States. Determining if the snake is an exotic species will help the care providers' ability to obtain antivenin in a timely fashion.

A directed patient history is important in the envenomed patient to better risk stratify those at higher risk of adverse events. Also, in the case of an unknown yet possible envenomation, the patient's history may be helpful to differentiate the different types of envenomation.

History of Present Illness

Although these patients are often anxious and the situation is stressful, it is important to get as much information as possible surrounding the envenomation. Use the OPQRST mnemonic to help evaluate complaints related to pain.

Several specific questions are helpful in the evaluation of the envenomed patient (Table 16-3).

Past Medical History

Past medical history is important to better risk stratify those patients who may be at risk for a worse clinical course or adverse events. For example, those patients with a bleeding disorder may be more at risk from bleeding complications

Table 16-3 History Taking for Bites and Stings

History that is helpful in the evaluation of the envenomed patient
• When did the envenomation occur?
• Where did this happen?
• Was there a prolonged evacuation?
• Did anyone see the (snake/spider/scorpion/etc.)?
• Did you have any symptoms initially?
• Have you ever been envenomed before?
• Have you ever received antivenin in the past? If so, how long ago and what type?
• Was there any care or treatment prior to prehospital arrival?

of snakebite. Although bleeding is rare, those patients with multiple abnormalities in their coagulation pathways, both pre-existing and from envenomation, may require further monitoring or treatment.

It is important for the Paramedic to ascertain allergies (food, medication, and environmental) in these patients. Those patients with a significant history of atopy, or allergies, may be more at risk from anaphylaxis to either the venom (or its components) or the antivenin.

The patient's history of prior envenomation is important in the evaluation. Prior antivenin use and tolerability may be reasonable indicators of the Paramedic's safety in using these agents. Prior antivenin use is not a contraindication of future antivenin use, especially with the use of antibody fragment antivenin. As with any medical or traumatic emergency, those patients with multiple comorbid conditions may be more at risk for complications secondary to their envenomation.

▶ CASE STUDY (CONTINUED)

The Paramedic obtains a set of vital signs on Mr. Bansky while her partner completes a physical examination. Mr. Bansky has a patent airway without breathing abnormality. His lungs are clear. The anterior lower third aspect of Mr. Bansky's left leg has two small puncture wounds. There is a small amount of oozing blood around the wound and surrounding ecchymosis. There does not appear to be any swelling away from the site. The Paramedic removes the patient's low hiking shoe and confirms distal pulses are there, as well as sensation and motor intact. The Paramedic records the first set of vitals as blood pressure of 138/90, pulse of 120 beats per minute, respiratory rate of 20, and a pulse oximetry reading of 98% on room air.

CRITICAL THINKING QUESTIONS

1. What are the elements of the physical examination of a patient with suspected envenomation?
2. Why is a distal neurocirculatory examination a critical element in this examination?

Examination

The Paramedic's initial evaluation of the envenomed patient should always include an evaluation of the airway, breathing, and circulation. These processes are rarely affected by the venom, especially soon after envenomation. However, anaphylactic or anaphylactoid reactions, or facial bites from crotalids, may incite airway obstructing edema. This can occur rapidly and with minimal warning. If the Paramedic suspects airway compromise, these patients require aggressive airway intervention including intubation or a surgical airway. Certain rattlesnakes, such as the Mojave sidewinder found in the desert areas of the United States and the coral snake in the southeast, possess a neurotoxin that can affect respiratory muscles if an envenomation evolves.

The Paramedic should frequently assess vital signs as there can be hypotension with snakebite envenomation as there is with the black widow spider. Most patients that are bitten or stung manifest a tachycardia that may be partially due to the venom's effect and partially from anxiety or pain.

The Paramedic should complete a careful exam of the affected area and reassess it throughout treatment and transport. If swelling is suspected, as in a crotalid envenomation, the Paramedic should mark and time the bitten area. It is helpful to outline the area with a pen, noting the date and

time, so progression can be monitored. If evaluation was delayed, such as in a wilderness setting, there can be significant progression of venom effect on presentation. A complete secondary exam is necessary to assure there are no other sites of envenomation or injury.

Examination of the Hymenoptera Bite

Clinical manifestations of Hymenoptera can be broken down by type of reaction. Local reactions are the most common and cause swelling, pain, erythema, and pruritus. Although these can extend past the bite site, most are self-limited and resolve. Larger areas of what seem to be localized reaction can occur with some mild systemic symptoms such as nausea and weakness. Although these also generally resolve, they can be more prolonged, lasting two to three days.

Anaphylaxis or systemic allergic reaction can occur quickly and with one sting, with or without prior envenomation. This is a medical emergency and the presentation can be quite dramatic. These patients can present with diffuse urticaria, erythroderma (widespread reddened areas), and angioedema. They can be hypotensive and have respiratory compromise including shortness of breath, bronchoconstriction with wheezing, and airway edema. These reactions are on a spectrum from very mild to life-threatening and can progress quickly. Death can occur from airway loss, hypotension, or cardiovascular collapse.

Multiple stings, such as will occur with Africanized honeybees, can cause systemic, non-allergic reactions. These can be from any other Hymenoptera. These patients can appear quite ill. Along with obvious multiple sting sites, they can be hypotensive, with nausea, vomiting, headache, seizure, and fever.

Patients can become sensitized to Hymenoptera venom at any time and it is difficult to predict who might have an allergic reaction. Although patients may be aware of a prior reaction, its severity may be different or a significant reaction may be present in a patient with prior uncomplicated stings.

Fire ant envenomation is primarily painful, similar to a burn, which is where it got the name fire ant. The bite causes pustules that can eventually rupture, potentially causing secondary infection.

Envenomation of other ants, such as the Harvester ant, can cause pain and local skin symptoms similar to, but not as extensive as, other Hymenoptera. The area can have erythema and edema, with ecchymotic areas.

Snake Identification

The Paramedic should not attempt to capture the snake or transport it to the emergency department even if the snake is thought to be dead. Some unwitting patients have been surprised by envenomation after approaching a snake that was thought to be dead.

Bite patients are often unable to identify the snake, and sometimes the snake is not even seen. Although a snake handler or collector may be able to identify the snake, he may be unwilling to do so for fear of losing the snake or facing law enforcement intervention.[7]

Although snake identification is often impossible, it is often helpful to know if the snake is indigenous to the United States (i.e., was the patient snakebitten when hiking in the woods) or if it is potentially an exotic, non-indigenous snake. In general, the tenets of care are the same; however, if the need for antivenin is indicated, exotic snake antivenin might require time to obtain. The local poison center can be a valuable resource in the allocation of exotic antivenin.

STREET SMART

There are documented cases of bee sting-induced myocardial infarction. These patients experienced a myocardial infarction despite the absence of coronary artery disease. The Paramedic should consider obtaining a 12-lead ECG for bee sting patients complaining of chest pain.[8,9]

Examination of the Snakebite

Bite sites can have one, two, multiple, or no fang marks. Depending on the strike, it may be a glancing blow that might resemble an abrasion, laceration, or other injury. The area between fang marks is not a good indicator of snake size, as local swelling may cause the fang marks to appear spread out.

The severity of clinical effects is variable based on the patient's age, comorbid factors, sensitivity to venom, amount of venom effects, and time since envenomation. Also, severity can differ between species, with less toxicity often associated with Agkistrodon than with some other Crotaline species.

Local effects are the most common following Crotaline envenomation. They include pain, progressive edema, and ecchymosis that can move proximally and distally from the bite site. The effects can be rapid, starting within minutes of the bite, or can be delayed with slower progression of symptoms.

Although coagulation abnormalities are not unusual after Crotaline envenomation, frank bleeding is not a common occurrence. These abnormalities are often not initially clinically evident but can cause bleeding or significant ecchymosis later in the course.

Systemic symptoms include nausea, vomiting, numbness/tingling, diarrhea, and metallic taste. These can be accompanied by tachycardia and hypotension that can worsen as hemoconcentration develops when intravascular fluid moves into the subcutaneous space.

Although airway compromise is unusual, it can occur either as a result of primary venom effect or as a result of the anaphylaxis noted previously. This can develop quickly and be in a location remote from the bite site.[10]

Coral snakebites often occur to hands and feet. Because these bites rarely cause significant local injury, there can be a false sense that the bite was a dry bite. These bites produce primarily neurologic effects: tremors, salivation, dysarthria, diplopia, and bulbar paralysis with ptosis, dysphagia, dyspnea, and seizures. This can progress to a flaccid paralysis that can be delayed in presentation. These effects can be difficult to treat even with antivenin and can last for days. The immediate cause of death is paralysis of respiratory muscles.[11]

Examination of the Black Widow Spider Bite

Often described as a pinprick, the black widow's initial bite may go unnoticed. The bite site may exhibit a red, halo type shape with localized piloerection and hidrosis (sweating). However, there may initially be only minimal physical findings.

Systemic symptoms can start within 30 to 60 minutes, although they can also be delayed by a few hours. Muscle pain and cramping, spreading proximally from the bite site to the large muscle groups contiguously, is the hallmark of *L. mactans* envenomation. A patient that was bitten on the leg may note muscle pain and cramping that extends up into the thigh, buttocks, and then to the back and trunk muscles. The pain can be very severe; in fact, the abdominal cramping caused by the venom has been mistaken for an intraperitoneal process. Patients will often have a waxing and waning course, describing the pain as coming in waves. The muscle pain can last from hours to a few days in severe envenomations.

An unusual and uncommon finding is a pattern of facial swelling and symptoms called **latrodectus facies**. This is manifest by ptosis of the eyelids, with rhinitis, conjunctivitis, and facial spasms. Although this can be confused with an allergic reaction, it is primarily a venom effect.

Bites can cause nausea, vomiting, hypertension, and tachycardia, although often it is difficult to differentiate these from similar physiologic responses to pain and anxiety.

It is exceedingly rare for bites to cause life-threatening hypertension and tachycardia. These rarely require specific treatment in the prehospital environment.

Examination of the Brown Recluse Bite

The bite from *L. reclusa* is generally painless, and a patient may go 6 to 12 hours before noticing a small red lesion or papule at the bite site. Although most lesions do not progress from this early state, the recluse can cause **necrotic arachnidism**, which is the formation of a necrotic lesion from the spider's venom. These necrotic lesions tend to become evident over 24 to 48 hours after envenomation.

After the initial papule formation, the lesion tends to blister or form bullae. Reddish bullae can be surrounded by a bluish area, with a narrow white, blanched area between the red and blue, giving a "bull's-eye" pattern or what has been called the "red, white, and blue" bite of the brown recluse. The central and surrounding skin and underlying tissue can proceed to have worsening necrosis, or tissue death. At this point, the wound is quite painful from the destruction of the underlying tissue. These lesions can take many months to heal and may be quite disfiguring.

There is a rare systemic response to a brown recluse bite. This tends to occur more in children and can cause joint aches, fever, rash, kidney failure, coagulation abnormality, and coma. When this does occur, it is usually after approximately 24 to 48 hours after the bite. Without a history of spider bite, diagnosis can be difficult.

Examination of the Scorpion Bite

Although U.S. scorpion stings generally do not cause local tissue destruction, they do produce pain at the envenomation site, with possible localized paresthesia, numbness, and tingling. This begins soon after envenomation and will often resolve within hours to days. A more significant envenomation, which is more likely to occur in infants and small children, can produce tachycardia, hypertension, nausea and vomiting, diaphoresis, and hypersalivation with significant secretions. Somatic complaints can include muscular hyperactivity with erratic, but bilateral, ocular movements; restlessness; muscular fasciculation; and ataxia.

Without known visualization of a scorpion, these clinical presentations, especially in children too young to communicate, can present a challenge for diagnosis.[12] Although patients are generally aware of an envenomation, it is possible to have been bitten without immediate effects and then later note the onset of symptoms. This is also not uncommon with a black widow or brown recluse spider envenomation.

Examination of the Cnidaria Sting

Most encounters with Cnidaria cause pain almost immediately after the envenomation. Although the pain can be significant, systemic toxicity is uncommon. An urticaria-like rash may also develop at the site of tentacle contact. Although this rash may resolve in a few hours, some rashes may progress to vesicles.

Chironex fleckeri can cause severe pain and is known to have significant systemic toxicity. Although likely the fatality rate is overestimated, patients can have severe pain, nausea, vomiting, muscle spasm, paralysis, pulmonary edema, hypotension, renal failure, and death. This represents the exception, and children may be at higher risk due to body mass versus venom load.

Irukandji syndrome is a severe systemic toxicity from the Cubozoa *Carukia barnesi* or box jellyfish. Although initial local symptoms are mild, within approximately 30 minutes patients note severe pain, described as a whole body spasm, with tachycardia, hypertension, palpitations, diaphoresis, restlessness, and other sympathomimetic-type symptoms. The hypertension can be severe, which can then lead to significant hypotension. Fatalities have occurred, associated with intracranial hemorrhage from the hypertension. Although *C. barnesi* is found off the northern coast of Australia, there have been similar reports from unknown species off the coast of Florida.

Physalia physalis (Portuguese man-o-war, bluebottle jellyfish) is the Hydrozoa responsible for most Cnidaria envenomations in the United States. The primary clinical effect is pain, although it can also cause generalized weakness, limb numbness and tingling, nasal and ocular discharge, muscle spasm, and, in severe cases, renal failure and death. Vesicles and bullae can be present, with the potential for skin necrosis in the affected areas.

The fire coral (*Millepora alcicornis*) is found off the coast of the southern United States. Also from the Family Hydrozoa, it appears similar to harmless coral. However, it causes a burning-type pain when touched. It may also cause an urticaria-like wheal reaction that can last one to two weeks.

The Scyphozoan true jellyfish, or lion's mane (*Cyanea capillata*), is the largest reported jellyfish with tentacles. It is found in the cold waters of the Arctic, northern Atlantic, and northern Pacific Oceans. They have been known to have tentacles that reach 30 meters. There are population blooms some years with large numbers of lion's mane in shallow waters. Their sting causes a burning type pain; however, it is not a significant systemic toxicity.

Seabather's eruption is a cutaneous, pruritic reaction to the larvae of the thimble jellyfish (*Linuche unguiculata*). The eruption typically occurs underneath the bathing suit, which is believed to trap the jellyfish larvae against the skin. Symptoms often start either while the patient is in the water, or soon after coming out. Symptoms can be delayed for five to eight hours. Skin lesions usually develop after the pruritis begins and are vesicles, pustules, and urticarial lesions. The severe pruritis is the primary feature, which can interfere in sleep and daily activities.

CASE STUDY (CONTINUED)

Mr. Bansky's envenomation appears to be localized to the one limb and there are no systemic signs. Though the fang marks indicate a venomous snakebite, the Paramedic thinks, "This may be a dry strike." The Paramedic decides the patient has a minor envenomation that she should treat conservatively. Nevertheless, she resists Mr. Bansky's suggestion that he "walk out."

CRITICAL THINKING QUESTIONS

1. What is the significance of the local symptoms only?
2. What diagnosis supports the decision to not have the patient walk out?

Assessment

Most Crotaline bites are subcutaneous and occur on the extremities, although they can be intramuscular and, in rare cases, intravascular. Intravascular envenomation can result in rapid venom effect that may be difficult for the Paramedic to distinguish from allergic reaction.

Most envenomations create localized trauma that is self-limiting. In the United States, approximately 20% of pit viper bites are "dry" bites, which means no venom is injected. These sites can have a small amount of erythema and edema around the bite site; however, the swelling and reddened area do not progress.

CASE STUDY (CONTINUED)

After marking the area of the bite site and placing a dressing over the wound, the Paramedic begins to splint Mr. Bansky's leg while her partner starts an intravenous line of normal saline. Mr. Bansky is complaining of significant pain, although he still has no shortness of breath. He is given 8 mg morphine sulfate. After assuring that Mr. Bansky and the Paramedic are secure in the back, her partner starts the 12-minute drive to the hospital without lights or siren.

CRITICAL THINKING QUESTIONS

1. What is the national standard of care of patients with suspected snakebite envenomation?
2. What are some of the patient-specific concerns and considerations that the Paramedic should consider when applying this plan of care that is intended to treat a broad patient population presenting with snakebite envenomation?

Treatment

Treatment for a suspected envenomation is focused on symptomatic care with safe transport to an appropriate facility. Initial treatment should always be directed toward airway, breathing, and circulation, especially in those patients that present with immediate systemic effects of envenomation or anaphylaxis. Patients presenting with an apparent allergic reaction should be treated similarly to other patients with anaphylaxis. These patients can have rapid airway edema and may require intubation or a surgical airway. The Paramedic should also initiate epinephrine, diphenhydramine, and intravenous crystalloids.

Treatment of Snakebites

Even without anaphylaxis, intravenous access is important in all but the mildest envenomations. Hypotension can occur as a primary venom effect, as well as hemoconcentration, which may be present soon after envenomation. It is not recommended that any type of venom extraction device be used. None of these devices have been proven to change a snakebite outcome and can potentially cause further tissue damage.[13,14]

Tourniquets should be avoided as they can cause significant tissue ischemia and necrosis. There have been multiple home remedies utilized for the treatment of snakebite including electric shock and freezing. These hold no therapeutic value and are also potentially harmful.

If a patient has a snakebite to the extremity, the Paramedic should immobilize it as if it were a fracture below the level of the heart. The patient should avoid walking or vigorous activity in an effort to decrease proximal venom movement. In Australia, there has been evidence to support the use of pressure immobilization to prevent systemic absorption. This has been studied with the Australian elapid snakes, creatures that do not generally cause significant tissue injury.[15,16] In the United States, with snakes that cause significant local injury, this is of unknown value and has been shown to cause worsening tissue injury. At this time, pressure immobilization is not recommended as a field treatment for snakebite. The Paramedic can cover the wound site with a sterile bandage and place an ice pack on the covered affected area for comfort.

Judicious use of narcotic pain medication may be helpful as these bites can be painful. If narcotics are utilized, it is important to monitor respiratory and ventilator status as these can become compromised.

As snake venom can cause coagulation disorders, bleeding may occur at the site. Although minimal bleeding is not of great concern and can be managed with usual techniques, significant bleeding may be a sign of significant venom effect and may be an indicator for the use of antivenin.[17]

Treatment of Arthropod Bites and Stings

There is no specific prehospital treatment for arthropod envenomation. Treatment is generally symptomatic and supportive.[18] Patients with a black widow spider envenomation or scorpion sting may benefit from judicious use of opiate analgesia for the significant muscle cramping or bite site pain. If this is utilized, it is important for the Paramedic to closely monitor the patient's respiratory and ventilatory status. Patients with a late presenting brown recluse envenomation that has a necrotic lesion should have appropriate wound care, with a dry sterile dressing, and be transported for further medical evaluation.

Treatment of Hymenoptera Stings

Hymenoptera exposures can be life-threatening situations that may cause death within minutes of an envenomation. As previously noted, patients should be treated aggressively for an allergic reaction. If not already done, the Paramedic should remove the stinger if still in place by scraping the stinger off the skin with an edged tool, such as a credit card.

If there are local findings, only diphenhydramine may reduce the scope of the reaction and improve symptoms. Ice packs may help with local discomfort. However, the ice should not be placed directly on the skin and it should be removed occasionally during transport to re-evaluate the site.

Those patients with either an allergic reaction or systemic non-allergic reaction should have intravenous access in case of medication need or hypotension. Those patients with known allergy may have an epinephrine injector device. Depending on their clinical presentation, this may or may not be indicated and the patient may require assistance from the Paramedic.

Treatment of Marine Envenomation

The prehospital treatment of Cnidarians initially involves decreasing the risk of further injury to the patient or rescuer. If a Paramedic is entering the water to rescue an individual, she should wear protective clothing to keep from being envenomed. In addition, this should only be attempted if the Paramedic is trained in water rescue.

Treatment should first be directed at preventing further firing of nematocysts. Vinegar or acetic acid (4% to 6%) is a commonly accepted treatment to prevent further nematocyst discharge. The Paramedic should pour the vinegar over the affected area with adherent tentacles for at least 30 seconds.

After treatment with vinegar, tentacle removal can be done. If no vinegar is available, this removal can also be done with an object that has an edge, such as a credit card or driver's license. The rescuer needs to be careful with tentacle removal, as nematocysts can remain active for many hours. Nematocysts from *Physalia* and *C. barnesi* can be inactivated by hot water that is 100°F to 113°F (37.8°C to 45°C). If unable to measure water temperature, the Paramedic should use the hottest water the patient finds tolerable. Hot water immersion, or rinsing in a shower, should continue for 20 minutes. There has been no better efficacy shown with using ethanol or urine instead. Therefore, they are not recommended over hot water immersion or vinegar.[19]

Wounds caused by stingray, coral, or lionfish may require immediate wound care, especially in the case of the stingray, as well as antibiotic therapy later. Bleeding may need to be controlled. Embedded foreign bodies should be stabilized and not be removed in the prehospital environment.

Use of Antivenin

Antivenin is a product used to halt the progression of, or reverse the signs and symptoms after, envenomation. Antivenin is made by inoculating animals (i.e., horse or sheep) with the venom of the target species. The animal is then allowed to create antibodies to the venom. Antibodies, created by the immune system to combat foreign proteins in the blood, are ubiquitous in the immune system and are necessary in order for the body to protect itself not only from things like bacteria and viruses, but from the proteins in venom as well.

After the animal creates appropriate antibodies to the injected venom, the antibodies are withdrawn from the animal, purified, and readied for human use.

Although many different antivenins are available for various envenomations, the most commonly used antivenin in the United States is **Crotalidae Polyvalent Antivenin (Fab) (CroFab®)**.[20] This antivenin is indicated for treatment of symptomatic North American Crotalid and should be initiated after symptoms have been noted to progress after envenomation. It is administered as an initial bolus of vials, and then as a maintenance infusion after the progression of symptoms has been halted.

Paramedics should be familiar with antivenin as it may be encountered during interfacility transfer. It should also be taken into consideration when determining the hospital destination for the patient if it is believed that antivenin may be indicated.

CASE STUDY (CONTINUED)

En route to Torristown Memorial Hospital, the Paramedic calls into the emergency department to report the patient and assess the availability of antivenin. Dr. Blevins assures her that Torristown has rapid access to appropriate amounts of antivenin if they are needed and that he awaits their arrival. Although the patient's pain is improved somewhat, the Paramedic notes increased swelling to the area, beyond the area they had marked about 10 minutes prior. On re-evaluation, his blood pressure is 125/88, heart rate is 100, respiratory rate is 18, and he seems calmer.

CRITICAL THINKING QUESTIONS

1. What are some of the predictable complications associated with snakebite envenomation?
2. What are some of the predictable complications associated with the treatments for snakebites?

Evaluation

The Paramedic must be vigilant in monitoring and reassessing a potentially envenomed patient. Both vital signs and physical findings at the site can change during evaluation and transport. The patient's airway must be continually reassessed, especially in those patients in whom there is concern for an allergic reaction. The Paramedic should always be ready to respond appropriately to a change in the patient's condition.

CASE STUDY CONCLUSION

Upon arrival at the hospital, Mr. Bansky's pain has returned. His vital signs are stable, and his airway remains intact. Both the swelling to his leg and the ecchymosis throughout his leg have worsened.

After noting the progression of the symptoms, in conjunction with recommendations from their regional poison center, Dr. Blevins gives the patient antivenin. After receiving the initial dose, Mr. Bansky is admitted to the hospital for further maintenance doses and close monitoring. The swelling stops at his knee.

CRITICAL THINKING QUESTIONS

1. What is the most appropriate transport decision that will get the patient to definitive care?
2. What are the advantages of transporting a snakebite victim to these hospitals, even if that means bypassing other hospitals in the process?

Disposition

Patients with suspected envenomation should be transported to the closest appropriate facility. Because symptoms from envenomations may not show up immediately, Paramedics must encourage patients, even if they are feeling well, to go to the hospital. Paramedics should also take into consideration the patient's status and antivenin availability when determining the hospital destination. A patient who is in extremis should always be brought to the closest facility. Patients requiring specific treatments may be transferred from a community hospital to a tertiary care center for specialty care not available at the community hospital. Alternatively, antivenin can be sent to the community hospital from the tertiary care center.

CONCLUSION

Although the vast majority of stings and bites are benign, these creatures tend to invoke a strong emotional response from the patient. The Paramedic is tasked with evaluating the patient, determining the level of emergency, and treating the patient accordingly, up to and including providing psychological first aid. The prudent Paramedic learns which snakes, spiders, and other "biting" creatures are common to the jurisdiction as well as which areas may have the presence of "exotic" pets.

▶ KEY POINTS:

- Death from venomous bites is usually due to anaphylaxis, not the venom.

- Hymenoptera bites are some of the most commonly occurring bites.

- Venomous snakes include rattlesnakes, cottonmouths, copperheads, and coral snakes.

- Although pit vipers have two fangs, a strike can produce two punctures, one puncture, or just "chew" bites. Not all strikes inject venom (i.e., dry strikes).

- Spiders are carnivorous arthropods. Only two are known to have medical importance: the black widow spider and brown recluse spider.

- There are 1,000 species of scorpions worldwide, but the only poisonous scorpion in the United States is the bark scorpion.

- Cnidaria, such as jellyfish, are venomous marine life forms that use nematocysts containing venom to sting.

- The safety of the Paramedic and patient are the first priority on the scene of a suspected envenomation.

- One antivenin is available for indigenous snakebites. Exotic snakebite antivenin must be specially ordered.

- The patient's past medical history of allergies, bleeding disorders, or use of anticoagulants impacts the effects of envenomation. However, frank bleeding is rare.

- Examination focuses on the symptoms of anaphylaxis.

- Localized reactions are generally self-limited and include swelling, erythema, and pruritus. However, systemic reactions, such as urticaria, erythroderma, and angioedema, can be life-threatening conditions.

- Latrodectus facies (i.e., ptosis, rhinitis, conjunctivitis, and facial spasms) are due to venom and not anaphylaxis.

- Nausea, vomiting, hypertension, and tachycardia may be systemic manifestations of anxiety and pain or of anaphylaxis from bites. It is difficult to differentiate.

- Spider bites can cause necrotic arachnidism, an ulceration that starts with blisters or bullae.

- Tourniquets and venom extraction kits (i.e., snakebite kits) are not proven to change the patient's outcome and can potentially be harmful.

- Most care of envenomation is supportive and symptomatic.

- Crotalidae Polyvalent Antivenin is the most commonly used antivenin in the United States.

► REVIEW QUESTIONS:

1. Can a person have a reaction from a bee sting the first time she is stung?
2. What is the toxic effect of black widow venom?
3. What is the toxic effect of brown recluse venom?
4. What is the toxic effect of a marine envenomation by a Portuguese man-o-war, and its treatment?
5. What are the symptoms of a scorpion bite?

► CASE STUDY QUESTIONS:

Please refer to the Case Study in this chapter, and answer the questions below:

1. What differentiates a poisonous snake from a nonpoisonous snake?
2. What is the rhyme for the coral snake?
3. What are the symptoms of a Crotaline envenomation?

► REFERENCES:

1. Bronstein AC, Spyker DA, Cantilena LR Jr, Green J, Rumack BH, Heard SE. 2006 annual report of the American Association of Poison Control Centers' National Poison Data System (NPDS). *Clin Toxicol (Phila)*. Dec 2007;45(8):815–917.
2. Spiller HA, Bosse GM. Prospective study of morbidity associated with snakebite envenomation. *J Toxicol Clin Toxicol*. 2003;41(2):125–130.
3. Richardson WH, Goto CS, Gutglass DJ, Williams SR, Clark RF. Rattlesnake envenomation with neurotoxicity refractory to treatment with Crotaline Fab antivenom. *Clin Toxicol (Phila)*. Jun–Aug 2007;45(5):472–475.
4. Boyer LV, Theodorou AA, Berg RA, et al. Antivenom for critically ill children with neurotoxicity from scorpion stings. *N Engl J Med*. May 14 2009;360(20):2090–2098.
5. Brush DE. Marine envenomations. In: Flomembaum N, Goldfrank LR, Howland MA, Lewin NA, Hoffman RS, Nelson LS. *Goldfrank's Toxicologic Emergencies* (8th ed.). New York, NY: McGraw-Hill; 2006:1629–1642.
6. Watters MR, Stommel EW. Marine neurotoxins: envenomations and contact toxins. *Curr Treat Options Neurol*. Mar 2004;6(2):115–123.
7. Hunsaker DM, Hunsaker JC 3rd, Clayton T, Spiller HA. Lethal envenomation: medicolegal aspects of snakebites and religious snake handlers in Kentucky: a report of three cases with comment on medical, legal, and public policy ramifications. *J Ky Med Assoc*. Nov 2005;103(11):542–556.
8. Rekik S, Andrieu S, Aboukhoudir F, Barnay P, Quaino G, Pansieri M, et al. ST elevation myocardial infarction with no structural lesions after a wasp sting. *J Emerg Med*. Mar 26 2009 epub before print.
9. Valkanas MA, Bowman S, Dailey MW. Electrocardiographic myocardial infarction without structural lesion in the setting of acute Hymenoptera envenomation. *Am J Emerg Med*. Nov 2007;25(9):1082.e5–8.
10. Cowles RA, Colletti LM. Presentation and treatment of venomous snakebites at a northern academic medical center. *Am Surg*. May 2003;69(5):445–449.
11. Norris RL, Bush SP. North American venomous reptile bites. In: Auerbach PS, ed. *Wilderness Medicine* (4th ed.). St. Louis: Mosby; 2001:896–926.
12. Sofer S. Scorpion envenomation. *Intensive Care Med*. Aug 1995;21(8):626–628.
13. Bush SP, Hegewald KG, Green SM, Cardwell MD, Hayes WK. Effects of a negative pressure venom extraction device (Extractor) on local tissue injury after artificial rattlesnake envenomation in a porcine model. *Wilderness Environ Med*. Fall 2000;11(3):180–188.
14. Bush SP. Snakebite suction devices don't remove venom: they just suck. *Ann Emerg Med*. Feb 2004;43(2):187–188.
15. German BT, Hack JB, Brewer K, et al. Pressure-immobilization bandages delay toxicity in a porcine model of eastern coral snake (*Micrurus fulvius fulvius*) envenomation. *Ann Emerg Med*. Jun 2005;45(6):603–608.
16. Norris RL, Ngo J, Nolan K, et al. Physicians and lay people are unable to apply pressure immobilization properly in a simulated snakebite scenario. *Wilderness Environ Med*. 2005;16(1):16–21.
17. Jordan GH, Deitch EA, Britt LD. Management of poisonous snakebites. *American College of Surgeons: Consensus Statement*. 1997.
18. Carlton PK Jr. Brown recluse spider bite? Consider this uniquely conservative treatment. *J Fam Pract*. Feb 2009;58(2):E1–6.
19. Currie BJ. Marine antivenoms. *J Toxicol Clin Toxicol*. 2003;41(3):301–308.
20. Offerman SR, Bush SP, Moynihan JA, Clark RF. Crotaline Fab antivenom for the treatment of children with rattlesnake envenomation. *Pediatrics*. Nov 2002;110(5):968–971.

EMS OPERATIONS

Maintaining an attitude of safety first is important in EMS operations. If Paramedics do not operate in a safe manner, they risk injury, thus rendering themselves unable to care for patients. This section leads off with a comprehensive chapter on EMS safety considerations. The next two chapters focus on aeromedical considerations and specialty care transport, respectively, and examine the provision of paramedicine in these specialized environments.

- **Chapter 17:** EMS Vehicle and Transport Safety
- **Chapter 18:** Air Medical Transport
- **Chapter 19:** Specialty Care Transport

EMS VEHICLE AND TRANSPORT SAFETY

KEY CONCEPTS:

Upon completion of this chapter, it is expected that the reader will understand these following concepts:

- The hazards associated with operating an emergency vehicle
- Means of optimizing vehicle safety

The two Paramedics are stunned as they respond to the reported motor vehicle collision involving an ambulance. Both understand the inherent danger of operating an ambulance under emergency conditions, but neither of them ever considered a collison would happen to one of their own.

CRITICAL THINKING QUESTIONS

1. What are the vehicle safety standards for ambulance construction?

2. What can be done to make the patient compartment safer for all of the occupants?

OVERVIEW

The Paramedic is most likely to remain safe if he applies a safety-first approach to the ambulance transport environment. Safe procedures regarding ground ambulance transport are unique in that they bridge public health, public safety, emergency Paramedic care, automotive safety, transportation systems safety, and also occupational health and safety. Thus, a "systems-based" multidisciplinary approach is necessary to address the safety of this complex environment. Someone may have the safest vehicle in the world, but unless safety issues are properly addressed in the transport system that vehicle operates in, there is a safety risk. There must be a global culture of safety across all elements of the transport process.

Recently there has been an increased focus—nationally, federally, and academically—on the issues pertaining to air ambulance safety. However, the safety issues pertaining to ground ambulance transport generally have not been part of this focus or oversight.[1-10] Nonetheless, a number of initiatives over the past two years have increased the attention given to ground ambulance transport, as well as provided opportunities for collaboration and access to information resources. The activities of the National Academy Transportation Research Board's new Ambulance Transport Safety Subcommittee and its recent November 2008 and October 2009 Ambulance Transport Safety Summits have provided a new platform for advancing interdisciplinary knowledge in ambulance transport safety. As a result, there is an increased focus on ambulance transport safety issues occurring in the EMS press and at EMS conferences. Additionally, a number of organizations and on-line platforms are now specifically addressing ambulance transport safety. There are also organized delegations designed to explore global best practices regarding ambulance transport safety issues. However, there is an absence of specific federal oversight, guidance, and infrastructure pertaining to the safety of the ground ambulance transport. This underscores the need for increased awareness of ambulance transport and vehicle safety issues among those Paramedics involved in ambulance transport as well as those in service director and administrative roles. Among the safety questions to be addressed are the following:

- What are the safety issues?
- What do we know of the risks and hazards?
- How can we measure these?
- How can we optimize the safety of this system?

The published research addressing these safety questions is very recent; in fact, the vast majority has only been published over the past five years. The relevant literature is found in a combination of multidisciplinary fields bridging epidemiology and public health, engineering, transportation, and ergonomic studies, as well as topics in the liability and risk management field.[7]

This chapter provides an outline of the known hazards and current safety challenges facing ground ambulance transport. It specifically addresses some of the multidisciplinary techniques designed for optimizing the safety of the ground ambulance transport system as a whole.

Background

First, and most importantly, the transport safety and occupational safety issues pertaining to ground ambulance transport have not kept pace with the related industry, vehicle, and occupational safety developments. Unlike the safety regulations established with air ambulance transport or commercial vehicle transport, ground ambulance transportation safety has developed largely outside the purview of most other arenas (automotive safety, transport safety, occupational safety and health), with the exception of its policies regarding biohazards.[9] Compounding this situation further is that ground ambulance vehicles are a very diverse fleet including type I, II, and III ambulances as well as Paramedic pumpers, industrial response vehicles, and recreational vehicles such as motorcycles, bicycles, all-terrain vehicles, snowmobiles, and so on. This fleet is largely exempt from the **Federal Motor Vehicle Safety Standards (FMVSS)**, the minimum safety performance requirements for motor vehicles, established for all occupants seated 60 cm behind the driver's seating position.[10] This is in stark contrast to other commercial fleets, which must abide by air medical transport safety standards and the FAA oversight and regulations.

Thus, ascertaining the safety of ground ambulance transport vehicles (and products used in that environment) remains limited to expert opinion and peer evaluation conducted in a piecemeal fashion. In both biomechanical and epidemiological studies, the rear patient compartment has been shown to be the most dangerous part of the ground ambulance vehicle in terms of occupant safety.[11–15] In addition, recent data suggests that ambulances are among the most hazardous vehicles on the road, both in terms of vehicle and per mile travelled. Unfortunately, since no reporting system or database exists that is specifically designed for identifying ambulance crash-related injuries and their nature, specific details as to which injuries occurred and what specifically were the mechanisms that caused them are currently scarce. Even the information pertaining to fatal ground ambulance injuries is lacking or very difficult to access.

A number of publications in the epidemiology literature have addressed ground ambulance transport morbidity and mortality crash-related statistics.[16-21] These publications reach very similar general conclusions regarding hazards with the use of high speed and lights and siren, as well as serious injuries and fatalities that occur due to failure to use seat belts in the rear patient compartment. Ground ambulance vehicle crashes are the most likely cause of an EMS work-related fatality.[14] In fact, these studies indicate an 83% fatality risk for unbelted providers in the rear compartment during an intersection collision.[9]

Ground EMS providers at an emergency rescue scene also face numerous risks, such as being struck by a passing vehicle due to poor visibility. Recent data suggests that one in five transportation-related fatalities among EMS providers occurs in this type of setting.[21] The **Worker Visibility Act**, an initiative requiring emergency personnel (among others) in highway zones to wear high-visibility garments and reflective bands to aid others in observing them, should have a positive impact on improving the safety of the highway rescue scene.

As mentioned earlier, peer-reviewed automotive safety engineering tests conducted for the EMS environment[11–15] have clearly identified some predictable and largely preventable hazards, particularly pertaining to the hazards present in the rear patient compartment. These tests demonstrate the benefit of all occupants (Paramedics and patients) using existing restraints, the importance of over-the-shoulder harnesses for the recumbent patient on the gurney, and the need to firmly secure all equipment at all times.[11–15] These studies also specifically identify hostile interior surfaces and hazardous head strike zones, poor design and interior layout of the rear compartment, and the uncrashworthiness of many ambulance rear compartments. The tests also point to the need for head protection.[11–15, 22–24]

Although the lack of seat belt use by EMS personnel is cited frequently in the literature as a predominant cause for the high injury and fatality rates in ground EMS crashes,[15] other reports describe serious hazards resulting from the failure to secure equipment in the patient compartment. For example, in a collision unsecured defibrillator/monitors have caused severe traumatic brain injury, and unsecured oxygen cylinders have caused serious and fatal head injuries.[8] These findings are supported by the engineering data from ambulance safety research involving crash tests,[11-15] as well as insurance and litigation records.[12]

Although some crashes may not have been preventable, EMS personnel connect many fatal and injurious ground ambulance crashes to risky driving practices, particularly during emergency mode. One paper cites that 80% of the ambulance crashes are caused by 20% of the drivers.[18] Failure to stop at intersections is an extremely high-risk practice,[12,23] particularly given the realities of real-world stopping distances (Figure 17-1). Some of the larger EMS services have clear policies that require ground ambulances to come to a complete stop at a red light or a stop sign at intersections.

Optimizing Safety

A systems approach to safety and risk management is key to optimizing safety for ground ambulance transport. These initiatives focus on such issues as selecting safer, more compact vehicles with nonhostile interiors; instituting practical policies on vehicle operation; integrating intelligent transportation systems (ITS) technology, specifically technology-driven auditory real time driver feedback devices; using personal protective equipment (PPE) that addresses identified injury hazards, and implementing a structured safety program, with formal safety management oversight.

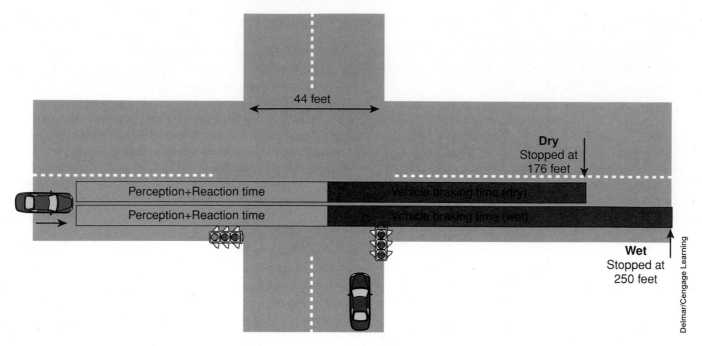

Figure 17-1 The stopping distance* at an intersection for a passenger car traveling at 40 mph on a dry and wet surface.

*Stopping distance:

Perception time + Reaction time + Vehicle braking time (varies with age, skill, agility, alertness + vehicle type, tire pressure, road, etc.)

The very recently developed **American National Standards Institute/American Society of Safety Engineers Z15.1 Fleet Safety Standard**[25] may be the only nationally approved safety standard in the United States that is now applicable to the safety management of ground EMS vehicle fleets. The implementation of this standard will likely provide more emphasis on EMS vehicle safety generally, enhance the data collected regarding EMS vehicle safety, and assist in bringing EMS vehicle safety more in line with state of the art automotive safety practices.

Vehicle Crashworthiness and Design and Occupant Safety Devices

Occupant safety engineering and crashworthiness design are based upon crash mechanics and injury biomechanics data. In the ambulance environment, such data is very limited, and some is even unreliable. Also, technical approaches that are developed for other circumstances, environments, or vehicles may not be effective or applicable. In fact, they may be harmful when applied to the ambulance environment when this ambulance crash and injury mechanics data is not considered.

Furthermore, unlike passenger vehicles or air paramedical craft, restraint systems for the rear compartment of ground ambulance vehicles have no specific design or safety standards to ensure that they perform safely in the ground ambulance environment. This environment includes very different forces and mechanics under crash and sudden deceleration circumstances.

There are different types of crash mechanisms (frontal, frontal offset, side, rear, and rollover) and a number of different orientations of occupants within an ambulance. This makes approaching the safety of occupants in the ambulance setting complex, not to mention quite different from routine passenger vehicles.

Routine passenger vehicles, as well as the front cabs of ambulances, are designed to create an "envelope of safety" within which an occupant has a maximal chance of survival during a collision. A number of engineering elements create this envelope of safety, including crumple zones and the seat design, which provides the occupant with a large degree of protection in the event of a crash. The purpose of the seat belt is to keep the occupant both in the envelope of safety and in the seat. However, in the rear ambulance compartment of the box and chassis style ambulance, there are no engineered crumple zones, and the only automotive style seating is usually the rear-facing captain's chair.

In a crash, the duration of the impact is generally 60 to 100 milliseconds. During this time (the time it takes to blink an eye), all the kinetic energy is transferred to the occupants (Figures 17-2a and b). Thus, there is no effective time to take any evasive action, and definitely no time to buckle a seat belt at that point. Not only is it important to wear a seat belt for one's own safety, but it also prevents the occupant from becoming a projectile and striking other occupants in the ambulance.

Regarding restraint devices, any restraint device designed to encourage an occupant to get up from the seat in a ground ambulance exposes that occupant to serious

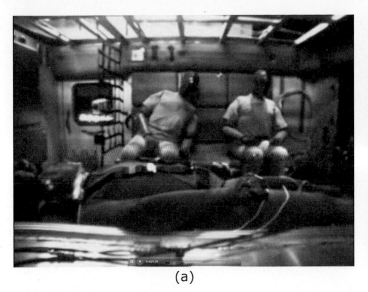
(a)

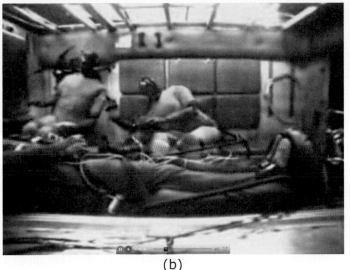
(b)

Courtesy of NIOSH

Figure 17-2 This shows how (a) the pre-crash configuration and (b) the moment of impact affect occupant kinematics.

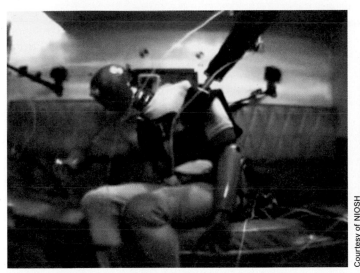

Courtesy of NIOSH

Figure 17-3 These providers, although restrained on the ambulance bench seat, are not well restrained.

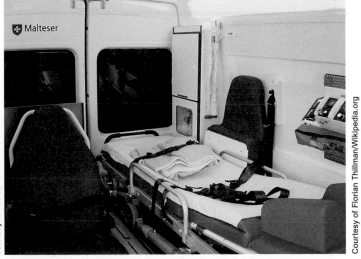

Courtesy of Florian Thillman/Wikipedia.org

Figure 17-4 The interior of this European ambulance shows the seating is either forward or rear facing. In addition, the seat on the left rotates to allow for increased loading and unloading access.

and life-threatening hazards and should be avoided. For example, technical information exists that clearly demonstrates a harness restraint system for a side-facing occupant in a frontal crash (Figure 17-3) exposes that occupant to hazardous and serious head and neck forces that can result in injury. This hazard is not present with the use of a standard lap belt system. Any device that is complex to secure—or worse, encourages the occupant to stand or move about in a vehicle in motion—places the occupant in a potentially serious and hazardous position, and thus should be avoided.

Forward- and rear-facing seating presents fewer hazards to the occupants, and also allows for easier patient care access. For these reasons, they are routine in European vehicles (Figure 17-4).

Patient access while seated is a constant challenge for the Paramedic in the larger box and chassis style EMS vehicles. The compact vehicles are inherently safer by eliminating this problem in their design. For the larger ground transport trucks, using a seat design that lets the Paramedic slide toward the patient can offer enhanced access to the patient, while still allowing the Paramedic to remain securely belted in the seat. However, the ergonomics of leaning forward to reach a patient or equipment is fraught with obvious challenges. Forward-facing or rear-facing seating alongside the patient addresses these problems very effectively.

Some serious concerns exist regarding the "trapeze" or "standing up" harnesses that are currently marketed. These harnesses are not only potentially dangerous, as they encourage the Paramedic to leave the safety of being securely belted in the seat, but they may even cause more injury than they protect providers from since they provide no support to the Paramedic's head or neck. They are also likely to increase the forces exerted across these regions. Since there are no safety testing standards for properly evaluating such "trapeze" harnesses (nor even crash dummies that are appropriately designed to test them), any claims regarding the "safety" of these devices may be flawed. In fact, such devices may not protect providers from injury in the real world and just might cause serious harm to those in the harness, not to mention the other vehicle occupants.

In general, purchasing products without established safety or design standards is problematic. Manufacturers can make whatever claims they desire. However, the only people qualified to truly evaluate the merits of such devices are independent experts regarding automotive safety in the EMS environment who have a solid understanding of impact biomechanics. In fact, there are numerous devices that, to the non-engineering expert, appear to be good solutions to safety concerns. However, they may actually be worse than the current practice.

Since this is a new field, EMS providers should focus their attention on new peer-reviewed scientific papers and on independent and objective evaluations rather than manufacturers' claims in this setting of absent safety standards. Safety and design standards are now under development, which should make this now-somewhat-challenging situation less problematic in the future.

Current automotive safety technical information suggests that using the lap belts that are fitted low and firmly over the pelvis for all seated occupants, and using the over-the-shoulder harnesses for recumbent patients on the stretcher (with the stretcher back in an upright or 45-degree angle where acceptable), will provide an optimal degree of safety. In addition, all loose equipment should be firmly secured and locked down. According to the peer-reviewed literature, this has been demonstrated to substantially enhance safety in both testing models and in data collected regarding real world EMS safety. In addition, the use of automotive grade energy-absorbing padding in "head strike" zones would likely assist in minimizing the inevitable injury that occurs in the event of a crash or sudden deceleration.

The issue of head protection is an important topic.[15,22] Air Paramedic transport providers use head protection in the aviation environment. However, these same providers are not using head protection devices in the ground vehicle, where the head injury risk may be even greater than that present in the air paramedical vehicle. Therefore, the issue of design and safety standards for head protection is currently being addressed, although the head safety needs in the ground

Table 17-1 Attributes Considered Important When Designing Head Protection

- Communications capability with patients and driver
- Stethoscope auscultation
- Effective in high horizontal G forces, such as those found in an automotive crash
- Ability to identify the responder
- Lightweight and low profile
- Biohazard protection
- Unobstructed visibility
- Internal visor
- Image enhancing

transport setting differ from those needed in air transport, due to a different risk and injury mechanism profile. Based on research conducted to date,[26] a head protection device for ground transport needs to be protective in a range of conditions and contain several specific attributes (Table 17-1).

Prototypes and a design standard are currently being developed for head safety equipment. EMS-specific PPE for head protection is already available on the market that integrates a number of these features; this PPE is used extensively in Europe.

An acceptable practice to optimize ground transport safety is to adopt the accepted air transportation practice of ensuring and confirming, before takeoff, that all equipment and passengers are safely secured, and translate that practice to ground transport. In addition, if any occupants become vulnerable or unsecured during transport (i.e., to attend to specific patient-care needs), the provider should notify the vehicle's driver of the situation immediately so that the driver can drive with extra caution until the occupant is again secured. Currently, it appears that the opposite practice occurs in ground ambulance transport (i.e., no notification of the driver), with largely predictable morbidity consequences.

Two recent studies published in the automotive and transportation literature highlight these biomechanics and systems approaches that are focused on the real world of operational safety issues in ambulance transport.[5,27] These papers highlight that the safety of this environment is a system, in which the safety of the occupants is interrelated and that safety determinants in a vehicle environment must be guided by objective technical data from technical experts in automotive safety.

Visibility and Conspicuity

Very few scientific publications have addressed the subject of visibility and conspicuity. A recent report compiled by FEMA summarized the information available, but even this document highlighted that the science was fairly minimal.[28] Along

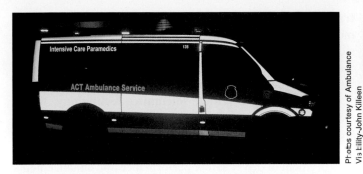

Figure 17-5 An effective, and also cost effective, visibility and conspicuity example from Canberra, the Australian capital territory.

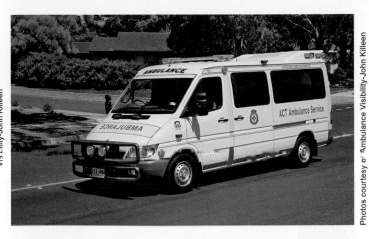

Photos courtesy of Ambulance Visibility-John Killeen

Figure 17-7 Repainting an ambulance enhances its daylight visibility.

with a number of other reports, that document highlighted that strong science does not support a number of "popular" approaches and that there is not much solid evidence behind practices such as **Battenberg visibility markings** (a cross-hatch reflective marking popular in Europe). A number of more effective approaches have been identified globally (Figure 17-5, which are also more cost effective than the increasingly questioned Battenberg approach.

Understanding the key elements of safety from a visibility and conspicuity perspective is paramount when determining the markup and color used on vehicles, as well as provider clothing (Figure 17-6).

For example, the Muskoka EMS in Canada applied the basic scientific principles of visibility and conspicuity to their ambulances in order to improve day and night visibility (Figures 17-7 and 17-8).

A proper understanding of the ergonomics of the workplace assist greatly in enhancing and optimizing ground ambulance vehicle design and safety. The complexities of tasks performed in the ambulance vehicle, particularly in the ground transport setting, lend it well to ergonomic evaluation. For example, where should the needle disposal container be positioned? And what is the optimal sharps disposal device to use in the ground transport environment? Where are the head strike regions, and how can they be engineered out? EMS should request assistance on these issues from experts in this particular field of ergonomics, particularly from the government agencies dedicated to safety in the workplace.

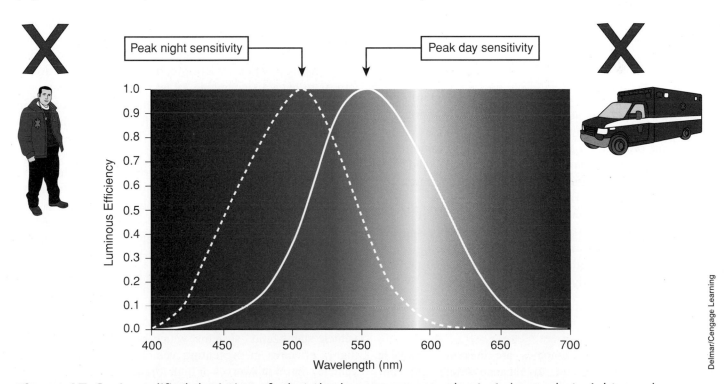

Figure 17-6 A modified depiction of what the human eye sees best at day and at night—and examples of poor choices for EMS vehicle color and personnel clothing.

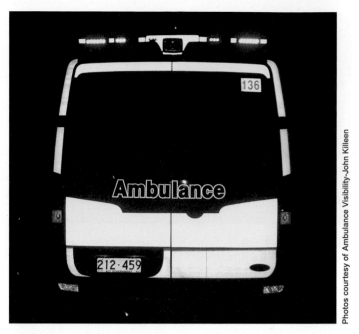

Photos courtesy of Ambulance Visibility–John Killeen

Figure 17-8 Changes in the reflective striping enhance night visibility.

The **National Institute for Occupational Safety and Health (NIOSH)** is an organization that is historically geared toward epidemiology, biohazards, and ergonomic research. However, even though there are millions of EMS transports each year; thousands of work-related injuries (many related to poor ergonomics in and around the ground ambulance vehicle), and even fatalities, there is not one published paper in the United States addressing ground ambulance operational ergonomics. This population-based epidemiological and ergonomic research, which is so needed in EMS, is also needed as a fundamental foundation in order for any automotive engineering and crashworthiness research to be conducted effectively.

Additionally, high visibility clothing will optimize the safety of providers at an emergency scene. Wearing such clothing, as mandated by the Worker Visibility Act, should be a routine practice for all providers. It is also important to ensure that the providers don't become "camouflaged" with the emergency vehicle and scene; this is another hazard of the Battenberg vehicle pattern.

Biohazard protection is primarily focused on biological PPE, more so than from a vehicle and transport perspective. However, it is important to ensure that vehicle design allows for proper decontamination from body fluids, and that surfaces are able to be easily and effectively cleaned.

Intelligent Transportation Systems (ITS)

A number of new technologies are currently available, with more on the horizon, to enhance safety and collision avoidance. These technologies, known as **intelligent transportation systems (ITS)**, pertain to driver behavior modification,[29–31] intelligent vehicle design,[27] and other roadside safety technologies.[32] ITS is a well-established field in the passenger vehicle safety industry, and in time may be an integral component in ground ambulance safety as well.

For example, **in-vehicle telematics technology**, which electronically offers real time driver monitoring and immediate auditory feedback, has been implemented in some regions in the United States. It has shown impressive and sustained improvement of driver safety performance and enhancements in vehicle fleet safety in a number of studies.[33,34] Driver performance data recording has shown great promise in optimizing safety in the EMS ground transport environment. These devices have reduced the number of seat belt and speeding violations by EMS personnel, decreased the number and severity of vehicle collision events, and also minimized vehicle maintenance costs. Additionally, these positive outcomes have been achieved with an improvement in response times as well. When properly implemented, these devices are not only cost effective, but pay for themselves within six months in vehicle maintenance savings alone. Thus, they have been scientifically shown to optimize safety, cost effectiveness, and response times.

Additionally, these devices have a role in the drivers' ongoing training. Therefore, they should not only be considered a valuable fleet and vehicle safety technology tool, but also a powerful and highly effective driver-training device. These systems should be regarded as the most effective safety intervention for addressing EMS transport safety challenges.

Other devices are available that provide video capture of the driver and vehicle. However, these other devices appear to be more intrusive and also require a very substantial administrative burden for monitoring and feedback. They also appear to have less impact on preemptively addressing risky driving practices. Therefore, these video devices do not appear to have a sustainable effect. Furthermore, there are no studies yet that have shown a sustained improvement in performance over extended periods. It is apparent that these devices create a negative impact on morale and the culture within the service. Furthermore, they have not yet been subjected to independent peer review. The only study addressing these devices was funded by the product's manufacturer and was of a brief duration. However, that study did show that there were some major concerns about the administrative burden and sustainability of effectively using the system.

ITS technologies that give the driver preemptive warnings of potential road or other vehicle hazards via dashboard warnings (or possibly projections onto the windshield, which are now fitted in some passenger vehicles) are still not features integrated into routine ground EMS vehicles. Enhanced vehicle stabilization systems, which have been shown to be highly effective in preventing vehicle roll and promoting vehicle control in swerves or high torque turns, also still have not been integrated into ground ambulance vehicles.

Other devices, such as systems that interact with the road signals, have been piloted in some regions with a certain amount of success. However, their applicability to other environments has not yet been demonstrated. There is also the very real concern that these devices will train drivers to anticipate that a stoplight will change color, thereby causing accidents if it does not. Another unresolved issue is that often more than one emergency vehicle is heading to an emergency, and these additional vehicles may be coming from different directions. This may cause a conflict with the signals. Thus, rather than preventing collisions, these systems have the capacity to increase the rate of collisions between emergency vehicles at intersections.

EMS Practice and Policy, and Fleet Management

To be effective, the translation of safety practice and oversight should address patient and provider safety as well as public safety and be smooth and consistent. It makes no sense to operate from well-understood safety precautions in patient care and then get into a vehicle where one does not have the safety features or the safety oversight that is warranted, creating risks for the patient, the provider, and the public. One aspect that makes addressing the system safety of ground ambulance transport more easily manageable than many other fleet work forces is that practice and policy are well structured in EMS providers' culture.

The personnel and patient safety awareness and practice model is well understood and applied in the air medical environment, an environment of structured safety practice and policy. Ironically, the stringent safety precautions, monitoring, and oversight that are so accepted as part of air medical services are not so readily translated to the ground transport environment, even though they are part of the very same program, have the same Medical Directors, and even use the same personnel for ground services.

Ideally, a culture of safety and a structured safety approach for ground ambulance transport will develop, with a rigor and focus that is comparable to air medical environments. EMS directors, managers, and decision makers should have a comprehensive understanding of the types of ground vehicles that are available and best suited to their environment or setting. They should also make themselves familiar with the safety issues that are important with respect to these ground vehicles. When formulating a safety program for their service in general, the ground vehicle safety issues should be encompassed within that safety program. The current data suggests that EMS services are 27 times more likely to be sued for their ground transport operations than they are for medical malpractice on the part of the Paramedic.

EMS providers are fundamentally responsible, as well as used to being routinely closely monitored, for their clinical and professional performance. They are also accustomed to following highly structured policy and procedure, particularly in reference to delivery of paramedical care. Because of this, they can expect close supervision and scrutiny. This scrutiny should also extend into the realm of ground vehicle operations and safety. Given the longstanding exemptions provided for ambulance vehicles from the FMVSS as far back as in 1979,[35] even in the face of the National Transportation Safety Board (NTSB) making recommendations to the contrary—identifying best practices with respect to vehicle safety has been a challenge for the ground EMS industry. However, there is now enough data available in the peer-reviewed literature to address the important elements of a data-driven safety culture and practice policies.

To optimize driver performance and fleet safety, a number of driver training courses are available. One course, the **Emergency Vehicle Operators Course (EVOC)**, is an expert panel-derived risk and safety awareness driver-training program, created as a result of the 1979 NTSB recommendations. EVOC is not mandated across the entire United States; in fact, until the ANSI/ASSE Z.15 standard[25] there was limited guidance provided nationally for general EMS fleet vehicle and driver performance safety management.

For example, the national EMS associations and accreditation organizations, the Committee on the Accreditation of Ambulance Services (CAAS), and the Committee on the Accreditation of Medical Transport Services (CAMTS) provide guidance and certification for the management of an ambulance service. The guidelines for these organizations cover the broad scope of what is involved in managing an ambulance service and also advance awareness for ambulance vehicle safety issues.

In Australia and Europe, specific ambulance vehicle safety standards exist: the AS/NZS 4535:1999 in Australia,[36] and the EN 1789:2007 in Europe.[37] Both are true safety performance standards and specifically address the design, restraint system integrity, safety performance testing, dynamic crash testing, and safety features of ambulance vehicles.

The only U.S. guidelines specifically addressing ambulance vehicles are the **KKK specifications**,[26] which are federal purchase specifications for a General Services Administration (GSA) Star of Life ambulance.[26] These are purchase specifications, not safety performance standards. As such, they do not address crashworthiness issues or any dynamic crash or impact performance testing, nor do they address equipment or occupant restraint safety or performance, in contrast to the international standards. Similarly, the Ambulance Manufacturers Division of the National Truck Equipment Association's AMD Standards[33] are not written by a standardizing body or an automotive safety organization, but rather the aftermarket ambulance retrofitters. In response to a number of catastrophic ambulance crashes with occupant fatalities in the past few years, the National Fire Protection Association (NFPA) has embarked on coordinating an ambulance vehicle standard. To date, integrating technical expertise from automotive occupant protection safety engineers into that initiative has not occurred. There is also the "do's and don'ts" guideline for transporting children in ambulances,[38] which was initially written with technical input from automotive safety and occupant protection expertise. However, these do not address vehicle design or safety

Table 17-2 Key Points for Optimizing Ground Transport Safety

Vehicle Crashworthiness and PPE	
Vehicle	• Compact OEM vehicles (i.e., vans)
	• Non-hostile interiors
	• Crumple zones
	• Ideally forward- and rearward-facing seating
	• Lockdown positions for routine equipment
	• Seat belts for all seated occupants
	• Over-the-shoulder belts for all patients on the stretcher
	• Attention to ergonomics
PPE	• Head protection
	• Visibility for providers and vehicles
	• Biohazard protection
Intelligent Transportation System (ITS) Technologies	
	• Driver/vehicle performance monitoring and feedback devices
	• Collision avoidance vehicle technologies
	• Roadside safety technologies
Safety Management	
Fleet management	• Safety program ANSI/ASSE Z15
EMS practice and policy	• Safe driving policy and practice
	• Seat belt use policy for providers and patients
	• Safety monitoring and feedback
	• Stop at red lights, stop signs
	• EVOC
	• Secure all equipment
	• Use portable communications
	• Notify driver if rear occupants are in vulnerable positions

performance; instead, they are practical guidelines to optimize the safety of transporting pediatric patients in ambulances.

Until the release of the American Society of Safety Engineers and American National Standards Institute[25] fleet vehicle standard (released March 2006), there was no U.S. standard specifically for fleet management that encompassed EMS fleets. The ANSI/ASSE Z15.1 fleet management standard is a major advance, as it provides a comprehensive template for the safety oversight and management of a fleet of vehicles. This most valuable adjunct specifies EMS-specific safe practices such as coming to a full stop at red lights and stop signs, and requiring EVOC training (Table 17-2).

One of the true challenges to optimizing ground ambulance transport safety is accessing safety information that is reliable and objective.[34] As this is a complex field that involves multiple disciplines, much of the relevant technical information and peer-reviewed literature is in the engineering, safety, and other non-EMS literature.[27,32] This makes it very difficult for EMS providers to keep abreast of current developments regarding ground ambulance vehicle safety.

Publications and presentations relating to ground transport safety given at scientific meetings are helpful, although it is important that the sources represented contain objective information based in the appropriate safety disciplines. The air medical discipline has established industry-based forums in a similar fashion which are also major steps forward.

Modeling initiatives such as this for ground transport, with representation from the different disciplines and infrastructure relating to ground transport safety (such as engineering, automotive safety, and crashworthiness), would be both an important and valuable approach. Specific ambulance transport safety summits—such as the National Academies Transportation Research Board's Inaugural 2008 event and the subsequent full day 2009 TRB Summit—provide a special opportunity to have the technical experts in transport and vehicle safety share data and safety information with the EMS providers. These resources are available for open and gratis access both live and as an on-line resource. A regular biennial or twice-decade summit to bring together both ground and air ambulance transport safety could provide an opportunity for those involved in fleet management to hear the latest in safety practice and management developments, and also provide an environment which facilitates the translation of safety practices in the aviation environment to ground transport.

In addition, use of web-based resources, such as the information portal http://www.objectivesafety.net, could assist in facilitating access to current practical and technical information.

Pulling up on-scene, the carnage is unbelievable. Apparently, the ambulance had "run the red," and was broadsided. It had rolled over and the patient compartment completely disassembled, leaving a gaping hole in the side of the "box." Fire department first responders are caring for the patient, who is still strapped to the stretcher, and the driver is outside the rig, talking loud and fast. To the side of the rig is one body with a blood-soaked sheet overtop.

Across the street, the Paramedics can see the other ambulance standing by while the fire department extricates the patient. Choking back tears, the two Paramedics close the horrible scene from their minds and proceed to take care of the visibly shaken patient.

CRITICAL THINKING QUESTIONS

1. What safety performance modifications to an ambulance would increase its crashworthiness?
2. What liability does the service hold in this crash and what is the likelihood that they will be sued?

▷▷▷▷▷▷▷▷▷▷▷▷▷▷
PROFESSIONAL PARAMEDIC

There are a number of websites with information and resources on ambulance safety. The two that follow are among the most notable:
www.objectivesafety.net

Visitors to this site can reference current peer-reviewed scientific papers and access recorded presentations from peer-reviewed and other symposia, as well as find links to other print and electronic resources. www.EMS SafetyFoundation.org

This collaboration, innovation, and knowledge transfer foundation-focused site is geared toward enhancing the systems safety of EMS for the patient, provider, and public.

Challenges in Emergency Vehicle Design

In contrast to the safety culture and the comprehensive safety oversight of the clinical aspects of EMS care, the comprehensive oversight of commercial vehicle and ground ambulance transport is lacking in both safety standards and safety oversight. Thus, it is important that the EMS provider be familiar with the risks and hazards involved in ground ambulance transport. In this way, she will have the knowledge and resources needed to minimize these hazards, as well

as optimize safety in terms of design, practice, and policy aspects.

Additionally, there are current challenges in the design, layout, and crashworthiness of ambulance vehicles.

Although it is very important to have the safest vehicle design that is feasible, the Paramedic can also take personal steps to improve ground transport safety. Failure of the providers and other seated occupants to use seat belts, failure to use over-the-stretcher shoulder belts for the patient, and failure to secure equipment have been identified as risks and hazards that have an impact on enhancing safety. Other identified risks relate to high speed driving and use of lights and siren, failure to stop the vehicle at a stop sign or red light, and driver performance history.

Simple solutions are available now to address the technology, practice, and policy of ground transport, as well as optimize design. Use of technologies such as the real time auditory monitoring and feedback devices to optimize safe driving and vehicle handling is one highly effective solution.

Implementation of a comprehensive safety program and basic policies such as those that ensure optimal use of seat belts, safe driving practices, and intersection policies that firmly support that the EMS vehicle come to a full stop before ever proceeding through any red light or stop sign, as well as policies that follow the air paramedical model of ensuring that all equipment and persons are secured prior to departure, are important and cost-effective enhancements to safety performance. In addition to these safety initiatives, use of personal protective equipment such as head protective devices and high visibility clothing should be implemented to enhance safety.

The new Z15 standard is a valuable tool in designing and maintaining a safety program, culture, and safety oversight for the ground vehicle component of a patient transport system.

CONCLUSION

Many useful tools are available to optimize the safety of ground ambulance transport that are readily available and valuable to implement. By creating a culture of safety and awareness of existing hazards and risks with strict safety oversight, EMS providers hold the key to a safe working environment.

▶ KEY POINTS:

- The ideal is to develop a global culture of safety in EMS.

- New initiatives are being developed for vehicle safety.

- The field of ambulance safety is relatively new and involves multiple disciplines, including public health, engineering, transportation, ergonomics, and liability and risk management.

- Ambulances have historically been exempt from Federal Motor Vehicle Safety Standards.

- Ambulances are considered the most dangerous vehicles on the road.

- The limited reporting systems for ground ambulance transport have produced limited data.

- Risks to Paramedics include collisions while en route to the hospital as well as providers being struck by passing motor vehicles at the emergency scene.

- The Worker Visibility Act has promoted scene safety for Paramedics.

- Three practices markedly increase ground transport safety while in transit: using safety restraints, securing all equipment, and using over-the-shoulder harnesses for the recumbent patient on a gurney.

- Failure to stop at a red light is a high-risk practice.

- The systems approach to safety includes non-hostile interiors, proactive policies on vehicle operation with enforcement, intelligent transportation systems, use of personal protective equipment, and establishment of safety programs.

- Three goals of the ANSI/ASSE Z15.1 fleet safety standards are increased emphasis on EMS vehicle safety, enhanced data collection, and bringing ambulance safety in line with automotive safety practices.

- Occupant safety in the ambulance compartment is complex.

- Use of helmets, similar to flight helmets, while operating in the back of a moving ambulance can dramatically reduce head injuries in ambulance crashes.

- Traditionally, the National Institute of Occupational Safety and Health addresses issues of ambulance safety.

- Intelligent transportation systems pertain to driver behavior modification, intelligent vehicle design, and roadside safety technologies.

- In-vehicle telematics technology provides ambulance drivers with auditory feedback in real time.

- The Emergency Vehicle Operators Course is one of many emergency driver training programs available.

- KKK specifications are ambulance purchase specifications, not safety performance standards.

REVIEW QUESTIONS:

1. What are the three practices that can immediately improve safety in a moving ambulance?
2. What is one driving practice that has been directly linked to an increased number of ambulance crashes?
3. What are the three goals of the ANSI/ASSE Z15.1 fleet safety standards?
4. What do intelligent transportation systems pertain to?
5. List three benefits of in-vehicle telematics technology.

CASE STUDY QUESTIONS:

Please refer to the Case Study in this chapter, and answer the questions below:

1. What driver behavior may have prevented this ambulance crash?
2. Why did the patient survive?
3. What is the most likely cause of death for the Paramedic and what could have prevented it?

REFERENCES:

1. Levick NR. Hazard analysis and vehicle safety issues for emergency medical service vehicles: where is the state of the art? *American Society of Safety Engineers, Proceedings* .June 2006-9.
2. Levick NR. A crisis in ambulance safety. *Emerg Resp Disaster Man.* 2002;4:20–22.
3. Levick NR, Editorial. New frontiers in optimizing ambulance transport safety and crashworthiness. *The Paramedic* (UK journal). December 2002;4:36–39.
4. Levick NR. Emergency medical services: a transportation safety emergency. American Society of Safety Engineers Technical Paper #628, Orlando, June 2007. Available at: **http://www.objectivesafety.net/2007ASSE628Levick.pdf.** Accessed February 23, 2010.
5. Levick NR. Emergency medical services: unique transportation safety challenge. Report No. 08-3010, Transportation Research Board. January 2008. Available at: **http://www.objectivesafety.net/LevickTRB08-3010CD.pdf.** Accessed February 23, 2010.
6. Baker S, Grabowski JG, Dodd RS, et al. EMS helicopter crashes: what influences fatal outcome? *Ann Emerg Med.,* 2006;47(4):351–356.
7. Levick NR, Mener D. Searching for ambulance safety: where is the literature? *Prehosp Emerg Care.* January/March 2006;10(1):138.
8. Maguire BJ, Hunting KL, Smith GS, Levick NR. Occupational fatalities in emergency medical services: a hidden crisis. *Ann Emerg Med.* 2002;40:625–632.
9. Becker LR, Zaloshnja E, Levick N, Miller TR. Relative risk of injury and death in ambulances and other emergency vehicles. *Accid Anal Prev.* 2003;35:941–948.
10. Federal Motor Vehicle Safety Standards (FMVSS). Dept. Transportation, National Highway Traffic Safety Administration (NHTSA). Docket No. 92–28, Notice 7.
11. Levick NR, Li G, Yannaccone J. Biomechanics of the patient compartment of ambulance vehicles under crash conditions: testing countermeasures to mitigate injury. Society of Automotive Engineering, Technical Paper 2001-01-1173. March 2001. Available at: **http://www.sae.org (type ambulance crash into search engine).** Accessed February 23, 2010.
12. Levick NR, Li G, Yannaccone J. Development of a dynamic testing procedure to assess crashworthiness of the rear patient compartment of ambulance vehicles. Enhanced Safety of Vehicles, Technical Paper series. Paper #454. May 2001. Available at: **http://www-nrd.nhtsa.dot.gov/pdf/nrd-01/esv/esv17/proceed/00053.pdf.** Accessed February 23, 2010.
13. Levick NR, Donnelly BR, Blatt A, Gillespie G, Schultze M. Ambulance crashworthiness and occupant dynamics in vehicle-to-vehicle crash tests: preliminary report. Enhanced Safety of Vehicles, Technical Paper series. Paper # 452. May 2001. Available at: **http://www-nrd.nhtsa.dot.gov/pdf/nrd-01/esv/esv17/proceed/00012.pdf.** Accessed February 23, 2010.
14. Levick NR, Grzebieta R. Development of proposed crash test procedures for ambulance vehicles. International Enhanced Safety of Vehicles Technical Paper 07-0254. June 2007.

Available at: **http://www.nrd.nhtsa.dot.gov/pdf/esv/esv20/07-0074-O.pdf.** Accessed February 23, 2010.

15. Levick NR, Grzebieta R. Crashworthiness analysis of three prototype ambulance vehicles. International Enhanced Safety of Vehicles Technical Paper 07-0249. Lyon, France. June 2007. Available at: **http://www-nrd.nhtsa.dot.gov/pdf/esv/esv20/07-0249-W.pdf.** Accessed February 23, 2010.

16. Auerbach PS, Morris JA, Phillips JB, Redlinger SR, Vaughn WK. An analysis of ambulance accidents in Tennessee. *JAMA.* Sept 1987; 258(11):1487–1490.

17. Centers for Disease Control (CDC). Ambulance crash-related injuries among emergency medical services workers United States, 1991–2002. *MMWR.* February 28, 2003;52(8):154–156.

18. Biggers WA, Zachariah BS, Pepe PE. Emergency medical vehicle collisions in an urban system. *Prehosp Disaster Med.* 1996;11:195–201.

19. Kahn CA, Pirrallo RG, Kuhn EM. Characteristics of fatal ambulance crashes in the United States: an 11-year retrospective analysis. *Prehosp Emerg Care.* Jul-Sep 2001;5(3):261–269.

20. Ray A, Kupas D. Comparison of crashes involving ambulances with those of similar sized vehicles. *Prehosp Emerg Care.* Dec 2005;9:412–415.

21. Heick R, Peek-Asa C, Zwerling C. Occupational injury in EMS: does risk outweigh reward? Abstract #121840. American Public Health Association, Dec 2005.

22. Levick NR, Garigan M. A solution to head injury protection for emergency medical service providers. International Ergonomics Association proceedings, July 2006.

23. Best GH, Zivkovic G, Ryan GA. Development of an effective ambulance patient restraint. *Society of Automotive Engineering Australasia Journal.* 1993;53(1):17–21.

24. Levick NR, Winston F, Aitken S, Freemantle R, Marshall F, Smith G. Development and application of a dynamic testing procedure for ambulance pediatric restraint systems. *Society of Automotive Engineering Australasia Journal.* March/April 1998;58(2):45–51.

25. ANSI Accredited Standards Committee. ANSI/ASSE Z15. 1-2006 Safe Practices for Motor Vehicle Operations. *ANSI/ASSE,* February 2006.

26. General Services Administration. Federal Ambulance Specification KKK-A-F 1822. Automotive Commodity Center, Federal Supply Service. 2007. Available at: **www.ntea.com/WorkArea/downloadasset.aspx?id=1352.** Accessed February 10, 2010.

27. Levick NR, Grzebieta R. Ambulance vehicle crashworthiness and passive safety design: a comparative vehicle evaluation. Society of Automotive Engineering. ComVec Technical Paper. October 2008-01-2695, Available at: **www.sae.org.** Accessed February 23, 2010.

28. Emergency Vehicle Visibility and Conspicuity Study FA-323. Federal Emergency Management Administration. August 2009. Available at: **http://www.usfa.dhs.gov/downloads/pdf/publications/fa_323.pdf.** Accessed January 27, 1010.

29. De Graeve K, Deroo KF, Calle PA, Vanhaute OA, Buylaert WA. How to modify the risk-taking behaviour of emergency medical services drivers? *Eur J Emerg Med.* 2003;10(2):111–116.

30. Levick NR, Swanson J. An optimal solution for enhancing ambulance safety: implementing a driver performance feedback and monitoring device in ground ambulances. Proceedings—49th Annual Conference of the Association for the Advancement of Automotive Medicine, 2005.

31. Levick NR, Wiersch L, Nagel ME. Real world application of an aftermarket driver human factors real time auditory monitoring and feedback device: an emergency service perspective. International Enhanced Safety of Vehicles Technical Paper 07-0254. Lyon, France. June 2007. Available at: **http://www-nrd.nhtsa.dot.gov/pdf/esv/esv20/07-0254-O.pdf.** Accessed February 10, 2010.

32. Levick NR, Grzebieta R. Engineering analysis of "safety concept" ambulances: poster presentation. NAEMSP. January 2009. Available at: **http://www.objectivesafety.net/NAEMSP2009SafetyConcept.pdf.** Accessed February 10, 2010.

33. Ambulance Manufacturers Division of the National Truck Equipment Association. Ambulance design standards 001–025. 2007. Available at: **http://www.ntea.com/WorkArea/showcontent.aspx?id=1350.** Accessed February 10, 2010.

34. Levick NR. Rig safety 911: what you need to know about ambulance safety and standards. *JEMS.* October 2008. Available at: **http://www.objectivesafety.net/JEMSRigSafety911.pdf.** Accessed February 23, 2010.

35. National Transportation Safety Board (NTSB). *Highway Accident Report.* NTSB Number: HAR-79/04, NTIS Number: PB-296889/AS. Adopted May 3, 1979. Available at: **http://www.ntsb.gov/publictn/1979/har7904.htm.** Accessed February 10, 2010.

36. Joint Standards Australia/Standards New Zealand Committee ME/48 on Restraint Systems in Vehicles. Standards for ambulance restraint systems. *AS/NZS.* 1999;4535.

37. European Ambulance Restraint Systems Standards CEN. *European Committee for Standardization.* 2002;EN 1789.

38. Federal guidelines child restraint for ambulance transport, do's and don'ts of transporting children in ambulances. *EMSC/NHTSA.* December 1999. Available at: **http://www.nhtsa.dot.gov.** Accessed February 10, 2010.

CHAPTER 18

AIR MEDICAL TRANSPORT

KEY CONCEPTS:

Upon completion of this chapter, it is expected that the reader will understand these following concepts:

- Indications and contraindications to air medical transport
- Effects of air medical transport on the patient
- Operational aspects of air medical transport
- Importance of safety to air medical services

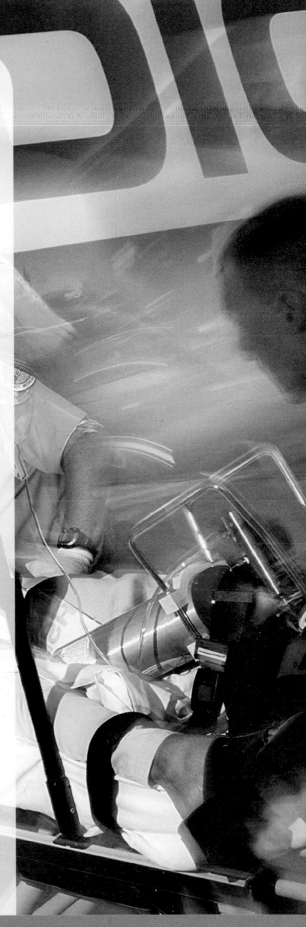

CASE STUDY:

The Paramedic notes the patient's facial droop, slurred speech, and inability to raise one arm as she completes her assessment. Looking at her watch, she asks, "Mrs. Johnson, can you tell me the last time you saw your husband act normally?" Knowing that the answer will mean the difference between destination hospitals, she calculates that the total time since the symptoms began is just under one hour.

Since there is a two-hour ground transport time to the nearest stroke center, the Paramedic asks her partner to begin moving the patient to the ambulance while she steps outside to make a phone call. "Dr. Bradley, this is Paramedic 946. I am on the scene of a 48-year-old man with an acute stroke onset just under one hour ago. I would like permission to request a helicopter for rapid transport to the stroke center."

CRITICAL THINKING QUESTIONS

1. What are some of the possible advantages of helicopter transport?
2. What conditions warrant air medical service?

OVERVIEW

Emergency transport of critically ill and injured patients by air has become an expectation within the emergency medical community in the United States today (Figure 18-1). Although not every area of the country has completely integrated air medical services into their existing transport system, it is very clear that progress has been made over the years.

Background

Wartime

As with ground-based EMS, air medical transport originated through wartime rescue efforts. The first reported air transport of a patient was in 1915 when a French pilot reportedly evacuated an injured Serb in an unmodified fighter plane. Through progressive conflicts, airplane evacuation of ill and injured patients became more common. The first medical use of a helicopter was seen in 1944 in Burma; however, the first large scale medical evacuation by helicopter was in Korea. This was accomplished largely with Sikorsky airframes outfitted with outboard stretchers. The UH-1H (Figure 18-2), or "Huey," was central to the medical efforts in Vietnam, as significant numbers of patients were flown to treatment facilities during this war. The use of helicopters to rapidly move injured patients was thought to contribute to the reduction in morbidity and mortality in subsequent conflicts. Not surprisingly, this improvement in care came to the attention of the American public.

Civilian Adaptation

In the early 1970s, feasibility studies suggested a tenuous economic viability existed for an air medical program. It was recognized that, in order to offer timely response, a dedicated medical configuration was needed in the airframe. Even in these early days of air transport, integration of air travel into the developing ground EMS systems was recognized to be an important part of a successful program.

In 1970, the Maryland state police aviation unit became the first U.S. agency to provide emergency air transport from the scene of an accident (Figure 18-3). Two years

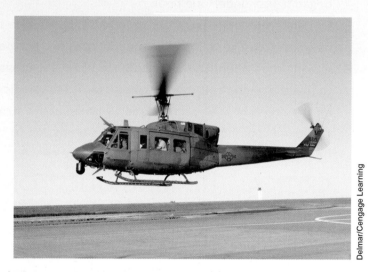

Figure 18-2 Helicopter evacuation was central to the rescue efforts in Vietnam.

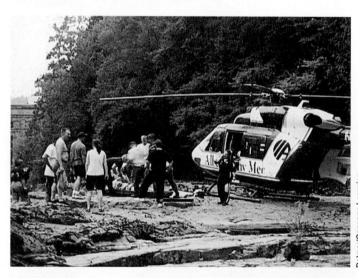

Figure 18-1 Air medical services work together with ground-based services to create an integrated approach to emergency medical care.

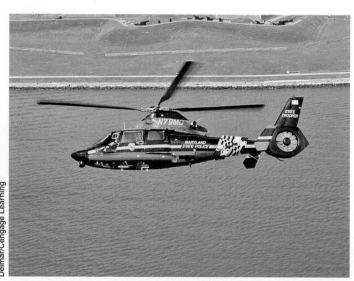

Figure 18-3 The Maryland state police aviation unit was the first U.S. agency to provide emergency air transport from the scene of an accident.

later, St. Anthony's Hospital in Denver, Colorado, began their own civilian air medical transport program, offering both on-scene and interfacility transports. Although these two agencies were the first to pursue dedicated air medical agendas, other law enforcement and fire agencies, such as the New York State Police aviation unit and Los Angeles Fire Department, also developed aviation components that would offer air medical transport in addition to their primary mission.

Ground EMS Development

Much like air medical transport, ground-based EMS developed as a result of wartime experiences. Multiple models of system operation were developed to meet the needs of different communities, including private contractors, fire department-based systems, private for-profit services, and municipal third service systems.

In addition to multiple models for operation, multiple levels of providers were developed based upon local needs. These tended to be regionally dependent and consisted of some form of basic (and later on, advanced) life support providers.

Integration of Ground and Air

Although ground and air medical services were developing at much the same time with seemingly the same goal in mind, they developed more in parallel than in conjunction with one another. This may have been because helicopter services were largely based at hospitals and EMS services were run through the Department of Transportation. Whatever the reason, the end result was that many areas had air medical services and ground services that coexisted but did not necessarily cooperate as well as they could have been. However, significant improvement has occurred in recent years in integrating ground and air EMS, with good results taking place in many areas. Air service is an integral component of the emergency transport system in any area and therefore should be utilized.

Current State of Air Medicine in the United States

During the last decade, there has been an incredibly rapid rise in the numbers of air medical services across the United States. This is likely due to many factors: an increased need for longer distance transports of more critically ill patients, more specialized time-dependent treatments offered at larger centers, and improved reimbursement rates for this air travel. Today, helicopter transport is expected in the appropriate circumstances in many communities. In 2006, the Association of Air Medical Services reported that 792 air medical helicopters were providing this service in the United States, and completing more than half a million patient transports annually. However, compared to the more than 16,000 ground EMS agencies, air medical agencies are still considered a limited resource that should be utilized appropriately.[1]

Program Types

As the numbers of transport agencies increased, the most common model of operation involved a hospital-based program in which some sort of cooperative effort existed between a helicopter vendor and hospital staff. Over the years, the structure of programs has continued to change, with the community-based model becoming more and more common.

Mission Profile

Nationally, the majority of air medical programs offer both on-scene and interfacility transports, with anywhere from 30% to 50% of the transports being on-scene responses. Each community has a slightly different need based upon its geography and hospital capabilities.

Since helicopters are most often called to care for the more significantly injured or more critically ill patients, the staff will usually have an expanded scope of practice when compared with typical ground transport agencies. They can be thought of as bringing the resources of the tertiary care hospital they are associated with to the patient's side wherever the patient may be located. This can be useful during both interfacility and on-scene medical care.[2]

Special Operations

Some helicopter programs have special operations units that provide search and rescue or extraction services. These services are useful and should be integrated into the local system's response to a given situation.

Staffing Configuration

The staffing configuration of an agency depends largely upon the expected patient population. If an agency only intends to respond to on-scene requests and not offer interfacility services, then they may choose to staff with Paramedics. On the other hand, if hospitalized patients will be included in the program mission, a nurse, physician, or respiratory therapist may be useful. The most commonly seen staffing pattern among U.S. programs is Paramedic/nurse. Those who utilize this crew mix believe it provides a useful mix of expertise for their agency's expected mission profile.

Paramedic

The Paramedic that is part of a helicopter staff will benefit from advanced training beyond the standard Paramedic curriculum. Although this additional training will vary depending upon local expectations and protocols, at a minimum this training must include flight physiology and flight safety. Typically, flight Paramedics have some range of expanded skills and at times a more independent practice. This is necessary due to the critical nature of the patients they are likely to see and the remote situations they may find themselves in. Skills such as rapid sequence intubation, surgical airway management, and advanced pharmacology are useful when managing a patient in this environment.

Many advanced training programs are utilized by air medical agencies around the nation. The **Air Medical Crew Curriculum**, established by the Department of Transportation in conjunction with multiple air medical organizations, is a good resource for this education. A document created by the **International Association of Flight Paramedics**, an organization that provides leadership development, educational opportunities, and advocates for critical care flight paramedics, also outlines minimum guidelines for flight Paramedic education.[3] Close medical oversight to any advanced training program is imperative.

Nurse

A flight nurse must be capable of independent practice in the prehospital environment. Typically, flight nurses have background in a critical care environment and are provided with training regarding EMS operations. Skills provided by nurses in a helicopter often exceed those performed by in-hospital colleagues, such as hanging blood and blood products. Appropriate training must be provided in order to assure competence.

Respiratory Therapist

Respiratory therapists are ideally suited to the patient population transported by helicopter services due to their expertise in airway and pulmonary pathophysiology. This is especially helpful as patients who may require advanced airway management are frequently transferred by helicopter rather than ground. In order to assure a broader experience base, some programs that staff respiratory therapists also require these providers to have Paramedic certification. If this is not the case, it would likely be necessary to expand the respiratory therapist's training to best suit the flight environment and the expected patient population.

Physician

Although in the minority, there are a few air medical programs that continue to staff a physician on the aircraft. Although it might logically appear more beneficial to have these highly trained providers on-board the helicopter, there does not seem to be that much of a difference in the interventions they offer. Some feel that appropriately trained nurses, Paramedics, or respiratory therapists can accomplish the same tasks at a fraction of the cost.

Specialty Team

Specialized mission profiles may require special team configurations. Some services offer response to very specialized patient populations such as neonatal or pediatric patients. In these cases, the team is comprised of staff whose expertise lies in those areas of practice.

On-Scene Missions

When utilized appropriately, helicopter transport from the scene of an accident can potentially improve the patient's outcome. This may seem intuitive when the concept of the "golden hour" is considered; however, the actual measured benefit continues to stimulate controversy.[4-6]

Indications for Air Medical Transport

Given the relative scarcity of helicopters when compared with ground units, it is imperative that the helicopters be utilized only in circumstances in which they are felt to offer the most benefit. Although every state and region should have guidelines to assist local providers in making this determination, the National Association of EMS Physicians has put forth its own "**Guidelines for Air Medical Dispatch**." Providers can utilize this document, considered a national standard, when creating local guidelines.[7]

The two main advantages to utilizing a helicopter are related to speed and capability. Helicopters can fly upwards of 150 mph in straight-line travel; that is, they have no need to follow roads. This can offer significant benefits when environmental obstacles or traffic pose a significant delay to rapid ground transport. The second benefit many helicopter services offer is an advanced level of care provided by the flight team. As previously discussed, depending upon the mission and staffing configuration, the interventions offered by the flight team may far supersede those available on the ground or even at small hospitals.

Triage

The concept of triage is well known to Paramedics. Even the most basic level of provider is adept at determining whether a patient meets certain criteria and the level of care most likely needed for transport. Triage is an inexact process, however, that is completed in a rapid manner with limited information. Although it is necessary in the case of a critically ill or injured patient, the triage process may result in some **overtriage**. That is, even if a patient meets specific transport criteria, he may not actually have a level of injury that is considered severe. This will not be definitively known until after a thorough emergency department workup is completed.

Undertriage occurs when patients that do meet specified criteria and have severe injuries are overlooked and not transported by helicopter based on their priority of needed care. A certain percentage of overtriage is accepted as necessary in order to avoid unacceptable rates of undertriage.

Dispatch

Once EMS dispatch determines that a helicopter is needed, based on a provider's request, they arrange for one to be sent to the scene. The individual requesting the air transport must provide certain basic information to the helicopter dispatch center (Table 18-1).

Table 18-1 Triage Flight Data

Information to provide when requesting a helicopter from dispatch
• Incident location
• Requesting unit and designated landing zone officer
• Radio frequency for contact
• Nature of the incident
• Number of patients
• Ages of patients
• Mechanism of injury
• Vital signs
• Specific injuries, if known

Table 18-2 Auto-Launch Criteria

• Flight distance > 10 minutes or > 29 miles
• Patient location > 20 miles from specialty hospital and condition is critical:
○ Including but not limited to:
• Prolonged extrication time
• Multiple patient incident
• Ejection from vehicle/patient entrapped
• Pedestrian struck with serious injury
• Death of occupant in same vehicle
• Critical burns > 10% TBSA
• Falls with serious injury
• Deep penetrating injury to head, neck, or torso
• Unstable vital signs
• Acute stroke

Auto-Launch

A commonly utilized tactic is for responding personnel to request a helicopter early based upon a potential expected need. Another way to decrease the helicopter's response time is to utilize an **auto-launch** policy. This involves simultaneous dispatch of the helicopter and the ground units based upon the dispatch information. Dispatchers can utilize predesignated trauma and/or medical indications set up by a local or regional EMS system to make these decisions. Depending upon the distances involved, some helicopter agencies will prepare the aircraft for response but not actually begin the flight until a confirmed need is reported.[8]

In the case of either early activation or auto-launch, if ground providers arrive on-scene and realize that the helicopter is not actually needed, they should immediately cancel the helicopter with no penalty to the patient or provider. Even though many such cancellations will likely occur if an auto-launch system is used, this is often felt to be acceptable in order to offer faster response in those cases where a helicopter actually is needed. The **Association of Air Medical Services** (a national association which serves both the air and ground medical transport community, providing its members services and encouraging its members to maintain safe operations and high-quality patient care) distributed a position statement describing early activation and auto-launch as effective means to decrease response time in certain circumstances. Other criteria were also suggested in this position paper (Table 18-2).[8]

First Responder Arrival

Although each air medical agency may have its own policy, and local guidelines may define who may request a helicopter, it is common practice for helicopter dispatchers to accept flight requests from any provider on a scene. This may include law enforcement officials, firefighters, industrial safety officers, ski patrol, certified first responders, EMTs at any level, nurses, and physicians. However, if the helicopter transport is cancelled, the highest level of medical provider on the scene should make that call. This should occur only after a care provider has made contact with the patient, reviewed her condition, and determined there's no need for the air transport.

Specific Conditions

Although a list of possible medical conditions that may benefit from helicopter transport may be endless, creating a list of specific conditions is useful to guide prehospital providers in practice. If certain clinical traumatic conditions are present in a given patient, they might be appropriate indications for air medical transport from a scene (Table 18-3). However, local protocols must prevail as local conditions vary.[9]

When considering whether to request a helicopter transport, a good rule of thumb is to determine if the patient's condition is urgent enough that it requires a decreased time to definitive care or services that are only available in certain areas. This type of decision requires knowledge of local geography, travel times, and hospital capabilities. Development of local guidelines is imperative to guide the Paramedic's decision making in a given region.

Nontrauma Considerations

Although the literature is certainly less robust in support of nontrauma indications for on-scene air medical transport, there are certainly situations where access to rapid transport could offer significant patient benefit. Situations that may fall into this category include time-dependent conditions such as ST-segment elevation myocardial infarction (STEMI) and acute stroke (Figure 18-4). Local protocols will govern if patients with these conditions are to be selectively transported to certain hospitals. If so, helicopter transport should be considered if it will result in a more timely arrival at the most appropriate facility.

Additional situations that might benefit from the advanced level of care brought by some helicopter services include obstetrical complications, neonatal emergencies, or other surgical or medical conditions in need of interventions

Table 18-3 Criteria for On-Scene Response

- Trauma—general and mechanism
  - Unstable vital signs
  - Significant trauma in young, old, or pregnant patients
  - Multisystem injuries
  - Ejection from vehicle
  - Pedestrian struck by vehicle
  - Death in same passenger compartment
  - Penetrating trauma to abdomen, pelvis, chest, neck, or head
  - Crush to abdomen, chest, or head
  - Fall from significant height
- Neurologic considerations
  - GCS < 10
  - Deteriorating mental status
  - Skull fracture
  - Spinal cord injury
- Thoracic considerations
  - Major chest wall injury
  - Pneumothorax/hemothorax
  - Suspected cardiac injury
- Abdominal/pelvic considerations
  - Significant abdominal pain after blunt trauma
  - Abdominal wall contusion
  - Obvious rib fracture below nipple line
  - Major pelvic fracture
- Orthopedic/extremity considerations
  - Partial or total amputation of a limb (exclusive of digits)
  - Finger/thumb amputation when emergent surgical evaluation is indicated and rapid surface transport is not available
  - Fracture or dislocation with vascular compromise
  - Extremity ischemia
  - Open long-bone fractures
  - Two or more long-bone fractures
- Major burns
  - > 20% TBSA
  - Involvement of hands, feet, face, or genitalia
  - Inhalation injury
  - Electrical or chemical burns
  - Burns with associated injuries
- Patients with near drowning injuries

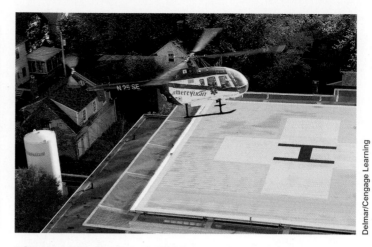

Delmar/Cengage Learning

Figure 18-4 Some EMS systems suggest helicopter transport in the case of a STEMI if arrival at a cardiac center will be accelerated by this mode of transport.

Logistical Considerations

In addition, patients with logistical issues might benefit from helicopter transport, such as patients in areas that are difficult to reach by surface transport or areas so remote that ground transport would take entirely too long. Other system considerations that might impact the decision to utilize air medical services include a scarcity of local ALS care, or any other situation in which local services are threatened or overwhelmed. Once again, it is crucial to develop local protocols to guide providers in this decision making. Interregional cooperation on such protocols is wise since air medical services often cover more than one region.

Interfacility Missions

Patients who need to be transferred from one facility to another may benefit from using air medical services in several circumstances. The most obvious relates to the speed of travel, which is primarily relevant in two circumstances. First, if the overall time to the receiving center can be minimized by using a helicopter for transport, the provider should consider it. This is especially relevant in time-dependent conditions in which a crucial therapy awaits the patient at the destination facility. Second, the prehospital time can almost always be shortened by helicopter transport when compared with ground travel. This can be extremely important in unstable patients or those patients with conditions that would prevent them from spending a prolonged amount of time in a moving vehicle.

Perhaps more commonly, air medical services are requested to transport patients between facilities for reasons related to the level of care that these facilities offer. Increasingly, hospitals are beginning advanced therapies as they work to stabilize patients prior to transfer. These therapies require trained hands to continue patient management

not offered by local ground agencies. Another category of patients in need of rapid transport are those needing organ transplants who have been called to respond to a transplant center or are having complications related to the transplant.

during the transport. Therefore, the patient needs a team with advanced capabilities present in the transport vehicle. In many areas, the most advanced teams are found on helicopters. If an area has a ground-based critical care transport team, they should be considered as an option if the travel time is less of an issue. Regardless of whether air or ground transport is used, the level of care for the patient must be maintained from the sending hospital to the receiving hospital.[10]

EMTALA

The **Emergency Medical Treatment and Active Labor Act (EMTALA)** is a section of the larger Consolidated Omnibus Budget Reconciliation Act (COBRA) that was originally passed in 1986. After several revisions, it remains one of the most important pieces of healthcare legislation in the United States. A section of this legislation requires hospitals to make arrangements for transfer that are appropriate for the patient's needs. For critically ill or injured patients, air medical transport should be considered.

Indications for Air Medical Transport

As with the guidelines for on-scene air medical transport, there are nationally recognized indications for interfacility transport as well. These can also be found in the National Association of EMS Providers (NAEMSP) position statement (Table 18-4). Although the literature is most abundant in support of air transport of the critically injured patient, there is building evidence that air transport provides benefits in other situations as well. In general, if the level of care needed or the nature of the patient's illness will benefit from the aircraft's speed or the provider's skill level, then the provider should consider air transport.

Contraindications for Air Medical Transport

As discussed previously, there are many fewer helicopters than ground ambulances. This fact, together with the helicopter's increased cost of operation and other risks involved, suggest that air transport should not be used unless a substantial benefit is likely to be derived. There are several circumstances in which use of a helicopter might be contraindicated. Of course, there could be exceptions to each of these circumstances, so every situation should be evaluated individually.

If a patient is known to be terminally ill and has no correctable medical problems, using a ground ambulance is likely more appropriate when a transfer is necessary.

Similarly, patients who have suffered cardiac arrest and have not achieved return of spontaneous circulation after the Paramedic's initial efforts are not likely to benefit from air transport. This is true of patients suffering from both medical and traumatic causes of arrest. A notable exception is the hypothermic drowning patient, as invasive rewarming measures might be beneficial.

Patients who are likely to die or decompensate en route and are in a facility capable of definitively managing the condition most likely should not be transferred at all. In a similar line of thought, patients in active labor should not be removed from a hospital capable of a controlled delivery if delivery is expected during transport. Although this is sometimes very difficult to predict, the provider should consider the risk of intra-transport delivery when deciding to transport a woman with ongoing contractions.

Patients who are prone to psychotic or violent behavior should not be placed into a transport vehicle without appropriate restraint in place. In some cases, that restraint may include chemical paralysis with intubation and appropriate sedation. This level of restraint obviously carries with it some risk; therefore, the care provider should carefully consider whether to embark upon such a treatment pathway. The patient's safety as well as the safety of the transport team should both be weighed against the risk of the procedure. At no time should a hospital initiate a transport if the care team's safety is at risk. The hospital's written policy and/or protocol should support this practice.

Flight Physiology

During the course of an air medical transport, the flight team and the patient are exposed to stressors related to the vehicle and environment that they might not experience during a surface transport. In order to best prepare for these and prevent potential injury, the flight Paramedic must be knowledgeable about how the flight environment affects her own physiology as well as that of her patient.

Gas Laws

A review of basic altitude mechanics is best accomplished by remembering that the atmosphere consists of many gasses. The two primary gasses are nitrogen and oxygen, which account for 78% and 21%, respectively, of the gaseous composition of the environment. The force exerted by the atmosphere at any point is known as the **atmospheric pressure**. Normal physiologic function is possible up to around 12,000 feet. This is known as the physiologic or efficient zone. People at higher altitudes require pressurization and temperature control for optimal physiologic function. This is relevant both for the patient as well as the flight Paramedic.

The decrease in physiologic efficiency at higher altitudes is related to the physical gas laws that were discussed in Chapter 15, specifically Boyle's and Dalton's laws. Reviewing these laws will help the Paramedic to predict the patient's physiologic response to altitude and take measures to prevent undesirable consequences of altitude changes.

Boyle's law describes the volume of a gas as the pressure exerted upon it changes. It predicts that the volume of the gas will vary inversely with the pressure. For example, as a balloon ascends and the atmospheric pressure upon it decreases, the gas within it will increase in volume (Figure 18-5).

Table 18-4 Interfacility Indications for Air Medical Transport

- Trauma
  - Any diagnostic consideration listed under the scene criteria that cannot be managed at the local hospital
  - Injuries or potential injuries that require evaluation or treatment beyond hospital capabilities
- Cardiac
  - Acute coronary syndrome with a time-critical need for urgent interventional therapy that is not available at the local hospital
  - Cardiogenic shock
  - Cardiac tamponade
  - Mechanical cardiac disease
- Critically ill medical or surgical patient
  - Pretransport cardiac/respiratory arrest
  - Continuous IV vasoactive medications or mechanical ventricular assist
  - Risk for airway deterioration
  - Acute pulmonary failure and/or requirement for sophisticated pulmonary intensive care during transport
  - Severe poisoning or overdose requiring specialized toxicology services
  - Urgent need for hyperbaric oxygen therapy
  - Requirement for emergent dialysis
  - Gastrointestinal hemorrhages with hemodynamic compromise
  - Surgical emergencies such as fasciitis, aortic dissection, or aneurysm or extremity ischemia
  - Pediatric patients for whom referring facilities cannot provide required evaluation and/or therapy
- Obstetric (minimized prehospital time must be weighed against risk of intratransport delivery)
  - Need for obstetric or neonatal care beyond the capabilities of the local hospital
  - Active premature labor
  - Severe pre-eclampsia or eclampsia
  - Third trimester hemorrhage
  - Fetal hydrops
  - Maternal medical conditions that may cause premature birth
  - Severe predicted fetal heart disease
  - Acute abdominal emergencies in third trimester
- Neurological
  - CNS hemorrhage
  - Spinal cord compression
  - Evolving ischemic stroke
  - Status epilepticus
- Neonatal (consider using air transport to get specialized team to patient)
  - Gestational age < 30 weeks, body weight < 2,000 grams, complicated neonatal course
    - Requirement for supplemental oxygen exceeding 60%, continuous positive airway pressure or mechanical ventilation
  - Extrapulmonary air leak, interstitial emphysema, or pneumothorax
    - Medical emergencies such as seizure activity, congestive heart failure, or disseminated intravascular coagulation
  - Surgical emergencies such as diaphragmatic hernia, necrotizing enterocolitis, abdominal wall defects, intussusception, suspected volvulus, or congenital heart defects
- Other
  - Transplant
    - Organ salvage
    - Organ recipient

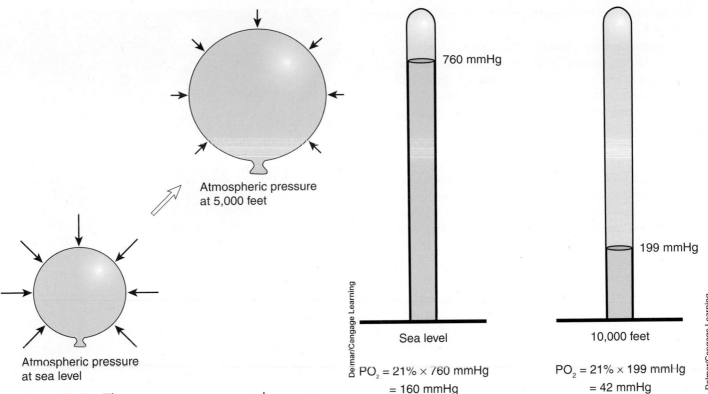

Figure 18-5 The pressure on a gas decreases during ascent, resulting in an increase in volume. The reverse is true during descent.

Sea level
PO$_2$ = 21% × 760 mmHg
= 160 mmHg

10,000 feet
PO$_2$ = 21% × 199 mmHg
= 42 mmHg

Figure 18-6 At increasing altitudes, the partial pressure of oxygen will decrease. The clinical relevance of this depends on the patient.

Dalton's law, states that the total pressure of a gas mixture is the sum of the individual or partial pressures of all the gasses in the mixture. In other words, as altitude increases and pressure decreases, gas expansion causes the available oxygen to decrease as gas molecules move farther apart (Figure 18-6).

Stresses of Flight

Both Boyle's law and Dalton's law offer explanations for some of the altitude-related physiologic changes seen in patients and, in some cases, team members. As stated, Dalton's law relates that, at increasing altitudes, less oxygen is available. This may result in hypoxia even in perfectly healthy individuals. These effects can become clinically apparent at altitudes above 10,000 feet with oxygen saturations dropping from 98% to 87% without supplemental oxygen. Conditions such as anemia, poor cardiac output, and poor oxygen utilization can compound this problem and can even lead to hypoxia at much lower altitudes. It is a good idea to fly at the lowest safe altitude if the patient has one of these conditions or if the patient becomes hypoxic upon ascent.

The expansion of gas in a given space described by Boyle's law suggests that a pneumothorax will increase in volume upon ascent. The higher the altitude, the more significant the problem becomes. Although many rotor wing flights are completed at a relatively low altitude, the Paramedic should remember that the degree to which this change affects a given patient is not as predictable as Boyle's law might suggest. It is wise to consider decompression of a pneumothorax prior

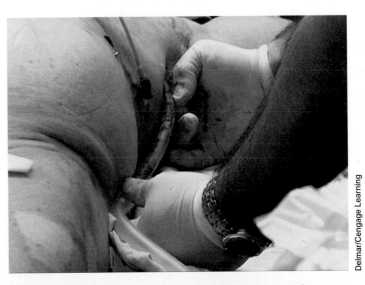

Figure 18-7 Prior to interfacility air transfer, giving consideration to decompression of a pneumothorax with a tube thoracostomy is appropriate.

to flight if the Paramedic believes it to be in the patient's best interest (Figure 18-7).

Other places in the body with pockets of air that may be subject to clinically relevant expansion include the gastrointestinal tract, the middle ear, the sinuses, and teeth. An increase in gastrointestinal gas volume can result in significant clinical consequences for patients if not properly managed.

Gastric decompression is often indicated when going to altitude with a patient in whom an increase in stomach or bowel gas is detrimental. If a nasogastric tube is in place, it should remain unclamped to allow for continued gas escape.

Ear, sinus, and dental pain related to expansion and/or retraction of gas in those spaces can be incapacitating if not adequately handled. Upon ascent, the gasses in the middle ear will expand and ordinarily equalize with the nasopharynx through the Eustachian tube. If this does not occur spontaneously, simple movement of the jaw—as occurs during a yawn or chewing motion—can facilitate this. During descent, the equalization happens spontaneously less often and active measures are required to prevent painful retraction of the tympanic membrane. In the presence of sinus disease such as occurs with upper respiratory infections, the air in the sinuses can become trapped, causing acute pain upon ascent or descent. Although a change in altitude can offer some relief, in most cases this is not possible during emergency transport. The best measure is to use topical vasoconstrictors prior to the flight to facilitate equalization of pressure or to avoid flight when sinus disease is prominent.

Occasionally after dental manipulation, tiny pockets of air remain in the root of the tooth for a day or two. If this tooth is then exposed to a change in barometric pressure, the air's change in volume can cause significant pain. Therefore, a Paramedic should avoid flight duty for one to two days after any significant dental work is completed.

At higher altitudes (i.e., > 10,000 feet), air inside medical equipment may expand, resulting in a problem (Figure 18-8). The cuff on an endotracheal tube, air inside an IV bag, or pressure inside MAST pants are examples of areas of concern that would require monitoring during changes in altitude.

Besides the changes in air volume and composition that occur with altitude, several other consequences of the flight environment may take a toll on both patients and flight team members. These include thermal changes, loss of humidity, noise, vibration, and fatigue.

Ambient temperature decreases with an increase in altitude. This occurs predictably with a decrease in temperature by 3.5°F (2°C) for every 1,000 feet increase in altitude. Although this cooling may feel great in the heat of summer, a significant change in ambient temperature may pose a problem for an at-risk patient. Many conditions alter the patient's ability to thermoregulate, which can impact the patient adversely if not countered. The flight Paramedic must always take measures to prevent heat loss in his patient by removing the patient's wet clothing and providing appropriate blankets. In addition, some therapies contribute to the patient's inability to maintain body temperature, namely the use of neuromuscular blockade. Combining chemical paralysis with intubation, ventilation, and unwarmed oxygen can result in a clinically significant drop in body temperature.

With increases in altitude, there is a notable loss of moisture in the air. This loss of humidity can be inconvenient for

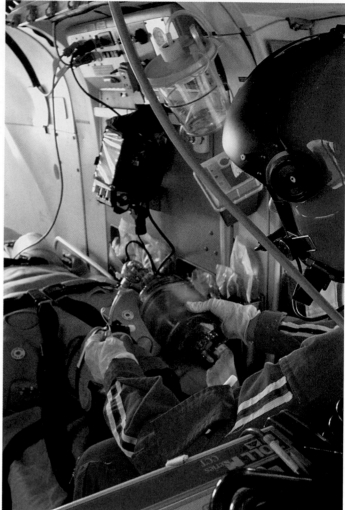

Figure 18-8 At higher altitudes, it may become necessary to monitor the pressure inside any air-filled piece of medical equipment such as the cuff on an endotracheal tube (ETT).

the flight Paramedic, producing chapped lips or a dry itchy throat if preventive measures are not taken. Perhaps more significantly, the unconscious patient may be injured if her eyes are not protected or if adequate fluid intake is not assured on longer flights.

The noise associated with aircraft flight may seem to be simply an annoyance, but it can significantly interfere with patient care as well as cause temporary and/or permanent hearing loss. Therefore, methods of patient assessment that do not rely upon the sense of hearing are needed. Additionally, proper hearing protection is imperative for both the flight team and the patient (Figure 18-9). The ability to verbally communicate can be impeded in this environment. Plans for effective communication between team members are crucial for the team's safety.

Vibration caused by the aircraft and the changes in air temperature can cause physiologic stress beyond simple motion sickness, sometimes significantly increasing a person's metabolic rate. In addition, some equipment may

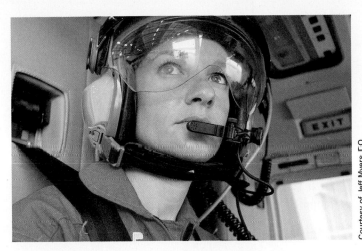

Figure 18-9 Proper hearing protection is necessary during all phases of flight.

Table 18-5 Physical Signs of Fatigue

- Sleepiness
- Difficulty concentrating
- Apathy
- Annoyance
- Increased reaction time to stimulus
- Slowing of higher-level mental functioning
- Decreased vigilance
- Memory problems
- Task fixation
- Increased errors while performing tasks

malfunction unless it is situated in such a way as to minimize exposure to vibration.

Fatigue is a state of exhaustion or a loss of strength or endurance that can lead to a decreased capacity for physical or mental work. All of the factors discussed so far can induce or contribute to fatigue. Additionally, self-imposed factors such as inadequate sleep, poor diet, dehydration, illness, or psychological stressors can contribute to the development of fatigue during flight duty (Table 18-5). With its many contributing factors, fatigue may manifest itself through poor decision making on the part of the flight team member. This must be avoided at all costs.

A great deal of effort is put into prevention and recognition of fatigue in the air medical environment. Knowing that the flight environment and duties themselves can be fatiguing, the flight Paramedic must do everything possible to come to work rested and well prepared. A Paramedic's coworkers must be constantly vigilant about recognizing the signs of fatigue and taking appropriate actions to alleviate an unsafe situation. Many programs have policies in place to encourage a team to remove themselves from duty if they feel that any one of the members is fatigued and potentially unsafe to continue to practice in the high stress environment.

In summarizing the stresses of flight, it is important to remember the effects of altitude on patients with regard to air in trapped spaces and the potential for hypoxia. Additionally, however, the noted effects of flight on the flight team cannot be ignored. Proper preparation for duty and recognition of the adverse consequences of flight on team members is crucial for a safe and healthy work environment.

Air Medical Practice

The aviation component of the air medical service is very clearly regulated at the federal level through the stringent Part 135 Federal Aviation Regulations pertaining to operations with a passenger on-board. Additional state regulation may be imposed as well. The regulation of the medical aspect of air medical services is much less standardized from one state to the next.

Scope of Practice

Many air medical teams enjoy the expanded scope of practice they maintain for management of their expected patient population. Obviously, if a Paramedic wants to practice at a level higher than he is currently trained, he will need additional training. Although this chapter offers an introduction to some of the facets of air medicine and the flight Paramedic's role in the process, more extensive training is likely mandated in order for a Paramedic to work for a particular agency. This training may be standardized for a given area or may be determined by an air medical agency based upon their known patient population and mission profile. Several standardized programs of advanced training are available for the Paramedic, as well as many more locally developed courses of education. The International Association of Flight Paramedics (IAFP) recognizes a certification exam leading to credentialing as a Certified Flight Paramedic (FP-C).[11] Many agencies may require this certification or a local equivalent as a condition of employment (Figure 18-10).

Protocols

Despite the extensive training required for practice at this level, Paramedics continue to function under the direction of a supervising physician. Although on-line medical control is available in most circumstances, flight Paramedics largely operate under a set of protocols that guide their practice in most circumstances. The physician's role in creation of these protocols is inherent in the concept of off-line medical control.

Quality Assurance

As with the practice of medicine in any environment, a continuous quality improvement plan is critical to maintain safe and effective practice. An active quality management program must involve regular review of all aspects of a program's function, from the dispatch all the way through to the final documentation of the flight. All aspects of practice and

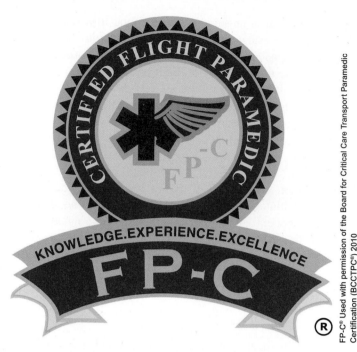

Figure 18-10 The Certified Flight Paramedic has successfully completed a standardized examination offered internationally by the IAFP.

patient care must be reviewed regularly in a systematic way in order to assure that the program is operating in the safest and most efficient manner possible. Perhaps the unique part about air medical quality assurance when compared to most similar ground-based system reviews is the attention given to more than just the medical aspect of each case. The operational aspects must be given just as much attention as the details of the medical care provided in order to assure safety.

Medical Direction

The Medical Director for a flight program must have an understanding of both the medical aspects and aviation considerations related to air medical transport. The Medical Director's specific training and qualifications should be appropriate to the program's specific mission. For example, a program that has a large neonatal patient base should have a Medical Director who is an expert in care of the critical neonate. If a flight program does not consider neonatal transport to be within its mission profile, having a Medical Director with expertise in neonatology is likely not as crucial. Most physicians do not have an extensive knowledge of aviation safety or flight physiology; therefore, they often require additional training in these areas.

The Medical Director should be an active part of the program's management team and must be empowered to make decisions related to the medical care provided by the service. She should have knowledge of the budgetary concerns, staffing issues, and reimbursement patterns. Additionally, she should take an active role in determining the criteria for appropriate utilization of the air medical service as well as in reviewing flights for compliance with these criteria.

Medical crew composition, training, and practice all fall well within the realm of a Medical Director's responsibility. As the medical provider under which the flight team practices, this person provides the program's overall medical control. If actual real time consultation via on-line medical control is to be designated to other providers, the Medical Director has a responsibility to assure that these providers are appropriately trained to provide this consultation. The Medical Director must also have a prominent role in the quality management and safety programs. As with every member of the flight team, it is imperative that the Medical Director have good communication skills.[12]

Continuing Education

Every healthcare professional should recognize the need to continually refresh his knowledge about his profession, specifically the situations that aren't frequently encountered. Situations that are only encountered every so often need to be reviewed more often than those the healthcare professional sees on a daily basis. Additionally, as new evidence and new equipment becomes available, it provides the provider with opportunities to improve the care offered to patients. All healthcare professionals have an obligation to remain current in their knowledge within their specific field of expertise. Many states have continuing education requirements for Paramedics that must be met for continued licensure or certification. This should take the form of both didactic style education as well as hands-on assurance of competence in all skills. There is some variation based on the program regarding the frequency with which skill competency is assured and the number of demonstrations that are required to assure competence. It is clear, however, that with skills as critical as endotracheal intubation, assurance of competence is mandatory.[13]

Landing Zone

If a helicopter is requested, the ground personnel must find a safe place for it to land, usually referred to as a **landing zone (LZ)**. A landing zone is an area intended for the purpose of landing and taking off in the helicopter. One person who is familiar with the landing zone's requirements should take charge of its preparation. Only this person, referred to as the LZ officer, should be in communication with the aircraft as it approaches.

When choosing an appropriate LZ, there are several things to consider. First, it should be located as close to the actual scene of the incident as possible while still being safe. Often, in the case of a car accident, the LZ can be in a field adjacent to the road or even in the road itself if traffic can be stopped. If a suitable area is not available close by, a more remote LZ may be chosen. In that case, the ground personnel should make arrangements to either bring the patient to the LZ or bring the helicopter crew to the patient.

Landing zones must be a certain size and have certain safety features. Most medical helicopters require a

touchdown area (the actual site where the aircraft will land) of between 75 square feet and 100 square feet. The preference is 100 square feet, since that is large enough for both day and night operations, as well as for landing the larger aircraft that the military and many police agencies routinely use.

The touchdown area should be fairly level and free of any obstacles such as trees, signs, posts, or markers. If the area is unpaved, shrubs, brush, grass, weeds, and so forth should not be higher than 24 inches. Any slope should not be more than 5 to 10 degrees.

The area above and around the touchdown area, called the **surrounding area**, should be free of any obstacles that may get tangled with the helicopter. When evaluating the surrounding area, the LZ officer should take note of any trees, poles, towers, signs, or wires that are in the surrounding area (Figure 18-11). These should be reported to the helicopter pilot as LZ hazards when the helicopter approaches the scene. The specific locations of such hazards must be made clear since it is sometimes difficult to see hazards such as wires from the air.

Additional information that is useful for incoming pilots includes a report of the wind direction and intensity and the condition of the touchdown area. For example, if there are moderate winds out of the southwest and the ground surface is muddy, the pilot should be made aware of these conditions when she is given the initial information about the LZ hazards.

Approach

Although a helicopter is capable of taking off and landing straight up and down, having a clear path for a more favorable approach angle is preferable. The approach path should be free of towers, poles, wires, trees and so forth.

Because of the confusing nature of many accident scenes, it is often helpful for the Paramedic to clearly mark the intended touchdown area with cones (Figure 18-12), flares, or other secured markers at its four corners. Any markers that are used should be carefully secured, since the wind created by the rotor blades (called **rotor wash**) can be quite forceful.

If appropriate markers are not available, emergency vehicles can be used on two or four corners of the LZ. Although headlights may be used to illuminate the LZ, they must never be directed at the helicopter (Figure 18-13). Bright lights, including LEDs and strobes, can temporarily blind the pilot, making a safe landing impossible.

Landing Zone Safety

As the touchdown area is prepared, the LZ officer must be sure to secure any loose debris, clothing, hats, or anything

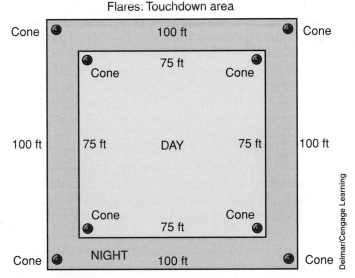

Figure 18-12 Cones marking the perimeter of the touchdown area clearly identify its boundaries for the helicopter pilot.

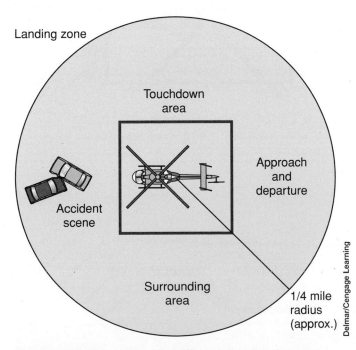

Figure 18-11 The LZ officer should choose a touchdown area that has an obstacle-free surrounding area and approach path.

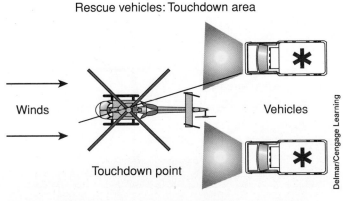

Figure 18-13 Emergency vehicle headlights can be used to mark a landing zone.

else that may blow around as the helicopter lands. A loose piece of debris can be blown into the helicopter's rotor blades and cause significant damage, which may render the aircraft useless.

As the aircraft is approaching the touchdown area, any nearby personnel should wear goggles or face visors to protect their eyes from winds created by the helicopter's rotor until the helicopter has landed and shut down.

If the accident is near the LZ, the patient and any exposed crew members should be appropriately protected from blowing debris during the aircraft's final approach. Doors and windows to nearby vehicles should be kept closed and any nearby traffic should be held if it has any potential for coming into contact with the aircraft in the LZ area.

Because a landing helicopter is certainly exciting to watch, rescues that involve helicopters often draw a crowd of onlookers. These people should be kept at a distance of at least 200 feet from the touchdown area for their own safety.

As the aircraft approaches the touchdown area, the LZ officer should continue to observe its descent from a safe distance of at least 100 feet. Nobody should be within 100 feet of the touchdown area until it is safe to approach, which will be indicated by the aircraft's pilot. If an unsafe situation develops during the final approach, the LZ officer should immediately and calmly contact the pilot with the information.

Landing Zone Hand Signals

The LZ officer really needs to know only two hand signals to communicate with the pilot. While facing the pilot at the edge of the LZ, the LZ officer simply stands with his arms outstretched, indicating that the aircraft approach is safe. The LZ officer should not be concentrating on how the aircraft is descending; rather, he should be looking around the aircraft for dangers.

If, for example, a wire strike suddenly seems possible, an individual runs out to meet the helicopter, or another danger under or around the helicopter arises, the LZ officer should signal the immediate danger to the pilot, using a vigorous crossing and uncrossing of his arms over his head (called

a **wave-off**). This will cause the pilot to quickly abort the landing.

Touchdown

Several rules also pertain to operations around the helicopter while it is on the ground. In general, nobody should ever approach the aircraft while it is running unless she is signaled to do so by the pilot. This includes the LZ officer. The pilot will usually direct the appropriate movement about the aircraft. If the pilot signals for a Paramedic to approach the aircraft, she should always approach from the front (the 12 o'clock position) within clear view of the pilot. Personnel should never approach a helicopter from the rear (the 6 o'clock position). Other danger zones also exist around the aircraft (Figure 18-14). The rear of the aircraft tail has a tail rotor that spins so fast that it is nearly invisible. This tail rotor is very dangerous. Any person who hits a spinning tail rotor will be very seriously injured and possibly even killed.

Due to the height of the main rotor blades, approaching personnel may need to duck down to avoid being struck by them. For this reason, Paramedics should wear a safety helmet whenever they are around an aircraft. When approaching a helicopter on a slope, the Paramedic should approach from the downhill side to avoid being struck by the main rotor blades on the uphill side (Figure 18-15).

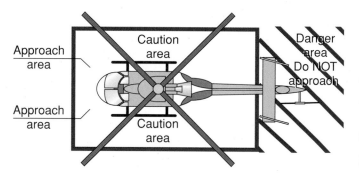

Figure 18-14 Ground personnel should be familiar with the danger zones around a helicopter.

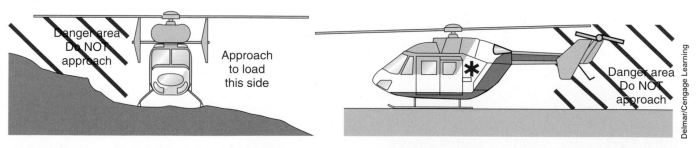

Figure 18-15 When approaching a helicopter that has landed on a slope, always approach from the downhill side to avoid injury. Never approach the aircraft from behind.

The LZ officer often designates an assistant who takes a position opposite the LZ officer at the edge of the landing zone. This assistant monitors activity in that area and radios problems to the LZ officer. The most dangerous place in the LZ is the area immediately behind the aircraft, near the tail rotor. No one should be allowed to approach the aircraft from that angle. It is the assistant LZ officer's job to ensure no one does so.

Most helicopter crews will come to the patient, away from the aircraft, to quickly assess the patient. After they initiate any necessary treatment, the pilot and helicopter crew will direct the patient's movement to the aircraft.

When carrying the patient to the waiting aircraft, the Paramedic should stay close to the patient's side, semi-crouched, and walk at a deliberate pace. The Paramedic should never run to the helicopter. Furthermore, the Paramedic should never carry anything, including intravenous fluids, over his head as he approaches the aircraft.

Liftoff

Once the patient has been safely loaded, all ground personnel should leave the landing zone in the direction indicated by the pilot or helicopter crew and should remain at least 200 feet away from the aircraft while it prepares to liftoff. A great deal of rotor wash will again be generated as the aircraft lifts off. Again, no one should aim any bright lights or flashes at the aircraft during this time, as they can create a vision problem for the pilot.

To save on-scene time, some helicopter pilots permit what is called a hot load. Whenever the helicopter's rotors are still spinning and the engine is running during a hot load, the potential for danger is increased. Therefore, only experienced crews should be permitted to hot load. If the patient is being hot loaded, the patient must protect his eyes with either safety glasses or a blanket. The LZ officer should also ensure that items like ball caps, hats, names tags, and linens such as blankets and sheets are secured.

Although general safety issues surrounding operation around helicopters are similar between agencies, ground EMS personnel should routinely practice and train with their local helicopter agencies so that safe operation around the aircraft becomes second nature.

The landing team should remain assembled for about five minutes after liftoff. If an in-flight emergency should occur, the aircraft may need to return quickly to the secured landing zone.

Aircraft Capabilities

In order to determine the most appropriate aircraft for a particular patient, multiple factors must be considered, such as the patient's condition and the distance that needs to be travelled. Within air transport, the choice of aircraft will depend upon local availability and types of services offered as well as the local geography, weather conditions, and aviation resources.

Rotor Wing

The majority of the aircraft currently dedicated to emergency air medical transport are **rotor wing** aircraft, or helicopters. Many different types of helicopters are utilized, depending upon the geography covered and the expected mission. They range from small single-engine, single-pilot aircraft up to extensively outfitted dual-engine, instrument landing-rated, dual-pilot helicopters. It is important to realize that more is not always better. An airframe is chosen by a program based upon its needs (Figure 18-16). Although there will always be controversy regarding what manufacturer or model aircraft is best, the Federal Aviation Regulations assure that each aircraft is safe to conduct the mission for which it is intended.

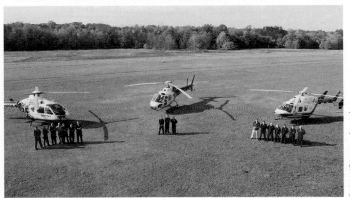

Figure 18-16 The airframe is chosen based on terrain and mission requirements.

Flight Rules

From the EMS perspective, the functionality of one helicopter over another may be distinguished by whether it is being operated under **visual flight rules (VFR)** or **instrument flight rules (IFR)**. Visual flight rules refer to aviation regulations that essentially permit a pilot to fly only when environmental conditions allow him to actually see with his own eyes well enough to safely navigate the aircraft. The Federal Aviation Administration (FAA) has established specific requirements for visibility, distance from clouds, and altitude to assure safe operations. Many air medical programs have created limitations more stringent than those required by the FAA in the interest of safety. This means that there will be some weather and visibility situations in which a pilot operating a VFR helicopter will not be able to accept a mission.

When operating under IFR, the pilot relies upon the aircraft's instruments for navigation, with additional instruction from air traffic control (ATC). Although IFR permits a planned flight in a broader range of environmental conditions, the pilot must file a flight plan, and each part of the flight into controlled airspace must receive ATC clearance. In addition, the pilot in an IFR-rated program must maintain additional certifications and the aircraft requires different equipment specifications.

Many VFR programs maintain pilot IFR credentialing and have equipment to allow for the use of instruments when visibility unexpectedly deteriorates during a flight. This safety measure allows the pilot to use every resource to safely navigate the aircraft to an appropriate landing zone. Every air medical program is mandated to conduct every flight according to stringent safety regulations regardless of whether they are VFR or IFR rated. At the scene operation level, both VFR and IFR pilots must have sufficient visibility to allow for complete identification of the intended landing zone and any hazards.

Weight and Balance

Another consideration when determining use of a helicopter is the issue of weight and balance. Every helicopter has a maximum lift capacity that must account for the combined weight of the crew, patients, equipment, and fuel. Although larger aircraft may be less limited with regard to weight, it must always be considered when using this mode of transport.

Speed

In general, rotor wing aircraft can travel at speeds two to three times faster than ground ambulances and have the advantage of straight-line travel. That is, they can fly from point A to point B without having to overcome surface obstacles. In some areas where ground time is extensive due to such obstacles, the use of a helicopter may translate into even more time savings. Knowledge of the local area, as well as estimated driving times and flight times, can help providers determine if using a helicopter is appropriate to consider in a given circumstance.

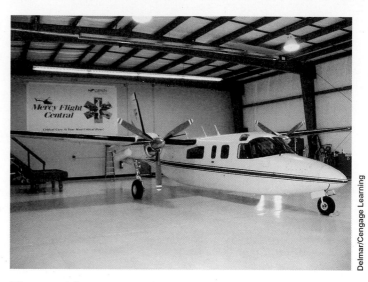

Figure 18-17 Fixed wing aircraft are used on longer range flights.

Fixed Wing

Fixed wing aircraft, or airplanes, are also used in air medical transport (Figure 18-17). Although they are able to travel at greater speeds and their range of travel is significantly longer than their rotor wing counterparts, the main disadvantage of fixed wing operations is the need to begin and end each transport at an airport.

The need for the patient and team on both ends of the transport to arrange alternate transport from the hospital to the airport adds time to the trip, sometimes negating the time saved by using the faster aircraft. On the other hand, the main advantage of this form of transport is the ability to complete long-distance transports in a much shorter time than a ground vehicle. Transports that are greater than 100 miles in length, in which there is an airport located within a reasonable distance to each end of the trip, should be considered for fixed wing travel.

Although many types of aircraft are utilized for fixed wing air medical transport, they are all instrument flight rated and most can travel in excess of 250 mph.

The cost of maintaining a fixed wing aircraft is more than needed to maintain a rotor wing. However, the cost for each mile of travel on a fixed wing transport is less, making an airplane a more economical choice for long distance flights. Additionally, the larger cabin offers an obvious advantage for patient care and crew comfort when compared to most helicopters. In addition, fewer restrictions with regard to weight and environmental conditions allow for a broader range of transports.

Cost and Reimbursement

Any discussion of air medical transport must touch upon the issue of cost. It should be evident that the cost to operate a helicopter and the personnel associated with it is significantly more than the cost required for a neighboring ground ambulance. The cost of these operations is handled differently depending upon the model of the program.

Although some very large independent organizations operate programs throughout the country, the majority of the dedicated air medical programs remain based at, and at least partially supported by, hospitals or hospital systems. Regardless of the program's model or size, the cost of business in air medicine is not small.

Typically, the air medical program bills a patient or insurance company a standard rate made up of a base cost for liftoff plus a per-mile fee for each loaded mile flown. Some programs have additional charges if high-priced items or services were utilized during the patient's care.

Many insurance companies have a rate that they believe to be acceptable. If they determine the flight was warranted after their own review, the program is reimbursed at the rate determined as appropriate.

Concerns regarding the cost of this type of transport are proper. However, if air medical transport is the most appropriate means of transport for a given patient, fears about cost should not affect the decision to do what is right. In fact, by making the decision to use this method of transport up front, money can potentially be saved in the long run if the patient has a decreased length of stay in the hospital from a better outcome than if the transport had been completed in a different manner. This is probably most clearly seen in the case of a trauma patient flown from a distant scene directly to a trauma center as opposed to being taken to a nontrauma center first, then requiring additional transport for definitive care.

Safety

The importance of safety during all phases of transport cannot be overemphasized. No matter the transport vehicle or the nature of the patient's illness, the priority of all involved must be to complete the task at hand in the safest manner possible.

History

In the early days of air medical transport and rapid growth within the industry, the rate of helicopter accidents was unacceptable. Although regulatory changes led to a temporary improvement, the late 1990s saw an alarming increase in the number of helicopter accidents encountered. Given the nature of the vehicle, incidents involving a helicopter tend to be more catastrophic than an incident involving a ground transport vehicle. Although a greater number of incidents occur with ground ambulances compared with air ambulances, the air ambulances tend to get more public attention. This attention and justified concern of the industry has led to increased regulation at the federal, state, and local levels, as well as an emphasis on a universal culture of safety within the air medical community.

Regulation

The Federal Aviation Administration has imposed stringent regulatory requirements on air medical helicopter operators. These requirements are designed to create as safe an environment as possible within the industry. Equipment specifications, maintenance policies, training requirements, and risk assessment tools are among the measures required under the regulations.

Culture of Safety

The Centers for Disease Control (CDC) has defined a **culture of safety** as the shared commitment of management and employees to ensure the safety of the work environment. It is important to note that a true culture of safety involves the active participation of every team member with the overarching goal of risk reduction. In air medical services, this means that both aviation and medical personnel are responsible for ensuring the team's safety.

Management support regarding safety is integral. Obstacles to a culture of safety include imposed pressures, risks, distractions, poor communication, and complacency, among other things. Awareness of the potential for each of these factors to result in unsafe practices must be a part of the safety culture. Identification of errors or near errors is mandatory; in fact, one of the best methods of error prevention available is having the entire team examine the details of each situation.

Air Medical Resource Management

Although the pilot in charge is given the ultimate responsibility over the aviation aspects of the flight, it is important to recognize that every member of the team can impact the mission's safety. This concept of entire team participation in a safety plan is fostered in the Air Medical Resource Management concept. This program involves training crew members on an aircraft to foster open communications, teamwork, and an overall awareness and participation in risk reduction.

Most accidents do not happen because of a single event, but rather result from a cumulative string, or chain, of events. Any of these events can be recognized by any member of the team and, if dealt with properly, can break the chain and hopefully prevent an accident.

Survival Training

Although safe operations are the goal of every program, safe does not necessarily mean without risk. In the case of an unavoidable incident, measures can be taken to improve survivability. Protective equipment such as helmets, flight suits, and safety harnesses can help an individual survive an accident (Figure 18-18). Specific training meant to help someone survive an incident is useful and mandated by many programs.

CAMTS

In 1990, the **Commission for Accreditation of Air Medical Services (CAAMS)** was formed as an accrediting body developed by the industry to validate its members' standards regarding safety, medical care, and utilization review. Although the name changed to the Commission for Accreditation of Medical Transport Services (CAMTS) to reflect the broader range of services seeking accreditation, the self-imposed

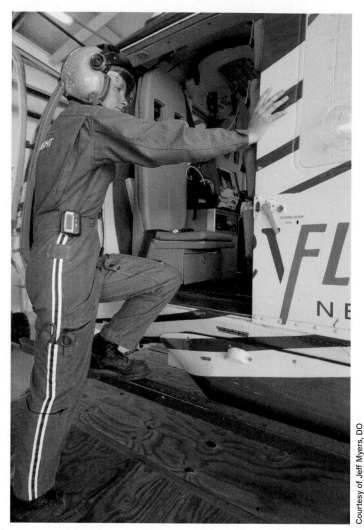

Figure 18-18 Protective clothing and equipment can improve the flight Paramedic's chances of survival in a crash.

Courtesy of Jeff Myers, DO

requirements reflected in the CAMTS standards are considered by many to be the national standard for practice in the air medical industry. Many states require air medical agencies operating within their borders to hold CAMTS accreditation or the equivalent. Excellence in patient care and safety of the transport environment are recognized as the pillars of the CAMTS standards. Continual review and revision of these standards, as appropriate, as well as the broad representation on the governing board, lend credibility to the accreditation process.

Individual Organizations

As with other professional groups, organization on a national level has far reaching benefits. In the case of the **International Association of Flight Paramedics (IAFP)**, the group draws its members from a worldwide base. The IAFP was founded in 1986 (originally named the National Flight Paramedics Association) and lists the following as their mission statement:

> _The purpose of the IAFP is to maintain an international organization of Paramedics which support and coordinate educational and research activities relating to its members and the flight Paramedic industry at large, and establish standard levels of training and performance for safe, efficient and quality patient care._

Holding true to that statement, the group has co-sponsored numerous educational conferences, position statements, publications, and research endeavors. They continue to offer support to members through creation of a certification exam and legislative initiatives, among other activities.

CASE STUDY CONCLUSION

The Paramedic explains to her patient's wife that she has requested a helicopter to respond in order to provide rapid transport to a distant hospital that is the regional stroke center. The Paramedic points out that this hospital is the only center in the area that can potentially offer specific therapies for acute management of stroke and that the treatment is very time dependent, making the air medical service a good option. While moving toward the arranged landing zone, the Paramedic places a peripheral venous access, monitors her patient's cardiac rhythm, and frequently reassesses his neurologic status.

CRITICAL THINKING QUESTIONS

1. What is the most appropriate transport decision that will get the patient to definitive care?
2. What are the advantages of transporting a patient with suspected stroke to these hospitals, even if that means bypassing other hospitals in the process?

Careers in Flight Medicine

According to the IAFP, approximately 277 programs fly with a Paramedic on-board. There are approximately 1,200 flight Paramedics in the United States. Because the practice of a flight Paramedic is usually fairly advanced and somewhat independent, most programs require between three and five years of experience in a busy system before considering a Paramedic as a viable applicant. Additionally, some advanced certifications and experience with interfacility and hospitalized patients is often looked upon as desirable in an applicant. Numerous resources are available for a Paramedic who is interested in finding more information about a career in flight medicine. Local air medical programs may be a good place to start. In addition, online resources such as the IAFP website can be invaluable when looking for industry information.

CONCLUSION

The air medical service is an integral part of EMS. With the majority of the U.S. population protected by air medical service, rapid transportation of critically ill patients by highly trained flight crews will positively impact on morbidity and mortality.

KEY POINTS:

- The predominant types of air medical services are community-based and hospital-based programs.

- Mission profiles are on-scene rescue and interfacility transfer.

- Staffing configurations include Paramedic/nurse (the most common), as well as Paramedic/respiratory therapist and Paramedic/physician.

- Primary advantages of air medical transport are its speed and the ability for special capabilities such as medication-facilitated intubation.

- Overtriage and undertriage are problems with air medical utilization.

- To achieve maximal efficiency, some air medical services have an auto-launch policy based on initial dispatch information.

- Although speed of transport is relevant for interfacility transfers, the more common reason for transfer is that the hospital of origin does not have the services that the destination hospital possesses.

- Altitude has a physiologic impact on the body, and the patient's disease and health must be factored into the decision to fly the patient.

- Both Boyle's law and Dalton's law affect flight physiology.

- Significant additional educational preparation is needed for air medical transportation.

- Since much of the medical control of the flight Paramedic is off-line, strict quality assurance is necessary to ensure proper patient care.

- Air medical services often have Medical Directors who are knowledgeable about flight physiology as well as critical care medicine.

- Landing zones must be carefully chosen for suitability according to criteria such as size, slope, and the surrounding area.

- The landing zone officer is responsible for safety, including eye protection from rotor wash, safety helmets for head protection from rotating blades, and crowd control.

- The pilot controls all aspects of the helicopter, including its approach.

- Air medical services include fixed wing aircraft as well as rotor wing aircraft.

- Visual flight rules and instrument flight rules affect which helicopter pilots can accept which missions.

- Fixed wing aircraft has the advantage of speed and distance over rotor wing aircraft, but the disadvantage of needing an airport and ambulance transportation to and from the airports.

- The growing culture of safety among air medical services is placing greater restrictions on flight operations for the betterment of patients and crew.

- The Commission for Accreditation of Air Medical Services helps assure the public about the safety, medical care, and proper utilization of air medical services.

- The International Association of Flight Paramedics represents flight Paramedics, advocates for their education and safety, and offers them certification.

REVIEW QUESTIONS:

1. Define overtriage and undertriage.
2. List some nontrauma indications for air medical transport.
3. List contraindications for air medical transport.
4. How do Boyle's law and Dalton's law affect flight physiology?
5. What is required for an adequate landing zone?

CASE STUDY QUESTIONS:

Please refer to the Case Study in this chapter, and answer the questions below:

1. How could the helicopter flight adversely affect the suspected stroke patient?
2. Would the patient qualify for an auto-launch of the helicopter?
3. If the air medical service was operating under visual flight rules, how would that affect the mission?

REFERENCES:

1. Air medical services: future development as an integrated component of the EMS system. A guidance document by the air medical task force of the NASEMSO, NAEMSP, AAMS.
2. Foundation for Air Medical Research and Education. Air medicine: the future of health care. Available at: **http://www.aams.org/MedEvac/Outreach/White_paper_translations/White_Paper_English.aspx.** Accessed September 2009.
3. Gryniuk J. *Certified Flight Paramedic Education Requirements.* Board for Critical Care Transport Paramedic Certification. Available at: **www.bcctpc.org.** Accessed September 2009.
4. Lerner EB, Moscati RM. The golden hour: scientific fact or medical "myth." *Acad Emerg Med.* 2001;8(7):758–760.
5. Butler DP, Anwar I, Willett K. Is the H or the EMS in HEMS that has an impact on trauma patient mortality? A systematic review of the evidence. *Emerg Med J.* 2010;27(9):692–701.
6. Newgard CD, Schmicker RH, Hedges JR, et al. Emergency medical services intervals and survival in trauma: assessment of the "golden hour" in a North American prospective cohort. *Ann Emerg Med.* 2010;55(3):235–246.
7. Thomson DP, Lerner EB, Thomas SH. Guidelines for air medical dispatch: position paper of National Association of Emergency Medicine Physicians. *Prehosp Emerg Care.* 2003;7(2):265–270.
8. Early activation of an air medical helicopter and auto-launch recommendations: Position statement of AAMS, 2006. Available at: **AAMS.org.** Accessed September 17, 2009.
9. Beebe R, Funk DL. *Fundamentals of Basic Emergency Care* (3nd ed.). Clifton Park, NY: Delmar-Cengage; 2010.
10. Tintinalli JE, Kelen GD, Stapczynski S. *Emergency Medicine. A Comprehensive Study Guide* (5th ed.). American College of Emergency Physicians. Irving, TX; 2000.
11. Board for Critical Care Transport Paramedic Certification. Available at: **http://www.bcctpc.org/.** Accessed March 12, 2010.
12. Blumen IJ, Lemkin DL. *Principles and Direction of Air Medical Transport.* Air Medical Physician Association. Salt Lake City, UT; 2006.
13. Air Medical Crew National Standard Curriculum. Available at: **www.flightParamedics.org.** Accessed September 17, 2009.

CHAPTER 19

SPECIALTY CARE TRANSPORT

KEY CONCEPTS:

Upon completion of this chapter, it is expected that the reader will understand these following concepts:

- Specialty care centers
- EMTALA impact on interfacility transfer
- Sending hospital responsibilities
- Receiving hospital responsibilities
- Paramedic responsibilities during transport

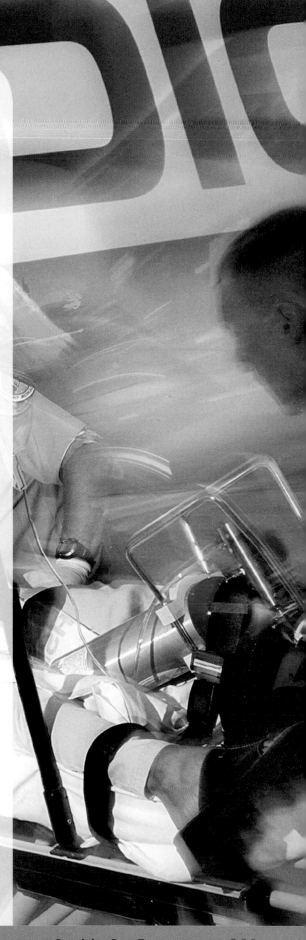

"Starr ambulance service, respond to Community General Hospital for an emergency interfacility transfer. . . ." Having just completed his specialty care course, the Paramedic is excited to be dispatched for his first independent interfacility transfer. While he and his driver are en route to Community General, their dispatcher tells them that they are responding for a 6-year-old boy who has been struck by a car. He is reported to have head, chest, and abdominal injuries. Additional information is that the child is intubated and on several medicated drips. The Paramedic acknowledges the information and feels a knot in his stomach. This child sounds pretty injured. He hopes his recent training has prepared him to safely transport this patient.

Upon arriving at the sending facility, the Paramedic and his driver move their stretcher and equipment to the patient's bedside. A nurse gives the Paramedic the patient report. This 6-year-old child was struck by a car and brought to Community General several hours prior. He requires intubation for respiratory distress and a chest X-ray indicates bilateral hemopneumothorax for which chest tubes have been placed. A CT scan indicates that the child also has an acute subdural hematoma and a Grade 4 splenic laceration. The child has experienced several episodes of hypotension and is currently on neosynephrine and getting transfusions of packed red blood cells. He has been chemically paralyzed and has a propofol infusion running for sedation. Orders have been written for all of these interventions to be continued during transport.

CRITICAL THINKING QUESTIONS

1. What are some of the possible complications that the Paramedic could encounter en route to the receiving hospital?

2. What is the "problem list" that the Paramedic must monitor?

OVERVIEW

Over the past several decades, the medical community has seen an increased need to move sick patients from one hospital to another. There are likely many reasons for this situation. Patients with complex illnesses or a need for a very specialized intervention may be moved to a hospital that can provide a higher level of care. Overcrowded hospitals may find it necessary to transfer patients to a hospital that has more available beds in which to house the patient. And patients may simply request to be moved to another locale for personal reasons.

In any case, when ill and injured patients need to move from one facility to another, a team is needed to complete the transfer. Since Paramedics have the most experience with prehospital patient transport in many communities, they are typically asked to participate in **interfacility transports** (moving a patient from one facility to another).

For the Paramedic, interfacility transport requires a different mindset and different training and protocols than those used at the typical emergency scene response. The patients being moved from one hospital to another usually have a specific diagnosis and often have interventions in place that are not typically encountered in the prehospital environment.

This chapter will review the history behind much of the regulation governing interfacility transport and outline the issues that are relevant to the Paramedic involved in such transports. This chapter is meant to be an introduction to the topic; by no means is it detailed enough to be the sole education for a Paramedic staffing an interfacility transport. In addition, local and regional protocols and guidelines will dictate the scope of practice (which is typically beyond the Paramedic's scope of practice) and advanced interfacility transportation skill set.

Specialization of Hospitals

In this era of highly specialized care being available for critical illnesses, advanced care for some conditions is only available at certain hospitals. The concept of specialization is familiar in the field of trauma, as the well-studied concept of trauma centers is accepted nationwide. Regional systems are set up in many areas that designate which hospitals will serve as the most appropriate facility to care for injured patients who meet specific criteria.

By designating a hospital for trauma, the resources for managing critically injured patients can be concentrated at strategically located centers in a given region. In this way, the staff at the designated center is experienced in caring for large numbers of injured patients, resulting in improved efficiency and decreased morbidity and mortality.

Rather than dispersing the resources utilized in managing trauma patients throughout a region, theses resources are concentrated at centrally located facilities. Although this makes sense on multiple levels, it means that an injured patient may initially be brought to a facility that does not have all the resources required to manage her injuries in a

definitive manner. The trauma system concept addresses this shortcoming through cooperation among hospitals in a given trauma region so that the care for all patients is streamlined. If a patient enters the system at a nontrauma center, the patient's management is standardized as a part of the system. Based on agreed-upon guidelines, if a patient has injuries that will benefit from care at a higher level trauma center, she will be transferred after the physicians complete critical stabilization.

Utilizing the trauma center concept, over the past decade many areas have been designating hospitals that specialize in the care of patients with other illnesses such as acute stroke or acute ST elevation myocardial infarction.

Although the concept of hospital designation is less extensively studied in these conditions than in the trauma example, it is reasonably clear that if specialized care known to improve an outcome is available for a patient with a time-dependent illness, the patient should be quickly taken to the center that is able to provide that care. This can only occur with coordination between hospitals and EMS systems.

Protocols that guide EMS agencies to transport patients to the hospital most appropriate for their condition are the first part of this system. It is also necessary to streamline the system to rapidly recognize these patients and have a plan in place to transfer them to the facility capable of providing definitive care for their condition.

In today's medical community, there are oftentimes very specialized treatments available for many conditions. Since the number of physicians trained in these interventions is small, it is impossible for every hospital to offer them. Patients in need of these interventions will require transfer in order to be evaluated for this care. Some examples of such interventions include certain neurosurgical, cardiovascular, and radiological procedures.

Transfer of Critical Patients

Many patients with an acute illness who are in need of emergent transfer are quite ill and not only need timely transport but also specialized care en route to the facility. It is interesting to review the federal regulation in place that governs the transfer of such patients.

EMTALA

In the early 1980s, it was not unusual for transfers to be motivated by both the need for a higher level of care and financial reasons. Hospitals might arrange to transfer a patient with less ability to pay simply to avoid expending their resources when compensation was not likely. Although these hospitals may have had the resources to handle the patient's medical needs, they may have recommended transfer for purely economic reasons. This practice, often referred to as "dumping," was obviously not in the best interests of the patient's medical needs in most cases.

In response to accumulating evidence of this economically driven denial of care throughout the country, in 1985 Congress enacted a law that was intended to prevent this unethical practice. The Emergency Medical Treatment and Active Labor Act (EMTALA) was established as a part of the Consolidated Omnibus Budget Reconciliation Act (COBRA).[1] Although EMTALA has been amended a number of times, it remains the most significant regulation ever enacted related to the emergency care and transfer of patients in the United States. In fact, it was the first law that provided a right to emergency medical care for every citizen.

The **Emergency Medical Treatment and Active Labor Act (EMTALA)** defines a hospital's responsibility to provide emergency care to anyone presenting with a request for help. It details the hospital's obligations with regard to initial evaluation and management as well as with regard to transfer arrangements. Hospitals are obligated to obey these guidelines under penalty of fine.

Shortly after this law was enacted, a new problem emerged. The original language of EMTALA mandated the care that must be provided at the hospital to which the patient presents but did not address the responsibilities of higher-level centers to which patients might be transferred. When hospitals attempted to transfer patients they felt were in need of care at another facility, they encountered difficulty in obtaining acceptance of these patients. This problem also appeared to have a financial motivation in some cases. This is sometimes referred to as "reverse dumping" and is just as big an ethical issue as the original problem.

In 1989, EMTALA was amended to include language that required higher-level hospitals to accept a patient in transfer when they had the ability to manage the patient's condition. The details associated with the many amendments of these laws are rather confusing; therefore, interpretive guidelines have been issued over the years clarifying hospitals' responsibilities under the law.[2]

Screen and Stabilize

The law requires that every hospital provide an appropriate screening exam to any patient who requests examination or treatment. This screening cannot be delayed for reasons that are financially motivated. If the screening exam reveals an emergency medical condition, the hospital is obligated to stabilize the patient. If stabilization is not possible, the patient must be transferred to a hospital that can stabilize the patient. The interpretive guidelines issued over the years are extensive and have clarified many of the details regarding these responsibilities.

Hospital-Owned Ambulances

Although a hospital-owned or operated ambulance service is considered an extension of that hospital according to the law, interpretive guidelines allow for the ambulance to follow local EMS guidelines with regard to patient transport without penalty under EMTALA. This is important when the most appropriate hospital for the patient in the ambulance may not be the base hospital. The basis of the law is to assure that patients get the best available medical care. If a system is set up to allow for that, then in most cases the hospital will be in compliance with the law.

Hospital Helipads

A common misperception is that, if a patient is brought by ambulance to a hospital-owned helipad, that hospital must provide the patient with a medical screening exam to be in compliance with the law. However, interpretations have detailed that if the intent of the patient's arrival at the hospital-owned helipad is to use it as a rendezvous location and not to request care from the hospital, then the hospital is under no obligation according to EMTALA.

However, if the patient, ambulance personnel, or helicopter team requests an examination or treatment, the hospital is then obligated to assess and stabilize as detailed in the law. Therefore, Paramedics should not hesitate to utilize hospital helipads as predesignated landing zones for incoming helicopters if they feel that is the safest option in a given situation. The Paramedic should work together with that hospital to assure that all appropriate safety measures are in place when using the helipad.

Sending Hospital Obligations

Sending hospitals must comply with a number of requirements when arranging the transfer of an unstable patient. The first is certification of medical necessity. This documentation may take many forms but must include a statement of the medical benefits expected from transfer as well as the risks that can reasonably be expected due to the transfer. The sending facility must certify that the expected benefits outweigh the potential risks of the transfer.

The sending hospital must always obtain consent for transfer, whether directly from the patient or family member or implied under the emergency doctrine. This consent must be informed and in writing and is often included as a part of the certification of risks and benefits. The sending hospital has an obligation to arrange an "appropriate" transfer.

Four components to this process are outlined in the law. First, the hospital must provide treatment within their capacity to minimize the risks of transfer. This might range anywhere from initiating venous access to intubation or chest tube placement if the hospital feels that these interventions will reduce the risk of the transfer.

Next, the sending hospital must arrange for another hospital to accept the patient in transfer. Simply transferring a patient without having another hospital identify that it is willing and able to accept the patient constitutes a violation of the law.

The sending facility is also legally required to assure that relevant data is sent with the patient for the receiving staff to use in continuation of care. This includes documentation of care, results of tests performed at the sending facility, and a copy of the radiographic studies performed at the facility, often in the form of a CD.

Finally, the transfer must take place through the use of qualified personnel and transportation equipment. It is important to recognize that the patient's needs are not simply what the patient needs at the time of the transfer, but must include potential needs if the situation changes during the move. This determination must be based upon the treating physician's best estimate of what the patient may need during transfer. For example, if a patient with an acute coronary syndrome is being transferred, there is a good possibility that the patient may experience an arrhythmia during transport. The team chosen to complete that transfer must be qualified and have the equipment necessary (i.e., medications and defibrillator) to effectively manage arrhythmias.

Similarly, a patient with an acute stroke may deteriorate and require intubation during transport. The team accompanying the patient should be qualified to perform an intubation and have the appropriate equipment available, if needed. The team should also utilize the vehicle determined to be most appropriate for the patient's condition, based on the judgment of the sending physician.

The sending facility is legally responsible for providing patient care (i.e., medical control) until care is assumed by the receiving facility physician. This includes the care provided by the transport agency. It seems imperative for the sending facility to have a good understanding of the transport team's capabilities. Good communication and preplanning between hospitals and transport agencies will facilitate this.

Stabilized Patients

EMTALA regulations regarding transfers relate to unstable patients, those whose conditions have not been stabilized. Once a patient has been stabilized, these regulations do not apply and transfers can be arranged for economic reasons, if desired. EMTALA defines "stabilized" as the point when a patient is *not likely* to deteriorate during transfer. This definition is clearly somewhat subjective and is best left to the treating physician to determine.

Receiving Hospital Obligations

Hospitals that offer specialized services have an obligation under EMTALA to accept patients in transfer if they have the ability and capacity to manage that patient's condition at that time. This must be done without any consideration of the patient's ability to pay for such care. Refusal to accept transfers is one of the largest areas of EMTALA violation investigations today. This has led to the development of very complicated algorithms in some hospitals to determine the hospital's capacity at any given time for any given condition. That way, if a hospital determines that it does not have the ability or capacity to manage a patient for whom transfer is requested, they can refuse without being in violation of the law. This seems to be very reasonable, as it is not safe to bring an unstable patient to a hospital that doesn't have the ability to safely handle the condition. In today's age of hospital overcrowding, overfull emergency departments and lack of hospital beds may result in interfacility transfers that bypass one or more institutions that would have otherwise been able to manage a patient's condition. This translates into what may be very long transport times for the interfacility transport team.

Transport Provider Obligations

Although the Paramedic's practice during interfacility transfer is not directly detailed in this regulation, it is helpful to understand the background behind the transfer process that exists today. There are clearly legal obligations for the transport agency and providers to affect a medically appropriate patient transport in the safest manner possible. However, these obligations are not detailed under EMTALA. Since these regulations may differ from state to state, the Paramedic who provides interfacility transport should be familiar with the relevant local regulations.

It certainly makes sense for a transport service to meet with local hospitals for the purposes of preplanning regarding interfacility transport needs. The transport service should educate the hospital regarding the transport team's capabilities and equipment. This knowledge will enable the facility to make appropriate decisions regarding staffing during a transfer. At times, hospital staff may need to accompany a patient during transfer. It is helpful to have some sort of collaborative training prior to this occurrence that enables the hospital staff to function safely in the transport vehicle. Clarification of the roles and responsibilities of each of the providers staffing the transport in this case is helpful.

Staffing

In general, the staffing required for an interfacility transport should be determined based upon the patient's expected needs during the transport. There may be local regulations that specify what type of provider must staff a given transport. The Paramedic should be familiar with any such guidelines.

Level of Care

As in any hospital environment, the level of training required of the caregivers for a particular patient will depend upon that patient's illness, the complexity of the interventions, and the frequency with which reassessments and changes in care are expected. For example, a patient who does not require ventilatory or hemodynamic support and whose condition is stable enough to not require reassessment more than every few hours might be appropriately situated on a non-intensive care unit of a hospital. The training level of the nursing staff is not at the critical care level and the ratio of patients to nurses is high.

Similarly, the patient who is more unstable, who has need of reassessment more frequently, or has interventions in place that require advanced training will require an intensive care unit (ICU) bed. Typically, the nursing staff on an ICU is credentialed by the hospital to perform additional advanced skills and the ratio of patients to nurses is much lower than on a non-ICU floor. This allows for the more unstable patients to be given more attention as their condition mandates.

Traditional EMS

Paramedics who hold a standard certification with no additional training specific to interfacility transport complete the majority of interfacility transports. Most patients who require transport from one hospital to another do not have needs that go beyond what a traditionally trained Paramedic is able to manage. However, a small percentage of patients will have more extensive needs during transport. In this case, the options include providing additional training to the Paramedic or adding additional staff to the transport team who are trained to a higher level.

Additionally Trained Providers

Knowing that traditional EMS training focuses on scene response, some may argue that an EMT at any level who intends to staff an interfacility transport should have some form of additional training to prepare for this new environment and patient population. This will likely be regulated at the state or local level.

Basic Life Support

An EMT who staffs an interfacility transport should have a basic knowledge of the laws surrounding the movement of patients between hospitals. The scope of practice and any relevant policies regarding the EMT's responsibilities during an interfacility transport are clearly of importance.

Basic knowledge of the common conditions likely to be seen during interfacility transport are helpful to the EMT whose training is classically based on symptoms rather than diagnoses. Finally, the EMT should have an understanding of the more common medical devices seen during these types of transports, including indwelling urinary catheters (Figure 19-1), nasogastric or gastrostomy tubes, and non-medicated intravenous access devices. Depending upon local training and policy, EMTs may be asked to move patients with these devices in place, even though they have not received training in their management.[2]

Advanced Life Support

As with the EMT, the Paramedic also should have an awareness of the relevant laws and policies regarding interfacility transport in the local area. Since Paramedic training prepares the student to provide the patient with initial assessment and management of a given condition, the Paramedic will likely benefit from some additional training in order to manage the hospitalized patient. Once again, a patient with an actual diagnosis rather than an undifferentiated complaint is managed differently. A good example is a patient who has chest pain and is diagnosed with an acute thoracic aortic dissection. Standard Paramedic training and protocols would indicate the administration of certain medications which might be contraindicated in this specific condition. Understanding the need for specific care guidelines based upon the hospital diagnosis is important.

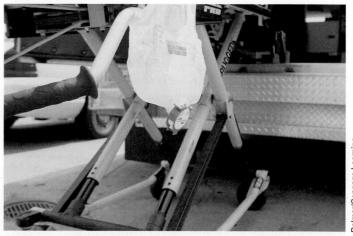

Figure 19-1 Urinary catheters are commonly encountered during interfacility transport.

Although the Paramedic will develop a broad knowledge base regarding pharmacology in a traditional training program, some medications commonly used during interfacility transport are not usually seen during on-scene response. The Paramedic staffing an interfacility transport should review these medications (Figure 19-2). Some common examples

Special Interfacility Formulary	
1. Albuterol	39. Lidocaine
2. Aminophylline	40. Lorazapam
3. Amiodarone	41. Magnesium Sulfate
4. Ampicillin	42. Mannitol
5. Aspirin	43. Meperidine
6. Atropine	44. Methylprednisolone
7. Benzocaine	45. Metoclopramide
8. Bumetanide	46. Metoprolol
9. Calcium Salts	47. Midazolam
10. Cefazolin	48. Milrinone
11. Cefotaxime	49. Morphine
12. Cefriaxone	50. Naloxone
13. Cistracurium	51. Nicardipine
14. Dexamethasone	52. Nimodipine
15. Dextrose	53. Nitroglycerin
16. Diazepam	54. Nitroprusside
17. Diltiazem	55. Norepinephrine
18. Diphenhydramine	56. Ondanestron
19. Dobutamine	57. Oxytocin
20. Dopamine	58. Prostaglandin
21. Epinephrine	59. Phenobarbital
22. Esmolol	60. Phenylephrine
23. Etomidate	61. Phenytoin
24. Fentanyl	62. Potassium Chloride
25. Flumzenil	63. Prednisone
26. Fosphenytoin	64. Procainamide
27. Furosemide	65. Promethazine
28. Gentamicin	66. Propofol
29. Glucagon	67. Racemic Epinephrine
30. Haloperidol	68. Ranitidine
31. Heparin Sodium	69. Rocuronium
32. Hydrazaline	70. Sodium Bicarbonate
33. Hydromorphone	71. Succinylcholine
34. Hydroxocobalamin	72. Terbutaline
35. Insulin	73. Trimentobensamide
36. Ipratropium	74. Vasopressin
37. Ketamine	75. Vecuronium
38. Labetolol	76. Verapamil

Delmar/Cengage Learning

Figure 19-2 An expanded formulary is common for the Paramedic providing care during interfacility transport.

are nitroglycerin or heparin infusions or administration of electrolytes or antibiotics.

Similarly, a Paramedic's knowledge of anatomy and physiology enables her to understand common interventions utilized in hospitalized patients. However, her original training most likely did not cover specific training regarding devices used in the hospital. However, such training is important to have prior to an interfacility transport in which the Paramedic may encounter such a device. Typical examples might include thoracostomy drainage tubes or ventilators.

Specialty Care Transport

The advent of the National Medicare Ambulance Fee Schedule on April 1, 2002, defined a separate category of reimbursement for interfacility transport patients requiring specialized interventions beyond the Paramedic's scope of practice. This level of reimbursement, labeled **specialty care transport (SCT)**, is to be provided by professionals with appropriate training such as emergency or cardiovascular physicians, nurses, respiratory technicians, or Paramedics with additional training.

Although the billing schedule coined the term, it should be clear to the medical community that a need exists for a class of provider that has special training to care for critically ill patients during interfacility transfer. Some might argue that the most appropriate staff to accompany a critically ill hospital patient during interfacility transport are those credentialed by the hospital to manage the condition. Others might point out that hospital staff are not trained to practice in the out-of-hospital environment and are not best suited for it.

The truth most likely lies somewhere in-between. It certainly is true that the Paramedic is more specifically trained to operate in the out-of-hospital environment. Yet, the Paramedic is not trained in the management of hospitalized patients. With this in mind, one might conclude that the ideal transport team would include both hospital-trained staff as well as EMS-trained staff. Some transport agencies staff nurses and Paramedics for this reason. Another alternative might be to have a nurse from the sending facility accompany the Paramedic from the transport agency on the transport. This is done in a number of areas and serves to offer the patient both levels of expertise. The hospital-trained nurses, however, should have some specialized training to be better equipped to provide care in this nontraditional setting.

Another option exists that is becoming more common as hospitals are experiencing nursing shortages and the training of Paramedics is being expanded in several areas to serve local needs. This involves expanding the Paramedic's scope of practice to specifically enable her to care for critically ill patients during interfacility transport. These Paramedics are provided specific training beyond the standard curriculum to help them care for the critically ill patient during interfacility transport. In keeping with the CMS terminology which was introduced in 2001, this level of care might be called **specialty care**.

Scope of Practice

The scope of practice is the extent to which a healthcare provider is permitted to perform medical procedures. This is defined differently from state to state and might be based upon the educational curriculum, protocols, or a stand-alone document detailing the procedures allowed. The Paramedic should be very familiar with the prescribed scope of practice for the region in which he practices. Performing procedures beyond that scope of practice is not appropriate without specific guidelines to allow it.

Paramedic with Additional Training

A Paramedic who is provided with additional training in a defined area might have an expanded scope of practice. This should be clearly defined by the governing body with authority over Paramedics so that the provider knows to what level he may practice. Simply attending training on a particular intervention does not necessarily enable the provider to perform that intervention, however. If the intervention goes beyond the usual scope of practice for that provider, an expanded scope of practice should be defined (Table 19-1). Although every state will handle this somewhat differently, the Paramedic who is attending training with the intent of providing care at a more advanced level than what his original certification allows should be knowledgeable regarding local regulations.[3]

The Paramedic should clearly know the ceiling of his "scope of practice" so that he will recognize when a patient's needs require training beyond the level that he can provide. In those cases, a higher level of care will be needed for the transfer. This will usually be provided by a nurse from the sending facility who is skilled in the intervention required.

Specialty Team

Some hospitals with specialized services provide a team that will go to outlying hospitals and provide care during transport back to the tertiary care center. It is not uncommon for a Paramedic to accompany that team to assist them with patient movement and assure their safety in the EMS vehicle. Pediatric and neonatal teams are probably the most common specialty teams encountered (Figure 19-3).

Initial Training

The training for a Paramedic intending to staff an interfacility transport for a critically ill patient should be expansive enough to cover the most commonly seen conditions and interventions. Many areas require a broad training program to cover a certain minimum standard, allowing agencies to expand upon that minimum depending upon that agency's needs. At a minimum, a training program should cover certain essential topics (Table 19-2).

Ongoing Education and Skill Maintenance

As with any training program, recurrent education is mandatory in order to keep the provider competent. Some patient types and conditions are seen quite often and other types and

Table 19-1 Example of an Expanded Scope of Practice for the Specialty Care Paramedic

- Specialty Care Transport Scope of Practice
  - Includes the standard skill set as defined in the EMT-P scope of practice and authorized by state and local protocols AND
  - Managing patients with chronic indwelling assistive devices including urinary catheters, gastrostomy tubes, tracheostomy tubes, peripherally inserted central catheter (PICC) lines, and other central vascular access devices
  - Assessment of hospitalized patients and transition of care according to federal guidelines
  - Airway management
    - Advanced mechanical ventilation
  - Venous access
    - Central venous catheter–insertion
    - Central venous catheter (implanted)–access
  - Pharmacology
    - Infusion pump operation
    - Parenteral bolus medication—outside Paramedic protocol
    - Parenteral infusion maintenance—outside Paramedic protocol
    - Parenteral infusion titration—outside Paramedic protocol
  - Neurology
    - Intracranial pressure monitor–maintenance
    - Ventriculostomy-maintenance
  - Pulmonology
    - Chest tube maintenance
  - Cardiology
    - Transvenous pacing–maintenance
    - Arterial line–maintenance
    - Swan Ganz–maintenance
    - Left ventricular assist device–maintenance
    - Intra-aortic balloon pump–maintenance
    - Pericardiocentesis
  - Hematology
    - Blood product transfusion–initiation
    - Blood product transfusion–maintenance

conditions are seen less frequently. A process should be in place to identify the low-volume, high-risk patient types to be certain that ongoing education is focused most appropriately. Similarly, Paramedics should demonstrate their ability to perform infrequently used skills on a regular basis in order to assure competence.

Quality Assurance

Interfacility transport should be incorporated into a total quality management plan just like what occurs in the more traditional on-scene responses. Quality indicators that are specific

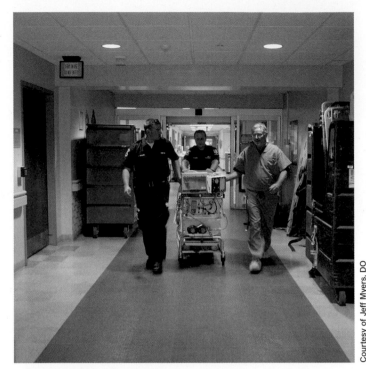

Figure 19-3 Pediatric and neonatal specialty teams offer specialized care to specific patient populations during interfacility transport.

Courtesy of Jeff Myers, DO

Table 19-2 Specialty Care Training for Paramedics

- Overview of specialty care transport
- Medical and legal responsibilities
- Neurological disorders
- Pulmonary disorders
- Gastrointestinal disorders
- Urogenital disorders
- Hematological disorders
- Infectious diseases
- Trauma
- Advanced airway management
- Respiratory therapy
- Special vascular access
- Blood administration
- Pharmacology
- Hemodynamic monitoring
- Biomedical devices

for interfacility transport should be applied during review of these transports. This should involve assuring that appropriate protocols or guidelines are followed and that appropriate care is provided. The QA process is a good way to identify areas that need further education or review.

Protocols

Protocols that are written for the standard prehospital EMS response are not suited to the care provided during interfacility transport. As identified previously, the patient being moved from one hospital to another most often has a clear diagnosis rather than undifferentiated symptoms. This makes protocols geared to symptoms inappropriate to use in some cases. Patient care guidelines meant specifically for the interfacility transport patient should outline the standard care provided to patients with the most common conditions seen during transport. Although in many cases the sending physician will provide written orders detailing the interventions needed during transport, the Paramedic should have a document to guide his practice in a given situation if it is not covered in the prescribed orders. These guidelines might take the form of a formal protocol or might be more of a general guide for the Paramedic to use in a given circumstance.

Although the format might be different depending upon the local regulations, the Paramedic should have some document to refer to when determining the best course of action for a given patient or situation. The protocol might also be used to define the provider's scope of practice. In that case, if an intervention is required that is not included in the protocol, it may not be performed by that provider. In a world of rapidly advancing medical technology, this makes it clear to the Paramedic what he will be expected to manage during a transport.

Medical Control

Out-of-hospital care, both on-scene and during interfacility transport, is most often provided by non-physicians. However, this care is often prescribed by physicians through protocols or guidelines, as previously discussed. Oversight of out-of-hospital care by physicians is important and necessary. The physician oversight that takes the form of written protocols and other guidelines is known as "off-line medical control." As the term indicates, the physician has control over a patient's care although he is not present, nor does he need to be, at the patient's bedside.

On-Line

In contrast, "on-line medical control" is required when the written guidelines do not provide the Paramedic with the guidance he is looking for. In this case, he should contact a physician directly and discuss the situation in order to obtain the needed direction. It is important that the Paramedic staffing an interfacility transport know who will be providing the on-line medical control for a given transport if the need arises. In many cases, this guidance will come from the sending or receiving physician; in other cases, from the agency Medical Director or other designated medical control physician.

Patients

Much of this chapter has been devoted to the Paramedic who will staff an interfacility transport. In order to understand the need for specific training, it is helpful to discuss the types of patients that will be encountered. Depending upon the local resources, the Paramedic may or may not encounter each of these patient types and may or may not staff such transports independently.

Types of Transfers

Patients require transfer for any number of reasons. These might include a need for specialized services not available at the original institution, a desire for care by a particular physician or care in a particular locale, or a need to move to a facility where a physical bed is available. Depending upon the patient's condition and reason for transfer, there are several categories of transfers that deserve mention.

Stabilized vs. Not Stabilized

Stabilized

As previously discussed, every hospital has an obligation pursuant to federal law to assess a patient who presents with a request for medical care. If the assessment reveals that the patient has an emergency medical condition, the hospital must provide stabilization. A patient can be considered stabilized if he has been treated to a point where deterioration is unlikely during transfer.

Not Stabilized

Depending upon the patient's condition and specific needs, the hospital may not have the ability to stabilize his condition, making transfer in an unstable condition necessary. In this case, the hospital staff has an obligation to do everything they can to make the patient as safe as possible for transfer. The patient who remains unstable, by definition, risks the possibility of deterioration during transport. The providers staffing the transport must have the training, equipment, and protocols to allow them to manage the predicted deterioration. An example of an unstable patient requiring transfer might be a patient with a ruptured abdominal aortic aneurysm who is at a hospital that does not have a vascular surgeon. This patient can be markedly unstable; however, despite that instability, transfer is necessary to offer definitive management. In this case, adequate intravenous access might be the necessary treatment provided by the hospital in order to best prepare the patient for emergent transfer. The transport team should be able to manage deterioration in this patient's condition and provide the appropriate treatment, which may include advanced airway management, additional intravenous access, and administration of crystalloid and blood products when necessary.

Conditions Requiring Transfer

Many conditions might require a patient to be transferred from one facility to another. This is largely dependent upon the resources available at the local hospital (Table 19-3).

Table 19-3 Specific Conditions That May Be Encountered in Interfacility Transfer

Trauma	Nontrauma	Pediatric	Obstetrical
Traumatic brain injury	Acute coronary syndrome	Epiglottitis	Preterm labor
Spinal cord injury	Acute stroke	Reactive airway disease	Premature rupture of membranes
Vascular injury	Status epilepticus	Sepsis	Pre-eclampsia/eclampsia
Thoracic injuries	Respiratory failure	Diabetic ketoacidosis	Placental abruption
Intra-abdominal injuries	Endocrine emergencies	Traumatic injuries	Trauma during pregnancy
Orthopedic injuries	Aneurysms, dissections, or vascular occlusions		

Needs during Transfer

Depending upon the patient's condition, the Paramedic may be required to perform different interventions during the course of the transfer. It is imperative that the Paramedic be appropriately trained and have the necessary equipment and authorization through guidelines to perform any skill that might be required during a patient transport.

Airway

Ideally, any airway concerns should be dealt with at the sending facility before the patient leaves. If the patient requires intubation, it should be accomplished in the controlled setting of the hospital rather than in a moving vehicle. There are, however, times when patient deterioration makes airway management during transport necessary.

Intubation

A Paramedic staffing an interfacility transport should be skilled at endotracheal intubation as well as use of secondary airway devices. Continuous waveform capnography is becoming the standard of care for tube confirmation, especially during movement of the patient (Figure 19-4).

Breathing

If a patient is intubated before or during a transport, the most consistent way to provide effective ventilations is by using a ventilator. Transport ventilators vary from the most simple unit offering only basic settings to fully programmable models with as many options as intensive care unit ventilators.

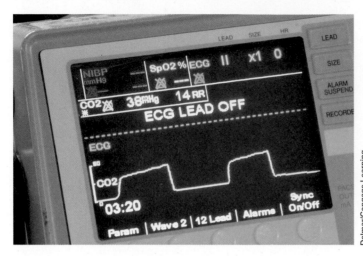

Figure 19-4 Continuous capnography is the standard of care for intubated patients during transport.

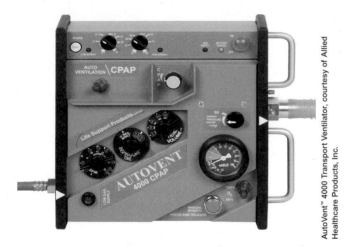

Figure 19-5 A Paramedic should be competent in the use of the ventilator utilized by his agency.

The Paramedic must be adept at managing the ventilator that she will be expected to use during a transport (Figure 19-5).

Chest Tube

A patient with a pneumothorax or hemothorax might benefit from decompression of the pleural space prior to transport. This is done via tube thoracostomy and is part of the stabilizing therapy a hospital may perform prior to transport. The Paramedic places a tube between the patient's ribs (most commonly in the 4th or 5th intercostal space at the anterior axillary line) in order to evacuate air or fluid from the pleural cavity. The tube is sutured in place and connected to a water-sealed suction device to allow continuous drainage. Evacuation of pneumo- or hemothorax can allow more effective pulmonary function.

Upon assessing the patient with a chest tube in place, the Paramedic should assess the insertion site to be certain that the drainage holes are not outside the chest wall. These drainage holes must be within the pleural cavity in order for the tube to be effective. (If the holes are found outside the chest wall, the tube must be replaced. A tube must never be inserted further into the chest wall once the original sterile field has been broken.) The Paramedic should dress the insertion site with an occlusive dressing and secure it well with tape.

The Paramedic should securely tape the connection between the chest tube and the evacuation system as well. There are several different brands of evacuation system. Some use water to measure the prescribed amount of pressure, whereas others are waterless. Generally, continuous suction and a position below the level of the insertion site is required to obtain adequate drainage. A chest tube or drainage system should never be clamped or allowed to become kinked. The Paramedic should familiarize himself with the drainage system most commonly used in his area of practice.

Circulation

Hospitalized patients may have vascular devices in place that the Paramedic does not commonly encounter. If the Paramedic's scope of practice is designed to manage patients with these devices in place, she should be provided training to become competent in their use.

Intravenous Devices

When peripheral intravenous access is impossible or simply insufficient for a patient's condition, the Paramedic may place central venous catheters. These can take many forms but are most commonly large bore and placed in the femoral, subclavian, or internal jugular veins. These catheters must be sterilely dressed and secured into place either with sutures, tape, or both. These centrally placed intravenous catheters, sometimes called "central lines," can be used to administer medications and fluids directly into the central circulation. In hospitals, they are also used for blood sampling.

Hemodynamic Monitoring

In addition to offering the Paramedic access to the central circulation for medication administration, central venous catheters can be utilized to measure the central venous pressure. This can be accomplished by attaching the line to a transducer, which is leveled at the phlebostatic axis, and utilizing an appropriate monitoring unit (Figure 19-6). Any transduced monitoring lines should be leveled, zeroed, and calibrated at the time of the initial assessment as well as whenever needed during transport. A pressure bag is typically applied to the flush solution and is set most commonly at 300 mmHg.

Arterial Line

Catheters can also be placed into an artery, most commonly the radial or femoral artery, for the purpose of monitoring intra-arterial pressure. This device allows the continuous

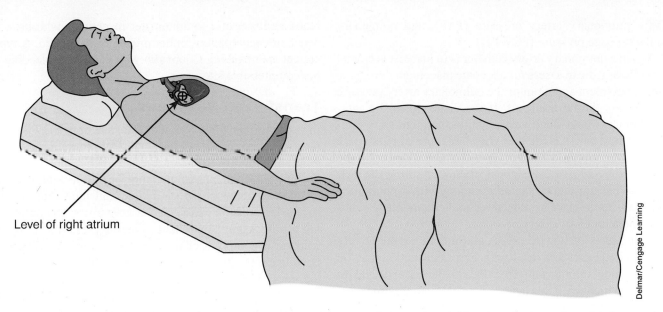

Figure 19-6 When monitoring an invasive line, the transducer should be leveled to the phlebostatic axis located at the level of the patient's right atrium.

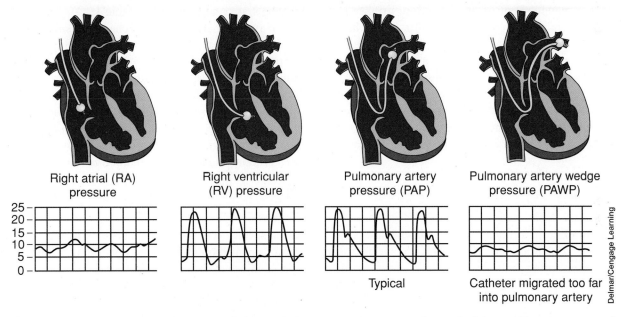

Figure 19-7 Continuous monitoring of the pulmonary artery waveform is imperative to recognize inadvertent catheter migration.

measurement of systolic, diastolic, and mean arterial pressures through monitoring of a waveform. When assessing the patient with an arterial catheter in place, the Paramedic should pay careful attention to the vascular function distal to the device. She should note any change and communicate them immediately to a physician. The Paramedic should sterilely dress the site and secure the line well with sutures, tape, or both. All arterial lines should be attached to a transducer and continually monitored. Tubing should remain free of air and all connections should be tight. At the time of the initial assessment, and occasionally during transport, the Paramedic should compare the arterial pressure with a cuff pressure to assure accuracy. If the waveform is crisp and the transducer is leveled and zeroed, the arterial pressure should be the most accurate means of determining blood pressure.

Pulmonary Artery Catheter

In patients who require continuous monitoring of various hemodynamic measures, the Paramedic may utilize a pulmonary artery catheter (Figure 19-7). This larger bore central catheter is placed in the subclavian or internal jugular vein and advanced through the right atrium, the right ventricle, and into the pulmonary artery. In this position, it can be utilized to monitor several parameters: central venous pressure

(CVP), pulmonary artery pressure (PAP), and pulmonary capillary wedge pressure (PCWP).

When a pulmonary artery catheter is in place, it is crucial for the Paramedic to assess for adequate placement during the initial assessment and monitor the pulmonary artery pressure continuously during transport. If the distal tip of the catheter migrates into a small vessel within the pulmonary arterial system, it can occlude that vessel, leading to pulmonary infarction or rupture of the artery. Migration can easily be recognized by a loss of waveform when monitoring the PAP. Under no circumstances should a patient with a pulmonary artery catheter in place be moved without continuously monitoring the pulmonary artery pressure.

The details of how to assess and monitor a pulmonary artery catheter are best dealt with in a dedicated course on hemodynamic monitoring. If a Paramedic is expected to manage a patient with this device in place, such training must be made available.

Urinary Catheter

Although the concept is simple, most Paramedic courses do not review the management of an indwelling urinary catheter. This device is placed within the urethra and is held in place with a saline-filled balloon located within the bladder. The catheter is typically attached to a drainage bag that should be hung at a level below the patient to allow for continuous drainage. During patient movement, the Paramedic should assure that the urinary catheter is well secured to avoid accidental displacement. During longer transports, the hourly urinary output is very useful in judging the patient's fluid status.

Blood Products

Regulations vary from state to state regarding Paramedic administration of blood products. If local laws allow for this practice, strict guidelines will likely be in place to assure appropriate monitoring and use of this scarce resource. Appropriate training and credentialing is imperative before the Paramedic becomes involved in transfusion of blood or blood products. Local guidelines are likely specific and should be abided by at all times. The goal should be to safely and appropriately utilize this resource to benefit the patient during interfacility transport.

Indications

The most common blood component administered in an emergency situation is packed red blood cells. A sufficient amount of red blood cells, the oxygen-carrying component of blood, is required to perfuse the body's vital tissues. A patient with witnessed or suspected blood loss with symptoms of hypoperfusion might benefit from infusion of one or more units of packed red blood cells.

Perhaps the next most common blood component required during interfacility patient transport is fresh frozen plasma (FFP). The plasma contains the clotting factors in the blood and is useful to administer to patients who have evidence of coagulopathy, either proven or suspected. A typical patient is one taking Coumadin who has active bleeding in a noncompressible site.

Transfusion Reactions

In order to recognize a transfusion reaction, the Paramedic must known the patient's baseline. Therefore, prior to beginning any blood transfusion, the Paramedic must assess and document the patient's temperature, heart rate, blood pressure, respiratory rate, oxygen saturation, and lung sounds. These parameters must be reassessed at least every 15 minutes during a transfusion. Any changes may represent a transfusion reaction or simply a change in the patient's condition. If a transfusion reaction is suspected, the Paramedic should stop the transfusion immediately and assess and document vital signs. She should then remove the blood bag and tubing and set it aside for delivery to the receiving blood bank for evaluation. The patient should be supported as indicated in local protocols.

Several types of transfusion reactions may be seen, with varying signs and symptoms (Table 19-4).

In order to minimize the chance of inappropriate unit administration, it is imperative that two persons confirm the patient's name and blood type, the unit's blood type, the unit number, and the expiration date prior to administration. Blood should be administered in a dedicated intravenous line with only normal saline solution running. Additionally, blood products must be packaged for transport in a way that maintains their integrity. Most blood banks certify the units for up to four hours when properly maintained in a cooler.

Disability

Monitoring of a patient's neurologic status is important in all patients; however, the details and means of monitoring this status become somewhat more specific in patients with neurologic injury during interfacility transport.

Neurologic Monitoring

Baseline assessment of a patient's neurologic status on the AVPU scale, as well as the Glasgow Coma Scale, should be a part of the Paramedic's initial assessment as well as the ongoing assessment of any patient, including those being moved between hospitals. More complex monitoring devices are sometimes utilized when more exact monitoring is required or sedation or chemical paralysis makes mental status and GCS impossible to monitor. These invasive monitoring devices are known as intracranial pressure monitors (Figure 19-8) and should only be managed by providers credentialed in their use. An intracranial pressure monitor includes a tube inserted into the cranial vault that is attached to a pressure tubing system. This device can be transduced in much the same way as the hemodynamic monitoring devices discussed earlier. This device should be monitored according to the patient-specific orders and changes responded to as indicated.

Table 19-4 Overview of Transfusion Reactions

Type	Onset	Cause	Signs and Symptoms	Treatment
Febrile	First 15 minutes	Presence of bacterial pathogens, sensitivity to leukocytes/platelets, hemolytic episode	Fever and shaking chills within 30 minutes Shock ensues	NSS infusion Tylenol Dopamine Systemic support
Allergic	15 to 30 minutes	Sensitivity to plasma protein	Hives Generalized itching Wheezing Anaphylaxis	Benadryl If patient has history of prior reactions, premedication considered
Septic	15 to 30 minutes	Contaminated with bacteria	Chills High fever Vomiting/diarrhea Hypotension	NSS infusion Dopamine Solumedrol
Hemolytic	30 minutes	Blood incompatible with patient	Chills Low back pain Headache Nausea Chest pain Fever Hypotension Vascular collapse	NSS infusion Dopamine

Exposure

Recent literature indicates that there may be some situations where controlled hypothermia might be of benefit to some patients. Outside of these specific circumstances, it is generally unwise to allow a patient to become hypothermic. During interfacility transport, patients are often wearing only a hospital gown and may or may not be covered in blankets. It is important for the Paramedic to take measures to prevent the patient from suffering a temperature loss during transport.

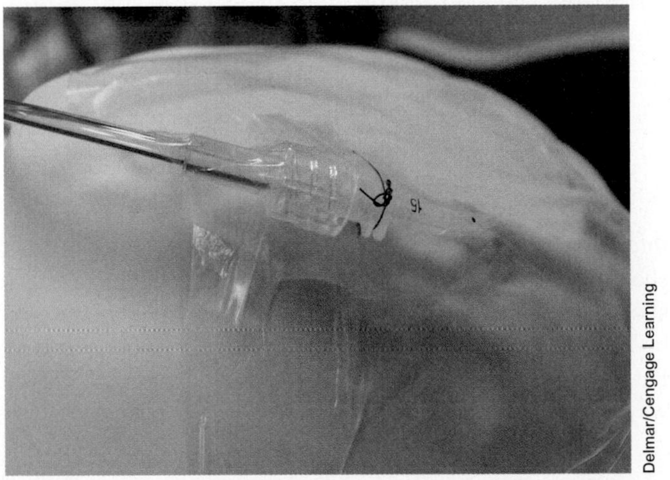

Delmar/Cengage Learning

Figure 19-8 An intracranial pressure monitor provides a quantitative measure of the intracranial pressure.

Simple measures such as covering the patient when exposure is not necessary and maintenance of a reasonable ambient temperature within the transport vehicle can help to prevent loss of body heat. This becomes very important during extremes of weather and during extended transports.[4]

Vehicles

The type of vehicle used to move a patient during an interfacility transport will depend upon the patient's condition, the distance to the receiving center, and the staffing configurations of local services.

Ground Ambulance

Most interfacility transports are completed by ground ambulance. The vehicle utilized must be large enough to accommodate the needed devices and staff and must be equipped with the necessary equipment for the patient's needs.

It should be intuitive, but is worth a reminder, that all personnel and equipment must be secured in the back of the vehicle when the vehicle is in motion. The patient's illness should never prompt a provider to make an unsafe decision for himself or his team.

Rotor Wing

Rotor wing transport vehicles are utilized when there is a need for emergent transfer of a patient in which out-of-hospital time must be minimized. The advantages of rapid flight without environmental obstacles make helicopter transport a good option when time is of the essence. Often, the providers staffing a helicopter service have advanced training and credentialing. The need for an advanced level of care during transport should be considered an indication for air medical transport when this is the case.

Fixed Wing

In cases where the transport distance is greater than the range of a rotor wing service, fixed wing transport might be considered.

System Considerations

As discussed earlier, system organization and planning is imperative to efficient functioning. As the need for more advanced care during interfacility transport has arisen, the planning for education and training of staff has lagged behind in some areas. The transport phase of care of a hospitalized patient must be considered when system planning is in progress.

Integration

Design of the interfacility transport system must be integral to both EMS system design as well as to hospital planning. Neither system should create this in isolation from the other. The ideal interfacility transport system has Paramedics training alongside hospital staff in order to best prepare them to care for hospitalized patients. This cooperative training will also provide hospital staff with an increased familiarity with the transport system and provider. This will be beneficial when a hospital staff member is needed to accompany a patient during a transport.

Preplanning

Cooperative training is one way to foster the relationship between the EMS system and the hospital system. Another important piece in the smooth operation of an interfacility transport system is preplanning. Physicians should be familiar with the capabilities of the transport system and understand the scope of practice of each provider involved. Written guidelines that detail the process of arranging and carrying out the safe transfer of a critically ill patient are helpful and lend to the system's efficiency.

CASE STUDY CONCLUSION

The Paramedic immediately recognizes that he needs help if he is going to safely complete this transport. He calls his supervisor and explains the situation. While the Paramedic completes his assessment of the child, his supervisor is able to speak with the sending physician. Once he explains that the patient's expected needs are more than a single provider can be expected to manage, the physician arranges for the emergency nurse who is caring for the patient in the emergency department to accompany the Paramedic on the transport.

CRITICAL THINKING QUESTIONS

1. What is the most appropriate transport decision that will get the patient to definitive care?
2. What are the advantages of transporting a patient with suspected significant head injury to a specialty care center, even if that means bypassing other hospitals in the process?

Future Directions

Consolidation of services will likely continue in the future, in an effort to make health care more efficient and cost effective. This will predictably result in an increased need for transfer of critically ill patients. Paramedics are ideally suited to practice in the transport environment and therefore are the most logical choice to staff such transports. Recognition of the interfacility transport as a time during which advanced care should be provided is important. The interfacility transport should be approached in such a way that the level of care will be maintained from one hospital to another. Advancement of Paramedic practice in cooperation with hospital staff is one way to accomplish that goal.

CONCLUSION

As regionalization of expensive medical therapies continues, the need for specialty care transportation will increase. Paramedics, trained above the standard Paramedic curriculum and practicing an advanced scope of practice, will be needed to take care of these complex patients while they travel between facilities.

KEY POINTS:

- Patients are transferred between facilities for several reasons: higher-level care, bed utilization, and personal preference.

- The concept of specialty hospitals (i.e., heart centers, stroke centers, trauma centers) have driven the need for interfacility transport.

- Centralization of hospitals brings together standardization of care, economies of mass, and higher level of care.

- The Emergency Medical Treatment and Active Labor Act provided the right to emergency medical care to every citizen regardless of ability to pay.

- All hospitals must "screen and stabilize" patients before transfer.

- Sending hospitals must provide certification of medical necessity that states the expected benefits outweigh the risks before transferring a patient.

- Consent must be obtained from the patient or healthcare proxy, or obtained under the emergency doctrine, before transfer.

- The sending hospital must arrange for appropriate transfer that includes stabilizing the patient to the extent possible given the sending hospital's resources, making arrangements with the receiving hospital for admission, transmitting data including medical images and laboratory results, and having appropriate personnel and supplies accompany the patient.

- The sending facility is legally responsible for the patient, including the care provided in transit, until the receiving hospital accepts the patient.

- EMTALA regulations pertain to unstable patients (i.e., those likely to deteriorate during transfer).

- Receiving hospital obligations include the ability and capacity to manage the patient's condition, regardless of ability to pay.

- Medically appropriate care during transfer includes staffing with personnel who have the level of training needed to manage complex unstable patients and who are credentialed to provide such care.

- Paramedics are not trained about hospital treatments and nurses are not trained to operate in the out-of-hospital environment. Cross-training is necessary to ensure the best patient outcomes during transfer.

- Even with additional training, the Paramedic may not have the expertise to care for special patient populations, such as neonates. In these cases, a specialty care team from the hospital is sent.

- Ongoing medical education is necessary for the specialty care Paramedic in order to maintain her proficiency and competency.

- Specialty care Paramedics still operate under on-line as well as off-line medical control (i.e., protocols and guidelines).

- During the transfer, the Paramedic must be able to manage the intubated airway, ventilators, chest tubes, intravenous devices including central lines, hemodynamic monitors, and even indwelling urinary catheters.

- Blood transfusions require special training and an ability to recognize transfusion reactions.

- Means of patient transfer are ground ambulance, rotor wing aircraft, and fixed wing aircraft.

- Preplanning is the key to a successful interfacility transfer.

REVIEW QUESTIONS:

1. Must a patient brought to a hospital helipad receive medical screening at that hospital before being permitted to lift off?

2. What are the obligations of the sending hospital before transferring a patient?

3. What does the certification of medical necessity provided by the sending hospital assure?

4. What skills must the specialty care Paramedic be able to perform?

5. Why must the Paramedic receive specialty care transport training?

CASE STUDY QUESTIONS:

Please refer to the Case Study in this chapter, and answer the questions below:

1. What impact would EMTALA have if the ambulance was hospital owned?

2. Does transfusion of blood complicate this patient's care?

3. What should the Paramedic do if he is not familiar with a drug such as propofol?

REFERENCES:

1. Bitterman RA. Providing emergency care under federal law: EMTALA. American College of Emergency Physicians, Irving, TX. 2001.

2. Beebe RW, Scadden J, Funk DL. *Fundamentals of Basic Emergency Care* (3rd ed.). Clifton Park, NY: Delmar-Cengage Learning; 2010.

3. NHTSA guide for interfacility patient transfer. Available at: **http://www.nhtsa.dot.gov/people/injury/ems/Interfacility/images/Interfacility.pdf.** Accessed September 2009.

4. Life Net of New York. Patient Care Guidelines 2007.

SECTION IV

EMERGENCY INCIDENT MANAGEMENT

Since Paramedics operate in a variety of conditions and situations, the Paramedic must be able to integrate medical care into a variety of special circumstances. This section begins with a general review of Incident Command and management, discussion of triage of patients in multiple-casualty situations, and review of paramedicine in the support of different operational situations, such as hazardous materials and Tactical Emergency Medical Services. These operational chapters provide the basics for the new Paramedic, but also demonstrate the breadth of paramedicine. During her career, a Paramedic may choose to specialize in one or more of these operational areas, deepening her knowledge and allowing her to serve as an expert for her agency.

CHAPTER 20

NATIONAL INCIDENT MANAGEMENT SYSTEM

KEY CONCEPTS:

Upon completion of this chapter, it is expected that the reader will understand these following concepts:

- Role of Paramedics at a large-scale incident
- Authority for the federal disaster response
- Elements of the federal disaster response
- The five essential elements of the National Incident Management System
- Elements of the federal disaster response

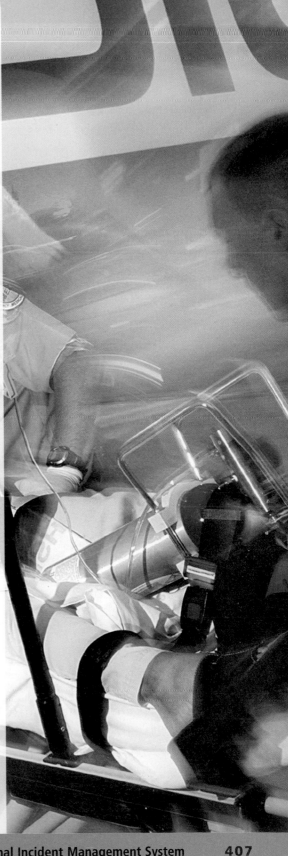

CASE STUDY:

"We've been called up by the Department of Health. They have activated the disaster response plan. I need volunteers, some to go to the quake center and others to work double shifts to cover those going to the quake center," Tom yells to the assembled workers. Even as Tom says the words, he realizes that he will not have enough resources to cover the call volume at home. Several of his employees, some as reservists and others as members of the disaster team, have already been deployed. The combination of layoffs from budget cuts and the hiring freeze has already left him strapped for providers.

CRITICAL THINKING QUESTIONS

1. What is the National Response Framework for a mass casualty incident?
2. What law empowers the federal government to activate reservists and disaster teams, as well as call for volunteers?

OVERVIEW

Paramedics need to understand their role when federal resources respond to a large-scale incident. Federal personnel, equipment, and training are necessary for local communities to effectively respond to, and recover from, catastrophic events. Although the concept that disasters in a certain area begin as local incidents remains valid, incidents that involve weapons of mass destruction, incidents that cross jurisdictional boundaries, or incidents that overwhelm local and state resources rapidly escalate into incidents of national importance.[1]

Several areas are called upon when there is a federal response to a local disaster. The first area, the authority that empowers the federal response, is found in law. The second, the **National Response Framework** (National Response Plan), describes the organization, concept of operations, and responsibilities of federal departments and agencies tasked to respond to a disaster. This includes the **Incident Command System (ICS)**, a flexible organizational structure that integrates personnel, facilities, procedures, and equipment to develop an effective response to emergencies, and the **National Incident Management System (NIMS)**, a system that coordinates emergency preparedness and responses between the local, state, and federal level. Finally, there are specific medical elements likely to support local responders during a federal response within the National Response Plan structure. Each one of these points will be explored within the chapter.[2]

Two additional concepts are also important to understand when discussing the federal disaster response. First, the federal government recognizes that disasters start as local events. The people who are affected will be the initial responders. Citizens and first responders will continue to be critical participants in the response and recovery after a disaster even when the scope of the problem exceeds local capacity.[3]

Second, the federal government has the authority to respond to catastrophic events that exceed local and state capability to mount an effective response. When a coordinated federal response is required, components of the National Response Plan are activated. In other words, local first responders and emergency managers need to be prepared to receive and coordinate with the hundreds or thousands of federal responders who will arrive when a National Response Plan response is activated.

STREET SMART

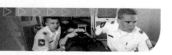

All EMS providers are expected to have taken the courses ICS-100-Introduction to Incident Command System and IS-700a-An Introduction to the National Incident Management System, and to keep that training up-to-date as updates come along.

Authority for Federal Disaster Response

The federal disaster response authority resides in various statutes, executive orders, and presidential directives. There are at least 15 principal emergency authorities and 20 presidential directives or orders that cover the federal response to date. Department of Defense resources used for disaster response are primarily addressed in eight separate authorizations. Although many authorities exist, three authorities are considered essential to the process (Table 20-1).

Table 20-1 Three Acts That Provide Federal Authority in National Disasters

1. Robert T. Stafford Disaster Relief and Emergency Assistance Act of 1974
2. Homeland Security Act of 2002
3. Post-Katrina Emergency Management Reform Act of 2007

Prior to 2002, the **Federal Emergency Management Agency (FEMA)** was the lead agency for federal emergency planning and response. However, that changed in 2002. The **Homeland Security Act (HSA) of 2002** established the **Department of Homeland Security (DHS)** and consolidated other federal components—including FEMA—into the DHS. Under the HSA, the DHS became the lead for the National Response Plan, and the National Incident Management System is now the FEMA administrator.

The Robert T. Stafford Disaster Relief and Emergency Assistance Act of 1974 (**Stafford Act**), as amended, covers all hazards and defines the processes for federal provisions of disaster assistance. For example, the Stafford Act defines the process a governor follows to request a presidential disaster declaration. The Stafford Act also allows for federal assistance without a governor's approval when necessary to save lives or if the incident is exclusively the responsibility of the United States.

The third core federal authority is the **Post-Katrina Emergency Management Reform Act (PKEMRA)**. In 2007, the PKEMRA modified the HSA to clarify FEMA's organization and responsibilities. Specifically, the PKEMRA required FEMA to coordinate precautionary evacuations including people with disabilities, children, pets, and service animals.

The roles of two military authorities are important to understand. The **Posse Comitatus Act** (18 U.S.C.) prevents the Army or Air Force from being used in a law enforcement capacity within the United States.[4] The Navy and Marine Corps are included in this directive through Department of Defense (DOD) regulations. However, exceptions to this policy may apply when specifically authorized by law or in the U.S. Constitution.

National Guard disaster authority is described in Titles 10 and 32 of the U.S.C. The National Guard may be called to national service under Title 10, U.S.C. In addition, governors are authorized to activate and command National Guard units under Title 32, U.S.C. Also under Title 32, U.S.C. National Guard units may be federalized while remaining under the governor's control. National Guard units activated under Title 32 U.S.C. are not subject to the restrictions of the Posse Comitatus Act.

Paramedics need to be aware of these laws because federal responders must perform within the restrictions or with the authority of the law. For instance, federal personnel are authorized to deploy into a potential disaster area prior to an incident and without the approval of local emergency managers when an incident is imminent, such as when a hurricane approaches landfall. Federal, state, and local public health coordination can begin without a formal disaster declaration.

Additionally, military restrictions can be difficult to understand. National Guard and active duty military wear the same uniforms, but can have different roles. National Guard personnel can be assigned law enforcement duties, whereas active duty personnel generally cannot assist with law enforcement activities. National Guard units will usually remain under the governor's command, whereas active duty units will remain under the military chain of command.

The federal response to disasters is complex. To be effective participants, Paramedics need to understand what is happening and why it is happening. All of the federal disaster authorities permit the federal government to push overwhelming resources into a local area. In disaster response, Paramedics work within a framework designed so that similar organization, terminology, and methods of communication are recognized regardless of where personnel are from.[5]

The National Response Framework

The National Response Plan represents the latest product in a dynamic and constantly evolving federal disaster planning sequence. In 1992, the **Federal Response Plan (FRP)** was signed and implemented as the guideline for a coordinated federal disaster response. The FRP, which was used for the response to Hurricane Andrew, can be considered the foundation of modern federal disaster planning documents. The Federal Response Plan was primarily designed to clarify the roles and responsibilities of the federal departments and agencies responding to catastrophic events.[6]

The Federal Response Plan evolved into the **National Response Plan** in 2004 after the terrorist attacks in September of 2001 demonstrated a need to integrate local, state, and federal disaster management and response concepts. The National Response Plan was published one year after the DHS became responsible for coordinating federal incident management. Hurricanes Katrina and Rita tested the policies and the lessons learned from these disasters resulted in the current National Response Plan.[7]

The National Response Plan is the federal all-hazards response guide required by **Homeland Security Presidential Directive (HSPD-5)**. National incident management policy and the mechanism for developing an operational structure for domestic incidents were refined into the National Response Plan because of HSPD-5 and feedback from emergency responders. The National Response Plan is built on a NIMS backbone so that there is incident management consistency across all jurisdictions. Following a disaster, federal responders expect EMTs from all parts of the country to interface using the principles established in NIMS.

Because the National Response Plan is flexible and scalable, a federal response can be limited to unique resources such as firefighting equipment for wildfires. However, when an incident has national or long-term consequences or results in catastrophic damage or loss of life, the weight of the entire federal system will be focused on the problem. The National Response Plan describes the way the federal resources will be organized and controlled regardless of the nature of the incident.

In anticipation of specific risks, the federal government is required under the National Response Plan to conduct plans for scenarios described in the **National Preparedness Guidelines** (Table 20-2).[8] These national planning scenarios are intended to focus local, state, and federal emergency managers on planning for incidents with potentially catastrophic consequences. The scenarios include both terrorist acts and natural disasters. Each community should have contingency plans including emergency medical services for the 15 scenarios.

The National Response Plan is activated when a state's governor requests federal disaster resources. Although catastrophic events require rapid interactions at all levels of government, movement of federal resources generally is delayed until the governor makes a request for assistance. Commonly, it is the perception of local first responders that communications between agencies are adequate to begin the process. Although mutual aid agreements existing between local and state jurisdictions can be used to mobilize local resources, the federal response requires specific notification and requests by the governor. Unfortunately, critical resources can be delayed unless the National Response Plan is activated appropriately.

Clearly, the local community retains the burden of recognizing that an event of national importance is occurring. A rapid, well-rehearsed local assessment of the situation is essential, and Paramedics have a central role in this assessment. Paramedics provide accurate, timely reports through the ICS to the **Emergency Operations Center (EOC)**, the centralized control facility responsible for emergency management

Table 20-2 The 15 Scenarios Found in the National Preparedness Guidelines

1. Improvised nuclear device
2. Aerosol anthrax
3. Pandemic influenza
4. Plague
5. Blister agent
6. Toxic industrial chemicals
7. Nerve agent
8. Chlorine tank explosion
9. Major earthquake
10. Major hurricane
11. Radiological dispersal device
12. Improvised explosive device
13. Food contamination
14. Foreign animal disease
15. Cyber attack

in the case of a disaster. When the local assessment indicates that resources will be needed from other jurisdictions, the chief presiding officer (i.e., mayor, chief executive) issues a disaster declaration which activates mutual aid plans and requests assistance from the state. The National Response Plan outlines the mechanism for federal plan activation and interaction with state, tribal, and local governments.

Although many first responders are government workers, the National Response Plan also recognizes the role of private businesses in disaster response. There is provision in the National Response Plan for information sharing and coordination of activities between the governmental responders and private entities. Prehospital medical equipment and personnel are parts of the local critical infrastructure and are important stakeholders in any disaster response regardless of whether they are in private or public organizations.

The National Response Plan provides a description of the roles and responsibilities of all federal departments and agencies. Although the secretary of homeland security is the federal official responsible for incident management, other departments will manage specific incident requirements. For example, the attorney general (AG) is the chief law enforcement officer of the country and retains responsibility for investigation of criminal acts such as terrorism. The attorney general typically performs this function through the Federal Bureau of Investigation (FBI).

When required, the secretary of defense provides military resources to support other federal departments and agencies. Defense resources are only committed with the approval of the secretary of defense or the president. A Department of Defense directive provides guidance for defense support to civilian authorities. Emergency managers must remember that military personnel deployed to a disaster remain under the command of the Department of Defense and perform tasks limited to those directed by the defense coordinating officer at the Joint Field Office (JFO).

Responders working in communities bordering Canada and Mexico should be aware of the secretary of state's role in managing international preparedness and response. Although most border communities have cross-border emergency plans approved by the state and federal governments, international solicitation of additional assistance not specified in existing international assistance agreements must be coordinated through the State Department.

The National Response Plan contains an **Emergency Support Function (ESF)** structure that provides the method for allocating federal resources during a disaster. The National Response Plan identifies 15 Emergency Support Functions (Table 20-3).[9] Each Emergency Support Function is associated with specific task-organized capabilities and is assigned a federal coordinating department or agency. The requirements for Emergency Support Function activation after an incident are determined based on responders' skills at gaining and maintaining situational awareness, assessment of the situation by emergency managers, and effective coordination of initial response actions.

Table 20-3 The 15 Emergency Support Functions

1. Transportation
2. Communications
3. Public Works and Engineering
4. Firefighting
5. Emergency Management
6. Mass Care, Housing, and Human Services
7. Resource Support
8. Public Health and Medical Services
9. Urban Search and Rescue
10. Oil and Hazardous Materials Response
11. Agriculture and Natural Resources
12. Energy
13. Public Safety and Security
14. Long-Term Community Recovery and Mitigation
15. External Affairs

Information about disasters is collected and analyzed at the National Operations Center (National Operations Center) managed by the Department of Homeland Security. Requests for federal assistance are routed to the National Operations Center using the Homeland Security Information Network. When an incident occurs, the National Operations Center notifies the other federal operations centers and coordinates information flow. Overall situational awareness and information collection is maintained at the National Operations Center.

Paramedics will be involved with several Emergency Support Functions. Emergency Support Function 8: Public Health and Medical Services includes public health, medical care, mental health services, and mortuary services. The Department of Health and Human Services (DHHS) is the designated coordinator for Emergency Support Function 8. The DHHS maintains the response plans for public health and medical emergencies. The National Disaster Medical System (NDMS) staff operates out of the DHHS. Paramedics should also be familiar with Emergency Support Function 4: Firefighting; Emergency Support Function 5: Emergency Management; Emergency Support Function 6: Mass Care, Housing, and Human Services; Emergency Support Function 9: Urban Search and Rescue; and Emergency Support Function 13: Public Safety and Security.

Paramedics in the disaster area must work closely with DHHS officials to coordinate an appropriate response to the incident. DHHS determines the federal medical resources required based on stated shortfalls, situation reports, and ongoing assessments from local emergency managers. When Emergency Support Function 8 is activated, local public and private medical departments and agencies should be prepared to assist DHHS in determining the Federal Capabilities needed to respond.[10]

A catastrophic event or an incident of national significance will be managed through a coordinating center established near the incident. Initially, the states communicate with the DHS/FEMA Regional Response Coordinating Center (RRCC) (Figure 20-1) to establish federal priorities for the response. There are eight DHS/FEMA regions, and each region maintains an RRCC at all times. As the response gains momentum, federal teams will be deployed in anticipation of

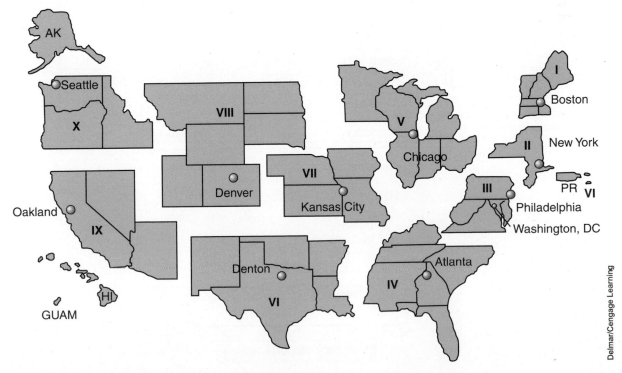

Figure 20-1 FEMA regional offices are located around the country.

establishing a **Joint Field Office (JFO)**, a shared command where two or more organizations pool their resources to put together an emergency response, using NIMS principles.

The structure for the federal disaster management organization in the affected region is based on National Incident Management System. In most cases, the federal organization will be a **Unified Command** (shared authority) because the disaster area crosses political boundaries and involves more than one agency with the authority to respond. For EMS personnel, an Incident Command, Area Command, and Local Emergency Operations Center will transmit information and make requests to the Emergency Support Function coordination site. Ultimately the Joint Field Office could include thousands of federal personnel, Figure 20-2, divided into geographically separate Emergency Support Function-based functional work areas (Figure 20-2). For instance, the Joint Field Office for Hurricane Andrew was located at the Miami International Airport and Emergency Support Function 8 operations were located in the South Dade Justice Center over 10 miles away.

The Joint Field Office is set up in a local secure facility or site to give federal, state, local, and tribal executives a place to conduct business related to the disaster. The Joint Field Office is a dynamic organization that adapts to the magnitude or complexity of the disaster. Multiple Joint Field Office's can be established when a disaster requires resources in several states or large metropolitan centers. Using NIMS span of control personnel management principles, the Joint Field Office can easily include thousands of people. The goal of the Joint Field Office is to provide the resources local commanders need to do their jobs. However, but the Joint Field Office does not manage on-scene operations.

A Joint Field Office coordinating group is assigned to assume functional authority for the incident. The Joint Field Office coordinating group contains several key people from the federal, state, and local jurisdictions. Policy conflicts, priorities of work, and decisions about allocating limited resources are brought to the Joint Field Office coordinating group. The chairperson, is the Principal Federal Officer (PFO), who is chosen by the Secretary for Homeland Security. The Principal Federal Officer coordinates federal incident management and assistance activities and is responsible for efficient coordination with the entire ICS/Unified Command structure. Generally, the Principal Federal Officer chooses the members of the Joint Field Office coordinating group.

The Joint Field Office coordinating group structure can expand to include a senior federal law enforcement official, a Federal Coordinating Officer (FCO), and other senior federal officials as required. Commonly, the Joint Field Office coordinating group includes state, local, and tribal officials as well as nongovernmental organizations and private-sector representatives. The work of the Joint Field Office is conducted by the Joint Field Office coordination staff.

A chief of staff leads the Joint Field Office coordinating staff. A large-scale incident requires a coordinating staff with liaison officers representing each member of the Joint

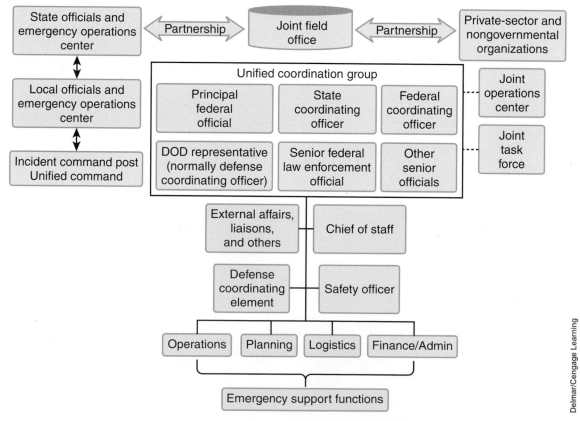

Figure 20-2 The JFO structure can include thousands of responders to an incident.

Field Office coordinating group as well as jurisdictional liaison officers. The staff typically includes a safety officer, legal affairs advisor, security officer, critical infrastructure liaison officer, defense coordinating officer, and external affairs officer.

The Defense Coordinating Officer serves as the Department of Defense's single point of contact at the Joint Field Office. All requests for Department of Defense assistance are routed to the Defense Coordinating Officer at the Joint Field Office. Since the Department of Defense supports all of the emergency support function operations, the Defense Coordinating Officer usually assembles a staff to coordinate directly with each emergency support Function. A request for Defense Support to Civil Authorities (DSCA) generated at the local level is generally driven through the officer in charge of the emergency support function to the Joint Field Office where the Defense Coordinating Officer assembles the requests and transmits them to the Director of Military Support (DOMS) in the Pentagon. The Director of Military Support assigns each requested and approved task to a service (i.e., Army, Navy, Air Force, Marines) where the appropriate material or personnel are allocated for transportation to the disaster area.

Since disasters are significant media events, responders need to understand the role of the public affairs officers.

The National Response Plan includes guidance for disseminating official information to the media. Generally, official information is released by the Joint Field Office to the **Joint Information Center (JIC)**, established by NIMS, where media representatives gather for press conferences and important messages. The joint information office is located near the Joint Field Office using Emergency Support Function 15 staff. Public affairs/public information officers (PA/PIO) meet at the Joint Information Center to provide official information and support to the media. The Joint Information Center is coordinated with state and local authorities. When an incident covers large areas, multiple JICs may be needed. Emergency personnel should refer media questions to the JIC for up-to-date and accurate information.

The National Incident Management System

The National Incident Management System (NIMS) operates within the National Response Plan and provides first responders with an interoperable approach to disaster management based on the ICS (Figure 20-3). Understanding NIMS makes it easier for first responders to scale their

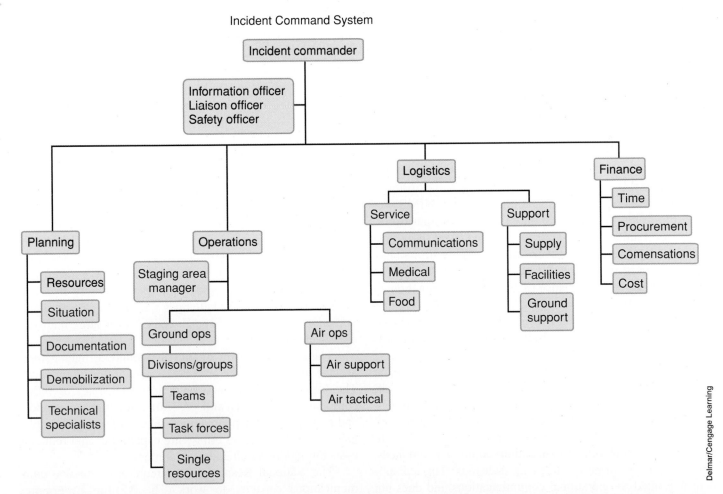

Figure 20-3 The ICS structure is the basis for NIMS interoperable approach to disaster management.

response up or down across jurisdictional and organizational lines. Since NIMS uses an "all-hazards" approach to preparedness, responders arriving at any type of disaster can expect to operate using the same doctrine, terminology, and command and control framework regardless of the type of incident.[11]

The National Preparedness Doctrine includes NIMS structure to ensure that unity of effort is applied through Unified Command. Regardless of the size of the event, each participating emergency responder should be coordinating activities in support of common objectives. This Unified Command concept is crucial for clarifying each responding organization's roles and responsibilities.

Unified Command allows all organizations to work with a single set of objectives regarding the preferred incident outcome. Using a collective strategic approach, responding organizations can establish clear priorities and restrictions. Unified Command improves communications and coordination between responders and jurisdictions without compromising responders' legal authorities. Finally, Unified Command optimizes the efforts of all responders under a single plan.

Conceptually, NIMS is proactive and includes five essential or key components: preparedness, communications and information management, resource management, command and management, and ongoing management and maintenance. Although NIMS institutionalizes these components for professional emergency managers, it is not a response plan. However, NIMS does offer principles allowing disaster responders and managers to establish an interoperable approach to communications and information management as well as standard procedures for coordinating resources.

Preparedness is an important component of NIMS, as it is related to all of the other key components. Mutual aid agreements including templates, types, and examples are described in this component. To understand the priority of resource allocation after a catastrophic incident, NIMS provides information on planning for **continuity of operations**, which will maintain national services in the event of a catastrophe, and **continuity of government**, which will maintain national leadership in the event of a catastrophe. Paramedics must recognize the importance of maintaining a functioning government and essential services. The preparedness component also describes the roles of nongovernmental organizations (NGOs) and the private sector in disaster preparedness activities.

The communications and information management (CIM) component of NIMS contains three sections. NIMS addresses the first responder requirement for reliable, redundant communications across the organizational spectrum. Emergency managers and responders are encouraged to establish standards for communications equipment and methods for using information to make decisions. This component is limited to operational communications and does not include public information.

The first CIM section is concepts and principles. This section deals with the importance of maintaining a clear communications concept of operations and interoperability. The NIMS emphasis is on establishing reliable and portable communications systems that include redundant networks. Anticipation that normal communications like landline telephones, cellular telephones, and daily emergency frequencies will be disrupted or destroyed is a principle particularly relevant to Paramedics.

The second CIM section is management characteristics. This section provides guidance for standardizing types of communications. Standards can include communications agreements between the stakeholders in the disaster plan as well as for communications training. The types of communications and the policies, plans, and procedures for their use in disasters are covered in this section.

The third CIM section in Communications and Information Management is organizations and operations. This section describes the way information is used and the format for transmitting information. First responders typically communicate using voice over radio or cellular telephone, but these messages can be transcribed, logged, and shared between operations centers in a disaster. Establishing standard formats for communications encourages timely decision making and allows information to be quickly shared between organizations.

The third component in NIMS is resource management. NIMS recognizes that resources need to be managed when preparing for, as well as while responding to, an incident. Since resources can be people, supplies, or equipment, their management can be complex as they flow between the federal, state, local, and private sectors. Disaster personnel organized under the federal umbrella require credentials. This component of NIMS describes the credentialing process as well, including diagrams demonstrating how resource requests flow between organizations in need and suppliers.

Command and management, the fourth component of NIMS, includes descriptions of the intelligence and information function, the incident command complex, area command, multiagency coordination, and public information. Much of this component deals with the realities faced during Hurricanes Katrina and Rita where multiple incidents in close proximity and challenges with multiple emergency operations centers and dispatch centers over large interstate areas were common.

The last component of NIMS is ongoing management and maintenance. There are two sections in this component. The National Integration Center is responsible for NIMS compliance, standards and credentialing, training support, and management of publications. The supporting technologies section focuses on improving capabilities and reducing costs through research and development.

The National Response Plan requires a massive communications capacity to work. The **Mobile Emergency and Response Support (MERS)** concept is the basis for maintaining federal communications in the field during a disaster response. Each of the MERS detachments can concurrently support a large JFO and multiple field operating sites within the disaster area. MERS is equipped with self-sustaining telecommunications, logistics, and operations support elements that can be driven or airlifted to the disaster location from six strategic locations.

MERS telecommunications assets can establish or reestablish communications connectivity with the public telecommunications system or government telecommunications networks. International Maritime Satellite (INMARSAT) and American Mobile Satellite Corporation (AMSC) satellite terminals provide immediate single voice channel capabilities. Line-of-sight microwave communications connect to the public network, and provide connection to other disaster management facilities. High frequency (HF) radio communication connects to federal, state, and local emergency centers via the FEMA National Radio Network and the FEMA Regional Radio Network. Very high frequency (VHF) and ultra high frequency (UHF) radios are used to connect to local emergency services communications systems.

Each MERS detachment supporting the JFO arrives with generators, as well as heating, ventilation, and air conditioning (HVAC) systems, adequate for a 16,000 square foot building. They also bring diesel fuel. Potable water is provided using reverse osmosis water purification units (ROWPU) that produce 300 to 480 gallons per hour.

Another special capability deployable by FEMA is the **Urban Search and Rescue (USAR)** task force (TF). These task forces contain local emergency services personnel who are equipped and trained to rescue patients of structural collapse as well as assist with other search and rescue missions. FEMA maintains 28 USAR task forces; they are established in such a way that they can be at an embarkation point within six hours of notification.[12]

The RRCC will deploy an **Incident Management Assist Team (IMAT)** to the state EOC and incident sites to assess the situation and determine immediate federal requirements. When the RRCC resources are overwhelmed, the Department of Homeland Security can deploy additional Incident Management Assist Team members. The Incident Management Assist Team contains subject matter experts and identifies facilities for potential federal field sites such as the Joint Field Office or Joint Information Center

Federal Medical Response Elements

Although the primary federal command and control structure is made up of the Joint Field Office, Joint Information Center, and Emergency Support Functions, there are many other federal teams and task forces able to rapidly move into a disaster area. Paramedics should be aware of federal teams specifically designed to deploy in support of Emergency Support

Function 8. Disaster Medical Assistance Teams, Veterinary Medical Assistance Teams, Disaster Mortuary Operational Response Teams, and National Medical Response Teams are examples of federal assets trained and equipped to respond to disasters.

The **Disaster Medical Assistance Team (DMAT)** is a component of the National Disaster Management System. The DMAT is designed to provide medical care during a disaster. A deployable DMAT usually includes about 30 volunteer personnel represented by physicians, nurses, pharmacists, Paramedics, logisticians, and administrators. DMATs are located in every state and may be the first federal medical response to a disaster when activated through local agreements. Paramedics will interface with the DMAT to provide evacuation of casualties to and from the site.

The DMAT concept includes both deployable teams with equipment and supplies and teams without equipment which are designed to augment or backfill previously deployed teams. Some DMATs are designed for special situations and are trained and equipped to support missions. For instance, some DMATs are uniquely capable of managing mental health concerns, crush injuries, or burns.

DMATs are designed to be quickly deployed to supplement local medical care. In fact, DMATs deploy to disaster sites with sufficient supplies and equipment for a period of 72 hours. Although many DMATs deploy with shelter systems, ideally the local emergency managers identify a building where the DMAT becomes operational.

In the event that a disaster results in overwhelming numbers of casualties, the DMAT may be required to establish an evacuation staging facility. One of the National Disaster Management System missions is evacuation of casualties from the affected area to unaffected regions of the nation. The DMAT is designated as a resource for managing the various evacuation medical staging facilities.[13,14]

The **Veterinary Medical Assistance Team (VMAT)** is also an National Disaster Management System resource. Veterinary Medical Assistance Team provides local emergency personnel with services unique to the effects of disasters on animals. In addition to the treatment of animals, Veterinary Medical Assistance Team conduct surveillance for animal disease outbreaks, assist with food and water inspections, and assist with animal decontamination. Veterinary Medical Assistance Team include veterinarians, veterinary pathologists, animal health technicians, disease specialists, epidemiologists, toxicologists, and support personnel.

The **National Pharmacy Response Teams (NPRT)** are located in each of the 10 federal regions. NPRTs assist in **chemoprophylaxis** (vaccination activities) when a disease outbreak or biological attack occurs. National Pharmacy Response Teams are composed of pharmacists, pharmacy technicians, pharmacy students, and support personnel. The National Pharmacy Response Teams is a National Disaster Management System resource.

A **Disaster Mortuary Operational Response Team (DMORT)** is also an asset of the National Disaster

Management System and serves to provide patient identification and mortuary services. DMORT is prepared to establish temporary morgue facilities; identify patients using forensic dental pathology and forensic anthropology methods; and process, prepare, and make disposition of remains. When deployed as part of a federal disaster response, the DMORT works under the guidance of local authorities, abiding by local laws regarding management of human remains.

DMORTs are composed of funeral directors, medical examiners, coroners, pathologists, forensic anthropologists, medical records technicians and transcribers, fingerprint specialists, forensic odontologists, dental assistants, X-ray technicians, mental health specialists, computer professionals, administrative support staff, and security and investigative personnel. To augment DMORT, FEMA maintains two Disaster Portable Morgue Units (DPMUs). The DPMUs contain a complete morgue with prepackaged equipment and supplies.

The **National Nurse Response Team (NNRT)** provides hundreds of nurses to assist in chemoprophylaxis, a mass vaccination program, or a scenario that overwhelms the nation's supply of nurses whenin responding to a disaster or terrorist event. The National Nurse Response Team is an asset of the National Disaster Management System. National Nurse Response Teams are identified in each of the 10 FEMA regions and contain about 200 nurses.

The **Strategic National Stockpile (SNS)** is designed to supplement and re-supply state and local public health agencies in the event of a national emergency. The Strategic National Stockpile contains antibiotics, chemical antidotes, antitoxins, life-support medications, IV and airway maintenance supplies, and other medical/surgical items. Strategic National Stockpile resources are prepositioned to be rapidly available by ground or air transportation.

The rapidly deployable Strategic National Stockpile packages are available anywhere in the country within 12 hours of a valid request by the state. When an incident exceeds the capability of the standard Strategic National Stockpile package, pharmaceuticals and/or medical supplies from vendor-managed inventory (VMI) are coordinated through the Strategic National Stockpile. Each state is required to have a plan to receive the Strategic National Stockpile and distribute its contents to the affected population within 48 hours of arrival.[15]

CHEMPACK, a component of the Strategic National Stockpile, establishes caches of antidotes for nerve agents and other toxins in selected cities. CHEMPACK supplies are controlled by the Centers for Disease Control (CDC) and stored by cooperating local health facilities. CHEMPACK resources may be released to Paramedics when local supplies are exhausted and criteria for their release have been satisfied. Local emergency managers are responsible for plans to mobilize and distribute the CHEMPACK to hospitals and first responders.

CHEMPACK is configured in two types of containers. One type of container is designed for EMS use, the other is designed for hospital use. The EMS container contains nerve agent antidote auto-injectors, whereas the hospital containers contain nerve agent antidote auto-injectors as well as bulk supplies with multi-dose vials and antidote administration sets. Each EMS container is configured to begin treatment for over 400 casualties. Each hospital container is configured to begin treatment for 1,000 casualties.

After the anthrax attacks on the postal system in 2001, the U.S. Postal Service (USPS) recognized the need to screen mail for biological warfare agents. The **Biohazard Detection System (BDS)** was designed to satisfy this mail surveillance requirement, as it. The Biohazard Detection System samples the air as mail is sorted to identify anthrax spores. USPS began deploying BDS to large sorting facilities in 2004, and plans to expand their BDS capability for other biological agents as well.

Emergency service personnel in communities where Biohazard Detection System is deployed are required to coordinate response plans in case of a Biohazard Detection System alarm. A Biohazard Detection System alarm kicks off a multiagency local, state, and federal response designed to contain anthrax in the postal facility, identify if the community is at risk, collect criminal evidence, and provide prophylaxis against anthrax infection to people who might have been exposed.

The federal government sponsors **Community Emergency Response Teams (CERT)** to augment emergency responders following a disaster. The Community Emergency Response Teams concept began in Los Angeles in 1985. Following an earthquake in 1987, authorities recognized the importance of training people in the community to meet their immediate needs before emergency responders arrive.

The original Community Emergency Response Teams materials were expanded by FEMA and the National Fire Academy to include all hazards and training materials that are available through the Emergency Management Institute.[16] Local programs are coordinated for the community by emergency services departments that provide equipment and training to volunteers. Volunteers who complete the training will be better prepared to respond to, and cope with, the aftermath of a disaster. Community Emergency Response Teams prepares people to help themselves, their families, and their neighbors in the event of a disaster in their community. Community Emergency Response Teams volunteers learn about disaster preparedness and basic disaster response such as fire safety, light search and rescue, and disaster medical operations. These Community Emergency Response Teams volunteers can provide critical neighborhood support by giving immediate assistance to patients before first responders arrive on the scene.

Community Emergency Response Teams can be a neighborhood, business, or government team that acts to augment responders. Community Emergency Response Teams provides immediate assistance in its area, organizes people to assist with rescue and scene safety, and assists emergency services with assessment of the extent of the disaster. Since 1993, when this training was made available nationally by FEMA, most states have conducted Community Emergency Response Teams training.[17]

The **Medical Reserve Corps (MRC)** program is a volunteer program for medical professionals administered by DHHS. Medical Reserve Corps. organizes public health, medical, and other volunteers who want to donate their time and expertise to prepare for, and respond to, emergencies. Volunteer Medical Reserve Corps. units accomplish this mission by supplementing existing emergency and public health resources during a disaster.[18]

CASE STUDY CONCLUSION

Tom continues, "While we are sending the ambulances, the equipment you will need is already there. The federal government has released the Strategic National Stockpile. Please keep track of what is being used."

Tom smiles as he looks over his shoulder. Several members of the Community Emergency Response Team have already shown up without being called. They will be a great asset in the days and weeks ahead, he thinks to himself.

CRITICAL THINKING QUESTIONS

1. What is the Strategic National Stockpile?
2. What is the Community Emergency Response Team?

CONCLUSION

Paramedics are on the front line of disaster response. When the disaster requires federal resources, familiarity with the National Response Framework, the National Incident Management System, and the Incident Command System will allow local Paramedics to integrate more effectively into the Unified Command structure. The national emergency response guidelines, policies, and procedures are dynamic and constantly evolving. Contemporary concepts are derived from past experience, current threats, and stakeholder input. Knowledge of the roles and responsibilities of responding federal resources will enhance emergency medical integration and effectiveness.

▶ KEY POINTS:

- The National Response Framework includes the Incident Command System and National Incident Management System.

- Disasters are, first, a local event. Local emergency responders will manage the problem until it exceeds local capacity.

- A multitude of authorities and directives permit federal response. Three key authorities are the Stafford Act, Post-Katrina Emergency Management Reform Act, and the Homeland Security Act of 2002.

- The Department of Homeland Security is the lead federal agency and includes the National Response Plan and National Incident Management System.

- State governors can declare an emergency, activating federal resources.

- The Posse Comitatus Act prevents the military from being used in law enforcement. The National Guard is exempted under Title 32 U.S.C.

- The National Response Plan, required by Homeland Security Presidential Directive-5, is the backbone of national preparedness and is an all-threats plan for 15 predictable disaster scenarios.

- Paramedic reports to the Emergency Operations Center, part of the Incident Command System, provide the chief executive with the information needed to declare an emergency and activates the federal response.

- The attorney general, through the Federal Bureau of Investigation, retains responsibility for criminal investigation.

- The defense coordinating officer, through the authority of the secretary of defense or the president, manages the response of federal troops via the Joint Field Office.

- The National Response Plan has 15 Emergency Support Functions. Each allocates specific federal resources. Emergency Support Function 8 is Public Health and Medical Services and is coordinated by the Department of Health and Human Services.

- The National Disaster Medical System functions under the Department of Health and Human Services as part of Emergency Support Function 8.

- Incident Command and/or Area Command, if one exists, and local emergency operations centers make requests for emergency support to the JFO, a shared or Unified Command under the JFO coordinating group. The principal federal officer is in command of the Joint Field Office coordinating group.

- The public affairs/public information officer in the Joint Information Center disseminates official reports about the status of the response to a disaster.

- Unified Command is part of the National Incident Management System and permits all organizations/services to operate with one set of objectives.

This collective strategy approach helps ensure adequate resources and proper priorities.

- The National Incident Management System consists of preparedness, communications and information management, resource management, command and management, and ongoing management and maintenance.

- Preparedness includes mutual aid plans, continuity of operations, and continuity of government. Preparedness also deals with the private sector (i.e., nongovernmental organizations such as the American Red Cross).

- Communications and information management includes emergency communications with an emphasis on reliability and redundancy.

- Resource management includes personnel and credentialing.

- Command and management deals with the incident command complex, multiagency coordination, and public information.

- Ongoing management and maintenance includes the National Integration Center, which deals with standardization and credentialing for interagency operability of supplies and equipment.

- A Mobile Emergency and Response Supports detachment is a self-sustaining telecommunications, logistics, and operations support unit strategically located in areas throughout the United States.

- An Urban Search and Rescue task force is a deployable FEMA unit used in building collapses.

- Federal disaster response, as part of the National Disaster Management System, includes the Disaster Medical Assistance Team, Veterinary Medical Assistance Team, National Pharmacy Response Team, Disaster Mortuary Operational Response Team, and the National Nurse Response Team.

- The Strategic National Stockpile divides supplemental supplies to the disaster and contains the CHEMPACK.

REVIEW QUESTIONS:

1. What is the federal government's authority during a disaster?
2. What act prevents the federal government from using the military for law enforcement?
3. What provides uniformity in the National Response Plan?
4. What Emergency Support Functions listed in the National Response Plan pertain to EMS?
5. How could "volunteers" from the community help at a disaster?

CASE STUDY QUESTIONS:

Please refer to the Case Study in this chapter, and answer the questions below:
1. What are the three conditions that would necessitate a federal response to a disaster?
2. What part of the National Response Plan is the "disaster team"?
3. What is the Strategic National Stockpile?

REFERENCES:

1. Kahsai D, Kare J. Prehospital disaster management; implications for weapons of mass destruction. *Top Emerg Med*. September 2002;24(3):37–43.

2. Hardin E. Disaster planning and management. *Top Emerg Med*. September 2002;24(3):71–76.

3. Auf der Heide E. *Disaster response: principles of preparation and coordination*. St. Louis: Mosby,1989.

4. Furman HWC. Restrictions upon use of the Army imposed by the Posse Comitatus Act. *7 Mil. L. Rev*. 1960;85:85.

5. Bullock JA, Haddow GD. *Introduction to Emergency Management* (3rd ed.). *Butterworth–Heineman Homeland Security Series*. Burlington, MA: Elsevier; 2008.

6. FEMA. Federal Response Plan (PL 93-288). *FEMA*. 1992.

7. Auf der Heide E. The importance of evidence-based disaster planning. *Ann Emerg Med*. 2006;47(1):34–49.

8. Department of Homeland Security, Accession number ADA506960, September 2007.

9. Emergency Support Function Annexes Introduction. June 2008. Available at: **http://www.fema.gov/pdf/emergency/nrf/ nrf-esf-intro.pdf**. Accessed September 29, 2009.

10. Ousley E, Syama A, Dang C. Public health issues of a disaster. *Top Emerg Med*. September 2002;24(3):56–60.

11. Bigley G, Roberts K. The Incident Command System: High-reliability organizing for complex and volatile task environments. *Acad Manage J*. 2001;44(6):1281–1299.

12. Phillip H, Sunshine W. Urban Search and Rescue. *Top Emerg Med*. September 2002;24(3):26–36.

13. Henderson A, et al. Disaster Medical Assistance Teams: providing healthcare to a community struck by Hurricane Iniki. *Ann Emerg Med*. 1996;23(4):726–730.

14. Cohen S, Mulvaney K. Field observations: Disaster Medical Assistance Team response for Hurricane Charley. Punta Gorda Florida. *Disaster Manag Response*. August 2004;3(1):22–27.

15. Esbitt D. The Strategic National Stockpile: roles and responsibilities of healthcare professionals receiving the stockpile assets. *Disaster Manag Response*. 2003;1(3):68–70.

16. Emergency Management Institute website. Available at: **http:// training.fema.gov/**. Accessed September 29, 2009.

17. Durham B, Williams J. Civilian preparedness: disaster planning for everyone. *Top Emerg Med*. September 2002;24(3):66–70.

18. Hoard M, Tosatto R. Medical Reserve Corps: strengthening public health and improving preparedness. *Disaster Manag Response*. 2005;3(2):48–52.

CHAPTER 21

EMERGENCY RESPONSE TO TERRORISM

KEY CONCEPTS:

Upon completion of this chapter, it is expected that the reader will understand these following concepts:

- Danger terrorism presents to emergency responders
- Definition of terrorism
- Categories of terrorist groups
- Paramedic responses to terrorism
- Types of harm caused by terrorism
- Specific forms of terrorism (B-NICE)
- Signs, symptoms, and emergency care of terrorism patients

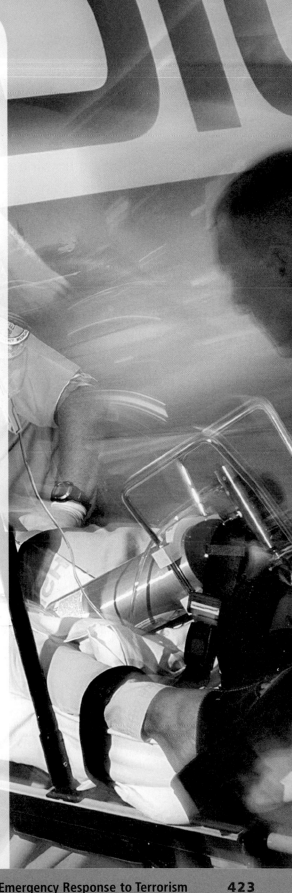

CASE STUDY:

The call comes in for "multiple patients with vomiting." The Paramedic turns to her partner and says, "Multiple patients, hmmmm. What do you think? Maybe we should stage and wait for the fire department hazmat to confirm?"

CRITICAL THINKING QUESTIONS

1. What is the implication of multiple patients presenting with the same symptom pattern?
2. Why did the Paramedic want to stage and await confirmation?

OVERVIEW

No matter the emergency, the Paramedic's first responsibility is always personal safety. Certain situations can put that to the test. On March 20, 1995, terrorists released sarin gas into a Tokyo subway, killing 12 people and injuring 5,498, including 135 firefighters. This event, among many others, illustrates the dangers terrorism presents to EMS.[1]

The lesson hit closer to home in January of 1997. Several responders, who had come to assist with care following a bombing at an Atlanta abortion clinic, became patients themselves when a second bomb detonated in the proximity of the command post, injuring several responders. The secondary device was specifically targeted at first responders.[2]

The death toll at Columbine High School in Littleton, Colorado, on April 20, 1999, may have been greater if any one of the several bombs placed in and around the high school had detonated, as they would have killed or severely incapacitated many of the first responders.[3]

However, the events of September 11, 2001, clearly drive home why it is important for the Paramedic to understand terrorism. Hundreds of emergency responders were injured that day and 450 died, one-sixth the total number killed at the World Trade Center.[4]

As illustrated by these examples, many of the nation's first responders may respond to what sounds like an ordinary call, only to find out later that they have been exposed to a terrorist incident.[5] Since September 11, 2001, the world in which the Paramedic works has changed in many ways. Those Paramedics who believed they were already in high-risk professions now find themselves faced with new, unknown threats.[4] The attacks on that infamous day changed how first responders and EMS organizations go about their daily routines, as many now feel especially vulnerable to terrorism.

Even before the events of September 11, experts in both the emergency response and national security fields had stated for years the need to increase the Paramedics' readiness to respond to potential acts of terrorism.[6] To do so, the Paramedic must possess an understanding of terrorism that extends beyond simply what actions can hurt the Paramedic.

What Is Terrorism?

Since the events on September 11, 2001, the word "terrorism" has become a household term. However, its roots go much farther back, deriving from the Latin term *terrere*, meaning "to frighten." In 105 B.C., the Cimbri, a Germanic tribe, along with the Teutones and the Ambrones, threatened the Roman Republic. The Romans, fearing for their lives, developed a sense of widespread panic along with a general state of emergency. This panic was known as the terror cimbricus.[7]

In the eighteenth century, the term "terrorism" was first used to describe the reign of terror that the Jacobins incited during the French Revolution.[8] The "Reign of Terror" lasted for 13 months (June 27, 1793, to July 27, 1794) and involved the recorded execution by guillotine of at least 16,594 people who had opposed the revolution or were considered enemies of it, the most well-known being Marie Antoinette.[9] To help entrench their revolutionary government, the Jacobins used public trials and executions to "strike terror in the hearts of all who lacked civic virtue."[8] From that point forward, people were *terrified* to speak against the revolution.

Defining Terrorism

Defining terrorism using a single phrase or paragraph is not an easy task. Over 100 different definitions of the word have been published throughout the years by numerous individuals.[7]

A philosophical definition, as cited by Per Bauhn in the article *Terrorism,* defines **terrorism** as ". . . performance of violent acts, directed against one or more persons, intended by the performing agent to intimidate one or more persons and thereby to bring about one or more of the agent's political goals."[8]

Another philosophical definition, created by C. A. J. Coady, is "the tactic of intentionally targeting non-combatants . . . with lethal or severe violence . . . meant to produce political results via the creation of fear."[8] The United Nations (UN) has also made numerous attempts to define terrorism, but to this point the member states have had difficulty coming to a consensus.

One of the main issues that arises when trying to define terrorism is that "one man's terrorist is another man's freedom fighter." Consider the actions of American soldiers during the Revolutionary War.[7] The British most likely considered them acts of terrorism. Yet, those labeled as a terrorist by one organization or government may not see themselves as evil but rather fighting a just fight for their cause using whatever means are possible.[10] The difference in perception comes from the individual defining the actions.

Freedom fighting is generally aimed at a government, as the attackers are hoping to destroy what they feel is an unjust social or political system. In contrast, terrorists are indiscriminant, often attacking the general population in order to obtain their goal. This confusion and grayness between freedom fighter and terrorist causes news services, such as Reuters, to avoid using either term, preferring to use "bomber" or "militants" instead.[7]

Alex P. Schmid, a Dutch terrorism scholar and former officer-in-charge of the Terrorism Prevention Branch of the United Nations, was instrumental in developing an academic consensus definition for terrorism in 1988:

> "Terrorism is an anxiety-inspiring method of repeated violent action, employed by (semi-) clandestine individual, group or state actors, for idiosyncratic, criminal or political reasons, whereby—in contrast to assassination—the direct targets of violence are not the main targets. The immediate human victims of violence are generally chosen randomly (targets of opportunity) or selectively (representative or symbolic targets) from a target population, and serve as message generators. Threat- and violence-based communication processes between terrorist (organization), (imperiled) victims, and main targets are used to manipulate the main target (audience(s)), turning it into a target of terror, a target of demands, or a target of attention, depending on whether intimidation, coercion, or propaganda is primarily sought."[8]

Schmid's simple, direct, and legal way of defining acts of terrorism as peacetime equivalents of war crimes has become legally recognized internationally.[11]

No matter how the term is defined or who defines it, each definition found typically includes the terms "violence" and "intimidation." Simply put, terrorism invokes images of violence. This violence is not used indiscriminately but, instead, is strategically designed to coerce or further someone's political, social, or religious agenda through intimidation.[8]

There is still a need to establish a base definition of terrorism for the purpose of discussion. Referencing the *Code*

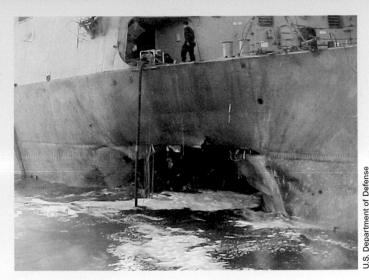

Figure 21-1 This damage was produced in the hull of the *USS Cole* as a result of terrorism.

of Federal Regulations (28 C.F.R. Section 0.85), the United States Department of Justice, Federal Bureau of Investigation (FBI), has defined terrorism as "the unlawful use of force and violence against person or property to intimidate or coerce a government, the civilian population, or any segment thereof, in furtherance of political or social objectives." Defining terrorism more specifically requires that the incident location as well as the terrorist's country of orgin be known.

Terrorism: International vs. Domestic

International terrorism is defined by the FBI as "violent acts to human life that are violations of the criminal laws of the United States . . . acts occur outside the United States or transcend national boundaries in terms of the means by which they are accomplished, the persons they appear intended to coerce or to intimidate, or the locale in which their perpetrators operate or seek asylum" (Figure 21-1).[12]

Domestic terrorism, however, is the result of an attempt by an individual or group to intimidate or coerce the government or its people in furtherance of political or social objectives. These groups are based and operating, without foreign direction, entirely within the United States or Puerto Rico.[12] After September 11, 2001, the passage of the USA Patriot Act further defined domestic terrorism in a much broader sense as any criminal acts that are dangerous to human life and appear to be meant to scare civilians or affect policy.[13]

Terrorism at Home

The idea of terrorism on the home front is not a new concept. In fact, it dates back over a century. For example, William McKinley, the twenty-fifth president, was shot by an anarchist named Leon Czolgosz shortly after McKinley began his second term as president in 1901.[13] Czolgosz's reasoning for assassinating President McKinley was that, in his opinion, one man should not hold office for more than one term as it prevents someone else from being president.[14]

The FBI reports that between 2002 and 2005 there were 24 terrorist attacks on domestic soil and that 23 of those attacks were perpetrated by domestic terrorists. Special interest groups such as animal rights and environmental activists perpetrated 22, whereas eight of the 14 thwarted attacks were from right-wing extremists such as the white supremacists.

Who Are the Terrorists?

Domestic terrorists are extremists[13] who believe that their views and beliefs are the way to a better world and that others should follow the same paths.[15] They use extreme measures to obtain their objectives, usually acting with violence. Domestic terrorists can be categorized by their views and beliefs into three categories: left-wing extremists, right-wing extremists, and special interest groups.[13]

Left-Wing Extremists

During the spring of 1886, anarchists joined several other groups in Chicago's Haymarket to protest in favor of an eight-hour workday. Violence erupted several times, causing police to shoot into the protestors, killing at least two. The crowd reconvened on May 4 and, when a speaker urged the crowd to "throttle the law" as police were attempting to disperse the crowd, someone threw a bomb at the officers, killing one. The ensuing battle caused additional deaths, wounded countless others, and raised fears among business owners that the labor movement was growing with radical influence.[16] These East European immigrants, sympathetic to the international anarchist movement, had started what is thought to be the first wave of domestic left-wing terrorism in the United States.[13]

The left-wing extremists are traditionally anticapitalists[13] with some having an anarchist philosophy, in which they reject the idea of private property and organized government.[17] In the mid- to late 1960s and early 1970s, left-wing extremism experienced a resurgence as groups such as the Weather Underground (WU), Symbionese Liberation Army (SLA), and Armed Forces for Puerto Rico National Liberation (FALN) began using terrorism to bring attention to their radical ideas.[13]

The Weather Underground, formally the Weathermen, were a violent offshoot of a 1960s group called the Students for a Democratic Society (SDS). Their goal was to promote social change, but their organization collapsed in 1969. However, the WU remained quite active throughout the 1970s as they used terrorism to promote communist ideologies while protesting against the Vietnam War and racism.[18] Their ultimate intentions were to place chemical and biological agents into urban water supplies, thereby disrupting government and temporarily incapacitating major U.S. cities.[19] By 1975, the WU claimed responsibility for 25 bombings, and orchestrated several more during the next several years.[18]

By the 1980s, the majority of the left-wing terrorism had begun to diminish, and they currently pose much less of a threat today. The FBI warns, however, that even though their activity level is down, these organizations still pose a potential threat. In fact, much of the damage that occurred from the street protests at the 1999 World Trade Organization meeting in Seattle, Washington, was the result of left-wing extremists.[13]

Right-Wing Extremists

On April 19, 1995, right-wing extremist Timothy McVeigh—who feared the increased involvement of the United Nations in domestic policies, opposed stricter gun legislation, and was angry over the events and outcomes of Waco and Ruby Ridge—parked a Ryder truck carrying agricultural fertilizer, diesel fuel, and other chemicals in front of the Alfred P. Murrah Federal Building in downtown Oklahoma City. At 9:02 a.m., the truck detonated, taking down one-third of the building. The blast killed 168 people and wounded countless others. Convicted of the crime, McVeigh—the ex-Army soldier and security guard—was sentenced to death and executed in 2001.[20]

During the 1990s, the right-wing extremist movement began to grow, blending political rhetoric with racial undertones. The right-wing cherishes individual freedoms over government regulations, and often declares a racist and radical supremacy while embracing antigovernment and antiregulatory platforms. Two of the most currently active right-wing groups are the anti-abortionists and the self-proclaimed militia. Although each has their share of nonviolent organizations to promote their ideals, the focus here is upon the violent, or terrorist, factions of these groups. Merely having these beliefs and expressing extreme right-wing political ideas does not make one a terrorist. Only when violence and intimidation are used does this description fit.[13]

Although terrorist attacks by right-wing extremists have steadily declined since September 11, 2001, as their anger shifted toward foreign entities, they are still active. Between 2002 and 2005, there were 14 thwarted terrorist attacks in the United States—eight by right-wing extremist groups. For example, there was an anarchist plan to bomb a Coast Guard Station, a prison-gang attempt to attack military and Jewish targets around Los Angeles, and a few persons who tried to establish ties with al-Qaeda.

STREET SMART

Emergency responders should note the anniversaries of major terrorist attacks, such as September 11, Ruby Ridge, and Waco, as well as federal holidays. These dates have a higher risk of terrorism.

Militia

Militia organizations are groups that, in most cases, violently oppose firearm legislation, income tax payments, and government in general. They feel government has gone out of control through their implementation of laws, taxation, repossession, and foreclosure.[21] The U.S. Department of Treasury, which is not only responsible for money, but is also responsible for the enforcement of Alcohol, Tobacco, and Firearms (ATF) matters, is often a target of these militant organizations. They use two well-known clashes between civilians and law enforcement—Ruby Ridge and Waco—to illustrate and gain support for their cause. These incidents serve as rallying points for the organizations, as they blame the FBI and the government for the violent outcomes and loss of civilian life that occurred at each of these incidents.[21]

White supremacist groups have a long history of violence, are often heavily armed, and have a strong dislike for law enforcement.[22] They often cite Adolf Hitler, who espoused beliefs that races should be segregated, as a model. However, the Aryan Nations may be best known for their violence. Over the years, associates of the Aryan Nations have committed numerous bank and armored car robberies to support their organization, allegedly killed a Jewish radio host, engaged in shootouts with police,[22] and injured five children after opening fire in a Jewish Family Center.[21]

Ruby Ridge

On August 22, 1992, a 12-day violent standoff in Idaho came to an end through surrender only after an FBI sniper shot and killed Vicki Weaver, the wife of the suspect, Randy Weaver, as she held her 10-month-old infant. The U.S. Marshals Service was attempting to apprehend Weaver after he missed a court date to answer to weapons charges. Weaver was later acquitted of all charges, excluding missing the court date. Through investigations, the FBI was found to have broken several rules for engagement, including firing upon non-threats as the Weavers were retreating.

Waco

David Koresh, the self-proclaimed prophet of the Branch Davidians Seventh Day Adventists, was suspected of child abuse and polygamy. On February 28, 1993, as the FBI attempted to serve a search warrant on the Branch Davidian ranch located nine miles from Waco, Texas, an exchange of gunfire ensued between the Branch Davidians and FBI agents. The siege lasted for 51 days, culminating in violence on April 19 as the FBI stormed the ranch. In total, four FBI agents died, and 16 were wounded during the initial raid. However, the greatest loss of life was inside the compound during the final raid as a fire raged through,[23] burning the compound to the ground. Koresh, as well as 76 of his followers (including more than 20 children) perished in the blaze.[24]

Special Interest Groups

Special interest groups are those that are on the far edge, or extremes, of certain social movements. They include animal rights activists and the environmentalists[13] and are the most likely perpetrator of domestic terrorism. These ecological terrorists, or ecoterrorists,[25] feel that they are advocates for animals and Earth, and use acts of violence to draw attention to their cause. Between 2002 and 2005, 22 of the 23 domestic terrorist attacks were committed by either an animal or environmental extremist group.[2]

Although violent, these groups are generally not out to harm people. Rather, their intention is to target facilities and materials that are perceived to be harmful to animals or the environment. They use vandalism, arson, and animal theft to deter those they feel are their "enemies."[13] These organizations are very difficult to prosecute, as they are made up of smaller individual groups that operate autonomously and have a high level of secrecy and security, making them even harder to infiltrate.[13]

Animal Rights Groups

The Animal Liberation Front (ALF) is the most extreme of the animal rights organizations and has an extensive history of violence. Research groups in areas such as health care, pharmaceuticals, and cosmetics often use animals to test their products. The Food and Drug Administration (FDA) requires that extensive testing, often using animals, must be performed before a drug moves into clinical studies. Even though the FDA states that, "Drug companies [are to] make every effort to use as few animals as possible and to ensure their humane and proper care,"[26] animal activists feel that other, more ethical methods of testing are available.[21]

Environmentalists

Not all environmentalists are terrorists. However, those that use violence to bring attention to their cause are terrorists. These ecoterrorists believe that the actions of government and industry are causing great harm to the environment, so they use vandalism and arson to draw attention to the need to preserve Earth's environment. These organizations typically do not target people but instead construction sites (especially new home construction), equipment and buildings at mining and logging companies, ski resorts, and waste disposal or nuclear power plants. They are also known to target personal property such as sport utility vehicles and the dealerships that sell them. Offshoots to the environmentalists are the anti-biotech organizations. As technology advances, science has found ways to genetically alter seeds to deliver better crops. These organizations are strongly against this practice, so they attack crops and storage facilities to demonstrate their opposition, as well as use the attack as a medium to deliver their message.[21]

Religious Extremists

Although a very generic title, religious extremists use scripture and teachings to form their beliefs in life and feel that all others should share their same views or they will most certainly perish. Each form of religion has these people on the fringe, some going so far as to use violence to convince others to convert.

One such religion that has become quite prominent is Islam. Although a peaceful religion, some have begun perverting the scripture from the Koran. In 1998, Osama bin Ladin and Ayman al Zawahiri published a fatwa, or an interpretation of Islamic law, issued in the name of a "World Islamic Front," in an Arabic newspaper in London.[27] They were appalled at the ways of the Western world and felt that America had declared war against God and his messenger by the way Americans live. They called for the death of all Americans, no matter their location, and that it was the "individual duty for every Muslim who can do it in any country in which it is possible to do it."[27]

As previously noted, the vast majority of terrorist attacks that the Paramedic may encounter will be the result of domestic terrorists. This still holds true when dealing with Islamic extremists, as there are numerous American-Muslim converts that hold many of the same beliefs as those in the Middle East. Several of these groups originated within the prison system, such as the Sunni Islamic extremist group known as the JIS, or the "Assembly of Authentic Islam." These groups often have no foreign ties; rather, they raise money through armed robberies to finance terrorist attacks against the "enemies of Islam," such as the United States and Israel. The worrisome part of these radical Muslim converts is that not only do they have expansive knowledge of the United States, but their appearance and diversity allows them to meld into their surroundings. These factors make them potentially quite dangerous.[28]

The Greatest Terrorist Threat

Although ecoterrorist groups have committed the vast majority of terrorist attacks domestically, they typically only target infrastructure. In contrast, the right-wing extremists, with their antigovernment or racist sentiment,[13] target people with the intent to bring about physical harm and death.[18] This "propensity for violence," as well as their tendency to amass weapons and explosives, are the reasons why the FBI considers right-wing extremists a constant threat.[18]

However, the most significant threat is also one of the deadliest and most difficult to detect: the "lone wolf" terrorist.[18] These individuals hold beliefs similar to the organization that they are associated with but operate on the extreme fringe, carrying out their attacks alone.[13]

Responding to Terrorism

In today's violent world, Paramedics should remain ever vigilant to the possibility that the emergency they are responding to may be an act of terrorism and they may actually be the targets. These additional factors that must be considered will greatly complicate the response, making it difficult to coordinate.

Many of these terrorist organizations attempt to create as much devastation as possible, thus causing a high number of casualties. This greatly stresses the EMS response capabilities. Casualties may be the result of an explosion, shooting, fire, or dissemination of an agent. They may often require specialized teams, such as hazmat or SWAT, for assistance. This adds another layer of complexity to the already stressful situation.

Still another layer of complexity is added since terrorism is considered an illegal act, punishable under the penal system.

Therefore, the incident location must be considered a crime scene, and the Paramedic must make every effort to preserve it as the evidence remaining is vital to the investigation.[2]

Suspecting Terrorism

Since many terrorist events appear as horrible accidents, Paramedics may not be aware that what they are in fact encountering is a terrorist event. Although Paramedics should always possess a high index of suspicion when responding to any call, they must have a heightened situational awareness when responding to a call whose location, nature, timing, and/or presentation displays the hallmark signs of a potential terrorist event.

Location

The location of the call may be one of the first clues that the Paramedic needs in order to determine if the event involves terrorism. Terrorist organizations often choose targets that are symbolic of their cause. The target may be an organization or event that is controversial or considered the source of the problem, and is therefore condemned by the terrorist organization.[2] ATF and IRS offices, abortion clinics, mosques, and temples are examples of these symbolic targets.

Since fear is one of the main weapons used by the terrorists, targeting public buildings or assembly areas not only creates a mass-casualty situation at the time of the event, but also has long-lasting effects as the public associates danger with the owner or operator of that building or assembly area. Other potential targets are large public gathering areas such as shopping malls, sports arenas, convention centers, tourist areas, and even entertainment venues.[2]

To create widespread fear and panic within society, terrorists may also target vital components of the infrastructure. They may attempt to destroy (or take off-line) power plants, contaminate water treatment facilities, or disrupt mass transit. In addition, hospitals may also be considered targets. No matter what the target, any disruption of the infrastructure can disrupt an entire region and possibly cost millions of dollars to rectify.[2]

Nature of the Event

As many terrorist groups use explosives and arson as their weapons of choice, any call that involves either of these—especially when combined with a relevant location—should be suspect. Other examples suggesting potential terrorism are large non-trauma-related mass-casualty incidents, unusual smells in an area, and even shootings. Terrorists know that a shooting not only becomes a media event but it brings out a large number of public safety responders who then may become the actual target.[2]

Timing of the Event

The goal of the environmentalists is not to cause harm to humans, but to disrupt infrastructure. Many of their attacks occur when the potential for human casualties is at its lowest, such as on weekends, holidays, and early morning or nighttime hours. Anniversaries of historical events are also important.[2] For example, April 19 is a significant date for right-wing extremists as it is the anniversary of the events at Waco and Oklahoma City. April 20 is relevant to the white supremacists as it is Adolf Hitler's birthday. Since the massacre at Columbine High School occurred on that same day, it is also a significant date to schools.

On-Scene Warning Signs

Upon their arrival at the scene of an event, Paramedics should not quickly rush to help; instead, they should cautiously and systematically evaluate the scene. Large numbers of fatalities or ill patients without obvious causes suggest a chemical, biological, or radiological event. There may also be low-lying clouds, fog, vapors, or mists as well as chemical containers, sprayers, or lab equipment in unusual places. Objects that seem to be out-of-place, such as a backpack or briefcase in the middle of a room, should suggest to the Paramedic a secondary or tertiary device meant to harm the incoming Paramedics. Fires that are behaving unusually or spot fires are also of concern. These will be discussed in greater detail later in this chapter.[29]

Protecting the Paramedic

Scene safety is important in every level of emergency services. With violence occurring so frequently, not only is evaluating the scene for safety required, but continual assessment of the scene safety is also important. **Situational awareness**, or being ever vigilant for potential dangers at the scene, is one of the most important steps that a Paramedic can take to remain safe. By instituting several self-protective measures, the first of which is using the senses, the Paramedic will greatly reduce the chance of unwittingly becoming a casualty or, worse yet, part of the forward body line (FBL), or first people killed at the scene of a potential terrorist event.

Time, Distance, and Shielding

Measures used to reduce the Paramedic's exposure to a harmful environment involve the concepts of time, distance, and shielding. The basic underlying premise is that the shorter the time of exposure, the farther away from the source, and the more objects (i.e., PPE, vehicles, buildings, etc.) between the Paramedic and the hazard, the less exposure the Paramedic will theoretically have.[29] The Paramedic must keep in mind that these measures will not eliminate the inherent risks in these types of responses, but should help to mitigate them.

Time

Regardless of the environment and their level of protection, Paramedics should spend the shortest amount of time possible exposed to the hazard.[29] This not only protects the Paramedic from chemicals and other forms of harm, but also limits the Paramedic's exposure to such dangers as secondary or tertiary devices and armed assaults. This practice also helps in preserving the crime scene by limiting contamination that the Paramedic may cause.[2]

Distance

The "rule-of-thumb" taught in many hazmat courses is that a Paramedic should consider himself far enough away from a scene if, when holding up his thumb in front of his eye, he can no longer see the scene. This concept holds true when responding to terrorist events as well. Not only the hazmat scene, but also the possibility of secondary devices placed in close proximity of the scene or command post, may pose additional risks to the responders.

Shielding

The most basic concept of shielding is that there should be something between the Paramedic and the hazard. Shielding may come in the form of vehicles, buildings, and chemical-protective clothing, perhaps as simple as gloves and a mask.[29] The type of shielding at hand may depend upon the system in which the Paramedic works and is often based upon the tasks she is expected to perform. For some, this may be as little as taking universal precautions, whereas others may have turnout gear with self-contained breathing apparatus (SCBA).

Fire-based services have turnout gear and SCBA that are effective in protecting them from fire or oxygen-deprived environments. However, depending upon the type of attack, this equipment may not fully protect them from the actual agent. Nonetheless, it should give them the opportunity to retreat once the danger is noted.[1] EMS personnel often do not possess such equipment; thus, by entering an incident scene they are not equipped to deal with, they may become part of the forward body line.

By using the knowledge and PPE that they already possess regarding infection control practices, Paramedics may be prepared and equipped to deal with a biological attack on a limited basis. However, they will still be limited when responding to a larger chemical attack.[1] Police may possess little, if any, protective equipment, and may be limited to wearing disposable gloves.[4] Therefore, hazmat teams are best suited to deal with these agents—specifically ones that are chemical, biological, or radioactive in nature—because of the equipment and education that they already possess.[1] However, they must still be aware of other potential threats such as secondary explosive devices, something that they are not equipped to handle.

Decontamination

Brushing and washing off chemicals or other hazardous materials is another form of protection. Decontamination reduces the amount of time the Paramedic is exposed to the material. It also increases the Paramedic's distance from the agent. Not only should the Paramedic be decontaminated, but the patient should be as well to prevent patient/caregiver cross-contamination. In some instances, patient care may be limited, or even impractical, until the patient is decontaminated. Therefore, by allowing the hazmat team to perform their jobs, the Paramedic creates, in one sense, a form of time, distance, and shielding.

Types of Harm

Paramedics use time, distance, and shielding most effectively when they know the different types of harm that they may encounter. These types of harm, identified by the acronym **TRACEM**, are **T**hermal, **R**adiological, **A**sphyxiation, **C**hemical, **E**tiological, and **M**echanical hazards.[29] Addressing the specifics of each of these harms, while stressing the use of time, distance, and shielding, will increase the Paramedic's safety and chances of survivability.

STREET SMART

Other mnemonics used to remember threat agents are CBRNE (**C**hemical, **B**iological, **R**adiological, **N**uclear, and **E**xplosive) and **B-NICE** (**B**iological, **N**uclear, **I**ncendiary, **C**hemical, or **E**xplosive). Each mnemonic has its advantages. The important issue is that the Paramedic chooses one and uses it to learn about the threat agents.

Thermal

Temperature extremes, either hot or cold, expose the Paramedic to the possibility of a thermal injury through direct contact, convection, conduction, or any of the other methods of temperature transference. At the scene of a terrorist event, the Paramedic will most commonly encounter extremes in heat as the result of a fire or explosion. Burning metals, embers, and liquids may be encountered at the scene as a result of the original event or due to secondary devices such as a Molotov cocktail (gas grenade made with a bottle filled with gas and a rag used as a fuse).[2]

Paramedics may also encounter extremes in cold through exposure to cryogenic materials like liquid oxygen, although these situations are rare.[2] This form of harm may be especially dangerous when combined with asphalt, as this combination involves one of the other components of TRACEM—explosion.

Radiological

Nuclear radiation exposure occurs when the Paramedic encounters alpha particles, beta particles, or gamma rays. Alpha particles, the least penetrating, are generally not dangerous unless ingested, at which point they can cause organ damage. Standard issue PPE with SCBA is enough to protect Paramedics operating within the environment.

Beta particles are more likely than alpha particles to cause damage to tissue, as they are able to penetrate more deeply into the skin. If they remain outside the body, any harm they cause will be cutaneous. Thus, PPE with SCBA is the best measure of protection.

In contrast, gamma rays are the most lethal of all types of radiation. They cause severe burns to the skin while inflicting internal injuries and long-term physical effects due to their high degree of penetrating power. Typical PPE will not protect responders from the dangers of gamma radiation.[2]

Asphyxiation

The atmosphere is composed of 21% oxygen. As the Paramedic breathes, oxygen is displaced from the air, making the environment less hospitable and even deadly. Asphyxiants (those means that cause the displacement of oxygen from air) can be broken down into two categories: simple and chemical.[2]

Simple asphyxiants occur as heavier forms of gas displace oxygen. These gasses are generally inert but are able to dilute the oxygen levels below the level required to live, inhibiting external respiration. These gasses may include hydrogen, helium, ethane, ethylene, nitrogen, neon, carbon dioxide, acetylene, argon, methane, propane, and propylene.[30]

Chemical asphyxiants are much more dangerous than simple ones as they inhibit or retard cellular respiration. These chemicals, often referred to as "blood poisons," include such gasses as hydrogen cyanide, cyanogen chloride, phosgene, carbon monoxide, aniline, and hydrogen sulfide, which is becoming a popular homemade chemical asphyxiant in itself.[2]

Chemical

Chemical harm comes in the form of toxic, corrosive, etiological, and mechanical mechanisms. Most people think of toxic chemicals, such as nerve agents, when dealing with terrorism. Exposure may be acute, as with dissemination of the agent, or chronic, as occurs when working in the incident scene or with contaminated patients.[29]

Some chemicals are corrosive, causing visible destruction or irreversible alterations to skin or tissue. Others affect steel or aluminum.[29] Strong acids, caustics, and blister agents are all examples of corrosives and should be dealt with using typical hazardous materials protocol.

Etiological

Etiological risks also supply the potential for chemical harm. These risks may include use of intentionally disseminated organisms such as bacteria, rickettsia, viruses, and toxins from other living organisms or from bloodborne pathogens that are common everyday risks.[29] The best protection is through use of standard universal precautions such as gloves, face mask with splash shield, and protective outerwear.

Mechanical

Mechanical harm, one of the most encountered forms of harm, occurs as the direct result of physical trauma, such as being shot while responding, facing explosions from secondary devices or other sources, and/or encountering fragmentation from the same.[29] In addition, spills, unseen objects, and uneven terrain cause numerous slips, trips, and falls with injuries every year and are common mechanical hazards that the Paramedic must be aware of when at the event scene.

Initial Response

Unless the nature of the call is obvious, the Paramedic may be unaware that she is responding to a terrorist attack. For this reason, every call must be approached with the same thought process as an MCI or hazmat scene, with the initial focus being to contain the incident while protecting the public.

This goal is accomplished, and made successful, by the first arriving units as they initiate the incident management system, establish a perimeter to the incident, and develop work zones. By focusing upon these areas early in the response, the Paramedic takes steps to protect the public by preventing unwitting civilians and responders from entering the work zone. This also helps control the mass exodus of panicked and potentially contaminated people. However, this task may be difficult in that the crowd will most likely overwhelm the first responders on the scene. Nonetheless, every effort at protection must be taken by using whomever and whatever means possible.

The Paramedic should realize that the perpetrator of the attack may still be at the scene. In fact, the terrorist may be lying in wait for the first responders to arrive, as they may be the actual target. The terrorist might also be among the patients. Therefore, the Paramedic should always have a high index of suspicion when triaging and treating patients found at such events.[2]

The Paramedic must also anticipate that the initial location of the incident may only be one of several locations. Prior to the Paramedic's arrival, before containment and establishment of a perimeter, patients may have walked away from the scene to go home, see friends, go to work, visit local doctor's offices, or even go to nearby hospitals. Such individuals may be in shock and looking for help or comfort, thus adding to the complexity of the response and containment of the situation. Several smaller command units may need to be established to deal with these multiple locations, coordinating with a central command center.

Another possibility is that the patients did not wander off, but rather were intentionally targeted by the terrorist so as to strain the response and resources of the system. This makes the situation difficult to manage, and thus helps create the sense of fear the terrorist so desires.[2]

The Paramedic's primary objective when responding to a potential terrorist event is the responders' safety. By understanding the goals and methods used to achieve the terrorists' objectives, the Paramedic should be able to maintain a constant state of situational awareness. These responders must be constantly alert to their surroundings and aware of their actual and perceived hazards.

Specific Forms of Terrorism and Response

Many different tools are available that allow terrorists to successfully create an environment of fear and intimidation. Depending upon the terrorist's objective, the tool may cause damage ranging from destruction of property to injuries and fatalities. These tools may be biological, nuclear, incendiary, chemical, or explosive in nature or may be appear in the form of armed attacks, assassinations, barricade or hostage taking, hijacking, suicide terrorism, or cyberterrorism. No matter the method used, the terrorist's goal is the same: to create a sense of fear.

Biological Terrorism

Biological terrorism may be one of the hardest forms of terrorism to recognize as it presents in two forms. The first is a focused emergency response where the incident is localized and the potential or actual dissemination point is located, thus allowing for containment. This form allows Paramedics to prevent—or at least minimize—damage.[2]

An event using the second form is not initially known or recognized. It may originally present as a few sick patients but then turn into a sudden surge that floods the healthcare system without any explanation.[2]

Infection by a biological weapon occurs much in the same way as any infectious disease is spread. Subjects may inhale the agent, which is then absorbed by the respiratory tract or lung tissue. They may also ingest the agent through contaminated food or drink, leading to subsequent absorption from the oral mucosa or gastrointestinal tract. Other agents have the ability to be absorbed into the body through the mucous membranes of the eyes, nasal tissues, or open skin.[31]

These agents may be in the form of bacteria, which are single-celled organisms that grow in many different types of environments. They have the ability to cause damage by living and multiplying within the host or living outside of the host and producing dangerous toxins.[31] Anthrax, for example, is a bacterium.

Smaller than bacteria but larger than viruses, rickettsia multiply within living cells.[2] *Coxiella burnetii* (Q fever) is an example of this highly infectious agent that can be disseminated through the air and then inhaled by humans, causing disease in a susceptible person.[32]

Viruses are the smallest known organisms that have the ability to replicate when in the cells of a host. Finally, toxins are poisons that are created by other living organisms, such as bacteria, fungi, flowering plants, insects, fish, reptiles, and mammals.[2]

Agents of Concern

When evaluating biological threats terrorists may use as weapons, the Centers for Disease Control and Prevention evaluates each agent to determine its ease of dissemination or transmission, the potential impact it may have upon public health such as mortality, and the degree of panic and social disruption it may cause, as well as what steps the public health system requires to be adequately prepared for a response.[33]

Bacillus Anthracis (Anthrax)

Anthrax is an encapsulated, aerobic, gram-positive, spore-forming, rod-shaped bacterium that is transmitted through direct contact, inhalation, and ingestion (Figure 21-2).[34]

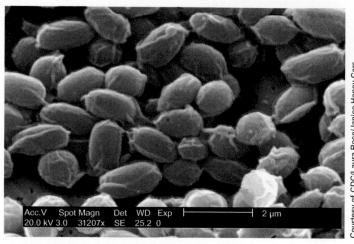

Figure 21-2 These *Bacillus anthracis* spores are seen under phase contrast microscopy.

Acc.V Spot Magn Det WD Exp | 2 μm
20.0 kV 3.0 31207x SE 25.2 0

Courtesy of CDC/Laura Rose/Janice Haney Carr

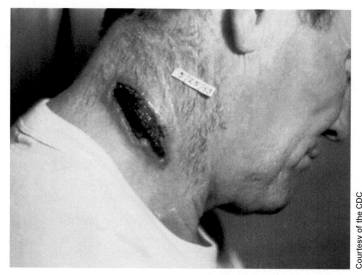

Figure 21-3 This anthrax lesion is caused by the bacterium *Bacillus anthracis*.

Signs and symptoms of exposure vary in onset and severity, depending upon the route of exposure.

Cutaneous exposure to anthrax occurs through direct contact with spores or bacilli. Signs and symptoms are localized to the area of contact and may develop immediately or within 24 hours. Itching is generally the first sign, followed by a papular lesion that turns vesicular. Within 7 to 10 days, the lesion will turn black (Figure 21-3)[34] and, if left untreated, can cause the patient to become septic.[2]

Although a much less likely route of exposure, anthrax may also be inhaled, thereby affecting the respiratory tract and lung tissue. Signs and symptoms of this exposure are not immediate, as the incubation period is typically between one and six days, and may be as long as two months. Initially, patients may develop low-grade fever, nonproductive cough, malaise, fatigue, myalgias, profound sweats, and chest discomfort. Although the lungs may be clear to auscultation, rhonchi may be present as well. Within one to five days of the onset of these

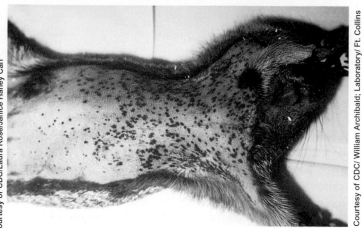

Figure 21-4 This photograph depicts the shaved anterior thoracoabdominal region of a plague-afflicted rock squirrel. Note the petechial rash, which is similar in appearance to those found on humans.

Courtesy of CDC/William Archibald; Laboratory/ Ft. Collins

symptoms, and possibly after a couple of days of improvement, the exposed patient will suddenly become significantly febrile and develop severe dyspnea with stridor. This leads to cyanosis, followed by shock and death within 24 to 36 hours.[34]

Anthrax may also be contracted through the gastrointestinal tract, although this is unusual. Initial signs and symptoms of exposure generally appear within a week and include nausea, vomiting, anorexia, fever, gradual onset of worsening abdominal pain, hematemesis, and hematochezia. Within a few days of onset, the patient's abdominal pain will decrease, ascites develop, and then shock occurs, followed by death.[34]

Courtesy of the CDC

Yersinia Pestis (Plague)

Yersinia pestis, or "the **plague**," is a bacterial disease that is found in rodents and their fleas (Figure 21-4).[35] To transmit the disease, an infected flea from an infected rodent bites a person, causing lymphatic and blood infections.[36] This form of plague, which is not transmittable between humans, is better known as the bubonic plague (the generic term often associated with the plague). However, pneumonic plague, which is transmittable from human to human, occurs if the *Yersinia pestis* bacterium is aerosolized, released, and inhaled.[35]

Within one to six days of inhaling the aerosolized plague, patients begin to exhibit signs of exposure such as fever, cough, weakness, shortness of breath, chest pain, and hemoptysis. They may also have what appears to be rapidly developing pneumonia. Gastrointestinal signs and symptoms may include nausea, vomiting, and abdominal pain. If left untreated, these patients will develop respiratory failure and shock, followed rapidly by death.[35]

Variola Major (Smallpox)

Smallpox is an extremely contagious viral illness that has no cure. The trademark signs of smallpox are small, raised bumps that appear on the infected person's body and face

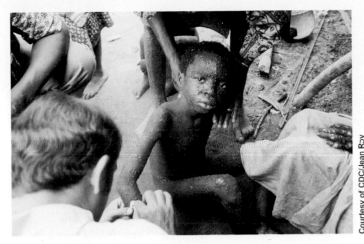

Figure 21-5 Smallpox lesions—small, raised bumps that appear on the infected person's body and face—are the trademark signs of smallpox.

(Figure 21-5).[37] Since there is no cure, the only treatment is prevention.

Because of worldwide efforts to vaccinate Earth's population against this disease. the world's last known case of smallpox was discovered in Somalia in 1977.[37] Currently, the only known samples of the *Variola major* virus are kept in secured labs. However, since the fall of the Soviet Republic there is fear that some of these specimens may be obtained by terrorists[37] and turned into a potentially devastating biological weapon, as routine immunizations against smallpox have not occurred for decades.[36]

Smallpox is only spread from human to human. It can be transmitted via droplets when close to an infectious source or through direct contact with infected bodily fluids or contaminated objects.[37] Although the potential exists for airborne transmission, this is unlikely unless the virus is disseminated in an enclosed setting such as a bus or train.[37] Symptoms resembling an acute viral illness such as the flu begin 7 to 17 days after exposure. Skin lesions appear but quickly turn from macules, to papules, to vesicles.[36]

Clostridium Botulinum toxin (Botulism)

Botulism is a toxin created by the *Clostridium botulinum* bacterium and classified as a neuroparalytic,[38] which can cause flaccid paralysis by preventing the release of acetylcholine.[36] Spores of this toxin are found throughout the world in soil and marine sediment.[38] Foodborne botulism is the most common disease in adults, generally presenting as gastrointestinal distress.[36]

Botulism is not contagious. However, if botulism is aerosolized and disseminated among a population, exposure can occur through inhalation. Patients infected through this method present nearly identically to the other forms of botulism exposure.[38]

Clues suggesting a biological attack using botulism include an unusual clustering of illness, such as people who attended the same public event and/or a large number of cases of flaccid paralysis in otherwise healthy individuals.[38] The incubation period may be another clue, as the onset of symptoms of inhalation botulism occurs in 24 to 72 hours, as opposed to foodborne exposure, which occurs in 12 to 36 hours.[36]

Signs and symptoms of botulism exposure generally present as symmetrical neurological deficits. These may include dysphagia, dysphasia, diplopia, blurred vision, mydriasis (dilated pupils), nonreactive pupils, and ptosis (drooping eyelid). As the disease process continues, the patient may experience general weakening of the respiratory muscles (causing hypoventilation) and descending flaccid paralysis. However, the patient remains conscious, alert, and without any sensory dysfunction as these symptoms occur. Since botulism is a toxin and not an infection, the patient will generally be afebrile.[39]

Francisella Tularensis (Tularemia)

Tularemia is a serious illness that naturally occurs in the United States through exposure to animals (rodents, rabbits, and hares) infected with the *Francisella tularensis* bacterium. Tularemia is not contagious between humans. Instead, exposure occurs when one is bitten by an infected insect such as a deerfly or tick, handles an infected animal carcass, eats or drinks contaminated food or water, or breathes in the *F. tularensis* bacteria.[38]

Incubation for the onset of symptoms is generally three to five days post-exposure, but may take as long as two weeks. Signs and symptoms of exposure are similar to those of other illnesses and include a sudden onset of fever, chills, headaches, diarrhea, muscle aches, joint pain, nonproductive cough, and progressive weakness. If left untreated, the patient may develop pneumonia, chest pain, bloody sputum, dyspnea, and eventually respiratory failure. Other signs and symptoms depend upon the route of exposure. Patients may have ulcers on the skin (Figure 21-6) or mouth, swollen and painful lymph nodes and eyes, as well as a sore throat.[38]

The most likely dissemination technique is also the most difficult to produce as the *F. tularensis* has to be aerosolized to be an effective biological weapon.[40]

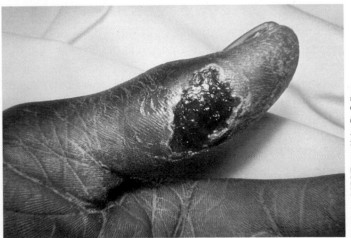

Figure 21-6 This patient's thumb has a skin ulcer from tularemia.

Viral Hemorrhagic Fevers

Viral hemorrhagic fevers (VHF) are zoonotic diseases that are generally spread from contact with infected animals and affect the body on a multisystem level. These diseases impair the body's ability to self-regulate, damage the vascular system, and sometimes cause non-life-threatening hemorrhages. There are four distinct families of these viruses, but the ones of greatest concern are filoviruses and arenaviruses.[41]

Filoviruses, including the Marburg virus and Ebola virus, are spread through contact with infected animals. The Marburg virus is named for the German city where an outbreak occurred in 1967. Patients were sickened after handling infected tissue of green monkeys. As a result, 31 laboratory workers became sick with hemorrhagic fever and seven died.

Two major outbreaks of the Ebola virus appeared in Africa in 1976: once in the southern Sudan and once in the country known as Zaire (now the Democratic Republic of Congo). Both of these outbreaks had high fatality rates of between 50% and 90%. Since then, there have been smaller outbreaks throughout the continent.[41]

Arenaviruses are quite prevalent in some areas of the world. They are spread through infected rodents and have been known to cause severe illness. There are several different types, with a new one being discovered about every three years. Transmission occurs through human contact with the infected rodent's waste products (fecal/urine). This may occur through ingesting contaminated food or water or by direct contact of non-intact skin with infectious materials. Inhalation exposure may also occur when particles containing urine or saliva become aerosolized.

Two specific forms of arenaviruses are known to spread between humans: Lassa and Machupo viruses. Transmission occurs through direct contact with bodily fluids from the exposed patient, secondary exposure from medical items used in the patient's treatment, and the airborne route.[42]

Although the transmission of viral hemorrhagic fevers from host to human is not quite understood, once a human outbreak occurs, it spreads rapidly among those who are in close contact with those infected. In general, it appears the risk of airborne transmission is minimal.[43]

Once a person is exposed, signs and symptoms generally begin to appear within 5 to 10 days. These include an abrupt onset of fever, myalgia, and headache, as well as nausea and vomiting, abdominal pain, diarrhea, chest pain, cough, and pharyngitis. A rash may also appear on the patient's trunk within five days of the first symptoms, with hemorrhagic signs—such as petechiae, ecchymosis, and various hemorrhages—appearing as the disease process progresses.[33]

Dissemination of Biological Weapons

Terrorists can use many different methods to disperse a biological weapon. However, the exact method depends upon the agent being used. Aerosolizing the agent is the most common and effective means, as it produces an airborne hazard that can easily be inhaled, causing rapid distribution throughout the body. Anthrax, for example, is an ideal agent for this form of dispersion.[2]

Contaminating food, water, or medicine is another means to disseminate a biological agent. Ingestion into the body allows the agent to be absorbed and distributed. Although terrorists may seek to contaminate reservoirs or water treatment plants, these take a great deal of planning and are difficult to accomplish due to their complexity. A more common target may be a salad bar or buffet at a local restaurant. A terrorist can simply sprinkle salmonella spores onto the food. Unwitting patrons then ingest the contaminated food, causing illness hours or even days later when they are all away from the source.[2]

Exposure to a biological agent may also occur through direct skin contact, as occurred when postal workers in New Jersey were exposed to anthrax sent by terrorists in anthrax-laced letters through the postal system. Other transmission methods include spreading the spores in public places such as seats in a theater or on playground equipment.[2]

Situational Characteristics, Clues, and Warnings

The biological attack may be one of the hardest forms of terrorism to recognize in that clues may be subtle or non-existent depending upon the agent and dispersal method used. The most obvious and ideal situation for the Paramedic is when a terrorist actually provides a warning regarding the attack via a written or verbal threat. However, this rarely occurs.

The Paramedic should assess the scene for industrial or agricultural sprayers, especially in an environment in which they appear out-of-place such as in a mall or non-agricultural area.[29]

Terrorists favor the use of biological agents as weapons because there is often a delay of signs and symptoms due to the agent's incubation period. This allows the exposed patients to leave the area; return to their home, work, or school; and, depending upon the agent, experience continued exposure through contamination.

In fact, since many of these agents resemble naturally occurring outbreaks in their early stages, such as influenza, the outbreak may go unnoticed for days.[33] The primary indicator of a biological agent's release is a clustering of illnesses in a single geographic area. Upon investigation, Paramedics may determine that the ill may have attended the same event, or been in the same area, as others who are affected. Symptoms shared in common between these patients may include a febrile illness that develops into sepsis, pneumonia, respiratory failure, rash, flaccid paralysis, or chicken pox-like illness in an adult. These symptoms are especially worrisome if they are found in otherwise healthy individuals.[33]

The healthcare community needs to be alert to patterns of illnesses and clues, called **clusters**, that may indicate an intentional release of a biological agent. If the target is a mass population, then the emergency may present itself as a public health emergency, such as occurs with a cholera outbreak or anthrax theat. The Paramedic must continually assess the immediate situation, but must also examine past and present calls in order to recognize unusual patterns of illness.

TRACEM Dangers to the Paramedic

When responding to a biological attack, the most obvious of all the TRACEM dangers to the Paramedic is the etiological danger. Paramedics must be aware that the agent they may be encountering can be highly infectious, with the ability to enter the body through many various routes including absorption, inhalation, ingestion, or injection.[2]

Protective Measures

One of the Paramedic's best protective measures is planning and being well-versed in hazard assessment, as well as exposure potential. Understanding the various levels of respiratory protection and equipment, under what conditions to enter and exit, as well as measures for decontamination are imperative if the Paramedic does not wish to become exposed.[34]

Preplanning a response to a biological agent's release requires that emergency first responders, public health officials, law enforcement, and other experts in this area meet to discuss these levels of protection, decontamination, vaccination, and treatment. They should base these plans off of the current recommendations and biological safety information published by the Centers for Disease Control and Prevention.

Further protection of the Paramedic revisits the concept of time, distance, and shielding. The Paramedic should spend the smallest amount of time in the incident zone as possible since some agents, such as ricin, can be fatal even with a small exposure.

The Paramedic should also keep in mind that he may be the actual target. Therefore, he should reduce his exposure to secondary devices. Similarly, the Paramedic should remain as far away from the incident as possible. The Paramedic must understand that the incident site of a biological attack may not only be large and in multiple areas, it may also be moving as contaminated persons flee the area.[29]

After planning, shielding is the next best form of protection available to the Paramedic. The choice of shielding depends upon the agent used. However, clothing made from materials that are impervious to the agent is essential for maximum protection.[34] The specific type of protective clothing to be donned, such as a Level A or B protective suit with the appropriate level of respiratory protection, depends entirely upon the agent's concentration and potential routes of transmission.[34]

Since many of these agents are most deadly when aerosolized, the risk of inhalation is present. Paramedics responding to and working at the scene of a suspected biological agent release must consider some level of respiratory protection. Minimum recommendations from the CDC include a half-mask or full facepiece. Air-purifying respirators with particulate filter efficiencies ranging from N95 to P100 provide a wide range of protection from pulmonary tuberculosis to the Hantavirus. In certain situations, especially when the situation is not understood, the use of a self-contained breathing apparatus (SCBA) offers the highest level of respiratory protection.[2]

In general, the CDC recommends that when responding to an incident where the type of airborne agent, dissemination method, duration of dissemination, or exposure concentration is unknown, those entering the scene should wear a **Level A protective suit** in addition to a NIOSH-approved pressure-demand SCBA.

A **Level B protective suit**, with an enclosed or exposed NIOSH-approved pressure-demand SCBA, can be used when the biological aerosol is no longer being generated and where conditions may present a splash hazard (Figure 21-7).

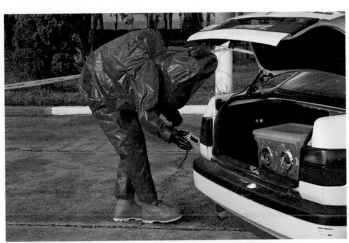

(a)

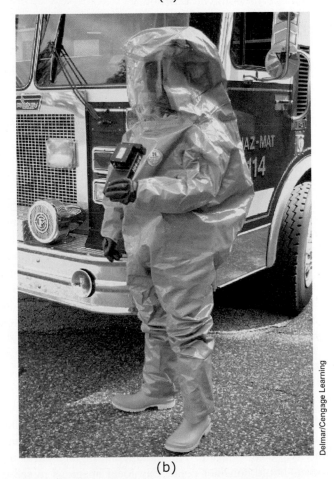

(b)

Figure 21-7 Both the (a) Level A protective suit and (b) Level B protective suit provide protection from biological agents.

Finally, if the aerosol-generating device did not create high airborne concentrations, or the agent's dissemination was by a letter or package that can easily be bagged, then using a full-face respirator with a P100 filter or powered air-purifying respirator is appropriate.

Treatment of Those Exposed to a Biological Agent

Although each agent requires specific treatment, the Paramedic is not likely to be involved in delivering any of these. In general, the Paramedic's attention will be focused on managing the patients' life functions, in particular their ventilatory status. The Paramedic should ready suction, both basic and advanced airway equipment, and prepare for respiratory arrest. These things must only be done once the patient has been fully decontaminated and, depending upon the agent used, once the Paramedic dons the appropriate CDC-recommended personal protective equipment.

Nuclear Terrorism

There is much fear that terrorists will either obtain nuclear material to create a bomb or attack a nuclear power station. To this day, however, there has not been a successful detonation of a nuclear bomb on U.S. soil.

Overview

There are three different potential forms of nuclear terrorism. The first is the detonation of a fission device similar to that of the atomic bomb. Due to the complexity of designing and constructing a device of this magnitude, it would not only take a sophisticated group of scientists but also an extraordinary amount of funding to accomplish.

Another method is to detonate a traditional large-scale explosive containing large amounts of nuclear materials (i.e., a **dirty bomb**) near a target.[2] These dirty bombs are relatively simple devices to construct as the radioactive material is easier to acquire (this is often accomplished by stealing or obtaining discarded radiographical equipment used to test bridges, buildings, or other structures for example).[2] These materials are then packed around conventional explosives and disseminated once the explosion occurs. This type of device produces immediate effects, such as radiation burns and acute poisoning, as well as long-term effects such as contamination of ground water, cancers, and forced mass evacuations.[2]

Situational Characteristics, Clues, and Warnings

The Paramedic should suspect a nuclear attack has occurred any time he finds an unusually high number of sick or dying people or animals, especially if they present with reddening of the skin and vomiting. The Paramedic, or incident commander, should consider contacting local hospitals to see if they are also observing large numbers of patients with similar signs and symptoms.[44] However, one must keep in mind that the severity of the signs and symptoms, as well as how quickly they appear, are directly associated with the type of radiological material used and the dose received. These symptoms may appear anywhere from hours, to days, to weeks post-exposure, making it even more difficult to recognize these patients as victims of a terrorist event.[44]

As the Paramedic continues to survey the scene, he may discover objects or containers with radiological symbols on them. He may also come across materials that seem to emit heat or are glowing, yet have no signs of an external heat source; these are signs that the objects may be highly radioactive.[44]

TRACEM Dangers to the Paramedic

The Paramedic responding to a nuclear attack will face several unique hazards, but the most significant and obvious is the radiological exposure. Not only will the radiation present an immediate problem, but it will also cause an ongoing hazard through contamination of the incident area. In addition, long-term health effects will result. The severity, of course, will be determined by the amount and type of radioactive material encountered.[2]

An often-overlooked danger at the scene of a nuclear attack is that there is not only a radioactive hazard but a chemical hazard as well. Radioactive materials are also hazardous chemicals and should be treated as such. Depending upon how the radioactive material was disseminated, the Paramedic needs to be aware of mechanical hazards, especially if a "dirty bomb" was used to disseminate the material.[2]

Protective Measures

The Paramedic's best method of protection when encountering a potential nuclear incident is to use radiological detection equipment.[2] Beyond that, the Paramedic should observe for any suspicious clues that a radiological agent has been used and follow the protective concepts of time, distance, and shielding. The severity of illness encountered as the result of exposure to radiation is dose dependant where short time/high radiation can equal long time/low radiation. The Paramedic needs to spend the shortest amount of time as possible exposed to the material to perform a rescue or deliver care.[29]

The Paramedic and patient start reducing their exposure time by shedding any and all clothing, as dust can collect in the clothing, thereby continuing to expose the wearer and those in close contact. Decontamination of the full body using showers or other water sources such as a fire hose is also advised, as this will again decrease the amount of exposure time.

Maintaining their distance is another way Paramedics are able to protect themselves. They should remain away from the area of detonation and only enter the surrounding areas to save lives, as the potential exists that these areas will have high levels of radiation as well.[39] Similar to the decontamination of clothing, all equipment, including ambulances, needs to be washed before leaving the incident site so as not to cause cross-contamination.[39]

Another method to reduce the radiological hazard is not eating, drinking, applying makeup, or smoking while exposed to potentially radioactive smoke or dust. Rehab may be necessary for those working in bulky protective clothing, so water should only be consumed if absolutely necessary and only if it comes from a canteen or other closed container.[39]

The amount and type of shielding is dependent upon the type of radiation involved, as discussed earlier in this chapter. The CDC recommends that the Paramedic should wear a full-face mask with a HEPA filter to reduce the risk of inhalation of radioactive dust. However, if such a device is unavailable, the Paramedic can also use a wet handkerchief or cloth to cover the mouth and nose while breathing. Since there is little danger from radioactive gasses, the use of SCBA is not necessary.[39] Protection from dermal exposure comes in the form of wearing loose-fitting garments that cover as much of the body as possible and covering all open wounds and abrasions to protect them from exposure to radioactive sources.[39]

Treatment of Those Exposed to a Nuclear Agent

Patients will quickly succumb to traumatic injuries, as compared to the gradual rate seen in injuries sustained by radiation. Paramedics should be prepared to treat conventional injuries first and then treat the contamination once the patient is stable.[39]

However, only those properly trained and working as part of the hazmat team should do this. Since the incident may have a large number of patients, it is not prudent to try to determine who is contaminated and who is not. Therefore, anyone who has dust on her must be considered contaminated. A decontamination facility should be established upwind from the incident and far from ground zero (the point of impact or explosion and the origin of the "hot zone") to prevent radiation levels from interfering with monitoring of patients.

The facility also needs to allow for the expeditious and effective movement of patients throughout. Areas should be established where patients can remove and discard their outer clothing and wash as thoroughly as possible. Afterwards, they should be given coveralls (those worn by painters work well) or covered in blankets to maintain their body temperature as well as modesty.[39]

As radiation can cause long-term effects, the Department of Health and Human Services requests that public health officials collect contact information from all patients involved so that they can perform long-term medical monitoring of these individuals. Although this record keeping should not interfere with patient care, the Paramedic may work with public health officials in collecting this information.[39]

Since many contaminated people may leave the incident scene before responders arrive and establish a perimeter, Paramedics should notify hospitals of the potential arrival of contaminated patients so they can prepare to initiate their mass-casualty decontamination plans.[39] Public authorities should also make public service announcements by radio and television, advising anyone who is potentially involved to bag their clothes, place them outdoors, and wash thoroughly. If they begin to experience nausea, vomiting, reddening of the skin, or unexplained lesions, they should report to a hospital immediately, requesting a checkup for acute radiation syndrome.[39]

Incendiary Terrorism

Terrorists rarely use fire in the form of arson as a weapon; in fact, it makes up only approximately 4% of terrorist activities.[45] It is a more popular method with the ecoterrorist groups as their purpose is to destroy property.

There are two general types of incendiary devices: those that are triggered and those that are delivered. **Triggered devices** allow the terrorist to be distant from the scene at the point of ignition. Triggers may be made using a chemical reaction such as an inside burning fuse. More sophisticated devices may involve electric or mechanical switches that may be activated remotely or on a timer. **Delivered devices** may be as simple as a hand-thrown Molotov cocktail or self-propelled such as a rocket or grenade.[2]

Materials used to make an incendiary device that are found easily throughout the home and garage include roadway flares, gasoline and motor oil, light bulbs, common electrical components, matches, household chemicals, fireworks, propane and butane cylinders, plastic pipes, bottles, and cans.[2] These items can be used to construct the ignition source, the combustible filler material that actually ignites, and then a container to house both of these.[2]

Situational Characteristics, Clues, and Warnings

This form of terrorism is often used by the ecoterrorist who generally goes out of his way to assure that no living creature is harmed in the perpetration of the attack. With that said, the first clue of an incendiary attack is the target in terms of its symbolism and location, such as with new construction or luxury cars. Multiple fires or an unusually large volume of fire for the structure may be a sign that the fire was intentionally set. Further evidence may be the use of accelerants, containers that hold flammable liquids, splatter patterns from a thrown device, fusing residue, signs of forced entry, and appliances that are out-of-place for the environment, like a gas stove.[2]

TRACEM Dangers to the Paramedic

Thermal injury from burns is the Paramedic's primary hazard. However, if accelerants or a hand-thrown device are used, the Paramedic must be aware of chemical hazards as well. A slow burning or smoldering fire will lead to incomplete combustion, resulting in the release of poisons like carbon monoxide and cyanide. As fire uses oxygen to burn, there is an asphyxiation risk as well.

Fires create numerous mechanical hazards, such as weakening the structure and creating the potential for a collapse. As with any fire, it is not always possible to know what the burning building contains. Therefore, the Paramedic needs to consider that explosions and secondary events may occur.[2]

Protective Measures

Similar to radiation, the severity of the burn depends upon the temperature and duration of exposure. Therefore, Paramedics should keep the time of exposure to an absolute minimum, especially if they do not have the proper PPE. Paramedics also need to be aware of potential collapse areas, even on the outside, as chimneys and other structures have been known to fall away from the structure. The best shielding is the use of structural firefighting turnout gear as well as the use of an SCBA.

Treatment of Those Exposed to an Incendiary Agent

If an accelerant is used, then the patient must be decontaminated as soon as possible. Patients rarely succumb to thermal injuries in the initial periods post-exposure; therefore, treatment of traumatic injuries takes precedence. Treatment of the burn patient involves assertive airway and ventilatory management, pain control, and fluid administration. Chapter 9 features more information regarding burn trauma and care.

Chemical Terrorism

Chemical agents are considered hazardous materials as exposure may cause injury or death. They can range from simple everyday household items to industrial and military-grade chemicals. These include nerve agents, vesicants, blood agents, choking agents, and irritants. Depending upon the agent used, the routes of entry into the body are inhalation, ingestion, absorption, and injection.[2]

Agents of Concern

Chemical agents can be classified based upon their effects on the human body. Although it is not required that Paramedics have expertise in this area, they must possess a basic understanding of how these chemicals can affect the body to assist patients exposed to these substances. This not only helps the Paramedic develop a course of treatment, but also alerts the individual Paramedic to the dangers that these chemicals pose to the provider.

Nerve Agents

Nerve agents are **organophosphate compounds** that attack the nervous system by impairing nerve impulse transmission through inhibition of acetylcholinesterase and preventing the re-uptake of excess acetylcholine.[46] Organophosphates are often found in farming communities and are commonly used as a pesticide.

However, these agents also have a darker history. For decades, they have been used in strengths 100 to 500 times more potent than usual as weapons.[46] Common examples of weaponized nerve agents are tabun, sarin, soman, thickened soman, and V agent.[46]

These agents are liquid at room temperature[46] and disseminated as an aerosol.[29] They are generally clear, colorless, tasteless, and may smell slightly fruity, although many have

Table 21-1 Mnemonics Used to Remember Signs of Organophosphate Poisoning

SLUD		SLUDGEM		DUMBELS	
S	Salivation	S	Salivation	D	Diarrhea
L	Lacrimation	L	Lacrimation	U	Urination
U	Urination	U	Urination	M	Miosis
D	Defecation	D	Defecation	B	Bronchospasm
		G	Gastrointestinal	E	Emesis
		E	Emesis	L	Lacrimation
		M	Miosis	S	Salivation

no smell at all.[46] Exposure to these agents often occurs by absorption through the skin, but may occur through any of the other routes. Even small amounts can be deadly.[46]

Symptoms can occur within minutes or hours, depending upon the dose received. Exposure to these agents affects the nerves that are associated with the central nervous system, those associated with the parasympathetic nervous system, some sympathetic nerves, and the somatic nerves, causing the patient to exhibit signs and symptoms associated with nervous sytem dysfunction.[1] Several acronyms are used when discussing these symptoms, such as SLUD, SLUDGEM, and DUMBELS (Table 21-1). Other symptoms may include anxiety, restlessness, convulsions, absent reflexes, coma, respiratory and circulatory depression, fasciculations, cramps, weakness, paralysis, cardiac arrest, tachycardias, bradycardias, hypertension, hypotension, and sweating.[1]

Besides the general clues found at the scene of a terrorist attack, the Paramedic should specifically look for small explosions that may have disseminated the nerve agent, an unscheduled or unusual spraying, abandoned aerosolizers, numerous dead animals and a lack of insects, a non-trauma MCI, numerous patients presenting with signs of organophosphate poisoning, and civilian panic in areas that are potential targets.[46]

The Paramedic should also take standard hazmat precautions—using time, distance, and shielding—while contacting the regional hazmat team. In the early stages of a response, or due to dissemination of an agent from a secondary device, Paramedics may unwittingly find themselves exposed to a nerve agent. If not prepared, the Paramedic may quickly become a patient and part of the forward body line.

Stockpiles of the antidotes for these types of agents are located throughout the United States and are ready for dispersal in mass quantities to the site of an attack. However, these stockpiles will do exposed first responders little good when they arrive hours after the event begins.[47] Currently there are at least three auto-injectors approved for civilian medical use by the FDA in the event of a nerve agent exposure: AtroPen, containing atropine; **pralidoxime chloride (2-PAM)**, packaged in the Mark 1 kits; and, most recently, the DuoDote, which is the previous two pens combined into one single injection.

Another available injector is for diazepam (Valium). Some of the poisoned patients may develop seizures, and the diazepam injectors can help limit the seizures, even though it is not an antidote.

Vesicants

Blister agents, such as mustard gas, are heavy, oily liquids that are colorless and odorless in their pure state. However, in their impure state they take on a darker color and often smell like mustard, onion, or garlic.[46] Exposure can occur if the liquid is aerosolized and sprayed or heated, thus creating a vapor.[2]

Vesicants are extremely toxic. They can cause severe burns to the eyes, leading to pain, reddening, tearing, and the sensation of grittiness, as well as edema and spasms of the eyelids. These symptoms appear within 30 minutes or as long as 12 hours post-exposure. Evidence of skin irritation appears early with itching followed by redness, tenderness, and a burning pain in the affected areas, with larger burns presenting as second degree burns with blisters.

Two to 12 hours post-exposure, the patient may present with respiratory complaints—including a burning sensation in the throat and nose, followed by hoarseness, a profusely runny nose, severe cough, and dyspnea. Gastrointestinal complaints can appear within two to three hours and include abdominal pain, nausea, vomiting blood, and passing bloody stool.[46]

Treatment is based upon the symptoms encountered; however, self-protection is the primary concern when encountering a blister agent. Similar to other clues found upon arrival, the Paramedic should be aware of explosions that dispense liquids, mists, or gasses, especially if the explosion just damaged the package or bomb itself. Unusual spraying, abandoned sprayers, non-trauma MCIs, injury patterns, and target selection are all clues to the use of such an agent.[46]

Blood Agents

Cyanides are cellular asphyxiants that inhibit the body's ability to exchange gasses. Examples include hydrogen sulfide and cyanogen chloride, which are generally liquid under pressure, and common chemicals found in industrial settings. Information about these types of chemicals may also be available from these settings as well. Exposure to blood agents can occur through the chemical in its liquid form or as a vapor which occurs once it is no longer under pressure.

Symptoms of patients exposed to a blood agent are associated with hypoxia. A high-concentration exposure may result in seizures and respiratory arrest followed by a rapid death. Low-concentration exposure may result in dyspnea, vomiting, diarrhea, vertigo, and headache. The patient may have noticed an odor of peach or bitter almond in the air; however, not all people possess the ability to smell these agents.[2,46]

Pulmonary Agents

Pulmonary (choking) agents are industrial chemicals such as chlorine and phosgene gasses. They are similar to cyanide in that they are a liquid when kept under pressure but rapidly vaporize when released.[46] If exposed, patients may present with coughing, choking, and severe irritation of the eyes and pulmonary tract.[46]

If enough of the vapors are inhaled, the patient may also develop acute respiratory distress syndrome (ARDS), resulting in pulmonary edema.[2] Witnesses and patients may state that, prior to their complaints, they may have smelled an odor similar to a pool or possibly freshly mowed hay or grass.[46]

Irritants

Irritants are generally non-lethal, but seem to act like asphyxiants for those exposed. These are the easiest chemicals to obtain and are commonly used in law enforcement. They include tear gas, mace, and pepper spray. Although these agents cause pain, burning, and discomfort on exposed skin and mucous membranes, their symptoms are transient.

Treatment is aimed at patient decontamination, especially to prevent cross-contamination of the responders who should be wearing gloves while treating patients exposed to these agents.[2]

Situational Characteristics, Clues, and Warnings

First, the Paramedic should look for the presence of life (or more specifically, death). This includes humans, animals, birds, fish, and insects. The Paramedic should then assess the scene for unusual liquid droplets on surfaces, especially if there has been no rain and they appear oily or there appears to be an oily film on objects or water. The Paramedic assesses the surrounding vegetation for discolored, withered, or dead trees, crops, shrubs, bushes, and lawns, especially in non-drought conditions. She should also take note of unexplained low-lying clouds or unusual fog-like conditions.

Upon exiting the ambulance, any unexplained odors such as fruity, flowery, sharp, pungent, garlic, horseradish-like, bitter almond, peach, newly mown hay, or any odor that is out-of-place for the surroundings should alert the Paramedic to chemical agent dispersal. Discovery of unusual metal debris, unexploded bombs, or munitions may also be a clue that a chemical agent has been used.

Next, the Paramedic should look for injury or illness patterns in patient presentations that may give the Paramedic clues as to the type of chemical used. Unexplained water-like blisters, wheals, miosis, choking and other respiratory complaints, and rashes, especially if there are a large number of patients experiencing similar serious health complaints, are common at the scene of a chemical release. The location of the patients may lead to additional information, as those in confined areas may be more symptomatic than those outside. However, due to the dissemination method used, the opposite may quite possibly hold true.[44]

TRACEM Dangers to the Paramedic

Exposure to the chemical is the Paramedic's primary danger. Each chemical is rated in terms of how much danger it presents. Relevant factors include the chemical's corrosiveness, reactivity, and health hazards. These are often rated on a zero to four scale.

The Paramedic may also encounter thermal dangers, since chemical reactions not only cause heat, but some chemicals are flammable and/or explosive in nature. Neutralization of chemicals is not performed when chemicals are present on a patient because of the potential creation of extreme heat from the reaction. As previously discussed, some chemicals present an asphyxiation danger in that they are either heavier than air, displacing oxygen, or prevent the exchange of gasses within the body. Finally, mechanical dangers occur as a result of secondary explosive/dissemination devices or through the weakening of structural elements due to the exposure of strong acids.[2]

Protective Measures

In general, all chemical attacks are hazardous materials incidents. The Paramedic must remain the maximum distance away from all contaminated areas and vehicles, uphill and upwind, based upon the recommendations published for that chemical in the ***Emergency Response Guidebook (ERG)***. Protective clothing worn should be based upon each chemical, as per the *ERG*, and worn by those who are trained in hazmat.

The Paramedic should remain as far away from the incident as possible unless she is part of the hazmat response team. In addition, she should only receive and treat patients once they have been decontaminated and cleared for transport. Even though a patient has been decontaminated, he still may pose a risk to the Paramedic.

Inhaled gasses may **off-gas** (the process where the chemical leaves the body through exhalation) and expose the Paramedic to the same chemical as the patient. Similarly, if the patient ingests the chemical and vomits, the Paramedic is also at risk for exposure.[48]

Treatment of Those Exposed to a Chemical Agent

When encountering patients exposed to a chemical weapon, the Paramedic should make every attempt to identify the hazardous material.[48] From a safe distance, the Paramedic should look at the shape of the containers (noting, for example, if they is pressurized). Although this may not completely identify the agent, it will allow the Paramedic to obtain a better understanding of the agent.

Placards, labels, and shipping papers are also ways to identify the agent; however, these may not always be present, especially if the chemicals were not in transit or storage but instead were brought by the terrorist. In that case, experts in identifying chemicals through analytical tests are needed to determine the agent.[48]

Treatment of these patients should never begin before they are decontaminated, which includes the removal of all clothing. Failure to follow this procedure will not only expose the Paramedic and crew to the chemical but the hospital as well, thus creating another hazardous incident location.[48]

Explosive Terrorism

Terrorists have used explosives as a tool for centuries. Anarchists used them in the 1800s, having the philosophy that dynamite made all men equal.[45] Today, explosives have reportedly been used in 57% of all terrorist attacks, as they are one of the most versatile tools available.[45]

Bombs can be small for an individual target, such as a letter bomb, or larger to create mass destruction and casualties, as with a large truck.[45] They may be an isolated event[2] consisting of a single device, oftentimes targeting infrastructure, or may consist of multiple devices set as booby traps to increase the scale of the attack.[2,45]

Types and Dissemination of Explosive Weapons

Many widely available materials can be used in making explosive weapons. They include commercially available explosives as well as improvised explosives, such as those used in Oklahoma City. Vehicle bombs are large, powerful devices that can hold a large quantity of explosive materials. They are often triggered remotely, by a timer, or driven into the target.[2] Pipe bombs are another common form of explosive.

To make an explosive device, a small amount of explosive material is packed into a pipe or metal container and then detonated by using a timing fuse, electric trigger, or remote triggers with motion sensors.[2] Bombs may also come in satchels or backpacks, allowing the terrorist to add nails, screws, or other shrapnel to the device to increase casualties.

Other forms of explosives are rocket-propelled grenades, mines, anti-personnel mines, and homemade grenades.[2]

TRACEM Dangers to the Paramedic

When responding to any of the aforementioned forms of terrorism, the Paramedic must understand that the responders may be the actual targets. They should not only assess for bomb damage but also for packages, backpacks, bags, and pipes that are left unattended and seem out-of-place, which might be a **secondary device** (weapon intended to attack the responders).

Post-explosion, the Paramedic should not typically have to be concerned with thermal hazards unless there are actual fires, as the primary heat generated from the explosion occurs at the time of detonation. Similarly, the mechanical threat occurs at detonation as well, involving blast overpressure, shock waves, and fragmentation. However, if the explosion occurs in or near a building, Paramedics need to consider the building's structural stability and be prepared for a partial or complete collapse, as well as the presence of secondary devices.

As previously noted, the terrorist's intent in using an explosive device may be to disseminate the actual agent.

Therefore, the Paramedic must be aware that radiological, chemical, and etiological dangers may also exist.[2] The Paramedic should be particularly wary if the explosion is small and does not cause significant damage.

Protective Measures

Planning is one of the best protective measures that the Paramedic can have. This may come in the form of general operating guidelines or preparation following a pre-blast warning. However, as pre-announced warnings of a terrorist event rarely occur, the response will typically take place after the blast.

Since the responding agencies may be the terrorist's actual targets, the Paramedic needs to spend as little time at the scene as possible. Most explosions occur in 100ths of a second, which does not provide the Paramedic with time to react or protect herself. If a bomb is discovered, the Paramedic should remain as far away as possible (Table 21-2). As explosives may be remotely detonated, Paramedics should not use radios in and around the scene.

Since secondary devices may be present and remotely detonated, the Paramedic should remain out of sight lines whenever possible. She should also realize that any remaining structure, either in whole or in part, may collapse, causing further injuries.[29]

By using buildings not damaged by the explosion or other nearby large structures, there should be adequate protection of the established staging areas, Incident Command, and any other operational areas. Depending upon the size of the structure, the use of vehicles for shielding may not be appropriate as falling debris or subsequent explosions can crush them.

Treatment of Those Exposed to an Explosive Agent

A terrorist event using explosives as the primary weapon will present with unique characteristics in terms of patient symptoms often not seen outside the combat theater.

One of the first unique components of this type of incident is that those who experience minor injuries will not be seen by EMS. Instead, they seek medical attention on their own, causing an influx of low priority patients at the emergency department. These low priority patients are then followed by the more critically injured who arrive at the hospital by EMS or other vehicles. Injuries are often both penetrating and blunt in nature and require continuous reassessment as patient conditions may change rapidly.

Bombs used as dissemination devices typically have a small amount of explosive material so as not to destroy or burn off the agent. The Paramedic's fear of radioactivity should not delay triage and treatment since the possibility of contamination is minimal and common universal precautions should suffice.[49]

Paramedics are most likely to encounter blast injuries when caring for a patient involved in an explosion. These injury patterns are the primary result of a sudden overpressurization force, or blast wave, that strikes the body. This, in turn, impacts hollow and solid organs, potentially causing catastrophic internal injuries.

Table 21-2 Bomb Threat Standoff Distances

Threat Description	Explosive Capacity	Lethal Air Blast Range	Mandatory Evacuation Distance	Desired Evacuation Distance
Pipe bomb	5 lbs (2.2 kg)	25 ft (8 m)	70 ft (21 m)	850 ft (259 m)
Briefcase or suitcase	50 lbs (23 kg)	40 ft (15 m)	150 ft (46 m)	1,850 ft (564 m)
Compact sedan	220 lbs (100 kg)	60 ft (18 m)	240 ft (73 m)	915 ft (279 m)
Sedan	500 lbs (227 kg)	100 ft (30 m)	320 ft (98 m)	1,050 ft (320 m)
Van	1,000 lbs (454 kg)	125 ft (38 m)	400 ft (122 m)	1,200 ft (366 m)
Moving van or delivery truck	4,000 lbs (1,814 kg)	200 ft (61 m)	640 ft (195 m)	1,750 ft (533 m)
Semi-trailer	40,000 lbs (18,143 kg)	450 ft (137 m)	1,400 ft (427 m)	3,500 ft (1,067 m)

Explosive capacity—Based on the maximum volume or weight of explosives (TNT equivalent) that could reasonably be hidden in the package or vehicle.

Lethal air blast range—The minimum distance personnel in the open are expected to survive from blast effects. It is based on severe lung damage or fatal impact injury from body translation.

Mandatory evacuation distance—The range to which all buildings must be evacuated. From this range to the desired evacuation distance, personnel may remain in the building (with some risk) but should move to a safe area in the interior of the building away from windows and exterior walls. Evacuated personnel must move to the desired evacuation distance.

Desired evacuation distance—The range to which personnel in the open must be evacuated and the preferred range for building evacuation. This is the maximum range of the threat from flying shrapnel/debris or flying glass from window breakage.

Source: Developed by the ATF, with technical assistance from the U.S. Corps of Engineers. Supported by the Technical Support Working Group (TSWG), a research and development arm of the National Security Council Interagency working group.

Pulmonary injuries may appear immediately post-blast or potentially 48 hours after the incident. These injuries are commonly found in patients who have suffered skull fractures, burns to greater than 10% of their body surface area, or penetrating injuries to the head or torso.[49] The Paramedic should suspect pulmonary involvement in any patient complaining of dyspnea or chest pain, or who has hemoptysis (cough). Initial treatment focuses upon the prevention of hypoxemia through the administration of high-flow, high-concentration oxygen by nonrebreather mask, CPAP, or endotracheal intubation. A pneumothorax may also be present and should be decompressed promptly in the face of a developing tension pneumothorax.[49]

The abdominal cavity contains numerous organs, both solid and hollow. Hollow organs, especially the colon, are most vulnerable. Bowel perforations, hemorrhages, shearing of the mesenteries, lacerations of solid organs, and testicular rupture are all potential injuries that may be sustained and should be suspected in any patient complaining of abdominal pain, nausea, vomiting, hematemesis, rectal pain, tenesmus, testicular pain, or unexplained hypovolemia. The Paramedic must perform a careful assessment as clinical signs may initially be subtle until an acute abdomen or sepsis develops.[49]

Other injuries that the Paramedic may encounter include tympanic injury or rupture evident with a complaint of hearing loss, tinnitus, otalgia, vertigo, otorrhea, or bleeding from the external canal. Patients may also suffer ocular injuries (very common), traumatic amputations, concussions, compartment syndrome, acute renal failure, or inhalation injuries/poisoning from released chemicals.[49]

Secondary injuries result from projectiles like shrapnel coming from the bomb material or other shrapnel added to the bomb by the terrorist. These cause penetrating injuries, fragmentation injuries, and blunt trauma. If the blast is strong enough, it may actually throw the patient, causing tertiary injuries such as fractures and traumatic amputations. Quaternary injuries are generally all other injuries sustained. These may be crush injuries, burns, asphyxia, toxic exposures, or the exacerbation of chronic illnesses.[45]

Other Forms of Terrorism

Although the elements of the mnemonic B-NICE are the most talked about forms of terrorism, they are not the only ones. Armed attacks, assassinations, hostage taking, hijacking, suicide terrorism, and cyberterrorism are other common forms of terrorism.

Armed Attacks

Armed attacks have a wide variability in their use and prevalence. Some studies have shown that this form of attack is used in anywhere from 7.5% to 30% of all terrorist incidents.[45,50] Some of these may be small attacks, such as the aforementioned 1999 World Trade Organization attack in Seattle, or may be more complex, such as the shootings at Columbine High School.

The types of weapons used may vary as well. Rifles, handguns, semi-automatic weapons, and automatic weapons are all possibilities, and the type chosen will depend upon the terrorist's objective. If the sole purpose is to kill the most people, then terrorists will select a weapon that can accomplish this in the shortest amount of time.[2]

The Paramedic may encounter several TRACEM harms when responding to an armed attack, such as mechanical (in the form of the fired projectile) and etiological (through contact with blood or bodily fluids).[2]

Assassination

When one typically thinks about assassinations by terrorists, key leaders are often the focus.[45] However, in recent years assassinations have become more prevalent as they bring about a high level of visibility, which sends a message to others in government, witnesses, investigators, and most recently, abortionists.[45]

The Paramedic responding to an assassination incident should take similar precautions as those used with an armed attack in terms of time, distance, and shielding. Paramedics should also be aware that the assassin may not want the patient to be cared for and may target the Paramedic to prevent anyone from entering the scene, caring for the patient, or even leaving with the patient. The Paramedic must work closely with law enforcement to safely mitigate the hazards.

Hostage/Barricade

There have been no recent incidents of domestic hostage taking or barricade cases of terrorism.[50] Generally speaking, terrorists use barricading and hostage taking to obtain publicity for a cause, achieve political demands, or negotiate leverage.[45]

In a barricade situation, the location of the terrorist and hostages is known.[45] They may be in a building, office, bus, train, ship, or other location. Another form of hostage taking occurs through kidnapping. In this instance, the location of the terrorist and hostage is often unknown.

Although the Paramedic's role will generally be post-rescue, Paramedics should still remain alert at all times for secondary devices. They also need to consider, as with any incident, that they may be the intended targets and could easily become a hostage themselves. Situational awareness throughout any incident is extremely vital to Paramedic protection.

Hijacking

Terrorists will often take and hold an aircraft, ship, car, or other form of transportation by force. This allows them to then use the vehicle and those on it as leverage to negotiate political demands or gain safe passage.

As increased security measures have been implemented on domestic forms of travel, this form of terrorism is still possible but highly unlikely. Similarly to hostage taking, the Paramedic must have continuous situational awareness, as ambulances are just another vehicle susceptible to hijacking.

Suicide Terrorism

Intentionally killing oneself in order to further a cause is more often seen with religious extremists than domestic terrorists and occurs frequently in the Middle East.

To kill oneself, one must either believe fervently in a cause, perhaps expecting to be rewarded handsomely in the afterlife, or be pressed into the situation through tactics such as kidnapping or hostage taking. Either way, the rate of suicide attacks has been increasing.

When people are willing to die for a cause it adds validity, but it is also an effective stealth tactic to create a large number of casualties in a crowded area.[45] The suicide terrorist often includes explosives, either by wearing the explosive and detonating it in a crowd of people or by driving a vehicle bomb into the target. This form of terrorism has been prevalent in the Middle East for many years and is expected to eventually arrive domestically.

Cyberterrorism

Civilization has become dependent upon computers. From television to ATMs, automatic doors to hydroelectric plants, the nation's infrastructure has become dependent upon computer networks.[12] Cyberterrorists are acutely aware of this and use cyber (hacking) tools to threaten the shutdown of critical infrastructures, actually shut them down, or create nuisance issues such as denial-of-service or other such attacks.[51]

Although terrorist groups have not used cyberterrorism to handicap any major U.S. infrastructures, they have been using their expertise in computer and electronic media for planning, fundraising, spreading propaganda, and communication.[12] These advances in technology have alarmed terrorist experts, causing concern not about if terrorists will use cyberterrorism, but when a cyberattack will occur.

This concern is so great that the National Infrastructure Protection Center in Washington, DC, was established to monitor for such attacks.[12] In 2008, there were 5,499 known breaches of the federal computer systems with hackers gaining access to such data as designs for a new fighter that is being built as well as computer networks that control three main U.S. electrical grids.[52]

Although cyberterrorism does not seem to pose an immediate threat to the Paramedic, the emergency services and public safety sectors are becoming more reliant on computers for communication, dispatch, organization, and even treatment. As these services often have little in terms of protective measures, they may soon become targets of the domestic cyberterrorist.

If hackers obtain access to such a system, they will have the ability to impede the entire operation of the public safety department. This could lead to response delays, improper responses, communication loss, and potentially a complete operational shutdown.

The Best Protection: A Change in Mindset

Throughout this chapter, a recurring theme has been stated: the Paramedic may inadvertently become a casualty of the incident or may actually be the intended target. The culture of public safety is to protect and rescue those in need and that danger is part of the job. This instinct is one of the greatest challenges Paramedics must overcome when responding to a potential terrorist incident.

The Paramedic's purpose is to save people when others are not able to. Many Paramedics feel that they are invincible and that their training has prepared them adequately for this mission. This is not entirely their fault, as the culture promotes "heroism" through awards and special recognition, instilling this behavior into the younger generation.

Terrorists not only know this, but also depend upon it. They depend upon the thought that responders will risk their lives for a complete stranger or one of their own, knowing that their "brothers" will rush in to their rescue. Terrorists have thus lured rescuers into their trap when rescuers have become casualties or even fatalities. This not only decreases the number of responders available, but paralyzes the response as well. This mindset of rushing in must change to prevent others from becoming patients. Accomplishing this will be extremely difficult and will take time. In fact, the possibility of the Paramedic being the actual target has already impacted future events, as responses may be delayed to assess the scene for safety.

▶ CASE STUDY CONCLUSION

"All units stand by for emergency traffic," barks the radio. The report is for multiple patients with exposure to an unknown chemical agent that produced patients with abdominal cramps, vomiting, and watering mouths. EMS has been detailed to the decontamination corridor to receive casualties in the cold zone.

CRITICAL THINKING QUESTIONS

1. What agent is likely to cause this symptom pattern?
2. Why is EMS involved in decontamination and what antidote is used to treat exposure to this agent?

CONCLUSION

The key concept Paramedics must realize about terrorism is that the goal is not necessarily to kill innocent people but to create such fear and dread that people can be coerced into following the terrorists' wishes. These methods are often low cost and low risk, but obtain high media exposure[45] such as the Atlanta Olympic pipe bombing. Alternatively, they may be much more involved, as with the September 11, 2001, attacks.

The Paramedic must maintain a high level of suspicion when responding to *any* call. As first responders, Paramedics must understand that terrorism is present domestically. Terrorism is not unique to foreign interests; domestic groups use it as well. These groups know that by causing first responders to become patients, they not only hinder the operations of the event, but also can psychologically impair the survivors and secondary responders. Provider safety must be the priority.

KEY POINTS:

- Provider safety is the first priority when responding to suspected terrorism attacks.

- Many definitions of terrorism have evolved.

- Terrorism can be either international or domestic.

- Domestic terrorists include left-wing extremists, right-wing extremists, militia, special interest groups such as the animal rights groups and environmentalists, and religious extremists.

- Suspicion of a terrorist attack is based on the location, the nature of the event, and the timing of the event.

- Principles of self-protection include time, distance, and shielding.

- The acronym TRACEM lists the injuries from terrorism.

- Agents of concern for biological terrorism include *Bacillus anthracis, Yersinia pestis, Variola major, Clostridium botulinum, Francisella tularensis*, and viral hemorrhagic fevers.

- Protective measures for biological attack involve the use of standard biohazard PPE.

- Nuclear weapons will most likely be dirty bombs.

- Protective measures for a nuclear attack will be time, distance, and most importantly shielding from radiation.

- Use of incendiary devices in terrorism is relatively low.

- Chemical agents depend on the same mechanisms as poisoning (i.e., inhalation, ingestion, absorption, and injection).

- Classes of chemical agents include organophosphates, vesicants, blood agents, and pulmonary agents (such as irritants and asphyxiants).

- Organophosphates are commonly used chemical weapons.

- The symptom pattern for organophosphate poisoning is highlighted in the mnemonic SLUDGEM.

- Armed attacks are also methods used in terrorism, and include assassination, hostage taking, hijacking, and suicide bombers.

- Cyberterrorism is the newest form of terrorism.

REVIEW QUESTIONS:

1. What differentiates a terrorist from a freedom fighter?
2. Who are the recognized domestic terror groups?
3. What does the acronym TRACEM stand for?
4. What are the biological agents of concern?
5. What are the types of armed attacks?

CASE STUDY QUESTIONS:

Please refer to the Case Study in this chapter, and answer the questions below:

1. What are the different classes of chemical agents used in terrorism?
2. What protective measures should a Paramedic take when confronted with chemical agents?
3. What does the acronym SLUDGEM stand for?

REFERENCES:

1. Bevelacqua A, Stilp R. *Terrorism Handbook for Operational Responders*. Albany, NY: Delmar Thompson Learning; 2002.
2. United States Department of Justice & Federal Emergency Management Agency. *Emergency Response to Terrorism: Basic Concepts*. Washington, DC: United States Fire Adminisration; 1997.
3. Nordberg M. When kids kill: Columbine High School shooting. *Emerg Med Serv*. 1999;28(10):39–46.
4. Jackson BA, Peterson DJ, Bartis JT, LaTourette T, Brahmakulam I, Houser A, et al. *Protecting emergency responders: lessons learned from terrorist attacks*. 2002. Available at: **http://www.rand.org/publications/CF/CF176/CF176.pdf**. Accesed December 16, 2003.
5. Touger HE. Weapons of mass destruction [Electronic Version]. *NFPA J*. July/August, 2001:63–65.
6. Maniscalco PM. EMS response to hazardous environments and its implications for the future of EMS education [Electroninc Version]. *Domain*. 2002;3(Winter):1–5.
7. Wikipedia. *Definition of terrorism*. 2009. Available at: **http://en.wikipedia.org/wiki/Definition_of_terrorism**. Accessed March 3, 2009.
8. Primoratz I. Terrorism. Stanford University Center for the Study of Language and Information. 2007. Available at: **http://plato.stanford.edu/entries/terrorism/**. Accessed January 14, 2009.
9. Wikipedia. The French Revolution. 2009. Available at: **http://en.wikipedia.org/wiki/French_Revolution#Reign_of_Terror**. Accessed February 26, 2009.
10. Terrorism Research. (n.d.). Goals and motivations of terrorists. Available at: **http://www.terrorism-research.com/goals/**. Accessed May 5, 2009.
11. Wikipedia. Alex P. Schmid. 2008. Available at: **http://en.wikipedia.org/wiki/Alex_P._Schmid**. Accessed March 3, 2009.
12. United States Department of Justice Federal Bureau of Investigation. (n.d.). Terrorism 2002–2005. Available at: **http://www.fbi.gov/publications.htm**. Accessed January 14, 2009.
13. Fletcher H. Militant extremists in the United States. Council on Foreign Relations. April 21, 2008. Available at: **http://www.cfr.org/publication/9236/**. Accessed March 23, 2009.
14. Rosenberg J. (n.d.) 1901–U.S. President William McKinley assassinated. Available at: **http://history1900s.about.com/od/1900s/qt/mckinleykilled.htm**. Accessed April 28, 2009.
15. Federal Bureau of Investigation. (n.d.). Famous cases: the Patty Hearst kidnapping. FBI History. Available at: **http://www.fbi.gov/libref/historic/famcases/hearst/hearst.htm**. Accessed April 2, 2009.
16. Thale C. Haymarket and May Day. *Encyclopedia of Chicago*. 2005. Available at: **http://www.encyclopedia.chicagohistory.org/pages/571.html**. Accessed April 25, 2009.
17. Nelson B. Anarchists. *Encyclopedia of Chicago*. 2005. Available at: **http://www.encyclopedia.chicagohistory.org/pages/49.html**. Accessed April 23, 2009.
18. Federal Bureau of Investigation. BYTE out of history 1975 terrorism flashback: state department bombing. Press room—headline archives. January 29, 2004. Available at: **http://www.fbi.gov/page2/jan04/weather012904.htm**. Accessed April 2, 2009.
19. Tucker JB. Historical trends related to bioterrorism: an empirical analysis. Centers for Disease Control and Prevention: Emerging Infectious Diseases. July 1, 1999. Available at: **http://origin.cdc.gov/ncidod/EID/vol5no4/tucker.htm**. Accessed March 23, 2009.
20. Federal Bureau of Investigation. Famous cases: terror hits home: the Oklahoma City bombing. FBI History. Available at: **http://www.fbi.gov/libref/historic/famcases/oklahoma/oklahoma.htm**. Accessed April 3, 2009.
21. Crawford M. Domestic terror: what it holds for the new millennium. MILNET. 2008. Available at: **http://www.milnet.com/domestic/Dom-Terror.htm**. Accessed March 5, 2009.
22. Federal Bureau of Investigation. (n.d.). Aryan Nation. Available at: **http://foia.fbi.gov/foiaindex/anation.htm**. Accessed May 5, 2009.

23. Wikipedia. Ruby Ridge. May 4, 2009. Available at: **http://en.wikipedia.org/wiki/Ruby_Ridge.** Accessed May 5, 2009.

24. Wikipedia. Waco seige. May 5, 2009. Available at: **http://en.wikipedia.org/wiki/Waco_Siege.** Accessed May 5, 2009.

25. United States Department of Homeland Security. *Ecoterrorism: Environmental and Animal-Rights Militants in the United States. United States Department of Homeland Security's National Preparedness Directorate.* Arlington, VA: Helios Global, Inc; 2008.

26. Food and Drug Administration. (n.d.). Animal testing. Available at: **http://www.fda.gov/CDER/HANDBOOK/animal.htm.** Accessed May 5, 2009.

27. The 9/11 Commission. *The 9/11 Commission Report: Final Report of the National Commission on Terrorist Attacks upon the United States.* New York: W.W. Norton & Company, Inc; 2004.

28. Mueller RS. Statement before the Senate Select Committee on Intelligence. January 11, 2007. Available at: **http://www.fbi.gov/congress/congress07/mueller011107.htm.** Accessed June 1, 2009.

29. United States Department of Justice & Federal Emergency Management Agency. *Emergency Response to Terrorism: Self-Study.* Washington, DC: United States Fire Administration; 1997.

30. Brown J. Confined space. October 10, 2003. Available at: **http://www.haz-map.com/NoEntry.htm.** Accessed May 5, 2009.

31. Centers for Disease Control and Prevention. Interim recommendations for the selection and use of protective clothing and respirators against biological agents. Emergency Preparedness and Response. October 25, 2001. Available at: **http://www.bt.cdc.gov/documentsapp/Anthrax/Protective/10242001Protect.asp.** Accessed March 23, 2009.

32. Centers for Disease Control and Prevention. *Q fever.* Viral and Rickettsial Zoonoses Branch. February 13, 2003. Available at: **http://www.cdc.gov/ncidod/dvrd/qfever/index.htm#Significance%20for%20Bioterrorism.** Accessed March 23, 2009.

33. Centers for Disease Control and Prevention. Recognition of illness associated with the intentional release of a biologic agent. *MMWR Weekly.* October 19, 2001;50(41):893–897.

34. Centers for Disease Control and Prevention. Fact sheet: anthrax information for health care providers. Emergency Preparedness and Response. March 8, 2002. Available at: **http://www.bt.cdc.gov/agent/anthrax/anthrax-hcp-factsheet.asp.** Accessed May 5, 2009.

35. Centers for Disease Control and Prevention. Frequently asked questions (FAQ) about plague. Emergency Preparedness and Response. April 5, 2005. Available at: **http://www.bt.cdc.gov/agent/plague/faq.asp.** Accessed May 5, 2009.

36. English JF, Cundiff MY, Malone JD, Pfeiffer JA, Bell M, Steele L, et al. Bioterrorism readiness plan: a template for healthcare facilities. Emergency Preparedness and Response. April 13, 1999. Available at: **http://www.cdc.gov/ncidod/dhqp/pdf/bt/13apr99APIC-CDCBioterrorism.PDF.** Accessed May 5, 2009.

37. Centers for Disease Control and Prevention. Smallpox disease overview. Emergency Preparedness and Response. December 30, 2004. Available at: **http://www.bt.cdc.gov/agent/smallpox/overview/disease-facts.asp.** Accessed May 5, 2009.

38. Centers for Disease Control and Prevention. Botulism facts for health care providers. Emergency Preparedness and Response. April 19, 2006. Available at: **http://www.bt.cdc.gov/agent/botulism/hcpfacts.asp.** Accessed May 5, 2009.

39. Centers for Disease Control and Prevention. Casualty management after detonation of a nuclear weapon in an urban area. Emergency Preparedness and Response. May 10, 2006. Available at: **http://www.bt.cdc.gov/radiation/casualtiesdetonation.asp.** Accessed March 23, 2009.

40. Centers for Disease Control and Prevention. Key facts about tularemia. Emergency Preparedness and Response. October 3, 2003. Available at: **http://www.bt.cdc.gov/agent/tularemia/facts.asp.** Accessed May 5, 2009.

41. Centers for Disease Control and Prevention. Filoviruses. Special Pathogens Branch. August 24, 2004. Available at: **http://www.cdc.gov/ncidod/dvrd/spb/mnpages/dispages/filoviruses.htm.** Accessed May 6, 2009.

42. Centers for Disease Control and Prevention. Arenaviruses. Special Pathogens Branch. August 22, 2005. Available at: **http://www.cdc.gov/ncidod/dvrd/spb/mnpages/dispages/arena.htm.** Accessed May 6, 2009.

43. Centers for Disease Control and Prevention. Viral hemorrhagic fevers. Special Pathogens Branch. August 23, 2004. Available at: **http://www.cdc.gov/ncidod/dvrd/spb/mnpages/dispages/vhf.htm.** Accessed May 5, 2009.

44. National Counterterrorism Center. (n.d. e). Indicators of a possible chemical incident. Available at: **http://www.nctc.gov/site/technical/chemical_incident.html.** Accessed April 2, 2009.

45. Lal R, Jackson BA. Change and continuity in terrorism revisited: terrorist tactics, 1980–2005. *The MIPT Terrorism Annual 2006.* Available at: **http://www.tkb.org/documents/Downloads/2006-MIPT-Terrorism-Annual.pdf.** Accessed August 18, 2009.

46. Buck G. *Preparing for Terrorism: An Emergency Services Guide.* Toronto, Ontario, Canada: Delmar; 2002.

47. Heightman AJ. Rude awakening. *JEMS.* 2001;26(11):10–11.

48. Agency for Toxic Substances and Disease Registry. Medical Management Guidelines for Unidentified Chemical. Medical Management Guidelines. September 24, 2007. Available at: **http://www.atsdr.cdc.gov/MHMI/mmg170.html.** Accessed April 10, 2009.

49. Centers for Disease Control and Prevention. Blast injuries: essential facts. Emergency Preparedness and Response. March 25, 2008. Available at: **http://www.bt.cdc.gov/masscasualties/blastessentials.asp.** Accessed April 10, 2009.

50. Lawson Terrorism Information Center. (n.d.). Terrorism incidents and significant dates. MIPT Library: Available at: **http://www.terrorisminfo.mipt.org/incidentcalendar.asp.** Accessed April 2, 2009.

51. Mueller III RS. Testimony of Robert S. Mueller, III, Director, FBI before the Select Committee on Intelligence of the United States Senate, February 11, 2003, "War on Terrorism." Congressional Testimony. February 3, 2003. Available at: **http://www.fbi.gov/congress/congress03/mueller021103.htm.** Accessed May 6, 2009.

52. Falk W, ed. The rise of the cyberspy. *The Week.* 2009;9(415):13.

PUBLIC HEALTH EMERGENCY PREPAREDNESS AND RESPONSE

KEY CONCEPTS:

Upon completion of this chapter, it is expected that the reader will understand these following concepts:

- The roles and responsibilities of public health
- The Paramedic's role in public health
- The similarities and differences between disasters and public health emergencies
- The challenges to public health

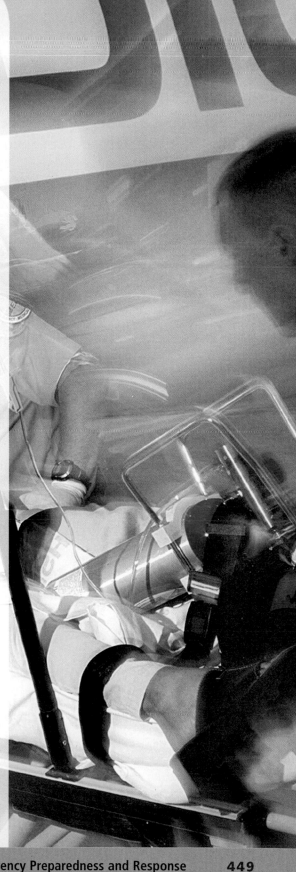

CASE STUDY:

"It seems like all we transport anymore is the flu, the flu, the flu," The Paramedic sighs. "Will it ever stop?" The hospitals are bursting at the seams. The only remaining beds are outside of the region and many hospitals seem reluctant to accept these "flu" patients for fear of spreading the disease.

CRITICAL THINKING QUESTIONS

1. How does a public health emergency differ from a mass-casualty disaster?
2. How might a Paramedic's role change during a public health emergency?

OVERVIEW

The public health system is comprised of many private and public entities including local, state, and federal health agencies that collectively promote wellness; prevent illness, injury, and premature death; and otherwise protect the community at large. Emergency Medical Services (EMS), a part of the public health system, are delivered by a wide assortment of diverse entities that each play a vital role in the public health system. The traditional EMS role of responding to day-to-day clinical emergencies throughout communities continues to expand in the twenty-first century. In addition to a broader medical scope of practice that may provide value-added care for individual patients, Paramedics have taken on increased responsibility in public health emergency responses involving—or potentially involving—multiple patients. Events like those of September 11, 2001; local and national foodborne and infectious outbreaks; chemical and radiation releases; and threats of bioterrorism are a few of the situations in which emergency responders have been called upon to assist public health agencies.

Local public health departments utilize various tools on a daily basis, such as disease surveillance; outbreak investigation; case finding; laboratory analysis; environmental protection; outbreak immunization; treatment and prophylaxis for infectious, chemical, and radiation exposure; isolation and quarantine; public health education; and health risk communication. During public health emergencies, these state and federal health agencies typically deploy these same tactics. The difference is that in larger scale public health emergencies these actions must occur faster, more robustly, and on a wider scale.

The challenge to current public health departments stems from the ongoing erosion of their infrastructure, in large part because of governmental belt tightening, especially at times when public health problems have not been at the forefront. These shortcomings become very apparent during public health emergencies. Utilizing Paramedics for support beyond their typical clinical care duties can be invaluable to help fill some of these public health emergency voids. Despite the logistical and practical challenges of the public health agency and EMS interface, the ability to strategically leverage these two branches of the public health system at a moment's notice can prove beneficial to protect and serve the public in times of crisis and tragedy.

Traditional Disasters and Public Health Emergencies

Public health has been defined as the practice and discipline of maintaining and improving the health of communities. This occurs through assessment of the population's health, assurance of health care including prevention services for all, and promotion of public policy designed to protect the public's health. Paramedics can play important roles in the implementation of these public health goals, especially in terms of surveillance and treatment. Care and access to the healthcare system frequently begins with EMS. In times of crisis, this access becomes even more crucial.

In general, traditional mass-casualty incidents (MCIs) and other disasters have been macro, confined, de-escalating events. In other words, a catastrophic event of a relatively sudden onset and defined duration causes effects that can be visualized in a fairly well demarcated geographic area, which then recede over time. These incidents include earthquakes, floods or other weather-related events, large multi-vehicle crashes, fires, explosions, and airplane crashes. Although the damage from these MCIs generally occurs fairly abruptly and may or may not involve humans, there is typically a definitive endpoint of the destruction, after which the event de-escalates. The geographic area involved is typically obvious, and the threat is easily visualized or otherwise recognized by responders and the community alike. Perhaps most significantly, the danger is not occult, which helps individuals put it into the proper perspective.

In contrast, incidents that might be defined as **public health emergencies** are typically micro, poorly demarcated, potentially escalating events that involve humans. These include incidents such as large foodborne illness outbreaks (e.g., salmonella, *E. coli*), bioterrorism (e.g., smallpox, anthrax), chemical and radiation release, and pandemic infections (e.g., influenza). Both the onset and endpoint of a public health emergency may be poorly defined and difficult to recognize, especially in real time. The offending agents often cannot be easily visualized or measured, and can spread in unpredictable manners throughout poorly demarcated geographic areas.

Because of these characteristics, management of public health emergencies can present challenges that are not encountered with more traditional disasters. For example, an infectious disease cannot be seen with the naked eye and can be readily transmitted from person to person by those patients who do not remain stationary. Containment of such a disease can be especially difficult. More importantly, these occult properties can lead to irrational fear and even panic among the masses who have little to no ability to personally recognize the presence or disappearance of the threatening agents as they can during more traditional disasters. It becomes very difficult for citizens and even responders to know where the danger is and, perhaps more significantly, where it is not.

In reality, even traditional disasters have public health implications, and vice versa. The distinction between traditional disasters and public health emergencies is artificial at best since there are typically roles to play for all agencies in most large-scale events. For example, during an early snowstorm in Buffalo, New York, in October 2006, many trees and tree limbs fell because of heavy, wet snow sticking to leaves that had not yet fallen (Figure 22-1). This resulted in widespread power outages, which led to other consequences including travel problems from nonfunctioning traffic signals; house fires from cooking and heating with stoves and grills; various other public safety issues; food, medication, and sheltering needs; and a near wide-scale water outage.

The Buffalo snowstorm response required expertise and resources from many disciplines including EMS and public health. As one example, many individuals began requesting assistance with symptoms of carbon monoxide poisoning after placing portable gas generators in unsafe locations (e.g., basements, garages, outside open windows and doors). Public health recognized this problem through various reporting channels and launched aggressive risk communication efforts. However, sharing of information via traditional

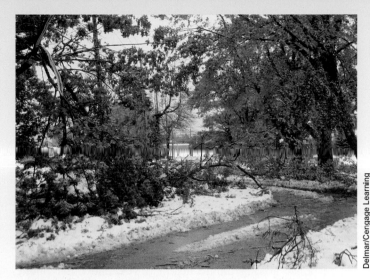

Figure 22-1 The widespread power outages and difficulty in road travel caused by a winter storm created a multitude of public health issues in Buffalo, New York.

methods such as electronic media was limited because of the lack of power. Therefore, public health workers placed brightly colored signs on gas pumps where citizens might go to purchase fuel for their generators. In addition to providing patient care and surveillance, EMS could also distribute signs, as well as engage in other creative risk communication actions, given its knowledge of local neighborhoods and their unique positions in them.

Responding to Public Health Emergencies

A public health emergency is likely to be more protracted than a typical incident. An outbreak of an infectious disease, for example, is likely to occur over several days, weeks, or even months. An **index case** (the first reported case) or several cases may go unrecognized for some time before a response is even initiated, and resolution of the matter may require protracted interventions over time. Events such as the contamination of peanut butter with salmonella in the United States in 2006 to 2007 and 2009 are examples of the slowly progressive nature of recognizing and responding to public health emergencies.[1] In each instance, several weeks elapsed before the cases were linked to each other and to a common source.

This presents a significant challenge to public health officials, especially in terms of isolation and prevention strategies. In contrast, a large incident involving bioterrorism or an intentional release of a chemical or radiological agent may occur over a period of hours, necessitating a rapid response from EMS and healthcare officials. Whether the onset is rapid or insidious, the same principles of prevention, isolation, and treatment apply.

In a mass-casualty or disaster event, "the needs of the many may outweigh the needs of the few."[2] In other words, individual illness and injury, while important to recognize and treat, may have to be of secondary importance compared to the safety and security of the population as a whole. Although this may lead to difficult ethical triage and treatment decisions for the Paramedic, the overall goal is to prevent the expansion of the public health incident.

In mass-casualty incidents, effective communication among public health, EMS, and all other public safety agencies is critical. EMS and other public safety agencies are likely to have superior communications technologies compared to those used by public health. Public health may appreciate the opportunity to share these resources.

In addition to shared communication, coordination of the response among public health, EMS, and other public safety agencies is vital. A clearly delineated Incident Command structure and hierarchy should be established according to the national response framework as soon as possible after an outbreak or incident begins. However, this may be complicated by the widespread nature of the incident, particularly if an airborne or otherwise communicable disease or agent is circulating. In some instances, cooperation between state, local, federal, and even international agencies may be required. Even so, establishing a clear, Unified Command structure may not be feasible given the multitude of overlapping jurisdictions.

The Paramedic's role may be expanded during a public health emergency, especially if the event requires rapid mobilization of evaluation and treatment services (Figure 22-2). In addition to providing initial patient evaluation and transport to an appropriate healthcare facility, the Paramedic may be called upon to perform duties outside his or her usual scope of practice. Patient triage, isolation, prolonged care, vaccination, and evacuation may become the Paramedic's responsibility, depending on the event's specifics and the availability of resources to meet the patients' needs. One example of this occurred in New York State in anticipation of the need for mass H1N1 influenza vaccinations. In this case, an emergency order enabled Paramedics to participate in providing vaccinations in public health mass clinics.[3]

In general, states or subdivisions thereof define Paramedics' day-to-day scope of practice. These official roles may need to be expanded or amended, however, if a situation arises in which the Paramedics are needed to help meet the response's increased and unmet demands. For example, Paramedics may be asked to provide or oversee manual bag-valve-mask ventilation of intubated patients in the setting of a severe respiratory illness outbreak and ventilator shortage. These same Paramedics may also be tasked to help provide comfort measures to moribund patients (those without the capacity to survive) when hospital resources are overwhelmed caring for potentially viable patients.

Triage during an outbreak scenario may be significantly different from what is practiced during a trauma MCI. For example, triage of patients is unlikely to occur at a single location. Unlike a trauma MCI where multiple patients are in one general area and require rapid triage to determine the extent of their injuries and viability, the patients of a public health emergency may be spread out across a large region. However, this is not always the case. In a simple scenario such as a food- or waterborne illness in a residential facility, the patients may actually be in a single location. In this situation, standard triage principles might apply. However, in a more widespread event such as a bioterrorism exposure like that seen with the anthrax cases in 2001, usual triage guidelines may not be applicable. The issue at hand may not be determining which patients are treated first, but rather which patients have been exposed and require decontamination, prophylaxis, and/or treatment at all. Additionally, the severity of the event may not be apparent at the outset, thus complicating the process of determining the order in which patients receive medical care. As more information becomes available or as the situation evolves, public health officials may add additional guidelines and practices to appropriately allocate resources to care for these patients.

Isolation is defined as the physical separation of individuals with a communicable disease from others, as opposed to quarantine where susceptible but not necessarily infected individuals are separated from others. This practice is not uncommon in medicine. For instance, patients diagnosed with illnesses such as influenza, chicken pox, or rotaviruses are usually advised to limit their contact with others to curtail the spread of their illness. This may include keeping children home from school or daycare, or missing work to prevent the infection of coworkers. When the number of patients is substantial or even unknown, the practice of isolation becomes extremely challenging. Under those circumstances, **social distancing** efforts may need to be invoked. Institutions within communities such as school systems, business or government offices, and religious organizations may be asked (or required) to alter or suspend normal activities to

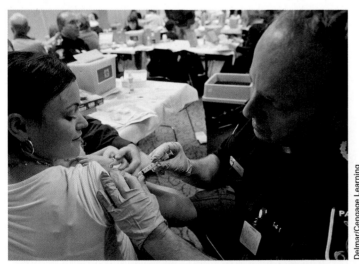

Figure 22-2 This Paramedic is administering H1N1 vaccine under an expanded scope of practice order during the 2009 season.

prevent unnecessary person-to-person contact. In these settings, Paramedics may be asked to help identify potentially infectious persons and aid public health officials in establishing and enforcing quarantine and isolation. Assistance may range from providing masks for respiratory protection, to full quarantine of infectious persons, depending on the risks and transmission routes of a particular disease.

In addition to providing patient isolation, Paramedics may be called upon to assist with prevention and/or treatment through vaccination and/or medication dispensing if public health officials determine that these actions are necessary to reduce risk in a given population (i.e., **ring vaccination**). Typically, these actions will be time dependent, and the need to serve large groups of individuals in a short time frame may exceed the resources of the local public health and medical community. As a means of increasing the number of patients screened, treated, immunized, or provided with prophylactic medications in a timely fashion, Paramedics may be utilized to assist with preparation or actual administration of vaccines or medications at a **point-of-dispensing (POD) site**. Within the POD site itself, patients will be moved through the process of being screened, examined, and treated, and Paramedics may be involved in any of these tasks (Figure 22-3). For

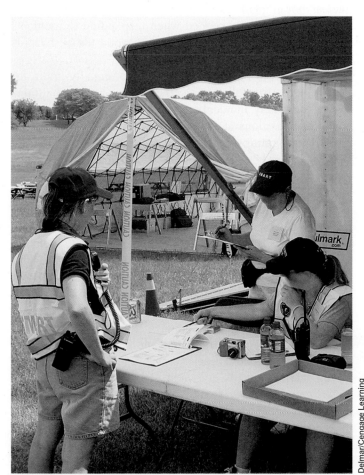

Figure 22-3 Paramedics can be utilized to perform many different functions during a POD deployment.

instance, they may help administer a screening questionnaire, take vital signs, or perform a basic health screen in addition to assisting with the intended treatment as previously described.

By providing these services at a centralized location, personnel and other healthcare resources are consolidated, thus increasing operational efficiency. In this situation, EMS providers may be asked to transport patients who are otherwise unable to get themselves to and from POD sites. Alternatively, EMS providers may deliver vaccinations and/or medications directly to these shut-ins. Of course, state and other laws will dictate what, if any, expanded scope of practice EMS providers will be allowed to perform.

Challenges of Public Health Emergency Response

Events in the United States such as the terrorist attacks of September 11, 2001, and Hurricane Katrina have highlighted some of the challenges associated with responding to public health emergencies. Perhaps the most striking challenge results from insufficient resources. Lack of funding, personnel, and medical equipment and supplies can quickly limit an agency's ability to mount an appropriate response, which may result in inadequate prevention or treatment of large numbers of individuals.

For most agencies, inadequate funding is a common theme in today's world. Budgets are lean for public and private agencies alike, and this leads to difficulties just meeting basic day-to-day operational needs. Additional expenditures for public health emergency preparations may quickly exceed available funds and, therefore, fall by the wayside. Further, costs incurred during actual responses are typically not included as contingencies in budgets. For EMS agencies, these expenses may include overtime pay for Paramedics and dispatchers, increased vehicle maintenance and fuel costs, and the cost of medical supplies and equipment replacement. Whether the agency is government sponsored or private, these additional expenses are likely to contribute to both immediate and long-term financial strain.

Inadequate personnel (human resources) is also likely to contribute to a delay in public health's response to a public health emergency or disaster. A significant rise in the number of patients seeking emergency medical care during such an event may not only exceed the resources of the local emergency departments, but will likely overwhelm the EMS system as well. In addition, if the Paramedics are serving expanded roles to assist with the public health emergency, it will further limit the number of Paramedics available on ambulances for triage, treatment, and transportation. Furthermore, the potential exists for rescuers to become patients in the line of duty, not only from exposure to the incident at hand, but also due to fatigue and burnout if called upon to work longer hours in strained environments. These complications effectively limit their ability to provide medical care and potentially worsen the provider shortage.

The scarcity of medical supplies may be the most ominous deficiency. Lack of medications, antidotes, vaccinations, immunizations, and supplies such as resuscitation equipment and ventilators may result in higher morbidity and mortality if the need becomes too great. Although stockpiling these supplies ahead of time will aid in ensuring the agency has adequate resources, there is no way to predict the potential needs of an emergency. Therefore, even the best preparedness efforts can fall short if the number of patients becomes too great. Moreover, if various supplies and medications are kept too long without restocking, they may pass their expiration date. This is another challenge public health officials must consider when planning and implementing a stockpile program.

Supplies can be quickly exhausted as a situation's needs become increasingly overwhelming. Sharing resources and making concerted efforts at cooperation between local, state, and federal agencies is one method of meeting the needs of a strained system. In a collaborative system, in which development and deployment of resources is a shared duty without duplication of efforts and funds and supplies are readily available, the result is an improved and streamlined response. An article published in 2003 highlighted a policy of pooling resources among several county health departments within a particular geographic area.[4] The result was better utilization and availability of resources without inappropriate duplication of services.

Communication between and within a variety of agencies may be difficult during a large event. Even when the event is limited to a single location, communication frequently breaks down. This challenge is magnified when the emergency extends beyond geographic borders. Even with the establishment of an excellent flow of communications and a flawless Incident Command structure, technical difficulties such as downed phone wires or cell towers, power outages limiting computer and electronic usage, and operator error are all potential sources of ineffective communication. Most agencies and organizations have a contingency plan that must be able to handle the increased and unique needs inherent in mass incidences.

Finally, the public's response to a public health emergency may present responders with a significant challenge. Most people will receive their information from the national or local media, including radio, television, newspapers, and Internet sources. Reporting by the media has the power to both incite and suppress public mass hysteria, depending on the tone thereof and how often information on a given topic is presented. However, reporting by even the most dedicated media outlets may contribute to inappropriate public panic if the information they are given is incomplete, false, or misleading. The responsibility for clear and accurate dissemination of information for a particular emergency or event lies with the public health officials at an appropriate level. This may include the World Health Organization, Centers for Disease Control, and/or state and local health departments.

In all cases, medical personnel including Paramedics should provide patient education and treatment in a manner consistent with published public health guidelines and statements for that particular incident. It is important for Paramedics to be well informed and stay updated, as events are often very fluid. Accordingly, changes occur frequently and suddenly. Failure to stay updated may lead to less-than-optimal outcomes.

Preparing for Public Health Emergencies

"Be Prepared!"

—The motto of the Boy Scouts of America[5]

This simple phrase should also be the mantra for EMS agencies and public health organizations alike. Although it is impossible to be fully prepared for every conceivable event or incident, taking an all-hazards approach to planning will provide Paramedics with the basic framework necessary to respond to any type of event. The all-hazards approach develops a general response plan that is applicable to all events and has appendices for specific situations that are pertinent to a geographic area. For example, a community that has a nuclear power plant close by will develop an appendix to cover specific actions needed when responding to incidents at the nuclear power plant that goes beyond the all-hazards response plan.

Individually, Paramedics should continually train for their response to public health emergencies just as one trains for mass-casualty incidents, typical medical calls for assistance, or operations at the scene of a motor vehicle crash. Training programs are essential to ensure that plans are well understood by all responders. A well-trained workforce will afford the best chance for a coordinated and successful response, especially when the unpredicted event occurs.

Many individual training courses exist to allow the Paramedic to gain new knowledge or reinforce current knowledge. Both the Federal Emergency Management Association (FEMA)[6] and United States Fire Academy (USFA)[7] offer on-line and on-site training programs for Paramedics. These sites also have resources the Paramedic can use in community education programs.

Tabletop exercises use either paper instructions or scale models to walk Paramedics and emergency managers through an incident. These exercises are logistically easier to run than live drills and help test and modify response plans or appendices without expending significant resources. Tabletop exercises may be used during the development of a multi-agency plan to allow leaders to think through actions during an incident and integrate knowledge of their specific agency's operational policies or habits. Tabletop exercises also help new officers or leaders in an organization develop incident management skills. Didactic or practical information may also be included in the tabletop exercise. As an example, a tabletop exercise on an influenza pandemic may include not only a didactic run-through of the steps to activate a vaccination POD, but also an injection demonstration and practice station.

Live drills are the next stage in testing a response plan. Live drills attempt to recreate an incident in compressed time with agencies performing the functions required at the scene of an actual response (Figure 22-4). These exercises should be progressive, unfolding with reasonable timing of an actual response to best test the system. Live drills are resource intensive and typically involve a significant amount of resources. In contrast to tabletop exercises which generally involve management and supervisory personnel, live drills involve the average street Paramedic in the process.

Live drills can be creative. For example, one county health department tests their smallpox immunization plan annually by holding seasonal influenza vaccination PODs to maintain proficiency in moving people through the system. A similar setup was used to test the anthrax post-exposure prophylaxis plan using boy scouts on jamboree who distributed M&M's candies to simulate ciprofloxacin and doxycycline packs. These regular drills helped maintain proficiency, which helped during the implementation of H1N1 vaccination PODs in the fall of 2009.[8]

Tabletop exercises and drills are important ways for EMS and public health organizations to combine preparation exercises and uncover preparedness strengths and weaknesses.

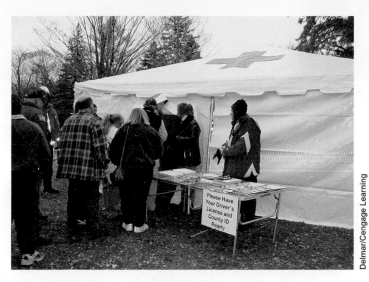

Figure 22-4 Live training drills allow public health departments to fully test their ability to handle large numbers of patients.

These exercises should occur as frequently as needed in order to maintain familiarity with the various plans and strategies. Continuing education to maintain appropriate skill levels can be integrated into these drills to help maintain proficiency with the response plan.

CASE STUDY CONCLUSION

The crew has been called to the Holiday Inn hotel on Route 66 to meet with the public health medical director. The public health agency has taken over the hotel as a temporary shelter and is reminiscent of the original hospitals, like the *hospitel-Hotel Dieu* in Paris. The county medical director assigns Paramedics to administer vaccinations at the grocery store in the next village over as part of a ring vaccination program.

CRITICAL THINKING QUESTIONS

1. What authority does a county medical director have to commandeer a hotel for use as a temporary hospital?
2. What is the purpose of ring vaccinations?

CONCLUSION

Citizens rely on the public health system to protect them and deliver the best care possible in times of public health emergencies. The Paramedic's role may be expanded during such events, and the need for effective communication and cooperation is never greater. With appropriate training and effective planning, the EMS response to a public health emergency may not only save lives, but can be an incredible and rewarding experience.

KEY POINTS:

- EMS is part of public health and its larger entity, health care.

- Paramedics may be more utilized in public health as a result of expanded roles and an enlarged scope of practice.

- Public health emergencies tend to be micro events that are poorly demarcated and have the potential to escalate.

- One of the largest challenges during a public health emergency is containing mass hysteria.

- Triage for a public health emergency differs from mass-casualty incident triage.

- Isolation and social distancing are practiced during a public health emergency.

- Prevention includes ring vaccination at points of dispersal.

- Challenges at public health emergencies include inadequate numbers of personnel, insufficient quantities of medical supplies, lack of interagency communications, and poor public notification. These problems are the result, in part, of insufficient funding.

- Public health training, as well as tabletop drills, can help prepare the Paramedic for an EMS response.

REVIEW QUESTIONS:

1. What are the roles of public health during a public health emergency?
2. What differentiates a disaster, such as an earthquake, from a public health emergency, such as a flu epidemic?
3. What are some examples of public health emergencies?
4. What principles do disaster management and public health management have in common?
5. What are some of the challenges the Paramedic faces at a public health emergency?

CASE STUDY QUESTIONS:

Please refer to the Case Study in this chapter, and answer the questions below:

1. What procedures might a Paramedic be called on to perform that are outside the Paramedic's usual scope of practice?
2. How would triage be different in this case than triage performed at a typical disaster?
3. What roles would the Paramedic perform while assisting public health officials?

REFERENCES:

1. Multistate outbreak of *Salmonella* serotype: Tennessee infections associated with peanut butter—United States, 2006–2007. *MMWR*. June 1, 2007;56(21):521–524.

2. Wolfson AB, ed. *Harwood-Nuss' Clinical Practice of Emergency Medicine* (4th ed.). Philadelphia: Lippincott Williams & Wilkins; 2005.

3. New York State executive order 29. Available at: **http://www.ny.gov/governor/executive_orders/exeorders/eo_29.html.** Accessed December 20, 2009.

4. Billittier AJ. Regional emergency preparedness efforts by local health departments in western New York. *J. Pub Health Practice and Mgmt*. 2003;9(5):394 400.

5. Boy Scouts of America. Emergency preparedness BSA. Available at: **http://www.scouting.org/scoutsource/Media/Publications/EmergencyPreparedness.aspx.** Accessed December 1, 2009.

6. FEMA independent study courses. Available at: **http://training.fema.gov/IS/crslist.asp.** Accessed December 20, 2009.

7. USFA campus and online course offering. Available at: **http://www.usfa.dhs.gov/applications/nfacourses/main/home.** Accessed December 20, 2009.

8. Personal communication. Craig Cooley, MD, Medical Director, Erie County Specialized Medical Assistance Response Team. December 20, 2009.

CHAPTER 23

TRIAGE SYSTEMS

KEY CONCEPTS:

Upon completion of this chapter, it is expected that the reader will understand these following concepts:

- The origin of triage
- Prehospital triage systems such as START, JumpSTART, SALT, and STM
- Evidence-based triage
- Computer-assisted triage
- Hospital triage

CASE STUDY:

"This is a National Weather Service warning," the radio blasts. Heavy downpours and tornados have been tearing down the eastern portion of the state. The Paramedics are already en route to a neighboring town where a small Category 4 tornado reportedly touched down in the center of town. The carnage is reportedly extensive with barely a building left standing. As part of the first-arriving ambulance crew, the Paramedic guesses that they will be doing triage.

CRITICAL THINKING QUESTIONS

1. What is the goal of triage? Has that changed over time?
2. What are some of the commonly used triage schemas?

OVERVIEW

Triage is the process of sorting patients into appropriate care categories. More specifically, triage can mean choosing an appropriate destination for the patient; for example, a trauma center for a patient with a life-threatening injury or a cardiac center for a patient experiencing an ST-elevation myocardial infarction. Triage in the setting of a **mass-casualty incident (MCI)** (a situation involving several potential patients) is a means of sorting patients by severity and condition. The goal remains to get patients to the most appropriate care. From an overall incident perspective, the Paramedic's objective is to do the greatest good for the most patients. The first step in this process is ensuring patients are treated in the order of their severity of injuries, based on available resources. During MCIs, the Paramedic determines prioritization of patient care by identifying the most severely injured patients who are likely to survive, even though these patients may not always be the most critically injured.[1] This chapter discusses the history of triage, practical considerations of triage, and several of the different triage methodologies used by EMS and the emergency department to sort patients.

Origin and History of Triage

The concept of triage dates back to the late eighteenth century and has been modified several times over the subsequent two hundred years. In 1797, Baron Dominique Jean Larrey, Napoleon's chief surgeon, designed the flying ambulance system for the specific purpose of transporting injured soldiers from the field of battle to the forward field hospitals at or near the time of their injury instead of waiting for each day's battle to end at nightfall. Prior to initiating this system, casualties waited, lying on the ground, until the fighting stopped for the day and then were moved to the field hospitals. That same year, Larrey described the process of *triage*, the French word for sorting, of the injured to maximize survivorship. Larrey stated,

> *"The best plan that can be adopted in such emergencies, to prevent the evil consequences of leaving soldiers who are severely wounded without assistance, is to place the ambulances as near as possible to the line of the battle, and to establish headquarters, to which all the wounded, who require delicate operations, shall be collected to be operated upon by the surgeon-general."[2]*

Relative to the medical aspects of the triage process, Larrey further stated,

> *"Those who are dangerously wounded should receive the first attention, without regard to rank or distinction. They who are injured in a less degree may wait until their brethren-in-arms, who are badly mutilated, have been operated and dressed, otherwise the latter would not survive many hours; rarely until the succeeding*

> *day. Besides with a slight wound, it is easy to repair to the hospital of the first or second line, especially for the officers, who generally have means of transportation. Finally, life is not endangered by such wounds."[2]*

Larrey's statement, "Those who are dangerously wounded should receive the first attention, without regard to rank or distinction," must be read in context to the entire description. Taken by itself, the concept of **worst first** (the most seriously injured are the first to receive treatment) makes sense and seems appropriate. In fact, this approach seems so logical that current triage schema advocate this approach. However, as Larrey's system was modified, the paradigm shifted away from the worst first concept.

In the mid-1800s, British Naval Surgeon John Wilson observed that, in order to be most effective in treating large numbers of casualties, physicians needed to focus on the group of patients who needed immediate treatment and in whom treatment was likely to be successful.[3] Wilson also observed that treatment of patients with less severe injuries should be deferred until after the group requiring immediate treatment was treated.

As weapons became more deadly in World War I, the number of casualties requiring triage and treatment grew tremendously. With the number of casualties far outpacing available resources, the worst first paradigm changed to the following:

> *". . . The greatest good for the greatest number must be the rule", recognizing that ". . . A single case, even if it urgently requires attention . . . may have to wait, for in the same time a dozen others, almost equally exigent, but requiring less time, may be cared for."[4]*

This paradigm shift brings about several ethical issues that are different from the normal provision of care.[5]

Triage continued to evolve within military medicine. With each war, the process continued to improve survival outcomes. In World War I, the triage system continued to require physicians to make the triage decisions once the wounded arrived at the clearing station. The less seriously injured were sent to evacuation hospitals, whereas the more seriously injured were sent to field hospitals. World War I physicians used a three-category system of triage (Table 23-1). It is important to note that the patients in Category 2 were the highest priority patients and received first aid before being moved to the next level of care.

Significant advances were also made during the Korean Conflict and the Vietnam War, primarily due to advancements in communications, transport, and the expansion of field care at the physician and physician extender levels. These advances in triage, rapid transport, and field care reduced battlefield death (Table 23-2).[6]

Development of Civilian Triage

In the mid-1970s, the U.S. Department of Navy at Camp Pendleton, California, contracted with a healthcare optimization and maximization consulting firm to solve the problem of inaccurate assessment of wounded sailors and soldiers. Upon studying the issues, they determined that, regardless of the amount of training provided, corpsmen and medics initially assessed the wounded by geography. The first time they were placed in a battlefield medical situation, they would assess and treat the first injured soldier they physically came upon, then the next, and then the next. Shortly thereafter, they would assimilate their training and knowledge and begin assessing those that needed care, thereby making decisions based on patient survival instead of location.

The Department of Navy also required that the assessment process include the knowledge and equipment already being provided to the medical teams. It was specified that the gear could not include anything that added weight to the medic's pack, required calibration, or required a power source. The team evaluated numerous additional factors in the assessment process including the physiological perimeters of pulse, pulse oximetry, respiratory rate, EKG, heart rate, mental status, and motor response, to name a few. After several years of evaluation and analysis, the final report focused on assessing the respiration rate, the pulse rate, and the best motor response to provide an accurate assessment. Each of the physiological measures was assigned a coded value that enhanced the accuracy of the patients' criticality at the time of the assessment. With this accurate, objective information, the triage officer was able to properly prioritize the wounded and increase their likelihood for a positive outcome.

Shortly thereafter, the local hospital and fire department in the nearby community of Newport Beach developed a civilian version based on this research and other information available at the time. The adapted protocol was named **Simple Triage And Rapid Transport (START)**.[7] Originally, START was promoted as a way to reduce the chaos at the scene of a disaster and thus increase prehospital scene effectiveness. Although the original work focused on blunt trauma, START has also been used to triage patients of penetrating trauma. Over the ensuing two decades, START became the de facto triage protocol across the United States and in many places around the world.[8]

Complications of Inappropriate Triage

Throughout the history of triage, issues of under- and over-triaging have continued to plague the application of the triage method and patient outcomes. **Undertriage** is commonly defined as underestimating the severity of a patient's injuries. It may also be defined as underestimating the expanse of the entire event. Undertriage may occur when the first-arriving rescuers instruct the patients who can move to relocate to a safer location. Whether from "adrenaline rush," a "fight-or-flight" response, or a primal survival response, some patients may move as instructed despite potentially life-threatening or life-altering injuries.

One documented example of undertriage occurred at the Pentagon on September 11, 2001. In this case, military personnel were acting as rescuers despite having significant injuries of their own. Paramedics had to take actions to assure that those injured were assessed before they were allowed to

Table 23-1 The Three-Category Triage Schema Used by U.S. Military Physicians in World War I

Category 1	These patients, who were unlikely to respond to treatment locally or to survive evacuation, were provided with palliative care and placed in a common area.
Category 2	These patients, who were capable of surviving the trauma of evacuation and required treatment or surgery which was only available at areas or facilities with higher levels of resources, were transported to the hospitals first.
Category 3	These patients, the "walking wounded," whose injuries were minor and within the capabilities of local treatments, were cared for and then sent back to their military units.

Table 23-2 Outcomes and Time to Care in the Major Twentieth Century Conflicts

Conflict	Time to Care	Mortality Rate
World War I	12 to 18 hours	8.5%
World War II	6 to 12 hours	5.8%
Korea	2 to 4 hours	2.4%
Vietnam	65 minutes	1.7%

assist in the rescue of their colleagues. These patients were undertriaged because of the chaos at the scene and because they were not typically assessed until the obviously critical patients received care.

Overtriage is the opposite process, whereby the seriousness of a patient's physiological or physical condition is overestimated. Children are commonly given higher levels of criticality. Many rescuers are overly cautious when assessing and caring for pediatric patients, as their maternal or paternal instincts take precedence. The cost in human lives lost and the wasting of resources are compounded by these circumstances, potentially affecting mortality.[9–12] Paramedics must minimize under- and overtriage to assure proper care is provided and the medical response system functions with the patients' best interests in mind.

Triage Systems

Many different triage systems or protocols have been developed in an attempt to strike a balance between under- and overtriage and between simplicity and accuracy. Three major triage systems are in use in the prehospital setting and two in the emergency department setting. This section discusses each of these methods.

START Triage

The START triage system is the most common system used throughout the United States.[8] Although the algorithm is somewhat standard, the operationalization of START triage varies from region to region. The START triage algorithm is based on the rapid assessment of the patient's respirations, pulse or perfusion, and mental status simplified from the original Department of Navy Research. The overall process has a number of common definitions that need to be understood in order to assure consistency (Tables 23-3 and 23-4). The START development group originally defined the operational aspects of their triage protocol as a process that should take 30 seconds or less per patient. Using the START triage algorithm (Figure 23-1), patients are sorted into one of five categories (Table 23-4).

Patients who have potentially life-threatening injuries affecting the airway, breathing, or circulation with an alteration of mental status or other clinical signs of shock are assigned to the **Immediate category**. Paramedics should treat and transport the patients who fall into this category to definitive care first by quickly identifying and moving them to the **casualty care area** for further assessment and care before moving them to the **transport area**.

Table 23-3 The RPM Assessment Schema Definitions

R =	Respiratory rate per minute
P =	Pulse or assessment of perfusion
M =	Mental status

Table 23-4 Triage Category Definitions

Category	Tag Color	Definition
Immediate	Red	Patients with critical, life-threatening injuries
Delayed	Yellow	Patients with potentially life- or limb-threatening injuries; patients who have a tourniquet applied to a limb
Minor	Green	Minor injuries, normal mental status, able to communicate and potentially ambulate
Dead	Black	Patients deceased on-scene
Expectant	Blue	Patients not dead at the time of triage but with mortal injuries that will probably cause them to die within a short period of time

Patients in the next category, the **Delayed category**, have injuries that require evaluation and treatment within 60 to 90 minutes. This includes patients who may have life- or limb-threatening injuries as well as patients who require

CULTURAL/REGIONAL DIFFERENCES

The Dead category has also been the basis of misinterpretation by the public. The deaths of a number of patrons at a night club in a predominantly ethnic neighborhood caused a public uproar following reports that the fire department was refusing to treat patients because of their ethnic origins. In reality, it was a misunderstanding based on terminology. Patients who fell into the Dead category were termed "Blacks," referring to the triage tag color for that patient rather than the patient's race. When the public observed firefighters stating, "This one's a black" and moving to the next patient, the perception was that there was racially related action instead of understanding the color-coding protocol. The firefighters were from a variety of ethnic backgrounds, but what the public saw became their truth. Separating those who are Dead from those who are Expectant and training personnel to use that terminology rather than color codes may help avoid similar misperceptions.

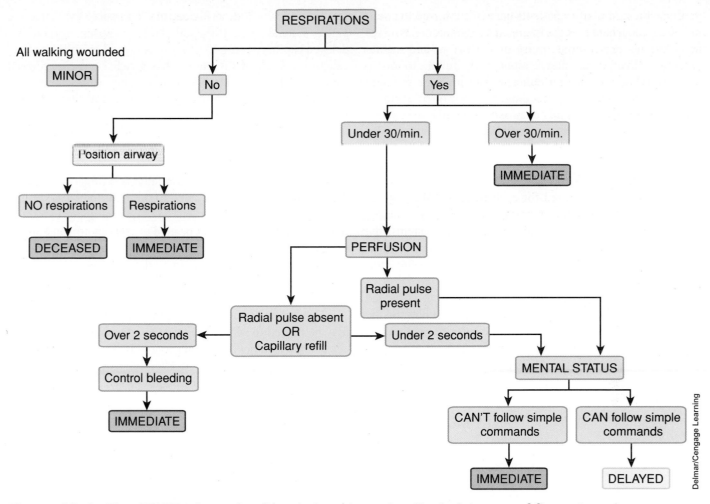

Figure 23-1 The START triage algorithm is used to sort patients into one of five categories.

tourniquet application to stop significant limb hemorrhage. Delayed category patients should be cared for and transported to definitive care after patients in the Immediate category, but before the least injured.

The **Minor category** consists of those people injured in the event who do not have any life-threatening or life-altering injuries. The term **walking wounded** is sometimes used to describe patients in this category as they are usually ambulatory to some degree and may be able to assist in the care of other, more severely injured patients.

The final category is those patients classified as part of the **Dead category**. These patients have either died from their injuries by the time rescuers arrive on-scene or are mortally wounded and expected to die prior to transport. These patients should be left where they are to preserve the scene for the subsequent investigation after the patients are cleared from the incident. If patients who fall into this category are relocated, they should be moved to an area physically separate from the other treatment areas.

A fifth category, the **Expectant category**, has been added to further identify the group of patients who are still alive, but expected to die within a short period of time. This separate category allows the Paramedic to avoid placing living patients in the Dead category during triage. During usual patient encounters, a Paramedic does not place a patient to the side or fail to deliver care. However, when resources are constrained, as they are during an MCI, this changes. For many Paramedics, this concept is difficult to embrace. Regardless of how often or how intensively these concepts are studied, some Paramedics simply cannot bring themselves to leave or ignore a person with some signs of life.

The other benefit of adding the Expectant category is that it identifies patients who will benefit from palliative care, including analgesia. These patients can either be treated once resources become more available or can be attended to by clergy or social workers that may be called to the scene to augment the emergency medical system's capabilities in a disaster. In some cases, willing volunteers who are less injured may elect to sit with these patients until they expire.

Following the START algorithm, patients who can ambulate are often directed to a meeting point away from both the incident and the treatment areas. These patients automatically are triaged as Minor category patients until they can be further triaged. The Paramedic still must formally triage these patients, however, as some patients who are able to ambulate can have injuries that place them in an Immediate or Delayed category and should be treated and transported as such.

Once the ambulatory patients have been moved to a separate area, the triage process begins. The Paramedic assesses each patient's respirations, pulse or perfusion, and mental status. At this point, interventions are limited to opening the airway and placing either a tourniquet or pressure bandage to control heavy bleeding. The Paramedic should assess each patient as rapidly as possible, ideally in less than 30 seconds. Triage is often accomplished in teams of two. One Paramedic can perform the assessment while the other is filling out the triage tag (Figure 23-2) or applying the limited treatments.

The first factor assessed for each patient is the respirations. If the patient is not breathing, the Paramedic makes one attempt to reposition the airway. In some systems, the Paramedic can place an oral or nasal airway at the same time. If the patient still has absent respirations after the Paramedic repositions the airway, the patient is tagged Dead. If the patient's respirations are restored, the patient is tagged Immediate. The Paramedic makes a rough estimate of the respiratory rate. If the respiratory rate is over 30 respirations per minute, the patient is triaged as an Immediate. If the respirations are under 30 respirations per minute, the Paramedic then assesses the patient's pulse or perfusion.

In assessing the perfusion, the Paramedic evaluates the patient's radial pulse. If the radial pulse is absent or there is a delayed capillary refill, the patient is tagged as an Immediate category patient. If the patient has a radial pulse or normal capillary refill, the patient's mental status is assessed next. Regardless of the triage category assigned at this step, the Paramedic should control any extremity hemorrhage with a tourniquet.[13]

The Paramedic performs an assessment of the patient's mental status by asking the patient to follow a simple command, such as showing the Paramedic two fingers. However, the simple command may need to be modified based on the patient's injuries. If the patient has bilateral upper extremity injuries, the patient will not be able to raise an arm and put up two fingers. If the patient cannot follow simple commands, the patient is triaged as an Immediate category patient. If the patient can follow simple commands, he is triaged as a Delayed category patient.

Depending on the amount of resources available, patients may be moved to separate treatment areas based on their triage category immediately after triage. If resources are scarce, then patients may be moved after all patients are triaged. The incident commander or operations sector leader usually

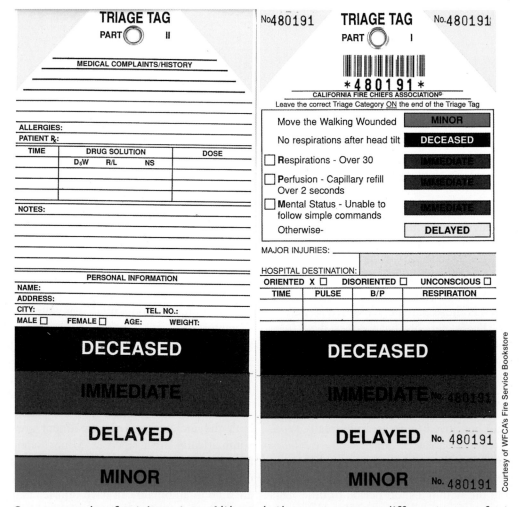

Figure 23-2 One example of a triage tag. Although there are many different manufacturers of triage tags, they generally contain similar information.

makes this decision. On arrival at the treatment area and before transport, patients should be re-triaged to ensure their triage category has not changed due to deterioration or improvement in their condition.

Although the START triage algorithm is one of the most widely used, its operational aspects may vary. A significant issue identified during a research evaluation of the protocol is that if the patient has a normal RPM, but does not ambulate away from the scene when instructed, the patient is deemed Delayed. Because many patients are placed in spinal restriction due to concerns of potential spinal injury, some patients may be overtriaged because of their inability to ambulate rather than because of their physiologic status. Some agencies have modified the respirations criteria to classify a patient as Immediate if his respiratory rate is greater than 30 or less than 10 respirations per minute. In assessing perfusion, some systems have adopted the "no distal pulse" criteria, whereas others use the capillary refill > 2 seconds as the criteria to assess perfusion. The Paramedic must assure interoperability with neighboring agencies is maintained whenever changes from the standard algorithm are made. Additionally, the change needs to be evaluated for medical validity to assure patient care is not being compromised. As the need for evidence-based science increases, the triage process has begun to come under scrutiny. As triage becomes more objective, the decision-making processes will evolve into an increasingly simple process with sophisticated knowledge and tools to support the event in the background.

The START triage algorithm has been studied in actual disaster use. The triage levels and outcomes for a 2003 commuter train crash outside Los Angeles were reviewed by the researchers based on the patients' triage, transport, and hospital records. In this incident, START triage demonstrated an acceptable level of undertriage for both the Immediate and Delayed categories. However, there was a significant amount of overtriage in which patients with less severe injuries were placed into more urgent triage categories.[8]

JumpSTART

In 1995, Dr. Lou Romig, a pediatric emergency medicine physician from Miami's Children's Hospital and Medical Director for Florida DMAT 5, developed the **JumpSTART triage tool** to incorporate pediatric physiologic parameters into triage decisions (Figure 23-3).[14] Dr. Romig was motivated to develop JumpSTART because of the gaps she observed between the adult application of the START algorithm and the unique needs of children in the disaster setting. A subsequent needs analysis for U.S. Disaster Medical Assistance Teams identified that pediatric patients comprised up to 85% of the patients during deployments over the prior five years.[15]

Similar to the START triage algorithm, JumpSTART begins with a segregation of those who can and cannot walk.

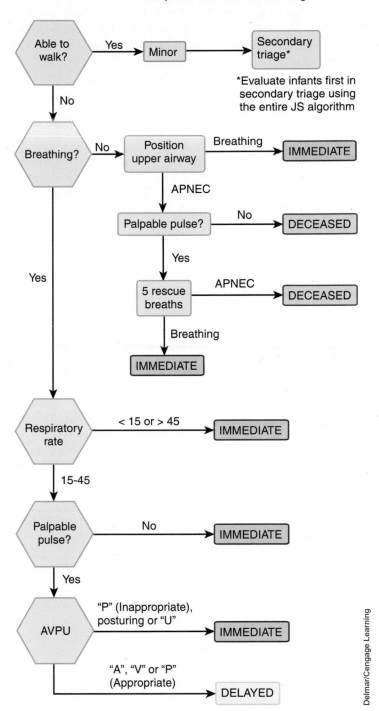

JumpSTART Pediatric MCI Triage

*Evaluate infants first in secondary triage using the entire JS algorithm

Delmar/Cengage Learning

Figure 23-3 The JumpSTART triage algorithm was developed to incorporate pediatric physiologic parameters.

A special note is made to re-triage infants and smaller children first in order to identify those who may have been carried by uninjured parents but who may themselves be more severely injured. These children may actually belong in a more severe triage category.

For those left after the ambulatory patients have moved away, the triage process begins with an assessment of respirations. The respiratory assessment in the JumpSTART algorithm differs from that in the START algorithm. It recognizes that in pediatric patients death is primarily secondary to respiratory causes. If the patient is not breathing, the triage officer is asked to reposition the airway. If the patient is still not breathing, then the triage officer assesses the pulse. If there is no pulse, the patient is triaged as part of the Dead category. If there is a pulse, the triage officer is asked to administer five rescue breaths and reassess the patient. If breathing starts, then the patient is triaged as an Immediate category patient.

After evaluating the breathing, the triage officer evaluates the patient's respiratory rate. If the respiratory rate is less than 15 or greater than 45, the patient is triaged as an Immediate category patient. If the patient's respiratory rate is within the range of 15 through 45, the triage officer moves on to assess perfusion by palpating a pulse. If a pulse is not palpable, the patient is triaged as an Immediate category patient.

If the patient has a palpable pulse, the triage officer assesses mental status using the AVPU classification scheme (Table 23-5). Patients who are responsive to painful stimulus only or who are unresponsive are categorized as an Immediate category patient. Those who are either completely alert or are responsive to voice are categorized as Delayed category patients.

SALT Triage

The **Sort–Assess–Lifesaving interventions–Treat/transport (SALT) triage system** (Figure 23-4) was developed by a task force commissioned by the U.S. Centers for Disease Control in an effort to develop a standardized triage algorithm to be used across the country.[16] The benefit of having a single unified triage algorithm is that it allows Paramedics from different areas of the country to work together during a disaster. The committee examined many of the existing triage systems along with literature evaluating those systems. The SALT triage system borrowed many concepts from these different algorithms in an effort to produce a standardized triage algorithm. To date, SALT has only been evaluated during mass-casualty exercises[17,18] and not during actual incidents.

Table 23-5 The AVPU Classification Scheme to Assess Mental Status

A = Alert
V = Responds to verbal stimulus
P = Responds to painful stimulus
U = Unresponsive

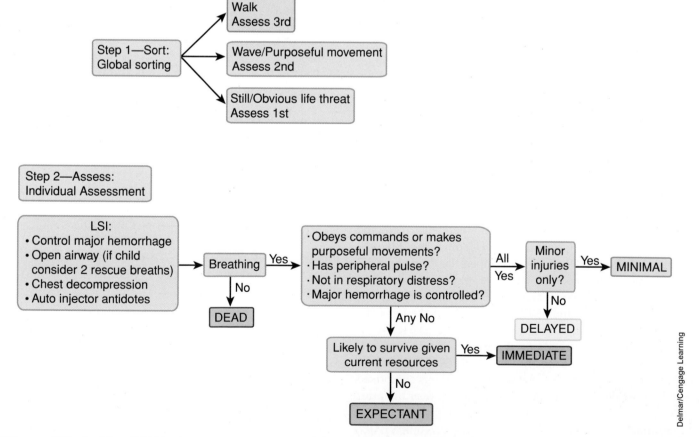

Figure 23-4 The SALT triage system; LSI = life-saving interventions.

The SALT triage system is a two-step process. In the first step, the Paramedic performs a global assessment to quickly divide the patients into three groups. First, the triage officer asks those who can walk to move to a collection point for evaluation. Once the ambulatory patients have moved away, the triage officer instructs, "If you can hear me, wave your hand or move your leg." This group becomes the second group of patients. The third group consists of those who cannot ambulate, cannot make a purposeful movement, or have an obvious external hemorrhage. These three groups are then prioritized for individual triage of each patient within the groups. Those in the last group (the ones who do not make purposeful movements or have an obvious external hemorrhage) are triaged first. The second group to undergo individual triage is the non-ambulatory group who showed purposeful movements. Finally, the third group to undergo individual triage is the ambulatory group.

The second step is an individual assessment of each patient. During individual assessment, the Paramedic first assesses each patient's need for a life-saving intervention (Table 23-6) before assigning a treatment priority. These life-saving interventions can be performed rapidly and may temporarily stabilize the patient. Once any appropriate life-saving interventions are performed, the Paramedic assesses the patient's breathing. If the patient is not breathing, the person is placed in the Dead category. If the patient is breathing, then the patient is assessed based on four criteria (Table 23-7) designed to identify high-risk patients. If any of these criteria are not met (e.g., the patient does not have a palpable pulse),

and he is not likely to survive given current resources, the patient is placed in the Expectant category. If the patient is expected to survive given the current resource constraints, he is placed in the Immediate category.

If all four criteria (Table 23-7) are met and the patient has only minor injuries, the patient is placed in the Minimal category. If the injuries are not minor, then the patient is placed in the Delayed category.

After the Paramedic completes triage, she carries out treatment and transport based on the priority categories assigned to the patients. The Expectant category identifies those patients who are still alive, although not salvageable given current resource limitations. These patients may be given comfort care when resources become available.[16]

Sacco Triage and Resource Methodology

The Sacco triage system was developed by Dr. Sacco and Mick Navin as an evidence-based triage methodology. The **Sacco Triage and Resource Methodology (STM)** is designed to maximize the number of expected survivors of a traumatic event through use of an objective, measurable, interoperable, and reproducible method. STM is based on research examining the initial assessment and outcomes of approximately 76,000 patients in a statewide trauma registry.[19] In contrast to an algorithm, STM determines a score based on the patient's respiratory rate, pulse rate, and best motor response (Table 23-8). The overall STM score is the sum of the scores for these three parameters.

The use of this triage methodology involves a five-step process. The first step is to evaluate and compute an STM score for each patient based on the respiratory rate, pulse rate, and best motor response. All patients are triaged and the scores reported to a central command post.

The second step is to organize patients into three general categories based on their STM scores. Group 1 is made up of all the patients with STM scores between 0 and 4. This roughly corresponds to the Dead and Expectant categories in the START triage algorithm. The second group consists of patients with an STM score between 5 and 8. These patients roughly correspond to the Immediate and Delayed categories in the START algorithm. The third group covers patients with an STM score between 9 and 12. This roughly corresponds to the Delayed and Minor category patients. Patients with STM scores of 11 and 12 are generally ambulatory.

The third step involves reporting the STM scores to a centralized location. The numbers are input into the proprietary

Table 23-6 Life-Saving Interventions in the SALT Triage System

- Control major hemorrhage
- Open airway
- If child, consider two rescue breaths
- Needle thoracostomy
- Auto-injector antidotes

Table 23-7 The Four Criteria Used during Individual Assessment of the SALT Algorithm

1. Does the patient obey commands?
2. Is the peripheral pulse present?
3. Is the patient not in respiratory distress?
4. Is major hemorrhage controlled?

Table 23-8 The Sacco Triage and Resource Methodology Assigns Scores for the Individual Parameters

	0	1	2	3	4
Respiratory Rate	0	1 to 9	> 36	25 to 35	10 to 24
Pulse Rate	0	1 to 40	41 to 60	> 121	61 to 120
Best Motor Response	None	Extends/flexes from pain	Withdraws from pain	Localizes from pain	Obeys commands

software that contains the STM programming model. The software analyzes the scores and determines the best treatment and transport strategy that will maximize survivability. Additionally, the software can take into account information about the status of regional hospitals and factor in emergency department volume at the time of the incident in formulating the strategy.

The fourth and fifth steps occur concurrently and involve constant re-evaluation. These steps involve carrying out the recommended treatment and transport priorities and constantly evaluating for changes in resources at the scene and at the receiving facilities. Treatment and transport priority change dynamically in response to the dynamic changes in resources available not only at the incident but throughout the entire system. As with SALT triage, the STM has not been evaluated in an actual disaster.

Secondary Assessment of Victim Endpoint

All of the previously mentioned triage systems are easy to implement for initial triage of patients who can be moved from the scene of an incident within a relatively short period of time. However, not all disasters occur in urban areas with multiple hospitals and transport resources. Some occur in less populated areas. In addition, some natural disasters (e.g., an earthquake) disrupt the basic infrastructure, thus prolonging evacuation from the scene. Furthermore, some incidents are open, meaning the incident is spread out over a large geographic area, creating many smaller MCIs. In an attempt to address these issues, the **Secondary Assessment of Victim Endpoint (SAVE)** was developed.[20]

After patients are triaged and divided into categories as previously described, the patients are reassessed and divided into three categories based upon the resources needed, the resources available, and the prognosis given the injury and the time expected to elapse until definitive care. Patients who are expected to die regardless of how much care they receive are placed into the first group. Patients who will survive regardless of care are placed in the second group. The third group is comprised of patients who are expected to benefit significantly from the interventions and resources that are available in the field.

These three groups of patients are then segregated into two physical areas. The first area is an observation area where minimal care is rendered. The second area is a treatment area where active treatment of patients occurs. Patients in the first and second groups are placed in the observation area, whereas patients in the third group are triaged to the treatment area. A patient is placed in the treatment area if she has a good prognosis given a minimal amount of treatment based on the resources available. Patients may also be triaged to the treatment area if treatment may reduce morbidity or mortality

and will not consume an inordinate amount of resources in the field. The SAVE process takes into account a situation in which movement to an appropriate hospital is delayed more than a few hours.

SAVE provides guidelines to help the secondary triage process for several common injuries in disasters,[20] including crush injuries, head injuries, chest and abdominal trauma, spinal trauma, burns, pediatric injuries, pre-existing illnesses, multiple-injury patients, and nontraumatic emergencies. These guidelines help triage officers better sort the patients who can benefit from treatment as well as those patients who have a high chance of death from their injuries. The SAVE guidelines also describe a treatment priority order that is based on resources (Table 23-9). The ordering of conditions as part of these priorities is based on studies that examine the mortality of trauma patients with similar conditions cared for in tertiary care centers. The SAVE guidelines recommend that pediatric patients be treated with higher priority, as research indicates seriously injured pediatric patients have a better chance of recovery than adults with the same injuries.[20]

Although the SAVE guidelines have been recommended for implementation in Australia[21] and in the Medical Disaster Response project, these guidelines have not been evaluated during an actual extended duration disaster.

Emergency Department Triage

On arrival at the emergency department, patients are re-triaged to identify changes in their status. During an MCI,

Table 23-9 Treatment Priorities for Several Specific Injuries as Described in the SAVE Guidelines (from Highest to Lowest)

1. Temporary airway management
2. Pressure dressings/tourniquet applied to bleeding
3. Simple pneumothorax
4. Treatment of shock after control of bleeding
5. Advanced airway management
6. Limb manipulation/treatment for vascular supply
7. Moderate burns with 25% expected mortality
8. Miscellaneous chest trauma
9. Spinal injuries
10. Fasciotomy/amputations when indicated
11. Open wound care/closure
12. Closed head injury — GCS = 6 to 7
13. Burns with 50% expected mortality
14. Burns with 75% expected mortality
15. Closed head injury — GCS = 3

some hospitals will utilize START or another triage system during the re-triage process. Most U.S. hospital emergency departments, however, use a system called the Emergency Severity Index (ESI). In Canada, the most commonly used system is the Canadian Triage and Acuity Scale (CTAS).

The **Emergency Severity Index (ESI)** algorithm sorts patients into five levels that not only look at the need for immediate, life-threatening interventions, but also for resource utilization (Figure 23-5).[22] The triage level is based on the answers to four questions (Table 23-10). Life-saving interventions include procedures like assisting ventilations, defibrillation, needle decompression, or administration of a select few medications that are used to treat life-threatening cardiac rhythms or improve decreased mental status. Conditions that place the patient in a Level 1 category include a patient who arrives intubated or in cardiac arrest, is in severe respiratory distress, is hypoxemic, has decreased mental status, or is unresponsive.

Patients who do not fall into a Level 1 category are assessed for high likelihood of deterioration, severe pain or distress, and altered mental status. These patients should not wait a long time to be seen by a medical provider. If the triage nurse feels the patient fits into one of these classifications, the patient is labeled as a Level 2 patient. For patients that do not clearly fit into a Level 2 category, the triage nurse makes a judgment regarding the amount of resources the patient may require. The fewer the anticipated number of resources the patient requires, the lower the triage level. The triage nurse is reminded to reconsider a Level 2 triage category for patients who may require many resources based on the patient's vital signs. The ESI has been shown to be valid and reliable in the emergency department.[23]

The **Canadian Triage and Acuity Scale (CTAS)** has been adopted across much of Canada as well as other countries.[24] First detailed in 1999, the CTAS is a five-level triage scale with the most critical patients designated as Level I and the least serious as Level V (Figure 23-6, Table 23-11).[25] Similar to the ESI, the CTAS attempts to identify patients who have higher acuity illnesses or injuries and will require a higher utilization of resources. The CTAS can also dynamically adjust based on the resources available at the specific facility and in the community.

Although both scales provide an improved sorting of patients into groups with similar prognoses, neither completely interfaces with the triage systems used in the field.

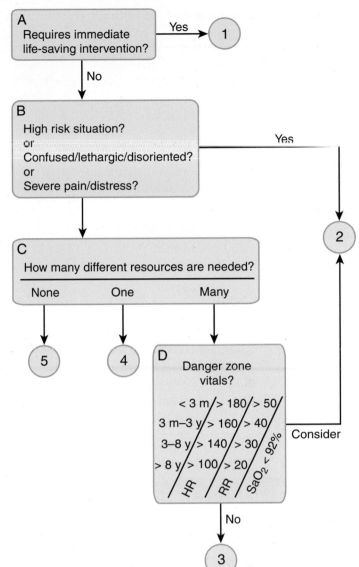

Figure 23-5 The Emergency Severity Index algorithm is used for triage decisions in many hospitals.

Table 23-10 The Four Questions the Triage Nurse Answers in Applying the ESI Algorithm

1. Is this patient dying?
2. Is this a patient who shouldn't wait?
3. How many resources will this patient need?
4. What are the patient's vital signs?

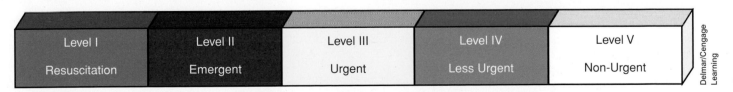

Figure 23-6 CTAS uses five category definitions to triage patients.

Table 23-11 Examples of Conditions That Fit into the Triage Classifications

Level I–Resuscitation	Level II–Emergent	Level III–Urgent	Level IV–Less Urgent	Level V–Non-Urgent
• Code/arrest • Major trauma • Shock states • Unconscious • Severe respiratory distress • Absent/unstable vital signs	• Altered mental status • Head injury • Severe trauma • Neonates • Eye pain • Chest pain (presumed cardiac or pulmonary embolism) • Overdose • Abdominal pain • GI bleed • CVA • Asthma • Anaphylaxis • Vaginal bleeding • Fever (young children), with lethargy • Acute psychosis/agitation • Diabetes	• Mild head injury • Moderate trauma • Mild asthma • Moderate dyspnea • Chest pain (not cardiac/PE) • GI bleed	• Head injury, GCS 15 • Minor trauma (isolated fractures/sprains) • Headache • Earache • Suicidal/depressed • Chronic back pain • Upper respiratory infection symptoms	• Minor trauma (soft-tissue injuries) • Sore throat, upper respiratory infection • Vaginal bleeding with mild pain • Vomiting alone, diarrhea alone • Other psychiatric issues

▶ CASE STUDY CONCLUSION

As the ambulance arrives there are additional reports of multiple tornados striking up and down "tornado alley." This may stress the emergency response system, perhaps to the breaking point. The area-wide command post has started to use SAVE triage to adjust destinations. They hope the communications system will stay up and that the storms quickly pass, enabling air medical evacuation.

CRITICAL THINKING QUESTIONS

1. What is SAVE triage?
2. How is hospital triage different from EMS triage?

CONCLUSION

Across the United States, the most commonly used triage protocol is START. Since variations occur locally and regionally, its interoperability continues to come into question. The latest research indicates that patient outcome is more important than clearing the event scene. Considerable work is being done to validate both the medical implications of triage as well as the operational function. Although a perfect triage system may currently be elusive, significant advancements are being made and are enhancing the care being provided by prehospital providers.

KEY POINTS:

- Triage is the categorization of patients according to the severity of their illness or sickness in hopes of improving their survival.

- The concept of triage was attributed to Baron Dominique Jean Larrey.

- The worst first paradigm in triage has shifted to the greatest good for the greatest number.

- The military has driven the refinement of triage.

- Simple Triage and Rapid Transport (START) triage was an adaptation of a military model for civilian use.

- Undertriage and overtriage both lead to increased morbidity and mortality.

- START triage has five levels, including Expectant (blue).

- JumpSTART is a triage tool developed for pediatric populations.

- The Sort-Assess-Lifesaving interventions-Treat/transport (SALT) triage system was developed by the Centers for Disease Control (CDC).

- The SALT triage system was an attempt to standardize triage across the United States.

- SALT consists of a two-phase process: global assessment and individual assessment.

- The Sacco Triage and Resource Methodology (STM) is an evidence-based triage system.

- The Sacco method quantified the RPM of START triage and involves the use of software for treatment and transport decisions based on probabilities.

- Secondary Assessment of Victim Endpoint (SAVE) was developed for prolonged evacuation and widespread MCI. SAVE is a three-level triage system that takes available resources into account.

- SAVE has a secondary triage process which is used in disasters.

- Hospital triage is based on an Emergency Severity Index or, in Canada, the Canadian Triage and Acuity Scale.

REVIEW QUESTIONS:

1. What was Baron Dominique Jean Larrey's original concept?
2. What is the difficulty with the worst first philosophy?
3. What is undertriage, and what is overtriage?
4. What is the concept behind Secondary Assessment of Victim Endpoint?
5. What triage systems do hospitals use?

CASE STUDY QUESTIONS:

Please refer to the Case Study in this chapter, and answer the questions below:
1. How does START triage work?
2. How does SALT triage work?
3. How does STM work?

REFERENCES:

1. Jenkins JL, McCarthy ML, Sauer LM, et al. Mass-casualty triage: time for an evidence based approach. *Prehosp Disaster Med.* 2008;23(1):3–8.
2. Larry DJ. *Memoirs of military surgery and campaigns of the French armies: vol 2.* Hall RW, trans. Baltimore, MD: Joseph Cushing; 1814.
3. Hogan DE, Lairet J. Triage. In: Hogan DE, Burstein JL, eds. *Disaster Medicine.* Philadelphia, PA: Lippincott; 2002.
4. Keen WW. *The Treatment of War Wounds.* Philadelphia, PA: WB Saunders; 1917.
5. Moskop JC, Iserson KV. Triage in medicine, part II: underlying values and principles. *Ann Emerg Med.* 2007;49(3):282–287.
6. Iserson KV, Moskop JC. Triage in medicine, part I: concept, history, and types. *Ann Emerg Med.* 2007;49(3):275–281.
7. Super G. *START: A Triage Training Module.* Newport Beach, CA: Hoag Memorial Hospital Presbyterian; 1984.
8. Kahn CA, Schultz CH, Miller KT, Anderson CL. Does START triage work? An outcomes assessment after a disaster. *Ann Emerg Med.* 2009;54(3):424–430.
9. Frykberg ER. Medical management of disasters and mass casualties from terrorist bombings: how can we cope? *J Trauma.* 2002;53(2):201–212.
10. Hirshberg A. Multiple casualty incidents: lessons from the front line. *Ann Surg.* 2004;239(3):322–324.
11. Hupert N, Hollingsworth E, Xiong W. Is overtriage associated with increased mortality? Insights from a simulation model of mass casualty trauma care. *Disaster Med Public Health Prep.* 2007;1(1 Suppl):S14–S24.
12. Armstrong JH, Hammond J, Hirshberg A, Frykberg ER. Is overtriage associated with increased mortality? The evidence says "yes." *Disaster Med Public Health Prep.* 2008;2(1):4–5.
13. Doyle GS, Taillac PP. Tourniquets: a review of current use with proposals for expanded prehospital use. *Prehosp Emerg Care.* 2008;12(2):241–256.
14. Romig LE. Pediatric triage: a system to JumpSTART your triage of young patients at MCIs. *JEMS.* 2002;27(7):52–58, 60–63.
15. Mace SE, Bern AI. Needs assessment: are Disaster Medical Assistance Teams up for the challenge of a pediatric disaster? *Am J Emerg Med.* 2007;25(7):762–769.
16. Lerner EB, Schwartz RB, Coule PL, et al. Mass casualty triage: an evaluation of the date and development of a proposed national guideline. *Disaster Med Public Health Prep.* 2008;2(Suppl 1):S25–S34.
17. Cone DC, Serra J, Burns K, et al. Pilot test of the SALT mass casualty triage system. *Prehosp Emerg Care.* 2009;13(4):536–540.
18. Lerner EB, Schwartz RB, Coule PL, Pirrallo RG. Use of SALT triage in a simulated mass casualty incident. *Prehosp Emerg Care.* 2010;14(1):21–25.
19. Sacco WJ, Navin M, Fiedler KE, Waddell RK, Long WB, Buckman RF. Precise formulation and evidence based application of resource-constrained triage. *Acad Emerg Med.* 2005;12(8):759–770.
20. Benson M, Koenig KL, Schultz CH. Disaster triage: START then SAVE—a new method of dynamic triage for victims of a catastrophic earthquake. *Prehosp Disaster Med.* 1996;11(2):117–124.
21. Nocera A, Garner A. An Australian mass casualty incident triage system based upon triage mistakes of the past: the Homebush Triage Standard. *Aust N Z J Surg.* 1999;68(8):603–608.

22. Gilboy N, Tanabe P, Travers DA, Rosenau AM, Eitel DR. Emergency Severity Index, version 4: implementation handbook. AHRQ Publication No. 05-0046-2, May 2005. Agency for Healthcare Research and Quality, Rockville, MD. Available at: **http://www.ahrq.gov/research/esi/.** Accessed December 10, 2009.

23. Wuerz RC, Milne LW, Eitel DR, Travers D, Gilboy N. Reliability and validity of a new five-level triage instrument. *Acad Emerg Med.* 2000;7(3):236–242.

24. Bullard MJ, Unger B, Spence J, et al. Revisions to the Canadian emergency department triage and acuity scale guidelines. *CJEM.* 2008;10(2):136–142.

25. Canadian Association Emergency Physicians. Canadian acuity and triage scale. Available at: **http://www.caep.ca/template.asp?id=B795164082374289BBD9C1C2BF4B8D32.** Accessed December 10, 2009.

CHAPTER 24

VEHICLE RESCUE AND EXTRICATION

KEY CONCEPTS:

Upon completion of this chapter, it is expected that the reader will understand these following concepts:

- Elements of scene size-up
- Safety equipment and the personal protective envelope
- Physical entanglement versus medical entrapment
- Alternative fuels and new motive forces
- Vehicle construction and extrication

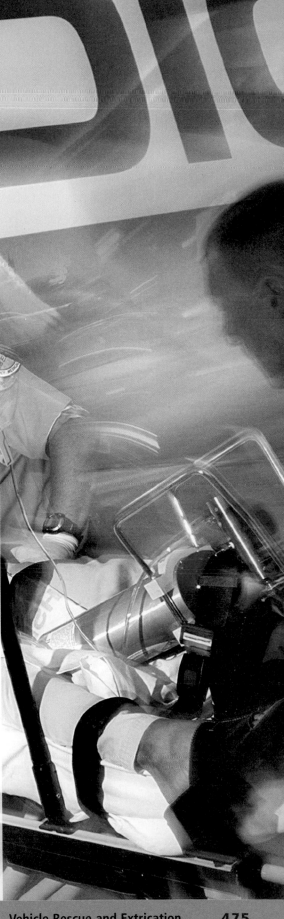

As the Paramedic pumper rolls up to the scene, the crew is awestruck by the carnage. "How can anybody survive a crash like that?" they mumble to themselves. The two vehicles were traveling in opposite directions when one apparently crossed the double solid line and ran square into the other one.

Getting out of the jump seat, the Paramedic prepares to declare one of the casualties dead when a patrol officer grabs his sleeve and says, "We got a live one!"

CRITICAL THINKING QUESTIONS

1. What are the Paramedic's first responsibilities at the scene of a motor vehicle collision?

2. What are the initial actions the Paramedic should take to stabilize the vehicle?

OVERVIEW

Throughout an EMS career, most of the Paramedic's rescue skill incident responses will be for motor vehicle crashes (MVC). In these rescue efforts, the patient is the focus. Rescue is a patient-care-driven skill, whether the rescue is for a trench or structural collapse, technical rope rescue, or vehicle rescue. In addition, all the emergency responders on-scene—the Paramedic providing patient care, the rescue technician wielding the power hydraulic rescue tool, the firefighter manning the hose line, and the incident commander managing hazards—play critical roles in producing a better patient outcome.

As part of the Paramedic's role of managing the patient's care, she not only needs to provide appropriate prehospital care, but must also understand the potential hazards on-scene, know how to size-up and read the wreck effectively, and understand how that knowledge plays a role with patient management.

The Paramedic must realize that, when responding to an MVC, she will be working in a much different environment than the typical EMS scene. Although in a perfect world the Paramedic would set up in the ambulance and wait for the patient to be delivered, in reality the Paramedic must access the patient in the vehicle (either directly or indirectly) and provide care (either directly or through an intermediary such as a EMS-trained firefighter) while the rescue effort is underway in order to provide a better outcome for the patient. This chapter will detail what should happen on-scene at the motor vehicle collision, the elements of the rescue effort, vehicle hazards, PPE, and patient management in the environment.

Three Levels of Vehicle Rescue Competency

National Fire Protection Association Standard 1670, *Standard on Operations and Training for Technical Search and Rescue Incidents* (2009), describes three levels of vehicle rescue: Awareness, Operations, and Technician. Depending on the Paramedic's role and responsibility, the level of individual competencies will vary.

Awareness

All Paramedics are expected to have Awareness level competencies (Table 24-1). Many extrication incidents will require

Table 24-1 Extrication Awareness Level Competencies

- Recognizing the need for a vehicle search and rescue
- Identifying the resources necessary to conduct operations
- Initiating the emergency response system
- Initiating site control and scene management
- Recognizing general hazards
- Initiating traffic control

the services of agencies and organizations that can deliver Operations or Technician level services. These local, regional, state, or national entities may need to be alerted once the Paramedic completes a scene size-up.

Operations

Paramedics working for organizations that respond to 9-1-1-generated incidents need to demonstrate Operations level competencies for vehicle rescue (Table 24-2). In addition, they are required to have the Operations level core competencies described in NFPA Standard 472, *Standard for Competence of Responders to Hazardous Materials/ Weapons of Mass Destruction Incidents* (2008), as described in Chapter 26.[1]

These are the first steps in establishing the Incident Management System that is described in Chapter 20.

The detailed descriptions of Operations procedures include patient management and hazard mitigation (Table 24-3). These steps are designed to both protect the Paramedic and facilitate the delivery of emergency medical care to the patient. This chapter merely provides an overview of this level; it is not within the scope of this chapter to prepare a Paramedic for certification at the Operations level of vehicle rescue.

Table 24-2 Actions Expected from Operations Level Personnel upon Arrival at the Scene of a Motor Vehicle Crash

- Scope and magnitude of the incident
- Risk-benefit analysis (body recovery versus rescue)
- Number and size of vehicles affected
- Integrity and stability of vehicles affected
- Number of known or potential patients
- Access to the scene
- Hazards such as disrupted or exposed utilities, standing or flowing water, mechanical hazards, hazardous materials, electrical hazards, and explosives
- Exposure to traffic
- Environmental factors
- Available versus necessary resources

Table 24-3 Detailed Patient Management and Hazard Mitigation Actions at an Extrication Scene

- Identifying probable patient locations and survivability
- Making the search and rescue area safe, including the stabilization and hazard control of all vehicles involved
- Identifying, containing, and stopping fuel release
- Protecting a patient during extrication or disentanglement
- Packaging a patient prior to extrication or disentanglement
- Accessing patients trapped in a common passenger vehicle
- Performing extrication and disentanglement operations involving packaging, treating, and removing patients trapped in common passenger vehicles through the use of hand and power tools
- Mitigating and managing general and specific hazards (i.e., fires and explosions) associated with vehicle search and rescue incidents
- Procuring and utilizing the resources necessary to conduct vehicle search and rescue operations
- Maintaining control of traffic

Technician

An emergency responder trained to the Technician level in vehicle rescue will be expected to handle more complex incidents that may involve larger vehicles. These duties include higher level and more specialized activities than Operations level personnel (Table 24-4).

Technical level responders staff Urban Search and Rescue (USAR) teams and specialized rescue or squad companies. They have additional training and equipment to handle extrication situations such as overturned vehicles, incidents requiring multiple extrications, and crashes involving commercial trucks or other large vehicles. Some Technical level vehicle rescue specialists are Paramedics.

Table 24-4 Technician Level Activities Employed at the Scene of an Extrication

- Performing extrication and disentanglement operations involving packaging, treating, and removing patients injured or trapped in large, heavy vehicles
- Stabilizing in advance of unusual vehicle search and rescue situations
- Using all specialized search and rescue equipment immediately available and in use by the organization

Scene Size-Up at the Motor Vehicle Collision

An MVC can be a very bewildering event. Although the vehicle is still the dynamic hazard in the equation, supplemental restraint systems (SRS), battery(s) and their subsequent locations, motive power, and vehicle glazing are all items that need to be considered. In addition, the Paramedic needs to do this scene size-up quickly and completely to ensure a safe and effective plan of action.

Immediately upon arrival, the Paramedic needs to ensure personal safety before even stepping off the vehicle. One way of ensuring safety is to position the response vehicle/apparatus in a "fend off" manner (Figure 24-1). This vehicle positioning helps to protect the Paramedic and the patients by placing the apparatus between the incident and traffic. The Paramedic must then begin to evaluate the incident and scan the area for scene hazards.

As the Paramedic approaches the vehicle(s) involved in the MVC, she must take in how the vehicle appears. For example, the Paramedic must consider the vehicle's orientation (for example, upright, on its side, or overturned), the type of stabilization required, and the type and amount of vehicle damage (such as crush) This information should provide the Paramedic with clues relating to potential entrapment and injuries.

Next, the Paramedic should see if any supplemental restraint system devices were deployed (i.e., front and side airbags). Approaching the vehicle from the front, the Paramedic should make visual contact with the patient(s), followed by verbal contact. Once the Paramedic finds the patient and establishes contact, she should maintain that contact and provide reassurance throughout the incident.

Next, the Paramedic should assess the scene to locate and begin to mitigate the hazards. When the Paramedic is assured that the scene is safe, she must perform three tasks: immobilize the vehicle, stabilize the vehicle, and disable the vehicle.

Immobilizing the vehicle can be as simple as placing the vehicle in park or taking it out of gear (Figure 24-2a). Another simple and quick technique is to chock the wheels. Cutting the valve stems on the tires can also immobilize the vehicle, but that makes it difficult for the wrecker (recovery service) to remove the vehicle later.

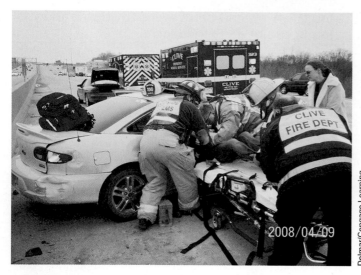

Figure 24-1 The Paramedic should position her vehicle in a way so that the scene is protected from traffic.

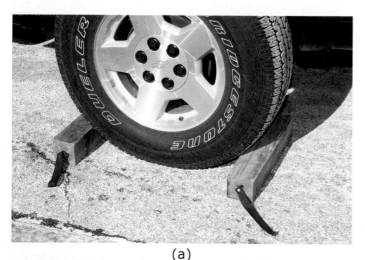

(a)

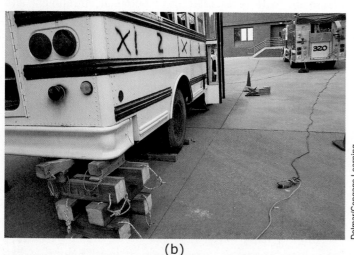

(b)

Figure 24-2 The vehicle should be (a) immobilized and (b) stabilized during initial contact to provide stability for the rescuers' entry.

Next, the Paramedic should stabilize the vehicle (Figure 24-2b) in order to prevent unwanted vehicle movement. Stabilization starts with turning off the engine, ensuring the vehicle is in park, and engaging the parking brake. This ensures a stable foundation for space-making evolutions (discussed shortly) and minimizes any patient movement that might potentially aggravate a spinal injury.

With the vehicle stabilized, the Paramedic enters the vehicle and begins hands-on patient management, manual cervical spine stabilization, primary assessment, and so on, as indicated. The Paramedic should take a good look at the vehicle's interior, observing for signs that might indicate the mechanism of injury (for example, whether the SRS devices were deployed or undeployed). While completing a 360-degree scan of the interior, the Paramedic should also look for damage to the interior that might cause any physical entrapment to the patient.

The vehicle's power needs to be secured as well, which effectively disables the vehicle. The Paramedic should ensure that the vehicle is out of gear and shut off by removing the vehicle's keys. With high-voltage vehicles, this is especially important. This topic is discussed further later in the chapter under the heading "Power Isolation." The officer in charge should document when power was shut down.

The Paramedic may need to make space to disentangle the patient, even if the patient is not physically pinned. The officer in charge of the rescue effort must devise a tactical plan of action based on the information presented at the crash and the information shared by the Paramedic. The tactical plan of action and various versions of it must take into account the many variables and be performed swiftly.

NFPA 1670 recommends that the officer in charge establish a 20-foot (6-meter) work area around the vehicle. If needed, the officer in charge can establish hot, warm, and cold zones to minimize rescuer exposure to hazards and to organize a complex vehicle extrication activity. Only essential personnel with appropriate personal protective equipment will be working in the hot zone. Medical and Technical rescue equipment is staged in the warm zone.[2]

Physical Entanglement versus Medical Entrapment

Once the scene size-up is complete, the Paramedic gains access to the patient within the vehicle. **Gaining access** is the process of creating a pathway to the patient. The initial path should allow the Paramedic to access the patient's face and neck to establish an airway and check the carotid pulse.

The pathway is established by making a space large enough to perform the tasks. Accomplishing this "gaining access" task involves displacing, disassembling, or removing exterior and interior vehicle components.

Once the initial patient assessment is made, the Paramedic works with the rescue sector officer to determine whether the patient requires disentanglement or extrication.

Disentanglement is the cutting away of a vehicle from a trapped or injured patient. In some cases, the patient may only have minor injuries but needs components of the vehicle displaced or removed in order to get out of the vehicle. This process may be as simple as using a hand tool to force open a passenger door, or as complex as removing a roof and displacing the dashboard using powered rescue tools.

In other cases, an injured patient must be disentangled and space made to facilitate medical care before the patient is removed from the vehicle. Stabilizing a fractured femur or decompressing a pneumothorax may require immediate in-vehicle intervention.

Extrication, or space making, is the creation of the path that will help remove patients from a crashed vehicle. Extrication requires the largest space, since the patient is unable or incapable of stepping out of the vehicle. Most patients requiring extrication will have spinal immobilization started in the disentanglement period, and will be removed on a backboard or other immobilization device. There may be airway control equipment, intravenous lines, and extremity splints to consider as well.

The size of the space and the speed of extrication will be governed by the patient's condition, environmental factors, and available resources. The Paramedic determines if the patient(s) need to be disentangled and extricated. Vehicle damage sometimes will intrude into the passenger compartment and physically constrict the occupant(s). Those instances will be easy for the Paramedic to identify.

Due to the smaller size of more recent model vehicles and construction considerations such as energy absorption, the "working" space inside the vehicle has shrunk considerably. Although the stronger construction and numerous supplemental restraint systems have improved safety and reduced serious injuries, they also make extrication efforts on-scene more complicated. Although the patient might not be physically entrapped or pinned, he can be entrapped by the nature of the injuries or perceived injuries and/or the sheer lack of usable space to extricate himself. In the past, the pathway to remove the patient often doubled as the initial access point. However, today such created access, such as a door displacement, does not offer enough space to safely disentangle the patient. Although a time-sensitive, critically injured patient will always need to be rapidly extricated, by whatever means and space are available, extrication of most patients is not time critical.

Personal Protective Equipment

Many times Paramedics overlook personal protective equipment when participating in a rescue on the scene of a motor vehicle collision. However, personal protective equipment (PPE) is essential to help the Paramedic inside the vehicle create a proper **protective envelope** (Figure 24-3), or layer of PPE used to shield himself from injury. A Paramedic working in a heavy rescue environment needs, at a minimum, head and eye protection. Some Paramedics use fire service

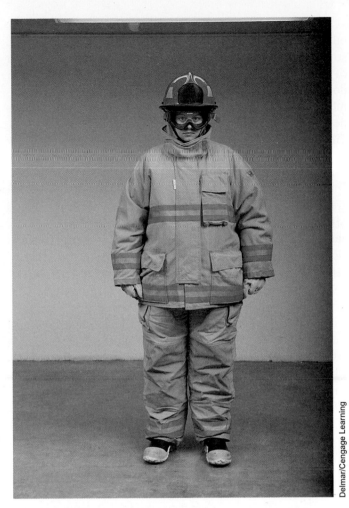

Delmar/Cengage Learning

Figure 24-3 Personal protective equipment is essential for the Paramedic to operate safely in the extrication environment.

helmets, which can be awkward and bulky. However, the Paramedic ideally needs close fitting head protection in the tight confines of the car's interior. The flip-down shields fitted to fire service helmets are acceptable for facial protection, although they are insufficient for eye protection. The Paramedic needs proper safety glasses or goggles, or must use the newer helmets with integrated flip-down goggles, just like those of flight helmets.

Proper hand protection is vital as well. The Paramedic should wear the proper gloves for the proper job. Although the Paramedic will utilize patient exam gloves during patient management, she also will need protective outer gloves when entering the vehicle and also during various stages of packaging and disentanglement. There are many options available. However, good form-fitting leather work gloves that can go over the top of exam gloves is a good base to start from.

The Paramedic may also be concerned about the various dusts and particles created during the rescue effort. Glass dust and certain vehicle materials such as carbon fiber, in a particle state, are a respiratory hazard. Although the patient may be protected by the high-flow, high-concentration oxygen mask, the Paramedic should have an N95 mask available.

Some controversy exists surrounding the Paramedic's outer layer of protection. In the past, Paramedics utilized structural firefighting gear (turnout gear) as the outer layer of their personal protective envelope. Although turnout gear does provide protection, it can be bulky and restrict movement inside the vehicle. In addition, the very gear that is designed to protect the Paramedic can also cause heat stress. Finally, in many cases turnout gear does not offer the protection from fluid contamination required by the NFPA 1999 standards for EMS protection.

New types of protective gear and even greater options are currently available to Paramedics. The outer layer should offer flash protection, protection from fluid contamination, and resistance to abrasions. Breathability in the garment is also important, as breathability reduces heat stress. Finally, visibility is a critical element for the Paramedic.

Federal regulations (23 CFR part 634) require that all workers, including emergency responders, that are operating within the right-of-way on federally subsidized highways must wear high-visibility safety apparel. This regulation is being extended to all public highways, so Paramedics are strongly advised to have any outer apparel, or safety vests, comply with ANSI standards for visibility. The ANSI/ISEA 207 (2006 ed.) standards call for a minimum of 450 square inches of fluorescent background material, over 200 square inches of reflective material, and complete 360-degree reflectivity.

Power Isolation

Regardless of the vehicle's make or model, the Paramedic at an extrication must ensure that the vehicle's power is shut down. Although power shutdown is important for safety reasons, the Paramedic must also consider the effect shutting the power down will have on the vehicle's power accessories. Modern vehicles have numerous power accessories (i.e., power seats, windows, hatches, sliders) which may be the only means to move a seat or lower a window. Therefore, before shutting down the vehicle's power, the Paramedic should make any needed adjustments to the power accessories.

Turning off the engine has also become more complicated. Besides "normal" ignition keys, today's vehicles may have proximity (wireless) keys (sometimes called smart keys). These keys must be kept more than 15 feet from the vehicle so that it does not accidentally start. After locating and removing the keys, the Paramedic should disconnect the battery. Depending on the vehicle, the battery (or batteries) may be hard to find. In more than 40% of vehicles, the batteries are located outside the engine compartment, often in the vehicle's trunk or rear area. Even if the battery is located in the engine compartment, it still may be hard to find; batteries are no longer located just in the front driver's side of the engine compartment.

In the past, many rescuers have felt that it wasn't important to isolate the vehicle's power. However, power isolation factors into the safety plan and provides protection for both the patients and rescuers alike.

Patient Considerations in the Extrication

Patient care is the first and primary consideration at every vehicle rescue. Good trauma care starts with good basic life support: airway management, manual cervical spine stabilization, application of C-collar, and so on. However, performing the primary assessment in contemporary cars can be a challenge. The dash and controls "wrap" around the driver and front passenger to form a "cockpit"-like configuration, and the seats are often bucket seats or racing styled seats. These innovations make for tighter spaces, leaving less room and less space for rescue equipment and personnel. Many times, in order to obtain the appropriate amount of space to access the patient and provide care, the rescue crew must displace vehicle components. In order to do this, the Paramedic needs to simultaneously provide patient care, help rescuers create more space, and help provide a pathway to remove the patient.

Space making is the process of creating a larger space around the patient for access, care, and egress. The rescue team performs tool evolutions to displace vehicle components and make appropriate space to remove the patient in an expedient manner. The Paramedic needs to be with the patient, not only to provide care but also to protect the patient while rescue tools are being used. The rescue team needs to understand both the issues and hazards surrounding the vehicle. Their power tools and how they will interact with the vehicle materials make vehicle rescue dangerous.

The Paramedic needs to provide prompt patient care simultaneously with spacemaking efforts. As part of those tasks, the Paramedic needs to be inserted into the interior of the wreck not only to provide patient care but also to assist in rapid patient removal. A better patient outcome can be produced when these operations are fused together. Personnel operating tools and performing spacemaking evolutions need to understand the current vehicle technology concerns. Paramedics also need to have proper background knowledge of these spacemaking techniques.

Interior Space Making

Vehicles have the inherent ability to absorb crash energy and redistribute it throughout the vehicle. For example, the vehicle compresses to absorb energy in engineered locations called crumple zones. When the crash exceeds the crumple zone's ability to absorb this energy, it is transferred into the passenger compartment. As a result, the vehicle deforms and components are displaced into the passenger compartment. This occurs more readily in today's vehicles than in those built a decade or more ago. Although this type of construction helps save lives, it also restricts and confines patients, thus limiting access to patients and hindering their removal from the wrecked vehicle.

Often the Paramedic is confronted with a motor vehicle collision with roof "impingement," resulting from a vehicle rollover or a severe impact in which the roof distorts and crushes around the patient. The goal is to remove or displace the roof, which is often in close proximity to the patient. The tools used may cause vibration or movement that might shift the roof even closer to the patient. Using a spreader is one way to provide space quickly. A spreader lifts the roof away from the patient by displacing the roof upward. Although this provides some space, the Paramedic may need even more space. The telescoping ram is an excellent tool for space making. The ram is simply placed vertically inside the vehicle and extended to lift the roof.

The Paramedic should place **hard protection**, a firm object such as a short board, between the tools and the patient, as well as between the tools and the Paramedic. When displacing the roof glass, patient management is also a concern. Often, the glass will break in the crash. If it is not broken, the Paramedic should consider what the glass will do when the roof is lifted. In addition to the glass already being "loaded" (stressed) from the crash's energy, use of the spreader or ram will add additional force, which will make broken glass a real possibility.

The Paramedic should also look at what the ram will be pushing against. The ends of the ram have a fairly small contact area that can fail catastrophically. Therefore, the Paramedic might want to increase that surface to spread the force more evenly.

One of the most effective methods to maximize interior space is the cross-ramming evolution in which the hydraulic ram is placed into the vehicle and then extended from one vehicle component to another. A key point in this evolution is to maximize the ram's surface contact area with cribbing at each end and thus spread the force of the ram over a larger area.

Depending on the vehicle damage and intrusion, the Paramedic may also consider removing the roof, which will enhance ramming efforts by weakening the vehicle's structural integrity. Cross-ramming may be an option when the vehicle's B-post is intruding into the occupants' cell. The interior trim should be stripped to check for safety system components such as seat belt pretensioners or gas generator cylinders used in side-curtain airbag systems. With the small size of some telescoping rams that are currently available, the Paramedic can effectively cross-ram space even in foot-well areas. As with any controlled displacement, however, the Paramedic needs to monitor the vehicle as it is displaced, manage that displacement by cribbing it, monitor the patient, and note any change in patient status as the extrication progresses.

Another possibility for maximizing interior space is displacing the steering column. In most vehicles, the steering column will tilt up to make more space; in some vehicles, the column can move or telescope as well. The Paramedic should look for and use these features prior to use of heavy rescue tools.

Seat movement is another spacemaking option. Although manually adjusting the seats can quickly increase the patient space, more vehicles now have power seats. As previously noted, the Paramedic should quickly cut off the vehicle's power at an extrication incident. However, before doing so, the Paramedic should consider whether the seats need to be moved before shutting down the vehicle's power. Seating configurations in minivans and SUVs may be removable or even "stowable" to maximize cargo space. If possible, the Paramedic should remove the vehicle's headrests, consoles, and armrests to get them out of the way.

Although the focus in extrication is on displacing the vehicle's exterior components (i.e., roofs, doors, and dashboards), the Paramedic needs to revisit "working" the interior. Current vehicle construction involves crash energy-absorbing and cab-forward design with a downsized exterior and maximized interior space.

Vehicles today may have "dissimilar" seating configurations and a structure that readily crushes inward. This makes extrication, which is already complicated by new external construction technology, even more difficult by reducing the space available to facilitate patient care. The Paramedic needs to employ varied extrication techniques, often simultaneously, to enhance the patient's outcome.

Motive Power Concerns

Motive power in the vehicles can take many forms. Although most vehicles are still propelled by a conventional drivetrain (i.e., gasoline or diesel fuel), many vehicles use other forms of fuel, or even combinations. Hazards are present with any of these fuels. However, some common sense and a little background information will keep the Paramedic safe.

Conventional Drivetrain

Gasoline and diesel drivetrains are the most common types of motive power the Paramedic will encounter at a motor vehicle collision. Fuel leakages and spills from these vehicles need to be managed on-scene, typically by the fire department.

Motor vehicle fires are a real threat. In 2007, fire departments responded to a vehicle fire on the highway every minute somewhere in the United States, and these fires resulted in one death every day.[3] The peak times for motor vehicle fires, according to the U.S. Department of Transportation, are between midnight and 3 a.m.[4] Therefore, the fire service should respond for fire suppression and spill control at all motor vehicle collisions.

Biofuels are also used, along with gasoline and diesel. Although the presence of biodiesel does not really provide any additional concerns, the gasoline and ethanol combinations do present additional problems associated with fire suppression and spill control.

Hybrids

Hybrid drivetrains use a combination of a gasoline or diesel engine with an electric motor, which uses a storage battery for electricity. The "conventional" engine not only supplies additional power but also runs a generator to supply electricity back into the storage battery. In some models, the drivetrain also recovers kinetic energy during deceleration and braking and converts it into electricity for storage in the vehicle's storage battery.

The hybrid vehicle has two electrical systems: a "normal" 12-volt system for the various vehicle operating systems and a high-voltage drivetrain system. The two systems do not cross. However, the high-voltage drivetrain system is controlled and regulated by a computer that is supplied with power from the 12-volt system. There are some basic rules of thumb for hybrids. The high-voltage (HV) power is direct current (DC), although some hybrids also generate 110 alternating current (AC). The HV power circuit is self-contained (i.e., it does not ground out to the vehicle chassis), and the HV drivetrain power is computer controlled. Perhaps most importantly, a crash and/or change in voltage results in a shutdown of the HV system.

All hybrids have a HV drivetrain circuit as well as a normal 12-volt automotive electric system. Even when the hybrid is shut down and secured there is always power in the HV battery. Although emergency responders should not need to interact with the HV battery, it can be identified by the cables. The automotive industry's electrical standards call for bright orange HV cables; this is consistent with the standards established by the Society of Automotive Engineers (SAE).[5]

Isolating the vehicle's power will shut down and secure the high-voltage drivetrain. This is doubly important in a hybrid vehicle as the Paramedic needs to secure the vehicle's various safety systems and its high-voltage drivetrain. Hybrid vehicles start off on electric power alone and travel up to certain speeds on the same power so the vehicle's motor will not make any noise. Therefore, it is vital to ensure the vehicle is secured, the power is shut off, the keys are removed, and the vehicle cannot move. The Paramedic cannot use the fact that the vehicle is not making any noise to determine that it is actually powered down or "off." Instead, the Paramedic needs to take proactive steps to ensure it actually is "off."

The high-voltage drivetrain has cabling between the storage battery and the electric motor. This cabling, along with its protective covering and connectors, are color coded. The high-voltage cabling is set up much like coaxial cable, in that the positive wire is surrounded by the negative wire and then surrounded by a protective covering. Regardless of the vehicle's power state, secured or not, the high-voltage cabling and connections should never be cut or damaged by the rescue team. Also, if the high-voltage system cabling is damaged during the crash, the high-voltage system will be shut down at the storage battery so that the vehicle does not become energized.

Plug-in hybrids are an outgrowth of the hybrid drivetrain. These vehicles can be plugged into the electric grid to charge the high-voltage storage battery and thus run longer on electric power alone. Otherwise, these vehicles are just like hybrids.

Electric vehicles are another motive power technology that is just emerging. Although Paramedics are likely to be familiar with electric specific-use vehicles, such as golf carts, larger electric vehicles are coming into play, especially in urban environments.

Original equipment manufacturers (OEM) that build hybrid vehicles produce an *Emergency Response Guide* for each type of hybrid vehicle. These guides are produced for emergency responders and give detailed information about the vehicle, specifically regarding how to secure the vehicle, extrication methods, fire suppression, and even towing.

STREET SMART

HV cable is never routed through posts, the roof, or inside any crumple zone. This prevents accidental damage to the cable that would energize the motor vehicle following a collision. Furthermore, automatic sensors stop electricity by opening relays whenever a collision occurs.

Hydrogen Cars

After powering London taxis for years, the use of hydrogen in U.S. cars is anticipated in the near future. Hydrogen is safe and lighter than air, so it dissipates quickly and burns without the typical by-products of combustion, providing a great safety margin for responders.

Another technology that uses hydrogen is **fuel cells**, hydrogen and methanol mixes, that produce electricity to power the automobile. Although currently in the development phase, the fuel cell holds a great deal of promise as the motive force for the future.

Vehicle Safety Systems

Vehicles today are equipped with a myriad of **supplemental restraint systems (SRS)**. Although many Paramedics are familiar with airbags, especially frontal airbags, SRS includes much more. Most vehicles today have six to eight devices, which protect occupants from impacts in all directions. These safety systems have made a dramatic difference in protecting occupants. However, they also have an impact upon the rescue activities post-crash.

The greatest danger to rescuers may be an undeployed airbag. Airbags deploy when an inertia sensor (a ball-in-tube device) detects a sudden deceleration. In some instances, these sensors malfunction and the airbag does not deploy. Although the likelihood of a post-crash accidental deployment is very low, the risk can increase over time due to a number of factors. The number of supplemental restraint systems, the condition of the batteries, and crash damage location are a few issues that increase the risk of post-crash deployment. However, the biggest factor is vehicle power. That is why Paramedics must not only remove the vehicle's keys but also find and disconnect the vehicle's power. This power interruption will drain the vehicle's electric storage capacitors in the supplemental restraint system computer within a short period of time and make the extrication process safer. In addition to performing power isolation, if possible the Paramedic should maintain a respectable distance from these devices. However, this is generally not possible if extrication is required.

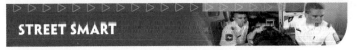

STREET SMART

The Paramedic should never place a hard object, such as a clipboard or pry tool, between the rescuer and the undeployed airbag. Even a small object, like a pen, propelled at 200 miles per hour can produce serious trauma.

Frontal Supplemental Restraint System

The **frontal impact supplemental restraint system** is a safety system located in the vehicle's steering wheel and dashboard to protect the front seat occupants during a frontal impact. The device is electrically activated and mixes two chemicals together to make nitrogen gas that then inflates the airbag. The initial generation of this device had one inflation module. However, contemporary vehicles have two inflation modules: one for high-speed crashes and one for low-speed crashes.

Casual observation of the deployed device will not tell the Paramedic if both modules have deployed or just one. Although this system is the least likely out of all the safety systems today to have an accidental post-crash deployment, the Paramedic should still use caution when working around the front seat occupants even if she observes that the airbag has deployed.

STREET SMART

Some responders have been told to "cut" the airbags. However, this practice is dangerous and should be discouraged. Cutting the airbag does not disable the airbag. If the airbag is accidentally deployed after being cut, then hot gasses are released to the vehicle compartment, potentially burning rescuers and patients.

Side-Impact Supplemental Restraint System

The **side-impact supplemental restraint system** is designed to protect occupants from a side impact. These SRSs are mounted either in the sides of the seat facing toward the vehicle's exterior or mounted in the door facing toward the occupants. Since these systems need to activate and deploy faster than any other devices, except the rollover protection system (ROPS), they use a different inflation method than the frontal supplemental restraint system (either pyrotechnics [gunpowder] or a gas cylinder).

Side-impact SRSs can usually be found in the front seat and/or door, and to a lesser extent in the rear seats/doors. Newer side-impact SRSs can have two side-impact bags, one to protect the pelvic region and one to protect the thorax region.

The **side-curtain supplemental restraint system**, as opposed to the side-impact supplemental restraint system, is a safety system that usually deploys downward from the roof edge along the interior of the vehicle's sides. The air curtain usually is found from the vehicle's first post to its last post, protecting the occupant's head and upper body from side impacts and from high-speed frontal impacts. Depending upon the crash and its location in relation to the vehicle, these systems might or might not be deployed.

The nature of the side-curtain SRS is that it must deploy in one-third of the time taken by the frontal SRS. The inflation module is a pressure vessel topped with a small pyrotechnic charge. Although the gas stored in the module is an inert gas, it is stored at approximately 3,000 to 10,000 psi. If these pressure vessels are accidentally cut, at a minimum, there is a release of high-pressure gas in close proximity to the tool operator and possibly the interior rescuer and patients. In the worst case scenario, the pyrotechnic charge deploys the side curtain and releases high-pressure gas. If the pressure vessel is cut, there is also the potential for creating debris and even shrapnel. Therefore, the Paramedic must avoid cutting these devices. Even disconnecting the battery and electrically disarming the system does not help if someone cuts through the device.

Another type of vehicle that can be equipped with side-curtain SRS is retractable roof convertibles. However, in these vehicles, instead of the curtain deploying downward from the roof edge, the device will actually deploy upwards from the top of the door.

A few years ago, the inflation device was in the rear roof post. However, that changed in 2002. They now can be found in any of the roof posts, the roof structure itself, or even in the vehicle body. These facts should at least alert the Paramedic

STREET SMART

Paramedics should be alert to the possibility of eye injury during an airbag deployment. Though statistically only 0.4% of airbag deployments result in severe sight-threatening injury, when eye injury does occur it is painful and anxiety inducing. One concern is the presence of sodium azide, the propellant, which can be corrosive to the cornea of the eye.

to use more caution when dealing with roof posts. However, the best approach is to strip interior trim before cutting the roof posts or the roof area.

Other Supplemental Restraint Systems

There are many places to place an SRS in a vehicle. In fact, even some motorcycles have airbags now. A common SRS is the **knee supplemental restraint system**, which deploys an airbag from the lower section of the vehicle's dashboard during a frontal crash. The device is designed to protect the front seat occupant's legs. It also helps protect the occupants from "submarining" and going under the vehicle's dash during a high-speed impact.

One hybrid model has a unique rear seat airbag system available. This system is mounted inside the bottom seat cushion of the rear seat. Upon activation, the seat belt pretensioner "fires," thus tensioning the seat belt. This draws the occupant into the seat (seat belt pretensioners are discussed shortly). Then the airbag deploys, inflating under the rear seat cushion and raising the cushion upward, creating a "hump" or "speed bump" under the occupant's thighs. This helps to keep the seat's occupant from moving forward.

Another new type of safety system that's rising in popularity is the pedestrian protection supplemental restraint system. However, not all of these systems use an airbag to protect the pedestrian. The system that is currently used in production vehicles takes the form of a "lifter" under the hood. This lifter is a combination of a small airbag and strut device that forces the rear of the hood upward, thus impeding the struck person from striking the windshield and rolling over the roof and rearwards.

Seat Belt Pretensioners

Seat belt pretensioners are powered devices that remove slack from the seat belt, ensuring that the occupant is seated properly when the airbag systems deploy. They are usually powered by a pyrotechnic charge, although some are powered by high-torque electric motors or even a gas cylinder.

These devices are used in all front, and most rear, seating positions in most vehicles. Looking for the accordion sleeve below the buckle fastener can identify the pretensioner. Although these devices are fairly benign to the rescuer, it is a good idea to cut the seat belts when working close to the belt. Even if the Paramedic disarms the pretensioner by

disconnecting the battery (just as with airbag systems), there is the potential for accidental deployment. Therefore, the Paramedic should avoid cutting through these devices during tool evolutions, especially in the area of the B-post.

Rollover Protection System (ROPS)

Current model convertibles are equipped with **rollover protection systems (ROPS)**. In some vehicles, the ROPS is a fixed device contained within the vehicle. However, most convertibles have deployable rollover protection. These devices are usually mounted as a pair in the rear of the occupant area. However, it can be a bar as well that spans close to the vehicle's width. The device is designed to deploy if the vehicle is potentially going to go on to its side or "roll over." The rollover, greater than 90 degrees, is detected using an electronic sensor. As with all electronically activated devices, there is a small potential for accidental deployment if the system is short-circuited, even if the vehicle is upright and the top is deployed.

Extrication with the Supplemental Restraint System

The combination of side airbags and seat belt pretensioners has made traditional extrication techniques (i.e., cutting roof pillars and displacing doors and roofs) dangerous. Therefore, several modified extrication techniques have been developed to avoid these hazards.

The first procedure is called a **modified dash roll**. After stabilizing the vehicle, the rescuer—with a charged safety line at standby and the battery disconnected—cuts the seat belt at the point closest to the door. The rescuer or Paramedic should never reach across the patient to do so. Using a short ram or spreaders, the rescuer rolls the dash forward after making several strategic cuts in the dashboard.

An excellent alternative is the use of a large ram on the opposite door. Not only does this roll the dash, it allows Paramedics access to the patient during the evolution. Note that it is not necessary to remove the door; in fact, it is desirable to leave the door in place to add structural strength to the A-post when using rams.

The final technique, called the modified jacking technique, uses spreaders to provide the desired lift. As the rocker panel tends to "bottom out" in all three techniques, it is prudent to place cribbing under the door. If the rocker panel buckles and bottoms out, it may pin the patient's legs under the dash.

Vehicle Materials and Construction

Vehicles are being constructed with an ever-enlarging list of materials including plastics, carbon fiber composites, baron steel, and so on. OEM is even using ultra-high-strength steels that cannot be cut with standard extrication cutters. This issue is now an everyday problem for the rescue crew. At a basic level, these materials and reinforcements add tremendous strength in key areas of the vehicle (roof posts, rocker panels, and foot-wells). Yet, the vehicle's construction allows the vehicle to crumple, crush, and absorb energy from the front and rear.

Not only does the structure and materials affect disentanglement and tool selection, but it also plays a key role in injuries and kinematics. Although the Paramedic will see a reduction in the severity of injuries at the motor vehicle collision, the Paramedic will also see an increase in the complexity of the extrication to disentangle occupants. In years past, a simple door displacement sufficed for patient access and extrication. Current vehicles do not afford a Paramedic the same amount of space, the same accessibility, or the same ease of extrication to facilitate access. This is owed, in part, to the large number of materials used in construction and the greater number of tools needed to dissemble the vehicle.

CASE STUDY CONCLUSION

The rescue squad arrives and starts to set up the tool staging area as well as an inner action circle. The Paramedic finishes donning the extrication gear and leans over to the rescue squad captain. Yelling over the din of the power tools, the Paramedic says, "Punch me a hole in the car so I can get in!"

CRITICAL THINKING QUESTIONS

1. What supplemental restraint systems should the rescue squad captain be concerned about?
2. What are the implications of new vehicle construction materials?

CONCLUSION

Although many of the incidents the Paramedic responds to share many of the same components, motor vehicle collisions have some unique issues. The basic operational cycle includes the following steps: size-up and scene management, hazard identification and control, vehicle stabilization and glass management, patient management, extrication evolutions, and return to service.

At every incident, command takes charge, ensures accountability, and develops a plan of action that includes hazard mitigation and a request for resources.

The Paramedic must assure vehicle stabilization to prevent unwanted movement of the vehicles involved, provide access into the wreck to begin patient management, create a pathway to remove the patient, and have the ability to send the patient to the appropriate medical facility.

The key to any successful vehicle extrication is to facilitate simultaneous operations on-scene; that is, extrication and patient care. The Paramedic needs to provide patient management as well as supply feedback to the IC and to the rescue team. The rescue team needs to accept the Paramedic's feedback as to what is going on with the patient and develop an action plan, as well as a backup plan, to displace vehicle components, as well as create space needed for patient care and a pathway to disentangle the patient from the wreck.

KEY POINTS:

- Vehicle extrication is a multidisciplinary effort with patient care as the focus.

- Safety remains the first priority at a motor vehicle collision.

- Three considerations regarding the vehicle are part of the Paramedic's scene size-up: orientation, stabilization, and damage.

- Stabilization of the vehicle starts with turning off the engine, ensuring the vehicle is in park, and engaging the parking brake.

- Interior assessment for damage that might indicate the mechanism of injury is essential prior to patient care.

- Physical entanglement is more common with newer vehicles.

- Paramedics need head protection and eye protection, as well as hand protection and even inhalation protection, to create the protective envelope.

- Regulation 23 CFR 634 requires Paramedics to wear bright, reflective apparel when working on the road.

- Space making is the process of opening the driver's 'cockpit' to permit access, care, and egress.

- Although heavy rescue tends to focus on displacing doors and dashboards or removing roofs, internal extrication (i.e., moving seats, displacing steering wheels) can be as helpful.

- Increasing numbers of vehicles are being powered by alternative fuels.

- Bright orange cable(s) indicate high voltage.

- Vehicle safety systems include the supplemental restraint systems.

- Airbags have two inflation modules for frontal impact, as well as side-impact curtains, under-seat and under-dash cushions, and even airbags for motorcycles.

- Vehicle construction materials (i.e., plastics, carbon-fiber composites, baron steel) make extraction more difficult than in the past.

- Successful extrication is the result of simultaneous operations on-scene.

REVIEW QUESTIONS:

1. What are the elements of the personal protective envelope?
2. Name three options for space making.
3. What are the motive power sources?
4. Name some vehicle safety systems.
5. What makes vehicle extrication more difficult with modern vehicles?

CASE STUDY QUESTIONS:

Please refer to the Case Study in this chapter, and answer the questions below:
1. What are the three considerations of the scene size-up?
2. What safety devices are in place to protect the patient in a crash?
3. How is the concept of spacemaking applied to this case?

REFERENCES:

1. NFPA 472. *Standard for Competence of Responders to Hazardous Materials/Weapons of Mass Destruction Incidents*, 2008 edition. Quincy, MA: NFPA; 2008.
2. NFPA 1067. *Standard on Operations and Training for Technical Search and Rescue Incidents*, 2009 edition. Quincy, MA: NFPA; 2009.
3. National Fire Protection Association. U.S. Vehicle Fire Trends and Patterns Report; 2007.
4. Nicholson J. Vehicle fire problem, *NFPA J.* 2007; issue 1: 460–471.
5. Cable Standards Committee, Society of Automotive Engineers. Available at: **http://www.SAE.org.** Accessed January 8, 2010.

CHAPTER 25

EMERGENCY INCIDENT REHABILITATION FOR FIREFIGHTERS

KEY CONCEPTS:

Upon completion of this chapter, it is expected that the reader will understand these following concepts:

- Standards related to firefighter fitness
- Importance of emergency incident rehabilitation
- Nine sections of rehabilitation
- Active and passive cooling methods
- Medical monitoring

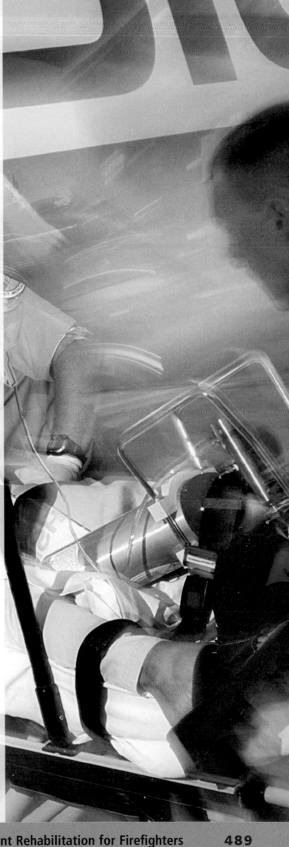

CASE STUDY:

The Paramedics can see the plume of smoke off in the distance. "We'll be going to that shortly," sighs Saul, the younger Paramedic. No sooner do the words spill out of his lips than the tones go off. What Saul witnessed is a major working fire with multiple responding fire companies, mostly volunteers. With the squad truck in gear, the two Paramedics discuss the rehabilitation sector and the likelihood that they will be doing the medical monitoring.

CRITICAL THINKING QUESTIONS

1. What are the standards related to firefighter fitness and, specifically, rehabilitation?

2. What are the nine sections of rehabilitation?

OVERVIEW

Firefighting ranks among the most physiologically demanding activities the human body can perform. Firefighting requires similar physical and mental exertion as is used when participating in marathon athletic competitions, yet provides the firefighter little to no opportunity to warm up. Often, firefighters are expected to awaken from a sound sleep and, within minutes, perform at maximal exertion. These demands, coupled with occupational hazards, make firefighting a dangerous and high-risk occupation. **Rehabilitation** is an intervention designed to mitigate the impact of the stressors of firefighting activities, restore the rescuers' work capacity, improve performance, and decrease risks for injury and death.

National Fire Protection Association Standards

Despite intensive efforts to reduce their incidence in recent years, **line-of-duty deaths (LODDs)** occur frequently among firefighters. Since 1977 when statistical data was first recorded by the U.S. Fire Administration, there has been an annual average of 100 firefighter deaths. Firefighters spend on average 10% of their time at the scene of a fire, yet half of all deaths and two-thirds of reported injuries occur at fires. Most likely three variables are connected to the significant numbers of injuries and deaths occurring during firefighting activities: medical condition, fitness, and rehabilitation.[1]

The **National Fire Protection Association (NFPA)** is a standard development organization that brings together key players in the fire and public safety industries to develop consensus on standards and guidelines. However, NFPA has no enforcement authority or ability to test, certify, or inspect for compliance with published standards and guidelines. At the behest of fire service organizations, NFPA sequentially developed standards designed to address each of the likely LODD culprits. The first of these was NFPA 1582, entitled *Standard on Comprehensive Occupational Medical Program for Fire Departments*, which provides detailed outlines for medical exams, testing guidelines for firefighter candidates, and continued requirements firefighters must meet throughout their career.[2]

The goal of **NFPA 1582** is to assist departments in maintaining a staff of medically qualified firefighters. By prescreening for conditions that might preclude an individual from safely performing the job of a firefighter, and early detection and subsequent intervention for conditions that arise during the course of a career, fire departments can identify conditions that might potentially harm a firefighter in the performance of the job.

The next NFPA standard introduced, **NFPA 1583**, entitled *Standard on Health-Related Fitness Programs for Fire Fighters*, provides guidelines for departments to create fitness programs that optimize the physical condition of firefighters to the degree necessary for performing their very strenuous duties. Several years ago, following the release of the first version of NFPA 1583, many fire departments purchased and installed workout rooms and exercise equipment for their members as a component of building their own comprehensive fitness programs.[3]

The most recent standard, **NFPA 1584**, *Standard on the Rehabilitation Process for Members During Emergency Operations and Training Exercises*, took the next logical step in protecting firefighters. Originally released as a guideline in 2003 (*Recommended Practices on the Rehabilitation of Members Operating at Incident Scene Operations and Training Exercises*), the evolution from the 2003 guideline version to the 2008 revision as a standard provided not only an update reflecting evolution in the science of rehabilitation but also more incentives to encourage compliance.[4]

The NFPA standards require not only industry-wide consensus for each recommendation, but also a strong evidence base when available. The legal system places significantly more weight on standards than guidelines when litigation arises questioning the appropriateness of department actions in protecting its workers.

It is important to understand that the standards for rehabilitation outlined in NFPA 1584 are premised on the belief that departments have already implemented a comprehensive approach to assure firefighters are medically qualified and have a proper level of fitness as outlined in NFPA 1582 and 1583. Otherwise, efforts at firefighter rehabilitation will amount to too little, too late.

There are two philosophical concepts to keep in mind when reading this chapter. First, implementation of NFPA 1584 is a constantly evolving process. The 2003 version of NFPA 1584 was perceived by many departments and firefighters as overly prescriptive and therefore difficult to implement. It was difficult to apply in all situations given the wide variety of climatic and work conditions encountered on various fire scenes. Implementation in a fashion that readily accounted for the wide range of health and physical conditions seen in personnel on the fire scene was also extremely challenging.

The 2008 version of NFPA 1584, however, is premised on the fact that firefighters need to make their own educated decisions about hydration, rest, and nutrition. Prescriptive volumes of fluids, specific medical treatments, and directions calling for use of specific commercial cooling devices were removed when the earlier version of NFPA 1584 was redeveloped into a standard.

Competitive athletes are not told when to rest or hydrate during a race or other athletic event. They know when and how much to drink and are very much in tune with their bodily needs for rest and nutrition. The first component of the 2008 edition of NFPA 1584 is that firefighters regularly perform at the same levels of exertion and endurance as professional athletes and should have the same insight and in-depth knowledge about their own needs for hydration, rest, and nutrition.[5]

From the first day in a fire recruit academy, firefighters need to be given the requisite education on these important components of rehabilitation. In addition, they need to understand the physiology of core body temperature regulation and must be able to recognize signs and symptoms of heat and cold stress. Emergency responders armed with experience and good information, like competitive athletes, will make the proper choices about hydration, rest, and nutrition to maximize their performance at emergency scenes. However, when a firefighter is too exhausted to recognize his needs, department procedures and fellow members of his team must provide a safety net to assure that the health and safety of every member is protected. That safety net includes a rehabilitation section.[6]

Chief officers also must understand the benefits of properly operated rehabilitation. There is a long-standing stigma in the fire service that rehabilitation is unnecessary and that rehabilitation operations deplete available personnel resources, leaving fewer firefighters to conduct fire scene operations. When rehabilitation is properly designed, established, and operated, however, it will have the exact opposite effects. Well-run rehabilitation increases the pool of available personnel and improves the performance of firefighters on-scene by allowing them to work longer, harder, smarter, and more efficiently. The end result, in addition to maximizing personnel resources, is ultimately a decline in injuries and, hopefully, a decrease in line-of-duty deaths.[7]

The second philosophical component is the significant tension that often arises between firefighters and Paramedics operating at a rehabilitation area on a fire scene. Most often, disagreements arise from differing points of view between fire officials and Paramedics about a firefighter's readiness or capability to return to firefighting operations. However, disagreements arise for many reasons. More often than not, Paramedics may not understand the intense physiological changes firefighters normally experience during firefighting activities. NFPA 1584 makes one point abundantly clear: Paramedics working in a rehabilitation area shall be delegated by the incident commander (IC) with the authority to keep a member in rehabilitation or transport for further medical evaluation or treatment if, in the Paramedic's professional judgment, the firefighter should not return to duty.

If NFPA 1584 stands a chance of being widely implemented by the fire and emergency services, then Paramedics working in rehabilitation areas absolutely need proper training and clearly defined protocols to assess, recognize, and make determinations about firefighter health and well-being. Without a comprehensive understanding of the physiological effects of firefighting on a firefighter and sound protocols to guide evaluation and decision making in the rehabilitation area, there will continue to be disagreements between Paramedics and fire service members that ultimately defeat the purpose of having a well-run rehabilitation operation on the emergency scene.

NFPA 1584 establishes minimum criteria for developing and implementing a rehabilitation process for emergency responders at an incident scene and at certain training exercises. The definition of an incident in which rehabilitation is required is any situation (emergency scenes or training exercises) that poses a safety or health risk to members, typically meaning those incidents lasting longer than one hour.

This standard applies to some organizations and not to others (Table 25-1). The organizations outside the scope of this standard have other federal or occupational standards that apply to them. EMS organizations may be surprised to learn that they are included in the scope of NFPA 1584 and should have **standard operating guidelines (SOGs)** in place delineating a systematic approach for how they intend to provide rehabilitation for their own members at incidents and certain training exercises. Likewise, law enforcement special operations teams are also included in the scope of NFPA 1584. In many parts of the country, either local fire service or EMS may be asked to provide rehabilitation for law enforcement operations given their lack of experience or expertise in running such an operation themselves.

The overarching requirement of NFPA 1584 is that every department will develop and implement a set of rehabilitation SOGs that spell out specifically how rehabilitation will be provided at incidents and training exercises. Ultimately,

Table 25-1 Organizations Impacted by NFPA 1584

Application of NFPA 1584 Rehabilitation Standard (2008 edition)	
Applies to Organizations Providing	**Does Not Apply to**
Rescue	Industrial fire brigades, also known as:
Fire suppression	
Emergency medical services	• Emergency brigades
Hazardous materials mitigation	• Emergency response teams
Special operations	• Fire teams
Other emergency services including:	• Plant emergency organizations
• Public fire departments	• Mine emergency response teams
• Military fire departments	
• Private fire departments	
• Industrial fire departments	

Table 25-2 Recommended Intervals for Firefighter Rehabilitation

Recommended Intervals for Firefighter Rehabilitation*
• Following use of the second 30-minute self-contained breathing apparatus (SCBA) cylinder
• Following use of a single 45-minute SCBA cylinder
• Following use of a single 60-minute SCBA cylinder
• Following 40 minutes of intense work without SCBA
*The company officer should assess the crew at minimum every 45 minutes for rehab.

SOGs need to delineate how the department intends to provide the equipment, supplies, necessary shelter, and medical expertise to firefighters where and when necessary. Ongoing education is expected so that members have a comprehensive knowledge of when and how to rehabilitate themselves. SOGs also need to incorporate a safety net mechanism that will provide for rehabilitation of members who are either unable or unwilling to recognize their own needs.

Although the NFPA 1584 standard suggests certain work intervals at which point rehabilitation might be recommended (Table 25-2), it is important to design SOGs that afford the company officer (the direct supervisor of the crew members operating a particular piece of fire apparatus) leeway to adjust time frames for the crew based on work or environmental conditions. In addition, the officer may have personal knowledge of the usual rehabilitation needs of individual firefighters.

Additional planning tools extensively described in the annex section of NFPA 1584 help chief officers and incident commanders make decisions about when a rehabilitation area should be established in the course of an incident. These include a National Weather Service (NWS) wind chill temperature (WCT) index as well as a U.S. Fire Administration heat stress index chart. These tools can be used to help plan when to initiate rehab operations during training or emergency responses.

Sections of National Fire Protection Association Standard 1584

There are nine sections of the NFPA 1584 rehabilitation standard: relief from climatic conditions, rest and recovery, cooling or rewarming, rehydration, calorie and electrolyte replacement, medical monitoring, EMS treatment according to local protocols, member accountability, and release.

Relief from Climatic Conditions

The rehabilitation area should be free from smoke (or other potentially adverse conditions present at the scene) and sheltered from extremes of heat or cold. Depending on environmental conditions, this may require a separate building, tent, vehicle, or other enclosed space where firefighters can rest away from wind, smoke, or dust. However, the area should not be located so far from the incident scene so that it is not readily accessible. In multistory building fires, for example, the rehabilitation area is often best located on the level just below the fire floor. Paramedics should be properly trained and wear firefighters' turnout gear inside any structure within a working fire.

Additionally, the rehabilitation area requires a vestibule or other segregated area where firefighters can remove their PPE (personal protective equipment, such as turnout gear and SCBA) prior to entering the rehabilitation area itself.[8] This assures that members in the rehabilitation area are not exposed to off-gassed toxins and chemicals carried on PPE from the incident scene.[9]

Rest and Recovery

Firefighters should be afforded the ability to rest for at least 10 minutes or as long as is needed to recover their capacity to continue working. Ordinarily, 10 minutes is sufficient time for an individual to rest in order to feel energetic enough to return to strenuous activity. If the firefighter does not feel adequately rested after 10 minutes, or is presenting to rehabilitation for the second or third time during an incident, he should rest for an additional 10 minutes. If after 20 minutes of rest a firefighter does not feel ready or appear able to return to operations, the firefighter should be assessed by EMS personnel in the rehabilitation area.[10,11]

Cooling or Rewarming

Firefighters who arrive in rehabilitation feeling cold should be allowed to add clothing (additional clothing may need to be included with rehab supplies), wrap up in blankets, or use other available means to rewarm. More often, firefighters will be warm or hot and require some form of cooling. There is considerable debate in the medical and sports literature about cooling. What is agreed, however, is that the normal core body temperature is 98.6°F (±1.8°F) or 37.0°C (±1°C). Multiple factors, both intrinsic and extrinsic, influence core body temperature in firefighters. Intrinsic factors include intense skeletal muscle work and increased metabolic rate, both of which contribute to an increase in core body temperature. Extrinsic factors include high environmental temperatures experienced when working in or around a fire and encapsulating PPE that traps heat near the body surface. The combination of these factors contributes to the increased core body temperatures often experienced by firefighters entering a rehabilitation area.

A variety of methods can be employed to cool firefighters in the rehab setting. These can be broken down into passive and active cooling techniques. **Passive cooling techniques** often involve "common sense" activities such as removal of PPE, evaporation of sweat, and moving to a cooler environment. **Active cooling techniques**, in contrast, use external methods of removing heat from the body such as misting

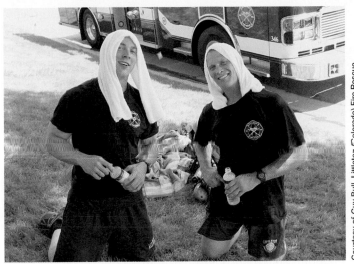

Figure 25-1 A firefighter seeks relief in a rehabilitation cooling station.

fans or tents, forearm immersion chairs, vacuum-assisted palm cooling devices, cooling vests, and cold towels. The use of passive cooling and active cooling devices such as misting fans or tents is limited by environmental conditions of increased temperature and humidity. The ability to cool when atmospheric temperatures exceed body temperatures or when humidity is extremely high is severely limited and, in many instances, can actually heat subjects rather than cooling them (Figure 25-1).

Studies comparing active cooling devices in firefighter rehabilitation find virtually all of the commercial devices (forearm immersion chairs, vacuum-assisted palm cooling devices, vest devices, and cold towels) fairly comparable in their ability to lower core body temperature. When compared to forearm immersion chairs and misting devices, cold towels were rated as more effective and refreshing in two separate studies. The low cost, portability, and ease of setup, coupled with the psychological appeal of being able to move around freely in the rehab area, makes cold towels an extremely affordable and effective means of cooling. Ice water and cold towels are recommended by the American College of Sports Medicine as the most effective means of cooling athletes with exertional heat illness.[12]

Cooling Towels

The supplies needed for a **cold towel cooling system** in rehabilitation include ice, water, bleach, towels, and plastic buckets. Five-gallon buckets that can be obtained from a local hardware or home improvement store work best for this operation. Initially, the Paramedic fills a bucket with water and adds ice until a comfortable temperature is achieved. If ice is not immediately available, cool water can be used alone. The Paramedic places dry towels into the water-filled bucket. Once wet, they should be wrung out until damp (not dripping). A single damp towel will hold slightly more than a pound (500 grams) or 500 milliliters of water and is able to remove thousands of calories of heat from a firefighter. When firefighters use cold towels according to personal preference, most will place the towel around the neck or over the head.

Following their use, towels require sanitizing prior to reuse. This is accomplished by mixing a bucket of bleach solution that consists of one-fourth cup of household bleach added to each gallon of water. After soaking in the bleach solution for a minute or two, the towels are sanitized. The Paramedic uses a separate bucket of water to rinse the bleach solution soaked towels. Once rinsed and wrung out, the towels are returned to the ice water bucket for reuse. The Paramedic should change the water as frequently as needed in order to maintain the function of each bucket. A system using 20 towels; one bucket each of ice water, bleach solution, and rinse water; with a 20-minute rehab cycle will supply sufficient cold towels to rehabilitate 60 people an hour. When kept resupplied, this system is capable of running indefinitely.

After use, ice water and rinse water can be dumped anywhere; bleach solution, however, should be discarded into a drain. The Paramedic should launder towels in hot water with bleach. A department can easily carry three buckets, a measuring cup, a small bottle of bleach, and 20 towels on virtually any piece of apparatus. Ice is easily obtained in the community. However, rehabilitation can proceed using cool water if ice is not immediately available.

Finally, consumption of cold water is a time-proven and highly effective active cooling method. The belief that drinking cold water somehow interferes with performance or results in indigestion is a myth without basis in the medical literature.[13] When consuming chilled water in the rehabilitation area, firefighters experience both active cooling and rehydration. The challenge in most rehabilitation operations is getting fluids chilled. Unless a department maintains a supply of cooled beverages or has a cooler installed and stocked on a rehabilitation support vehicle, there is often not enough time to prepare chilled beverages during rehab operations (Figure 25-2).

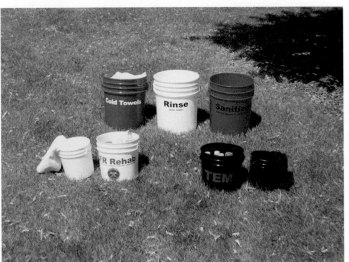

Figure 25-2 The cooling bucket system is an effective active cooling technique.

Rehydration

Firefighters, like other public safety workers, are often dehydrated when compared to the population as a whole. In recognition of this, coupled with the inability for firefighters to replace fluids as quickly as they may be lost during firefighting activities, NFPA 1584 recommends that firefighters prehydrate within two hours of planned events by drinking 500 milliliters (16 ounces) of fluid. In most circumstances, water is the best fluid for hydration.

After the first hour of intense work, or when an incident extends beyond three hours' duration, sports drinks may be added to the hydration fluids consumed. It is important to remember that the typical gastric emptying time for most adults limits the total volume of water that can be consumed to 1 liter (1,000 milliliters or 32 ounces) per hour. On the fire scene, this dictates that frequent consumption of small amounts of water (60 to 120 milliliters) is the best practice in order to rehydrate and prevent nausea from exceeding the stomach's ability to empty.

Sports drinks usually contain electrolytes and carbohydrates. A complete discussion about use of sports drinks is beyond the scope of this chapter, so readers interested in more in-depth information on choosing appropriate sports drinks for use in rehabilitation are encouraged to consult a rehabilitation textbook.

One important consideration for consumption of sports drinks is osmolarity, also referred to as concentration. Manufacturers adjust the osmolarity of sports drinks to maximize absorption of their drinks (i.e., gastric emptying time). Concentrating or diluting sports drinks outside of the manufacturer's recommendations (e.g., serving half-strength Gatorade®), will alter the osmolarity of the sports drink, affecting its absorption. This may lead to nausea and vomiting in firefighters. Sports drinks used to replace electrolytes and carbohydrates should be used conservatively, only when required, and should be served as recommended by the manufacturer to avoid nausea and vomiting. Nonetheless, water is the most ideal fluid for hydration. A recommended ratio of sports drinks to water consumed (when sports drinks are utilized) is one sports drink for every 2 to 3 liters (64 to 96 ounces) of water.

During the intense work of firefighting, it is fully possible to lose 2 liters of fluid or more each hour. This occurs primarily through sweating and respiratory losses. Dehydration significantly impairs work performance. Mild dehydration, defined as loss of up to 5% of body weight, can decrease work capacity by up to 30%. It is readily apparent that a dehydrated firefighter is more prone to injury, illness, and mistakes, not to mention less effective on the fire scene. Since it is often difficult to replace fluids at the same rate as a firefighter loses them, rehydration must continue post-incident.

There is currently no practical means of assessing hydration status of firefighters on the fire scene. The National College Athletic Association (NCAA) uses urine-specific gravity to assess hydration status in athletes. Urine-specific gravity, probably the most simplistic and accurate means of assessing hydration status in healthy adults with normally functioning kidneys, is commonly tested by dipping a urine test stick into a container of urine collected from the subject being tested. However, such a practice is impractical for use on the fire scene.

Weight is sometimes used to assess hydration status since water losses can be readily calculated from changes in weight before and after a period of intense work. Weighing firefighters before and after every fire is also impractical and requires that the weights be done without firefighters wearing sweat-soaked clothing. A new technology that holds promise for rehabilitation is a **saliva osmolarity monitoring device** that analyzes saliva collected on an oral sampling stick that is inserted into a companion machine, much like a portable glucose monitor. The analysis provides reliable hydration values. Other technologies are also in development.

The best available hydration monitor for the rehabilitation setting is thirst. Because other more reliable methods of assessing hydration are impractical, thirst is the only readily available means for use in the rehabilitation setting. NFPA 1584 recommends that firefighters drink to satisfy their thirst. Therefore, until a more reliable tool can readily be deployed on the fire scene, thirst will remain the sign by which the need for rehydration is indicated.

Water is the preferred hydration fluid and, as previously mentioned, sports drinks are helpful during incidents of prolonged duration. However, virtually all references warn against use of carbonated, caffeinated, and high carbohydrate-containing beverages in a rehabilitation setting. Shortly after publication of NFPA 1584, new evidence on the effects of caffeine appeared in the medical and sports literature.

Caffeine has long been recognized for its diuretic properties. Athletes have been advised to avoid caffeine based on studies that questioned caffeine's effects on hydration status. Recently, researchers have re-examined the effects of caffeine on hydration status and demonstrated that increases in urine output induced by caffeine (or carbonated soda) consumption are offset by the volume ingested, with a net effect of no change in long-term hydration status. These most recent studies were undertaken because competitive athletes, like some firefighters, believe caffeine consumption may enhance performance. The current state of the science has no evidence to support restricting caffeine intake on the basis that it may impair hydration.[14]

Calorie and Electrolyte Replacement

During prolonged incidences or when firefighters are working strenuously and continuously, calorie and electrolyte replacement may be desirable during rehabilitation. Longer duration events are typically defined as those lasting more than three hours or those where members are expected to (or actually do) work continuously for more than one hour. Paramedics are encouraged to consult a rehabilitation textbook for more indepth information on calorie and electrolyte replacement. Some basic recommendations for calorie and electrolyte replacement include: eat readily available carbohydrate sources such as meal replacement bars or fruit, drink 250 milliliters (8 ounces) of a sports drink (which contains approximately 15 grams of carbohydrate), and eat carbohydrate-containing foods ranging from 30 to 60 grams of carbohydrate per hour.

Foods that should be avoided in rehabilitation include high fat foods such as pizza or doughnuts. Additionally, NFPA 1584 appropriately requires that in any setting where food is available, firefighters must have the means to wash their hands and faces. This is easily accomplished with supplies of alcohol-based hand gel or with prepackaged wipes.

Medical Monitoring

It is important to differentiate between medical monitoring and emergency medical treatment in the rehabilitation setting. **Medical monitoring** refers to the observation of members for adverse health effects of firefighting including heat or cold stress, physical and psychological stress, and environmental stress. Emergency medical treatment refers to EMS treatment of an ill or injured person in the rehabilitation process. It is important that Paramedics performing medical monitoring have a thorough understanding and are equipped with protocols and guidance to understand the profound physiologic effects of firefighting on the human body.

Protocols or guidelines governing medical monitoring in rehabilitation should be established with explicit criteria for identification of individuals who require immediate EMS treatment and transport. Protocols are also needed for those who require close (or closer) medical monitoring in the rehabilitation areas and are subsequently able to leave the rehabilitation area and return to full duty on the fire scene.

These protocols must be contextual. That is, the tremendous physiologic changes seen with the exertion of active firefighting and the wide range of ages and physical conditioning levels encountered in a typical firefighter population must be recognized. Collaboration between fire department medical or occupational medical physicians and local EMS physicians is imperative so that medical monitoring protocols developed for rehabilitation address the specific needs and are not merely general population protocols translated for use on the fire scene. Failure to develop medical monitoring protocols specifically tailored for use in a rehabilitation area is a significant cause of disagreements that arise between Paramedics and fire officers.

NFPA 1584 provides some specific recommendations on medical monitoring. The first is that a trained EMS provider assess each member entering the rehab area for, at minimum, six conditions: (1) complaints of chest pain, dizziness, dyspnea, weakness, nausea, or headache; (2) general complaints including cramps, aches, or pain; (3) heat- or cold-related stress symptoms; (4) changes in gait, speech, or behavior; (5) level of alertness and orientation to person, place, and time; and (6) any vital signs considered abnormal by local protocol.

A close review of these six conditions translates into a simple "look test." Essentially, on entering rehabilitation, the Paramedic should assess each firefighter's general overall health and well-being, much like the primary impression formed during a medical or trauma assessment.

The next logical component of medical monitoring in rehabilitation is assessment of vital signs. There is considerable variation in the vital signs measured during rehabilitation and very little evidence demonstrating any value of the vital signs in determining when emergency treatment is necessary or what type and duration of rehabilitation a firefighter may require. As a consequence, many fire department rehabilitation protocols for medical monitoring do not routinely assess vital signs. On the other hand, some fire department physicians and medical directors find measuring vital signs is a helpful tool to set parameters for monitoring, treatment, transport, and release from rehabilitation.

NFPA 1584 provides some recommendations to consider when using vital signs to establish parameters. Some vital signs will not be available immediately. As soon as practical, EMS personnel should assess any vital signs recommended by local protocol. There is little value in measuring any vital signs prior to a firefighter being able to remove his or her PPE and being able to rest for a few moments in the rehabilitation area. NFPA provides some guidance for measurement of vital signs when departments choose to do so in rehabilitation.

Temperature

The most accurate measure of heat or cold stress on the body is core body temperature. As previously noted, the normal core body temperature is 98.6°F (±1.8°F) or 37.0°C (±1°C), varying between individuals by time of day and by activity level. Measurement of core body temperature is best done rectally or by swallowing a temperature transmitter capsule, neither of which are practical in rehabilitation situations. The most common methods used in rehabilitation to measure body temperature are oral or tympanic (ear) thermometers, both of which typically read lower than the actual core body temperature. Oral thermometers are about 1°F (0.55°C) lower and tympanic thermometers about 2°F (1.1°C) lower than the core body temperature.

Multiple factors can affect accurate measurement of oral and tympanic temperatures, including operator error, storage of the device in hot or cold environments, and external cooling of the temperature measurement surface (such as direct sunlight elevating a tympanic temperature or hyperventilation falsely decreasing an oral temperature measurement). Even with these limitations, elevated temperatures obtained by oral or tympanic devices suggest possible heat-related illness. Touch by a Paramedic has also been shown to accurately assess the presence of fever. However, normal temperatures obtained by touch or with an oral or tympanic thermometer cannot be reliably used to exclude heat-related illness.

Multiple recent studies have found that the core body temperature of firefighters will continue to rise during the first 20 minutes following cessation of physical activity, even with active cooling measures. Although the effects of heat stress are well documented, a danger level for core body temperature has yet to be established. No clear guidance exists on what constitutes an acceptable temperature for release from rehabilitation. Studies on performance athletes and individuals who have acclimatized to higher temperature climates have not conclusively demonstrated impaired performance at higher-than-normal core body temperatures.[15]

As temperature assessment is fraught with the potential for error, no clear guidance on upper core body temperature limits exists. As firefighters continue to experience increases in their core body temperatures despite active cooling measures, there is little utility to temperature measurement in a rehabilitation setting at this time.

Heart Rate

Given the exceptional demands of firefighting, heart rates should increase and in all likelihood will exceed 100 beats per minute. Because age, physical conditioning, medications, the degree of physical exertion, hydration status, pain, and psychological stress affect heart rate, it is imperative to interpret heart rate in the context of the individual firefighter. With rest, heart rate should return to near normal pre-exercise rates.[16]

To keep heart rate assessment contextual, some departments record baseline resting heart rates on personal identification tags or store them in a computerized reference database. Variations can then be interpreted as a percentage of deviation from normal for each individual (i.e., greater than 20% above or below normal). In rehabilitation, recovery of heart rate may be more significant than the actual heart rate itself. Any firefighter with a sustained heart rate above 100 beats per minute after 20 minutes of rest needs further medical monitoring and assessment, especially if a readily identifiable cause (such as dehydration or fever) cannot be determined. Heart rate can be measured quickly and accurately with a pulse oximeter or CO-oximeter.

Respiratory Rate

Firefighters entering rehabilitation will more than likely exhibit tachypnea as a normal physiologic response to exertional stress and elevated core body temperature. Before a firefighter is cleared to leave rehabilitation, his respiratory rate should return to normal.

Blood Pressure

Blood pressure is the most frequently measured, and most poorly understood, vital sign. As a consequence of difficulty interpreting changes in blood pressure, many medical authorities no longer routinely measure blood pressures in rehabilitation. As with heart rate, blood pressure must be interpreted in the context of the individual. Knowing an individual's baseline resting blood pressure can help with interpreting values obtained in rehabilitation, but may present difficulties with interpretation as the firefighters presenting to rehabilitation are certainly not rested and relaxed. NFPA 1584 recommends that individuals with systolic blood pressures above 160 or diastolic blood pressures above 100 not be released from rehabilitation.

Blood pressure measurement also has significant error potential related to incorrect cuff size and mispositioning on the extremity being measured. Accurate assessment requires a cuff that spans two-thirds of the distance between the elbow and shoulder; larger cuffs lead to falsely low measurements and smaller cuffs to falsely high readings. The extremity in which blood pressure is being measured must be positioned at mid-heart level during assessment. Any elevation above mid-heart level will yield falsely low readings, whereas positioning below mid-heart level will falsely increase pressures.

When using electronic blood pressure measuring devices, only heart rate and mean arterial pressure (MAP) are actually measured by the device, which then calculates systolic and diastolic blood pressures using heart rate and MAP. If there is any difference between measured and actual heart rate, the calculated systolic and diastolic pressures are likely incorrect.

Finally, and most importantly in a rehabilitation setting, blood pressure measuring equipment must be thoroughly decontaminated between use on each individual to prevent the spread of bacteria. There is probably no better environment for transmission of antibiotic-resistant organisms between individuals than by repeated reuse of sweat-soaked blood pressure cuffs on multiple individuals.

Pulse Oximetry

Pulse oximetry has been described extensively elsewhere in this textbook. Although oximetry can be a helpful assessment tool and may detect hypoxemia that is not otherwise discovered, it has significant limitations. For example, black, blue, and green nail polish cause falsely low oximetry readings. When in doubt, remove the nail polish or change the probe site. Bright external lighting and sunlight will sometimes falsely lower oximeter readings; by covering the probe and digit being measured, the Paramedic can eliminate this interference. Most oximeters are unable to differentiate between oxyhemoglobin and carboxyhemoglobin. In a rehabilitation setting, this could easily result in a carbon monoxide poisoned firefighter appearing to have normal oxygen saturation. Firefighters with oxygen saturations of less than 92% measured on room air should not be released from the rehabilitation area.[17]

Carbon Monoxide Assessment

Carbon monoxide (CO) is the leading cause of poisoning deaths worldwide, and is a common cause of death in victims at fire scenes. It has repeatedly been documented as an environmental hazard for firefighters. Medical monitoring conducted in the rehabilitation area must include assessment for symptoms of CO poisoning. Unfortunately, symptoms of CO poisoning are vague, often appearing as viral illness or other medical problems, and are often missed.

Any firefighter in rehabilitation who was exposed to CO or who complains of headache, nausea or vomiting, or shortness of breath should be assessed with a medical device designed to screen for CO poisoning. Examples of two devices for noninvasive CO assessment are a Pulse CO-Oximeter™ (a pulse oximeter designed to measure noninvasively measure blood constituents, including carboxyhemoglobin–Figure 25-3) and a portable exhaled breath CO monitor.

CO attached to hemoglobin in the bloodstream is reported as a percentage of blood carboxyhemoglobin (COHb %). In nonsmokers, normal COHb ranges from 0% to 5%. For smokers, levels range from 5% to 10%. Individuals in rehabilitation with COHb levels between 10% and 15%, need further assessment for CO poisoning signs and symptoms and, if present (or if they desire to reduce their COHb levels more rapidly), given high-flow, high-concentration oxygen. Any individual with a COHb level above 15% requires further assessment and evaluation by EMS. To be released from rehabilitation, firefighters should have a normal COHb level as determined by local protocol. Nearly all protocols require a COHb level of ≤ 5% in order to be released from rehabilitation for return to the fire scene.

EMS Treatment According to Local Protocols

When a firefighter in the rehabilitation area is identified as needing emergency medical care or transportation, the Paramedic should provide care according to local, state, or regional EMS treatment and transport protocols. This recognizes that medical monitoring protocols may well differ significantly from local emergency medical treatment protocols. Record keeping should also be maintained separately, with medical monitoring during rehabilitation logged with rehabilitation documentation. Records for members transported to a hospital or given emergency medical treatment should be documented on the patient care reporting system used by the treating EMS unit (Figure 25-4).[18]

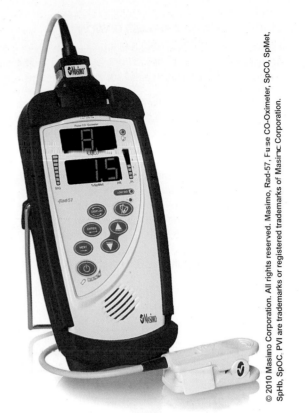

Figure 25-3 The Masimo Rad-57® Pulse CO-Oximeter™ allows clinicians to noninvasively measure oxygen saturation (SpO$_2$) and carboxyhemoglobin (SpCO) levels in the blood, in addition to methemoglobin (SpMet), total hemoglobin (SpHb), oxygen content (SpOC), Pleth Variability Index (PVI), perfusion index (PI), and pulse rate using a small finger sensor.

Member Accountability

NFPA 1584 specifies that members entering and leaving rehabilitation will be accounted for through the personnel accountability system being used by the incident commander in charge of the scene. The firefighters' progress should also be tracked through rehabilitation.

One potential solution is to utilize a rehabilitation tag system, similar to the triage tags used to track the flow of patients during prehospital multiple patient incidents (Figure 25-5).

Release

In a similar fashion to the evaluation conducted when a member enters the rehabilitation area, a Paramedic should evaluate each member prior to leaving rehabilitation to ensure the member is able to safely return to active duty on the fire scene. On release, the member's status should also be confirmed with the accountability system in use.

EMERGENCY INCIDENT REHABILITATION

The following guidelines are intended for use at events where fluid loss is a concern for participants or spectators. These guidelines may also be used at fire scenes to treat firefighters.[a]

At fire scenes, the "rehabilitation area" should be located near the SCBA bottle changing, triage, or staging areas.

1. When the person arrives in the "rehabilitation" area for the **first** time:
   A. If fire scene, remove firefighter PPE prior to entering the rehabilitation area.
   B. Encourage the person to drink water to satisfy thirst.
   C. A Paramedic should do a visual evaluation for signs of heat/cold illness or excessive fatigue. If the person exhibits any signs of heat/cold illness or excessive fatigue, take vital signs. If no s/s heat/cold illness or excessive fatigue, rest for 10 minutes.
   D. If person feels rested and able to return to event or duty, assess heart rate and, if fire scene, SpCO. If heart rate and SpCO are within criteria[b], release from rehabilitation.
   E. If vital signs are not within the criteria[b] listed below, the person should rest for at least 10 minutes with continued oral rehydration.
   F. If SpCO is outside normal limits (fire scene), consider high flow O_2 to accelerate carbon monoxide clearance.
   G. If vital signs return to criteria limits, the person shall be released to return to the event or to duty.
   H. If vital signs are still beyond criteria limits, continue rehabilitation for another 10 minutes and determine if further intervention may be needed.
   I. If after 30 minutes, vital signs remain outside limits listed below, ALS transport to the hospital should be initiated.

2. When a person arrives in the "rehabilitation" area for the **second** time:
   A. All steps listed above except initial rest period should be extended to 20 minutes.

[a] The use of this protocol assumes that the person has no significant complaint. If a person arrives at the rehabilitation area complaining of chest pain, shortness of breath, or has an altered mental status, keep the patient NPO and follow the protocol appropriate to the complaint.

[b] **Vital Signs Criteria**

Blood Pressure: Systolic $<$ 160 mm Hg or Diastolic $<$ 100 mm Hg
Respirations: $<$ 24 per minute
Pulse: $<$ 100 per minute
SpO_2: $<$ 92%
SpCO: $\leq$ 5%

An irregular pulse mandates ALS intervention, EKG monitoring, and removal from duty or the event.
A. Names and vital signs for each rescuer should be recorded on a log sheet for the incident.
B. A full PCR should be written on any transported person.
C. Electrolyte solutions are encouraged.
D. More aggressive treatment should be used during extremes of temperature.
E. Consider carbon monoxide poisoning during prolonged exposure to smoke.
F. Other agency procedures may be used in place of these guidelines as appropriate.
G. Contact Medical Control for advice if any issues arise with use of this protocol.

Figure 25-4 A model emergency incident rehabilitation protocol.

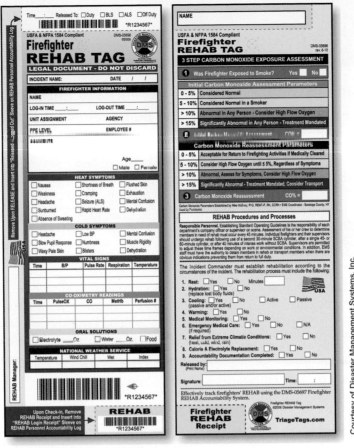

Figure 25-5 A rehabilitation tag can be used to track the flow of patients through rehabilitation.

Courtesy of Disaster Management Systems, Inc.

CASE STUDY CONCLUSION

A mutual aid company, Northside Elmwood Fire District, has already set up the rehabilitation sector in the building adjacent to the fire scene. The firefighters requested Paramedics to the scene because several firefighters are "high risk" and the chief wants Paramedics available, just in case. The two Paramedics set up their equipment next to the auxiliary services, which is putting out coffee and donuts.

CRITICAL THINKING QUESTIONS

1. Where should the rehabilitation sector be established?
2. What hydration and nutrition should be offered to rescuers?

CONCLUSION

Emergency incident rehabilitation has the potential to mitigate the danger to firefighters that exists from strenuous and demanding work and can reduce the number of line-of-duty deaths that occur on fire scenes.[19] Common sense, coupled with some simple techniques and knowledge of physiology, can ensure firefighters comply with rehabilitation protocols.[16,20]

KEY POINTS:

- Firefighting is stressful to the body and is associated with line-of-duty deaths.

- Three NFPA standards relate to a firefighter's fitness to fight fires: NFPA 1582, 1583, and 1584.

- NFPA 1584 is an evolving document that has been updated to reflect a less prescriptive standard.

- Paramedics, using professional judgment, can keep a firefighter out of service.

- NFPA 1584 pertains to all emergency operations, including training and law enforcement.

- The NFPA 1584 contains nine sections that include guidelines on environmental relief, rest and recovery, cooling or rewarming, rehydration, calorie and electrolyte replacement, medical monitoring, EMS treatment protocol, member accountability, and release.

- Firefighters should be afforded 10 minutes of rest and recovery time, and 20 minutes during their second rehab. Any firefighter requiring more than 20 minutes should be evaluated.

- The cold towel cooling system is very effective for rehabilitation.

- Prehydration can prevent heat exhaustion.

- Osmolarity is important when choosing a sports drink to avoid dumping syndrome.

- Mild dehydration, considered 5% of body weight lost, can reduce work capacity by 30%.

- Vital signs checked during rehabilitation include temperature, heart rate, respiratory rate, blood pressure, and pulse oximetry).

- Carbon monoxide levels greater than 15% should be evaluated. The firefighter remains in rehabilitation until the COHb is < 5%.

REVIEW QUESTIONS:

1. What three NFPA standards relate to a firefighter's fitness to fight fires?

2. What errors in the 2003 version of NFPA 1584 were corrected in the 2008 version?

3. What three tools are contained in the annex of the NFPA 1584?

4. What are the nine sections of the NFPA 1584 rehabilitation standard?

5. What is the lower range of carbon monoxide (COHb) that is acceptable?

CASE STUDY QUESTIONS:

Please refer to the Case Study in this chapter, and answer the questions below:

1. What are three indicators of dehydration and which is the most practical on a fire scene?

2. Medical monitoring is required for what conditions?

3. What is the acceptable range of heart rate during rehabilitation?

REFERENCES:

1. Kales SN, Soteriades ES, Christophi CA, Christiani DC. Emergency duties and deaths from heart disease among firefighters in the United States. *N Engl J Med*. 2007;356(12):1207–1215.

2. NFPA 1582. *Standard on Comprehensive Occupational Medical Program for Fire Departments*. Quincy, MA: NFPA; 2007.

3. NFPA 1583. *Standard on Health-Related Fitness Programs for Fire Department Members*. Quincy, MA: NFPA; 2008.

4. NFPA 1584. *Standard in the Rehabilitation Process for Members During Emergency Operations and Training Exercises*. Quincy, MA: NFPA; 2008.

5. NFPA 1584. *Recommended Practices on the Rehabilitation of Members Operating at Incident Scene Operations and Training Exercises*. Quincy, MA: NFPA; 2003.

6. Espinoza N, Contreras M. *Orange County Fire Authority Safety and Performance Implications of Hydration, Core Body Temperature and Post-Incident Rehabilitation—Final Report*. Orange County Fire Authority; December, 2007.

7. Missoula Technology and Development Center. *Wildland Firefighter Health and Safety Report*. 2006;10(Spring):1–10.

8. Selkirk GA, McClellan TM, Wong J. The impact of various rehydration volumes for firefighters wearing protective clothing in warm environments. *Ergonomics*. 2006;49:418–433.

9. Jankovic J, Jones W, Burkhart J, Noonan G. Environmental study of firefighters. *Ann Occup Hyg*. 1991;35:581–602.

10. Smith DL, Petruzzello SJ, Chludzinski MA, Reed JJ, Woods JA. Effects of strenuous live-fire firefighting drills on hematological, blood chemistry, and psychological measures. *J Therm Biol*. 2001;26:375–380.

11. Smith DL, Petruzzello SJ, Manning TS. The effect of strenuous live-fire drills on cardiovascular and psychological responses of recruit firefighters. *Ergonomics*. 2001;4:244–254.

12. Wilcox IM, Cronin JB, Hing WA. Physiologic response to water immersion—a method for sports recovery? *Sports Med*. 2006;36:747–765.

13. Armstrong LE. Assessing hydration status: the elusive gold standard. *J Am Coll Nutr*. 2007;26:575S–584S.

14. Ganio MS, Casa DJ, Armstrong LE, Maresh CM. Evidence-based approach to lingering hydration questions. *Clin Sports Med*. 2007;26:1–16.

15. McLellan TM, Selkirk GA. *The Management of Heat Stress for the Firefighter*. Canada: Defence Research and Development; 2005.

16. Shireffs SM, Maugham RJ. Rehydration and recovery of fluid balance after exercise. *Exercise and Sports Reviews (ACSM)*. January 2000;28(1).

17. McEvoy M. Averting oxygen hazards with oximetry. *Fire Engineering's FireEMS Magazine*. June 8–11, 2005.

18. Dickinson ET, Wieder MA. *Emergency Incident Rehabilitation* (2nd ed.). Upper Saddle River, NJ: Brady/Pearson; 2004.

19. U.S. Fire Administration (USFA). *FA-314, Emergency Incident Rehabilitation*. Emmitsburg, MD: USFA; 2008.

20. Smith DL, Petruzzello SJ. Selected physiological and psychological responses to live-fire drills in different configurations of firefighting gear. *Ergonomics*. 1998;41:1141–1154.

CHAPTER 26

HAZARDOUS MATERIALS OPERATIONS

KEY CONCEPTS:

Upon completion of this chapter, it is expected that the reader will understand these following concepts:

- Definition of hazardous materials
- Training requirements for each level of responder
- Use of container type, placards, and shipping papers in the scene size-up
- Use of the *Emergency Response Guide* and the NFPA 704 placards to identify the hazardous material
- Chemical properties associated with hazardous materials
- Toxicology concepts associated with hazardous materials
- Integration of the incident command system into a hazardous materials response
- Hazmat control zones
- Medical surveillance
- Decontamination principles
- Treatment planning for the exposed patient

Shortly after the Paramedics complete the morning equipment check, the sound of the alert tone fills the apparatus bay. "Medic 245, respond to state route 44 for a single vehicle motor vehicle collision, witness reports large tanker vehicle on its side. Injuries are unknown at this time." As the Paramedic scrambles to assemble her turnout gear, she begins to think about what might be inside the tanker. Could this be a hazardous materials incident? As she drives toward the accident, she considers a variety of possible situations. Is the scene safe? What material, if any, is inside the tanker? Is it safe to enter the scene to assess the patient?

Arriving on-scene, the Paramedic safely positions the ambulance upwind of the incident. Looking through binoculars, she sees a large tanker truck lying on its side. The Paramedic relays that additional information directly to dispatch, who informs the Paramedic that local fire and CBRNE response teams are en route. The first support unit to arrive on-scene is the district fire chief.

CRITICAL THINKING QUESTIONS

1. What will help the first responder identify the contents of the tanker?
2. What are the elements of a "first due" report?
3. How does the Paramedic use the *Emergency Response Guide*?

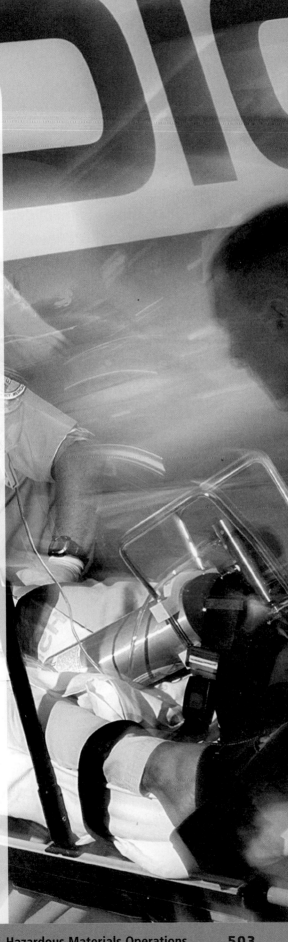

OVERVIEW

Hazardous materials are defined as any substances (solid, liquid, or gas) that, when released, are capable of causing harm to people, the environment, or property. This definition includes an extensive list of substances used as part of industrial manufacturing, as well as products found within the average home. Additionally, this definition includes a variety of naturally produced substances that pose a threat to those exposed. Toxins are poisonous substances that are produced by living organisms, such as plants, animals, bacterium, or fungi.[1] When these substances are injected by a bite, we describe them as venom. "Hazardous materials" is a general term used to alert Paramedics to a vast number of dangerous substances.

Historically, events involving hazardous materials have been referred to as hazmat incidents. In recent years, the abbreviation **CBRNE**, referring to Chemical, Biological, Radiological/Nuclear, and Explosive events, has been favored when describing such incidents. This change has resulted from an increased awareness of how hazardous substances may be used in terrorist attacks. Bacterial and viral agents can be used as a form of biological agent, with anthrax being an example of one such agent. When responding to any event involving a weapon of mass destruction (WMD), the CBRNE acronym helps providers maintain a wide differential of possible etiological agents.

This chapter shows why the Paramedic must be aware of the specific risks present when responding to a hazmat incident. In addition, it will address methods to best protect the Paramedic and the general public from exposure to dangerous substances.

Epidemiology

The U.S. Department of Transportation (DOT) has compiled data regarding the number of hazmat incidents in the United States since the 1970s. This data, which is currently available through the Pipeline and Hazardous Materials Safety Administration (PHMSA), includes the number of incidents, locations, type of substances released, and number of patients affected by the releases.

In 2007 alone, more than 19,000 hazmat incidents were reported in the United States. These events occurred in all 50 states and involved substances stored in fixed facilities as well as those in transit. Of these, 479 were defined as serious incidents, with reports of 41 hospitalized patients and 10 fatalities. Of the casualties listed, five emergency service employees were hospitalized, and 31 others were evaluated for hazmat exposure. Most injuries resulted from incidents involving corrosive materials, whereas most fatalities occurred from incidents involving flammable-combustible liquids.[2]

This data indicates that hazmat/WMD incidents are common, and injuries can often be severe if not fatal. Therefore, Paramedics should remain alert to the possible danger to themselves and other first responders at incidents involving hazardous materials.

Training Requirements

The original regulatory authority for hazardous material response training stemmed from the **Comprehensive Environmental Response Compensation and Liability Act (CERCLA)**, also known as the super fund. CERCLA, in broad terms, addressed the need for specially prepared personnel with advanced training in hazmat response.

In 1986, CERCLA was updated by the **Superfund Amendment and Reauthorization Act (SARA)**, which provided more details about hazardous materials operations including the "community right to know." It also established the State Emergency Response Commissions (SERC) and Local Emergency Planning Committees (LEPC). Armed with material safety data sheets (MSDS) provided to the LEPC by industries, emergency services can be proactive and plan for predictable emergencies.

In the late 1990s, pursuant to the federal regulation (29 CFR 1910.120 regulations) more commonly known as the **Hazardous Waste Operations and Emergency Response (HAZWOPER) standards**, OSHA spoke to the need for training, personal protective equipment (PPE), and medical monitoring among all responders, in addition to other issues. The Environmental Protection Agency's (EPA) 40 CFR 311 mirrored the OSHA regulations to include all agencies not covered by OSHA and to ensure comprehensive coverage of all responders.

The first level of training commonly recognized is the Awareness level. **Awareness level** is required of all emergency responders who are likely to witness a potential hazmat incident. The key to the Awareness level is an understanding of the risks of hazmat, the ability to recognize the presence of hazmat, and, by using the *Emergency Response Guide* (*ERG*), the ability to recognize the need for additional resources.

The next level, **Operations responder**, is primarily tasked to take defensive actions such as containment and control of the scene. With a minimum of eight hours of training, these responders are also expected to understand basic decontamination procedures. They may be further trained in specialized programs for the medical aspects of Operations level activities.[3]

The **Technician level** responds to the scene of a hazardous materials incident, dons special protective clothing (described later in the chapter), and enters the hot zone to stop the release. The Technician uses advanced control and containment techniques.[3]

Supporting the hazmat Technician is the Specialist. The **Specialist level** is familiar with the local emergency response plan, created by the LEPC, as well as the state's emergency response plan, created by the SERC. The Specialist may also be capable of implementing decontamination procedures and may be responsible for contributing to the site safety plan by working closely with the safety officer. See Chapter 20 for further discussion of the safety officer's role.[3]

National Fire Protection Association Training Standards

To lend support to OSHA/EPA regulations and to provide further assistance to all emergency responders, the National Fire Protection Association (NFPA) provides a number of standards.

The NFPA standard series 471 to 473 provide voluntary minimal training competencies for emergency responders to hazmat incidents. **NFPA 471** establishes competency standards for each level of responder, whereas **NFPA 472** expands on the previous OSHA standards.[3] Paramedics should particularly be interested in **NFPA 473**, which relates to EMS response and describes two levels, EMS/HM1 and EMS/HM2.[4]

NFPA EMS/HM1, described in NFPA 473, details the duties of the EMS/HM1 responders including Awareness level training (described earlier) as well as some other cold zone responsibilities, dealing specifically with medical surveillance.[4]

NFPA EMS/HM2 standards have four core objectives that are particularly important for Paramedics. First, the Paramedic should be able to analyze a hazmat incident to determine potential health risks as part of an incident survey and to collect data about the hazard based in part on available on-scene information.[4]

Next, the Paramedic should plan to deliver advanced life support as part of a local emergency response plan and identify strategic resources. These resources include those in the Strategic National Stockpile (SNS) and Metropolitan Medical Response System (MMRS).[4]

After analyzing the scene and planning the response, the Paramedic should be able to implement the treatment plan. Part of that treatment plan is an understanding that a hazmat incident may also be a criminal investigation. Therefore, evidence preservation must be included in the plan. Coupled with casualty care is medical monitoring of hazmat Technicians, which is a part of the rehabilitation of emergency responders.[4]

Finally, the Paramedic is expected to participate in the termination of the event. This includes incident debriefing, preparation of an incident critique, and medically documenting all exposures.[4]

Scene Size-Up

As an emergency unit arrives at the location of a possible hazmat incident, Paramedics should follow several steps to help identify the risk posed by a release of chemicals, particularly gasses. The Paramedic should make every attempt to stay upwind from the incident and away from the gasses. However, this may be difficult or impossible, depending on the Paramedic's access to the scene. By observing environmental cues, as well as smoke or gas plumes, one can quickly identify the general direction of the wind and the probable area of contamination.[3]

A key piece of equipment the Paramedic should use during initial scene size-up is a pair of binoculars, since the arriving unit should make every effort to avoid close contact with the release of chemicals until specific information about the substance can be obtained. Binoculars allow the Paramedic to determine the characteristics of the vehicle and locate liquid pools or solid dispersions from a safe distance. Additionally, the Paramedic may be able to identify any placards located on the involved storage or transport carrier. Maintaining a safe distance, a "standoff" position, away from the spill is important for the Paramedic's health and safety.

Transportation Containers

The **Hazardous Materials Transportation Act (HMTA; 49 CFR)** standardized containers, markings, and the mode of transportation used for materials, including hazardous materials. This makes it easier for Paramedics to grossly ascertain the nature of the contents being transported when they first arrive on-scene.

For example, oval tankers designated Motor Carrier 306 or **MC306 (DOT406)** (Figure 26-1, no. 131), carry approximately 9,000 gallons of liquids, in one or two internal compartments, that are not under pressure. These tankers, oval or elliptical on cross-section, are single-shell aluminum construction and are prone to rupture. They typically carry motor fuels or nonvolatile materials such as milk or water.

Rounded tankers, **MC307 (DOT 407)** (Figure 26-1, no. 137), are double-hulled, low-pressure chemical tanks. The flattened ends of these tankers give rise to their nickname,

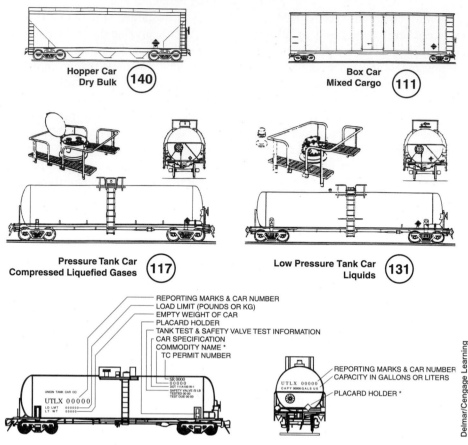

RAIL CAR IDENTIFICATION CHART*

Hopper Car
Dry Bulk (140)

Box Car
Mixed Cargo (111)

Pressure Tank Car
Compressed Liquefied Gases (117)

Low Pressure Tank Car
Liquids (131)

REPORTING MARKS & CAR NUMBER
LOAD LIMIT (POUNDS OR KG)
EMPTY WEIGHT OF CAR
PLACARD HOLDER
TANK TEST & SAFETY VALVE TEST INFORMATION
CAR SPECIFICATION
COMMODITY NAME *
TC PERMIT NUMBER

REPORTING MARKS & CAR NUMBER
CAPACITY IN GALLONS OR LITERS

PLACARD HOLDER *

Figure 26-1   Materials can be carried in many types of railcar and road trailer containers.

"blunties." Sometimes stiffening rings can be appreciated, particularly if the tank is not insulated. However, these tanks are often insulated and covered with a smooth aluminum skin.

The **MC312 (DOT 412)** (Figure 26-1, no. 137) tanker carries approximately 5,000 to 6,000 gallons of corrosive liquids under low pressures (35 to 50 pounds per square inch). Because of the dangerous nature of these chemicals, the tank is typically constructed of stainless steel or carbon steel and has reinforcing outer rings.

Another bulk tanker commonly seen on the road is the **MC331**, a high-pressure tank that carries liquefied gasses such as propane or anhydrous ammonia. The **MC332** has elaborate relief valves that vent the gas to the environment rather than risk an explosion, specifically a boiling liquid expanding vapor explosion (BLEVE).

The **MC338** has the classic "thermos bottle" construction (i.e., double-walled construction with insulation and relief valves) (Figure 26-1, no. 117). The MC338 is used to transport liquid oxygen, liquid nitrogen, liquid hydrogen, and liquefied natural gas, to name a few gasses compressed into liquids. It has the characteristic circular, rounded edges. Another danger inherent with compressed gasses that is somewhat specific to these tankers is the risk of cryogenic-induced frostbite.

Tube trailers are easily distinguishable by their permanently mounted cylinders (Figure 26-1). Tube trailers carry gasses, such as hydrogen, helium, and argon, under very high pressure.

Some bulk containers on the highway (Figure 26-1, no. 134) carry dry bulk materials. These bulk containers are often distinguishable by the V-shaped unloading compartments on the bottom of the trailer.

Paramedics must realize that any tractor-trailer can be carrying hazardous materials. Smaller quantities of dry chemical can be carried in boxes or 55-gallon barrels. Chemicals can also be carried in tight or closed head drums for liquids or solids or bottles for liquids. If the drum is plastic, it may be carrying corrosives; if it is metal, it may be carrying solvents/fuel.

Cylinders almost always carry gas under pressure. The DOT, in 49 CFR 1.G sec. 173.300, describes a compressed gas as having an absolute pressure of greater than 40 pounds per square inch (psi) and requires that the tank be free of defect and clearly marked with its contents. Although a distinctive cylinder color, such as green for oxygen, may be used, cylinder color has not been universally adopted. For example, green can mean oxygen or chorine. The Paramedic should instead look for the hazardous materials placard (Figure 26-2).

The placard, required under 49 CFR 173, indicates the nature of the material: flammable gas, flammable liquid, nonflammable gas, corrosive, poison gas, poison, or oxidizer (represented by the flaming circle).

ROAD TRAILER IDENTIFICATION CHART*

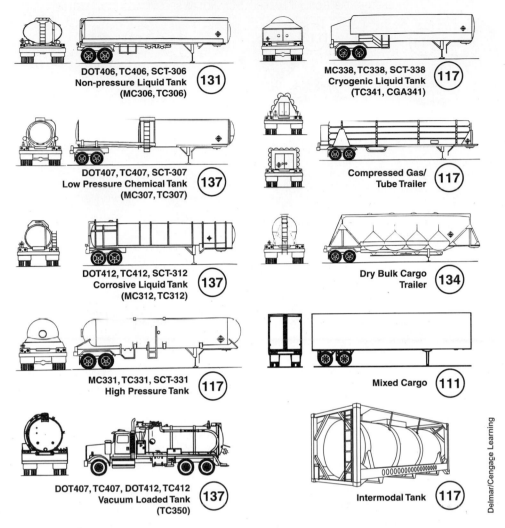

DOT406, TC406, SCT-306
Non-pressure Liquid Tank
(MC306, TC306) (131)

MC338, TC338, SCT-338
Cryogenic Liquid Tank
(TC341, CGA341) (117)

DOT407, TC407, SCT-307
Low Pressure Chemical Tank
(MC307, TC307) (137)

Compressed Gas/
Tube Trailer (117)

DOT412, TC412, SCT-312
Corrosive Liquid Tank
(MC312, TC312) (137)

Dry Bulk Cargo
Trailer (134)

MC331, TC331, SCT-331
High Pressure Tank (117)

Mixed Cargo (111)

DOT407, TC407, DOT412, TC412
Vacuum Loaded Tank
(TC350) (137)

Intermodal Tank (117)

Delmar/Cengage Learning

Figure 26-1 (continued)

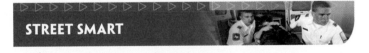
Emergency Response Guide

Specific information related to placards can be found in several quick reference guides. One of the most commonly used resources is the ***Emergency Response Guide (ERG)***, which defines the U.S. Department of Transportation (DOT) placard system and houses a wealth of information related to the potential health risk of hazardous materials. This reference is a collaborative effort between the United States, Mexico, Canada, and Argentina. The *ERG* is updated periodically and is available on-line as a reference as well. In addition, downloadable applications with versions of the *ERG* are available for personal computers and palm-based devices.

The *ERG* has several color-coded sections: yellow, blue, orange, and green. The yellow section contains a list of identification numbers that can be matched to the placard on the container. Next to the ID number is the chemical name and a three-digit number that can be cross-referenced to the initial response guide section highlighted in orange. Note that those substances highlighted in green within the yellow section are also cross-referenced in the green section and require special treatment.

If the placard is not visible, then the Paramedic should attempt to locate the shipping manifest (shipping papers). These documents will help to quickly identify substances stored in poorly labeled containers or containers without placards. The shipping manifest is usually kept in the truck's cabin, the ship's pilothouse, or the train's engine.

With the chemical name taken from the shipping manifest, and using the *ERG* guide, the Paramedic should reference the blue section for a list of chemical names and try to cross-match

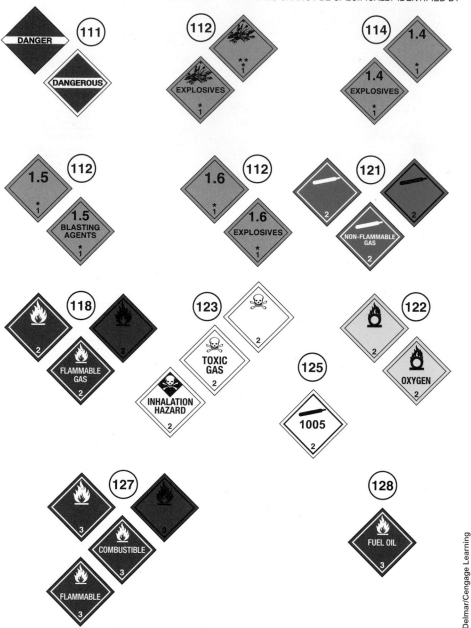

Figure 26-2 Standard hazardous materials placards indicate the nature of the gas inside the container.

the names. Attention to detail is important. Many chemicals have similar spellings and can be easily confused. Like the yellow section, those chemicals highlighted in green are also cross-referenced in the green section and require special treatment.

The Paramedic should remember to remain at a safe distance from the released material until the substance can be properly identified. Therefore, the Paramedic should only attempt to locate these resource guides if they are located safely away from the released substance or can be obtained without risk of exposure. For example, one means of obtaining the information from the shipping manifest may be to contact the shipping company.

STREET SMART

Along the border of both the yellow and blue sections is a special hazards listing. If the letter "P" is present, then it means the chemical may undergo polymerization if exposed to heat or to contamination with other chemicals. When polymerization occurs, heat and pressure can build up to explosive levels.

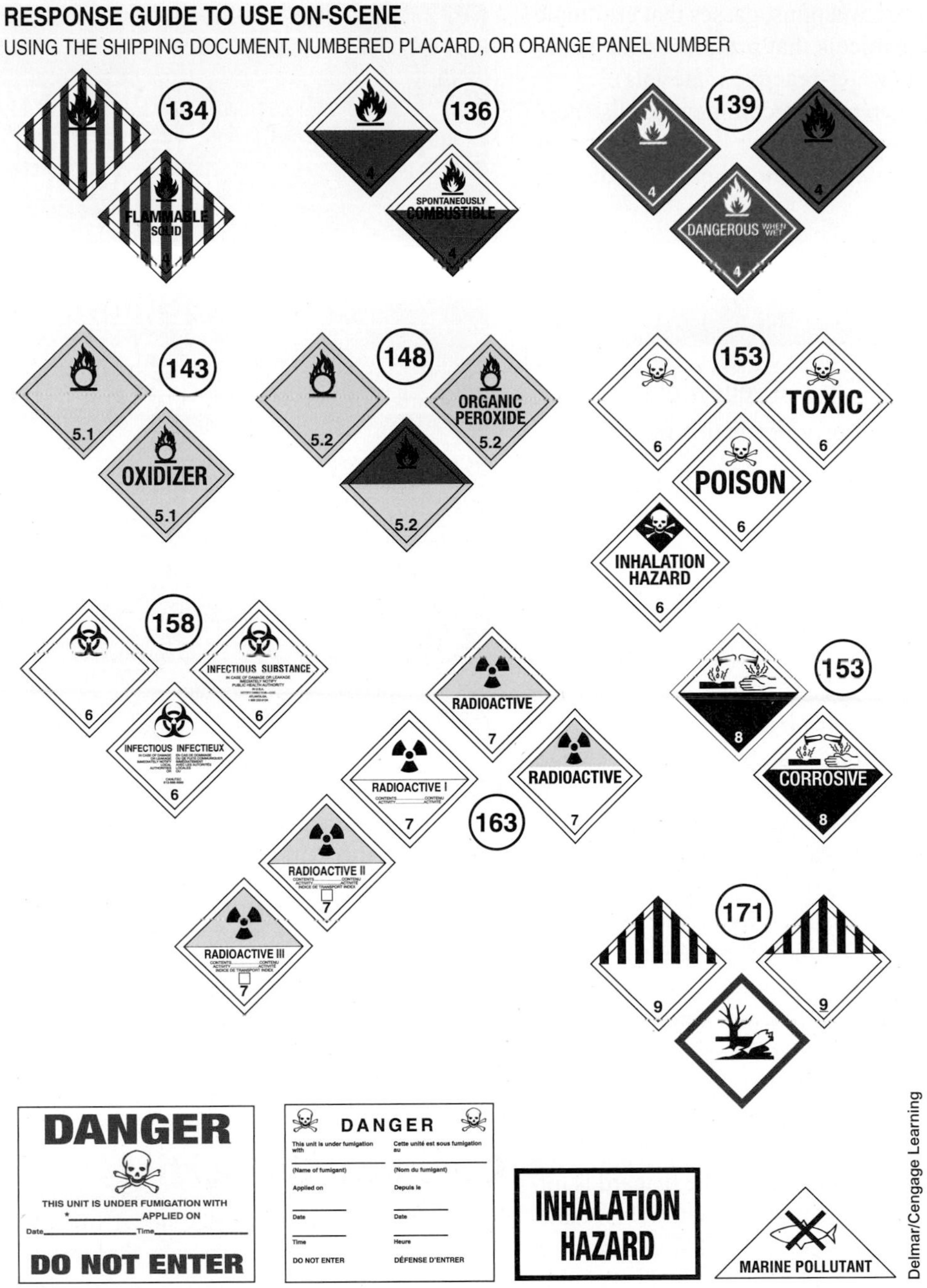

RESPONSE GUIDE TO USE ON-SCENE
USING THE SHIPPING DOCUMENT, NUMBERED PLACARD, OR ORANGE PANEL NUMBER

Figure 26-2 (continued)

Having used either the green section or the blue section, the Paramedic should have a cross-referenced guide number in the orange section. The orange section should provide the Paramedic with all of the information needed to start the initial phase of an emergency hazmat incident response.

The orange-bordered guide section contains information about potential hazards of explosion and fire as well as health hazards. In addition, the orange section contains public safety information such as minimal protective clothing and evacuation distances, which are cross-referenced to the green section. Finally, the orange section contains emergency response information for fire and EMS, such as first aid.

The Paramedic should not solely depend on the *ERG* for instructions on emergency medical care. The instructions provided are generally intended for first aid only in the first minutes of an emergency. As an exposure is a toxicological emergency, the Paramedic should consider contacting medical control and/or calling the poison control hotline to speak to a toxicologist.

Green Section of the *Emergency Response Guide*

The green section of the *ERG* contains the initial isolation and protective action distances to protect both Paramedics and the public from potentially lethal gasses. The chemicals listed can be chemical warfare weapons, gasses that are "toxic by inhalation" (TIH), or chemicals that produce toxic gasses when in contact with water (water-reactive materials).

These distances, which are only recommended distances for the first 30 minutes of an event, may be increased over time as conditions, particularly atmospheric conditions, change.

STREET SMART

If the product is highlighted in the yellow or blue section of the *ERG*, and the product is not on fire, then the Paramedic should go to the green section. If the product is on fire, then the Paramedic goes to the orange section.

Fixed Facilities

Additionally, the **NFPA 704 standard** describes the four-diamond hazard placard warning system for fixed storage tanks and buildings. The four diamonds provide information to Paramedics about the general health risks, the chemical's flammability, and its stability to shock. In addition, special hazards are illustrated in the bottom diamond of the placard. These hazards include warnings against water and oxidation, for example. A quick review of some of the features of the NFPA 704 will demonstrate its utility to the Paramedic.[3]

The upper red diamond in the placard represents flammability. A rating of zero indicates that the material inside is nonflammable, whereas a rating of four indicates that rapid vaporization will occur if the material is exposed to air and that the material burns readily.[3]

The yellow diamond on the right side of the placard is for reactivity. A rating of zero indicates that the material is stable under normal conditions, whereas a rating of four indicates that the material is capable of detonation or explosive decomposition at even normal temperatures.[3]

The third diamond, the blue diamond to the left side of the placard, is for health hazards. A rating of zero indicates that there is no health hazard even in the presence of fire. A rating of one indicates that exposure may cause minor irritation and may leave some minor nonpermanent residual effects, such as a rash. A rating of two means that there may be some temporary incapacitation of the exposed patients, which has implications for self-rescue.[3]

The ratings of three and four are ominous. Three means disability with risk of permanent injury on even short exposure. Four means that major permanent disability or even death is possible with even short exposure; in fact, sometimes only a whiff is necessary to cause death.[3]

The Paramedic should also note the white diamond at the bottom of the placard. This space is reserved for special

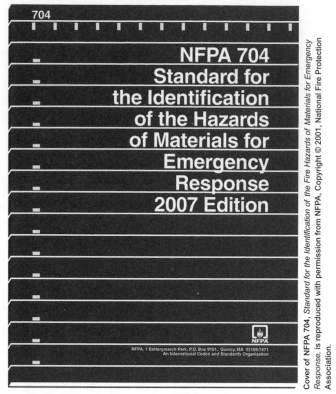

Figure 26-3 NFPA 704 describes the four-diamond hazard placard warning system for fixed storage tanks and buildings.

designations, such as reactive with water (noted by the letter W crossed out) or an oxidizer (the letters OX/OXY).[3]

Although this system can be very helpful to Paramedics, there is no law or regulation requiring its use. Therefore, it is not universally followed. Rather, it is a suggested standard, and its adoption is subject to local laws (Figure 26-3).

Chemical Properties

It is impossible to memorize all of the chemical properties of the thousands of chemicals that exist. However, there are some basic chemical principles of which the Paramedic should be aware. Many of these properties are listed on the chemical's **material safety data sheets (MSDS)**.

There are three common states of matter that the Paramedic may encounter on-scene of a hazardous materials spill: solid, liquid, or gas.

All liquids and gasses flow. The ability of a liquid to flow is based on its viscosity. The higher the viscosity (the thicker the fluid), the slower it will flow. Flow is also affected by gravity and by friction loss. A solid, which does not flow, can become a liquid when it reaches its **melting point**, typically under conditions of heat/fire.

When a liquid reaches its **boiling point** and becomes a gas, there is a danger of vapor formation. The faster a liquid evaporates (its volatility), the more vapor it creates, which creates a pressure inside a confined space, such as a tanker. This pressure, called the vapor pressure, can become explosive if released. These explosions, called a **boiling liquid expanding vapor explosion (BLEVE)**, can be devastating.

Chemical Movement

One of the first priorities at the scene of a hazardous materials spill is containment. As both liquids and gasses are capable of flowing, knowing the material's specific gravity or vapor density can help predict its flow.

The **specific gravity** is used to describe the difference between another liquid and water. Water has a specific gravity of one. Any substance with a specific gravity of less than one (e.g., flaming gasoline) will float and be carried on the surface. Any liquid with a specific gravity of greater than one (e.g., mercury, which has a specific gravity of 13.56), will sink.

Similar to specific gravity, any vapor with a **vapor density** (the concentration of a gas when compared to air) greater than hydrogen (though air is often used as the standard) will sink, whereas a gas with a vapor density less than hydrogen will be "lighter than air." It is estimated that 70% to 80% of hazardous materials, in gas form, are heavier than air. That means that these gasses will accumulate near the ground, where an unconscious patient might collapse, displacing air and making an oxygen-poor environment. Heavier-than-air gasses, those with a high vapor density, would also accumulate in low-lying areas, such as ditches and storm sewers. Understanding of this concept gives rise to the common instruction to "stay upwind and uphill" of any hazardous materials spill.

Hazardous Materials

Some chemical spills involve inert materials that pose little danger, or are no longer a danger, to Paramedics, first responders, or the environment. The problem then is simply one of containment and cleanup. However, the term "hazardous" pertains to those material spills that are potentially dangerous to life or the environment. The immediate danger to Paramedics and first responders when responding to incidents involving those materials often involves the material's flammability, corrosiveness, and/or reactivity.

The flammability of a chemical is typically dependent on a fuel/flammable chemical-air mixture and an available ignition source. **Flammability** is actually a range of conditions in which a flame can be initiated or sustained. The **flashpoint** is the minimum temperature whereby the chemical evaporates at a rate sufficient to form an ignitable fuel/air mixture. Although many chemicals are stable at ambient temperatures, the presence of fire can markedly increase the chance that the chemical will reach its flashpoint.

If there is too little vapor in the fuel-air mixture (the mixture is too lean), then ignition will not occur. This concentration is referred to as the **lower explosive limit (LEL)**. Alternatively, if the vapor/fuel-air mixture is too rich (the concentration of fuel to air is too high), called the **higher explosive limit (HEL)**, then the vapors cannot be ignited.

Any fuel-air mixture between these levels is potentially ignitable. If the chemical continues to emit sufficient volumes of flammable gasses, it will reach the **fire point**, the point at which fire will continue to burn after ignition.

A chemical's flashpoint is of particular concern to Paramedics and first responders. An ignition source such as a spark from a radio, or even the electromagnetic energy from a radio transmission, can be sufficient to ignite the vapors and sustain combustion.

Although fire is dangerous, it is often an obvious danger. The greater danger may be hidden and in the form of corrosivity. Any corrosive has the ability to permanently destroy any substance with which it comes into contact. A seemingly benign contact with a corrosive can cause irreversible damage to the skin (if exposed), the lung (if inhaled), or the gastrointestinal tract (if ingested).

These chemical burns are broadly categorized through the EPA's definitions as either **acid burns** (i.e., chemicals with a pH of less than 2) or **caustic burns** (i.e., chemicals with a pH of greater than 12.5). The pH range is 0 to 14, with 7 being neutral. The effects of acids and caustic bases are discussed in Chapter 9 on burn trauma.

Many chemicals can also become reactive upon exposure to other chemicals, depending on certain conditions. At one extreme, these reactions may be mild (e.g., the production of heat from an exothermic reaction). At the other extreme, these reactions can be violent, or even explosive.

Water-reactive materials may react, sometimes violently, on contact with water, whereas **air-reactive materials** will react and rapidly decompose on exposure to air. The placards for water-reactive chemicals may have the symbol W crossed out, indicating that the chemical is reactive to water. Therefore, water should not be used on the chemical, even in the presence of fire.

Some chemicals, called **pyrophorics**, have flammable vapors that will self-ignite when exposed to air (i.e., these chemicals do not need an ignition source). The by-products of these reactions (clouds of acidic gas) may be more dangerous than the self-limited burn that is created by exposure to either water or air.

Other chemicals, although they do not create heat, can support combustion. These chemicals, called **oxidizers**, release oxygen that in turn supports combustion, increasing the potential for a small fire to rapidly expand. The symbol OXY may be seen on the placard, warning the responders that the chemical is an oxidizer.

Finally, some chemicals undergo polymerization when inadvertently mixed with other chemicals. **Polymerization** can be a violent reaction as the two chemicals' molecules combine to become one larger molecule. If this reaction occurs in a closed container or a small space, the result can be explosive.

Toxicology

Although entire books have been written about the toxicology of hazardous materials, which the Paramedic should consult when preparing a plan of treatment, there are some basic toxicology principles that the Paramedic needs to understand that are common to all hazardous materials.

Any substance, including water, can be a poison. What makes a substance a poison is the dose—more specifically, the patient's response to that dose. This **dose/response** relationship is the basis of toxicology, the study of the effects of poisons on the body.

In general, the smaller the dose of chemical the patient is exposed to, the less likely that the patient will have a negative response to the exposure. However, this is not universally true. Some exposures, even in minute amounts, can cause cancer (known carcinogens). Therefore, every chemical exposure should be documented.

The dose is critical to determining potentially toxic exposures. An exposure which would be lethal to 50% of the patients exposed (as determined in animal studies) is called the **lethal dose 50%**, abbreviated as LD50. However, this concept has a limited application at the scene of a hazardous materials spill because most exposures on-scene are from inhalation.

The better measure may be the **lethal concentration 50%**, abbreviated LC50. This is the concentration of the chemical in the air that would be lethal to 50% of those exposed. These concepts provide a better understanding of the amount of exposure that is acceptable. However, zero exposure is optimal.

The federal government, toxicologists, and occupational medicine and industry experts have developed a system of threshold limits. **Threshold limits** balance a philosophy of zero tolerance to exposure with one of acceptable risk provided proper PPE is worn. This way of thinking shows an understanding that dangers exist and exposure can occur.

These levels are called the **permissible exposure limits (PEL)** and reflect those levels that are allowable during an average 40 hour work week. What may be of more utility on the scene of a hazardous materials spill may be the threshold limit values–short-term exposure limit. The **threshold limit values–short-term exposure limit (TLV-STEL)** is the maximum acceptable exposure a person can tolerate, without apparent ill effects, for 15 minutes of exposure. These levels may help the Paramedic predict the immediate or short-term risks to the patient while on-scene. The TLV–STEL is based on a 15-minute exposure.

The other, potentially more useful PEL is the **threshold limit value–concentration (TLV-C)**, the concentration of exposure that should not be exceeded in any exposure.

Another system for evaluation of hazardous materials exposure is called the **Immediately Dangerous to Life and Health (IDLH)** system. The IDLH system, developed by the EPA and National Institute for Occupational Health and Safety (NIOSH), defines concentration levels that cause unconsciousness, incapacitation (and an inability to self-rescue), or adverse health effects during a 30-minute exposure.

The IDLH system defines levels whereby a person can escape from an exposure, within 30 minutes, without immediate impairment or irreversible harm. This concept is helpful in determining triage priorities.

The Paramedic should understand that other references, such as the Emergency Response Planning Guidelines from the American Industrial Hygiene Association, or the Level of Concern developed by the EPA, may also be helpful during the risk analysis at a hazardous materials spill.

Special Problem of Illicit Drug Labs

Paramedics should also be able to identify less obvious hazardous materials exposures during emergency responses. An example would be the identification of an illicit drug lab within a residential dwelling. These locations contain large numbers of toxic and volatile chemicals that create an unsafe environment for the patient and the Paramedic.[3]

Paramedics should remain cautious when entering structures that contain large quantities of chemicals, including those with large gas storage tanks. Additionally, calls to scenes with multiple patients stating similar complaints should cause the Paramedic to consider the possibility of hazardous materials exposure. Furthermore, these clandestine labs are often booby trapped, presenting another danger to responders.

Initial Report

If the first-arriving responders determine that a scene possesses a potential hazmat threat, then the responders should obtain additional information about the scene. They should identify and note safe entry and exit routes. Again, entry and exit routes should always be established from the upwind side. The rescuers should also note the location of the release in relation to residential areas or other industrial sites. This information should be provided in the Paramedic's initial, or "first due," report to emergency communications. This information is then shared with all emergency responders, including fire and law enforcement.

Providers should also be prepared to contact one of several technical response centers for additional medical information. One of these is the **Chemical Transportation Emergency Center (CHEMTREC)**, a public service center used by firefighters, law enforcement, and other emergency responders to obtain information and assistance for emergency incidents involving chemicals and hazardous materials. Other centers include the Canadian Transport Emergency Centre (CANUTEC), Mexican Emergency Transportation System for the Chemical Industry (SETIQ), and poison control centers.[3]

Public Safety Critical Incident Management System

Once additional support arrives on-scene, Paramedics should be prepared to operate within the ICS. Chapter 20 provided additional detail related to the basic structure and operations of a multiagency response plan. ICS, also known as Public Safety Critical Incident Management (PSCIM), provides for command and control of operations on the scene of a hazardous materials incident.

It is important to remember that the Paramedic may be the first-responding unit to a hazmat incident. Any information relating to the scene, involved materials, and possible patients should be forwarded to the commander upon initiation of ICS operations.

Additionally, the Paramedic may find that she is the highest trained medical provider on-scene. As a result, the Paramedic may be assigned to a variety of tasks other than direct medical care or transportation, depending on the type of incident. However, these tasks are equally important and essential to the safety of both Paramedics and patients.

Isolation and Protection

Once a hazmat/CBRNE incident has been identified, emergency response personnel should be prepared to establish isolation or evacuation of potential patients. It is important to remember that the Paramedic's safety is a first priority. A Paramedic experiencing ill health effects from exposure will be unable to help additional patients and will require additional assistance to care for himself. The Paramedic in this state may even be a danger to other personnel.

After acquiring important information from the initial scene size-up, the Paramedic should be able to establish a basic perimeter around the incident. The Paramedic will need to identify a safe entry route from the upwind side of the scene. Once an entry point has been established, Paramedics should create an initial control zone called the initial isolation zone.[3]

The inner perimeter of this area is established by referring to the *ERG* for initial isolation distances (found in the green section). This guidebook provides the Paramedic with solid information on which to act with regard to specific chemical hazards and the establishment of a cold zone.

If the chemical is not known, then the Paramedic should refer to guide 111. Guide 111, the guide for unspecified cargo, is considered the universal guide when the chemical is unknown or a mix of chemicals may be present. For example, the guide may show a diagram of an initial isolation zone (cold zone) (Figure 26-4).[3]

Next, the Paramedic should consider establishing a protective action zone. A protective action zone includes the area where a person exposed to the chemical might be incapacitated or experience ill health effects. A protective action zone is both downhill and downwind of the spill. The majority of gaseous chemicals are heavier than air and thus are carried on the wind into low-lying places. This area is created by using the evacuation table found in the *ERG* and is subject to wind conditions, concentrations of gas in the air, and even the time of day.[3]

The distance for the protective action zone is found in the green-bordered section under "then protect." This fan-shaped area is subject to variations in terrain and atmospheric conditions as well as time of day (Figure 26-5).[3]

The Paramedic then either evacuates all persons within the protective action zone or he may choose, for various logistical reasons, to protect the public "in place." Protect in place (i.e., shelter in place) is a technique wherein buildings

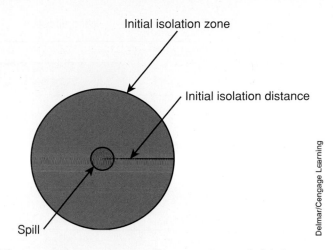

Figure 26-4 Paramedics create an initial isolation zone once an entry point has been established.

are shuttered and ventilation closed to prevent contamination of the occupants inside.

STREET SMART

Software is available that can plot toxic gas clouds or plumes and the distance that they can cover in a period of time so that isolation distances can be established and evacuation plans generated. Some of these programs interface with atmospheric data and topographic maps.

Response Preplanning

The federal SARA regulations require that there be a **Local Emergency Planning Committee (LEPC)**, which should have representatives from emergency services (fire, police, and EMS), as well as local industry. The LEPC may also maintain copies of the MSDS sheets for known hazardous materials within the area, which are made available during an emergency. These MSDS sheets can also be used to preplan the medical care necessary upon exposure. The LEPC then becomes part of a larger **State Emergency Response Commission (SERC)**. The SERC serves as the interface between federal response agencies, such as the Environmental Protection Agency, and the LEPC as well as providing technical support to the LEPC.

Federal regulations also call for a "**Process Safety Management**" plan (29 CFR 1910.119). These regulations require a site action plan for fixed facilities in the event of an accidental spill, including emergency shutdown procedures and failure mode analysis. A review of these plans can provide the Paramedic with valuable insight into the nature

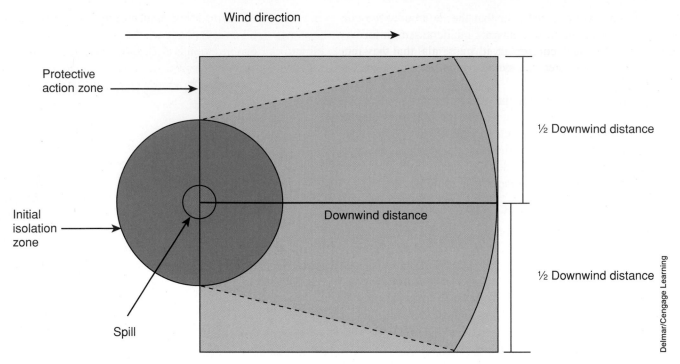

Wind direction

Protective action zone

½ Downwind distance

Initial isolation zone

Downwind distance

½ Downwind distance

Spill

Delmar/Cengage Learning

Figure 26-5 A protective action zone includes the area where a person exposed to the chemical might be incapacitated or experience ill health effects.

and likelihood of a hazardous materials incident, which is invaluable information when creating a preplan.

Hazmat Control Zone

Hazmat personnel have specific training in the organizing and implementation of three separate control zones that are contained within the initial isolation zone and arranged in a concentric circle around the site of the spill. These zones are described as the hot zone, the warm zone, and the cold zone.

The **hot zone** is identified as the area involving the material release. This zone possesses the greatest chance of additional exposure to those within its circumference. Special protective equipment, described shortly, must be used to enter this area.[3]

The **warm zone** is the area immediately outside of the hot zone. This area contains staging and support for the hazmat team within the hot zone. Additionally, this area will house the decontamination units, which will decontaminate hazmat team members, their equipment, and any patients they evacuate from the hot zone. Again, special protective equipment must be worn within the warm zone.[3]

Finally, the outer perimeter is referred to as the **cold zone**. The cold zone contains the command center/post, additional hazmat support personnel (such as physicians), and the boundary of the decontamination corridor. No contaminated personnel or equipment should enter the cold zone. Special protective equipment/apparel is not worn in this area, so people can become contaminated if they are in

contact with responders from within the hot zone or the warm zone. Additionally, medical support and emergency incident rehabilitation for the hazmat team will be located within this zone.[3]

Paramedics should not enter the warm or hot zones without specific hazmat training and equipment. In addition, no civilians should be allowed within the cold zone. This is a protective area for staging of additional resources including evacuation and transportation.

Once the three control zones have been established, personnel should only be allowed to enter or exit via specific points of entry. This is referred to as the access corridor. The decontamination corridor starts at the border with the hot zone and ends at the external border of the warm zone, with an exit to the upwind side of the incident. Absolute control must be maintained at these points of access and egress to prevent the unwanted spread of hazardous material.

Hazmat Team Personal Protective Equipment

Paramedics responding to hazmat incidents need to be aware of the variety of PPE used by hazardous materials team members. It should be noted that there is no single ensemble that can fully protect hazmat Technicians and responders from all possible exposures. For this reason, OSHA and the EPA have developed standard levels of PPE.

There are four levels of PPE, from A to D. Each has a unique set of respiratory and skin protective qualities for which it is rated. The specific threat of a given substance being released will dictate the appropriate level of protection worn by hazmat personnel. Though most Paramedics will not be trained to use such equipment, it is essential that they recognize the level of protective equipment being utilized during a response.[3]

Paramedics and other emergency medical personnel often perform on-scene medical rehabilitation for the hazmat Technicians. Chapter 25 features more information on emergency incident rehabilitation. A Technician wearing Level A PPE will likely suffer from greater levels of exhaustion and heat exposure than one wearing Level C PPE. It has been suggested that wearing Level A PPE raises the responder's endogenous heat load by as much as 500%. This increase can rapidly lead to heat exhaustion and dehydration.

Understanding the difference in levels of PPE will provide the Paramedic with valuable information related to the type of substance the patients may have come in contact with. An example is a patient removed from a scene that requires Level A PPE. These patients will have a high likelihood of respiratory exposure regardless of undergoing complete decontamination of the exterior body surface.

Medical Surveillance

By their nature, hazardous materials incidents have serious and potentially life-threatening consequences for Paramedics and first responders. Any single chemical or combination of chemicals can be a respiratory irritant, nephro- or hepatotoxic, a carcinogen, or a poison to any organ system. The results of an exposure can be immediate and/or delayed.

For these reasons, a program of medical surveillance is part of every hazardous materials response plan. A **medical surveillance** plan typically has three elements: baseline, exposure specific, and on-scene rehabilitation.[4]

A baseline examination not only ensures that the responder is physically fit to enter into the high stress and physically demanding environment of a hazardous materials incident, but also provides the responder some protection in the event of future claims of incident-specific injury. Beyond the obvious musculoskeletal injuries that are inherent with special operations, a baseline examination can help to establish the absence of specific conditions such as asthma or cancer. If these conditions develop later, the baseline examination can be used to trace the possible connection between the incident and the injury. For this reason only, baseline examinations should be done initially, annually, and upon entry into the scene, if possible.[4]

Toxin-specific treatment of responders is part of the overall medical plan established on-scene once the Paramedic knows the offending substance(s). Research of the toxicology of chemicals and the medical care necessary to care for the exposed patients was described earlier. The treatment plan should be instituted when patients suffer exposures above the permissible exposure limit (PEL).[4]

Finally, an integral part of the exposure plan is the on-scene rehabilitation. As mentioned earlier, the high stress and physically demanding nature of a hazardous materials response will leave responders exhausted and in need of rehabilitation. Rehabilitation is critical for this subset of specially trained responders because of their knowledge of hazmat operations.[4] Further information on rehabilitation is available in Chapter 25.

Decontamination

Decontamination is the process of removing excess hazardous material from emergency providers and patients. This is performed as all exposed individuals leave the warm zone through the access corridor. Only with thorough decontamination can emergency providers limit the amount of **secondary exposure**; that is, indirect exposure to the hazardous material as a result of contact with a contaminated patient.[3]

If large numbers of patients are exposed to a substance, the Paramedic will need to arrange mass decontamination. These systems range from large-scale portable shower systems to irrigation by multiple fire suppression nozzles. If the release is more confined, with only a few exposed individuals, irrigation with a simple hose line and brush may be adequate. When possible, all contaminated clothing should be removed prior to entering the cold zone.[3]

Improperly decontaminated patients can lead to extensive secondary exposures during their subsequent medical care. If transporting a patient believed to be contaminated by a hazardous material, the Paramedic should notify the receiving hospital immediately. The crew and patient will need to enter the hospital though the designated decontamination area. Once inside, the patient and EMS providers need to be decontaminated by hospital staff wearing appropriate PPE.

The patient should enter into the treatment area only when decontaminated. Removal of the patient's outer clothing, down to undergarments, can remove up to 75% of all contaminants. Unfortunately, despite the decontamination crew's best efforts, some residual contaminant is bound to remain on the patient. For this reason, many Paramedics prefer to wear Level C protective clothing and respirators.

Most Paramedics do not wear self-contained breathing apparatus (SCBA) or supplied air respirators, as these are bulky and unwieldy when caring for a patient. An acceptable alternative which Paramedics may use is an air-purifying respirator. These masks come in both full-face and half-face systems.

Some hospital personnel performing decontamination may be using a powered air-purifying respirator (PAPR). Although not an SCBA, these PAPR are effective.

Some of these air-purifying respirators are high-efficiency particulate air (HEPA) filters, whereas others use NIOSH-approved canisters. These masks should not be used for more than eight hours.

For the air-purifying respirators to be effective, the atmospheric air must be at least 19.5%. The airborne concentration of the chemical must be known and must not exceed the **maximum use concentration (MUC)** (the largest concentration of a chemical in the atmosphere that a rescuer is protected from when wearing the appropriate respirator). As a function of the PEL and the respirator's protection factor (PF), the mask must fit properly.

Paramedics should first be **fit-tested**, using either quantitative or qualitative methods, to ensure a proper face seal. The Paramedic's facial hair must not interfere with the mask's seal. Fit-testing should be done again if the Paramedic has lost more than 20 pounds or has had dental/facial surgery that alters the facial features.

The EPA has established levels of chemical protective clothing (CPC). The first two levels, Level A and Level B, are high-level protection and are generally worn in either the hot or warm zone. Level C CPC is for possible airborne contamination as well as accidental skin contamination.

Level C PPE generally includes a full-face air-purifying unit, often with canisters, chemical-resistant clothing (such as Tyvek® coveralls with a hood), and chemical-resistant gloves (such as Neoprene® overgloves). The NFPA 1993 standard speaks to the PPE worn by support personnel, such as Paramedics, outside the hot zone, including its chemical resistance and heat transfer characteristics.

Level D PPE is essentially a work uniform. Level D PPE is generally not acceptable until the patient is completely decontaminated.

During the decontamination period, medical care may be limited due to the use of PPE. As a result, this should be completed thoroughly but in a time-efficient manner. Following the patient's release to the hospital staff, all patient care equipment will require either decontamination or disposal. The ambulance must also be decontaminated.

STREET SMART

Some hazmat teams carry escape-only respirators. These limited air supply hoods are designed to minimize the patient's exposure to the chemical during the rescue. These special respirators are not intended for extended operations or for first responder entry into a hazmat scene.

Treatment

After the offending chemical is identified, and after the patient is decontaminated, the Paramedic must then develop a treatment plan. Although the *Emergency Response Guide* (*ERG*) is helpful in starting first aid, the treatment listed is limited. Fortunately, other resources exist for the Paramedic.

The first place to start is the MSDS sheet, which is provided on-site or as part of the preplan developed by the LEPC. The MSDS provides detailed information specific to the offending chemical.

If the MSDS is not available, or the Paramedic chooses, he may refer to the shipping papers. Department of Transportation (DOT) regulations require that all shippers of hazardous materials—by land, sea, or air—must list a 24/7 emergency contact telephone number where information, including health information, can be obtained.

The sources of information that can be used to develop the treatment plan are numerous and include written sources, telephonic advice, and computer databases. Examples of written sources include clinical toxicology textbooks and emergency response manuals. Examples of telephonic advice include CHEMTRAC (Chemical Manufacturers Association, phone number 800-424-9300), regional poison control centers, and even the Centers for Disease Control (for infectious disease exposures) (404-633-5313).

The richest source of information about the treatment of chemical exposures may be computer references available either on-line or on a CD-ROM. Some of these databases contain as many as 80,000 MSDS and many interact with other databases.

Air Monitoring

In some instances, the Paramedic may be responsible for monitoring air quality in the treatment area, the rehabilitation area, or in the general vicinity of the cold zone. The air monitoring is to ensure that responders can work safely and that chemical exposures are below the permissible exposure limits.

Paramedics are already somewhat familiar with patient-specific gas monitors (i.e., pulse oximetry and capnography). Air monitors sample the ambient air in the environment. The most commonly used air monitor may be the combustible gas indicator, which is generally used to test for the explosive limits.

The Paramedic is more likely to use gas meters, such as oxygen meters that read the percentage of oxygen in the air. The minimum acceptable oxygen level according to OSHA is 19.5%; oxygen levels below 19.5% require an SCBA or other type of compressed gas respirator.

Other commonly used sensors include gas-specific meters (CO, for example) and colorimetric indicator tubes. Colorimetric indicator tubes and field test kits are used to test gas or liquid for the presence of specific chemicals. These devices are growing in popularity because of the ease of operation and because military devices, such as the chemical agent monitor used to test for nerve agents, are being used for civilian purposes.

A special detector unit is the radiation meter, made famous by the Geiger–Mueller device. These radiation detection units can detect gross contamination but do not detect exposure. The OSHA minimum acceptable radiation level is 0.2 millirads (mR) per hour; levels above 0.2 mR require Paramedics to take special protective measures, such as distance and shielding.

CASE STUDY CONCLUSION

After briefing the district fire chief of all information relating to the scene, the Paramedic moves the ambulance safely upwind and within the cold zone. Additional units arrive on-scene and the CBRNE team dons Level C PPE. After several minutes, the entry team is witnessed pulling a patient from the vehicle. Prior to arrival into the medical triage area within the cold zone, the patient and team are preparing to undergo decontamination by support personnel.

As the patient is advanced through the decontamination sector, all contaminated clothing is removed. Additionally, the patient is irrigated with water and an unknown solvent. The Paramedic examines the patient to see that adequate decontamination has been completed. The Paramedic works to quickly evaluate the patient and identify any toxidrome displayed by the patient.

CRITICAL THINKING QUESTIONS

1. Why is it important for the patient to be decontaminated?
2. What are the advantages of transporting a patient with suspected hazardous materials exposure who has been decontaminated to a hospital capable of decontamination even if that means bypassing other hospitals in the process?

CONCLUSION

Hazardous materials and CBRNE incidents provide a number of challenges to the Paramedic. By following basic ICS protocols, one can quickly identify the appropriate role in the initial response. Most Paramedics will play supportive roles during these types of responses. However, all Paramedics need to be prepared to identify potentially hazardous situations and appropriately isolate these scenes. Additionally, Paramedics should know how to identify specific information related to a chemical release and efficiently relay this to the appropriate personnel.

KEY POINTS:

- Hazardous materials are included under the larger umbrella of weapons of mass destruction (WMD). The acronym CBRNE is used to describe classifications of hazardous materials.

- The type and shape of a vehicle or container can help identify the load.

- Use of the *Emergency Response Guide* is an essential tool for the Paramedic who is first on-scene.

- The Public Safety Critical Incident Management system is used for command and control of operations on the scene of a hazardous materials incident.

- Isolation and protection are the first priorities for Paramedics.

- Paramedics have roles in incident rehabilitation of responders as well as medical monitoring and emergency care of patients following decontamination.

REVIEW QUESTIONS:

1. What does the acronym CBRNE stand for?
2. What are the four levels of hazardous materials responders as defined in the HAZWOPER standards?
3. What are the three NFPA standards pertaining to hazardous materials incidents?
4. What do the four diamonds of the NFPA 704 placard mean?
5. What is the difference between lethal dose 50% and lethal concentration 50%?

CASE STUDY QUESTIONS:

Please refer to the Case Study in this chapter, and answer the questions below:
1. What implications does the shape of the container have to the hazardous materials?
2. What are the three clues to the container's contents?
3. What are the four sections of the *Emergency Response Guide*?

▶ REFERENCES:

1   Walter FG, et al. Personal protective equipment and decontamination. In: *Advanced HAZMAT Life Support, Providers Manual* (3rd ed.). Phoenix, AZ: University of Arizona; 2003: Chapter 4, p 69.

2. Data and Statistic, U.S. Department of Transportation, Pipeline and Hazardous Materials Safety Administration. Available at: **http://www.phmsa.dot.gov/hazmat/library/data-stats.** Accessed January 22, 2009.

3. NFPA 472. *Standard for Competence of Responders to Hazardous Materials/Weapons of Mass Destruction Incidents*, 2008 edition. Quincy, MA: NFPA; 2008.

4. NFPA 473. *Standard of Competencies of EMS Providers Responding to Hazardous Materials/Weapons of Mass Destruction Incidents*, 2008 edition. Quincy, MA: NFPA; 2008.

CHAPTER 27

URBAN SEARCH AND RESCUE

KEY CONCEPTS:

Upon completion of this chapter, it is expected that the reader will understand these following concepts:

- Definitions of Urban Search and Rescue
- Teams and deployment protocols
- Search and rescue principles
- Signs, symptoms, and emergency care of crush injuries

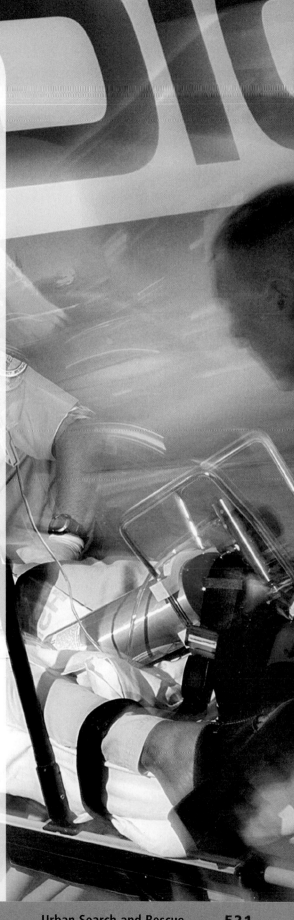

CASE STUDY:

While browsing the web, Stefan finds the local USAR team's website. He wants to see if there are any openings on the team. Recent events in Mexico City, then Haiti, have made him realize that he can contribute to the rescue efforts using his special training as a Paramedic. In addition, he is a veteran and understands the "federal" system, plus he is bilingual, which can be helpful in certain situations. He knows that selection for USAR is very competitive, but he nonetheless fills out the application.

CRITICAL THINKING QUESTIONS

1. What is the configuration of an Urban Search and Rescue team?
2. How does Stefan's special skills and experience help his application to the USAR team?

OVERVIEW

Urban Search and Rescue (USAR) is the science of locating, reaching, medically treating, and safely extricating deeply entombed survivors of collapsed structures[1] and confined spaces. The medical component of the team is involved from mission creation and protocol development through patient treatment and the decision to terminate rescue efforts. The USAR system evolved from the need for specialized rescue efforts for patients involved in structural collapses. War, terrorism, and earthquakes are the most commonly encountered types of disasters that can result in the collapse of heavy construction structures such as buildings and bridges. Of these, earthquake damage has accounted for the most need for USAR since World War II, although terrorism events have increased in recent years.

Definitions

As with other fields, a standard nomenclature is used to ensure all responders are speaking the same language. The following list contains some of the key terms, with illustrations, that the Paramedic must understand.

Confined space. This is an enclosed area with limited access and/or egress that is not designed for human occupancy and has the potential for physical, chemical, or atmospheric injury.[2] Examples include a void space inside a collapsed structure, the interior of a silo, or a tanker car (Figure 27-1).

Heavy construction. These structures are designed to withstand shear forces typical of earthquakes and heavy winds. For the purposes of this chapter, the term encompasses a variety of structure specifications which all have several of the following criteria in common: structures built with concrete and/or steel-reinforcing bars (rebar), "box type" structures, reinforced or unreinforced masonry, and fire-resistant exterior walls. Upon collapse, these types of structures require specialized search and rescue capabilities. Typical structures include office buildings, parking garages, schools, hotels, hospitals, freeway bridges, and apartment buildings (Figure 27-2).

Light construction. These structures are built to withstand vertical load forces. They generally include wood and brick construction (Figures 27-3 and 27-4). Upon collapse, the debris may be shifted by hand for search and rescue. Typical structures include single family residences.

History of Heavy Rescue

In the United States, heavy rescue has traditionally been part of the realm of local fire and EMS services. However, the tools and skills available in these organizations are increasingly inadequate for the task of search and rescue in collapses of heavy construction structures, which are becoming more prevalent in large urban settings worldwide. Rescue and government personnel discovered this in the early 1980s

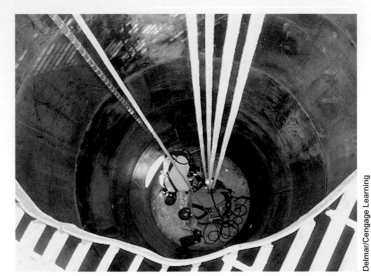

Figure 27-1 Example of a confined space, an enclosed area with limited access and/or egress.

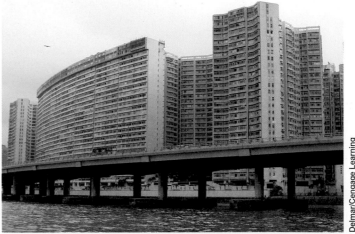

Figure 27-2 Example of a building classified as a heavy construction structure.

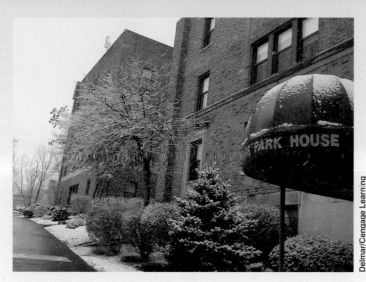

Figure 27-3 Example of a building classified as a brick light construction structure.

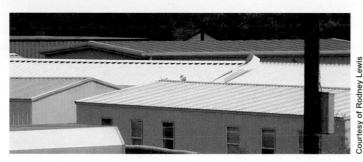

Figure 27-4 Example of a building classified as a light construction structure.

when several international disasters underscored the need for specialized search and rescue teams in the United States. In 1985, an 8.1 magnitude earthquake in Mexico caused serious or total collapse of over 3,500 buildings in Mexico City, killing over 9,500 and injuring over 30,000 people.[3] In 1986, a massive earthquake in Armenia left over 25,000 people dead. American rescuers involved in both these disasters found the responses very difficult and poorly organized.

Therefore, in order to send aid to the Philippines after a catastrophic earthquake in 1990, the U.S. Office of Foreign Disaster Assistance (OFDA) formed the first semblance of a modern USAR team. The team was comprised of a variety of specialists including rescue specialists from Fairfax County, Virginia, and Metro-Dade County, Florida; medical specialists from the Special Medical Response Team in Pennsylvania, search canines, and structural engineers.[4]

As described in Chapter 20, the Federal Response Plan (or National Response Framework [NRF], as it is now known) created the 15 Emergency Support Functions (ESFs) to organize the federal response to national disasters. USAR falls under ESF 9, Urban Search and Rescue. As the FEMA website states, "[The NRF] is built upon scalable, flexible, and adaptable coordinating structures to align key roles and responsibilities across the nation, linking all levels of government, nongovernmental organizations, and the private sector."[5]

USAR teams respond in an all-hazards manner. This means that they are equipped to respond to a variety of types of threats, from natural disasters to man-made incidents. As a result, the teams have responded to a wide range of incidents, including the Northridge earthquake in northern California in 1989, the tornadoes in Oklahoma in 1990, the collapse of the World Trade Center in 2001, and the floods after Hurricane Katrina in 2005.

Teams and Deployment

Upon their inception, there were 25 USAR teams strategically distributed throughout the continental United States. Currently there are 28 teams comprised of 70 personnel and four search canines each, as well as an extensive cache of specialized equipment.

All positions are rostered **three deep**, meaning there are three people to each station or post to guarantee availability and facilitate rapid deployment. The teams are referred to as task forces (TF) because they are a single unit composed of multiple subspecialties. Unlike other task forces, each USAR task force is designed to operate as a single well-coordinated unit.

The teams are distributed geographically over the 10 FEMA response regions (Figure 27-5). Their distribution is calculated to allow for the most rapid deployment of teams to areas most likely to require USAR interventions. Of the 28 teams, California has six, or 22% of the national capability. This is because the frequency and likelihood of earthquakes are relatively high along the San Andreas and nearby fault lines. There is a similar clustering of teams in the northeast due to the high concentration of urban populations in this part of the country. The teams deploy only within the United States and its territories, except for Virginia Task Force One (VATF-1) out of Fairfax, Virginia, which deploys internationally as well.

All teams are supported dually by federal funding and local sponsoring agencies. The majority of local sponsoring agencies are fire services, but many are state government agencies. Sponsoring agencies provide funding for equipment maintenance and training. The teams exist as local/state resources until activated on the national level. When a team is deployed to a national incident, all personnel become federalized and all expenses are funded through the federal government. This requires activation through channels delineated in the Stafford Act, described in Chapter 20.[6] This involves the local incident commander requesting federal assistance through the local authority having jurisdiction (AHJ) and up to the state emergency management agency (EMA), the governor, and then to FEMA. Activation through other channels would require the considerable expenses to be paid by the local authority having jurisdiction.

Teams are deployed first by proximity and second by call roster (i.e., personnel to post). This means that teams closest

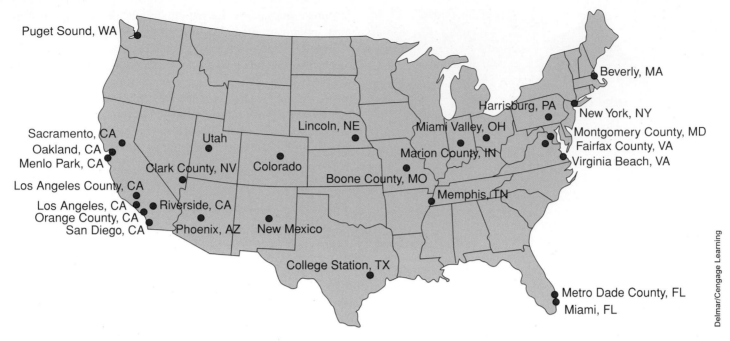

Figure 27-5 FEMA USAR task force base locations are found across the United States.

Delmar/Cengage Learning

to an incident are typically deployed first to that incident. For an incident in Washington DC, teams in Virginia (VATF-1) and Pennsylvania (PATF-1) would be first due. If further assistance is required, teams are then deployed according to a nine-month rotating call roster. Nine teams are allocated to the western, central, and eastern divisions of the country each, and then rotate monthly through a call schedule. This means that each team is typically first-due twice a year.

When called for deployment, there are three stages: advisory, alert, and activation. An **advisory** is issued to notify the system that there is an emerging or potential incident. This typically is a written communiqué detailing the current time, the duration of the alert, some information about the incident or event, and the status of all teams. This is sent to each team's administrative headquarters, which then alerts the team members as needed. An **alert** is issued when activation is expected. This allows team members time to take care of any necessary duties at home and prepare to be activated. However, there is not always an alert phase, such as happened with the events of September 11, 2001. **Activation** means that a team is being sent to the scene of a disaster for a search and rescue mission. Upon receipt of an activation order, a team has two hours to report to team headquarters and four more hours, for a total of six hours, to be en route with personnel and equipment. Because of this short activation time, a team can be at the scene and ready to start 24-hour operations in as little as 6 to 12 hours.

Teams must be able to deploy quickly and then be self-sufficient for up to 72 hours, although it may be even longer than that before support is available, depending on the site and situation. Being self-sufficient involves having sufficient food and water for both drinking and washing, and being able to run operations 24 hours a day. All of this occurs in some form of austere or potentially dangerous environment; for example, New Orleans after Hurricane Katrina in 2005, or the deployment to the Haiti earthquake in 2010.

There are two types of responses: Type I and Type III responses. A **Type I response** deploys the full 70-person team, four canines, and a full equipment cache. This type of team is typically deployed for structural collapse scenarios, such as the Murrah federal building bombing in Oklahoma City in 1995.

A **Type III response** deploys a team of 28 personnel, two canines, and a limited equipment cache. These teams are typically deployed to natural disasters not involving structural collapse, such as the floods after Hurricane Katrina in 2005 when all 28 teams were deployed to the Gulf Coast.

When deployed to the field, the USAR teams are aided and coordinated by **incident support teams (ISTs)**. These are 21-person teams of highly qualified specialists. As stated on the FEMA website, "The mission of the USAR incident support team is to provide Federal, State, and local officials with technical assistance in the acquisition and utilization of ESF #9 resources through advice, incident command assistance, management and coordination of USAR task forces, and obtaining ESF #9 logistic support."[7] There are three incident support teams nationally, and each is on call for emergency response every third month. The goal of the incident support team is to facilitate the field response. It is never to usurp authority from the local jurisdiction, but instead to support and enhance their efforts.

The USAR teams and the incident support team operate under the incident command.[8] It has since been adapted and mandated as the incident management system to be used in all domestic U.S. disaster response activities (see Chapter 20 for more details about the National Incident Management System).[9]

Personnel and Training

USAR team positions are filled by application. Available positions are posted on the FEMA, USAR, or individual team websites. Team members are local to the region served by the team and may come from any private or public sector, though the majority come from the fire and EMS services. There are six main subgroups of personnel: search, rescue, medical, technical, logistics, and command. Logistics and command function much the same as they do in any command structure and will not be discussed separately here.

Safety is an important topic when considering the missions of these subgroups. USAR teams, by their nature, are often working in inherently unsafe situations. ICS and USAR both have a specific safety officer position, but the same principle applies in USAR as in day-to-day field activities: safety is everyone's job. This is particularly important with a team that may be spread out over a geographically large scene with multiple areas of active operations and multiple hazards at any given moment. Hazards encountered can range from hazmat or oxygen-depleted environments to secondary structure collapse to infectious disease exposure.

All USAR team members undergo extensive initial and continuing education in order to function at the cutting edge of their fields. Although certain elements of team training must be gained through federal channels, much of it is available through federally sanctioned or federal-equivalent private courses. For instance, the Hazardous Waste Operations and Emergency Response (HAZWOPER) training standard is set by OSHA but is taught by any number of nonprofit and for-profit private entities. There are also private companies, for example Texas Engineering Extension Service (TEEX), that offer a variety of courses and exercises designed to enhance USAR personnel field capabilities.[10]

Search

Although not required, the majority of search and rescue personnel, with the exception of canines and their handlers, come from the fire services. The mission of the search specialists is to locate patients in confined spaces in order to facilitate medical treatment and extrication. Within the search specialty there are two subspecialties: technical search and canine search. **Technical search operators** use specialized computer equipment, microphones, listening devices, fiberoptic cameras, and vibration detectors to search for and locate entrapped patients (Figure 27-6). These pieces of equipment allow the technical search personnel to observe where they cannot see with direct line of sight, such as around inaccessible corners or through layers of concrete.

Canine search teams use highly trained dogs to locate entrapped survivors. These canines and their handlers undergo years of rigorous training before they are nationally certified as FEMA search canine/handler teams. The canines used in USAR are usually smaller animals, like beagles, so they can get into the tight areas commonly encountered in confined

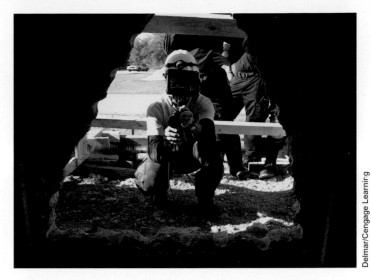

Figure 27-6 This technical search specialist is using a fiberoptic search camera to explore through a breach made in the concrete wall of a confined space by a rescue specialist during a training exercise.

space rescue. This is different than wilderness search and rescue where the canines are often larger animals. The canines are able to quite accurately differentiate between living and dead persons, which saves time and effort, and improves safety. As noted in the US&R Response System Rescue Specialist Training Manual, "No single tactic is sufficiently effective on its own to ensure that a complete search has been conducted. The most effective search strategy should blend all viable tactical capabilities into a logical plan of operation. The combined use of physical, canine, and electronic search tactics will enable the task force to better establish priorities and focus emphasis on the most important rescue activities."[11]

Rescue

The goal of the **rescue specialist** is to create a safe ingress to and egress from the entrapped patient. This involves the ability to rapidly and safely breach heavily reinforced structures. Rescue specialists use powerful breaching tools such as diamond chain saws, core drills, exothermic torches, and breakers. A core drill, for example, drills a hole through reinforced concrete to allow insertion of a hinged fiberoptic camera and microphone that allows the search or medical component to visually evaluate a possible survivor, or to communicate with the patient. A diamond chain saw can rapidly cut through steel-reinforced concrete to allow rescue or medical personnel to physically gain access to or extricate a patient.

Technical Specialties

The **technical team** is comprised of the following specialists: hazardous materials, structural, and heavy equipment and rigging. Hazardous materials specialists are trained in weapons of mass destruction response as well as traditional

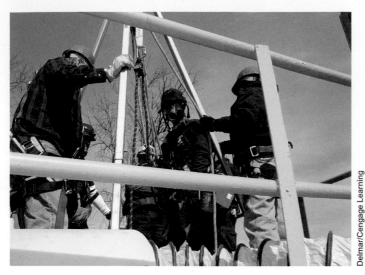

Figure 27-7 An example of rope rigging with personnel preparing to enter a simulated hazardous environment during training.

hazardous materials response. Their primary goal is evaluating the safety of the confined space environment in order to ensure the safety of the rescuers and the patient (Figure 27-7).

Structural specialists are structural engineers who evaluate both intact and damaged structures for active and potential collapse threats. They further triage the locations for probability of having survivors within a collapsed structure, and evaluate safe access routes within a collapsed structure.

Structural engineers are involved with the ongoing rescue efforts, particularly with ensuring safe movement of debris.[12] Heavy equipment and rigging specialists work with rescue personnel to move and stabilize debris. The tools of their trade include airbags for lifting, and ropes and rigging equipment to lower rescuers and raise patients safely as needed.

Medical

The **medical team** is composed of physicians and Paramedics. Physicians are ideally emergency medicine-trained physicians or trauma surgeons. This is because those specialties offer the most relevant training for situations and medical conditions encountered in the field during structural collapse search and rescue.

Physicians serve as **medical team managers**, coordinating the entire medical response including physicians assistants, nurses, and Paramedics as **medical specialists**; traditionally Paramedics work in the field but under disaster conditions may supplement hospital personnel. There are only eight Paramedics on each team, so the selection criteria are rigorous, allowing the best people to rise to the top. Many medical specialists on the teams have worked in critical care transport or aeromedical transport, although this is not necessary.

In addition to the requirements common to all personnel, such as ICS training and physical fitness requirements,

medical team members must fulfill certain basic medical prerequisites such as holding an active medical license or Paramedic certificate, and having BLS, ACLS, CPR, and PALS certificates (for all medical personnel), as well as Advanced Trauma Life Support (ATLS) certificates (for physicians).

Over and above that, the medical component undergoes a week-long classroom and field exercise-based training program, which focuses on evaluation, stabilization, and treatment of medical conditions that are more frequently or uniquely encountered in confined space and structural collapse situations. They also undergo confined space safety, hazardous materials, psychological, and swift water rescue training. This is in addition to training that all USAR personnel receive, including GPS, safety, and leadership training.

The medical component is trained not only in care of human patients, but also in rudimentary emergency canine veterinary care in order to care for the team canines in austere environments where professional veterinary services may not be readily available. The mission of the medical component is first to care for task force members, then for civilian patients, then for task force canines.

Medical Decision Making

One of the most difficult decisions an incident commander will ever have to make in a mass-casualty situation is the decision to transition from a rescue mission to a recovery mission.

Rescue signifies efforts to save living or presumed living patients. It is the driving force behind every member's participation in USAR and, as such, is a powerful motivator, driving people to work 24 hours a day in all kinds of weather and safety conditions. **Recovery**, on the other hand, is the search for deceased patients. This is usually a less pressured situation in which considerations like evidence preservation, resource conservation, the need for rest, and even finances take a more prominent role.

The decision to transition from rescue to recovery is difficult. Making it too early potentially leaves patients alive and trapped, and can be more demoralizing than making the decision too late. Making the decision too late, however, can unnecessarily endanger the safety and well-being of the rescuers. The medical component contributes a knowledge and understanding of the natural history of trauma and illness as well as the potential for survival at a given time to the decision-making process.

As an example, consider a patient pinned with a crushing force to both arms. Initially, there may be time to attempt to release the patient and possibly save his life and limbs. However, the longer he is entrapped, the further the injury progresses, and the sicker he will become. A trained medical provider is able to predict from the known injury and patient's clinical condition what time frame the rescue team is looking at as far as rescue versus amputation. In this case, the patient became altered and hypotensive, necessitating bilateral amputations to save his life but not his limbs.[13] This decision was made by the incident commander but with the critical input of the medical section chief and the understanding of all section chiefs involved in the rescue.

One study showed that there is a time when there is essentially no chance of finding a viable patient after an earthquake.[14] Knowing this can aid the incident commander in making the decision to transition to recovery.

Crush Syndrome

Certain medical conditions are seen more commonly in structural collapse situations than in everyday medical practice. These include contaminated wounds, dust impaction in the airway, and, most importantly, crush syndrome. Crush syndrome is a form of rhabdomyolysis and is seen exclusively in traumatic situations. According to Dario Gonzalez, "The earliest modern reports (1910) of rhabdomyolysis appear in German literature and, at that time, the classic triad of a syndrome (Myer Betz) of 'muscle pain, weakness, and brown urine.' The World War I medical literature described situations in which similar signs and symptoms were seen in German soldiers who were buried and rescued from trenches."[15]

A physician in London coined the term "crush injury" in World War II. **Crush injury** involves prolonged crushing force applied to a large muscle mass, causing tissue damage and release of intracellular toxins that then cause cardiovascular instability, kidney failure, and eventually death if left untreated. The following paragraphs examine each component of crush injury individually.

The first necessary criterion is the application of a prolonged crushing force. Prolonged means at least one to six hours, although on rare occasions crush syndrome has been seen after only 20 minutes of injury. Crushing force means pressure sufficient to cause muscle damage. The higher the pressure, the greater the damage.

The second criterion is that this force be applied to a large muscle mass. A sufficiently large volume of muscle tissue must be crushed in order to release enough toxin to cause cardiac and renal impairment. One could leave 1,000 kilos of pressure on a relatively small area like a person's hand for 10 hours without developing crush syndrome (however, the hand would be destroyed). Crush syndrome usually develops from injury to the muscle masses of the thighs and lower legs. Compartment syndrome, discussed in Chapter 8, can also develop from injury to these areas.

The third criterion is the release of intracellular toxins. The crushing force itself damages muscle cell membranes, releasing toxins such as potassium, acid, and myoglobin. Calcium precipitates locally, causing hypocalcemia. While the crushing force is being applied, damage is being done. However, toxins are being released primarily to the local vasculature, with a slow leak to the systemic circulation. This means that while the force, such as a slab of reinforced concrete, is being applied, there is usually little damage to the heart or kidneys. However, once the pressure is released, such as by rescuers removing the slab of concrete, the toxins that, until that time, have been locally sequestered now flood the systemic circulation and reach the heart and kidneys within seconds to minutes.

This is when the real damage is done to the patient. When the myocardial membranes are exposed to the elevated potassium levels, the patient can develop hypotension, dangerous cardiac dysrhythmias, or cardiac arrest almost immediately. When the myoglobin and acid hit the kidneys, they form a gel consistency that plugs the renal filtration system and shuts down the kidneys. Fatal damage can take days to have their effect in this manner. The crushing force also damages local vasculature, causing third spacing of fluid. Enough fluid can be extravasated to cause significant hypotension.

An untreated patient, when released from a prolonged crush injury, can go from awake, alert, and talking to dead within the time it takes to complete one volume of circulation, or less than a minute. Thus, the importance of recognizing the potential for, or the active presence of, crush syndrome is to counteract the potentially fatal pathophysiology by rapid medical intervention. Treatment consists of forced diuresis, alkalinization of the urine, and buffering and removal of potassium from the system.

Forced diuresis is achieved by infusion of massive volumes of intravenous fluids without potassium, such as normal saline. The goal is urine output of 100 to 200 mL/hr. This flushes the myoglobin gel from the kidneys, preventing renal damage. Alkalinization of the urine and the blood is achieved by infusion of sodium bicarbonate. A recommended dose is 3 amps of sodium bicarbonate in 1 liter of D_5W infused at 200 mL/hr after an initial push of 1 to 2 amps of sodium bicarbonate IV, although local protocols vary. Calcium chloride IV can be used as a temporizing measure to stabilize the cardiac membranes against the cardiotoxic effects of hyperkalemia. All these therapies can be instituted in the field. Indeed, if they are not, the patient may not survive to reach the hospital. Treatment must be started prior to release of the crushing force or, if that is not possible, as soon as possible after release in order to save the patient's life. It is the medical sector's responsibility to ensure that, in the rush to free the patient from the collapse, he or she does not then die.

Anatomy of a Rescue

Time zero of a rescue refers to the onset of the incident. This might be an explosion causing a single building collapse, such as in Oklahoma City in 1995, or an earthquake that destroys half the buildings in a city, as occurred in Mexico City in 1985. At this point, the 9-1-1 system will be activated and local responders will begin arriving on the scene. Most situations that require a federal USAR response will be immediately apparent. However, some will not be so obvious, and will become apparent only after hours of rescuer effort. Either way, at some point the local incident commander will call for help from the local AHJ, up to the state EMA, and finally the governor's office. FEMA will activate the USAR system upon a presidential disaster declaration. All this coordination takes time, so the earlier the need is recognized, the sooner it can be met.

Once a USAR team arrives, they will begin preparing for operations immediately while the command staff is briefed on the situation and meets the key local players. The hazmat component evaluates for environmental hazards and mitigates as possible. The structural and heavy rescue component assesses the scene and begins moving immediately accessible dangerous debris. One key thing the structural engineers do is to evaluate for the risk of secondary collapse, which is a huge risk when working on a collapsed structure. This was unfortunately demonstrated by the secondary collapse of the World Trade Center towers in New York City following the terrorist attacks in 2001.

The technical and canine search teams begin exploring the rubble to locate survivors. Debris is carefully shored up during the search process. Once a patient is located, rescue specialists begin creating a path to the patient to allow medical evaluation and extrication.

The medical team will have been preparing equipment and communicating with local hospitals and trauma centers throughout the initial search. Once contact has been made with the patient, medical evaluation begins immediately by speaking with and listening to the patient. Even when the patient cannot speak and is not fully accessible, the medical

component can listen to the patient's breath sounds with microphones, evaluate an exposed limb for indications of shock or trauma, insert an IV and begin treatment, and even assess mental status by the patient's response to touch and voice. A medical specialist may have to enter the rubble pile to evaluate, stabilize, and treat the patient while rescuers are working on making an egress.

Technical specialists work seamlessly in concert with the other components to facilitate rapid and safe patient extrication. Thousands of pounds of debris may have to be moved or cut through to allow extrication. Information from the scene is continuously being relayed to command in order to coordinate the response. There may be multiple rescue attempts at different areas of the rubble pile at once. Careful coordination is critical to preventing destabilization at one site by movement in another.

The logistics component works constantly at preparing, maintaining, and delivering equipment to the scene. They also ensure there is adequate lighting, heat, water, and food to allow self-sufficiency for 72 hours. If operations are expected to go beyond one operational period, they will also organize bunking arrangements to allow rescuers to rest and prepare for further operations.[16] During the response, the USAR command staff and incident support team work closely with local responders and AHJs to optimize the integration of the USAR teams and local responders.

▶ CASE STUDY CONCLUSION

Stefan quickly receives his answer. He will be interviewed within the next 30 days and he should expect to go to training within the next six months. The training is a week-long session at the TEEK facility in Texas. Afterwards, he will be placed in the third level of the roster.

Bursting with pride, he announces his interview to his coworkers. Bill, his supervisor, offers a caution about getting too excited. "I am sure you are one of a dozen they are going to interview. But I wish you the best of luck in the interview and, of course, you can use my name as a reference. You can practice for the interview right now. First, what is your name again?" Everyone chuckles.

CRITICAL THINKING QUESTIONS

1. What special training does the Paramedic on a USAR team receive?
2. What special conditions must the USAR Paramedic prepare to treat?

CONCLUSION

The federal USAR system is designed as a rapidly deployable, highly specialized resource of experts in search and rescue in the new urban setting. It was designed to respond to the after-effects of earthquakes and bombings and has been extremely valuable and life-saving in both settings. The need for the expertise of these teams must be recognized and called for as soon as possible by local responders using established channels. Since skilled personnel are needed for these teams, opportunities are available for participation in this elite system in areas throughout the country.

KEY POINTS:

- Urban Search and Rescue consists of locating, reaching, treating, and extricating patients.

- Urban Search and Rescue evolved from heavy rescue following structural collapses.

- The National Response Framework called for search and rescue under number 9 of the Emergency Support Functions.

- USAR teams are dually supported by federal and local agencies and are activated via the mechanisms detailed in the Stafford Act.

- USAR teams have either Type I or Type III responses and are supported by incident support teams.

- Positions within the USAR team are search, rescue, medical, technical, logistics, and command.

- Technical search operators and canine search teams augment physical search.

- Technical specialists, such as structural specialists, assist the USAR team.

- Medical teams are part of the USAR team.

- Command decisions include determining whether a mission is a rescue or recovery operation.

- Crush syndrome is a medical condition that USAR medical teams commonly treat.

REVIEW QUESTIONS:

1. What are the six groups of personnel in a USAR team?
2. What are the two search subspecialties?
3. A technical team is comprised of what members?
4. What are the three levels of the response system?
5. How many USAR teams are there available in the United States and what is their team composition?

CASE STUDY QUESTIONS:

Please refer to the Case Study in this chapter, and answer the questions below:

1. What is the Paramedic's role in the USAR team?
2. What training must a Paramedic undergo to be part of the medical team?
3. What incident support teams might be utilized?

REFERENCES:

1. Barbera JA, MacIntyre A. Urban Search and Rescue. *Emerg Med Clin North Am. 1996;*14(2). p. 399–412.
2. Schwarzenegger A, Renteria H, Zagaris K. *California Fire Service and Rescue Emergency Mutual Aid System.* Urban Search & Rescue Program. Governor's Office of Emergency Services report, revised January 2004.
3. USGS Historic Earthquakes archive. Available at: **http://earthquake.usgs.gov/regional/world/events/1985_09_19.php.** Accessed February 2009.
4. FEMA. *About US&R*, History. Available at: **http://www.fema.gov/emergency/usr/about.shtm.** Accessed March 2009.
5. The National Response Framework. January 2008. Available at: **http://www.fema.gov/good_guidance/download/10220.** Accessed March 2009.
6. Robert T. Stafford Disaster Relief and Emergency Assistance Act, as amended, and Related Authorities. FEMA, June 2007.
7. FEMA. *Urban Search and Rescue (US&R) Incident Support Team (IST) Operations Manual.* January 2000. Available at: **http://www.fema.gov/pdf/emergency/usr/ist_ops_manual.pdf.** Accessed March 2009.
8. FIRESCOPE, California. Past, Present, and Future Directions, A Progress Report. October 1988. Available at: **http://www.firescope.org/firescope-history/past%20present%20future.pdf.** Accessed March 2009.
9. Homeland Security Presidential Directive-5: Management of Domestic Incidents. Department of Homeland Security, modified August 25, 2008. Available at: **http://www.dhs.gov/xabout/laws/gc_1214592333605.shtm#.** Accessed January 28, 2009.
10. Available at: **http://www.teex.com.** Accessed March 2009.
11. FEMA. *FEMA National US&R Response System Rescue Specialist Training Manual.* Available at: **http://www.fema.gov/pdf/emergency/usr/appen_a.pdf.** Accessed March 2009.
12. FEMA. *FEMA National US&R Response System Rescue Specialist Training Manual*, Appendix A. Available at: **http://www.fema.gov/emergency/usr/sctc.shtm.** Accessed March 2009.
13. Personal communication from David Jaslow, MD, MPH, regarding field case.
14. MacIntyre AG, Barbera JA, Smith ER. Surviving collapsed structure entrapment after earthquakes: a "time-to-rescue" analysis. *Prehosp Disast Med.* 2006;21(1):4–19.
15. Gonzalez D. Crush syndrome. *Crit Care Med.* 2005;33[Suppl.]: S34–S41.
16. FEMA. Profile of a Rescue. 3/21/06. Available at: **http://www.fema.gov/emergency/usr/profile.shtm.** Accessed March 2009.

CHAPTER 28

WATER RESCUE

KEY CONCEPTS:

Upon completion of this chapter, it is expected that the reader will understand these following concepts:

- Types of fast water
- Types of ice
- Types of surf
- Levels of rescuers
- Personal protective equipment used in water rescue
- Phases of a water rescue
- Methods of shore-based water rescue

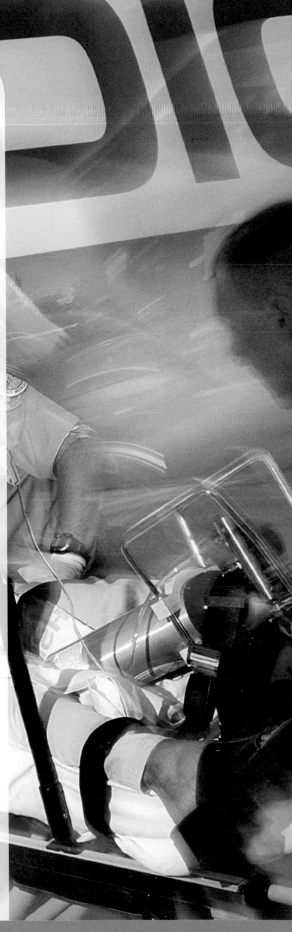

"9-1-1, what is your emergency?" the telecommunicator asks.

"Yes," the caller replies. "A boat went over the dam at Schuylerville. One man is on the far shore yelling that another man is in the water."

"Can you see the other man?" the telecommunicator asks.

"No," comes the reply.

"I understand, sir. Help is on the way. Could you please help direct rescuers to the water-edge? I would just like to confirm your address again." As the first telecommunicator takes the additional information, another telecommunicator begins the process of dispatching, "releasing the tones," for fire rescue and the special operations dive team as well as the state police rescue helicopter.

CRITICAL THINKING QUESTIONS

1. What are the phases of a water rescue?
2. What is the equipment used in a water rescue?
3. What is the Paramedic's role in a water rescue?

OVERVIEW

One of the many duties of EMS rescuers is water responses. Paramedics may not only expect to treat patients from water missions, but may also find themselves actively involved in the rescue attempt. Compounding this situation is the fact that many agencies send a medic unit out the door first in the response sequence. Simply put, the Paramedic may very easily find herself as one of the first rescuers on the scene. However, proper preparation and training will ensure that the proper rescue method, sequence, and scene safety are all intertwined into the mission.

Water Rescue

A "water response" call may represent any number of situations. In the same way that an "ill person" might refer to an individual with any number of diseases, water rescue comes in a few different forms and is very dynamic in that rescue attempts can change during the run. For example, a person trapped in a car in a swift water rescue might jump off of the car during the rescue attempt and be submerged downstream, thus requiring a dive rescue. Alternatively, the same person might make it downstream to an area of calm water and then be too tired to make it to shore, thus requiring a surface or boat rescue. The following text will discuss the common types of water rescue and some hazards and details of each.

Subdisciplines

The National Fire Protection Association (NFPA) 1006, *Standard for Technical Rescuer Professional Qualifications,* divides the various types of water rescues into subdisciplines, with each subdiscipline having Level I and Level II rescuer standards. Each type of water rescue has its own characteristics, hazards, and "personality," so teams often develop unique and specialized methods to deal with them. NFPA 1670, *Standard on Operations and Training for Technical Search and Rescue Incidents* provides the recommended techniques and practices. Another aspect of these broad water operations is that water rescues can range from a situation in a small swimming pool to severe flooding that will affect thousands of people and require hundreds of rescue personnel. The NFPA now divides water rescue into five main areas: surface water, swift water, ice rescue, surf rescue, and dive rescue.

Types of Water Rescue

Surface Water

Surface water is a catchall term for any flat, calm water found in a lake, pond, or waterway. **Calm water** is defined as water that moves at a speed of less than one knot. This can be anything from a very large inland lake or harbor to a small swimming pool in a backyard to major flood operations dealing with millions of acres.

Many surface waters are considered contaminated in this day and age, and most have some degree of chemical or biological contamination. During flood stages, many places become a toxic mixture of water, petroleum products, industrial and farm chemicals, and many other contaminants.

Flood responses also present hazards such as submerged electrical lines, sewer overflows, natural gas and propane leaks, washing out of the actual earth itself, and a very dangerous condition called differential pressure (Figure 28-1). **Differential pressure** is the force of two bodies of water at different elevations trying to equalize, and can easily be found in storm drainage systems. Rescuers can be easily sucked into culverts or a storm drain and drown in the process. Therefore, even though the surface of the water may appear calm, differential pressures under the water surface can present a drowning hazard to rescuers.

Swift Water

Terminology

Without common water rescue terms, directions and instructions can be confusing, especially when dealing with larger scenes or when teams of rescuers that do not normally work together are performing rescue operations. For example, a rescuer might ask, "Was that the *right* bank, or the *right bank*? Most swift

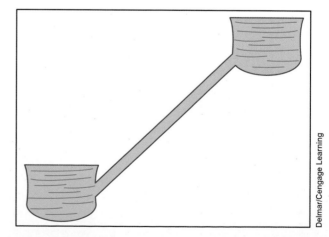

Figure 28-1 Differential pressure is the force applied to the drain when two bodies of water at different heights try to equalize.

Table 28-1 Definitions of Currents on Moving Water

Upstream	Where the water is coming from, collectively
Downstream	Where the water is going to, collectively
River Left	Looking downstream, the left-hand shore
River Right	Looking downstream, the right-hand shore

Current speed mph/knots	Force on legs, lbs 5.7 per mph	Body 11.3	Swamped boat 56
3 mph/2.6 knots	16.8	13	64
6 mph/5.2 knots	67.2	134	672
9 mph/7.8 knots	151	302	1512
12 mph/10.4 knots	269	538	2688

Delmar/Cengage Learning

Figure 28-3 Current force chart used to determine the velocity of water.

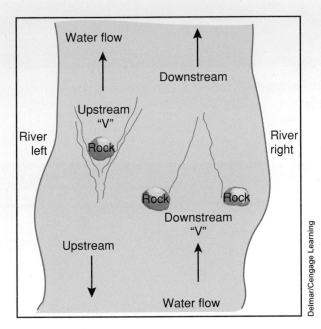

Delmar/Cengage Learning

Figure 28-2 Directional terms used on moving water.

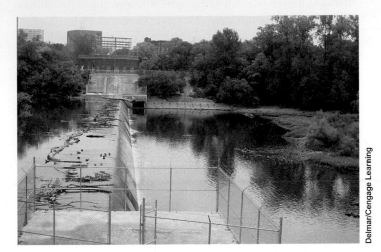

Delmar/Cengage Learning

Figure 28-4 A typical low-head dam is a simple wall across a waterway.

water rescue practices use the terms "upstream," "downstream," " river left," and "river right" (Table 28-1, Figure 28-2).[1]

Swift water, as defined by NFPA standards, is any water moving faster than one knot, or 1.15 miles per hour. A quick guide to figuring out this speed is timing a floating object as it moves 100 feet. If it takes approximately one minute for the object to cover a distance of 100 feet, the current is moving about one knot. This can be quickly adjusted in the field to reflect shorter distances or quicker times.

Many untrained rescuers greatly underestimate the force of moving water and do not understand that moving water never rests. Though Level I rescuers are not entering the environment directly, a good understanding of the power they will face should prevent any thought of jumping in when they shouldn't. The larger the object in the water, the more force that will be applied to it, since larger objects have more surface area which the flowing water will push upon. Current velocity also figures into the force of the current in that if the speed of the current doubles, the force applied quadruples (Figure 28-3). As few as six inches of moving water can take the legs out from under a rescuer, and most automobiles will float off the roadway in just 24 inches of water.[2] Many rescuers find themselves on missions because drivers didn't take heed of the high water sign in the road, or because they thought the vehicle could handle the water.

Low-Head Dams

Many recreational areas, flood control reservoirs, and public water sources are formed by damming streams and rivers, which contributes to improved living conditions. However, one type of dam has proven to be more dangerous than the others. The **low-head dam** is a simple wall across a waterway, usually less than 12 feet tall, with no way of controlling the flow over it (Figure 28-4). The water flowing over it creates a hydraulic current that will ensnare the patient. A **hydraulic current** is formed by water flowing over the dam and being pulled back into the dam face, creating a rolling boil of water. Hydraulic currents are made worse because not only can people be trapped in the boil but debris can, too, to the point of entire trees being circulated with the patient. Docks, ropes, stumps, or anything else that floats can be trapped, making it very possible the patient might sustain trauma along with the potential for drowning.

Ice Rescue

Ice can refer to either frozen water or ice-laden areas. The cardinal rule when dealing with ice is that it may fail to sustain weight at any time. By keeping this in mind, the rescuer will be prepared if the ice does give way. If a patient is already in the water, that should indicate the ice is weak and should not be trusted. Rescuer safety is always the first rule of any rescue.

Ice Types

Rescues often occur on newer, thinner ice; older, rotten ice; or where conditions on the ice change and leave no evidence of it. Ice sheets that are several inches thick may not offer the same thickness just a few yards away. In addition, weather changes, underwater currents, animals, and shore runoff can all change ice conditions. However, a good understanding of how ice is formed, the different types of ice, and environmental effects on ice will be beneficial to the rescuer (Figure 28-5).

Clear ice is the strongest ice that can form (Figure 28-6). Good clear ice can be transparent in thicknesses of many inches, supports the largest amount of weight relative to thickness, and is somewhat predictable when it fractures. Clear ice thicker than two inches is recommended if people wish to walk on it, but only if they are spaced out so as not to concentrate their weight together on the ice. One key point to remember is that ice, and anything placed on it, is floating on the water surface. If an air space exists between the ice and the water, the ice sheet may break.

Rotten ice is what rescuers normally have to deal with. Rotten ice has been thawed slowly, refrozen, and is very weak. It has a milky or opaque look, can fail without warning, and can be a very difficult surface to operate on (Figure 28-7). Rotten ice also may break into larger pieces, which may hinder forward movement when rescuers are trying to travel on it. Some pieces can be so large the rescuer must push them behind his body to advance farther along.

Ice on rivers, or **river ice** (Figure 28-8), is very dangerous, especially if it is exposed to stronger currents. Currents

Delmar/Cengage Learning

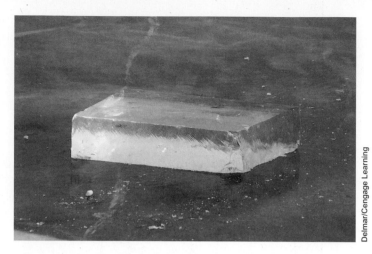

Figure 28-6 Clear ice can support the largest amount of weight by thickness.

Delmar/Cengage Learning

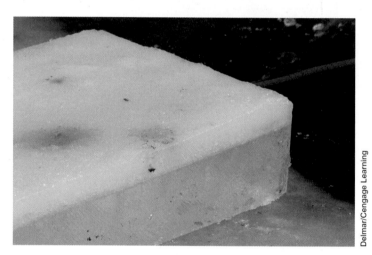

Figure 28-7 Rotten ice is weak and can fail without warning.

Recommended Minimum Ice Thickness
for New Clear Hard Ice.
No ice is without some risk.
Be sure to measure clear hard ice in several places.
3" (7 cm) or less
STAY OFF!
4" (10 cm)
ice fishing
walking
cross country
skiing
5" (12 cm)
one vehicle –
snowmobile
or ATV
8–12" (20–30 cm)
one vehicle – car or
small pick-up
12–15" (30–38 cm)
one vehicle –
medium truck
Delmar/Cengage Learning

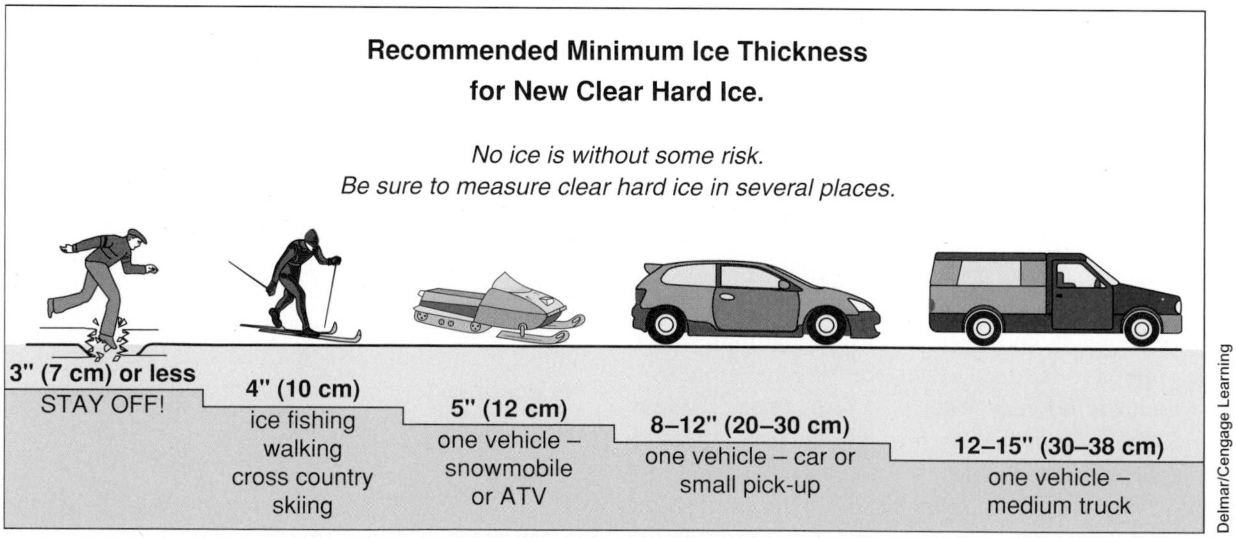

Figure 28-5 A minimum ice thickness is needed to support the weight of various methods of transportation.

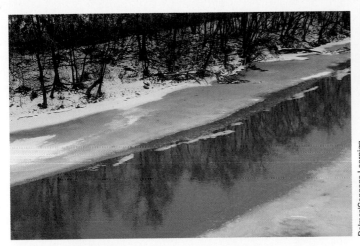

Figure 28-8 River ice forms around the banks of a river where the current is slower.

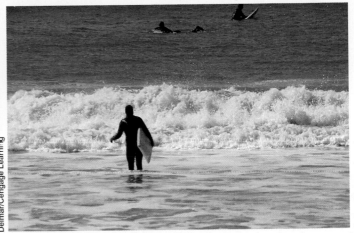

Figure 28-9 Spilling waves wash up on the shoreline, making a lot of foam from the agitated water, but do not crash into the water or shore from an elevated position.

erode ice from underneath, so rescuers may not be able to easily see the thickness of the ice. River levels rise and fall with rain and snow. As the river rises, the ice will be stressed as it moves upward, and as the water recedes it may leave dead air space in between the river water and the remaining ice. This is extremely hazardous to rescuers. If someone goes through the ice, the current may sweep the person under the ice downstream. It may be thicker at the bank, but thinner at the center of the channel, as faster currents found in the center erodes the ice.

Snow ice is ice with a layer of frozen snow on top of it. Melting snow can degrade the ice layer, and may insulate the ice enough to cause melting from underneath. It can also trap air in the mix, weakening the ice.

Environmental Effects on Ice

From day to day, ice can be affected by forces of nature or by man-made influences. The warmer air temperatures of spring can cause snow melt to coat the ice, and cooler temperatures at night cause new ice to form in thinner sheets on top of the old ice. Ice can melt because of the presence of animal feces as well. Geese and ducks can change the ice drastically by distributing droppings in a concentrated area, thereby causing patchy melt holes.

Wind blowing across the ice can also "churn up" or flex the ice surface, causing fractures. Wave action on any open water will fracture and pound the ice edges as well.

Human factors affecting ice include dock bubblers. When ice freezes it expands, causing a lot of damage to structures such as docks. Dock bubblers blow air into the water to create bubbles that in turn churn the water and keep it from freezing in order to protect docks or boats.

Other factors affecting the ice conditions are underwater springs; recreational vehicle travel, such as snow machines; and man-made holes used for training or recreation, such as ice fishing. Underwater springs can present a special hazard in that they erode ice from below, leaving no visible signs of erosion on the surface.

Warmer runoff waters from large industrial complexes or warmer areas can greatly affect ice conditions where that flow enters the water area. The warmer parking lots and rooftops warm the water that has run off, thus melting the ice in the retention pond in the outflow area. There will usually be an area of thinner ice, or even open water, near the runoff drain.

Surf Rescue

Surf areas are water areas that are showing wave action. The NFPA mainly deals with wave heights of up to six feet, measured from the low trough of the wave to the crest just before it collapses.

Spilling waves are waves that flow up and onto a gently sloping, mostly unobstructed surface, such as a beach that gradually gets shallower as the waves travel inshore (Figure 28-9). As the wave rises, the crest of the wave rises slowly enough that the wave simply collapses gently on itself, spilling into the shore where it dissipates.[3]

Plunging waves are much more dramatic and are associated in most people's minds with the sport of surfing (Figure 28-10). The wave passes over the bottom ground much faster, forcing the wave up and over onto itself so fast that the crest collapses on the wave. These waves mix a lot of air and water to form lots of foam, and can slam a person down into the water or down onto the bottom surface with incredible force. This also compounds rescue problems because these forces can easily injure rescuers and patients.[3]

Surging waves are waves that do not break on shore, but instead are pushed into rocks, cliffs, seawalls, or other large objects. The energy of the wave does not dissipate on a beach, but rather gets bounced into other waves and objects, making the seas very choppy and rough (Figure 28-11). The spectacular scenes of ocean water meeting rocky shores and spraying high into the air are examples of surging waves.[3]

Suicides are common on these spots where surge waves are found because of the cliff heights. Intentional or accidental

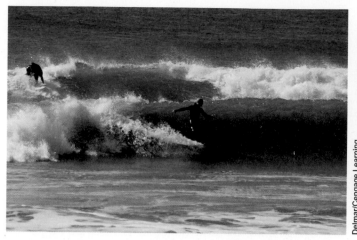

Figure 28-10 Plunging waves present a lot of energy from above when the wave actually breaks ahead and falls down on itself.

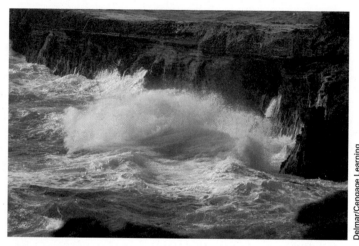

Figure 28-11 Surging waves do not have obstructions to dissipate their energy and can strike with enormous power.

falls from cliffs into the surge waves require a longer response time for rescuers to get to the patient. Many of these rescues are so dangerous that rescue crews will often attempt to rappel to the patient from the cliff, rather than try to get close to the patient in the water next to the rocks or cliffs.

Rip currents, or "rips," are the result of the waves or currents pushing water up the shore (Figure 28-12). The water must go somewhere, and a rip current involves this water draining back to the open water from which it came. They can be marked by a foamy or stained area on the water, with a reduced wave-breaking action, but this is not always the case. Rips can appear in different locations as the waves approach from different areas. Rip currents can also form when the incoming water hits the shore, travels laterally with it, and flows back offshore along a pier or shore break. They are also somewhat predictable, and many agencies are familiar with locations that present them on a regular basis. A large problem is that much of the general public, especially tourists, are not aware of where the rip currents may be found, so they

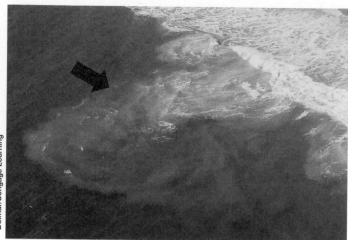

Figure 28-12 Rip currents are responsible for the majority of surf rescues.

venture into rip-current areas without knowing or recognizing the power or the danger.[3]

Dive Rescue

Dive rescue is any subsurface rescue operation in which rescuers wear self-contained underwater breathing apparatus (SCUBA). Dive rescue is complicated and requires advanced training; therefore, Paramedics are not expected to participate in a dive rescue without this training. However, Paramedics can anticipate caring for patients with a dive emergency.

Preplanning

Bodies of water, whether a beach or lake, have certain waterfronts to which the population tends to gravitate. Lakes and reservoirs have beaches, boat ramps, and gathering places such as restaurants and bars. Ice-covered water may have skating areas, fishing locations, or even racetracks for snow machines. Surf areas have beaches, sometimes crowded with thousands of people. Paramedics should be aware of these locations and account for them during preplanning. Resources should be allocated to these high-risk, high-life hazard areas.

Water Conditions

Water conditions play a role in preplanning for water emergencies. The agency having jurisdiction (AHJ) is the group or team that approves equipment, training, and procedures for a response area that intends to respond to water emergencies. Water conditions in the AHJ's locale might differ with various amounts of water present. These changing water conditions might also affect the response by closing streets and bridges, in addition to boat ramps and staging areas.

Low water levels frequently present problems for rescuers in terms of transporting gear and personnel to the patient's side. Since areas with normally navigable water might not be so easy to maneuver through in periods of extreme drought, this makes getting to a patient via water difficult. Rescuers should be aware of any change in water access and water use due to low water levels.

Normal water conditions exist in the range between high and low water conditions and are expected to be seen during times when neither drought nor flooding is present. Even normal water conditions can change from high to low, however, depending on currents, tides, flood control measures, and so on.

High water is the condition typically present when a rescue is required. High water periods are not a truly unusual event, and actions and preplans should reflect this understanding. Generally, waters will be contained to a known area, with predictable flows that the Paramedic can use to preplan the rescue.

Floods and **floodwater** often present major challenges to rescue teams, particularly in flood-prone areas. With the growth of urban areas and all the impervious surfaces, such as parking lots and roadways, that are drained quickly into culverts and drainage systems, many streams and creeks quickly rise beyond their banks.

Major flooding often results in contaminated water, secondary to sewage overflow. Flooding presents other risks to responders as well, such as submerged electrical wires, gas leaks, structural instability in buildings, and even terrain hazards like unstable banks or shore washouts.[4,5]

Yet another problem, especially in flash flooding, are citizens who disregard flood warning signs and road closures. Every year people die after driving around a road closed sign and trying to cross moving water.

Agency Response

The agency having jurisdiction must be aware of not only its capabilities as it relates to equipment and personnel, but also the status of surrounding agencies or teams that will be called in to assist in the event of a water emergency. Through shared resources, the rescuer can anticipate the greatest chance of success in a rescue operation.

Personnel Capabilities

Each agency having jurisdiction must ensure that the rescuers that will work a mission are properly trained for the task at hand. The fire service uses standards from the NFPA for group rescuers and the level of training required for different levels. For technical rescue, there are two standards: **NFPA 1670**, which deals with team operations and training, and **NFPA 1006**, dealing with individual rescuers. For this text, we will deal mainly with NFPA 1006 standards for technical rescuer professional qualifications.

Awareness level training, a term found in NFPA 1670, addresses training which responders and support personnel should receive at the most basic level. Awareness training can consist of classroom-type information only and should be offered to any person or agency that might be used in a water response, especially those in peripheral or first responder-type roles.

For example, a police officer would typically have very little ice rescue equipment in the cruiser, but should recognize a need for rescue and how not to get hurt when attempting a rescue. The responder trained to the Awareness level should know how to prevent anyone else from getting injured and, most importantly, where and how to get help. Officers trained at the Awareness level, in the case cited, should realize the risk of venturing onto the ice surface, know that specially trained rescuers with proper training and equipment are needed, prevent anyone else from turning into a patient, and call for assistance (usually fire or EMS).

Previously called Operations level, **Level I rescuers** are generally trained to use, deploy, and support surface-based or shore-based rescues, using some specific tools that are key to the mission being undertaken. Simply put, Level I rescuers do not directly enter the environment the patient is trapped in, but can use different means to effect rescue from a safe location, such as a boat or shore. Reaching the status of Level I rescuer also gives a person the needed prerequisites to attain the further training and expertise needed to reach Level II. Level I rescuers also act as mission support for Level II rescuers during "Go" rescues.

Level II rescuers can operate as Level I rescuers or, if needed, can enter the hazard the patient is trapped in. **Level II rescuers** use specific equipment and wear specific PPE that will protect them from that environment, and they also receive training on how to extricate a patient from the hazard. Level II rescuers are also expected to be able to lead and plan operations on missions and act as liaisons for Level I rescuers.

Generally speaking, all three levels can operate and complement each other on a scene. For example, a police officer arrives on a scene and provides scene security, sets up a command post, and notifies the local fire and EMS department. The first-arriving Level I trained members may try to use ropes unsuccessfully to rescue the patient, but instead end up controlling the line a swimming Level II rescuer uses to swim to and rescue the patient. The NFPA documents are guidelines for the agency having jurisdiction, and team members who wish to be called "Technical rescuers" are expected to follow them.

Mutual Aid Response

With a current trend toward "intra-operability," and the federal government imposing the required National Incident Management System training on all emergency services providers, teams can be "typed" into "operational groups." Different teams are equipped and trained and have a variety of missions, with each having different designations. For example, a Type 1 swift water team will have a very large gear cache, with many members trained to Level II, whereas a Type 4 emergency first response team may only have a few members at Level I training, and use as little equipment as some ropes and personal flotation devices.

Mutual aid or automatic response should be planned before the mission, with the capabilities of each team or department being considered. The water types and expected conditions should also be taken into consideration.

Logistics

Many times teams fail to adequately plan how to get these teams to a location when the water is unexpectedly high and blocking the travel route. For example, losing two bridges to fast moving water can create obvious problems of access and egress. A good plan has alternative routes available. This plan should be made available to mutual aid responders as well. Staging resources should also be considered. In addition, responders who are not actively assigned tasks should be prepared in case of need.

The staging officer should consider such questions as: "Where will they stage?" "How long?" and "What do they need?" At larger incidents, accountability, food and shelter, fuel, and communications will also have to be considered. In addition to rescuers, patients being evacuated also need food, water, EMS treatment, and shelter.

Training

Skills are honed by training and practice. Many times, especially in areas that do not see much flooding or water response, the mission becomes haphazard as a result of lack of training and practice.

A course on current forces, a review of the preplan for areas that have frequent calls, or a mockup tabletop exercise are acceptable methods for training indoors. Many county and state emergency management agencies (EMA) use graphic information systems that can show where floodwaters will run, or where the water will go if a dam breaks. Topographic maps, while requiring some adjustment to actually read, will give a lot of information on low areas. Even researching historic archives may reveal water levels that many have never realized possible. These "chalk talks" can help increase rescuer awareness of hazards and initiate preplanning for predictable missions.

Swimming pools are clean, clear, and easily managed training locales. Many recreation centers and resorts are now using "lazy river" type pools. These provide realistic swift water, as some lazy river pools are capable of delivering water up to seven knots. Use of freshly filled or unheated pools will also give rescuers some real-life feelings of hypothermia after a time in the water and will teach rescuers to respect water temperatures.

To maximize the training impact, the rescuer should implement the response plan. Open water trainings are also a great way to build mutual aid capabilities and knowledge, as well as to educate the public as to the water hazards that exist in every community.

Common Personal Protective Equipment

The first responsibility of every Paramedic is personal safety. Personal protective equipment (PPE) should be utilized for any water response and is common to all of the water rescue subdisciplines.

Personal flotation devices (PFDs) are grouped by the U.S. Coast Guard into five types, each providing the wearer with a different type of protection.[6] When properly used and worn, they will allow the wearer to float in the water with no effort. Some will even turn an unconscious wearer face up to protect the airway. However, a PFD must be properly worn to be effective. Following is a list of each type of PFD along with a brief explanation of its benefits and uses.

Type 1 PFDs are the horse-collar life jackets that fasten to the wearer by hanging around the neck. They also have a waistband strap. Type 1 PFDs are used primarily on commercial and offshore craft (for example, cruise ships) and are used in heavy seas when rescue may not arrive quickly. They should turn an unconscious patient face up while floating, and must deliver a minimum of 22 pounds of buoyancy. They are not considered rescue crew PFDs. Note: The PFD provided for oceanic flights generally consists of Type I vests.

Type 2 PFDs are the same basic design as a Type 1, but they only provide 15 pounds of buoyancy for an adult (Figure 28-13). These smaller, more common PFDs are used on smaller, noncommercial pleasure craft.

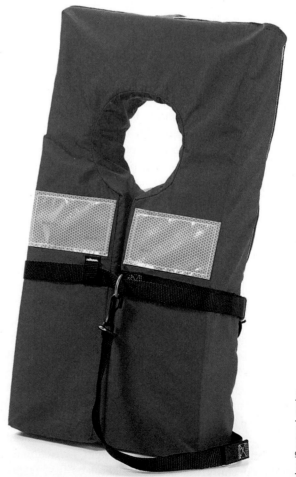

Delmar/Cengage Learning

Figure 28-13 Type 2 PFDs are lighter and smaller than Type 1 PFDs.

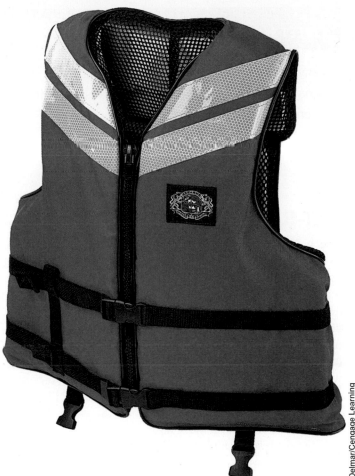

Figure 28-14 The typical Type 3 PFD is found on many EMS, fire, and law enforcement vehicles.

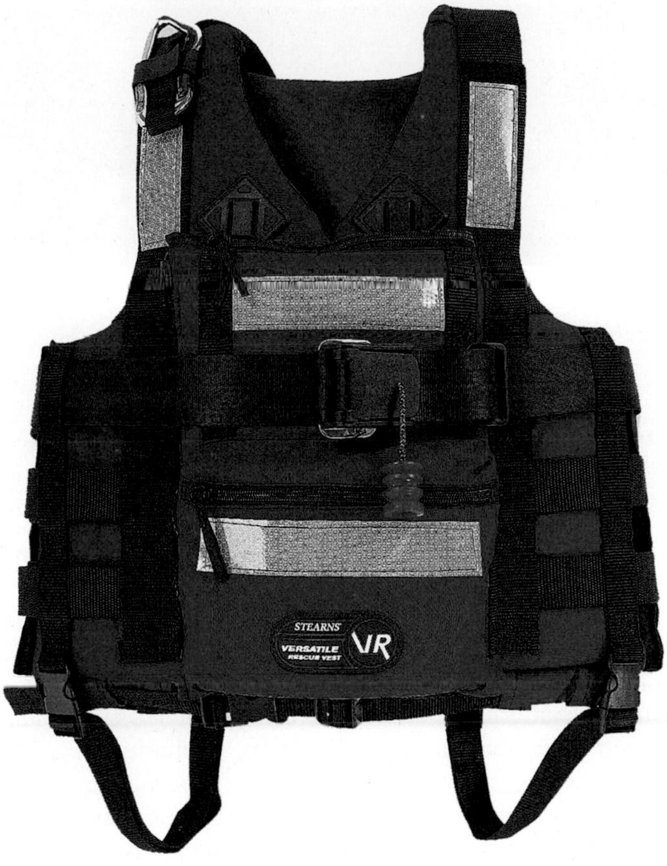

Figure 28-15 Type 5 PFDs are specialized, job-functional PFDs that can include float coats, work vests, paddling PFDs, and swift water rescue PFDs.

Type 3 PFDs, the typical "ski-vest" style PFDs, are found on many EMS, fire, and law enforcement vehicles (Figure 28-14). This class also includes the auto-inflated, suspender-type PFDs favored by sailors and hobby fishermen, although newer technology can place these into other classes as well. The Type 3 PFD does not necessarily turn unconscious wearers face up, but they are comfortable to wear, and provide the same 15-pound buoyancy as Type 2 PFDs.

Type 4 PFDs are not actually worn, but are meant to be thrown to a patient in distress in order to assist flotation until a very quick rescue is performed. They include throw ring buoys, seat cushions, and the like. Ring buoys are circular foam flotation devices with rope around the outside for gripping and are thrown to a patient. Most watercrafts over 16 feet of length are generally required to have one on board.

Type 5 PFDs are specialized, job-functional PFDs that can include float coats, work vests, paddling PFDs, and swift water rescue PFDs (Figure 28-15). These specialized PFDs are suited to the environment in which they are protecting the wearer. In addition, they will provide the buoyancy of a Type 1, 2, or 3 PFD (the buoyancy will be marked on it). These can only be considered U.S. Coast Guard (USCG) approved if worn for the purpose for which it is tagged.

Additional PFD Equipment

Some companies and most water rescue teams will purchase and use a Type 5 swift water rescue vest. However, the higher cost of these makes them somewhat less common than other PFDs. Regardless of what type of PFD a team buys, the best PFD is the one that will be worn. Various items are available to use with the PFD, including chemical light sticks, dye packs, throw bags, and knives. Knives are handy because becoming entangled in a line, whether in or around a boat, puts a rescuer in a potentially dangerous position. If this happens, rescuers must be able to cut themselves or other rescuers loose from such a predicament.

There is always the possibility that a rescuer may move quickly into the water, either by choice or by accident, and face hazards such as rocks, docks, or debris, especially in moving water. **Water rescue helmets** are light and have minimal foam padding inside so water is not absorbed (Figure 28-16).

Eye protection can be a very important part of boat-based water rescues for two primary reasons. Water spray or debris hitting the eye at fast speeds can damage the eye. In addition, blinding glare is another concern. If facing westward on a

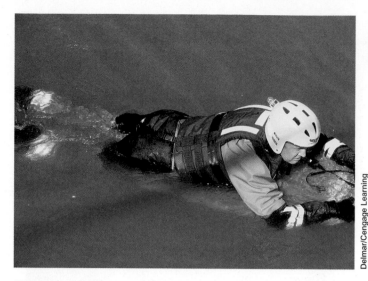

Figure 28-16 Water rescue helmets provide the rescuer with protection from head injury.

sunny late afternoon, the rescuer can be blinded by the sun's reflection on the water. Alternatively, operating on a lake surrounded by snow can cause snow blindness. Many good water goggles are now on the market that are specially made for the personal watercraft (PWC) market. These goggles work well for water rescuers. A set of tinted safety glasses can work as well.

Many swift water rescuers carry a **personal throw bag** for use on the water. Personal throw bags are just a smaller version of the typical throw bag, but can fit in a pocket or a hip belt. Because the bag is smaller, it can be worn comfortably and not present too large of a profile on the wearer. However, they must be properly secured to the wearer to reduce entanglement. Although they can be used from the shore, they also provide the ability to throw a rope from another place on the river that is out of reach from the shore.

The prospect of having to rescue another rescuer should always be considered as well. Sometimes getting a quick throw rope to a rescuer in trouble is all that is required for a rescue, especially in wider rivers; for example, a swimmer standing by in an eddy can throw a rope to a rescuer who is caught in current too strong to permit swimming. Short tether leashes can be attached to the rear of the PFD and used for support on steeper banks, but should also be stowed so as to minimize the entanglement risk.

Every rescuer who is working near or in water should carry cutting tools, as the risk of getting caught in a line or needing to assist another rescuer caught in a line is very real. A short, blunt-tip, straight-blade knife is considered the best type of tool. Folding knives need to be manipulated in order to open them, and pointed tips can injure a rescuer, thus decreasing their effectiveness. Trauma shears also require a fair amount of dexterity to use. When in the midst of a swift water entrapment, rescuers need a quickly accessible blade.

Many rescuers carry a whistle that allows them to signal others at a great distance. Water and radios often don't mix. The whistle is also useful as a "location identifier" if a rescuer goes into the water.

Self-Rescue

The goal of any rescuer should exceed simply being able to rescue someone. Rather, rescuers should be comfortable enough in the water environment so as to operate safely and with confidence. A rescuer that cannot extricate herself from a hazard should not attempt a patient rescue. Even if the rescuer does not plan on entering the water, there is always the possibility of falling in. Rescuers should know some methods of mitigating problems that might be encountered. Of course, wearing the proper PFD is the best means of self-preservation.

Some rescuers who lack swimming skills may find themselves in a water scenario. If they enter the water without a PFD, flotation is paramount. Flailing around in the water will only tire the rescuer, and can possibly make the rescuer hypothermic, since water conducts heat away from the body much faster than air.

The rescuer forms the **heat escape lessening position (HELP)** by drawing up his legs and knees to the chest, and wrapping his arms around them.[1] This position lessens heat loss, and can delay hypothermia if movement is kept to a minimum.

Anyone in water deeper than one's head without a PFD must make some sort of effort to keep her head above water. Treading water is very common, but less-experienced or out-of-shape rescuers will quickly fatigue. One problem is rescuers who jump in deep water with heavy-duty fire service boots on. The boots themselves might not be an issue, but treading water with water-laden boots will wear out the rescuer's muscles surprisingly fast. This can also cause the rescuer to panic, and create a reduction in the rescuer's effectiveness in using motor skills and proper technique. The easiest way to try to stay above water is to float (Figure 28-17). Large, deep inhalations of the lungs will help provide buoyancy, as will positioning the body face up and arching the back slightly. The rescuer should drop any heavy objects (multipurpose tools, large knives, radios, and so on). Relaxation, although probably not easily achieved at this point, will do much to help flotation. Some easy kicking or treading of the legs can be done, which may even start some movement toward safety.

The natural weight of one's arms and legs explains why some people have difficulty staying vertical in the water. The human head is also much heavier than most people realize, so it can take quite a bit of strength to keep it upright for long

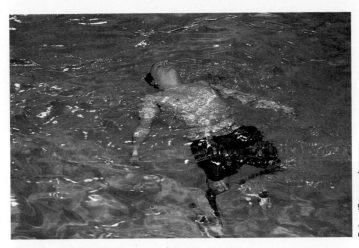

Figure 28-17 By calmly floating on one's back if swimming is difficult or not possible, the rescuer may buy time for help to arrive.

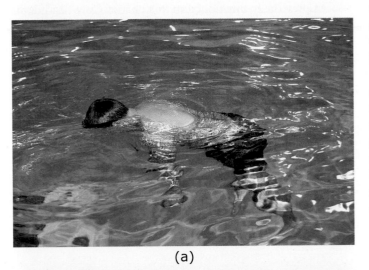

(a)

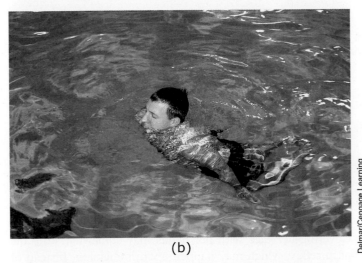

(b)

Figure 28-18 (a) The drownproofing position saves energy while floating. (b) Breathing while drownproofing is accomplished by raising the head just above the water surface.

periods of time. Another way to survival float is drownproofing. **Drownproofing** is performed by laying face down in the water, without moving the hands and legs, and letting the head hang. The person in the water holds her breath, and when she needs to breathe she raises her head just enough to exchange air, then holds her breath again for a few seconds (Figure 28-18). Relaxation is the key to survival using this technique.

Anything that floats may help a rescuer. Logs, buoys, and even basketballs or soccer balls will float and offer some buoyancy. By using any of these makeshift aids, the rescuer's flotation problem is at least partially solved, and egress to shore can be considered. Some flotation devices, such as boogie boards, will allow the rescuer to lay on the stomach area, which allows the legs to kick for forward motion. It also frees the head to scan the area in front of the individual. Other flotation devices, such as a horse-collar style PFD, will be easier to manage with the rescuer lying on the back, keeping the head and airway protected that way.

Once the rescuer has achieved adequate flotation and can keep her airway clear of water, she can make some kind of effort to get to safety. Although one would hope the other rescuers might notice someone in the water or missing, in a worst case scenario the rescuer may buy the time needed to be rescued by floating.

Water conditions can affect where a rescuer trying to swim to safety should travel. Much of this decision depends on where the rescuer is located in the water. Getting to shore is half the battle, but getting ashore can be the other half, and swimmers without flotation devices may fatigue and go under before being rescued. For example, in surf rescue, the best place to go may be, in fact, farther offshore. The following text describes some specific methods to self-rescue from other water environments.

Swift Water Self-Rescue

In and of itself, swift water is a tough location for a rescue, given the force of the water present. However, there are a host of additional hazards other than the moving water—many unseen—that the rescuer can encounter.

Water moving through, rather than around, any object creates a **strainer**. Trees, cars, bridge pilings, and many other items can form strainers (Figure 28-19). Rescuers and patients alike can end up in, under, or on top of these strainers. In any case, the force of the water flowing through the strainer can very easily trap someone underwater and pin him there. If the rescuer is swimming and cannot avoid a strainer, it is best to actually swim forward to build up speed before reaching the strainer. Just before hitting it, the rescuer should kick both of his legs and try to get up and onto the strainer, which is a better option than being swept under or into it. If the water keeps pushing the rescuer, he should get over the strainer and prepare to defensive swim again. Staying put on top of it until rescue arrives is a good option if the strainer is stable.

Pillows form on the water when water piles up against a submerged object, making the water appear to be a raised

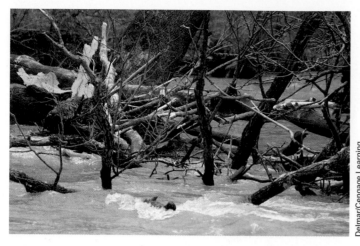

Figure 28-19 These trees form a strainer in the moving water.

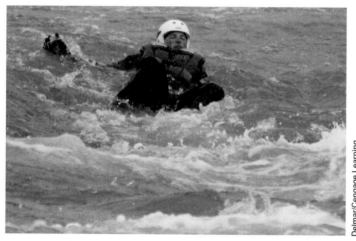

Figure 28-20 The defensive swimming position provides the rescuer with good visibility, head protection, and shock absorption.

area. These pillows may signal a shallow object that can injure someone striking it.

An **upstream V** in the water indicates an object which the water is flowing around, with wake disturbances found on each side. The V, pointing upstream, marks the hazard. A **downstream V** usually signals a path between two objects, with the V pointing downstream. The rescuer should try to position himself in the downstream V, and stay away from the upstream V (Figure 28-2).

The safest places in flowing water are eddies. An **eddy** is a relatively calmer pool of water formed behind an object when moving water flows around a large object. A rescuer that inadvertently ends up in the water can try to get to an eddy as a safe haven.

The rescuer assumes the **defensive swimming position** by lying on the back, facing downstream (Figure 28-20). The head remains up for visibility and protection, the feet are used as bumpers, and the knees are used as shock absorbers. The rescuer "rides" the river current using the increased visibility afforded by the position to identify and to work around

hazards or obstacles such as rocks or strainers. When the time comes to swim for positioning to avoid an obstacle, the rescuer must swim hard, try to keep his head up, and continually monitor his progress.

Ferry swimming means using the river's current to help push oneself or an object to one side of the river or the other. As a swimmer turns her body to angle against the current, it will guide her to the shore she is intending to reach. This angle, called a ferry angle, can increase or decrease the movement laterally in the water. Although there will still be downstream movement in faster currents, swimmers, boats, and patients can all use ferry angles to move laterally in the water, and it can be done while maintaining the defensive swim position.

One very large risk rescuers face in shallower rivers with a fair current is foot entrapments, which can frequently cause ankle fractures. Large rocks create holes and crevices among the floor, and when rescuers plant a foot to step, the loss of balance coupled with the current force can pull the rescuer downstream while pinning the foot between the rocks.

As previously mentioned in this chapter, low-head dams create an especially dangerous feature, the hydraulic. If a rescuer enters the hydraulic, there are not a lot of options. Escaping any hydraulic will likely involve some luck. The best course of action is to try to get downstream of the boil line (Figure 28-21).

Even wearing high flotation PFD may not be enough to stay on top of the water. It is very likely the rescuer will be sucked into the face of the dam and pushed back underwater. Once forced under, the rescuer should try to swim downstream while underwater. Another option is to time a heroic surface swim effort while as close to the downstream edge of the boil as possible. Once the water sucks the rescuer back into the boil, he will likely be fighting a losing battle and will probably be rolled underwater again.

Ice Self-Rescue

Similar to fast water rescue, the prepared rescuer can self-rescue from ice provided she uses a few simple techniques. Falling through the ice is a problem, but it is possible to escape this situation. Many times those who fall through the ice make the mistake of trying to pull themselves back up onto the ice by locking their arms and pushing up. If they make it that far, then they try to stand again. The key to ice self-rescue is to spread out one's body weight and stay spread out until one reaches stronger ice or even the shore.

The steps for emergency self-rescue on an ice shelf are basic (Figure 28-22). First, when the patient starts to feel the ice break underneath, she needs to concentrate on the fall. Covering her face with her hands may somewhat stifle the gasp reflex, which may happen upon immersion. Instead of thrashing around and flailing her arms, she should float on her stomach while resting her arms on the ice shelf. This may allow her legs and feet to float to a more horizontal position. If this happens, the patient should kick her feet and try to

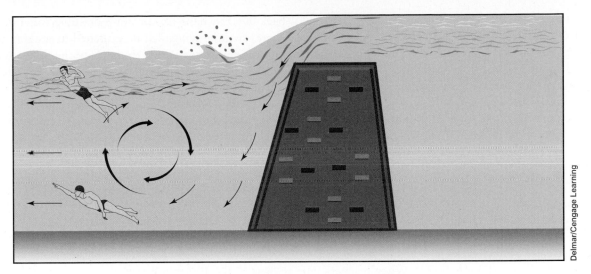

Figure 28-21 Two possible escapes from hydraulics are to surface swim very hard from the downstream edge of the boil line or to swim downstream underwater at the bottom of the boil.

Delmar/Cengage Learning

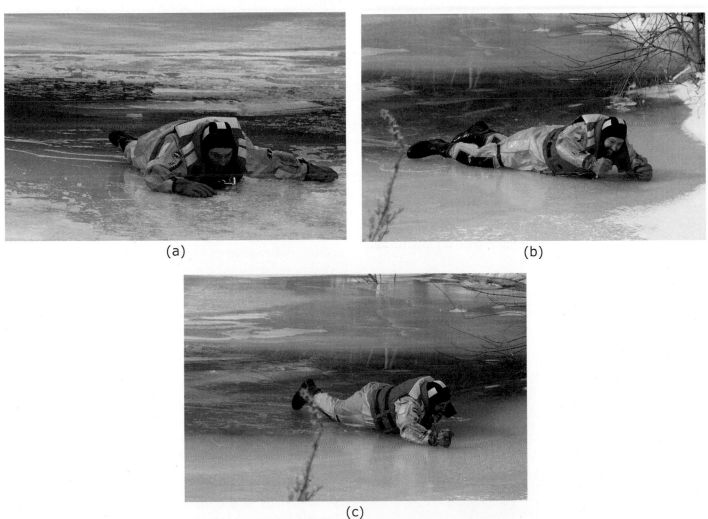

(a)

(b)

(c)

Delmar/Cengage Learning

Figure 28-22 Ice self rescue. (a) First, the person should try to get up onto the ice shelf on his stomach. (b) Next, he should reach out slowly to pull himself onto the ice shelf. (c) Once moving, the person should either keep moving or roll away from the open water.

"beach" up onto the ice. Lying prone may let the patient exit the water. If this is successful, it is important that she does not immediately stand up. Since this same ice just failed, it will likely fail again. The key in this situation is spreading the body weight on the ice surface to minimize any concentrated loading. Rolling away from the hole will keep the weight spread and also minimize the force of re-entry if the ice fails again. Rolling should be done until the patient is fully confident in the ice strength or makes her way to shore.

Using Ice Awls or Picks

Other than the correct PFD, the next most important piece of gear with which rescuers can equip themselves in ice environments is a set of ice awls. **Ice awls**, or picks, are simple tools that mostly consist of two ice picks attached to the rescuer or to each other with a leash (Figure 28-23). When rescuers fall through the ice, the main problem is getting a grip on something to pull them up and back onto the ice enough to roll out. The ice awls are used to stab the ice and provide that grip.

The ice awls need to be driven into the ice itself. One common mistake users make is to try to set the picks as far away from them as possible. By doing this, the rescuer is unable to effectively use the chest muscles. Instead, the picks should be planted into the ice closer to the hole, in order to use the pectoral muscles to pull the load. Once the rescuer has gained a few inches, he removes one pick and resets it a bit farther away until the rescuer gets moving out of the hole. Once out of the hole, the rescuer should stay on his belly and keep using the awls for movement. With some practice, rescuers can become quite proficient and actually move very fast across the ice.

Surf Self-Rescue

The most common surf entrapment rescuers face is getting caught in a rip current.[3] Rip currents are formed when water that is pushed perpendicularly inshore finds a place to drain

back out. Since the rip current is draining water back out offshore, swimming against it is likened to running on a treadmill. To beat this, people in the "rip," as they are frequently called, must swim parallel to shore until they are out of it. Then, swimmers can choose to swim to shore or possibly even farther offshore. This may seem odd, but the surf line is the line where swells start to break over and may become crashing waves. It is better to swim farther offshore and wait on rescue than to try to get through the wave action and be injured. This is especially true if there is known backup en route or other rescuers are aware of the situation.

When returning to shore, rescuers must also be aware of holes in the sand (from wave action) and the backwash (water draining back into the water, but along the bottom surface). Backwash can easily knock people off their feet, so any self-rescue in the surf is not complete until the rescuer is in the boat or on shore.

The Rescue Response

The first decision a rescuer makes during a rescue attempt is identifying the problem and determining the action to immediately follow (i.e., whether or not a viable rescue can take place). This decision has to be made before any operation is underway and, with experience, can often be made in just a few seconds. After taking a quick look at the conditions of the water upon arrival (i.e., what type of water is involved), the reported timeline, and the resources on-scene, the rescuer determines whether a rescue attempt can safely be made, or if a recovery situation has developed.

Paramedics may find it hard to change to a recovery state of mind, and even harder to actually start out in one. It is simply not in the makeup of the rescuer's job or mentality to start a mission in recovery mode. However, it is a necessity. There have been many examples of very good rescuers who come very close to dying while attempting rescue for a person who had no chance whatsoever of survival. On the other hand, patients have survived hazards from which survival was never thought possible. Only experience and the application of the following principles can help the rescuers make the best decision.

The **timeline** is critical in any rescue. The rescuer must determine when the incident occurred and whether rescue actions can be taken. For example, does the caller reporting the incident have a patient in sight or is this a third-party, good-intent call? Rescuers have died on runs that a witness will swear just happened but is actually hours old. The length of time the patient has been underwater also plays into the picture. Most traumas are treated under what EMS terms the "Golden Hour" (60 minutes), and water rescue is no different.

Timelines can be investigated through family members or persons around the area. If a boat is found floating, when did it actually launch? Is there a trailer in the parking lot? If there is, is the car engine warm or cold, or can law enforcement try and run the license plates and contact the owner? However, if a watercraft is found on a larger body

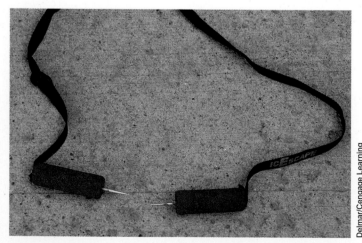

Figure 28-23 Ice awls are driven into the ice and provide a good method for pulling rescuers along on their stomach.

of water, with no witnesses, it becomes difficult to determine a timeline or even if there is a patient. A better choice may be to run a sonar grid and do some very good shore investigations.

Almost every water response can have the needed initial information boiled down to the following parameters.

Who? This not only means the name of the patient, but identifying the clothes or flotation devices worn, the strength of the patient's swimming ability, any patient disabilities or medical history, and whether the person was alone or with someone else. Even a patient's shoe can come into play; for example, a fisherman wearing large, heavy waders makes the tennis shoe footprint found on the shore irrelevant.

Where? The location of the incident is very, very important, and must be pointed out or explained from the point of view of the witness who watched things happen. Viewpoints vary wildly on larger bodies of water, so the witness must give the best visual clues possible to recreate the incident from where he actually saw things happen. **Triangulation** means using different lines of sight to narrow down a location, and is very effective if multiple witnesses are interviewed from where they saw the events (Figure 28-24).

How? This seems elementary, but includes such patient actions as struggling, shouting, or swimming. The act of shouting for help shows at least some proficiency in keeping one's head above water, which may allow the possibility of movement in the water. A sudden there-one-second-and-gone-the-next incident may indicate a seizure or other medical injury preceded the event, or even that the patient exited the water without being noticed by bystanders.

How long ago? Did the witness leave to find help? Did the witness have to drive to get help or was he able to walk? How far away was the help? Did he call from a cell phone and stay at the scene? This information will help the rescuer make the rescue/recovery decision.

Active and Passive Search Measures

Patients who are actually seen in the water by a witness will normally require what is termed an **active search measure**. This occurs when rescuers actually have determined a **point last seen (PLS)**, the exact location the person was last seen in the water.

Passive search measures can be more frustrating to rescuers, in that some resources, including rescuers who are ready to go, may be kept in a holding pattern while more investigation is done. **Passive search measures** usually do not involve an intense, quick search, as there are generally no witnesses to these events. Although incidents like people not reporting in from a boat ride at an expected time or finding a lone boat floating in a lake would be enough to warrant investigation, they most likely will not provide enough information for the rescuer to decide exactly where to begin an active search.

One of the ways rescuers arrive at the rescue or recovery decision is by using risk versus benefit judgments. Risk versus benefit describes what can be accomplished at what price. Responders make this decision on many runs, and hopefully that decision allows them to safely return home the next day. Whichever way the mission goes, the most important factor is safety. Even if a plan of action is considered, there could very well be another solution that keeps everyone safer. For example, a boat-based rescue is normally safer than a swim-based rescue, but can take longer to deploy.

Shore-Based Rescue Sequence

A common form of water rescue is a no-entry rescue, the types of rescues that are commonly orchestrated from the shore. Each subdiscipline mentioned previously will be examined. Some tools, such as throw bags, are used in each type of rescue but are applied through different techniques in each case.

Many rescuers have heard something of the old adage: "Reach, throw, row, and go." This refers to the types of rescue attempts, in order from the least risk rescue to the highest risk rescue. Some rescue instructors prefer to insert "Yo!" in front of that adage to include patient self-rescue. Sometimes patients can be directed to a safer spot or just reassured that help is on the way. The person clinging to a bridge pylon, but otherwise stable, might try to jump unless a rescuer can make it known a boat is on the way. Simple shouts, bullhorns, or vehicle public address systems can all be used for this purpose.

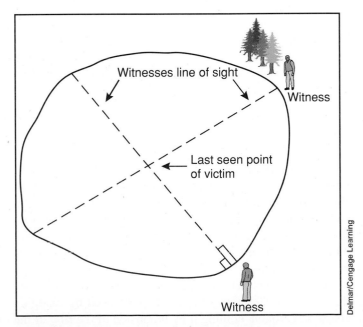

Figure 28-24 Triangulation uses witnesses at different vantage points to narrow down the patient's location.

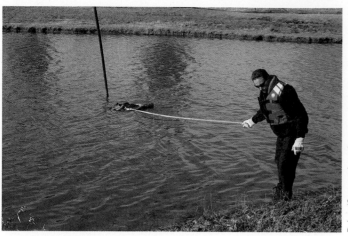

Delmar/Cengage Learning

Figure 28-25 This rescuer is using a pike pole to reach a patient in the water.

The safest, most direct way for the rescuer to reach the patient without actually entering the water is to reach for the patient (Figure 28-25). Fire trucks carry tools that are easily used to reach patients, or makeshift aids can be utilized on-scene. Pike poles, long poles with a hook on the end, work well, but are somewhat heavy, especially when extended fully to the patient. Trying to hold a 16-foot pike out to someone in the water by holding just the tip is difficult.

Shepherd's crooks, which are found at many pools and swimming sites, work very well. This large hook is used to actually sweep the patient toward shore, and the half-circle design will hold a patient in the hook when being pulled. Modified tools can include extension ladders with floats attached, or strapping a PFD onto the end of the pike pole to provide some flotation assistance to the patient. Hose inflator systems are primarily thought of as an ice rescue tool, but can also be used very successfully in swift water and surface rescue work.

Items found on-scene that are used in a pinch to help with the rescue are only limited by the rescuer's imagination and safety. Tree limbs, paddles or oars, and even long-handled tools can all be used. The important thing is to remember the patient will pull back. Sometimes the patient pulls so hard that the rescuer will end up in the water, too. Civilians will most likely use the reaching rescue method unless they have some specialized equipment available to them at the water's edge.

Throw Bags

Many rescuers use **throw bags** (Figure 28-26), comprised of a length of rope stuffed into a bag that is thrown. Some bags are equipped with a small float in the bottom of the bag that allows the bag to stay at the surface. The smaller diameter lines, around 7 millimeter, deploy better through the air and let the user throw them longer distances than large diameter lines, which create a lot of drag through the air. Although there are other throwing devices, including line guns, rescue rockets, ring buoys, and even Frisbee-style devices, throw bags are probably the most common water rescue tool. They

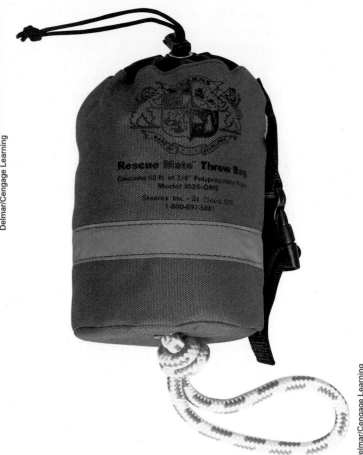

Delmar/Cengage Learning

Figure 28-26 A typical water rescue throw bag, which is commonly used throughout the United States.

are found on many watercraft, rescue trucks, EMS units, and frontline fire apparatus throughout the country.

The rescuer needs practice to accurately use a throw bag. It is not normally thrown like a football, but instead is thrown underhanded. One end must stay with the rescuer in order for the rescuer to pull the patient in. With some practice, throw bags can also be rapidly redeployed in case of a missed throw (**Skill 28-1**).

For a step-by-step demonstration on Deploying a Throw Bag, please refer to Skill 28-1 on page 554.

Ring buoys can also be attached to throw bags or lines and used in a throw rescue. Although they are bulkier than other throw devices and the added weight can cause a slight injury if it hits the patient in the head, the patient really has no choice in the matter. The added weight can give the rescuer some better distance with the throw and the device provides better flotation assistance for the patient. The sidearm lob is the most common method used to throw this device correctly and accurately. Throwing the ring is performed by swinging it back and around, holding it by the inside of the ring or the rope attached to the sides. By using a body swing and releasing the device at the correct time, the ring will travel straight. However, this technique takes practice.

Boat-Based Rescues

If a patient is beyond the reach of a surface swimmer, using some type of watercraft may offer rescue crews more safety and speed when responding. Safety, for rescuers, is increased in a number of ways when using a boat, the most obvious being flotation. Rescuers don't have to swim when a boat is available, and less fatigue equals better performance from the crews. Although hypothermia, chemical exposure, debris, and currents can all injure or kill improperly equipped rescuers, watercraft can allow crews to deal safely with all these issues. Lighting can be carried and utilized on the water. Finally, and even more importantly, patient care can begin more quickly on a watercraft, even to the point of ALS measures being administered while en route back to shore.

Every watercraft has specific terms used to describe the areas or makeup of the boat. This holds true regardless of the model or type of boat (Table 28-2).[7]

The most common boats seen for rescue work in smaller inland waterways are inflatable boats and metal-hulled johnboats. **Inflatable boats** are exactly what the name implies, boats inflated with air. They have shorter gunwales, or sides, which can make it easier for a patient or rescuer to be parbuckled or retrieved into the boat, and also make it easier to deploy rescuers into the water. Inflatable craft are generally very light, making them capable of being carried to remote locations by rescuers. Even though they are smaller, they have a lower center of gravity compared to most rigid-hulled boats. This low-riding operation, coupled with an inflatable boat's main flotation being around the outside of it, makes these boats very, very stable in many types of water.

Many teams also use johnboats (aluminum "johns" are the most durable craft commonly in use). **Johnboats** are often made from aluminum, but may be constructed of fiberglass, or even steel in older models. The aluminum presents the best durability. Johnboats can range from 10 feet to upward of 16 or 18 feet, and are fairly easy to move with rescuers through tough terrain. Since aluminum is naturally light, they are also easy to slide, both on land and over ice. Johnboats can be rigged to carry sonar units, toolboxes, PFD lockers, and so on. However, every permanent modification adds more weight to the boat, making it harder to keep truly portable.

Swift Water Rescue

Swift water rescue can be especially hazardous to rescuers, due to the sheer force the water presents while moving. If a person falls in, there may be no quick jump back to the shore, and by the time the rescuer truly reacts, he may be yards downstream. Imagine the problem when a rescuer throws a line, and ends up being tangled to a large tree still moving downstream. Safety personnel play a very key part, not only to act as a safety net to rescuers, but to also give the patient one last chance at a rapid rescue should things go wrong upstream.

Most swift water evolutions are done with a primary crew and a backup crew to assist the rescuers if something goes wrong. Upstream spotters can be utilized to warn of larger debris sweeping into the rescue zone and should have radio or voice contact with the incident commander or the crews operating near the patient. Upstream spotters should also be placed far enough upstream that the rescuers have the needed time to adjust or move in case of a warning.

Downstream safety teams have the responsibility of being the backup rescuers in case someone is washed downstream. These positions should be placed on both banks if possible, or even on bridges or boats. Downstream safety personnel are the safety net in the operation, and should have the proper training and experience to be able to think quickly and safely during an emergency.

The throw bag is deployed in the same way, but the rescuer might now have to face a slippery bank or overhanging trees. A throw from the bank will let the rescuer then tension the line slowly, and use the force of the river to let the patient swing into the shore. This is called belaying, or simply holding the rope firm. If there is adequate space along the bank, a gentler way to swing a patient into shore is to manage the rope with a **dynamic belay** (Figure 28-27). The rescuer on shore

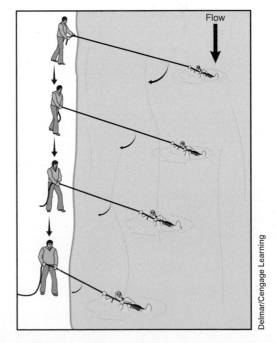

Figure 28-27 When using a dynamic belay technique, the rescuer moves downstream with the patient.

Table 28-2 Boat Terminology

Bow	The front of the boat
Stern	The rear of the boat
Gunwale	The vertical side of the boat
Port	The left side of the boat, looking to the bow
Starboard	The right side of the boat, looking to the bow

walks downstream along the bank, easing the tension on the line. Taking a short walk downstream may allow the patient to come ashore much closer to a shallow, calmer area.

Bridges are commonly found around water channels. For rescuers, they provide a location with good visibility of the water and normally good access to the water line. Smaller, vertically shorter spans give even better access. However, many rescuers will base a single line throw off the bridge. This leaves the patient hanging in the current with no place to go and possibly fighting anything that may wash downstream into him. If the rescuer throws the bag off the upstream side of the bridge, the line may be pulled so hard under the bridge decking that it cannot be moved along the bridge. Another option for rescuers, especially when operating off bridges or spans, is to use a droop line. A **droop line** is a rope held by two rescuers, one at each end of the span, or a distance apart, and used to literally drop a line onto the patient. Once the patient grabs the line, one of the rescuers lets go, and the patient will swing into shore. It is important that one rescuer let go, as the patient will be held in the water fighting current until one side is released.

A **ferry line**, which can also be called a **tension diagonal**, is simply a line stretched across moving water that is used to direct an object's movement to one side or the other (Figure 28-28). By setting the line at an angle to the current, and fastening the object to the line, the moving water will actually push the object laterally while pushing downstream. Ferry lines can be used as downstream safety lines for rescuers, for getting somewhere else to set up another aspect of the operation, or for reaching a patient who has made it to an island in the water. The line should be tight and may require a mechanical advantage system on one shore to accomplish this. The rescuer holds onto a pulley and carabiner, or even just a carabiner, clipped on the line at the upstream point, and lies on the back, with the arm holding the carabiner held above the head. The water will then push the body, but the angle of the rope will push the rescuer laterally to the other bank. A rescuer can be staged and waiting on a ferry line, and when the patient is secured the pair can be brought to shore. An even better technique is to add a short piece of netting that hangs from the line and is controlled with a rope from each bank. This way the patient can grab the netting, and the force of the water ferrying the patient will make the pull to shore very easy.

Two-line taglines are a good way to deploy and control a flotation object from each side of moving water. A line is deployed and operated on each side of the current, and each line is connected to the flotation device, which will be moving in the water flow (Figure 28-29). A low-head dam entrapment is a prime example of a tagline operation.

Operations on the water just upstream of the dam are normally a last-ditch effort, and are very risky to anyone in that area. Working below or downstream of the boil line, though, can provide a place of protection, even to the point of being able to ferry a line across the flowing water. Boats are commonly used to do this. Rescuers will need to be staged on either side of the water. In addition, safety personnel—either equipped with proper equipment or staged in watercraft—will provide a backup downstream and safety crew for the rescuers working upstream.

The line should be positioned across the water with a flotation object attached to the end of it. Ring buoys can be used in shorter, tamer rivers, as can several PFDs that are strapped together. Many teams and departments will fill a truck inner tube with expansion foam and add some webbing for handholds. These homemade rings will take a lot of abuse, offer great flotation, and cannot deflate. Another line is attached to the flotation device, and the original line is then hauled from the far bank. The near bank crew feeds their line out as the buoy is pulled into the flow. Moving upstream will place the buoy closer to the dam. If a patient is able to grab it, pulling quickly

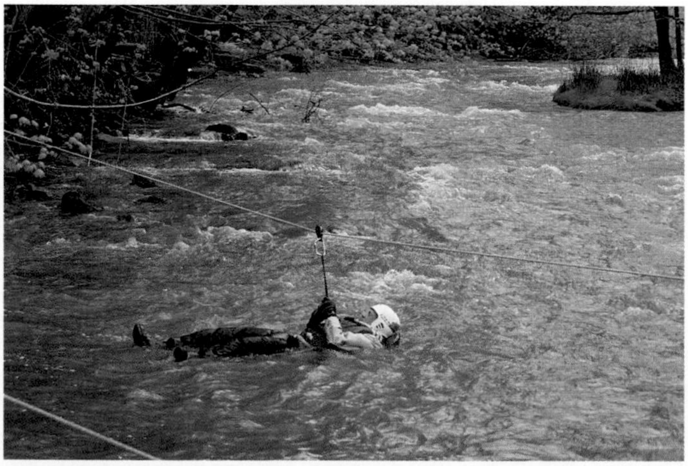

Figure 28-28 This rescuer is crossing a river on a ferry line.

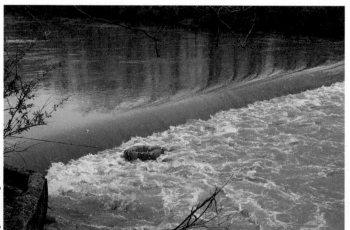

Figure 28-29 Two-line tethers often utilize some type of flotation device controlled with opposite lines from shore. The flotation device can be moved into the hazard by pulling or slacking each line.

downstream can usually get the patient and the flotation device out of the recirculation of the boil. Once this occurs, the patient can be laterally hauled to shore, or one line can be dropped or slackened to let the patient swing like a pendulum to shore.

A rescuer or patient experiencing a foot entrapment may be able to wiggle loose, especially if she has a walking pole. Leaning into the pole and forcing her body back upstream may allow the rescuer to slip the foot loose. However, if the rescuer or patient can't loosen the foot, there are other options using a throw bag or rope.

The first step is to stretch a rope immediately downstream of the rescuer or patient for support. Narrow rivers or channels can be spanned with a personal throw bag, and manned on each bank by other rescuers. This should take the initial pull off of the trapped foot and may allow the rescuer to be freed. In wider spans, rescuers staged in safe areas upstream may be able to float a loop of rope down to the rescuer, and control it from there. If needed, another rope can be deployed, low in the water. This rope is held low, and is pulled under the trapped patient's or rescuer's knees, in hopes of snagging the foot (Figure 28-30). Once the foot is snagged with the low rope, it might be possible to pull it loose by pulling upstream.

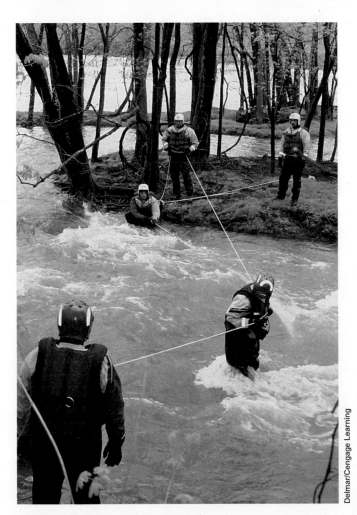

Figure 28-30 After supporting the trapped rescuer, a snag line can be lowered and pulled upstream to try to free the foot.

Surf Rescue

Because of the sheer size of the surf environment, the shore-based rescuer does not normally have a good situation for a rescue. Primarily, ring buoys or flotation devices may be thrown off piers to distressed swimmers, or at a very sharp shore dropoff the rescuer may use a throw bag. Most surf rescues will take place by highly trained lifeguards or rescue personnel, watercraft operators, or both.

Ice Rescue

Several shore-based techniques can be used for ice rescue. With a minimum of equipment, these rescue systems can be set up very quickly. The use of **hose inflator systems** is becoming more and more common, as fire companies get a productive tool that works with equipment every firefighter should know (Figure 28-31). A 50- or 100-foot section of two-and-one-half-inch or three-inch hose, and a self-contained breathing apparatus (SCBA) bottle, are the minimum tools used with an inflator system. The system consists of a threaded cap for the male end of the hose, most likely with an eye ring bolted through it, and a plug with an inflation valve or quick connect hose installed for the female end of the hose. A quick connect hose or valve system that uses air from an SCBA cylinder to inflate the hose completes the setup. Most systems have a pressure relief valve installed that limits working pressures to around 110 psi. There are a few key points to remember when using a hose inflator system, the first of which is someone needs to carry and control the SCBA bottle. A hose inflated to the maximum pressure will be very stiff, making a straight push into the water much easier. The rescuer controlling the SCBA bottle may have to open the valve occasionally to keep the pressure up.

The ring buoy is a great addition to the inflated hose. Ring buoys can be attached in such a fashion that the hose end is held up, keeping it from digging into loose snow or ice and jamming up. Webbing can then be used to lash the buoy to the hose with a clove hitch and a few half hitches. The

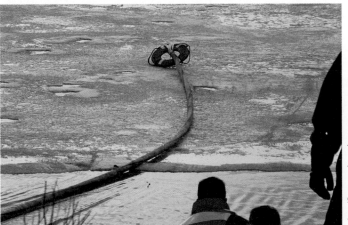

Figure 28-31 A typical hose inflator system is being used to push a buoy out onto the ice.

key is getting the buoy attached tightly. The rescuer should lash the buoy onto the hose before it is fully inflated. A tight attachment to the hose with the ring buoy lets the rescuers twist the hose and literally flip the buoy to either side on the ice, moving it laterally as needed. If taglines are attached and used as guides, remember that the harder the pull on the tagline to direct the hose end, the harder it will be to push the hose out. This may put "S" bends in the hose, instead of allowing it to move in a nice straight line.

Throw bags can be deployed in ice rescue as they are in any other water incident, with one twist. Due to the hypothermia, the patient may not be able to hang on to the bag, and rescuers may end up using the throw bag to provide time while other rescuers respond to the patient. The rescuer should deploy the bag as usual, with the knowledge that the patient will have to be pulled up and onto the ice shelf in order to be brought in. With the patient wearing heavy clothing, or lacking flotation assistance, it may be a difficult process for the rescuer. Most of the patient is below the direction of the pull, and it takes a great amount of leverage to "flip" or "pop" the patient up and onto the ice. Also, the cold water will make gripping the rope harder for the patient. If she cannot grip the rope, there is virtually no chance of getting her in on a line. In that event, the rescuer can try to get the patient to wrap an arm around the rope and then apply gentle pulling pressure. This will pin the patient to the ice shelf and buy some time while a boat or "go"-type rescue is performed.

Boat-Based Ice Rescue

Ice rescue is frequently done by way of pushing or pulling a boat out to the patient. Since the watercraft will float, the rescuers do not have to deal with the water. However, the boat must be tethered to the shore. This will let the shore crews pull the boat back in, making things faster and easier on the boat crews. Once arriving at the patient's location, the patient is extricated, generally from the stern of the boat, since that offers better stability than the sides. Often times, ALS care is actually initiated in the boat on the way to shore. Rescuers must remember to stay low and balanced, be wary of applying too much weight to the sides of the boat, and always wear a PFD.

Patient Treatment

Although the water environment is not truly suited to performing patient care, some procedures need to be started immediately regardless of the patient's location. However, there are still precautions to take. Often getting the patient out from the water is a challenge in its own right.

A **rescue tube**, a small foam tube, not only holds a patient up, but can also be used under a backboard to keep the patient floating (Figure 28-32). It should be remembered that once the patient is on a backboard, that patient has no way to protect his own airway, and he is now totally dependent on rescuers to keep them above the water surface.

Patients with cervical spine injuries are frequently encountered in water areas. Diving, water skiing, tubing, jumping off cliffs and bridges, and other events such as boat or vehicle accidents can result in injuries that present in the water. However, there are ways for the rescuers to maintain at least some cervical spine protection while packaging the patient.

One of the quickest ways to initially take care of the patient's head and neck is to simply extend the patient's arms up over his head and hold the arms together. This is sometimes known as the vise grip hold (Figure 28-33). This keeps the head from moving from side to side and/or rotating. If the patient—such as a water skier or swimmer—is wearing a PFD, it makes this entire scenario much easier in that the patient provides his own flotation assistance.

Backboards are a crucial part of cervical spine restriction, and they can be used in the water. Although some backboards do float, the majority of them do not supply enough flotation

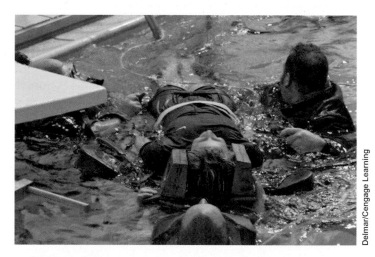

Figure 28-32 A rescue tube is used to assist with buoyancy of the patient on a backboard.

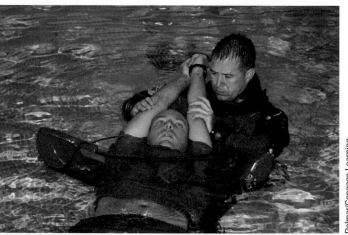

Figure 28-33 The patient is being held by the swimmer in the vise grip hold, which utilizes the patient's arms to provide spinal motion restriction.

for the patient. The way the patient lies on the board itself tends to present problems when the patient floats on them. They do not envelop the patient very well, and the backboard can get very tipsy in the water. The patient presents a very high center of gravity on the board, and the patient can easily slide off one side. In wave conditions this will be even more pronounced.

Often it takes several rescuers to properly immobilize the patient to the backboard. One rescuer should be specifically assigned to manually stabilize the patient's head and neck area and make sure the patient's head is not submerged. This rescuer also usually provides instructions to others while trying to keep the patient's body as straight as possible and in line from head to toe. Other rescuers can then move or float the backboard into place and position it under the patient. Moving the board into place from the feet keeps the rescuers in place on each side of the patient, resulting in better flotation. A key point for the rescuer to remember is to let the board float up to the patient, not sink the patient down to the board.

Flotation aids can be used with a backboard even more effectively, since the flotation device will support the board, which is supporting the patient. PFDs, ring buoys, or rescue tubes can all be used. Rescue tubes are very effective since they can be easily slid or forced under the backboard and create a natural sling effect. The rescue tube will also take on a crescent shape while floating, which cradles the backboard. The ring buoy can be used, but since the flotation device doesn't extend as well to the sides of the backboard, the backboard will have a tendency to tip or roll over in the water.

Stokes Basket Use

A piece of equipment that most rescue companies carry, or is sometimes found on ladder trucks, is the Stokes basket. The use of floating Stokes type baskets makes it easier to package any patient. The basket flotation is usually built in or attached around the sides of the basket, and the patient lies deeper in that basket, keeping him there.

The Stokes basket is used and maneuvered just like the backboard, in that one rescuer must control the patient's head and neck, and the other rescuers bring the basket to the feet of the patient, partially sink it, and move it underwater to a point under the patient. By releasing the pressure needed to sink the basket, the device will float into position and cradle the patient. A big concern is the flotation of the Stokes litter itself. There are ready-made, factory kits to provide flotation to the basket, but many agencies have adapted flotation on a litter by strapping or tying foam tubes or sealed plastic pipes to the sides of their basket. This is not a problem and can work very well, but it has to be tested in the water with sufficient weight before placing a patient on it.

The next step is moving the patient to the boat or dock. Some boats are equipped with small cranes that enable patients to be lifted onto the deck. This simplifies the process of lifting and moving the patient. Some rescue protocols state that once a patient is in the Stokes basket and secured to the backboard, the entire assembly goes to the emergency department until cleared by a physician.

▶ CASE STUDY CONCLUSION

The rescue is a success at several levels. First, no one on the rescue team is hurt. Although some folks got their "feet wet," that will be discussed in the post-incident debriefing. The patient, rescued by a shore-based water rescue team, has just a few abrasions. Although he is semiconscious, which many attribute to hypothermia, he seems no worse for the adventure. Nonetheless, the state police helicopter air-lifts the patient to the trauma center, just in case. All in all, the crew can celebrate a successful mission. Now it is time to pick up the equipment and put it back in service.

CRITICAL THINKING QUESTIONS

1. What personal protective equipment was needed by the rescuers?
2. What level of training is needed for shore-based water rescue?

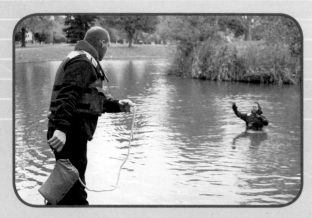

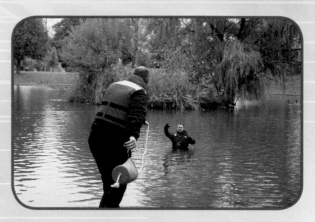

1 To make a proper throw, the rescuer first loosens the drawstring at the top of the bag. This lets the line in the bag deploy smoothly out in the air. If the string isn't loosened, the line inside may bind or ball up and stop the bag in midair before it gets to the patient. There should be a looped end on top of the stack of rope in the bag. The rescuer keeps this end either by gripping it or placing it under one of his feet. The rescuer should not place an arm through the loop, as the line may become entangled in something flowing downstream and might pull the rescuer into the water. Rather, the rescuer should keep hold of the end of the rope.

2 The rescuer holds the end of the rope and throws the bag underhanded, like a softball pitch.

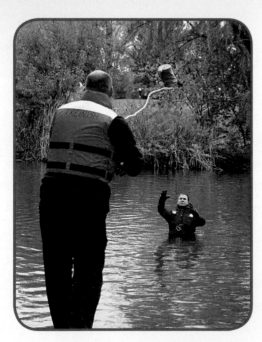

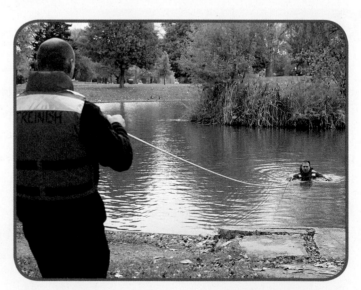

3 The rescuer obtains good aim and distance by relaxing a bit. The rescuer should aim for the patient but try to throw the bag past the actual location. It is generally a good idea to shout "ROPE!" when throwing. This noise may get the patient's attention so that she can see the rope being thrown.

4 A good throw places the rope on the patient's shoulder or at arm's length away. By aiming directly at the patient, the rescuer will likely place the rope short of him. By aiming past him, the rescuer lets the patient grab the rope directly, or the rope can be pulled in with the patient grabbing the bag and float as it passes through his hands. Grabbing the rope and pulling straight back a few steps will let the rescuer back away from the water's edge, so as to avoid being pulled into the water by the patient.

Delmar/Cengage Learning

CONCLUSION

The water rescue environment has many facets to it. From the largest floods to the smallest ponds, each rescue presents its own challenges and risks. Therefore, rescuers are urged to secure the best training and equipment that will be needed to keep the rescuers safe and give the public a thorough, well-trained team. It is important to remember that water conditions can change very quickly and a host of different problems can be encountered. Teams are well advised to complete advance planning to ascertain potential problems before the call comes in.

KEY POINTS:

- Response to water emergencies is part of the EMS duties.

- Water response is divided into surface water, swift water, dive rescue, surf rescue, and ice rescue.

- Identifying and preplanning for predictable water rescues improves rescuer performance.

- Agency response is a function of personnel, training, and equipment.

- Personal protective equipment includes a personal flotation device, water helmet, and personal throw bag.

- Self-rescue, using HELP or drownproofing, is a critical survival skill.

- Search and rescue includes active and passive search measures.

- Water rescue starts with the phrase: "Yo!, reach, throw, row, and go."

- Throw bags are an essential part of shore-based water rescue.

- Rope work is used extensively with swift water rescue.

- Spinal cord injury is a constant concern with all types of water rescue.

REVIEW QUESTIONS:

1. What are the four swift water directional terms?
2. What is the danger of a low-head dam?
3. What are the four types of ice?
4. What are the three types of waves in the surf?
5. What are the three water conditions?

CASE STUDY QUESTIONS:

Please refer to the Case Study in this chapter, and answer the questions below:

1. What are dangers of water rescue to the rescuer?
2. What are dangers of water emergencies to the patient?
3. Why would the patient be airlifted to a trauma center?

REFERENCES:

1. Ray F. *Swiftwater Rescue: A Manual for the Rescue Professional*. Ashville, North Carolina: CFS Press; 1997.

2. National Severe Storm Lab. Questions and answers about floods: flood basics. Available at: **http://www.nssl.noaa.gov/primer/flood.** Accessed April 15, 2010.

3. Brewster BC, ed. *Open Water Lifesaving, the United States Lifesaving Association Manual* (2nd ed.). Boston, MA: Pearson; 2003.

4. Naval Sea Systems Command. Guidance for diving in contaminated waters. 2008. Available at: **http://yosemite.epa.gov/r10/oea.nsf/Investigations/Dive%20Team%20Safety/$FILE/Navy%20Contaminated%20Dive%20Guidance.pdf.** Accessed April 18, 2010.

5. United States Navy. United States Naval Diving Manual Rev. 5. 2005. Available at: **http://www.uscg.mil/FOIA/healy/Number%20101-218/num_181.pdf.** Accessed April 18, 2010.

6. United States Coast Guard. Personal floatation device selection, use, wear & care. Available at: **http://www.uscg.mil/hq/cg5/cg5214/pfdselection.asp#DEFINITIONS.** Accessed April 18, 2010.

7. Maloney ES, ed. *Chapman Piloting and Seamanship* (65th ed.). New York, NY: Sterling Publisher; 2006.

CHAPTER 29

WILDERNESS SEARCH AND RESCUE

KEY CONCEPTS

Upon completion of this chapter, it is expected that the reader will understand these following concepts:

- Levels of search and rescue training
- Direct and indirect search methods
- Search principles
- ICS in search and rescue

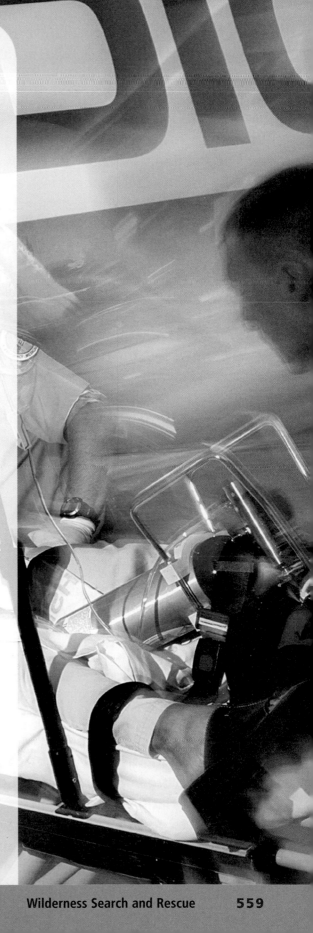

CASE STUDY:

In early June of 1990, 38-year-old David Boomhower set out on the 133-mile-long Northville-Lake Placid (NLP) trail in upstate New York. He intended to take a south to north route, which is the common direction of travel for NLP thru-hikers. Mr. Boomhower intended to complete the entire length of the NLP trail in 10 days, which would have him contacting his family sometime on June 15. On June 8, he encountered another person in the West Canada Lakes area of the trail. This was the last time David Boomhower was seen alive. On June 17, two days after his intended completion date, his family alerted the authorities.

CRITICAL THINKING QUESTIONS

1. What are the four goals of a search and rescue?
2. How is EMS involved in a wilderness search and rescue?

OVERVIEW

When searching for a lost person, time is a critical element. A study of 2,302 wilderness search and rescue (SAR) missions published in the *Journal of Wilderness and Environmental Medicine* in 2007 indicated that "time alone was the strongest predictor of survival."[1] Paramedics may be called upon to respond and participate in a wilderness search and rescue.

Search and rescue missions can be labor intensive and have many phases. Even so, despite the rescuers' best efforts, the lost person may not be found. Search and rescue incident management is no different from that used in mass-casualty incidents, fire scene operations, or large law enforcement incidents. In fact, a search and rescue mission may encompass all of those across multiple jurisdictions and multiple agencies. The incident described in the case study required government agencies, local law enforcement, formal established volunteer search teams, individual untrained volunteers, and even psychics. Without a solid management system, this group of people would operate under conditions of mass chaos that may have put searchers at undue risk, not to mention diminish the chances for a successful mission.

As discussed previously, the common management system or Incident Command System (ICS) used in the United States for any complex incident is the National Incident Management System (NIMS). NIMS and ICS for wilderness search and rescue will be discussed specifically later in this chapter.

With the publishing of the first National Search and Rescue Plan in 1956, the U.S. Coast Guard was designated the federal agency responsible for maritime search and rescue, whereas the U.S. Air Force was designated the federal agency responsible for federal level search and rescue for the inland regions.

In order to meet the need for trained Coast Guard and Air Force search and rescue (SAR) planners, the joint service National Search & Rescue School was established at Governors Island, New York, in April of 1966. This facility was devoted exclusively to training professionals to conduct search and rescue. In 1999, the government launched the National Search and Rescue Plan (NSP). The National Response Framework, a part of the all-hazards response plan, has since replaced the NSP.[2]

This updated and more comprehensive plan is a road map for all federal agencies involved in U.S. search and rescue operations and outlines how a U.S. response dovetails with their international commitments to provide aid abroad. Along with the NSP, the government also formed the **National Search and Rescue Committee (NSARC)**. The primary federal agencies on the NSARC are the Department of Transportation, the Department of Defense (DOD), the Department of Commerce, the Federal Communications Commission (FCC), the National Aeronautics and Space Administration (NASA), and the Department of the Interior. Additionally, there are several non-governmental organizations that provide training and organizational assistance to search and rescue teams across the United States, such as the **National Association for Search and Rescue (NASAR)** a nonprofit association dedicated to advancing professional, literary, and scientific knowledge in fields related to search and rescue, and the **Mountain Rescue Association (MRA)**, a critical mountain search and rescue organization that is among the oldest SAR associations in the United States.

The Four Goals of Search and Rescue

The goal of all search and rescue operations can be summed up in the mnemonic **LAST**: **L**ocate, **A**ccess, **S**tabilize, **T**ransport. Locating a patient can be a simple task with quick results and little financial cost, or a very complex operation over an extended time utilizing many resources at very high cost. Access to a patient can involve anything from the ability to walk right up to him unimpeded to complex technical rope systems for low to high angle or swift water rescue. Stabilization may require medical personnel at the basic or advanced levels. The patient's condition many times may dictate transportation as well as extrication methods. Other factors relating to how a patient is to be accessed and transported are weather, terrain, available manpower resources, equipment, and—most importantly—risk to searchers and patients.

Search and rescue missions are diverse in nature and are subject to variables such as weather, terrain, local hazards, and resources. The key questions that need to be asked are what resources are available and how can these resources be used most effectively?

Wilderness Search and Rescue Standards

The National Fire Protection Agency (NFPA) addresses wilderness search and rescue in its standard on operations for technical search and rescue incidents, NFPA 1670. **NFPA 1670** stresses the need for the agency having jurisdiction (AHJ) to preplan and break preplanning down into three steps.

The AHJ must perform a hazard analysis of its environment including assessment of areas where there is a high probability of lost persons (popular camping or hiking areas) or high life hazard (mountainous terrain). After an evaluation of the environmental and physical factors, the AHJ must consider hazard mitigation, which is a part of risk management; for example, the AHJ may create a technical rope team to support a search and rescue operation in mountainous terrain.

As a part of preplanning, the AHJ should establish a set of clear operational procedures in a formal written document. Often it is best if the incident response plan is vetted among all potential responders, whether they are police, fire, or EMS, as well as rangers and local search and rescue. This helps to ensure intra-agency cooperation and prevents confusion at the scene.

Finally, the AHJ should proceed with preparations, such as procuring equipment and training responders. Preparations and training should include consideration of locally driven conditions that may affect a search and rescue situation (Table 29-1).

Although some of these factors (such as altitude) are constant and predictable, others (such as weather) are not. Therefore, the AHJ's standard operating procedures (SOP)

Table 29-1 Factors Affecting a Search and Rescue

- Temperature
- Weather
- Terrain
- Flora and fauna
- Altitude
- Travel time
- Patient care
- Duration of incident
- Logistics
- Communications
- Navigation
- Management needs

NFPA 1670:10.4.6.

must take into consideration variables that can impact the operation. For example, although medical evacuation by helicopter might be expeditious and desirable, it may not be an option if weather prohibits flight. Some SOPs fail to take into consideration that a search and rescue may be protracted for days or weeks. These missions, sometimes involving hundreds of responders, may require resources (e.g., food, lodging, and logistical support) that are beyond the capabilities of a local fire department or rescue squad. In those instances, it is essential that state and even federal resources be included in the SOP. Many searches have used the valuable services of the National Guard, an organization that is prepared for prolonged operations and has excellent logistical support.

Search and Rescue Training

Like other technical operations standards, NFPA 1670 breaks training into three levels: Awareness, Operations, and Technician. At the **Awareness level** the Paramedic is expected to recognize the need for a wilderness search and rescue and initiate a rescue response. Following notification, the Awareness-trained Paramedic will establish Incident Command, including scene control. With knowledge of the potential hazards unique to the area, the Paramedic will put into motion resources to mitigate those hazards. Finally, the Paramedic will identify, isolate, and interrogate any witnesses or persons with knowledge of the lost person.

At the Operations level, the Paramedic starts the process of establishing a wilderness search and rescue with a set of SOPs. This might include "size-up" of the situation and a request for additional or specialized resources (e.g., technical rope teams). Part of the size-up involves deciding whether the operation is a rescue operation or a recovery.

The Operations level Paramedic is expected to obtain information about terrain. This includes procuring navigation aids such as topographic maps and weather forecasts for Incident Command. Beyond providing medical care to the patient, the Operations-level Paramedic may become involved in the search and rescue using **land navigation (landnav)** techniques, including map and compass, as well as **geographical information systems (GIS)**, which utilize global positioning satellites (GPS). The Paramedic must be trained in personal survival as well as equipped with the personal medical and support equipment required for wilderness search and rescue operations.

The Paramedic trained as a **search and rescue Technician** must also be trained to the Technician level for rope rescue and to the Awareness level for water rescue. The search and rescue Technician is capable of executing a search and rescue. It should be noted that this level does not automatically assume capabilities in rescues such as cave or alpine, for example.

Starting with participation in preplanning, the search and rescue Technician is able to participate in all phases of a search and rescue. This includes termination, incident critique, and debriefing.

Search and Rescue Operations

Regardless of the type of incident, all search and rescue missions should have several components in common. This is called the search and rescue incident cycle and the components are preplanning, notification and response, call-out and check-in, briefing, assignment, debriefing, check-out, and incident critique.

Preplanning and Preparation

Preplanning is a critical first step in mitigating serious issues and risk to searchers and patients. The preplanning phase takes into account the type of incident(s) anticipated: cave, high angle, woodland search, swift water, open water, and so on.

Potential resources need to be identified or developed locally and proper searcher training needs to be in place for searchers to maintain both initial and ongoing skill proficiency. Training in many technical disciplines is available at the Awareness, Operations, and Technician levels, as discussed earlier. Searchers need to acquire equipment equal to the anticipated mission, environment, and hazards likely to be encountered, and they need to be thoroughly trained in its use, handling, storage, and maintenance as well.

Once acquired, equipment will need to be "cached" or stored in accessible areas for mission deployment. This means that it is possible for a search and rescue team to have more than one equipment cache depending on the area covered and the hazards/risks anticipated.[3]

Notification and Response

When a person is reported as lost, the first step in notification is deployment. Accuracy and completeness of information provided in the notification leads to a successful search and rescue mission.

This information is obtained, sometimes by the Paramedic, from the person reporting the incident and from witnesses on-scene. The use of a **Lost Person Questionnaire** is recommended by NASAR and other organizations as a way to focus rescue personnel on important information that will speed the potential rescue of the subject (Figure 29-1).

The information gathered in the Lost Person Questionnaire includes the person's name, age, detailed physical description, and past medical history. The questionnaire also includes what the person was last seen wearing and items the person possessed or carried. In a wilderness setting, the items the person has is critical information. First, if these items become discarded along the subject's path, they become clues. In many instances, searchers are not looking directly for the patient but for clues that will help the searchers determine the subject's movement and direction. This helps to narrow the focus of the search to a smaller area. This area, called the **probability of area (POA)**, is determined by knowledge of the patient and the statistical probability that the subject is within an area (this concept is expanded shortly). Second, these clues can help rescuers decide what equipment to carry (e.g., clothing, food, and medical supplies).

An important question is whether the lost person has a cell phone. Many search and rescue missions in state and national parks are significantly aided with the use of cell phones. As a matter of fact, many times a "lost" party will call 9-1-1 and be able to be talked out of the predicament. Furthermore, cell phone calls can be triangulated to reveal the caller's location.

An important question pertains to the subject's **point last seen (PLS)**. The searcher can use the place last seen and the subject's age, physical condition, experience in the wilderness, and so on, to help determine the search perimeter. Even the subject's type of footwear is very important.

Once the initial detailed information is gathered, appropriate resources need to be called out. Having the Lost Person Questionnaire completed prior to the call-out is important to determine what resources are needed (e.g., a team with technical rope skills, water rescue, or cave rescue teams).

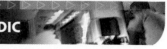

PROFESSIONAL PARAMEDIC

The rescuer should protect the point last seen. The subject's footprints and other signs may suggest the direction of travel, among other information. Therefore, the rescue team must keep well-meaning responders from trampling the trail. Even car exhaust can obscure a scent trail.

Lost Person Questionnaire

Investigator

Date	Time	District Mission Number	Recording Official

Source of Information

Name	Address	Town	St

Relationship to Subject	Phone Number	Second Phone

How / Where to Contact Now	How / Where to Contact Later

What Informant Believes to Have Happened

Subject Information

Name	Age	Sex	Nickname(s)

Home Address	Town	St	Zip

Local Address	Town	St	Zip

Home Phone	Local Phone	D.O.B.	Birthplace

Physical Description

Identification	Clothing / Style	Color	Size	Health
Height:	Shirt / Sweater:			Overall Health:
Weight:	Pants:			Physical Condition:
Age:	Outer Wear:			Medical Problems:
Build:	Inner Wear:			Psychological Problems:
Complexion:	Head Wear:			Medication:
Distinguishing Marks:	Rain Wear:			Amounts:
Eyes:	Gloves:			Consequences of Loss:
Hair Color:	Extra Clothing:			Eyesight w/o Glasses:
Hair Style:	Footwear:			Medic-Alert:

☐ Beard ☐ Jewelry
☐ Mustache ☐ Photo Available?
☐ Sideburns ☐ Return Photo?
☐ Glasses ☐

☐ Sole Sample Available
☐ Scent Articles Available
☐ Scent Articles Secured
☐ Clothing Visible from Air?

☐ Smoker ☐ Hitchhiker
☐ Alcohol ☐ Religious
☐ Drugs ☐ Educated
☐ Gum ☐ Local Hero
☐ Candy ☐ Extravert
☐ A Leader ☐ Introvert
☐ A Survivor ☐ Loner
☐ Legal Problems ☐ Depressed
☐ Personal Problems ☐

Youth / Child

☐ Afraid of Dark
☐ Afraid of Animals
☐ Afraid of Strangers
☐ Cry When Hurt
☐ Cry When Scared
☐ Hides When Afraid
☐ HUG-A-TREE Trained
☐ Has a Safety Word

Equipment

☐ Pack ☐ Stove ☐ Skis
☐ Tent ☐ Fuel ☐ Snowshoes
☐ Sleeping Bag ☐ Compass ☐ Money
☐ Ground Cloth ☐ Map ☐ Credit Cards
☐ Fishing Gear ☐ Food ☐ Other Documents
☐ Climbing Gear ☐ Knife ☐ Rope
☐ Liquid Container ☐ Camera ☐ Camp Tools
☐ Fire Starter ☐ Lens ☐

Continue ➡

Page 1

ICS SAR 201B

Rev. 6-17-97 ICS Forms Online

Figure 29-1 The Lost Subject Questionnaire is a way to focus rescue personnel on important information that will speed the potential rescue of the subject.

Place Last Seen

Date	Time	Common Name / Description

Description	Additional Comments
Subject Last Seen by:	
Talked to Subject About:	
Weather at That Time:	
Weather Since:	
Subject's Direction of Travel:	
Subject's Attitude:	
Subject's Condition:	

Subject's Trip Plans

Itenerary	Transportation	Additional Comments
Started At:	Transported By:	
Date:	Vehicle Location:	
Time:	Make / Model:	
Destination:	License:	
By Way of:	Vehicle Location Confirmed by:	
Purpose:	Time Confirmed:	
Length of Stay:	Additional Vehicles at Scene:	
Size of Group:	Alternate Plans / Routes:	
Has Subject Made This Trip Before:	Discussed With:	

Subject's Outdoor Experience

General Experience		Additional Comments
☐ Familiar With Area	☐ Travels Alone	
☐ In Area Recently	☐ Stays on Route	
☐ Formal Outdoors Training	☐ Travels X-C	
☐ Medical Training	☐ Lost Before	
☐ Scouting	☐ Will Stay Put	
☐ Military	☐ Keeps on Move	
☐ Overnight	☐ Climber	
☐	☐ Athletic	

Contacts Upon Reaching Civilization

Name of Person That Subject Would Contact	Relationship	Phone	Who Is There Now

Overdue Groups

Description	Group Characteristics
Kind of Group:	Personality Clashes:
Leader:	Actions If Separated:
Experience of Group / Leader:	Competitive Spirit:
Local Point of Contact:	Intragroup Dynamics:

Actions Taken So Far

By Family / Friends	By Others

ICS SAR 201B

Rev. 6-17-97 ICS Forms Online

Lost Person Questionnaire Page 2

Figure 29-1 (continued)

Call-Out

With the information on the subject, and information about the type of search incident, the next step is to assemble searchers. The basic information that should be communicated to searchers in the call-out is the basic subject information, type of incident, how long the subject has been missing, descriptions of the terrain, current and forecasted weather conditions for the search area, the staging area to report to, and the check-in procedure. This can include designation of radio frequencies for tactical operations as well as command frequencies.

The size of the search area exponentially increases with each hour of delay. Therefore, the AHJ should not delay nor be afraid of false alarms. If the subject is found quickly, with or without the help of responders, it was a successful mission.

Strategy and Planning

Once all of the subject information is in hand, the searchers are notified. The next step for the search manager is to plan a search strategy. Determining where to deploy the first searchers and who to use is an important initial decision. Generally, it is best to do a **hasty search** first (i.e., a search of the "high probability" areas). The high probability areas are where the subject is likely to be found and is discussed in more detail shortly. If none of these initial attempts are fruitful, it becomes necessary to plan for a more detailed, resource-intensive operation.

Check-in

Personnel accountability is a key concept for all emergency operations, and search and rescue incidents are no different. Once a call-out has been initiated, responding searchers must respond to a designated location and, in most incidents, formally check-in with Incident Command or a designee. Often, the check-in is at a trailhead or parking lot proximal to the place last seen. The searcher will usually be assigned to a group or team and sent for a detailed briefing on the specific tasks that will be required.

Briefing and Assignment

Briefings, consisting of general information shared with the searchers about the incident and the objectives, as well as specific information gained from the Lost Person Questionnaire, should be factual and concise. During this briefing, additional information about the specific areas a searcher will be working in—including terrain, hazards, and expected weather, as well as group and personal equipment needed—will be conveyed to the searchers. The searchers should discuss communication methods, including radio frequencies, any codes necessary for the operation, and times for radio check-in.

Once assigned to a team and given an objective, searchers need to be self-sufficient in terms of personal equipment and appropriate clothing for the season and environment. They should be skilled in the tasks they have been assigned and physically as well as mentally prepared for the task.

Typically, the operational period for a team is during the hours of daylight due to obvious safety concerns. However, dawn-to-dusk operations have their own perils. If the team is in the field for more than 12 hours, the searchers become exhausted and the search becomes compromised. Many search managers will put a team in the field for 10 hours, with eight hours spent in active search activities and one hour each of briefing and debriefing with the search manager and the command staff.

Debriefing and Check-Out

Debriefing is the process of relating all information gained by a searcher during an assignment to the search management. All observations made by a searcher should be related such as search area description, field of vision, and size of area covered, as well as any areas that were assigned but not covered. After debriefing, if there are no other assignments, the searcher should formally "check-out" with Incident Command.

Critique

A **mission critique** is best done shortly after the incident. This affords the best recollection of events and the best opportunity for searchers to express factual information regarding improvement of the process or review of something that worked particularly well during the incident. Searchers should also do a personal critique which should include a review of the gear needed but not provided, gear carried but not used, personal skill review, and physical condition.

Search and Rescue Incident Management

As mentioned earlier, a system of management is necessary for several reasons: someone needs to be in charge, each participant needs to know what to do and when to do it, resources need to be acquired, and their location needs to be made known. An incident management system needs to have many characteristics including flexibility, simplicity, and cost effectiveness.

An incident may change after the initial response. As time goes on, the mission may grow, be scaled back, or redirected to another area altogether. Every search mission needs to be scalable and, therefore, flexible.

A management system needs to be a simple, easily understood structure that can be used consistently by any agency, in any area, for any type of emergency. A complex or confusing search management system will only lead to confusion and lost efficiency.

A search and rescue mission can quickly grow, so keeping costs on par with the expected outcome is critical. If the probability increases that the subject is deceased, the mission becomes one of recovery rather than rescue. A recovery is not as time-sensitive, and far fewer personnel and resources are needed.

The search manager must make efficient use of resources and obtain the most coverage for the man-hours spent searching. Sometimes it is more cost effective to have a helicopter perform an aerial search over a broad area, though this can be expensive, as opposed to having dozens of searchers on foot ("ground pounders)."

Efficiency is the key to the modern search. As mentioned earlier, many search managers have started to use geographical information systems (GIS) instead of outdated topographic maps. The GIS integrates the most current digitally enhanced topographic maps with satellite imagery as well as real-time aerial photography. Some GIS systems even combine handheld global positioning satellites reporting to provide real-time displays of searchers in the field. This feature not only improves search assignments, by preventing overlap, but can also enhance searcher safety by identifying potential hazards before the searchers are in peril.

Search and Rescue and NIMS

The system used for incident management in the United States, the Incident Command System (ICS), was developed in the 1970s and meets all of the previous criteria. More recently, the terrorist attacks of September 11, 2001, led to the creation of the Department of Homeland Security and the formation of the National Incident Management System (NIMS).

NIMS establishes ICS as a standard incident management organization with five functional areas—command, operations, planning, logistics, and finance/administration—for management of all major incidents, as discussed previously in Chapter 20.

To ensure further coordination, and during incidents involving multiple jurisdictions or agencies, the principle of Unified Command has been universally incorporated into NIMS. This Unified Command not only coordinates the efforts of many jurisdictions, but provides for and assures joint decisions on objectives, strategies, plans, priorities, and public communications.

Communications and Information Management

Since standardized communications are essential during an incident, NIMS prescribes interoperable communications systems for both incident and information management. Responders and managers across all agencies and jurisdictions must have a common operating picture for a more efficient and effective incident response.

Preparedness and Interoperability

Preparedness incorporates a range of measures, actions, and processes and is accomplished before an incident happens. NIMS preparedness measures include planning, training, exercises, qualification and certification, equipment acquisition and certification, and publication management.

All of these measures serve to ensure that pre-incident actions are standardized and consistent with mutually agreed upon doctrine. NIMS further places emphasis on mitigation activities to enhance preparedness. Mitigation includes public education and outreach, structural modifications to lessen the loss of life and destruction of property, code enforcement in support of zoning rules, land management and building codes, and flood insurance and property buy-out for frequently flooded areas.

Joint Information System (JIS)

NIMS organizational measures enhance public communications. The NIMS advocates the Joint Information System (JIS) and provides the public with timely and accurate incident information and unified public messages. This system employs Joint Information Centers (JIC) and brings Incident Command and staff together during an incident to develop, coordinate, and deliver a unified message. This will ensure that federal, state, and local levels of government are releasing the same information during an incident.[4]

Search Theory and Tactics

The NASAR textbook *Fundamentals of Search and Rescue* states: "**Search theory** is a mathematical approach to determining how best to find that which we seek, and the principles of search theory apply to any situation where the objective is to find, in the most efficient manner, a person or object contained in some geographic area."[5]

Much of search theory originated from World War II. In the 1950s, the U.S. Coast Guard developed a methodology for search theory that was published in the first edition of the U.S. National Search and Rescue manual in late 1959. The principles described in the manual have been adapted for use in inland search operations and are the standard from which modern day search tactics are modeled.

Once a search plan has been established, the team must determine what tactics or specific actions are needed to carry out the plan in the most efficient and successful manner. Search tactics include all the actions employed by the search manager. These actions are progressive and are either indirect or direct.[5]

Indirect Search Tactics

Most searches utilize **indirect search tactics**, which are actions that do not take place in the search area itself. Nonetheless, these are some of the first actions taken. During this time, information is gathered and a further assessment of the situation can be made with this new data. It is possible that indirect tactics alone may result in finding the subject. Indirect tactics focus on fact finding, attraction, and containment.

Those managing the search usually carry out fact finding. Information can be gathered in a variety of ways, although the Lost Person Questionnaire mentioned earlier serves as the basis. Fact finding as an indirect tactic continues throughout the operation and long after the formal search has concluded.

Attraction is a method of encouraging the patient to come to the searchers or move to a specific location. The use of whistles, public address systems, and sirens are methods of attraction. It is important for the searchers to provide for periods of silence during the search, as this gives the subject the chance to respond in some fashion, such as by yelling. However, attraction does not work with some search subject types who may intentionally try to avoid searchers, such as despondent persons or psychotics.

Containment techniques are critical to mission success. **Containment** involves establishing a best guess perimeter to contain the subject and limit the search area. Often roads and trails are used to create a containment area. This will be discussed shortly.

Direct Search Tactics

The search manager's objective is to maximize the **probability of success (POS)** (i.e., chance of finding the patient) by bringing all available resources together, defining the search area (probability of area or POA), and determining which area has the highest **probability of detection (POD)** (i.e., chance the subject is in the area searched). The manager then creates a direct tactic to achieve that goal.

Direct tactics, or searches targeted toward actually finding the missing individual, are typically thought of as **ground searching** (conducting the search on foot). However, that is not always the case. **Aerial reconnaissance** (using aircraft to conduct a search) can be part of the direct search tactics. These are all actions taken inside the search area. These tactics include hasty searches, loose grid searches, and tight grid searches.

To constitute a search, the area must be effectively swept after clues to the subject's presence have been eliminated. A measure of the area that is effectively searched is a function of search speed, endurance, and effective search width, which will be discussed shortly.

Factors affecting how effective a search is can include coverage and search width. **Coverage** is the measure of a search area effectively swept versus the area searched and is a reflection of thoroughness. Good coverage means that no clues were found where none existed and the subject is not in the area. Effective **search width** is a measure of the effectiveness with which a particular sensor (person or dog) can detect a particular object under specific environmental conditions.

Based on search width and coverage, the search manager can project the probability of detection, assuming the subject was in the segment searched.[5]

It should be emphasized that in many cases the searchers are not looking for the subject but rather for clues indicating the subject's direction of travel and general location, as a means to narrow down the search area. It is critical that searchers note and document the location of clues, using GPS whenever possible. These clues determine the subject's

last known position (LKP), as opposed to the place last seen, and help to narrow the search perimeters, increasing the probability of detection in the process. The last known position helps the search manager establish the subject's general direction and speed of travel, which helps establish a new starting point for the search.

Hasty Search

Although some would advocate holding off a search, for fear of ruining scent trails, among other disruptions, every search is an emergency and should be undertaken as soon as possible. However, there are searches, such as a hasty search, that have a high probability of success with low risk of disruption to track and trail.

A hasty search, as the name implies, is a fast search of high probability areas such as trails, roadways, and along streams. In general, a hasty search is done wherever there is a probable line of travel.

The goal of a hasty search is to find either clues or the subject in the first minutes to hours before more complex, resource-intensive search tactics are employed. Hasty searches have a high probability of success and are conducted by small (two to four searchers), highly mobile teams of skilled searchers (these are formally referred to as **Type I searchers**). Type I searchers are often trained to the Awareness and/or Operations level and their searches are conducted by local resources. Hasty searches start at the last known point (LKP), or the point last seen (POS), and follow common paths, roads, and so on. These searchers often move at a fast pace, checking areas where a subject might go if injured as well as looking for clues (i.e., footprints, broken branches, pieces of clothing, etc.).

It is important that a hasty search does not "go off trail," as searchers may unwittingly trample signs or disturb scent trails. Often a hasty search is performed until a perimeter is established. At that point, the search manager establishes posts with sentries looking for the subject to come out of the area. This, in effect, creates a containment area.

The containment area is determined by time, the subject's physical condition, weather, and so on, and limits the search area. Searchers in easily identifiable vehicles, such as those equipped with flashing lights, and a pair of binoculars can monitor a long stretch of straight woods.

Bastard Search

Some consider the bastard search part of the hasty search. However, a **bastard search** involves looking for any place that can provide food, water, shelter, or medical attention. Typically, law enforcement officers, who are highly mobile and have good communications, go to locations where the subject might turn up or be delivered. Examples of these locations include hospital emergency departments, local shelters, police or fire stations, and even homes in the vicinity of the place the subject was last seen.

Many subjects seek shelter in storm drains, buildings, and other shelters. However, these structures may not be safe. Using USAR methods, these structures should be searched and then properly identified using the standard symbols.

Grid Searches

When a search is shown on television, the searchers are often seen walking in lines through the brush. These were referred to as **Type II searchers** in the past. These searchers cover more specifically defined areas, with searchers organized into search lines with specific boundaries, which are usually drawn on a map. Many times the searchers use terrain features such as ridges, water, and roadways as guidelines. Each searcher is responsible for a search lane, an area parallel to adjacent searchers and continually scanned by the searcher in that lane. Spacing between searchers and the method used by searchers to scan an area are different depending on the type of grid search employed. Grid searches are of two types: loose grid and tight grid.

Loose grid searches are usually done in teams of no more than seven search and rescue Technicians (three searchers is the ideal number). They are tasked with quickly covering an area larger than that searched by the hasty team. This is a much less thorough type of search and is designed to yield clues over a wide area in a relatively short period of time (Figure 29-2).

Searchers deployed for a loose grid type search form up on a search baseline and are widely spaced. They take random paths in the same general direction and visually scan between themselves and their adjacent searchers. They should remain in either voice or, if possible, visual contact as the terrain allows. This type of search also requires the searcher to have some skill at land navigation with GPS and/or map and compass because specific search guides are often based on map coordinates.

Loose grid searches are generally the next logical step after a hasty search has taken place and are especially important if clues were found during the hasty search. Clue consciousness is especially important for participants in a loose grid search. As the name implies, **clue consciousness** is high awareness of potential field clues and the mindset that clues can come from unexpected sources. Clues can be organized into various categories (Table 29-2). There are usually more clues than search subjects, so the first search priority is detecting clues. This process requires experience and practice.

When a clue is found, it must be preserved and recorded. Some searchers use waterproof sketchpads to document

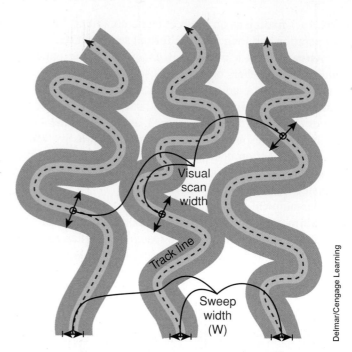

Figure 29-2 Example of a loose grid search pattern where the three-person team is free to follow a widely varying path to cover a significant amount of territory in a short period of time.

Table 29-2 Clue Categories

- Physical
  - Footprints
  - Clothing
- Documents
  - Trail head logs or registers
  - Summit flags
- Testimony
  - Witnesses
  - Family
- Events
  - Flashing light
  - Smoke
  - Reflective surfaces (mirrors)
- Rational
  - Obvious trails

the time, position, object, and so on. With the advent of personal cell phone cameras, some searchers have turned to photographing the evidence and then transmitting the photograph to the search manager. Both a closeup photograph, with a common object such as a coin used in the picture for comparison, as well as a distance shot, showing terrain, are desirable.[5]

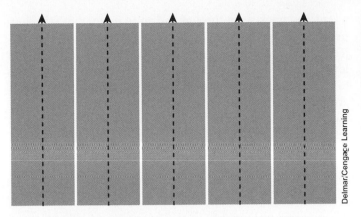

Figure 29-3 Tight grid searches are more methodical and time and resource intensive than loose grid searches.

Table 29-3 Sign Cutting

- Natural
  - Depressed stone in the soil
  - Disturbed soil
  - Disturbed plants
  - Scratches on rock
  - Bruised or broken vegetation
  - Embedded soil on underside of leaf
  - Disturbed animal droppings
  - Path in the frost or dew
- Man-made
  - Cigarette butts
  - Candy wrappers
  - Articles of clothing

PROFESSIONAL PARAMEDIC

In some cases, a clue is actually evidence of a criminal event. As such, the evidence should be preserved for law enforcement. Preserving evidence can save investigators hours of time.

Tight grid searches are very slow, methodical, and thorough, yielding high coverage of the search area. In a tight grid search, personnel, formerly called **Type III searchers**, are aligned in a parallel or echelon formation of equal spacing as the terrain allows (Figure 29-3). Each searcher has a specific field of view for the search area between himself and other searchers called a **sweep width**. The field of view generally extends half way between the searcher and adjacent searchers.

Thoroughness as opposed to speed is the key aspect of tight grid searches. Because this type of search involves more people in a given area, particular attention needs to be paid to searcher movement, line formation, and preservation of clues. This type of search is used when the faster methods of hasty and loose grid searches have not been successful. Tight grid searches are also used when the subject, such as an autistic child or an elderly person with dementia, may be avoiding searchers or if the search has changed from a rescue mission to one of body recovery.

Tracking

Tracking dates back to Native American trackers, wilderness guides, and Cavalry scouts, to name a few historical figures noted for their tracking skills. **Tracking** is looking for evidence that a subject has been in a given area, rather than looking for the subject himself. Tracking is performed by both humans and dogs. Humans are looking for visual evidence, what is referred to as a **sign**. A sign can be broken twigs on a limb of a tree, scuff marks in vegetation, trampled vegetation, a stone pushed into the soil, or anything else that does not look natural or looks out of place compared to the surrounding environment.

Of course, one of the best signs is an impression of the subject's footwear left in soft soil. The National Park Service SAR teams will actually create "track traps" to try and capture this sign. Built out of sand, these track traps are raked smooth and then frequently checked for evidence of tracks. Although tracking is a difficult skill in which to become proficient, track awareness is something that all searchers should be trained in.

The best time of day to track is during the early morning or evening, when tangential light highlights the contour of a sign. It is even possible to track at night provided that the trail can be illuminated. Heat, sunlight, rain, and wind can all alter signs; in other words, signs are temporary.

Sign cutting is the actual search for evidence that a subject has been in the area, thereby establishing a point from which to track (Table 29-3). Once a sign has been established, then the lead or point sign cutter is positioned on the opposite side of the sign and looks for the next sign. Often, as a sign is established, it is marked with indicators in the soil or even paper flags, such as the type used by surveyors. This is done to alert other searchers to avoid the area and to not "trample on the sign."

The common methods of tracking are jump tracking, step-by-step, and bracketing. Jump tracking is the fastest of the three and involves finding obvious, well-defined signs and then following along the presumed direction of travel to the next obvious sign. Jump tracking is used in time-sensitive missions.

Step-by-step tracking is a slow, methodical approach that looks for each step in succession using the measured stride length to search for the next print. In this method, the searcher(s) move no further than the last identified print. Using a **sign cutting stick**, an approximately 40-inch long stick, the length of a person's stride is determined. After finding a sign the searcher places an indicator on the stick, such as marking it with a rubber band. The next sign is then found and another rubber band is placed on the stick, marking the distance from the last sign to the current sign. This distance represents the subject's stride. The stick is then moved in an arc until another sign is found. This step-by-step method may be laborious but it accurately provides a direction of travel. Trackers will use heel-to-heel stride length along with location information to determine the subject's speed and direction of travel.

Tracking teams are typically made up of three searchers. The searcher with the sign cutting stick is often referred to as the **pointer**. Flankers often accompany the pointer. The pointer moves forward along the assumed direction of the subject's travel with the flankers slightly behind and off to each side. The pointer looks for each successive step based on the subject's stride length and the flankers look to the sides for other tracks that may cross and possibly confuse the tracking operation.

Bracketing is used to supplement the step-by-step method when the next successive print cannot be located. Bracketing uses stride length to skip a step when a sign cannot be found and to determine where the next step might be located.

Important information for trackers to note is the size (length and width) of a print and the type of sole (with a drawing or picture, if possible). For example, a hiking boot sole differs from a flat moccasin shoe sole.

All searchers should know what to look for, how and where to find it, and how to preserve it. Contamination of signs is a problem for the search effort and can cause significant delays or even mislead searchers. Track traps are soft areas, such as sand, snow, or mud, upon which a footprint is easily made.

STREET SMART

Some search and rescue Technicians will alter the soles on their boots to provide a "sole signature." This signature is copied to paper, in a manner similar to fingerprinting, to be distributed among searchers. Thus, when a sign is found it can be compared to the sole signature so rescuers know it was made by one of the rescue team and not the victim.

Scent Dogs

While humans search for visual evidence, specially trained dogs track by scent. Air **scent dogs** track by following the human scent through the air. These dogs work freely, not on

a lead, and track scent through the air to its source. Tracking/trailing dogs are exposed to an object that contains the subject's scent and, while on the lead, follows the scent at ground level and on vegetation. Dogs and their handlers take years to master their craft and communication between the two is critical to success. The handler must be able to recognize that the dog has picked up the scent. The dogs used in search and rescue need to be well trained not only in tracking but also in general acceptable behavior.

High-Tech Equipment

A new search technique being used to explore confined spaces and thickets is **infrared thermal imaging cameras**, which create pictures based on heat radiation rather than exposure to light. Thermal cameras are carried on many fire apparatus and can be especially valuable in finding a patient at night or a subject who is concealed.

Another technology now in use for search and rescue is **night vision goggles**. The military has utilized night vision for helicopter pilots for many years. Night vision technology amplifies available light from the moon or stars to enhance an image, allowing the user to distinguish between different objects. This capability hypothetically extends a search and rescue mission so as to permit execution 24 hours a day. This is a valuable consideration in a time-sensitive situation.

Aircraft are also used to supplement ground crews. Aircraft may be used in an initial scan of a search area before ground crews are deployed, such as in searching for a presumed downed aircraft. The military has vast experience with search and rescue missions for downed pilots which can also be applicable in the civilian sector.

Lost Person Behavior

People become lost for many reasons, some of which are accidental and some intentional. Elderly people with Alzheimer's disease many times wander away from caregivers. Children wander as well. Hikers, skiers, and hunters get "turned around" and become disoriented. Despondent patients may intentionally become "lost," sometimes in an effort to end their lives.[6]

Each of these patient categories has different behavioral characteristics (i.e., **lost person behavior**), leading to differences in search tactics needed to find them. Therefore, one of the search manager's first responsibilities is to match the lost person to a type of subject. Much of the approach will be dictated by the information obtained in the Lost Person Questionnaire. The lost person is then matched to one of 33 categories developed by Koester, who developed these classifications from reports of thousands of previous lost persons. This form of behavioral modeling has been demonstrated to be very effective.[7] Once the subject is matched to a category, with time factored in and starting from the point last seen (PLS), the search manager can determine the search area that will maximize the POS.

Children 1 to 3 Years Old

Children this young do not understand the concept of being lost. Their movement is very unpredictable because they do not have skills to navigate in the outside world or a sense of direction. Fortunately, small children move slowly. When tired, small children may seek out a comfortable place to sleep. Searchers need to be meticulous in their tactics to find small children because they tend to hide and can be tucked away in any small space available. Hollows under boulders or logs, abandoned buildings, and vehicles are all good hiding places for the small child.

Children 3 to 6 Years Old

These children do understand the concept of being lost and many times will try to find their way back to home or a campsite they left. They can be very mobile and are easily distracted by sounds or animals. Children in this age group may be very aware of their parents' and teachers' admonishment to stay away from strangers. For this reason, they may avoid or move away from searchers. Similar to very young children, 3- to 6-year-olds may try to find a cozy place to sleep or hide.

Children 6 to 12 Years Old

Children in this age group will generally be more aware of direction; however, they are easily confused when in an unfamiliar area. Searchers should remember that these children may have intentionally run away to gain attention or avoid punishment and may not respond to the calling of searchers. Their awareness of their fears, particularly darkness and strange sounds, may eventually cause them to be more receptive to searchers' efforts.

Adults Over 65

A couple of the significant issues with adults in this age group are the possibility of dementia and the probability of general health problems. Elderly people suffering from dementia, particularly due to Alzheimer's disease, are easily distracted and may wander away while following something like a butterfly's path, or the subject may attempt to travel to find a residence or friends from earlier life.

Alzheimer's patients generally continue forward, albeit slowly, and will continue to move forward until they reach a physical impediment. Unfortunately, even then the drive to find something familiar may cause them to cross dangerous streams or scale steep terrain, leading to many deadly mishaps.

The more active and physically fit subjects may continue moving until exhausted, exacerbating pre-existing medical conditions. Alzheimer's patients generally do not respond to searchers, nor do they have the ability to leave clues or make their whereabouts known.

Mentally Retarded and Autistic Children

The terms "mentally retarded" and "autistic" must be viewed with caution. Although these subjects may have the mental capacity of a child of younger age, they may have the physical capabilities of an adult.

For a variety of reasons, the lost person behavior of these subjects is difficult to determine. Most are not aware of being lost, and thus are not likely to call out. Furthermore, many will not respond to their name being called unless the voice is familiar. Instead, such subjects may become frightened and hide from view. In some cases, the subject will be found in a place like thick brush where refuge was sought, and will have been there for days.

One study showed that the median distance from the initial point of the search to the location of the subject is only 0.8 km in all terrains (i.e., mountainous, flat, and urban), with a maximum distance being 4 km.[8] These statistics support the need for an intensive search of the area where the subject was last seen.

Psychotic and Despondent

Psychotic subjects many times walk off from day trips and other social outings, but do not enter deep, thickly wooded wilderness areas. They are often found along roadways or in open areas. Despondent persons, on the other hand, are another category that becomes intentionally "lost," sometimes with the intention of suicide. Often they seek solitude in an effort to get away from everyone around them. For this reason, they will not respond to searchers' attempts to attract them.

Despondent persons are usually located in somewhat idyllic spots such as overlooks, scenic areas, or bodies of water used for the backdrop of suicide attempts. Rarely are they found in thick brush. The location may be just out of sight or somewhere specific that has meaning in the subject's life. Because of this, travel distances can vary greatly.

Hikers, Hunters, and Skiers

Outdoor recreationalists are not usually hampered by problems of age, health issues, dementia, or impaired mental facilities. They are generally more fit than the earlier described subjects. However, when an otherwise fit, capable individual realizes he is lost, the phenomenon of woods shock can set in.

Woods shock describes the sudden onset of overwhelming panic and confusion a person may feel after initially realizing he is lost. It is responsible for bizarre behaviors in otherwise rational people. An example of behavior exemplifying wood shock is a hiker succumbing to the elements despite having a backpack full of clothing, food, and shelter.

Hikers become search subjects in two ways: someone intentionally splits off from his companions because of fatigue or becomes slower than the rest of the group, or a solo hiker becomes disoriented in an unfamiliar area, possibly off trail. Many times hikers veer off-trail in search of the "short-cut" and become disoriented in unfamiliar ground. If emotions override rational thinking and woods shock takes over, the subject's survival instincts may disappear.

Of the categories discussed, hikers are the most mobile and can cover large areas in a relatively short time. Two miles per hour is not unreasonable, as an expert hiker can cover 12 to 20 miles in a day, even while carrying a pack. These subjects want to be found and will respond to the searcher's attraction tactics.

Hunters, on the other hand, tend to cover smaller distances than hikers but are focused on game and not necessarily land navigation. Hunters may also be less fit than hikers and are usually carrying less usable gear for an extended stay in the woods. Typically they have a good "woods sense" (a sense of direction in the woods). Hunters may tend to follow natural terrain features such as drainages in order to find escape.

Skiers are generally young, fit individuals who are well equipped. Often they do not become lost in the true sense but instead fall victim to extreme weather, cold, avalanche, or injury, and are unable to escape, thus prompting the search and rescue mission.

EMS in Search and Rescue

Emergency medical service is an integral part of search and rescue for both the subject and the searchers. A study reviewing search and rescue missions in the White Mountain National Forest published in the *Journal of Wilderness Medicine* in 2004 reported that searchers accounted for 4.7% of all search and rescue mission injuries. 41.7% of patients needed carryout, 25% were air evacuated, and one-third required transport to a hospital. Most injuries were orthopedic, primarily involving the lower extremities, and hiking was the most common activity requiring EMS in a search and rescue operation.[9]

Another aspect of EMS's involvement in search and rescue operations is that of **searcher rehabilitation**. Searchers work long hours, sometimes in extreme temperatures and harsh weather, carrying heavy equipment. The need for fire scene rehabilitation for firefighters is well documented and there are well-established protocols for this. However, searcher rehabilitation is not as formalized and work needs to be done to establish a similar set of protocols for this rescue activity.

Wilderness Medicine

Paramedics in search and rescue operations need to have specialized skills to be able to treat and transport patients in remote environments. This branch of emergency medicine is referred to as wilderness medicine. **Wilderness medicine** is defined as medical care rendered to patients who are at least one hour or more from definitive (medical facility) care.

Wilderness medicine skills blend long-term patient care and management, improvisation of medical equipment appropriate for the patient and environment, survival skills, and specialized patient packaging. Caring for a patient in a remote environment, and doing so for longer periods of time, requires considerations of comfort for orthopedic injuries, warmth and shelter, and attention to patient hydration, nutrition, and elimination. These skills can be learned from a number of excellent programs in wilderness medicine found around the United States. See Chapter 14 for more information about wilderness medicine.

▶ CASE STUDY CONCLUSION

What ensued was a massive search effort through early July of that year involving over 10,000 man-hours, hundreds of searchers, and several hundred aircraft hours. Despite this massive effort, few clues were found. Later, in October of 1990, hunters in the general area spotted something red in the forest. Upon approaching the red object, they found several pieces of bright clothing (seemingly used as signals), a tent, and other items. Several yards away in a dry streambed, they found David Boomhower. What is puzzling about this case is that a diary Mr. Boomhower kept was also found, and it seems to indicate that he may have survived until at least mid-August.

CRITICAL THINKING QUESTIONS

1. Why does it appear that the subject didn't try to make his way out of the wilderness?
2. Why did the intensive search efforts fail David Boomhower?

CONCLUSION

As the author noted regarding rescue, "Time alone was the strongest predictor of survival." Therefore, it is important that the Paramedic assisting with wilderness search and rescue be able to quickly establish the incident management system and prepare to perform a hasty search. In cooperation with other emergency services, the Paramedic can help achieve the goals of search and rescue: locate, access, stabilize, and transport (LAST).

Personal involvement in wilderness search and rescue of a lost person, whether that person is a patient with Alzheimer's or a child, is a very rewarding experience, as well as a highly valuable additional skill set for Paramedics.

▶ KEY POINTS:

- Wilderness search and rescue uses ICS, which is a part of NIMS.

- The National Response Framework replaced the National Search and Rescue Plan.

- Lead non-governmental agencies for search and rescue are NASAR and MRA.

- Goals of search and rescue are summarized in the mnemonic LAST: locate, access, stabilize, and transport.

- NFPA 1670 addresses wilderness search and rescue standards.

- There are three levels of training for search and rescue: Awareness, Operations, and Technician.

- Elements of the search and rescue operations include preplanning, notification and response, check-in and briefing, assignment and search, debriefing and check-out, and critique.

- The Lost Person Questionnaire narrows the probability of area for search.

- NIMS mandated ICS calls for five functional areas: command, operations, planning, logistics, and finance/administration.

- Indirect search tactics include information gathering, use of attraction, and containment.

- Direct search tactics start with determining the area with the highest probability of detection, which maximizes the probability of success.

- Direct search tactics include ground searching (ground pounders and scent canines), aerial reconnaissance, loose grid searches, and tight grid searches.

- Often the hasty search and the bastard search are the initial search methods.

- Some searchers search for clues rather than the subject (i.e., clue consciousness).

- Loose grid searches feature rapid moving teams, whereas tight grid searches are a slow, methodical, shoulder-to-shoulder type of search.

- Tracking involves looking for signs and using trackers for sign cutting.

- An effective old technology is using scent dogs, whereas new technologies include infrared thermal imaging cameras and night vision goggles.

- Koester classifications list expected lost person behaviors based on thousands of previous cases.

- Woods shock is a form of hysteria and confusion experienced by a subject when lost.

- Search and rescue workers need rehabilitation sectors.

REVIEW QUESTIONS:

1. What are the goals of search and rescue?
2. Are there any standards for wilderness search and rescue?
3. What are the three levels of search and rescue training?
4. What are the five functional areas in NIMS ICS?
5. What is the difference between a hasty search and a bastard search?

CASE STUDY QUESTIONS:

Please refer to the Case Study in this chapter, and answer the questions below:

1. What are the elements of a search and rescue operation?
2. What factors affect a search?
3. What is the difference between place last seen (PLS) and the last known position (LKP)?

REFERENCES:

1. Adams AL, Schmidt TA. Search is a time critical event: when search and rescue missions may become futile. *J Wilderness Environ Med.* 2007;18(2):95–101.
2. Available at: **http://www.fema.gov/emergency/nrf.** Accessed May 10th 2007.
3. National Association of Search and Rescue. *Managing the Lost Person Incident* (2nd ed.). Chantilly, VA: NASAR; 2007.
4. NIMSOnline, *NIMS Integration Center.* Available at: **www.nimsonline.com.** Accessed May 10th 2007.
5. Cooper DC, National Association for Search and Rescue. *Fundamentals of Search and Rescue.* Sudbury, MA: Jones and Bartlett; 2005: 228.
6. Cooper DC. *The Application of Search Theory to Land Search: The Adjustment of Probability of Area.* Cuyhoga Falls, OH: Private publication; 2000.
7. Koester RJ. *Lost Person Behavior: A Search and Rescue Guide on Where to Look—for Land, Air, and Water.* Charlottesville, VA: Dbs Productions; 2008.
8. Stoffel R. *The Handbook for Managing Land Search Operations.* Cashmere, Washington: Emergency Response International, Inc.; 2001.
9. Ela GK. Epidemiology of wilderness search and rescue in New Hampshire, 1999–2001. *Wild Environ Med*: 2004;15(1):11–17.

CHAPTER 30

TECHNICAL ROPE RESCUE

KEY CONCEPTS:

Upon completion of this chapter, it is expected that the reader will understand these following concepts:

- Phases of a technical rescue
- Slope analysis
- Technical rescue equipment
- Rappelling
- Lowering
- Hauling
- Carries

"Rescue 2, Engine 5 for manpower, and Ambulance 3, respond to High Falls for a man fallen in the ravine," crackles the radio. "That is the second rescue in that ravine," the Paramedic sighs to himself. The last rescue did not go so smoothly. The patient had multiple fractures and didn't get pain medication until he was out of the ravine. To prevent this from happening again, all Paramedics were trained to rappel. "Well, this is going to be a first," the Paramedic thinks.

CRITICAL THINKING QUESTIONS

1. What are the phases of a technical rescue?
2. What is the equipment used in a technical rescue?
3. What is the Paramedic's role in a technical rescue?

OVERVIEW

Rescue, by definition, is to free someone from danger and implies that one person is coming to the aid of someone who is in peril of loss of life or limb. Paramedics, as part of the public safety team, are frequently a part of that rescue. In some cases, the Paramedic is embedded in the rescue team, whereas in other cases the Paramedic is called to the scene to render medical care during the rescue. In every case, the Paramedic should be aware of the tools and techniques that professional rescuers use.

This chapter discusses techniques and tools used in technical rescue. **Technical rescue** is a broad term that applies to the use of ropes and rigging by specially trained personnel to effect a rescue. It encompasses rope rescue, confined space rescue, cave rescue, trench rescue, tower rescue, and structural collapse rescue, to name a few of its many applications.

Phases of a Rescue

Like every emergency operation, there are three phases to the technical rescue: preplanning, operations, and termination of operations. Perhaps the most important phase to an efficient and effective operation is the preplanning phase.

Preplanning

The first step in the preplanning phase is to request the AHJ. Or authority having jurisdiction (fire, police, or EMS), to perform a **hazard analysis** of the community to assess for any risk. As the definition of technical rescue suggests, any tower, multistory building, farm silo, cave, or sewer system has the potential for a person to become trapped, thereby requiring a technical rescue. Therefore, every community has a need for some form of technical rescue team, either local or via mutual aid. When reviewing the terrain—whether on foot, by map, or by Earth satellite photographs—a **slope analysis** is performed to determine the degree of hazard in the jurisdiction and the need for specialized rope rescue teams.

When most Paramedics think of technical rescues, they think of cliff rescue. However, a technical rescue need not involve a cliff. Slopes can vary from rough terrain with a slight incline to a vertical cliff. Technical rescue divides these terrains into four levels. The first level, called **low angle**, or sometimes slope rescue, includes inclines up to 30 degrees. In the first level of terrain, the majority of the Paramedic's weight is on his feet during a rescue, although the terrain is uneven and presents a fall hazard to rescuers. A Level I slope rescue typically only requires a single rope to protect the rescuer.

The second level of slope rescue involves any terrain with an incline of 30 degrees or greater that requires the use of both the rescuer's hands and feet to ascend. This **steep angle** can range from a scramble over scree (loose

rock covering a slope) to talus (loose rock at the base of a cliff) to a more traditional rock climb (rated Class 5 in climb rating).

The third level, **high angle**, is generally greater than 60 degrees and ranges from steep climbing with multiple pitches to a vertical wall. When the provider is unable to independently stand, even using his hands for balance, it is considered high angle. High angle rescue requires specialized equipment along with extensive training.

The fourth level, **highline**, is rescue over a chasm or ravine where the rescuer or patient is suspended in mid-air with only the rope for protection from a fall. Highline rescue is very technical and is performed only when no other viable alternative exists.

Needs Assessment

After the completion of the hazard analysis, the AHJ should make a **needs assessment**, a review of human resources as well as equipment. This needs assessment should address personnel needs for training (discussed shortly) as well as equipment needs. These resources may come from within the community (such as federal and/or state park services), from private concerns (such as volunteer search and rescue organizations), or from mutual aid from other communities.

Although it may not be possible for every community to support all forms of technical rescue, an incident management plan should be in place to ensure that the provision of care needed for all forms of rescue is available. In many instances, the local fire, police, or EMS departments are trained as "first responders." These first responders to an incident establish the incident management system and may perform rudimentary rescue. In other cases, caches of special equipment are maintained locally so that trained technical rescuers can go directly to the scene and immediately start operations (Figure 30-1).

Many utility companies have personnel who are trained on rope rescue as a function of their jobs. Another untapped resource can be FEMA Urban Search and Rescue (USAR) teams.

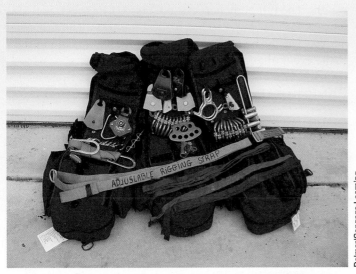

Figure 30-1 Preplanning includes maintaining equipment caches so rescuers can immediately provide assistance.

Every incident management plan should include the provision of medical care to rescuers (rehabilitation, see Chapter 25) and patients alike. In some cases, the Paramedic is included in the incident management plan and is trained as a part of the rescue team. In other cases, the untrained Paramedic may be asked to descend to the patient, render care, and be hauled up along with the patient. As a part of the rescue, the Paramedic should be familiar with the technical rescue equipment. Every incident action plan should include technical rescue training for Paramedics.[1]

The National Fire Protection Association in its *Standard for Technical Rescuer Professional Qualifications* (**NFPA 1006**, 2008 ed.) calls for a tiered training format: Awareness, Operations, and Technician.[2] Minimally, every Paramedic involved in a technical rescue should have an Awareness level of training. This level includes identification of high life hazard incidents that mandate higher trained operators, simple or non-entry rescue, and scene management. The Paramedic should preferably be trained to the Operations level and be capable of providing patient care and packaging as a part of the Operations team.

Operations

Like other rescues, technical rescue relies on the incident management system. This system, discussed in Chapter 20, includes those elements to which nontechnical rescue responders can contribute including, but not limited to, triage, transportation, rehabilitation, and so on. A schematic of the typical incident management system might be established for a technical rescue (Figure 30-2).

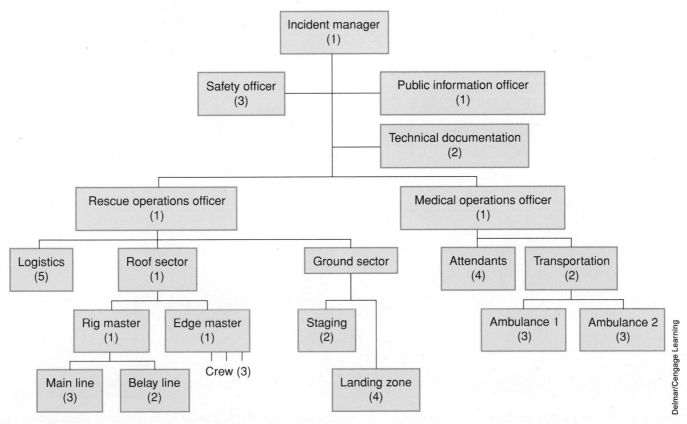

Figure 30-2 This example shows an incident management system for technical rescue.

Safety

The first priority in technical rescue is safety and redundancy, as exemplified by **NFPA 1670**, *Standard on Operations and Training for Technical Search and Rescue Incidents*. From the buddy system to the use of whistle stops, safety comes first (Figure 30-3).

The concept of safety is manifest in the system safety factor. The **system safety factor** is a ratio of the projected load (i.e., rescuers, equipment, and patient) on the system, including ropes and hardware. Like a chain, the system is only as strong as its weakest link. The force needed to break that link is called the **minimum breaking strength**. Although this calculation is complicated, and is an entire conversation by itself, the system safety factor emphasizes the importance of safety during any technical rescue.

As in any other situation, the Paramedic's first concern is personal protective equipment (PPE). PPE typically worn by a Paramedic during any technical rescue is a helmet, gloves to protect the hands from rope burns and the like, a safety harness to tie into the system, and a pair of sturdy boots.

The typical technical rescuer's safety helmet need be nothing more than a bump cap with a chinstrap and a pair of goggles, though more elaborate helmets are available. The general purpose of the helmet is to protect the Paramedic's head from falling debris or from a head injury during a fall.

A piece of PPE unique to the technical rescue arena is the harness. The harness is the means by which the Paramedic is tied into the rope system. The most common harness, the seat harness, is listed as a **Class II harness** by the NFPA in **NFPA 1983**, *Standard on Life Safety Rope and Equipment for Emergency Services*, (Figure 30-4). In contrast, the **Class I harness** is an emergency self-rescue harness that is not capable of holding more than one person's weight. The full body harness, a **Class III harness**, includes the seat harness but also has a chest harness.[3] The full body harness has the advantage of keeping the Paramedic upright in the event of a fall.

Equipment

A rope rescue system is made up of ropes, webbing, and hardware, but the core of any rope rescue system is the rope. There are many varieties of ropes and each has its purpose. The Paramedic should be familiar with the general classifications of ropes and their primary use.

Ropes can be made from nylon, polyester, and even Kevlar. Early ropes were made of twisted hemp; although

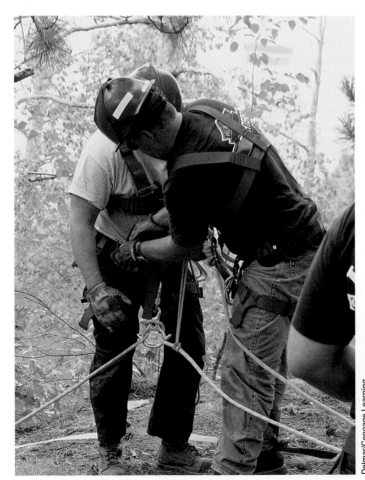

Figure 30-3 A buddy and/or safety officer performs a safety check before the rappel.

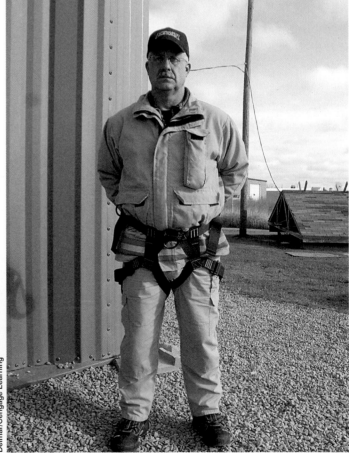

Figure 30-4 A Class II harness is also known as a seat harness.

these "natural" ropes can still be found, they are considered undesirable for rescue. Only ropes that are designated as **life safety ropes**—that is, designed to support a life load during an emergency—should be used in rescue. For example, escape ropes or throwlines are not considered life safety ropes by the NFPA 1983 standards.

A newer material used for rescue ropes is polyester. Being slightly stronger than nylon, it remains strong even when wet, unlike nylon. However, polyester ropes have less stretch (discussed shortly) than similar nylon ropes and thus are less forgiving when a load is suddenly placed on them, such as occurs during a fall.

Nylon, first invented in 1930 by DuPont, is still the predominate material used for life safety rope. Nylon 6 (i.e., perlon) is favored by the rock climbing community, whereas the rescue community prefers the more abrasion-resistant nylon 6.6. Although nylon has elasticity, which permits it to be bent and twisted without damage, it does tend to break down in the presence of light, particularly ultraviolet light. To prevent this breakdown, the nylon rope is often carried loosely in a **rope bag** (Figure 30-5).

There are two varieties of ropes: dynamic and static. A **dynamic rope**, which is popular with rock climbers, has stretch and thus is more forgiving to the climber during a fall. However, during a rescue, stretch is generally not desirable. Therefore, static rope is used.

Static rope is further divided into two categories. A true static rope has less than 6% elongation with a load. However, there are some conditions when a little stretch is desirable. For those times, there is low-stretch rope (rope with more than 6% but less than 10% elongation when a load is placed on it).

The predecessor of modern ropes was the twisted rope, which is still used by the military today. Most ropes now used in rescue operations are **kernmantle**, a nylon core with a fabric sheath often made of polyester. It is critical that these ropes be maintained in excellent condition. Most services regularly perform inspection and maintenance of their ropes and document their findings in the rope log, with one rope log per rope. If the rope displays any signs of wear, such as fraying or stains, it must be discarded.

Hardware and Software

A staple in technical rescue is webbing. **Webbing** is flat woven rope that has great strength and durability. Webbing can either be flat or tubular, and the webbing used by many rescue professionals is stronger than standard webbing

Webbing is used for anchors (discussed shortly), slings, and any number of uses where a short rope is helpful. Webbing comes in a large number of colors. Some rescue professionals have "codified" the colors; for example, green means a five-foot length whereas blue means 15 feet. This coding makes it easier for rescuers to differentiate them in an emergency (Figure 30-6).

Another short rope is the prusik. The **prusik** is a small diameter (usually 7, 8, or 9 mm) rope that is knotted, forms

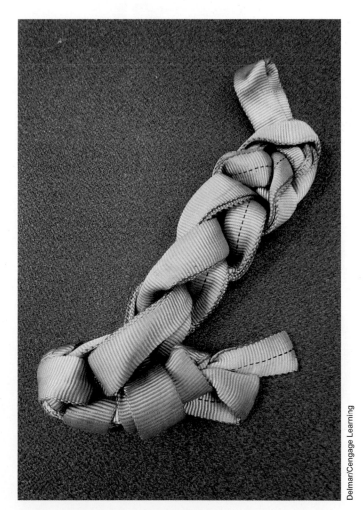

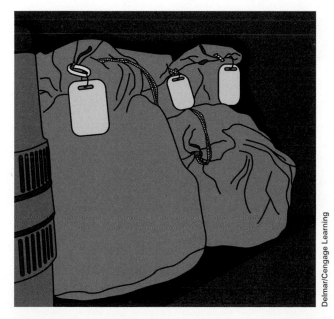

Figure 30-5 Rescue rope can be safely stored in a rope bag.

Figure 30-6 Webbing is flat woven rope that has great strength and durability.

a loop, and is then wrapped around a larger diameter rope. When a force is applied to the prusik, it binds up and locks the device being used. In essence, a prusik acts like a break during a catastrophic failure of the rope rescue system (Figure 30-7).

The most commonly used, and probably most easily recognized, piece of rescue hardware is the carabiner. A **carabiner** is a metal ring that is used to attach a sling or rope to another part of the rope rescue system. Carabiners can be made of either steel or aluminum. Although steel is arguably stronger in some rescue situations (e.g., wilderness rescue), a compromise is made in strength in favor of lesser weight. That is not to say that safety is compromised but, rather, that alternative methods are used to help ensure safety.

Carabiners are either oval, D-shaped, or some variation of either (Figure 30-8). The long axis of the carabiner has the greatest strength, whereas the short axis is more likely to fail under a heavy load. Carabiners also have a "gate." The gate opens, permitting the rope to be placed in the carabiner

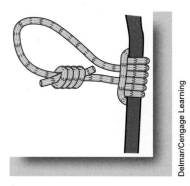

Figure 30-7 Prusik is a small diameter rope that is knotted, forms a loop, and is then wrapped around a larger diameter rope.

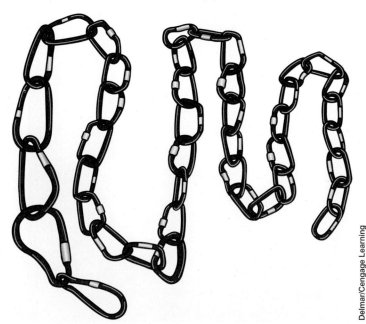

Figure 30-8 Rescue hardware includes locking and standard oval and D-ring carabiners.

without threading the entire length of rope through the carabiner like a thread and needle. Some gates have a pin-and-latch mechanism, whereas others have a claw-and-lock mechanism.

A cause of catastrophic failure is when the gate opens and the rope falls out. To prevent this failure, the Paramedic can either place two carabiners with the gates opposite and opposing, or use a carabiner with a "locking" gate. Locking gates can either be manually screwed closed or have an automatic spring mechanism.

Although it would seem that the rope is the weakest link in the rope rescue system, and ropes do fail on occasion, hardware is also prone to failure, especially if it is overloaded. To alert rescuers to the capacity of a piece of hardware, such as a carabiner, the NFPA established minimum standards for rescue hardware. Most rescue hardware has the NFPA 1983 notation stamped into the hardware as well as the load limit/breaking strength.

The next category of rescue hardware is broadly called descent control devices. A **descent control device** either provides the Paramedic with an ability to rappel safely to the patient or for a basket or other patient carrier to be lowered to the patient.

For the first purpose, most rescuers use a figure eight descent control device. This device depends on a load being placed on the rope, usually the weight of the rescuer, and uses the resultant friction as the rope runs over the metal to slow the speed of the rope (Figure 30-9).

To control the descent of a basket and/or rescuers, a rescuer may elect to use a brake bar. Like the figure eight descent control device, the brake bar depends on friction to slow the descent. An advantage of a brake bar is that additional bars can be placed across the rope when an additional load is placed on the system, such as a patient or rescuers. Often an open rack brake bar is used for rappelling, whereas a closed rack brake bar is used for lowering a basket (Figure 30-10).

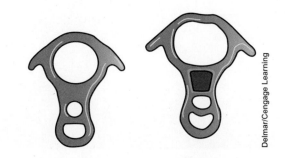

Figure 30-9 One example of a descent control device is the figure eight descender.

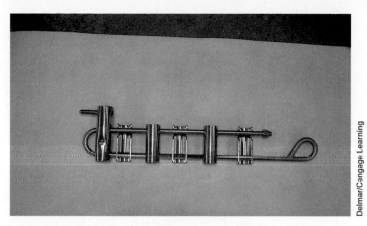

Figure 30-10 An open rack brake bar is used for rappelling.

Rope grabs, devices intended to prevent a rope from slipping, are a key component in an ascending or hauling system. These ascending rope systems utilize mechanical advantage, a mechanism that increases the effect of force put into the system by the use of pulleys. Many rescuers use the prusiks (described earlier) as an emergency brake in an ascending system. The use of a prusik knot is referred to as a "soft cam." However, once the prusik has "locked up" it can be very difficult to release. To replace the prusik, some rescuers use an ascender device. As the name implies, an **ascender device** allows the climber to climb the rope. Use of an ascender in this fashion is referred to as a "hard cam." These ascenders are easier to release and reset than a prusik (Figure 30-11).

Pulleys are frequently used to change the direction of a rope or, like a block and tackle, to provide a mechanical advantage. Some pulleys are specifically designed to allow a knot to pass through the pulley (Figure 30-12).

The final piece of rescue hardware is the rigging plate. The **rigging plate** permits multiple carabiners to be attached to a single solid plate of metal. A rigging plate is particularly helpful when multiple anchors must be used (anchors are discussed shortly). A rigging plate may be part of a preset descent system (Figure 30-13).[4]

Anchors

The heart of every rope rescue system is the anchor. An **anchor** is a point of fixation that permits a load to be applied to it without movement. An anchor can be natural (such as a tree) or artificial (such as a steel expansion bolt or a set of stakes placed in a row called a picket). Even a roadside guard rail, using a beam clamp, can be used as an anchor.

The simplest anchor technique may be wrapping the rope around a tree or post. This anchor, called a **tensionless hitch**, depends on the strength of the rope to hold the load (Figure 30-14). The load capacity of a rope is often printed at the end, or "sharp end," of the rope.

Another common anchor technique is to use a loop of webbing. The webbing is wrapped around the anchor three times and then two loops are pulled out. A carabiner is

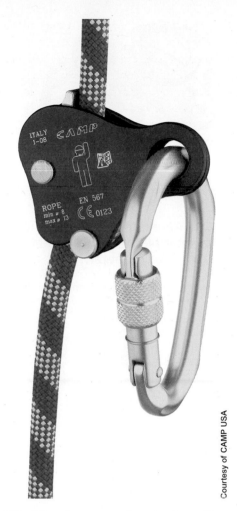

Figure 30-11 An ascender device allows a climber to climb a rope.

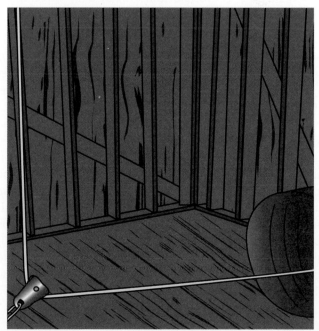

Figure 30-12 A pulley is frequently used to change the direction of a rope or to provide a mechanical advantage.

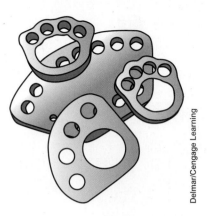

Figure 30-13 An example of a rigging plate, which permits multiple carabiners to be attached to a single solid plate of metal.

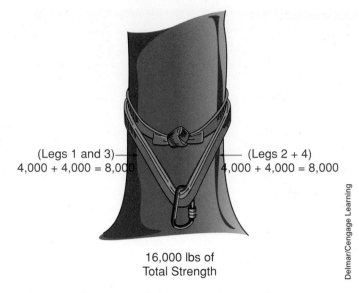

(Legs 1 and 3)⎯ ⎯ (Legs 2 + 4)
4,000 + 4,000 = 8,000   4,000 + 4,000 = 8,000

16,000 lbs of
Total Strength

Figure 30-15 Webbing can be used to create a wrap three, pull two anchor.

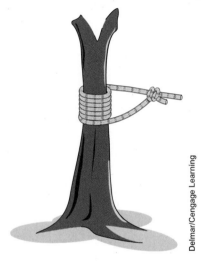

Figure 30-14 A tensionless hitch only uses the rope to secure the system to the anchor.

connected to the loops and the rope is clipped in. Usually a figure eight knot is tied on the end of the rope and a carabiner can be attached. This configuration is called a **wrap three, pull two anchor** (Figure 30-15).

A good anchor will not move under normal conditions and loads. If the rescuer has reservations about the anchor, then a second, third, or fourth anchor may be added. This redundancy increases the safety factor in the event of a sudden load on the first anchor. Rather than line anchors in a row, allowing each to sequentially fail, it is preferable to establish a load-distributing anchor. A **load-distributing anchor** spreads the load (i.e., the patient's weight) over multiple anchors simultaneously. Often a rigging plate (i.e., anchor plate) is used to maintain the "fall line" of the rope in line with the direction of the anticipated load.[5]

Rappel

The first step of a rescue is to get to the patient. With a rope and anchor system in place, the rescuer may rappel to the patient. A **rappel** (also known as abseiling) is a technique

wherein the rescuer descends to the patient. The rappeller uses a friction device to slow and control the descent. In the case of uneven ground or even low angle rescue, the Paramedic may elect to use an arm as a friction device (i.e., **arm rappel**) (Figure 30-16) or a **body rappel** (i.e., Dulfersitz) (Figure 30-17).

In most cases, the steep angle of the face requires that the Paramedic wear a harness, either Class II or III, and be connected to a descent control device along with a carabiner, which is in turn attached to the rope. Rescuers may then rappel using a figure eight descent control device (Figure 30-18).

Although most climbers will use a single rope to descend, for purposes of a rescue it is preferable for the rescuer to have a second rope attached. This second rope, called a **belay**, is used to protect the rescuer from a fall. Originally the word "belay" meant to make fast (i.e., to secure), or prevent a rope from moving. In this case, a belay is meant to make the rescuer secure.

A belay may be established by another rescuer who is secured to an anchor and uses a rope to connect to the rescuer. The belayer uses either the body as a friction device or, preferably, a descent control device to provide a belay.

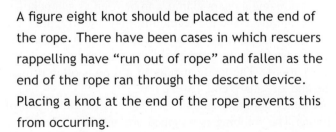

STREET SMART

A figure eight knot should be placed at the end of the rope. There have been cases in which rescuers rappelling have "run out of rope" and fallen as the end of the rope ran through the descent device. Placing a knot at the end of the rope prevents this from occurring.

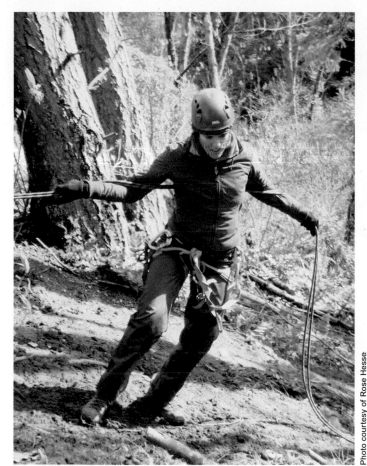

Figure 30-16 During an arm rappel, the rescuer uses an arm as a friction device.

To start the rappel, the rescuer may choose to either roll over the edge when rappelling from a vertical face or to walk over the edge. Once over the edge, the rescuer proceeds to "walk" down the face. Small jumps are used only to get over an obstacle.

Some Paramedics prefer to rappel nearby to the patient and establish a foothold before moving to the patient. This prevents the patient from grabbing the Paramedic. This also prevents debris, which might be accidentally dislodged, from raining down on the patient. Others prefer to rappel until directly above the patient and then to "lock off." A **lock off** is a technique in which the rope is wrapped securely around the descent control device, thus allowing the hands to be free to assess the patient, render aid, use a radio, and so on.

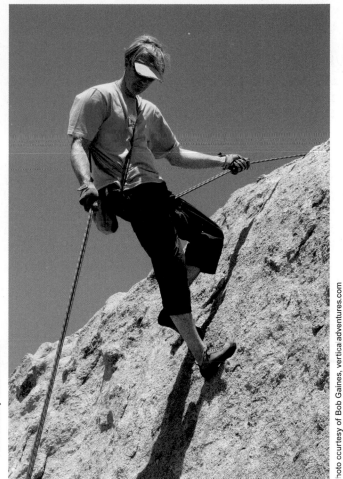

Figure 30-17 During a body rappel, the rescuer uses the body as a friction device.

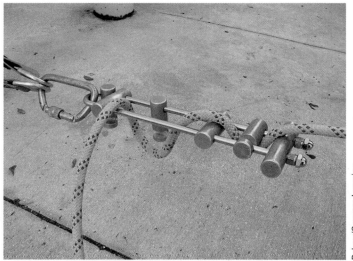

Figure 30-18 A figure eight descender is often used in rappels.

Some rescuers have been taught a rescue technique called the pick off. During a **pick off**, the patient is taken off her rope system after she has been clipped into the rescuer's rope system. This technique takes practice and the rope rescue system must be capable of sustaining the additional load. Sometimes a pick off strap (webbing with clips) is used.

Commands

Communications between the belayer and the rescuer are important. Use of a standard nomenclature helps to ensure clear communications. The following commands are commonly used in communication. "**On rappel**" is used as an interrogative, meaning "Are you ready for me to rappel?" The command "**rappel on**" means the belayer is ready for the rescuer to rappel and she may proceed to rappel. The rescuer may, as the need arises, either call out "**slack**" or "**tension**," referring to the looseness or tightness of the rope. Once the rescuer has reached the patient and has sound footing, the command "**rope free**" tells the belayer that the rescuer is safe. However, in most cases the rescuer remains on belay for the duration of the descent and ascent.

Lowering System

Once the Paramedic is at the patient's side and rendering care, other rescuers need to turn their attention to packaging the patient and hauling the patient up. To get the basket to the patient, the team uses a lowering system.

A **lowering system** uses a descent control device to lower patient care supplies and rescue equipment to the Paramedic at the patient's side. Therefore, the "**basket**" is an essential piece of equipment. A wide variety of baskets are available. The classic basket, in use since before World War II, is the wire **Stokes basket**. Solid form baskets, using fiberglass, Kevlar, or plastic, are available. These baskets have either an internal rail, which means the outer surface is smooth and can slide on snow, ice, and so on, or an external steel rail that permits multiple handholds. There are even frameless baskets (i.e., SKED) that form around the patient (Figure 30-19).

Packaging

Once the basket has been lowered to the Paramedic, the patient must be transferred to the basket (i.e., **packaged**). If the Paramedic suspects spinal injury, the patient may need to be secured to a long backboard, with cervical collar and straps

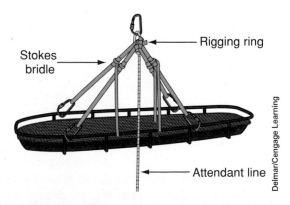

Figure 30-19 This open frame plastic basket has a handrail for added security.

in place, and then transferred to the basket. Often additional rescuers are lowered with the basket to assist with the transfer.

All of the patient's needs must be met when the patient is in the basket. A basic need is warmth. Using two blankets, the patient is folded into the blankets in a papoose fashion. In cold weather, an outer vapor barrier or reflective rescue blanket may be used to help keep the patient warm.

If the patient is nauseous, the rescuer may place a rope bag next to the patient's head in case of vomiting. Prophylactic antiemetics should also be considered. In some cases, it may be prudent to secure the patient on his side in case of vomiting.

If an intravenous access has been established, it should either be capped off (converted to a saline well) or the solution placed in a pressure bag to maintain the flow. The pressure bag must then be "tied into" the basket to secure it.

In some cases, the patient is intubated. Without a transport ventilator, it will be necessary for the Paramedic to be hauled up along with the patient in order to continue patient ventilation. Use of a length of corrugated tubing and a one-way proximal to the endotracheal tube will provide distance between the patient and the Paramedic and permit the Paramedic to "attend" the patient.

To prevent the patient from falling out of the basket, the patient must be secured to the basket. For low angle ascents, the patient may be "zippered" into the basket with webbing (Figure 30-20). Taking a long length of webbing secured by a hitch at one end, the two free ends of the webbing are weaved back and forth over the rails and tied off at the top.

However, in most cases the patient is secured into the basket with a seat harness (often improvised) and even a chest harness. These harnesses are especially important in high angle or vertical ascent. (Vertical ascent may be necessary in confined space.)

When the patient is strapped into the basket, the patient cannot protect himself. For this reason, the patient should have either a helmet and goggles or a litter shield to protect the eyes from falling debris or from head injury in case of an inadvertent fall.

Hauling

Next, the patient is either raised to the anchor for evacuation or lowered to a safe evacuation point. If the patient is being lowered, it can be helpful to have an "attendant" line. A rescuer on the ground uses this extra line to help guide the basket over obstacles.

Raising a patient in a basket, with an attendant, is a labor-intensive procedure. In some cases, sufficient personnel are on-scene and permit the patient to be hauled up directly using no mechanical advantage (the "Armstrong method)."

Using pulleys, it is possible to create the mechanical advantage seen in traditional block and tackle techniques used at the dock to lift heavy loads from a ship to shore. **Mechanical advantage** is a simple machine that multiplies the force put into it. The formula is length of arm divided by length of resistance arm. Simply by placing a rope through a

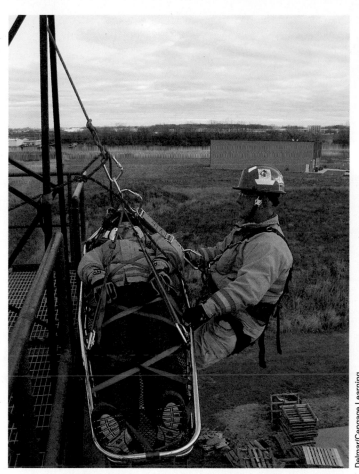

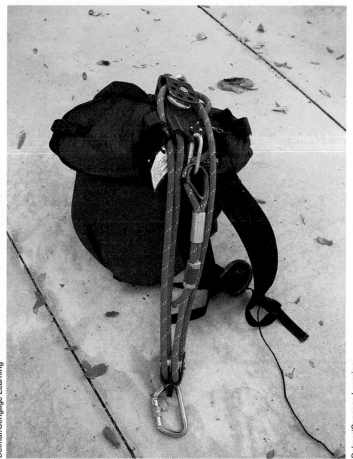

Figure 30-20 This patient is secured to a basket with a harness and webbing.

Figure 30-21 A prerigged hauling system saves time and prevents errors.

single movable pulley, for example, a mechanical advantage of two is achieved. Although the distance that the load must be hauled is twice as long, the weight to be lifted is cut in half.

Although many variations of mechanical advantage exist, perhaps one of the most common is the **3:1 Z rig**. The rope forms a Z pattern as it winds between two pulleys that are pulled closer together. Thus, a moderately efficient pulley (friction always plays a role in efficiency) can make lifting 200 pounds feel like lifting 91 pounds. A 3:1 simple pulley system is so commonly used that many rescuers "preset" the system in a hauling system (Figure 30-21). This preplanning saves time and prevents errors.[6]

Haul Commands

Similar to rappelling, a series of commands are used to direct the "haul team." Because of the distance between the rescuer(s) and the team, the members use a whistle. One short blast means stop the haul, whereas two short blasts means start the haul or raise. When a basket must be lowered and an obstacle such as a rock outcropping is encountered, then three short blasts of the whistle indicate lower or down. When the patient and basket are safely either on the ground or at the anchor, four short blasts of the whistle mean the "rope is free." One long and continuous blast signals trouble and that the rescuer(s) need help.

Overland Carry

Once the patient arrives on the ground or at the anchor, the patient may need to be carried out to the awaiting ambulance, helicopter, or other transport. Cross-country litter carries are physically demanding. With all rescuers facing forward, a team of four each takes either a corner (i.e., **four-corner carry**) (Figure 30-22) or one on each side and each end (i.e., **diamond carry**) (Figure 30-23). The choice of which carry to use is dependent on the terrain and the width of the trail. Additional rescuers can be added in the middle of the basket.

One rescuer is usually the trail finder, who clears out obstacles or calls out hazards. Another rescuer may be following the litter, carrying oxygen bottles and/or intravenous solutions, among other tasks. These rescuers are often used to relieve fatigued litter attendants.

When the team comes to an obstacle, rather than having all of the members of the team struggle over the obstacle, the patient is passed over the obstacle. This transfer of the litter, called a **caterpillar pass**, requires that the rescuers have their feet firmly planted before the litter is transferred (Figure 30-24).

To help with the burden, loops of webbing can be attached to the basket with a hitch. These loops of webbing, called a **sling**, help the litter bearers balance the load over their shoulders (Figure 30-25).

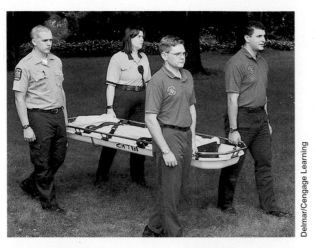

Figure 30-22 In a four-corner litter carry, each rescuer takes a corner of the litter.

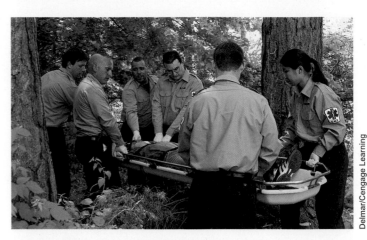

Figure 30-24 A caterpillar pass involves passing the litter over an obstacle.

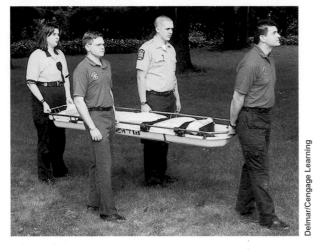

Figure 30-23 In the diamond litter carry, each rescuer takes a side or end of the litter.

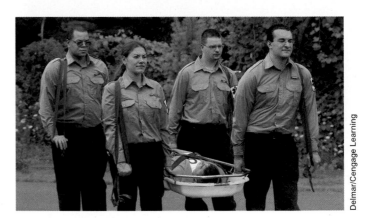

Figure 30-25 A sling is used with a basket to help the litter bearers balance the load over their shoulders.

Termination

Following every rescue operation, the team should reassemble and debrief. These "after action" reports can identify problem areas that hampered the operation and obtain suggestions in order to improve performance. These after action reports are not intended for critical incident stress debriefing.

CASE STUDY CONCLUSION

The team has rappelled to the patient, provided patient care, packaged the patient, and is prepared to haul the patient to the top of the cliff. With everyone in place, the slow and laborious process starts. After several starts and stops, as the rope system is reset, the patient makes it to the top.

Next, the patient is carried out of the woods to the awaiting ambulance. Fortunately, there are fresh responders at the top, with slings in hand, willing to start the hike out.

CRITICAL THINKING QUESTIONS

1. What precautions need to be taken to prepare the patient for the haul?
2. What are some of the patient concerns during the carry?

CONCLUSION

Whether the Paramedic is embedded in the rescue team or is an addition to the rescue team, it is important that the Paramedic be aware of basic rescue operations and the equipment that will be encountered. Although safety conscious rescuers perform most technical rescues, safety is everyone's job. Having another pair of eyes (those of the Paramedic) looking for potential problems means everyone is safer.

KEY POINTS:

- The three phases to technical rescue are preplanning, operations, and termination.

- Preplanning starts with hazard analysis and slope analysis.

- Slope analysis consists of determining if the slope angle is low, steep, high angle, or highline.

- Following the hazard analysis, the rescuer makes a needs assessment.

- NFPA 1006 describes three levels of training: Awareness, Operations, and Technician.

- Paramedic safety is paramount as represented in the system safety factor.

- Ropes are either static or dynamic; static ropes are used in rescue and dynamic ropes are used in sport-climbing.

- Equipment used for rescue includes twisted or kernmantle rope, webbing, prusik, carabiners, descent control devices, ascenders, rigging plates, and pulleys.

- Every rope system starts with an anchor that must be steadfast and immovable.

- Rescue starts when the rescuer, often protected by a belay, rappels to the patient.

- Lowering systems that bring equipment and the basket to the patient occur after the rescuer rappels to the patient.

- After the patient is packaged, the patient is hauled to safety by either raising or lowering the basket.

- Following the haul, the patient is then either air lifted or carried overland out of the woods.

REVIEW QUESTIONS:

1. What are the four angles in the slope analysis?
2. What is the difference between static and dynamic rope?
3. A "bomb-proof" anchor is great, but many times a load-distributing anchor is all that is available. What is a load-distributing anchor?
4. What is a mechanical advantage rope system?
5. What are the overland carries?

CASE STUDY QUESTIONS:

Please refer to the Case Study in this chapter, and answer the questions below:

1. What is the optimal harness for use during a rescue?
2. What is a lowering system?
3. What considerations should be taken when packaging the patient?

REFERENCES:

1. NFPA 1006. *Standard for Technical Rescuer Professional Qualifications* (2008 ed.). Quincy, MA: National Fire Protection Association; 2008.

2. NFPA 1670. *Standard on Operations and Training for Technical Search and Rescue Incidents* (2004 ed.). Quincy, MA: National Fire Protection Association; 2004.

3. NFPA 1983. *Standard on Life Safety Rope and Equipment for Emergency Services* (2006 ed.). Quincy, MA: National Fire Protection Association; 2006.

4. Brown M. *Engineering Practical Rope Rescue Systems*. Delmar/ Cengage Learning; Clifton Park NY, 2000.

5. Frank JA, ed. *CMC Rope Rescue Manual* (3rd ed.). Santa Barbara, CA: CMC Rescue, Inc., 1998.

6. Matthews J. *Rope Levels I and II*. Delmar/Cengage Learning; Clifton Park, NY, 2010.

CHAPTER 31

MASS-GATHERING MEDICINE

KEY CONCEPTS:

Upon completion of this chapter, it is expected that the reader will understand these following concepts:

- The nature of mass-gathering events
- The need for event planning
- Integration of the Incident Command System into event planning

"Brian, you have been assigned to be the liaison to the county event planning committee," Brian's supervisor informs him. "We need to cover this position because we have been notified by the County Office of Emergency Management that, in three months, our little town will be the site of The Concert of Peace and Love. The plan is to start the event on a Friday morning, July 21, and end that Sunday night. We are expecting over 90,000 attendees who will start arriving earlier in the week preceding the concert. As the contracted 9-1-1 EMS provider, we have been tasked with providing all emergency medical treatment at the event."

CRITICAL THINKING QUESTIONS

1. What is the mission of EMS at a mass gathering?
2. What should be discussed at the preplanning meeting and who should attend the meeting?

OVERVIEW

A mass gathering can be a fair, a concert, an air show, or a marathon race. Alternatively, a mass gathering can be "Black Friday" at the local shopping mall or a multidenominational prayer meeting. Almost every community has a mass gathering of one type or another in their jurisdiction. Regardless of the venue or the event, emergencies may develop, and people will expect Paramedics to provide EMS care at these mass gatherings under austere and sometimes difficult circumstances. Therefore, Paramedics need to have the ability to predict, prepare, and respond to these emergencies. The EMS motto might be, "Hope for the best but prepare for the worst." When good times go bad, the public expects the Paramedic to be there to help.

There are various definitions of what constitutes a mass gathering. The National Association of EMS Physicians and the American College of Emergency Physicians define a **mass gathering** as a group of more than 1,000 people. However, similar to a multiple-casualty incident, it is not the size of the crowd but the potential for medical emergencies and the ability of local EMS to respond to those emergencies that dictates the use of the descriptor "mass gathering."

The goal of mass-gathering medicine is to mitigate the predictable problems associated with these events and, when that is not possible, to provide timely emergency medical care. To meet that goal, Paramedics must make plans for the mass gathering.

Event Preplanning

In almost every case, there will be a greater volume of EMS calls for people at a mass gathering than for similar numbers of people in the general population.[1] Because of this increased volume of calls, the Paramedic must alter and/or adapt her normal operating procedures. To preplan for these operating procedures, the Paramedic must consider the event's biomedical, psychosocial, and environmental factors. The timeline for preplanning and preparation can be years (as in the case of the Olympics), months (as in the case with a marathon or iron man competition), or days (as in the case of a presidential visit).

Since EMS is the mission of Paramedics, the first factor to consider is the biomedical aspect. Specific types of medical emergencies can be anticipated at certain types of events. For example, alcohol abuse and illicit drug use are expected at a rock concert or motorsports event based on case studies. A review of the literature reveals hundreds of descriptive case studies on different types of events. These can help the Paramedic prepare for the anticipated emergencies by reviewing a historical record of similar events.

Even the age of the anticipated attendees comes into play when planning for a mass-gathering event. Young people often attend hardcore rock concerts complete with a mosh pit, slam dancing, and crowd surfing. As a result, head trauma, musculoskeletal trauma, and drug abuse can be anticipated among these attendees. Older people, in contrast, may attend

an easy listening-type festival or symphony concert and will more likely have another set of emergencies, such as sudden cardiac death. Each age group brings with it a unique set of pre-existing medical conditions.

Besides these biomedical factors, the Paramedic must take into consideration the psychosocial aspect of a mass gathering. By definition, a mass gathering is a social event, and social events tend to excite certain emotions. For example, the crowd at a championship football game is likely to feel and behave differently than the crowd welcoming the pope for a visit or protestors at a war rally. Therefore, the Paramedic should take into account the **crowd sentiment**, the emotional tone set by the event and by the crowd.

The Paramedic should be especially attuned to the availability of alcohol and the likelihood of drug trafficking during these social events, as these drugs tend to magnify people's emotions. Some event planners purposely set up a highly visible law enforcement presence in an effort to curb alcohol abuse and drug trafficking. To control the consumption of alcohol, event planners have enacted policies such as banning alcohol at the gate, banning the entrance of obviously intoxicated individuals, limiting the times alcohol is sold on-site, limiting the portions of alcohol served, and restricting sites for the sale of alcohol to designated areas. The problem of alcohol abuse should not be underestimated. At one rock concert, 48% of the patients seeking medical attention were estimated to be intoxicated. Paramedics should be familiar with the efforts and policies that venue management and law enforcement have made to control alcohol and drug abuse.

One way to enforce alcohol policies is to train the event staff in **techniques for effective alcohol management (TEAM)**, an educational program that teaches a concessionaire, or a Paramedic, the skills needed to identify an intoxicated individual and to intervene in a "non-confrontational way" to ensure the safety of the attendee and the staff.[2]

The most obvious of the three factors involved in event planning is the environmental factor (Figure 31-1). The first environmental factor is the location of the event. Public facilities, such as stadiums, generally are designed to support the mission of public safety, whereas public spaces, such as a park used for a protest or the streets used for a demonstration, are not. However, a preplan can still be developed for these locations. Protests and demonstrations often have to obtain a permit, and their organizers tend to choose high visibility locations, such as the front steps of the city hall, for their activities. Community intelligence by law enforcement can anticipate these events. For this reason, it is important that EMS work with its partners in law enforcement and the city/county clerk's office to optimize the public's safety.

The next environmental factor is whether the event is indoors or outdoors. Indoor events tend to provide amenities, such as bathrooms and public phones, for the convenience of the attendees. The Paramedic should make note of where these amenities are located as medical emergencies often arise at these locations.

Indoor venues often have specified positions that allow Paramedics and other safety officers to provide a rapid response through designated routes of access and egress. They also often use physical barriers for crowd control, thus limiting crowd size.

Outdoor events are often more problematic for the Paramedic. Weather can play a major role in the number and types of medical emergencies. For example, the Paramedic can anticipate heat emergencies if there is a lack of shelter from the sun and high temperatures and humidity. The use of alcohol by attendees magnifies that potential.

Some event planners recognize the potential for heat emergencies and have pallets of bottled water brought to the event. They may also have the fire department set up "fog streams" to cool the crowd.

Crowd migration in outdoor venues must also be considered. Some outdoor venues, such as open-air concerts and outdoor stadiums, have natural or man-made barriers in place that control crowd migration. However, other venues are nothing more than a large open field. The Paramedic must anticipate the flow of the crowd, particularly when the event ends, in order to plan routes to access patients.

Even the direction of the wind can come into play. Something as innocent as a change of wind direction during a fireworks display can cause problems as the fireworks rain ash into the eyes of the upward-looking attendees and smoke into the crowd. The Paramedic may anticipate subsequent EMS calls for shortness of breath and eye irritation. Extended forecasts, as well as up-to-the-minute weather reports, are useful during event planning.

The most obvious variable in event planning is the anticipated size of the crowd. Although estimates are, by definition, inexact (and sometimes inaccurate), estimating the anticipated crowd can help the Paramedic predict the needed EMS coverage.[3] Using historical data, either from previous events on-site or from reports from similar events held elsewhere, the Paramedic can predict the **patient load**, the number of patients expected based on the type of event and size of the crowd (Table 31-1) For example, according to some reports, there will be 0.3 to 1.6 medical emergencies per 1,000 attendees at a sporting event, 24 EMS calls per 1,000 participants at a marathon, and 0.96 to 17 calls for EMS per 1,000 people at a rock concert, with many of these calls involving alcohol and/or drug abuse.[4,5]

Preparation and Preplanning

After gathering biomedical, psychosocial, and environment data, EMS should plan a meeting of the key public safety officials to preplan and prepare and/or review the public safety plan. Since the goal of the plan is to improve operational preparedness, all of the key "players" should be invited to the preplanning meeting.

The first people to be invited should be the event planners and venue management. These two entities (sometimes they are the same person) have an interest in limiting life hazards and their **litigation profile**, the chance that they will be sued. The event planner/venue management is also responsible for obtaining permits for these public events. In many states, the organizer must obtain a permit before any large public event. Often the party requesting the permit is required to notify law enforcement. Unfortunately, in most cases there is scant consideration given to notifying EMS. In those cases when EMS is considered, it is generally only to note a list of minimum equipment that must be maintained on-site.

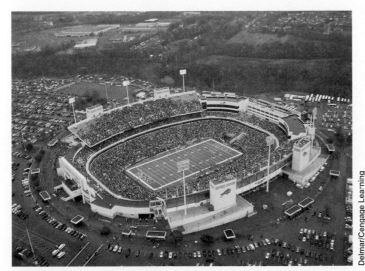

Figure 31-1 The physical structure and layout of the venue can affect the preplanning process.

Delmar/Cengage Learning

Table 31-1 Number of Medical Encounters for a Variety of Major Events

Event	Location/Date	Number of People	Medical Encounter/10,000	Reference*
Live Aid Concert	Philadelphia July 1985	90,000	33	1
Rock Music Concert	Toronto, Ontario August 1980	30,000	167	2
Rock Music Concert	Holland, Vermont September 1982	35,000	69	3
Rock Music Concert	Devore, California September 1982	410,000	64	4
National Football League	Denver 1978 season	72,000 per game	4 average 10 games	5
Crosby Golf Tournament	Advance, North Carolina May 1987 (4 days)	80,000	22	6
World's Fair	Knoxville, Tennessee May–Oct 1982	11,000,000	23	7
World Exposition	Vancouver, British Columbia May–Oct 1986	22,100,000	39	6
Summer Olympics	Los Angeles 1984	3,450,000	16	8
"The Open" Golf Championship	Several Venues, United Kingdom 1981 to 1990	1,568,833 (10-yr period)	51	9
Special Olympic Games	Galveston, Texas Spring, 1989	777 (athletes)	347	10, 11
Indianapolis 500 Road Race	Indianapolis 1983–1990	400,000 per year	3.5 average for 8 races	12
Winter Olympics	Calgary, Canada February 1988	1,800,000	15.2	13

Source: Copyright ©1996 American College of Emergency Physicians. All rights reserved.

References

Numbering has been modified from the original source references list to reflect that only the references that are relevant to this table are provided.

1. Mariano JP. First aid for LIVE AID. *J Emerg Med Serv.* February 1986:47–57.
2. Chapman KR, Carmichael FJ, Goode JE. Medical services for outdoor rock music festivals. *Can Med Assoc J.* 1982;126:935–938.
3. Osler DC, Shapiro F, Shapiro S. Medical services at outdoor music festivals. Risks and recommendations. *Clin Pediatr.* 1975;14:390–395.
4. Ounanian LL, Salinas C, Shear CL, et al. Medical care at the 1982 US festival. *Ann Emerg Med.* 1986;15:520–527.
5. Pons PT, Holland B, Alfrey E, et al. An advanced emergency medical care system at National Football League games. *Ann Emerg Med.* 1980;9:203–206.
6. Leonard RB, Nuji EK, Petrilli R, Calabro JJ. Provision of emergency medicine care for crowds. *American College of Emergency Physicians Information Paper.* 1990.
7. Gustafson TL, Booth AL, Fricker RS, et al. Disease surveillance and emergency services at the 1982 World's Fair. *Am J Public Health.* 1987;77:861–863.
8. Baker WM, Simone BM, Niemann JT, et al. Special event medical care: The 1984 Los Angeles Summer Olympics experience. *Ann Emerg Med.* 1986;15:185–190.
9. Additional reference missing from new list: Hadden WA, Kelly S, Pumford N. Medical cover for "The Open" Golf Championship. *Br J Sports Med.* 1992;26(3):125-127.
10. Year estimated from publication date.
11. From new list of references.
12. Boch HC, Cordell WH, Hawk AC, et al. Demographics of emergency medical care at the Indianapolis 500 Race (1983–1990). *Ann Emerg Med.* 1992;21:1204–1207.
13. New York State Sanitary Code, Part 18: Public Functions with Attendance over 5,000 People. *Public Health Law Section 225.* 1991.

Some event planners/venue managers will also have a risk manager present. In most cases, the **risk manager** represents the insurance company that is providing coverage for the event. These risk managers have a wealth of knowledge and experience from insuring similar events and can be an invaluable asset to the preparation efforts.

Some larger event planners even bring in psychologists and/or sociologists to the meeting. These experts in crowd behavior are familiar with how people act in large groups and how these crowds can be influenced and directed. The goal is to prevent death and injury by **human stampede**, compressive forces that result when people are trampled by a closely pushed together mass of people. Human stampedes have been reported at soccer stadiums, rugby tournaments, and even religious revivals. The power of a stampede should not be underestimated. Compressive forces from "penned in" participants can be greater than one-half ton as people pile on, either vertically or horizontally. Severe traumas and trauma arrests from **compressive asphyxiation** (known as crowd crush), a situation in which the patient lacks oxygen due to compression of the chest cavity, are not uncommon during a human stampede. Along with theories of crowd dynamics and crowd behavior, the input from these consultants can reduce serious injuries and fatalities from human stampedes.

The other meeting participants are typically the members of the public safety triad: police, fire, and EMS. Each participates according to her role. However, there is a great deal of crossover in those roles (as explained shortly). Therefore, it is in the best interests of all parties to listen to one another.

Preplanning can be broken down into prevention and response. Both public health and the fire service play a major role in prevention. Public health is responsible for establishing safety standards for on-site food preparation. With an eye on preventing waterborne and/or foodborne illness, public health inspectors can ensure that foods are wholesome, water is safe, and that waste management capacities are not exceeded. One outbreak of shigellosis can put an event into the media spotlight and result in a call for investigation into its preparation.

Similarly, fire inspectors inspect buildings and facilities to endure they comply with safety codes. Safety codes are established to reduce life hazards from fire and building collapse. Fire and smoke may represent one of the greatest potentials for mass casualty. Death and injury can also occur from panic and stampede or exposure to smoke and fire.

Security is often the first responder to the scene of a medical emergency "on the property." Although some of these security officers are medically trained, many are not. Furthermore, security can consist of a number of different private and public law enforcement entities with overlapping jurisdictions. A clear distinction must exist of the roles of these different law enforcement officers in terms of assistance to the public and support of the EMS team. For example, private security officers may be responsible for escorting responders, whereas police officers are responsible for on-scene crowd management.

The key to a timely response is the link between first responders and event communications. In some instances security personnel, in their role as first responders, alert event communications, who in turn activates the EMS system. Conversely, people may call in to event communications, transferred from public safety answering points (PASP) or via on-site telephone systems, to alert telecommunicators of a medical emergency. Event communications then activates EMS.

In some instances, particularly the smaller events, the PSAP and event communications are one in the same. In many instances, on-site communications occur through a separate system that is contained at or near a Command post. In this case, it is important that event communications and the PSAP have clear communication. This prevents dispatch from sending multiple responders to the same event or, worse, failing to send any responder.

During the planning meeting, the participants should consider all aspects of the **chain of communications**, the method by which concessionaires and vendors contact EMS in an emergency as well as notify hospitals of the impending arrival of patients.

Event planners must consider the possible need for **mass evacuation**, an organized effort to remove all individuals from a certain area, as there is the ever-present danger of a terrorist using weapons of mass destruction (WMDs) at a mass gathering. Following a credible threat of WMDs, the first step in mass evacuation is warning the public. The use of pre-existing public address systems is an option, as is use of the media. It may be possible to use the sound system set up at entertainment events. In those instances where public address systems are not available, however, telecommunicators will need to use existing resources to notify the public, such as the public address feature found on the siren of an ambulance or patrol car. EMS can give carefully prepared scripts to strategically placed units that will control the movement of the crowd and help to prevent crowd surge.

Part of the preplan should be the creation or review of policies that are likely to be used during the event, such as policies on the care and treatment of juveniles and policies on the level of sobriety at which an attendee can be treated and released. In terms of convenience, standardized algorithms and instructions should be prepared for the treatment and release of patients with minor complaints. These treat and release policies should be reviewed by a physician prior to use.

Paramedics are often approached with requests for Band-Aids®, aspirin, and even sunscreen. The event planners should establish a procedure that offers the Paramedic guidance on where to direct attendees requesting such items. In some instances, the event planners strategically place vending machines around the event. In other instances, a local pharmacy may provide a concession stand stocked with OTC medications and preparations.

The Paramedic should have an adequate supply of patient encounter reports, patient care reports, and patient refusal forms on hand. Patient encounter reports are used when a request for an over-the-counter medicine is made. In some instances, Paramedics use triage tags in addition to patient care reports to help track patient movement.

Operations at a mass gathering can use elements of the Incident Command System (ICS) or the entire ICS system. The goals of operations at a mass gathering and ICS are congruent (i.e., to establish a "set of personnel, policies, procedures, facilities and equipment, integrated into a common organizational structure designed to improve emergency response operations").[6]

There are several advantages to using ICS during a mass-gathering event. For example, ICS is understood and practiced by all three public safety teams. In this way, ICS provides for unity of command, a common terminology, and coordination of resources using an incident action plan.

In the event of a disaster, the flexible and modular organization allows ICS to be expanded and additional elements to be easily integrated. However, the greatest advantage to using ICS for a mass-gathering event is comprehensive resource management. Use of comprehensive resource management helps to ensure a timely response to medical emergencies.

Often a building is designated as the **Emergency Operations Center (EOC)**. This building is used to coordinate all the resources needed for an emergency response at the event. In some cases, a mobile EOC is brought to the scene (Figure 31-2). Other personnel in the EOC, other than the incident commander, may be the **public information officer (PIO)**, who distributes relevant data about the event to the media, and the **safety officer**, who oversees the well-being of attendees and may be part of the venue's risk management team.

Mutual aid plans in case of disaster must be in place as well. In some systems, the local mutual aid system is "exercised"—that is, put on alert—so that neighboring EMS can be prepared in case of activation. Minimally, the event planners should provide briefing packets along with maps of the grounds marked with the staging area and directions to the field hospital and/or local hospitals to all mutual aid partners.

Every mass-gathering event is an opportunity for the Disaster Medical Assistance Team (DMAT) and/or the Medical Reserve Corp. (MRC) to "drill" their skills as well. These teams are created to provide medical care, often under austere conditions, in circumstances such as those that might be encountered at a mass-gathering event.

EMS Operations

Although some 80% of patients reporting to EMS at one event complained of simple maladies like headache, blisters on the feet, and sunburn, a number of predictable medical emergencies may occur as well. For example, there is a higher incidence of asthma-related complaints at a mass-gathering event. Also, as mentioned earlier, some events have

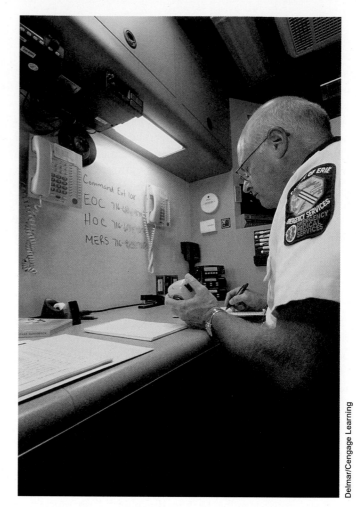

Delmar/Cengage Learning

Figure 31-2 A centralized communication center in a larger event helps coordinate EMS field units.

"event-specific" medical emergencies. The Paramedic should estimate, preferably based on past experience, the "vulnerable populations" and what medical emergencies are most likely to present to EMS.

While preparing for predictable patient presentations, the Paramedic should also prepare for high life hazard events, such as sudden cardiac arrest. Although rare, these events mandate a tiered medical response, including use of first responders, CPR, and AED, to maximize the patient's survivability.[7] EMS needs to be prepared. The media is likely to report any deaths that occur at one of these events, which will cast a spotlight on the EMS response.

Although the science is in dispute, there are some recommended staffing levels for mass-gathering events that are based, in part, on predicted patient presentation rates. The suggested ratio is one EMS team, usually consisting of an EMT and a Paramedic, for every 10,000 attendees (Figure 31-3). For every 50,000 attendees, research suggests that a physician also be available, although there has been some debate if the physician needs to be on the grounds or simply available for consultation.

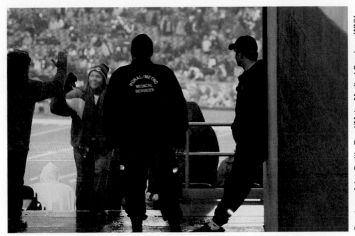

Figure 31-3 EMS field units are distributed throughout the venue.

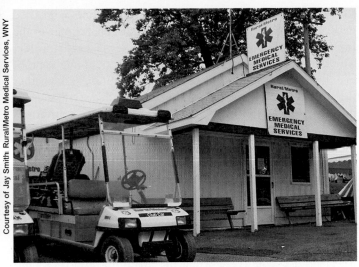

Figure 31-4 A fixed base of operations is essential to the team's coordination and operation during an event.

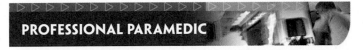

PROFESSIONAL PARAMEDIC

Although EMS team members may at times wear short-sleeved shirts or even special T-shirts to stay comfortable, it may be advisable to have these EMS teams wear the standard service uniform, including identification tags, while they are in public. This not only helps to establish a professional image, it also makes them identifiable to civilians and fellow responders alike.

In addition to supplies used for routine medical care, additional or special equipment and supplies may be needed at a mass gathering. For example, the event planners should provide hearing protection to all EMS personnel at a rock concert as part of their PPE. Some supplies are event specific. Ice and ice machines are often available at events, such as marathons, where musculoskeletal injuries are predictable. Likewise, additional intravenous solution should be on hand for heat emergencies on hot and humid days.

Ambient noise in the crowd makes it difficult for Paramedics to hear radio calls. For these special circumstances, some Paramedics prefer hands-free microphone/headsets that use Bluetooth® technology, earphones, or ear buds similar to the type used by the Secret Service. Paramedics can also use remote speaker/microphones, sometimes referred to as "parrots," that clip onto a short collar or radio sling while the radio transmitter remains on the belt or in the holster.

The focal point for EMS at a mass gathering is usually at a fixed point, such as a field hospital or forward aid station (Figure 31-4). These facilities can be permanent, such as designated buildings dedicated to EMS, or temporary shelters such as tents and portable shelters like the type used by the

DMAT and the military that are put up for the duration of the event. For some events, such as induction day at the Baseball Hall of Fame in Cooperstown, New York, specially equipped tractor-trailers are brought in. These mobile medical trailers, used by **Disaster Assistance Response Teams (DART)**, groups of trained personnel that can be rapidly called upon to provide aid during an emergency, have up to 1,000 square feet of treatment area. They come equipped with portable medical imaging equipment and mobile labs for point of care testing. Some even have a half-dozen critical care beds complete with monitors and ventilators.

Often personnel report to these facilities to receive their assignments and equipment before going "onto the property." In other instances, separate facilities, distant from patient care, are provided for personnel. These "collection points" often have refreshments as well as sanitary facilities. Similar to the rehabilitation efforts that occur on a fire scene, providing incident rehabilitation for providers is part of the emergency plan.

Some event plans call for a "split shift," meaning that the Paramedic cares for patients, or is part of a roving patrol, for four hours out of eight. This gives the Paramedic time to recuperate before the next tour.[8]

PROFESSIONAL PARAMEDIC

Personnel reporting for duty should be provided with directions to special event parking for EMS as well as given any special identification that will be required to gain entrance. Providing these simple materials can help an operation run more smoothly.

All EMS personnel should receive a briefing, a detailed description of the event and EMS operations. As part of the briefing, EMS personnel should receive an event profile. The **event profile** contains information about the type of event, such as whether it is indoors or outdoors, and whether it is restricted (such as fenced in) or extended (with a capability of expanding beyond the grounds). Crowd information should also be provided such as whether the crowd will be seated or mobile and the anticipated sentiment of the crowd (passive, active, or energetic). The teams should also be provided with expectations of crowd size, estimated from ticket sales as well as expected gate turnover based on past practice.

The Paramedics should be provided with published information about the duration of the event and the times for special events (e.g., when the headliner at a rock concert is expected to perform). Policies regarding alcohol consumption should also be furnished in the event profile brief.

Finally, the Paramedic should be provided with the extended forecast for the day of the event, which includes the expected high temperature and humidity, along with a map of the grounds. This map should clearly mark the location of crowd barriers, pathways, exits, and access points to bounded areas.

After securing supplies and equipment, as well as staffing, the Paramedic should next consider transportation. Transportation can be categorized as on-site or off-site. On-site transportation, from the incident location to forward aid stations or field hospitals, can be accomplished in a number of ways, depending on the event location. Wheelchairs and stretchers can be useful for shorter distances, whereas longer distances may require special four-wheeled carriers. These powered four-wheeled patient carriers include modified golf carts, special flatbed trucks, modified ambulances, and "quad" all-terrain vehicles (ATV).

Ambulances that are dedicated to the event generally transport patients off-site. These ambulances are usually parked in proximity to the field hospital or placed at predesignated access points. In many instances, additional ambulances are staged away from the event but close enough for rapid response. These ambulances remain in service and are available to respond to the event in cases of sudden and unexpected numbers of casualties that exceed the site's ability (i.e., **surge capacity**). They also can respond to emergencies that occur "off-grounds" but are associated with the event, such as motor vehicle collisions that occur at the end of the event.

The Paramedics should also consider using helicopters for medical evacuation (Medevac). Helicopters permit the timely evacuation of patients to more distant hospitals, thereby freeing up beds in closer hospitals. They can also be utilized as part of the surge capacity. Perhaps the greatest advantage of a helicopter is its ability to fly over gridlocked traffic that would immobilize an ambulance.

EMS Response

EMS at a mass-gathering event can be categorized using the points of the Star of Life: early detection, early reporting, early responses, on-scene care, care in transit, and transfer to definitive care. Early detection is usually provided by a combination of surveillance equipment and human surveillance.

Modern technology (e.g., in the form of reconnaissance cameras) can help provide electronic surveillance of crowds with surprising efficiency. However, these systems are generally expensive and are used at fixed facilities such as stadiums. Untrained civilians, such as concessionaires or minimally trained security forces, can accomplish human surveillance. To improve human surveillance, many plans call for "spotters," individuals with binoculars who are strategically stationed and scanning the crowd. For example, spotters might be stationed at or near the sound stage at a concert. Another technique of human surveillance is "roving teams" made up of security officers. These easily identified security officers detect and report medical emergencies.

The methods of reporting an emergency at an event are as varied as the types of events. In many instances, mobile cell phones are readily available, as are "pull boxes" at stadiums. Regardless of the PSAP that answers the call, it is imperative that the information is seamlessly transferred to on-site communications at the event. These communicators in turn lead to the dispatch of first responders.

The responders' goal is getting medical assistance to the patient in a timely manner. EMS responders should be strategically placed so that BLS responders can be at the patient's side within four minutes and Paramedics can arrive within eight minutes. The briefing packets containing maps that were provided to the Paramedics should indicate potential barriers. Security officers, who have the keys to locked gates, should anticipate opening the gates, permitting EMS access. Simultaneously, security forces should be dispatched to the scene for crowd control. To help locate the scene, some first responders are given location flags to wave down responders.

After treating immediate life threats, responders should triage the patients to the appropriate care. In some instances, the patient can be assessed, treated, and released on-scene. In other cases, the patient will need to be evacuated to a forward aid station. Forward aid stations should be strategically placed about one-eighth of a mile apart or about a five-minute walk through the crowd.

The advantage of using a forward aid station is that the patient can be further stabilized out of sight of onlookers and away from the rush of curiosity seekers. Paramedics are often staged, with their equipment, at these forward aid stations while awaiting the patient's evacuation from the scene.

In some cases, performers (the "talent") or VIPs with a security detachment will make provisions for private medical care that is organized apart from the event's EMS staff. During the planning meeting, these special provisions should be discussed with the event's EMS staff to clearly delineate their role, if any.

Care in transit refers to the care provided before a patient arrives at a hospital. At a small event, this is routine ambulance care. However, the sheer number of patients at a large event may overwhelm the capacity of local resources. In those cases, the care in transit is performed at a field hospital. Since the field hospital provides urgent treatment care, transportation to the emergency department may not be necessary in all cases. With good triage, and consultation with medical control, it may not even be necessary to have a physician on-scene.[9]

Since many events are time-limited, and the subsequent surge of patients is limited to the duration of the event, the field hospital can serve as a "holding area" until beds and ambulances become available or the patient is ready to be discharged. Use of the field hospital in this case is a form of "surge protection" for the local emergency department.

If transfer to definitive care is necessary because of the patient's condition, then the patient should be expeditiously transported to local facilities. Increased efficiency is obtained by using preplanned exits and special routes. In some instances, these exits and routes are longer than the more direct routes. However, they may avoid traffic and gridlock. If gridlock does occur, air medical services should be summoned and the patient airlifted to the hospital.

▶ CASE STUDY CONCLUSION

At the current meeting, in addition to finalizing plans for the Department of Health to provide food inspectors and the fire department to set up a Command post, Brian's idea of having medical treatment centers with roving patrols is well received. The team decides that there should be a total of four treatment centers: three located around the edge of the farm to the right, left, and the far end, with easy access to the road. The fourth will be the backstage treatment center. Additional staff for this center, which will be located footsteps away from the Emergency Operations Center, will come from the concert's travelling medical unit.

Staffing the treatment centers will be a collection of volunteer physicians and nurses along with paid EMS crews from Brian's agency, who will staff the transport vehicles. Assisting these crews will be EMS volunteers from the local ambulance corps and fire department. The word is already out and people can hardly wait for The Concert of Peace and Love.

CRITICAL THINKING QUESTIONS

1. What are the advantages of using forward aid stations, field hospitals, and mutual aid?
2. What groups of EMS providers might be invited to participate in a mass-gathering event?

CONCLUSION

The ability to provide high-quality medical care at a mass-gathering event is predicated on the Paramedic's ability to prepare for the foreseeable medical emergencies, to mitigate those hazards where possible, and to prepare for the inevitable patient workload. Utilizing ICS structure, with an understanding of the dynamic nature of this type of potential mass-casualty incident, the Paramedic can have the policies and procedures in place to handle any foreseeable event. Every community has a mass gathering of one type or another during the year. With a goal of providing high-quality medical care, and in the spirit of performance improvement, Paramedics need to critically analyze past history, share their findings with others, and use more evidence-based practice for planning for the next mass gathering.[10]

KEY POINTS:

- The goal of mass-gathering medicine is to mitigate predictable problems and to provide timely medical care in the event those problems occur.

- Preplanning involves consideration of biomedical, psychosocial, and environmental factors. Timelines for preplanning can vary from days, months or years.

- Alcohol distribution and consumption control among attendees can help to mitigate some of the incidents of alcohol-related emergencies at a mass gathering.

- Environmental factors include the physical location of the mass gathering; the available facilities, including aid stations; the weather; and so on.

- Indoor facilities provide amenities such as toilets, water fountains, and telephones, and are often designed with crowd control in mind. Outdoor venues are more problematic from an environmental standpoint.

- Patient loads can be estimated based on the size of the crowd and the type of event.

- Preplanning helps to decrease the litigation profile by bringing safety officials and event planners together to identify and mitigate predictable hazards.

- Compressive asphyxiation or crowd crush occurs with a human stampede.

- Security is often the first responder that activates EMS.

- The chain of communications should include interoperability.

- Mass evacuation is part of the response to a threat of weapons of mass destruction.

- The Incident Command System is often used at a mass-gathering event.

- In addition to an incident commander, there should be a public information officer and a safety officer in the Emergency Operations Center.

- Mutual aid agreements should be in place and implemented as needed.

- Fixed facilities include field hospitals, forward aid stations, or even mobile medical trailers such as those used by Disaster Assistance Response Teams.

- On- and off-site transportation must be considered, including staging ambulances.

- Intelligence, such as human surveillance and reconnaissance cameras, can help to monitor the crowd and improve EMS response.

- Transport to forward aid stations, performed after removing the patient from the crowd, helps to ensure patient privacy and uninterrupted care.

- Performers, athletes, and other talent may have personal healthcare providers who should be instructed on the on-site provision of emergency services.

- Field hospitals help to evenly distribute patient loads to local hospitals according to triage standards to prevent overloading.

▶ REVIEW QUESTIONS:

1. What effects would a large concert have in a small town with limited resources?
2. What is an event profile?
3. What are treatment centers?
4. Where should the emergency operations center be located?
5. Who would staff a treatment center?

▶ CASE STUDY QUESTIONS:

Please refer to the Case Study in this chapter, and answer the questions below:

1. What are some means of controlling alcohol consumption at a mass gathering?
2. What is the concept of "TEAM"?
3. What can be done if there is a sudden increase in patients?

▶ REFERENCES:

1. Thompson JM, Savoia G, Powell G, et al. Level of medical care required for mass gatherings: the XV Winter Olympic Games in Calgary, Canada. *Ann Emerg Med.* 1991;20(4):385–390.

2. Techniques for Effective Alcohol Management Coalition. Available at: **http://www.teamcoalition.org/.** Accessed December 27, 2009.

3. Milsten AM, Seaman KG, Liu P, Bissell RA, Maguire BJ. Variables influencing medical usage rates, injury patterns, and levels of care for mass gatherings. *Prehosp Disaster Med.* 2003;18(4):334–346.

4. De Lorenzo RA. Mass gathering medicine: a review. *Prehosp Disast Med.* 1997;12(1):68–72.

5. Arbon P, Bridgewater FHG, Smith C. Mass gathering medicine: a predictive model for patient presentation rates. *Prehosp Disaster Med.* 2001;16(3):109–116.

6. Auf der Heide E. Disaster response: principles of preparation and coordination. Online edition. Center of Excellence in Disaster Management and Humanitarian Assistance. Available at: **http://orgmail2.coe-dmha.org/dr/static.htm.** Accessed December 27, 2009.

7. Wassertheil J, Keane G, Fisher N, Leditschke JF. Cardiac arrest outcomes at the Melbourne Cricket Ground and Shrine of Remembrance using a tiered response strategy—a forerunner to public access defibrillation. *Resuscitation.* 2000;44(2):97–104.

8. Zeitz KM, Zeitz CJ, Arbon P. Forecasting medical workloads at mass gathering events: predictive models as an adjunct to retrospective review. *Prehosp Disaster Med.* 2005;20(3):164–168.

9. Salhanick SD, Sheahan W, Bazarian JJ. Use and analysis of field triage criteria for mass gatherings. *Prehosp Disaster Med.* 2003;18(4):347–352.

10. Arbon P. Mass gathering medicine: a review of the evidence and future directions for research. *Prehosp Disaster Med.* 2007;22(2):131–135.

CHAPTER 32

TACTICAL EMERGENCY MEDICAL SUPPORT

KEY CONCEPTS:

Upon completion of this chapter, it is expected that the reader will understand these following concepts:

- Tactical EMS as one aspect of paramedicine
- Special weapons and tactics used by tactical medics
- Tactical medicine
- Zones of care
- Care under fire
- Prolonged operations and occupational health care
- Weapons of mass destruction and tactical EMS

"Recruits for SWAT team are to report to occupational health for a preliminary screening at 0600 hours. That includes you, Doc. Sweet dreams, gentlemen!" yells the first sergeant. Settling into the rack, the rookie looks at the ceiling and thinks to himself, "I have five years of street experience. What can they throw at me? I have been preparing for this day." The rookie doubts he will get any sleep.

CRITICAL THINKING QUESTIONS

1. What is the mission of a tactical medic?
2. What are the physical demands placed on a tactical medic?

OVERVIEW

In an increasingly complex world where radical groups and terrorists threaten civilian populations, there is an increasing need for law enforcement operations to intercept, interdict, and interfere with these groups. Whenever conflict occurs, however, casualties often follow. In an effort to ensure the safety of citizens and law enforcement alike, as well as to care for combatants, Paramedics have been attached to these special operations groups.

Tactical Emergency Medical Support

Certain police operations, particularly **Special Weapons and Tactics (SWAT)** missions that involve skills beyond typical law enforcement, have a high life hazard. To mitigate those hazards for civilians and law enforcement alike, and to improve officer survival, special Tactical Emergency Medical Support (TEMS) teams were created to assist the SWAT teams. Since the onset of SWAT teams in the mid-1960s, special TEMS units have slowly been growing as a subspecialty of EMS.

Tactical Emergency Medical Support (TEMS) can be defined as the medical support tailored for tactical law enforcement operations. It is further described as a non-military EMS system designed to provide and maintain medical services for all law enforcement special operations.[1] This includes preventative medical care for law enforcement officers, medical threat assessment prior to operations, emergency medical support during operations, and medical direction/oversight of law enforcement special operations.

Paramedics should realize that, in referring to TEMS, this discussion is making a clear distinction between medical providers specifically trained for the tactical environment (i.e., **tactical medics**), and EMS units that have simply been called out in support of tactical operations. Ideally, the tactical medic should be able to provide any and all emergency medical care to the members of the tactical team (i.e., tactical operators) prior to, during, and immediately after a law enforcement operation.

It is apparent that this medical care is best accomplished by a combination of providers participating in the TEMS unit, ranging from EMT-level medics to physician-level medical direction.[2] As part of this unit, tactical medics are used to provide care in the field to SWAT technical operators (Figure 32-1).

Types of Tactical Emergency Medical Support Units

There are currently three general types of TEMS units in operational use in the United States: law enforcement-based, fire/EMS-based, and hospital-based TEMS units.[2] It is important to note that any combination of these three types of units

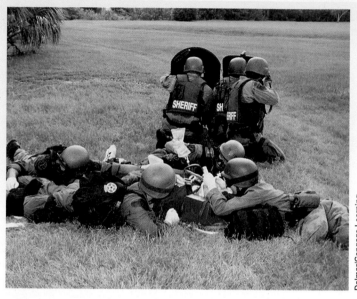

Figure 32-1 Paramedics integrated into tactical teams provide care to operators under fire.

may be at a single operation, and the type of unit used in any particular jurisdiction can depend on local laws, availability of resources, and so on.

The law enforcement-based TEMS units rely on sworn officers who are already members of the special operations team. These **law enforcement officers (LEO)** are responsible for acquiring and maintaining some degree of emergency medical training. The level of training can range from EMT-Basic to licensed physician, depending on the individual officer and the requirements of the specific team or law enforcement agency. The primary advantage of this model is that a medical care provider is present who is also a member of the tactical unit. The LEO with medical training is well trained in law enforcement special tactics as well as emergency medical care. These officers can perform in either capacity as required by the mission, allowing flexibility. Obviously, this also allows the medical provider to be in immediate proximity to those requiring care (i.e., care under fire, described shortly). There is an additional advantage found in the level of trust and camaraderie that exists between law enforcement officers; therefore, the LEO with medical training may be more readily involved in all aspects of mission operations than a typical Paramedic.

Fire/EMS-based TEMS units are a very common model. This type consists of members from local fire or EMS units who have received special tactical medical training to help support law enforcement operations (i.e., medic with tactical training). One of the advantages of this model is having medical providers who are experienced in patient packaging and transport. Unfortunately, many jurisdictions consider an adequate TEMS model to have Paramedics who are untrained in **tactical medicine** (treatment provided while in a hostile environment) on standby. However, an untrained Paramedic standing by, out of harms way, is not a tactical medic. In 1996, 69% of SWAT teams used civilian EMS on standby as their primary medical support, and 94% of those EMS units had no tactical training.[3] Many SWAT teams reported that their only plan for medical support was to call 9-1-1 if an injury occurred. By 2008, those numbers had decreased significantly, but the need for medical personnel to be familiar with tactical medicine remained crucial.

Hospital-based TEMS units often have several levels of medical provider, which may include nurses, nurse practitioners, physician assistants, and physicians. Often these team members will receive some form of specialized tactical medical training. One of the main advantages of this model is the benefit of having on-site physicians who can provide medical direction for the law enforcement team. A disadvantage is the fact that many of these teams are not very familiar with pre-hospital medical support.[3]

Mission of TEMS

According to FBI statistics, there were 33 injuries per 1,000 SWAT missions per year from 1996 to 1999.[4] In 2003, there were more than 58,000 assaults on police officers, 16,000 injuries, and 52 deaths that occurred in the line of duty.[3] One of the most important advantages to tactical medical support is the early intervention it provides to injured individuals, both law enforcement and civilians at the scene, leading to decreased morbidity and mortality. Greater than 80% of those fatally wounded from a gunshot die within the first 30 minutes, thus demonstrating the need for early interventions.

The importance of this early intervention can be demonstrated by both recent events and examples from the past. By the time of the Vietnam War, the concept of casualty care under fire and rapid evacuation and resuscitation, coupled with appropriate field triage, helped reduce mortality rates to 1%, down from 4.7% in World War II.[5] More recent examples include a SWAT raid in Dallas, Texas, in October 2007, in which an officer was shot in the neck while entering a house. The physician on-scene was able to perform an emergency cricothyrotomy and save the officer's life. On a larger scale, in the Columbine incident and the Virginia Tech shootings, there may have been multiple opportunities for tactical medics to intervene earlier than the time it took for SWAT to secure the area and bring the injured people out. In general, SWAT teams are asked to face unique challenges, including sniper attacks, terrorist

Table 32-1 Special Body of Knowledge of a Tactical Paramedic

- Weapons safety
- Psychological counseling
  - Barricades
  - Hostage situation
  - Critical incident stress management
- Evidence preservation
- Occupational health
- Hazardous materials
  - Weapons of mass destruction

attacks, and drug lab raids, all of which present specific threats and dangers.

Many differences exist between tactical and conventional EMS (Table 32-1). In tactical medicine, one must remember that the goal is to complete the law enforcement mission, which may at times override the medical mission if someone is injured. Although in traditional EMS one is taught self-preservation before helping others, the tactical medic may be called upon to conduct operations in unsafe situations, thereby putting himself at risk. The tactical medic should have specialized training on how to deliver efficient medical care while in a hostile environment.

Another difference is the idea of scene safety. Conventional Paramedics do not enter a scene until it is secure. In contrast, tactical medics often function in areas that are not secure, in all zones of the scene, including the hot zone. Tactical medics must also be prepared to provide care with limited supplies. There may not always be an ambulance in close proximity to supply all the medical instruments one would usually have while operating in an ambulance. Tactical medics should also have secure medical direction, if needed. However, tactical medics should also be able to operate independently, using good clinical judgment, at an advanced scope of practice if the situation prevents on-line medical control and communications. In addition, as the on-scene medical provider, there are several other aspects of medicine that the tactical medic must practice to keep the SWAT team functioning at a peak performance level. These additional duties include preventative medicine/occupational health care, as well as on-scene medical care for protracted operations (some SWAT operations can go on for days or even weeks).

The tactical medic also plays an important role in remote medical care. These medics should be able to communicate across any barricades, and thereby be able to direct others in how to provide medical care in the event they are not physically able to administer care themselves.

The Goal of TEMS

The goal of TEMS is to enhance mission success by focusing care on officers, civilians, and perpetrators through promotion of team safety and on-site medical care. This goal is achieved by fulfilling a set of defined roles and responsibilities.

Perhaps the most important responsibility of the TEMS unit is to maintain current tactical and medical training and to regularly participate in refresher courses, man-down scenarios, and any other regular training required by SWAT. Both the tactical medics and the SWAT team usually agree upon these training standards.

Prior to the mission. the TEMS unit must provide the SWAT team with a **medical threat assessment**, which includes assessing the potential for combat-related injuries to SWAT technical operators, perpetrators, and civilians, as well as the chances of accidental injury during the mission.

The threat assessment also considers potential environmental, chemical, biological, or animal (i.e., dog bites) exposure. The threat assessment usually includes a listing of the nearest hospitals and trauma centers, possible helicopter landing zones, and other important information (Figure 32-2).

In addition to the medical threat assessment, the TEMS Paramedic must keep and maintain current health information on members on the tactical team. This may include records of vaccinations as well as routine health screening results. This medical preplanning provides the tactical medic with information to make a better medical threat assessment, particularly in prolonged operations.

The TEMS unit also must provide members of the SWAT team with ongoing medical education, specifically regarding self-care and buddy care, two concepts borrowed from the military. This is important because the SWAT members are often the first caregivers on-scene who can render first aid and administer potentially life-saving interventions.

The core mission of the tactical medic is to provide medical care during all SWAT operations and training exercises. It is very important for the TEMS Paramedic to be present at all training exercises because historically there is a high potential for injury during these exercises, just as there is during actual law enforcement deployments.

The tactical medic must coordinate all medical communications for the SWAT team. This includes establishing clear communication with all EMS units that may be used during missions, providing information to any hospital that may be used for injured patients, and coordinating any air medical evacuation (Medevac).

The TEMS unit must provide occupational health care to members of the SWAT team. This includes caring for a wide variety of medical complaints ranging from simple sunburns and ankle sprains to more complex medical issues such as acute myocardial infarction. This aspect of TEMS responsibility can grow exponentially as the duration of the SWAT mission lengthens. For example, it is unlikely that the technical operator with diabetes will have issues of glucose control when the mission is only two hours in length; however, if it is drawn out into many hours, problems could arise.

Equipment

Tactical medics have specialized personal protective equipment (PPE). This includes, but is not limited to, a ballistic helmet, combat boots, Kevlar gloves, shatterproof eye protection, body armor, and gas masks (Table 32-2). If functioning in an outside environment, the tactical medic should have the appropriate clothing for that environment as well.

Personal body armor or ballistic vests may be the most distinctive difference in PPE for the tactical medic. Body armor is capable of preventing some gunshot wounds. For example, between 1980 and 1992, it is estimated that 330 of the 1,012 officer deaths that occurred may have been prevented by the use of body armor.

Since the tactical medic is called upon to function in a wide variety of situations, the medical equipment needed

Table 32-2 Features of the Tactical Medic's Uniform

- Identifiable uniform
  - Cargo pants, padded joint protection
- Ankle-high, combat-style boots
  - Good ankle support, good all-around traction, and waterproof
- Cold weather clothing
  - Hats, gloves, insulated clothing, parkas, and boots
- Wet weather gear
  - Poncho or raincoat
- Personal protective equipment
  - Ballistic vest
    - Level III threat protection
  - Helmet
    - Ballistic, Kevlar®
  - Black balaclava
    - Fireproof, Nomex®
  - Eye protection
    - Shatterproof, polycarbonate lenses
  - Ear protection
    - Foam plugs, shooting muffs
  - Over gloves
    - Leather, Nomex®
  - Medical PPE
    - Face mask/shield
    - Gloves
  - Additional
    - Knee pads
    - Gas mask
    - NBC protective filter

Dallas Police Department SWAT Team
Medical Threat Assessment

Operational Information

Location

Type of Operation	Hostage #	Suspect #	Warrant #	Protection #	Open Terrain Search #	Terrorist #
Other Teams	Tactical	EMS/Medics	K9	Patrol	Detective	FBI/Other

Trauma Centers

Parkland Memorial	5201 Harry Hines Blvd		(214) 590-8108 (590-8000)
Baylor University Medical Center	3500 Gaston Avenue		(214) 820-0111
Methodist Dallas	1441 N Beckley Ave		(214) 947-8181
BIOTEL			(214) 590-8848

Hospitals

Charlton Methodist Hospital	3500 W. Wheatland Road	214-947-7777
Children's Medical Center of Dallas	1935 Motor Street	214-640-2000
Dallas Veterans Affairs Medical Center	4500 S. Lancaster Road	214-742-8387
Doctors Hospital of Dallas	9330 Poppy Dr	214-324-6100
Medical City Dallas	7777 Forest Lane	972-661-7000
North Texas Hospital for Children	7777 Forest Lane	972-566-8888
Presbyterian Hospital of Dallas	8200 Walnut Hill	214-345-6789
RHD Memorial Medical Center	7 Medical Parkway	972-247-1000
St. Paul Medical Center	5909 Harry Hines	972-879-1000
Texas Scottish Rite Hospital for Children	2222 Welborn	214-521-3168
Zale Lipshy University Hospital	5151 Harry Hines	214-590-3000

Helicopter Plan

CareFlight *(800) 442-6260*	Other:	**Coordinates**	
Landing Zone	Address:	Latitude	Longitude
	Obstructions:	Debris:	

Weather

Temp Hi	WB Temp	<60	60-78	78-82	82-85	85-88	88-90	>90	Sunrise:		AM
Temp Low	H_2O $Qt/_{Hr}$	0.5	0.5	0.5	0.5-1.0	1.0	1.0-1.5	2.0	Sunset:		PM
Rain %	Rest $Min/_{Hr}$	0	0	0	10	15	30	40	Night Ops:		
Wind: MPH	Cold Casualties		Y/N		Work Cycles Yes / No		Duration:				
	Heat Casualties		Y/N								
Humidity %	Uniform Adjustments		Y/N		Shelter: Y/N		Location/type:				

Animal Threats

Y/N	Animals Present?	Yes No	Police Dogs Y/N	#		#
	Types of animals		Number:	Do you anticipate wild Animals?	Yes No	What type?
	Poisonous Snake Exposure: Yes No		Veterinarian Address		Vet Phone:	
	Animal Control: 3-1-1 or (214) 670-5111	Poison Control: 800-222-1222				

Plant Threats

Y/N	Exposure to poisonous plants likely?	Yes No	Type
	Uniform Adjustments Needed?	Yes No	Recomendations

Public Works

EMS/Fire Department Standby	Yes No	Unit # and location
Street Closings	Yes No	Where?
Gate Access	Yes No	Where?

Courtesy of Dallas Police Department

Figure 32-2 A sample medical threat assessment from the Dallas, Texas, TEMS unit indicates possible concerns for the team's safety.

Table 32-3 Tactical Medical Aid Packs

Primary Tactical Medic Pack	○ Face mask with eye shield
• Assessment	○ Trauma scissors
○ Stethoscope	○ Knife, folding style/utility
○ Nitrile rubber gloves	
• Airway management	○ ET tube (6.5 and 7.5) or supraglottic airway
○ Cricothyroidotomy hook with scalpel	○ Stylet
○ Mouth–mask valve	○ Oropharyngeal airway
○ Cook® pneumothorax kit	○ Laryngoscope with #3 curved blade
○ Hemostats	○ Asherman penetrating chest trauma seal
• Bleeding control	○ Cloth tape
○ Compression trauma bandages	○ Duct tape
• Minor wound kit	○ Triple antibiotic ointment
○ Steri-strips	○ Band-Aids®
○ Benzoin	○ 2 × 2 bandages
○ Betadine prep pads	○ Medical tape
• Minor medical emergency kit	
○ Acetaminophen and/or ibuprofen	
Secondary Tactical Medical Backpack	○ Additional trauma dressings, gauze bandages
• Second advanced airway management kit	○ Collapsible one-man stretcher
○ Set of above airway supplies	○ SAM splints
○ Magill forceps	○ Universal protection supplies (gloves, masks)
○ Laryngoscope #1 and #3 blades, full assortment of ET tubes	○ Disposable flash camera (documentation/forensic evidence)
○ Large curved hemostats	○ List of each team member's medical history/allergies
○ Scalpels	○ 50 feet of 400-lb parachute cord
○ Intravenous solution bags	○ Emergency thermal blanket
○ Venous access starter kits	○ Flashlight
○ Blood tubing	○ GPS unit
○ Pressure IV bag	○ ACLS medications: atropine, epinephrine, lidocaine
○ Disposable hot pack (optional)	○ MARK I kits, optional
○ Change-out catheter set—seven French	

may change given the specific circumstance. However, there are basic equipment requirements that are routine to most missions. These basic equipment requirements can be met in a number of ways, including individual or self-care first aid kits, entry bags, tactical medical aid packs (Table 32-3), and then more remote advanced medications/backup supplies.

Every member of the team, including people without medical training, should have an individual or **self-care first aid kit**. This typically includes gloves, tourniquet, trauma dressings, and rolls of gauze. In addition, police officers should have **tactical medical aid packs**, which include a variety of equipment and supplies needed for a medical emergency, as recommended by the American College of Emergency Physicians. Individual teams may decide to supplement these kits with other supplies, as they feel necessary.

Some tactical medics elect to use an **entry leg bag**, a slightly more equipped bag containing the same elements

as the individual first aid kits with the addition of a venous access device and chest decompression needle.

An **advanced emergency medical pack** (Table 32-4) contains more advanced airway supplies, IV setups, saline, dressings, splinting, drug box, AED with monitor, oxygen with pulse oximetry monitoring, suturing materials, and a method of safely disposing of sharps.

The Paramedic should consider using a GPS system, especially if in a remote area. In a hot area, extra hydration supplies may also be needed. Hydration is also important in that body armor and uniforms can markedly increase the endogenous heat load the SWAT member experiences, potentially leading to heat exhaustion and heat stroke. If the team determines during the risk assessment that children may be on-site, pediatric supplies should also be stocked.

If functioning at a remote area for a long period of time, the tactical medics should take into consideration the need for

Table 32-4 Advanced Emergency Medical Pack

- Syringes and needles, alcohol wipes
- Suture kits (2) and minor surgical emergency supplies
  - Gauze, basin, sterile gloves, suture material, Betadine swabs, and so on
- Dermabond® skin laceration tissue glue
- Additional IV fluid and IV lines, IV starting kits
- Anderson blast gauge
- Sterile saline bottles for irrigation/cleaning wounds
- Dental kit
  - Mirror, dental floss, clove oil, topical anesthesia, tongue blades, stoma wax, temporary filling material
- Additional trauma supplies
  - Antiseptic wipes, compression elastic bandage, trauma pads, eye dressing, Q-tips, SAM splints, triple antibiotic ointment, Band-Aids®, tape, non-stick gauze, gauze pads, moleskin/ blister kit, irrigation syringes/solution, scrub brushes, cold packs, heat packs, cling wrap, two Cook® pneumothorax kits
- Assessment equipment
  - Extra stethoscope, penlight, trauma scissors, knife
- PPE
  - Exam gloves, sterile and nonsterile
  - Face mask with eye shield
- Additional supplies
  - Pencil marker, waterproof paper, medical records of unit members
  - Patient ID/triage tags, emergency thermal blankets, portable strobe light
  - Medical waste bags, disposable sharps hard plastic container
- Medications
  - Cold/flu symptoms
    - Cough drops
    - Entex PSE decongestant
    - Neosynephrine nasal spray
  - Minor pain control
    - Ibuprofen 400 mg tablets
    - Tylenol 500 mg tablets
  - Severe pain control
    - Morphine sulfate 10 mg
  - Allergy/anaphylaxis
    - Epinephrine 1:1000
    - Benadryl 25 mg
    - Prednisone 20 mg
    - Albuterol inhaler
  - GI ailments
    - Imodium tablets
    - Pepto-Bismol® tablets
    - Mylanta® tablets
  - Unresponsive patients
    - Ammonia capsules
    - Dextrose 50%
    - Oral glucose syrup
    - Narcan
  - ACLS drugs
    - Lidocaine 1%
    - Atropine
    - Epinephrine 1:10,000
  - Seizure control
    - Diazepam
  - Medication-facilitated intubation
    - Diazepam
    - Ketamine
    - Vecuronium
    - Rocuronium
  - Ear/eye ailments
    - Gentamycin ophthalmologic ointment
    - Cortisporin otic suspension
  - Skin ailments
    - Lotrisone cream 10 gm
    - Triamcinolone 0.1% cream
    - Sunscreen, 30-SPF
  - Infection treatment
    - Cephalexin 500 mg tablets
    - Ancef 2 gm IV
    - Rocephin 2 gm IV
  - Other medications
    - Nitroglycerine spray
    - Oragel ®(dental analgesic)

utilities such as heat, light, and electricity. The tactical medic also needs to prearrange a way of communicating in the event that a person needs to be evacuated. Transportation for sick or injured people should also be in place before undergoing the mission. There may be many forms of evacuation devices, such as armed rescue vehicles and revised military ambulances. If ambulances are used and are near the hot zone, one must be careful due to their lack of armor and consider protective measures like covering oxygen with body armor.

Care under Fire

The primary role of TEMS is to provide medical support during SWAT operations. However, the vast majority of time dedicated to maintaining a TEMS unit will involve non-combat or non-operational duties and training. It is crucial to always remember the primary role of TEMS and it is equally important to grasp several concepts relating to tactical medical operations.

Zones of Care

The Committee on Tactical Combat Casualty Care (TCCC) has established the concept of **zones of care**. Essentially, this means care of the wounded occurs in three separate zones: green (cool), yellow (warm), and red (hot) (Figure 32-3 and Table 32-5). This was originally designed as a military model but has been adopted by civilian tactical medicine.

The **cool zone** is considered a relatively safe zone where staging and deployment occur. This area is typically farthest away from where traumatic injury is most likely to occur and is out of the line of fire. To be out of the line of fire, the tactical medics must have **coverage**, an impenetrable object that shields them from projectiles, and **concealment**, an obstruction blocking the view between the tactical medic and any potential gunfire.

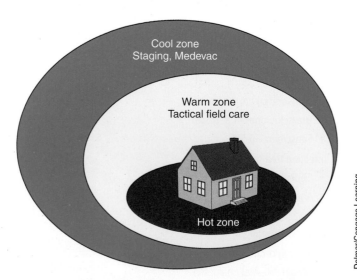

Figure 32-3 The zones of care were adopted from a military model and indicate the increasing levels of danger at a scene.

Table 32-5 Procedures Performed within the Zones of Care

- Cool zone
  - Staging
  - CPR
  - Wound care
  - Fracture management
  - Evacuation including Medevac
- Warm zone
  - Immediate life-saving interventions (circulation, airway, breathing)
  - Tactical field care
- Hot zone
  - Tourniquet
  - Protection
  - Care under fire
  - Rapid evacuation

The cool zone is where tactical medics will stage their support vehicle and advanced medical supplies, receive mission briefings, provide medical direction for the SWAT team, and coordinate medical evacuation of the wounded (Medevac). Ambulances and air medical transport will operate within the cool zone. Specific medical procedures that are performed in the cool zone and in no other zone are CPR, splinting of extremity wounds, and wound dressing.

The **warm zone** is defined as the area where tactical field care occurs. This is a zone where the provider may be relatively exposed. Therefore, medical care in this zone must also include some form of security for the provider, either in the form of **suppressive fire** (gunfire from the SWAT team that provides a deterrent for assailants who might attack the provider) and **armed protection** (keeping an individual carrying weapons near the provider to repel attackers), or cover.

The warm zone is where the provider must apply the **concept of CAB (circulation, airway, breathing)**. It is vital to recognize the difference here between the concept of ABC management and the tactical prioritization of circulation over airway and breathing. This is a result of several important realizations: The patient's chances of surviving a significant traumatic injury to the airway is much less than that of surviving a traumatic hemorrhage. This is largely due to the difficulty of managing a traumatic airway in the field as compared to the relative ease of applying pressure to active bleeding. Also, traumatic airway management is time-consuming and may place the provider in a situation where he is unable to move rapidly to a safer zone. Therefore, circulation must be addressed first.

Addressing circulation first is accomplished by attempting to control any active hemorrhage, often through the use of tourniquets or haemostatic agents. The tactical medic may also attempt to gain intravenous (IV) access or intraosseous (IO) access and administer intravenous fluids in this zone.

Through airway evaluation, the tactical medic will assess the need for airway management (such as chin-lift or jaw-thrust maneuvers, nasal airway insertion, and possibly orotracheal intubation) by clearing any possible obstruction. The tactical medic may assess the patient's breathing and address any issues found. This may include providing positive pressure ventilation by bag-valve-mask; performing a needle thoracostomy to decompress the chest in the setting of pneumothorax; and in rare cases inserting a chest tube for massive hemothorax.

The **hot zone** is considered a "care under fire" situation. Unless the tactical medical provider is also a sworn officer, there should be few (if any) circumstances that would require a tactical medic to be in the hot zone. The care in this zone of operation is simple: scoop and run. The provider should identify the wounded and remove them to the warm zone immediately. There should be no stabilization attempted in the hot zone. In all zones of care, provider safety is the top priority. Therefore, there should be no reason for a tactical medic to knowingly put herself at risk. It is also important to realize that tactical operations are dynamic and zones of care can fluctuate rapidly. A warm zone can quickly become hot if a perpetrator attempts to flee, for example.

Medical Evacuation

A vital duty performed by the tactical medic is coordination of medical evacuation or **Medevac**. Patients will be transported to hospitals outlined in the medical threat assessment. The decision whether to send patients by ground EMS or air medical transport is a complex one. Many factors contribute to the decision-making process including the patient's severity of injury and stability (i.e., triage), the distance to the nearest appropriate medical facility, the remoteness of the location where the injury occurred, current weather conditions, and many other factors. In some cases, the tactical medic and patient remain under cover while care is provided (a **protect-in-place** scenario) as opposed to Medevac. The medical director of the TEMS unit, in conjunction with the SWAT commander, will often make this decision.

Regardless of the decision, the tactical medic must ensure a safe transition of patient care to ground/air EMS personnel. Air medical transport will require a coordinated effort with other public safety agencies to ensure a secure landing zone.

The tactical medic should stabilize the patient's airway before departure. This may require early preventative intubation, using medication-facilitated intubation (MFI), if there is any doubt as to the possibility of airway issues en route. The rationale for using MFI and aggressive airway management is that it is much more difficult to intubate in the confines of a helicopter. If an airway is lost while the helicopter is airborne, it could be many minutes before the helicopter can land and advanced airway management can be attempted.

Debriefing

After the conclusion of a SWAT operation, the tactical medic should provide an after action report. The purpose of this report is to outline all tactical medical measures employed during the mission. This includes not only those measures that proved successful, but also any failures in the medical component of the mission. The report should also attempt to identify future risk and areas in need of possible improvement. This is an important duty of the TEMS unit and can lead to increased mission success in the future.

Special Circumstances

Although most tactical missions in a city region take minutes to hours to execute, there are some circumstances in which a little more planning should be instituted. Some of these include sustained operations, operations that may involve chemical or biological warfare, or instances in which the medic is unable to reach a patient and must deliver care through the instruction of others.

Sustained medical operations can be broken up into two broad categories. Short-term missions are those lasting approximately one week, whereas long-term missions are any missions lasting longer than one week. In planning for these missions, one must take into consideration both the environmental aspects as well as the physiologic aspects.

Many people on long-term missions can experience sleep deprivation. This can lead to many undesirable side effects including mood changes, difficulty making decisions, and cognitive impairment. In order to accommodate for this, one should be sure to have an evacuation plan.

On the other end of the spectrum is heat-related illnesses. If tactical medics are providing care for those at risk for these illnesses, they should be trained to recognize a wide variety of presenting signs and symptoms ranging from heat cramps and heat syncope (both of which are treated with removal from the environment, passive cooling, and fluids) to the more serious heat exhaustion and heat stroke. People who have these more severe heat-related illnesses initially present with more vague systemic symptoms (e.g., nausea, vomiting, dizziness), and then progress to central nervous system dysfunction with coma and death. Treatment for these people involves cooling, evacuation, and fluids. Paramedics should plan for the number of people and attempt to have supplies on hand to treat heat-related problems as well as to prevent them.

Tactical medics must be prepared in the event weapons of mass destruction are being used. Biologic and chemical agents have long been used as weapons; in fact, chemical agents were used in World War I. More recent chemical and biological attacks include using sarin in the Japanese subways and placing anthrax in letters in the United States. Tactical medics may also be exposed to unintentionally harmful materials, such as by-products of drug manufacturers or hazardous materials spills. The tactical medic should be trained on how to assess for the possibility of such threats, how to recognize them, and how to treat patients if the need arises.

The management of biochemical warfare begins with assessment of the situation for dangerous materials. Tactical medics must use PPE during this assessment. Gas masks are useful in the prevention of inhalation injuries. If an exposure is suspected, any person who may have been exposed should be decontaminated to prevent further exposure and to prevent exposing others that will be treating the patient later. Specific antidotes for chemical agents and antibiotics for biologic agents are dependent upon the agent used. Tactical medical providers will be familiar with these after training.

Tactical medics working with law enforcement agencies may be called upon to provide care in mass-casualty incidents as well. This may involve planning evacuation routes, providing preventative medicine, and obtaining enough medical providers to treat the casualties. In addition, the rescuers should have open lines of communication, extrication plans, appropriate triage skills, and enough equipment. Drills are helpful in planning for these scenarios. One should assume that the provider might be rendering care while still under fire.

Yet another challenge facing tactical medics is giving **care behind the barricade**, which means directing others on how to give medical care without seeing the patients themselves. This might happen, for example, in a hostage situation when one of the hostages is injured. In this circumstance, the tactical medic must establish a reliable means of communication, such as a phone or radio, and identify herself as a Paramedic. Both the hostage and hostage takers' medical problems should be addressed. This includes taking a history and description of any injuries. At that point, the tactical medic should determine the level of medical training possessed by the person taking care of the patient. The tactical medic then attempts to guide the person in contact with the patient through the initial treatment until a more trained caregiver can have access to the patient.

Operational Security

The concept of operational security cannot be overemphasized. SWAT operation success and team safety depend on a high level of security. This translates into the need for all members of the TEMS unit to maintain a high level of secrecy regarding any and all missions. Discussions of mission details should only occur during official operational meetings. No documentation should be left unsecured at any time. The danger of perpetrators discovering times and places of upcoming SWAT activity is obvious. A simple rule to follow is to keep silent regarding missions unless at an actual briefing. Silence is crucial as many lives may depend on it.

Armed versus Unarmed Paramedics

The most controversial issue related to TEMS is the debate on whether or not to arm tactical medics. The leading argument in favor of arming is that tactical medics should not be placed in dangerous situations in which they cannot adequately protect themselves. In addition, if they are not armed, other members of the SWAT team must provide security for the tactical medic while in the warm zone. This can seriously deplete SWAT team strength.

The argument against arming tactical medics addresses several issues. Armed TEMS unit members must have legal authority to carry a weapon and maintain a level of current weapon training comparable with that of other SWAT team members. This level of training can be difficult to maintain when many TEMS members are not law enforcement officers. There is also the concern that arming medics can lead to confusion about the primary role of the TEMS Paramedic, whether to be an officer or a medical provider. This does not, however, seem to present a significant problem because TEMS unit members must always consider both the tactical and medical aspects of every mission.

Many SWAT teams have chosen not to arm the TEMS unit members for various reasons and simply keep the TEMS members functioning primarily in the cool zone. If they enter the warm zone, it is under the protection of the tactical team. The decision whether to arm tactical medics must be made by each tactical team and is often based on the availability of SWAT resources, local laws, TEMS members' commitment to maintaining weapons training, and many other factors.

► CASE STUDY CONCLUSION

As the last bullet leaves the pistol's chamber, the rookie puts his weapon down. He will have to wait to see if he is now weapon qualified. He has successfully completed the tactical medic course, which was strangely similar to the combat casualty course he took when he was a military medic.

Turning to his right, he looks down the firing line and thinks to himself, "Someday the life of one of these guys may be in my hands." He resolves to re-read all of the manuals before reporting to his first day of duty with the metro police.

CRITICAL THINKING QUESTIONS

1. What are the most life-threatening injuries that technical operators may sustain?
2. What are the advantages of the tactical medic being "weapons qualified"?

CONCLUSION

Tactical Emergency Medical Support (TEMS) is one of the newest subspecialties of EMS, and as such it is constantly and rapidly evolving. Many individual jurisdictions are developing very effective protocols, methods, and training techniques for TEMS. National standardization of TEMS training remains a future goal. With proper training, cooperation, and equipment, TEMS can provide a true benefit to law enforcement operations by improving officer survival and "protecting the protectors."

KEY POINTS:

- TEMS refers to Paramedics trained to operate in a hostile environment as opposed to the EMS units assigned to standby for a SWAT team.

- Three types of TEMS units exist in the United States: law enforcement based, fire/EMS based, and hospital based.

- By providing casualty care under fire and rapid evacuation, TEMS has been shown to reduce combat morbidity and mortality.

- Tactical medics are responsible for the medical threat assessment, medical monitoring of the team, and medical education for SWAT team members regarding self-care and buddy care.

- Tactical medics are also responsible for medical communications with civilian EMS as well as occupational health care.

- The tactical medic wears special personal protective equipment.

- Medic supplies include personal aid kits, tactical medical aid packs, secondary tactical medical packs, and in certain cases a leg bag. The advanced emergency medical pack contains ALS equipment.

- Tactical medics adhere to the zones of care concept.

- Tactical medics participate in debriefings.

- Sustained medical operations require another set of skills for the tactical medic that includes occupational health care as well as exposure to weapons of mass destruction.

- Care over the barricade, providing instructions to another who does the hands-on treatment, is another special aspect of tactical EMS.

- Tactical medics may be armed in some circumstances.

REVIEW QUESTIONS:

1. What are the three types of TEMS units?
2. What items do the medical aid pack and the advanced emergency medical pack contain?
3. What is the zones of care concept?
4. What is the CAB concept of medical care?
5. What are sustained medical operations?

CASE STUDY QUESTIONS:

Please refer to the Case Study in this chapter, and answer the questions below:

1. What are the qualifications of the tactical medic?
2. What are the similarities and differences between a tactical medic and a combat medic?
3. Does a tactical medic need to be proficient with firearms?

REFERENCES:

1. Heiskell LE, Carmona RH. Tactical Emergency Medical Services: an emerging subspecialty of emergency medicine, *Ann Emerg Med*. 1994;23;778–785.

2. Eastman A, Sharma N, Huebner K. *Tactical Emergency Medicine: Section 1 Tactical Concepts*. Lippincott, Williams & Wilkins, Philadelphia, PA. 2007. P. 352–490.

3. Heck JJ, Pierluisi G. Law enforcement special operations medical support. *Prehosp Emerg Care*. 2001;5(4):403–406.

4. Jones JS, Reese K, Kenepp G, Krohmer J. Into the fray: integration of Emergency Medical Services and Special Weapons and Tactics (SWAT) teams. *Prehosp Disaster Med*. July–September 1996;11(3):202–206.

5. Kennedy K, et al. Triage: techniques and applications in decisionmaking. *Ann Emer Med*, 1996;28(2):136–144.

ACRONYMS

AAPCC American Association of Poison Control Centers

ABC Airway, breathing, circulation

ABCDE Airway, breathing, circulation, drugs, and ECG preceding extrication

AC Alternating current

ACL Anterior cruciate ligament

ACS American College of Surgeons

ADH Antidiuretic hormone

ADL Activities of daily living

AG Attorney general

AHJ Authority having jurisdiction

AICD Automatic implantable cardioverter defibrillator

ALS Advanced life support

AMS Acute mountain sickness

AMSC American Mobile Satellite Corporation

ANSI American National Standards Institute

AP Anteroposterior

ARDS Acute respiratory distress syndrome

ARF Acute renal failure

ASAM Arrestee Drug Abuse Monitoring

ASIA Anterior superior iliac spine

ATC Certified athletic trainer

ATF Alcohol, Tobacco, and Firearms

ATFL Anterior talofibular ligament

ATLS Advanced Trauma Life Support

ATV All-terrain vehicles

AVM Arteriovenous malformation

AVN Avascular necrosis

AVPU Alert, voice, pain, unresponsive

BDS Biohazard Detection System

BLEVE Boiling liquid expanding vapor explosion

BLS Basic life support

BMD Bone mineral density

B–NICE Biological, nuclear/radiological, incendiary, chemical, and explosive

BSE Bioengineered skin equivalent

CAAMS Commission for Accreditation of Air Medical Services

CAAS Committee on the Accreditation of Ambulance Services

CABG Coronary artery bypass grafting

CAGE Cerebral arterial gas embolism

CAMTS Commission on the Accreditation of Medical Transport Services

CANUTEC Canadian Transport Emergency Centre

CAT Combat Application Tourniquet

CBF Cerebral blood flow

CBRNE Chemical, biological, radiological, nuclear, explosive

CDC Centers for Disease Control

CERCLA Comprehensive Environmental Response Compensation and Liability Act

CERT Community Emergency Response Teams

CFL Calcaneofibular ligament

CHEMTREC Chemical Transportation Emergency Center

CIM Communications and information management

CK Creatine kinase

CMC Carpometacarpal joint

CMS Chronic mountain sickness

CO Carbon monoxide

COBRA Consolidated Omnibus Budget Reconciliation Act

COG Continuity of government

COOP Continuity of operations

COPD Chronic obstructive pulmonary disease

CPAP Continuous positive airway pressure

CPC Chemical protective clothing

CPP Capillary/cerebral perfusion pressures

CSF Cerebral spinal fluid

CTAS Canadian Triage and Acuity Scale

CVP Central venous pressure

DAI Diffuse axonal injury

DAN Divers Alert Network

DART Disaster Assistance Response Teams

DC Direct current

DCAP BTLS Deformity, contusions, abrasions, punctures, burns, tenderness, lacerations, swelling

DCI Decompression illness

DCO Defense coordinating officer

DCS Decompression sickness

DDH Developmental dislocation of the hip

DHHS Department of Health and Human Services

DHS Department of Homeland Security

DIP Distal interphalangeal

DMAT Disaster Medical Assistance Team

DMORT Disaster Mortuary Operational Response Team

DOC Drug of choice

DOD Department of Defense

DOE Dyspnea on exertion

DOMS Director of military support

DOT Department of Transportation

DP Dementia pugilistica

DPG Diphosphoglycerate

DPMU Disaster Portable Morgue Units
DSCA Defense Support to Civil Authorities
DSD Dry sterile dressing
DUMBELS Diarrhea, urination, miosis, bronchospasm, emesis, lacrimation, salivation
ECMO Extracorporeal membrane oxygenation
ECR Extracorporeal core rewarming
EHS Exertional heat stroke
EMA Emergency management agency
EMS Emergency Medical Services
EMT Emergency and Military Tourniquet
EMT Emergency Medical Technician
EMTALA Emergency Medical Treatment and Active Labor Act
EOC Emergency Operations Center
EOM Extraocular movement
EPA Environmental Protection Agency
ERG *Emergency Response Guide*
ESF Emergency Support Function
ESI Emergency Severity Index
ETT Endotracheal tube
EVOC Emergency Vehicle Operators Course
FAA Federal Aviation Administration
FACTS Function, arterial pulses, capillary refill, temperature, and sensation
FALN Armed Forces for Puerto Rico National Liberation
FAST Focused Abdominal Sonography in Trauma
FBI Federal Bureau of Investigation
FBL Forward body line
FCC Federal Communications Commission
FCO Federal coordinating officer
FDA Food and Drug Administration
FEMA Federal Emergency Management Agency
FFP Fresh frozen plasma
FMVSS Federal Motor Vehicle Safety Standards
FOOSH Fall on outstretched hand
FP-C Certified Flight Paramedic
FROPVD Flow-restricted oxygen-powered ventilation device
GCS Glasgow Coma Scale
GIS Geographical information systems
GPS Global positioning satellites
GSA General Services Administration
GSW Gunshot wound
HACE High altitude cerebral edema
HAPE High altitude pulmonary edema
HAZWOPER Hazardous waste operations and emergency response
HBO Hyperbaric oxygen
HEENT Head, eyes, ears, nose, and throat
HEL Higher explosive limit
HELP Heat escape lessening position
HEPA High-efficiency particulate air

HF High frequency
HIPAA Health Insurance Portability and Accountability Act
HIV Human acquired immunodeficiency virus
HSA Homeland Security Act
HSPD Homeland Security Presidential Directive
HTS Hypertonic saline solutions
HV High voltage
HVAC Heating, ventilation and air conditioning
IAFP International Association of Flight Paramedics
ICP Intracranial pressure
ICS Intercostal space
ICS Incident Command System
ICU Intensive care unit
IDLH Immediately Dangerous to Life and Health
IED Improvised explosive devices
IFP Interstitial fluid pressure
IFR Instrument flight rules
IM Intramuscularly
IMAT Incident Management Assist Team
INMARSAT International Maritime Satellite
IO Intraosseous
IOM Institute of Medicine
IPE Immersion pulmonary edema
ISMM International Society for Mountain Medicine
IST Incident support teams
ITS Intelligent Transportation Systems
IV Intravenous
IVC Inferior vena cava
JFO Joint Field Office
JIC Joint Information Center
JIS Joint Information System
JVD Jugular venous distention
KVO Keep vein open
LAST Locate, access, stabilize, transport
LEL Lower explosive limit
LEO Law enforcement officers
LEPC Local Emergency Planning Committees
LKP Last known position
LMA Laryngeal mask airway
LODD Line-of-duty death
LSI Life-saving interventions
LZ Landing zone
MAL Mid-axillary line
MAP Mean arterial pressure
MAR Mountain Rescue Association
MAST Military anti-shock trousers
MCI Multiple/mass-casualty incident
MCL Medial collateral ligament
MCP Metacarpophalangeal
MERS Mobile Emergency and Response Support
MESS Mangled Extremity Severity Score
MFI Medication-facilitated intubation

MMRS Metropolitan Medical Response System
MRC Medical Reserve Corps
MRSA Methicillin-resistant staphylococcus aureus
MSDS Material safety data sheets
MUC Maximum use concentration
MVC Motor vehicle collision
NAEMSP National Association of EMS Providers
NASA National Aeronautics and Space Administration
NASAR National Association for Search and Rescue
NCAA National College Athletic Association
NDMS National Disaster Medical System
NEMSIS National Emergency Medical Services Information System
NFPA National Fire Protection Association
NGO Non-governmental organizations
NIBP Noninvasive blood pressure
NIMS National Incident Management System
NIOSH National Institute for Occupational Safety and Health
NNRT National Nurse Response Team
NOAA National Oceanic and Atmospheric Administration
NOC National Operations Center
NPRT National Pharmacy Response Teams
NRB Nonrebreather mask
NRF National Response Framework
NSAID Nonsteroidal anti-inflammatory drugs
NSARC National Search and Rescue Committee
NSP National Search and Rescue Plan
NSS Normal saline solution
NTDB National Trauma Data Bank
NTSB National Transportation Safety Board
NWS National Weather Service
ODC Oxyhemoglobin dissociation curve
OEM Original equipment manufacturers
OFDA Office of Foreign Disaster Assistance
OPQRST Onset, provokes, quality, radiation, severity, time
ORIF Open reduction and internal fixation
OSHA Occupational Safety and Health Organization
OTC Over-the-counter
PAP Pulmonary artery pressure
PA/PIO Public affairs/public information officers
PAPR Powered air-purifying respirator
PASG Pneumatic anti-shock garment
PCWP Pulmonary capillary wedge pressure
PEA Pulseless electrical activity
PEEP Positive end-expiratory pressure
PEG Polyethylene glycol
PEL Permissible exposure limits
PF Protection factor
PFD Personal flotation devices
PFO Patent foramen ovale

PFO Principal federal officer
PHMSA Pipeline and Hazardous Materials Safety Administration
PICC Peripherally inserted central catheter
PIP Predictable injury patterns
PIP Proximal interphalangeal
PKEMRA Post-Katrina Emergency Management Reform Act
PLS Point last seen
P-NAG Poly-N-acetyl glucosamine
POA Probability of area
POD Point of dispensing
POD Probability of detection
POS Probability of success
PPE Personal protective equipment
PSAP Public safety answering points
PSCIM Public safety critical incident management
PSI Per square inch
PTFL Posterior talofibular ligament
PWC Personal watercraft
REMO Remote emergency medical oxygen
RICE Rest, ice, compression, and elevation
ROM Range of motion
ROPS Rollover protection system
ROWPU Reverse osmosis water purification units
RRCC Regional Response Coordinating Center
SAE Society of Automotive Engineers
SAH Subarachnoid hemorrhage
SALT Sort-Assess-Lifesaving interventions-Treat/transport
SAMPLE Symptoms, allergies, medications, past history, last oral intake, events preceding
SAR Search and rescue
SARA Superfund Amendment and Reauthorization Act
SAVE Secondary Assessment of Victim Endpoint
SBP Systolic blood pressure
SCBA Self-contained breathing apparatus
SCI Spinal cord injury
SCIWORA Spinal cord injury without radiological abnormality
SCT Specialty Care Transport
SCUBA Self-contained underwater breathing apparatus
SDH Subdural hematoma
SERC State Emergency Response Commissions
SERM Selective estrogen receptor modulator
SFLEO Senior federal law enforcement official
SFO Senior federal officials
SI Sacroiliac
SIS Second impact syndrome
SIT Surface interval time
SLE Systemic lupus erythematosus
SLUD Salivation, lacrimation, urination, defecation

SLUDGEM Salivation, lacrimation, urination, defecation, gastrointestinal, emesis, miosis

SMT Scapular manipulation technique

SNpr Substantia nigra pars reticulate

SNS Strategic National Stockpile

SOB Shortness of breath

SOG Standard operating guidelines

SOP Standard operating procedures

SRS Supplemental restraint systems

START Simple Triage and Rapid Transport

STEMI ST-segment elevation myocardial infarction

STM Sacco Triage and Resource Methodology

SVC Superior vena cava

SWAT Special Weapons and Tactics

SWB Shallow water blackout

TBI Traumatic brain injury

TBSA Total body surface area

TCCC Tactical Combat Casualty Care

TD Tetanus and reduced diphtheria

TdP Tetanus, reduced diphtheria, and pertussis

TEAM Techniques for effective alcohol management

TEMS Tactical Emergency Medical Support

TF Task force

TIH Toxic by inhalation

TLV-STEL Threshold limit values–short-term exposure limit

TMT Tarsometatarsal

TRACEM Thermal, radiological, asphyxiation, chemical, etiological, mechanical

TSWG Technical Support Working Group

UCL Ulnar collateral ligament

UHF Ultra high frequency

UN United Nations

USAG U.S. Coast Guard

USAR Urban Search and Rescue

USFA United States Fire Academy

USPS U.S. Postal Service

VFR Visual flight rules

VHF Very high frequency

VHF Viral hemorrhagic fevers

VMAT Veterinary Medical Assistance Team

VMI Vendor-managed inventory

VRE Vancomycin-resistant enterococci

WCT Wind chill temperature

WMD Weapon of mass destruction

GLOSSARY

Abrasion A superficial soft-tissue wound that does not extend below the epidermis.

Acclimatization A process through which the body adjusts to atmospheric changes, specifically the lack of oxygen found at higher elevations.

Acetazolamide A carbonic anhydrase inhibitor that assists with the process of acclimatization.

Acid burns Tissue damage caused by exposure to chemicals with a pH of less than 2.

Activation A notification that a USAR team is being sent to the scene of a disaster for a search and rescue mission. Upon receipt of an activation order, a team has two hours to report to team headquarters and four more hours, for a total of six hours, to be en route with personnel and equipment.

Active cooling techniques Methods used for reducing firefighter heat during rehabilitation that utilize external methods of removing heat from the body such as misting fans or tents, forearm immersion chairs, vacuum-assisted palm cooling devices, cooling vests, and cold towels.

Active rewarming Techniques used to externally add heat to the body, such as hot packs, in an effort to raise the core body temperature.

Active search measure Procedures intended to rescue a person actually seen in a certain area.

Acute mountain sickness (AMS) A transient illness that occurs as people travel to higher elevations. It usually begins 6 to 24 hours after arrival, possibly due to cerebral edema.

Acute stress reaction A psychological response to a traumatic event.

Advanced emergency medical pack A package of medical supplies containing advanced airway supplies, IV setups, saline, dressings, splinting, drug box, AED with monitor, oxygen with pulse oximetry monitoring, suturing materials, and a method of safely disposing of sharps.

Advisory A statement issued to notify the USAR system that there is an emerging or potential incident. This typically is a written communiqué detailing the current time, the duration of the alert, some information about the incident or event, and the status of all teams.

Aerial reconnaissance Using aircraft to conduct a search for a lost person.

After drop phenomenon A situation that occurs when cold extremities are warmed, causing cold, acidotic, and hyperkalemic blood to surge to the body's core. The result is an actual drop in body core temperature (after drop) which—combined with the acidotic, hyperkalemic blood—can lead to ventricular fibrillation and sudden cardiac death.

Air Medical Crew Curriculum An advanced training program established by the Department of Transportation in conjunction with multiple air medical organizations.

Air-reactive materials A chemical that will react and rapidly decompose upon exposure to air.

Akinetic mutism A condition that may present similarly to a patient in coma (i.e., no facial expression, mute) but eyes open and able to fix a gaze on a person. Akinetic mutism occurs with frontal lobe trauma, such as contusions or anterior cerebral artery damage, and specifically the destruction of the cingulate gyrus.

Alert A statement issued to the USAR team when activation is expected. This allows team members time to take care of any necessary duties at home and prepare to be activated. However, this stage will not always occur.

American National Standards Institute/American Society of Safety Engineers Z15.1 Fleet Safety Standard The only current nationally approved safety standard in the United States that is now applicable to the safety management of ground EMS vehicle fleets.

Amperage The amount of electrical current that flows through an object. As an example, the amount of current flowing through a lighted 100-watt bulb is approximately 1 ampere.

Amputation The separation of a limb or digit by a shearing force which leaves a clean line of demarcation.

Analgesia Pain management.

Anchor A point of fixation during a technical rescue that permits a load to be applied to it without movement. An anchor can be natural (such as a tree) or artificial (such as a steel expansion bolt or a set of stakes placed in a row called a picket).

Angiogenesis The wound healing process that occurs during wound contraction in which new blood vessels provide the growing tissue with nutrients.

Anhydrosis A failure of the sweat glands to produce sweat.

Anthrax An encapsulated, aerobic, gram-positive, spore-forming, rod-shaped bacterium that is transmitted through direct contact, inhalation, and ingestion.

Apneustic breathing A profound bradypnea (abnormally slowed breathing) with periods of apnea (temporary absence of breathing). The patient actually pauses during inhalation, as if to hold the breath, for periods of two to three seconds before exhaling. These breaths are then followed by equal length periods of apnea.

Arc A high voltage light flash that can produce temperatures as high as 4,000°C. These pale blue-violet flashes are formed when electricity goes between two objects of greatly different electrical potentials, such as a high power line and a person.

Armed protection Keeping an individual who is carrying weapons nearby the provider to repel attackers at a violent crime scene.

Arm rappel Use of the climber's arm as a friction device during a technical rescue descent.

Ascender device Equipment that allows a climber in a technical rescue to climb the rope. These ascenders are easier to release and reset than a prusik.

Association of Air Medical Services An international association which serves providers of air medical transport systems. This group distributed a position statement describing early activation and auto-launch as an effective means to decrease response time in certain circumstances.

Atmospheric pressure The force exerted by the atmosphere.

Attraction A method of encouraging the lost patient to come to the searchers or move to a specific location. The use of whistles, public address systems, and sirens are methods of attraction.

Auricular hematoma Commonly referred to as a cauliflower ear, bleeding within the cartilage and soft tissues that make up the ear due to blunt trauma.

Auto-launch A policy that involves simultaneous dispatch of a helicopter and the ground units based upon the dispatch information and assumed severity of the incident. This allows the helicopter to respond faster, in the event it is needed.

Avulsion A separation of a body part, usually caused by a tearing force that rends the limb from the body, often leaving a jagged or tattered stump behind.

Awareness level (Hazmat) (1) In chemical responses, the level of training required of all emergency responders. Those at the Awareness level must have an understanding of the risks of hazmat, the ability to recognize the presence of hazmat, and the ability to recognize the need for additional resources. (2) In wilderness search and rescue, the Paramedic at Awareness level is expected to recognize the need for a wilderness search and rescue and initiate a rescue response.

Awareness level training A term found in NFPA 1670, which addresses training that responders and support personnel should receive at the most basic level.

Background pain Pain that occurs while at rest, which is a constant in the burn patient's experience and will remain until the inflammatory response subsides.

Bandage Any clean material used to support a sterile dressing. Triangular bandages, also called cravats, have long been used by Paramedics.

Baroreceptors Sensors located in the carotid bodies and aortic arch that sense the blood pressure in the central arterial vessels through the stretch in the arterial wall at these locations.

Barotrauma A condition that occurs in divers from changing pressures. As the pressure on the lungs drops, the lungs expand proportionately. Since the lungs have a limited ability to expand, they tend to rupture, after which a pneumothorax can develop.

Basket An essential piece of technical rescue equipment, which may either be used to lower supplies to a rescuer or carry a patient to safety.

Bastard search A technique of looking for a lost person in any place that can provide food, water, shelter, or medical attention, where he might be likely to go if lost.

Battenberg visibility markings A cross-hatch reflective marking that is popular in Europe.

Battle's sign A discoloration behind the ear that represents hematoma formation.

Belay A second rope used during a technical rescue to protect the rescuer from a fall. Originally the word "belay" meant to make fast (i.e., to secure), or prevent a rope from moving. In this case, a belay is meant to make the rescuer secure.

Bennett's fracture An injury to the thumb's carpometacarpal joint (CMC), which can occur as a result of direct trauma or a fall on an outstretched hand with the thumb slightly flexed.

Bigelow method A common technique used for closed reduction of the hip. With the patient supine, one Paramedic provides posterior traction along the anterior superior iliac, in effect pinning the hips to the stretcher and stabilizing the hips. Another Paramedic then grasps the lower leg at the bent knee and applies steady longitudinal traction, levering the femur into the acetabulum by abduction and external rotation.

Bioengineered skin equivalent (BSE) A human skin substitute that consists of dermal cells seeded into a bovine collagen matrix and grown in the laboratory.

Biohazard Detection System (BDS) A system utilized to screen mail for biological warfare that samples the air as mail is sorted to identify anthrax spores or other chemicals.

Biomechanics The study of the forces muscles exert upon the skeleton.

Biot's breathing Sometimes called ataxic breathing, a pattern of irregularly irregular gasping breathing or breathing that is arrhythmic in nature. Biot's breathing is generally a premorbid sign and is often missed by Paramedics who have been assisting respirations before this phenomenon occurs.

Black widow spider The most well-known spider, which has a reputation for its powerful, neurotoxic venom.

Blunt trauma An internal injury caused by a force that does not penetrate through the skin and into the body.

B-NICE A mnemonic used to recall agents that may cause harmful exposure: Biological, Nuclear, Incendiary, Chemical, or Explosive.

Body rappel Sometimes called a Dulfersitz, use of the climber's body as a friction device during a descent.

Boiling liquid expanding vapor explosion (BLEVE) A situation in which liquid evaporates quickly, creating vapor, which creates a pressure inside a confined space, such as a tanker. This pressure, called the vapor pressure, can become explosive if released.

Boiling point The temperature at which liquid becomes a gas.

Bone mineral density (BMD) A system used to diagnosis osteoporosis and predict a patient's risk of fracture. A BMD, reported as a "T-score," of (−) 1.0 or greater is normal, translated as a low risk of fracture. A score of (−) 2.4 to (−) 1.0 is considered osteopenia, or a moderate risk of fracture. Any T-score less than (−) 2.5 is osteoporosis and poses a great risk of fracture.

Botulism A toxin created by the *Clostridium botulinum* bacterium that can cause flaccid paralysis by preventing the release of acetylcholine. Foodborne botulism is the most common disease in adults, generally presenting as gastrointestinal distress.

Boxer's splint A gutter splint modified to immobilize the fourth and fifth metacarpals.

Boyle's law A gas law that states when a gas is placed under pressure, assuming a constant temperature, the volume of gas will change inversely to the change in pressure; in other words, the greater the pressure, the smaller the volume.

Bracketing A technique used to supplement the step-by-step method during a search and rescue when the next successive print cannot be located during tracking. Bracketing uses stride length to skip a step when a sign cannot be found and to determine where the next step might be located.

Braden risk assessment scale An evaluation tool used to help identify and quantify risk factors for pressure sores, in order that appropriate treatment plans may be initiated. This scale is used extensively in the long-term care industry and includes evaluations of sensory perception, moisture, activity, mobility, nutrition, and friction/shear.

Briefings General information shared with rescue searchers about the incident and the objectives, as well as specific information gained from the Lost Person Questionnaire, which should be factual and concise.

Brown recluse spider One of the most commonly found spiders, so named because of the brown violin-shaped marking on the dorsum of its body. They are nocturnal hunters, and prefer to live in dark spaces such as in garages, in outhouses, under rocks, or in woodpiles.

Brown-Sequard syndrome A partial transection of the spinal cord which reduces position sense and motor control on the side with the injury (ipsilateral) and reduces pain and temperature sense on the other side (contralateral).

Buckle fractures A bone break that typically occurs in younger children when force is applied as an axial load to the humerus at the elbow. This causes a deformity in the softer bone similar to what occurs when a stick of butter is dropped from the dinner table onto the floor.

Buddy taping The process of taping an injured finger to the next finger. To add rigidity to the assembly, the Paramedic can insert a tongue depressor between the fingers.

Calm water Water that moves at a speed of less than one knot.

Canadian Triage and Acuity Scale (CTAS) A five-level triage scale adopted across much of Canada, with the most critical patients designated as Level 1 and the least serious as Level 5. The CTAS attempts to identify patients who have higher acuity illnesses or injuries and will require a higher utilization of resources.

Canine search teams Specialized rescuers who use highly trained dogs to locate entrapped survivors of a structural collapse.

Carabiner A metal ring that is used to attach a sling or rope to another part of the rope rescue system during a technical rescue. Carabiners are either oval, D-shaped, or some variation of either.

Carbonaceous sputum A combination of secretions, mucosal slough, and smoke residue that provides evidence of facial burns that may involve smoke inhalation.

Cardiac tamponade A condition in which the space between the epicardium and the pericardium fills with blood or fluid after an injury. Since the pericardium encasing this sac does not stretch, the accumulation of fluid does not allow the heart to refill with blood after a contraction because the heart chambers cannot dilate in the compressed space.

Care behind the barricade Situation that occurs when medical providers direct others regarding how to give medical care without actually seeing the patients themselves. This might happen, for example, in a hostage situation when one of the hostages is injured and the medic cannot get to him.

Care in transit The care provided before a patient arrives at a hospital. At a small event, this is routine ambulance care.

Casualty care area The location where patients are initially taken to provide further assessment and care after an incident.

Caterpillar pass A transfer technique in which a patient on a litter is passed over an obstacle by team members rather than having all the team members climb over it.

Cauda equina syndrome A syndrome involving neurologic deficits caused by compression of the lower end of the spinal cord as can occur from a lumbar spine fracture. This is a true surgical emergency.

Caustic burns A burn that destroys organic tissue through a chemical process, involving chemicals with a pH of greater than 12.5.

CBRNE An abbreviation used to identify hazardous materials: **C**hemical, **B**iological, **R**adiological/**N**uclear, and **E**xplosive events.

Central cord syndrome The most common partial cord syndrome, which usually involves a central tract injury with a mechanism of hyperextension.

Central herniation A supratentorial herniation during which increasing intracranial pressure exerts a force upon the diencephalon (at the midline of the brain above the brainstem), the thalamus, and the hypothalamus, as well as the temporal lobes. The classic triad of symptoms of a central herniation is coma, fixed and dilated pupils, and posturing.

Central neurogenic hyperventilation Sustained hyperventilation, at respiratory rates of 40 to 60 breaths a minute, caused by pressure on the pulmonary receptors within the brainstem that control respirations and represents midbrain dysfunction.

Cerebral arterial gas embolism (CAGE) One of the most serious forms of decompression illness, which occurs when a patient attempts a too-rapid ascent through water (i.e., panic ascent) without exhalation. A nitrogen gas bubble is created and passes into arterial circulation.

Chain of communications The method by which concessionaires and vendors at a mass gathering contact EMS in an emergency as well as notify hospitals of the impending arrival of patients.

Charles' law A gas law that states if the volume is held constant, the pressure will decrease proportionate to the decrease in temperature. If the pressure is held constant, the volume will decrease with a decrease in temperature.

Chemical Transportation Emergency Center (CHEMTREC) A public service center used by firefighters, law enforcement, and other emergency responders to obtain information and assistance for emergency incidents involving chemicals and hazardous materials.

Chemoprophylaxis Vaccination activities and/or distribution of medications carried out during or before a disease outbreak or biological attack to reduce morbidity and mortality.

Chemoreceptors Sensors located in the medulla oblongata, carotid, and aorta that sense pH, carbon dioxide, and, to a lesser extent, oxygen content in the blood and cerebrospinal fluid.

CHEMPACK A component of the Strategic National Stockpile (SNS) that establishes caches of antidotes for nerve agents and other toxins. CHEMPACK is configured in two types of containers: one designed for EMS use, the other for hospital use.

Cheyne–Stokes respiration Periods of hyperpnea (increased depth of breathing) followed by periods of apnea (temporary absence of breathing).

Cingulate herniation A supratentorial herniation during which an accumulation of blood from the expanding hematoma, particularly at the frontal lobe, creates a mass effect that pushes the cerebral cortex at the medial brain, called the cingulated gyrus, under the falx cerebri at the midbrain. As a result, the patient experiences problems of memory, particularly short-term memory, as well as problems with emotions such as anger or confusion.

Class I harness An emergency self-rescue harness that is not capable of holding more than one person's weight.

Class II harness The most common rescue harness, known as the seat harness.

Class III harness A combination that includes the seat harness along with a chest harness. The full body harness has the advantage of keeping the Paramedic upright in the event of a fall.

Clear ice The strongest ice that can form. Good clear ice can be transparent in thicknesses of many inches, supports the largest amount of weight relative to thickness, and is somewhat predictable when it fractures.

Clue consciousness High awareness of potential field clues during a search and rescue, as well as the mindset that clues can come from unexpected sources.

Clusters Patterns of illnesses occurring in the same general location that may indicate an intentional release of a biological agent.

Cnidaria The phylum that includes jellyfish, corals, and sea anemones. There are four classes within the phylum: Hydrozoa (Portuguese man-of-war, fire coral), Cubozoa (box jellyfish), Anthozoa (sea anemone), and Scyphozoa (true jellyfish).

Coagulation In Jackson's thermal burn theory, the center of the burn wound, which is the area of direct tissue destruction.

Coagulation necrosis The process of hydrolysis that changes proteins into their base amino acids, thereby destroying them in the process. Coagulation necrosis causes acid burns to be self-limiting.

Cold diuresis Excessive urination due to decreased temperatures.

Cold towel cooling system In rehabilitation, a process that uses towels soaked in cool water applied to the firefighter's face and neck to relieve the body of excessive heat.

Cold water reflex (Mammalian dive reflex) The physiological result of hypothermia. According to this theory, when the human body is suddenly exposed to cold water, the body's defense is to immediately shut down all but the vital organs.

Cold zone The outer perimeter of a chemical spill. The cold zone contains the command center/post, additional hazmat support personnel (such as physicians), and the boundary of the decontamination corridor.

Colles fracture A distal radial fracture that follows a fall on an outstretched hand, or an MVC in which the driver grabs the steering wheel. The resultant fracture produces a characteristic "silver fork" deformity. The wrist and hand are displaced dorsally compared with the forearm.

Commission for Accreditation of Air Medical Services (CAAMS) An accrediting body developed in 1990 by the industry to validate its members' standards regarding safety, medical care, and utilization review, which later became the Commission for Accreditation of Medical Transport Services (CAMTS).

Commotio cordis Latin for commotion of the heart, a type of sudden cardiac death that involves disruption of the contraction cycle without structural damage. To take place, a blunt impact must occur at the correct location on the chest and at the correct time in the heart's depolarization/repolarization cycle. This event is most often observed in young athletes who experience a direct blunt injury to the anterior chest, such as a collision with a baseball or other projectile.

Community Emergency Response Teams (CERT) A group of trained people in the community that augments emergency responders and helps meet an area's immediate needs before emergency responders arrive.

Compartment syndrome A painful condition caused by the compression of nerves and blood vessels in a particular location of the body.

Complete cord transection A situation in which bundled nerve cells that travel in the spinal column are severed by a displacement of the vertebra, presence of a foreign object, or potentially by being stretched (distraction). This can occur at any level and will eliminate the transmission and reception of all messages below the area of the insult.

Comprehensive Environmental Response Compensation and Liability Act (CERCLA) The original regulatory authority for hazardous material response training which addressed the need for specially prepared personnel with advanced training in hazmat response.

Compressive asphyxiation Sometimes known as crowd crush, a situation in which a patient lacks oxygen due to compression of the chest cavity, which often occurs during a human stampede.

Concealment An obstruction blocking the view between the tactical medic and any potential gunfire at a violent scene, but not protecting the Paramedic from projectiles.

Concept of CAB (circulation, airway, breathing) Philosophy often followed at a violent scene instead of traditional ABC assessment. In the tactical environment, more casualties are caused by significant bleeding than airway or breathing issues, therefore the first priority is stopping bleeding.

Conductor An object that electricity can freely flow through.

Confined space An enclosed area with limited access and/or egress that is not designed for human occupancy and has the potential to cause physical, chemical, or atmospheric injury.

Containment Establishing a best guess perimeter of where a lost patient may be located to contain the subject and limit the search area.

Continuity of government (COG) A plan designed to maintain national leadership in the event of a catastrophe.

Continuity of operations (COOP) A plan designed to maintain national services in the event of a catastrophe.

Contrecoup injury An injury to the opposite side of the brain than where the force was applied to the skull caused by the brain rebounding off of the inner surface of the skull.

Conus medullaris syndrome An altered mental status secondary to traumatic brain injury and incontinence associated with sacral cord injury.

Cool zone In the zones of care model, a relatively safe zone where staging and deployment occur. This area is typically farthest away from where traumatic injury is most likely to occur and is out of the line of fire.

Copperhead snake Snakes that have rust and copper color bands on the body with a prominent copper-colored head.

Coral snake A brightly colored snake found in southern, temperate areas of the United States, identified by the red, yellow, and black banding that runs along their body.

Core temperature The temperature in the body's vital organs (heart, lungs, and brain) and core organs (liver, kidneys, and spleen).

Corticospinal tract Descending tracts that send motor nerve instructions to the muscles, which are found in the anterior portion of the spinal cord (from the cortex to the spine).

Coup injury An intraparenchymal hemorrhage that results from acceleration-deceleration forces that cause the brain to strike the inner surface of the skull.

Coverage (1) The measure of a search area effectively swept versus the area searched, which is a reflection of search thoroughness. (2) Protection at a violent area provided by an impenetrable object, such as a building, that shields a rescuer from projectiles.

Crotalidae Polyvalent Antivenin The most commonly used antivenin in the United States, administered as an initial bolus of vials, and then as a maintenance infusion after the progression of symptoms has been halted.

Crowd sentiment The emotional tone set by the mass-gathering event and by the crowd.

Crush injury Syndrome that involves prolonged crushing force applied to a large muscle mass, causing tissue damage and release of intracellular toxins that then cause cardiovascular instability, kidney failure, and eventually death if left untreated.

Crush syndrome A condition that occurs in crush injury, in which the massive forces that compress the limb cause extensive damage to muscle cells.

Culture of safety As defined by the Centers for Disease Control, the shared commitment of management and employees to ensure the safety of the work environment.

Curling's ulcer A stress ulcer caused by electric shock.

Cushing's triad A symptom complex of hypertension, bradycardia, and altered respiratory pattern, which is suggestive of herniation syndrome.

Cutis marmorata A condition associated with decompression sickness in which the skin takes on a marbled appearance.

Dalton's law A gas law that states if pressure is exerted on a mixture of gasses, the individual gasses will all compress the same and the proportion of the pressures will all remain constant.

Dead category In the START triage system, those patients who have either died from their injuries by the time rescuers arrive on-scene or are mortally wounded and expected to die prior to transport.

Debriefing The process of relating all information gained by a searcher during an assignment to the search management team.

Decerebrate rigidity The second stage of posturing, which generally indicates upper brainstem injury and is often a premorbid finding. With decerebrate rigidity, both the hips and shoulders extend and internally pronate while the forearms hyperpronate. This is the most noticeable characteristic of decerebrate rigidity.

Decompression illness (DCI) An umbrella term that covers problems related to the pressure changes that occur with changes in depth. In DCI, air-filled spaces like the lungs and the intestines create a host of symptoms.

Decontamination The process of removing excess hazardous material from emergency providers and patients.

Decorticate rigidity The initial stage of posturing, in which the patient with increasing intracranial pressure demonstrates adduct of the shoulders, as the shoulders rotate internally with slight flexion while the forearms pronate and the wrist and fingers flex. Simultaneously, the lower extremities will demonstrate "triple flexion" of the hip, knee, and ankles.

Decubitus ulcers A pressure sore that extends into the deeper muscles and even into the bones. A decubitus ulcer can lead to osteomyelitis, necrotizing tissue fasciitis, and muscle necrosis.

Deep burns A classification used by some medical experts that groups partial and full thickness burns together.

Defensive swimming position A self-rescue water technique a rescuer performs by lying on his back, facing downstream. The rescuer's head remains up for visibility and protection, his feet are used as bumpers, and his knees are used as shock absorbers.

Dehiscence A condition in which a formerly closed wound reopens. As a result of decreased granulation, delayed epithelialization, and poor neovascularization, the "healed" tissues become friable and fragile.

Delayed category In the START triage system, those patients who have injuries that require evaluation and treatment within 60 to 90 minutes.

Delayed primary wound healing A lengthy process of wound healing that occurs if the wound is contaminated, preventing close approximation of the wound edges, during which macrophages wall off foreign material.

Delivered devices Explosives that may be as simple as a hand-thrown Molotov cocktail, or self-propelled explosives such as a rocket or flare gun that a person has to directly launch or ignite.

Denature To break down, such as proteins.

Dental malocclusion Disruption of the patient's teeth caused by forces applied to the mouth that causes abnormal closure of the mouth.

Department of Homeland Security (DHS) The department established by the Homeland Security Act of 2002 that became the lead agency for implementing the National Response Plan.

Dermatomes Areas of the body innervated by specific spinal nerves (nerves that leave the spinal cord). In the cervical spine, they are described consecutively in descending order from C1 to S-5.

Descent control device Equipment that either provides the Paramedic with an ability to rappel safely to the patient or allows a basket or other patient carrier to be lowered to the patient.

Dessication A process through which the body extracts water from cells.

Dexamethasone (Decadron®) An anti-inflammatory and immunosuppressant from the steroid family that is used to treat HACE.

Diamond carry A cross-country litter carry technique in which four rescuers are used, all facing forward, with one on each side and one on each end of the litter.

Diaphragmatic herniation Damage that occurs when abdominal contents are forced upward into the thoracic cavity, as may happen in motor vehicle collisions.

Diaphragmatic rupture Damage that occurs when abdominal contents are forced upward into the thoracic cavity, as may happen in motor vehicle collisions.

Differential pressure The force of two bodies of water at different elevations trying to equalize.

Diffuse axonal injury (DAI) A wound that occurs as a result of the rapid acceleration-deceleration of the brain within the skull. This movement of tissues over and away from other tissues as a result of shearing forces. This movement disrupts neural connections.

Dilutional hyponatremia A lack of sodium in the blood caused by excessive water intake.

Direct tactics Search methods targeted toward actually finding a missing individual.

Dirty bomb A traditional large-scale explosive containing large amounts of nuclear materials.

Disaster Assistance Response Teams (DART) Groups of trained personnel that can be rapidly called upon to provide aid during an emergency. They generally have up to 1,000 square feet of treatment area, and come equipped with portable medical imaging equipment and mobile labs for point-of-care testing.

Disaster Medical Assistance Team (DMAT) A group of volunteer personnel represented by physicians, nurses, pharmacists, Paramedics, logisticians, and administrators designed to augment or backfill previously deployed teams.

Disaster Mortuary Operational Response Team (DMORT) A group that serves to provide patient identification and mortuary services. DMORT is prepared to establish temporary morgue facilities; identify patients using forensic dental pathology and forensic anthropology methods; and process, prepare, and make disposition of remains.

Disentanglement The cutting away of a vehicle from a trapped or injured patient.

Dislocation Also known as luxation, the complete movement of a bone out of the joint. The resulting disarticulation of the joint results in loss of range of motion as well as concurrent tendon and ligament damage.

Dive rescue Any subsurface rescue operation in which rescuers wear self-contained underwater breathing apparatus (SCUBA).

Divers Alert Network (DAN) A group that has been working on recommendations relating to divers, such as how long to wait to fly in an airplane after diving.

Domestic terrorism An attempt by an individual or group, based and operating without foreign direction and entirely within the United States or Puerto Rico, to intimidate or coerce the government or its people in furtherance of political or social objectives.

Dose/response The concept that when the dose increases, so does the individual's response to that compound.

Double sugar tong splint An immobilization device that prevents both pronation and supination. The two "sugar tongs" are preformed from malleable splint material.

Down-and-under pathway A condition in which, during a motor vehicle collision, the occupant's lower body travels under the dashboard.

Downstream V An indication in water that usually signals a path between two objects, with the V pointing downstream. The rescuer should try to position himself in the downstream V, and stay away from the upstream V.

Droop line A rope held by two rescuers, one at each end of the span, or a distance apart, which is literally drooped onto the patient. Once the patient grabs the line, one of the rescuers lets go, and the patient will swing into shore.

Drownproofing A self-rescue water technique performed by laying face down in the water, without moving the hands and legs, and letting the head hang. The person in the water holds her breath, and when she needs to breathe she raises her head just enough to exchange air, then holds her breath again for a few seconds.

Dry drowning A condition in which the patient asphyxiates but the lungs stay dry.

Dynamic belay A water rescue technique. Belaying means simply holding a rescue rope firm to swing the patient in water to the shore. In a dynamic belay, a rescuer on shore walks downstream along the bank, easing the tension on the line. Taking a short walk downstream may allow the patient to come ashore much closer to a shallow, calmer area.

Dynamic rope A type of rope popular with rock climbers that has stretch and thus is more forgiving to the climber during a fall. These are generally not used for rescue, as stretch is not desirable.

Dynamic tension lines Tension that exists along the body's planes of movement, in which the underlying muscle creates the tension. An example of dynamic tension lines is when wrinkles appear on a person's forehead during a frown.

Dysbarism Disorders that result from changes in pressure, either from high altitudes or from ascending and descending under the water. Dysbarism consists of decompression sickness, arterial gas embolism, and barotraumas.

Ear squeeze A feeling of fullness in the ear, which originates in the middle ear as the Eustachian tubes equalize the middle ear with the external environment.

Eddy A relatively calm pool of water that forms behind an object when moving water flows around a large object.

Ehlers–Danlos syndrome A condition in which people are born with a congenital abnormality of collagen formation. This leads to fragile skin prone to injury with seemingly minor trauma and poor wound healing that invariably leads to extensive scarring.

Elapidae An animal classification that contains some venomous snakes in the United States, such as coral snakes, which are mostly found in the southeastern United States.

Ellis classifications A categorization of fractured teeth based on the amount of tooth involved. Ellis I tooth fractures only involve the enamel. Ellis II tooth fractures run through the enamel into the dentin. Ellis III fractures extend down to the pulp.

Emergency Medical Treatment and Active Labor Act (EMTALA) A section of the larger Consolidated Omnibus Budget Reconciliation Act (COBRA) that was originally passed in 1986, which remains one of the most important pieces of healthcare legislation in the United States. It defines a hospital's responsibility to provide emergency care to anyone presenting with a request for help, as well as the hospital's obligations with regard to initial evaluation and management and transfer arrangements.

Emergency Operations Center (EOC) The centralized control facility responsible for coordinating emergency management in the case of a disaster.

Emergency Response Guide (ERG) A publication that defines the U.S. Department of Transportation (DOT) placard system and contains information related to the potential health risk of hazardous materials.

Emergency Severity Index (ESI) An emergency department triage algorithm that sorts patients into five levels that not only looks at the need for immediate, life-threatening interventions, but also for resource utilization.

Emergency Support Function (ESF) A structure for allocating federal resources during a disaster. The National Response Plan identifies 15 Emergency Support Functions, each associated with specific task-organized capabilities and assigned to a federal coordinating department or agency.

Emergency Vehicle Operators Course (EVOC) An expert panel-derived risk and safety awareness driver-training program, created as a result of the 1979 NTSB recommendations.

Enophthalmos A condition marked by a depressed eyeball.

Entry leg bag A slightly more equipped first aid bag containing the same elements as individual first aid kits with the addition of a venous access device and chest decompression needle.

Epidural hematoma Created by intracranial bleeding between the dura mater and the skull, bleeding that typically occurs in the temporoparietal region, although it can occur anywhere in the central nervous system covered by the dura mater.

Eschar From the Greek word for scab, a layer of blackened necrotic tissue that prevents deeper penetration of acid into the skin and thus limits the depth of a burn.

Escharotomy A surgical incision performed by a surgeon into the depth of a burn patient's burnt tissue, generally in parallel lines along the mid-axillary line and horizontally along the plane of the diaphragm, which allows for expansion and movement.

Evaporative techniques Actions taken to reduce a patient's temperature by applying moisture that will draw heat away as it is evaporated.

Event profile A document that contains information about the type of mass-gathering event, such as whether it is indoors or outdoors, and whether it is restricted (such as fenced in) or extended (with a capability of expanding beyond the grounds). It also includes crowd information.

Exertional heatstroke (EHS) A form of hyperthermia, an abnormally elevated body temperature with accompanying physical and neurological symptoms, that results from strenuous physical activity.

Exophthalmos A condition marked by a protruding eyeball.

Expectant category In the START triage system, those patients who are still alive, but expected to die within a short period of time. This separate category allows the Paramedic to avoid placing living patients in the Dead category during triage.

Exsanguinate From the Latin term *sanguis*, meaning blood, to drain of blood.

Extensor posturing A posture where both the hips and shoulders extend and internally pronate while the forearms hyperpronate. This is the most noticeable characteristic of extensor posturing. This finding generally indicated upper brainstem injury and is often a premorbid finding.

Extreme altitude Any elevation above 18,000 feet.

Extrication The creation of a space-making path that will help remove patients from a crashed vehicle.

Exudates Fluid that weeps from an injured site. Blood-tinged liquid drainage is called serosanguineous, whereas clear fluid is just serous.

Fasciotomy A surgical procedure performed by a surgeon, where the fascia is cut to relieve tension on the limb compartment.

Fatigue A state of exhaustion or a loss of strength or endurance that can lead to a decreased capacity for physical or mental work.

Federal Emergency Management Agency (FEMA) Until 2002, the lead agency for federal emergency planning and response.

Federal Motor Vehicle Safety Standards (FMVSS) The minimum safety performance requirements for motor vehicles.

Federal Response Plan (FRP) The foundation of modern federal disaster planning documents, which is primarily designed to clarify the roles and responsibilities of the federal departments and agencies responding to catastrophic events.

Felon A purulent infection that results when bacteria-laden foreign material is injected into the pulp of the finger, most commonly the thumb or index finger. These infections are very painful and require careful incision and drainage by a physician in most cases.

Ferry line A line stretched across moving water that is used to direct an object's movement to one side or the other.

Field dressing A combined bandage and dressing in the same unit, usually stored in a waterproof pouch.

Field triage criteria An algorithm that includes anatomical issues, physiological issues, and mechanism of injury as decision parameters designed to aid Paramedics in making treatment and transportation decisions for injured patients.

Film dressing A thin, transparent, semipermeable membrane that permits moisture to escape and oxygen to enter. Because these dressings "breathe," they prevent the maceration (a softening of the dermis as seen when skin is submersed in water for a long time) that is associated with more traditional first aid strips.

Finger splint An immobilization device that should maintain the proximal interphalangeal (PIP) joint at an approximate 15 to 20 degrees of flexion.

Fire point The point at which a fire will continue to burn after ignition.

Fit-tested Using either quantitative or qualitative methods to ensure a proper face seal for a rescuer's respirator. The Paramedic's facial hair must not interfere with the mask's seal.

Fixed wing Airplanes used in air medical transport.

Flail chest Two to three ribs broken in two or more places that demonstrate paradoxical movement.

Flammability A range of conditions in which a flame can be initiated or sustained in a substance.

Flashpoint The minimum temperature whereby a chemical evaporates at a rate sufficient to form an ignitable fuel/air mixture.

Flexor posturing Seen with the patient with increasing intracranial pressure demonstrates adduct of the shoulders, as the shoulders rotate internally with slight flexion while the forearms pronate and wrist and fingers flex when stimulated. Simultaneously, the lower extremities will demonstrate "triple flexion" of the hip, knee, and ankles. Also called decorticate posturing.

Floating sternum A complete sternal dislocation from the costochondral joints (with the ribs) that results in paradoxical motion of the sternum.

Floodwater An overflow of riverbanks or other natural bodies of water, resulting in water flowing into normally dry areas.

Fluid creep A phenomenon that results from overly aggressive fluid administration (overresuscitation), which can lead to increased burn edema formation, abdominal compartment syndrome, and acute respiratory distress syndrome.

Flutter valve A one-way valve used when treating a pneumothorax to prevent air from returning.

Foam dressings A sterile gauze that absorbs exudate while protecting the skin. Foam dressings have high absorbency, conform to all body shapes, and provide protection from further trauma by cushion.

Focused Abdominal Sonography in Trauma (FAST) An exam used to detect the cause of shock by placing an ultrasound probe in the right and left upper quadrant, suprapubic, subxiphoid, and left and right upper chest. The FAST is used to detect free peritoneal or pelvic fluid, pericardial tamponade, or pneumothorax.

Forced diuresis Increase in urination through administration of fluids and/or diuretics.

Formication A condition associated with decompression sickness in which nitrogen under the skin makes the skin "feel" as if it is crawling. It is associated with a variable paresthesia as well as itch (pruritus).

Four-corner carry A cross-country litter carry technique in which four rescuers, all facing forward, each takes a corner of the litter.

Fracture A broken bone, which frequently occurs because of either direct force or an indirect force.

Frontal impact supplemental restraint system A safety system located in the vehicle's steering wheel and dashboard to protect the front seat occupants during a frontal impact.

Frostbite A localized cold injury that involves the freezing of tissue. Frostbite can occur because of prolonged exposure to cold temperatures or a sudden exposure to a cold-producing agent.

Frostnip Superficial tissue damage that involves just the epidermal layers of the skin.

Fuel cells Hydrogen and methanol mixes in hydrogen-powered cars that produce electricity to power the automobile. Although currently in the development phase, the fuel cell holds a great deal of promise as the motive force for the future.

Full thickness burn Tissue damage that extends past the skin's protective barrier and exposes the body to infection and insults from the environment. The appearance can range from a white, waxy look to a black, leathery surface consistent with charred flesh.

Gaining access The process used at a motor-vehicle collision to create a pathway to the patient. The initial path should allow the Paramedic to access the patient's face and neck to establish an airway and check the carotid pulse.

Galeazzi fracture A midshaft radial fracture with a dislocation of the radioulnar joint.

Gamow bag A sleeping bag-like device with a foot pump that can be inflated to mimic the hyperbaric chamber and is used to care for people stricken with HAPE. This device effectively raises the pO_2 and, over time, allows the patient to recover sufficiently to descend from an elevation on his or her own.

Geographical information systems (GIS) Technology used for helping one find directions which utilizes global positioning satellites (GPS).

Globe rupture A loss of the eyeball's integrity, often caused by direct force applied to the globe.

Glycogen debt A condition that occurs when the body uses all of its glycogen stores.

Granulation A healing step in wound care during which fibroblasts start to form a bed of collagen and rudimentary tissue replaces the fibrin clot. Granulation starts on the inside and pushes the scab up and out.

Greenstick fracture A bone break injury that occurs when the force applied to the bone causes one side of the cortex to break while the other side bends or deforms. Greenstick fractures get their name from resembling what happens when a fresh twig in spring is bent.

Gross hematuria Visible blood in the patient's urine.

Ground An area of zero potential voltage.

Ground searching Conducting a search for a lost person on foot.

Guidelines for Air Medical Dispatch A document issued by the National Association of EMS Physicians that is considered a national standard, which departments can reference when creating local guidelines.

Gustilo–Anderson system A classification system based on the patient's amount of soft-tissue injury, which is used for prognosis of fracture healing, risk of infection, and probability of amputation.

Haddon matrix A tool used to illustrate factors contributing to the outcome of an event that leads to an injury and illustrates that injuries are a result of many factors, not just random events. Three rows in the matrix list the phases of an event: pre-event, event, and post-event, whereas four columns contain information concerning the host, vector or agent, physical environment, and sociocultural environment.

Hard body armor Apparel made with a thick ceramic or metal plate hard enough to deflect the force of a projectile. It provides much more protection than soft body armor, but it also is much more cumbersome to wear.

Hard protection A firm object such as a short board placed between tools and the patient, or tools and the Paramedic, during an extrication.

Hasty search A quick search of the "high probability" areas where a lost subject is likely to be found. The goal of a hasty search is to find either clues or the subject in the first minutes to hours before more complex, resource-intensive search tactics are employed.

Hazard analysis An assessment of any risk factors that may be present in a community. Any farm silo, cave, or sewer system that has the potential for a person to become trapped in an oxygen poor environment, for example.

Hazardous materials Any substances (solid, liquid, or gas) that, when released, are capable of causing harm to people, the environment, or property.

Hazardous Materials Transportation Act (HMTA; 49 CFR) Legislation that standardized the containers, markings, and the mode of transportation used for materials, including hazardous materials.

Hazardous Waste Operations and Emergency Response (HAZWOPER) standards A standard that refers to five types of hazardous waste operations conducted in the United States under OSHA Standard 1910.120. It contains the safety requirements employers must meet in order to conduct these operations.

Healing by secondary intention Secondary wound healing that occurs when the wound is purposefully left open to air and the body is allowed to close the wound itself via granulation. Healing by secondary intention involves a more intense inflammatory response and is seen as more useful in grossly contaminated wounds.

Heat cramps Muscle spasms due to loss of water or sodium, which often accompany heat exhaustion (in as many as 60% of cases). These occur when the patient works at a sustained pace for several hours, sweats profusely, and drinks large volumes of water.

Heat escape lessening position (HELP) A self-rescue water technique in which the swimmer draws up his legs and knees to the chest and wraps his arms around them. This position lessens heat loss, and can delay hypothermia if movement is kept to a minimum.

Heat exhaustion A condition of generalized weakness, poor muscle coordination, and alterations in mental status following exposure to excessive heat.

Heat fatigue A decline in coordination and difficulty with task performance due to exposure to excessive heat. Weakness may also be a symptom.

Heat index Sometimes called the misery index, a function of ambient temperature and humidity. Combining these factors creates a "perceived" temperature.

Heat syncope A warning sign of heat exhaustion. When exposed to heat, the patient's body initiates actions to compensate. If the patient was previously dehydrated, has impaired hemodynamic regulation vis-á-vis cardiac disease, or takes medications such as diuretics or beta blockers, these compensatory mechanisms may be insufficient, leading to loss of consciousness.

Heat wave A period of two days with high heat over 90° F.

Heavy construction Structures designed to withstand shear forces typical of earthquakes and heavy winds. These structures are built with concrete and/or steel-reinforcing bars (rebar), are "box type" structures, have reinforced or unreinforced masonry, and have fire-resistant exterior walls.

Heimlich valve A device that may be attached to portable suction to allow complete re-expansion of the lung during transport.

Hematopoietic system A body system that increases production of red blood cells, gradually replacing red blood cells lost during hemorrhage.

Hemolysin A component of Harvester ant venom which can cause breakdown of red blood cells.

Hemopneumothorax An accumulation of air and blood in the pleural cavity, which leads to lung collapse. The presence of blood and air in the pleural cavity leads to an increase in intrathoracic pressure.

Hemostasis stage The first stage of wound healing during which bleeding is controlled.

Hemostatic agent A substance that facilitates the coagulation of blood to stop hemorrhage by collecting clotting factors.

Hemothorax An accumulation of blood in the pleural cavity.

Henry's law A gas law that simply states that the amount of gas dissolved into blood and tissues is proportional to the partial pressure of that gas.

Herniation A process in which intracranial pressure increases within the brain's compartment, making the mass effect greater. This causes the entire brain to start moving toward the foramen magnum.

Hertz (Hz) Cycles per second, a reference to the transmission of electricity.

High altitude Any elevation between 12,000 feet and 18,000 feet. Many mountains in the United States—including the ranges in Alaska—as well as the Canadian Rockies reach these heights.

High altitude cerebral edema (HACE) A life-threatening condition caused by increased intracranial pressure (ICP) due to reduced pO_2 at altitude and the resulting leakage of fluid that compresses brain tissue.

High altitude pulmonary edema (HAPE) A noncardiogenic edema caused by increased pressure in the pulmonary capillaries caused by fluid shift into the alveoli.

High altitude retinal hemorrhages Minor bleeding in the retina that frequently occurs at altitudes above 14,000 feet and is caused by a lack of oxygen to the retina. Some researchers believe that retinal hemorrhages are a sign of poor acclimatization.

High angle Rescue on any terrain that is greater than 60 degrees and ranges from steep climbing with multiple pitches to a vertical wall. When the provider is unable to independently stand, even using his hands for balance, it is considered high angle.

Higher explosive limit (HEL) A concentration in which the vapor/fuel-air mixture is too rich (the concentration of fuel to air is too high), so that the vapors cannot be ignited.

Highline Rescue over a chasm or ravine where the rescuer or patient is suspended in mid-air with only the rope for protection from a fall.

High water The condition of increased water levels, possibly due to a flood or a sudden rush of waves, that is typically present when a rescue is required. High water periods are not an unusual event, and actions and preplans should reflect this understanding.

Hippocratic method The original method of shoulder reduction, which uses a form of countertraction. With the patient supine, the Paramedic grasps the wrist of the extended arm, then places a foot into the patient's axilla and applies steady countertraction.

Hippus A rapid alternating constriction and dilation of the eyes to bright light as the pupil tries to adjust. Hippus is an early sign of an uncal herniation.

Homeland Security Act (HSA) of 2002 Legislation that established the Department of Homeland Security (DHS) and consolidated other federal components—including FEMA—into the DHS.

Homeland Security Presidential Directive (HSPD)-5 Legislation that refined national incident management policy and the mechanism for developing an operational structure for domestic incidents into the National Response Plan.

Hose inflator systems A water rescue technique using a 50- or 100-foot section of two-and-one-half-inch or three-inch hose and a self-contained breathing apparatus (SCBA) bottle. A quick connect hose or valve system that uses air from an SCBA cylinder inflates the hose to complete the setup.

Hot load A situation in which the medical transport helicopter pilot keeps the helicopter running while the patient is loaded, which creates additional hazards from the whirling rotors.

Hot zone (1) The area involving the chemical material release. This zone possesses the greatest chance of additional exposure to those within its circumference. (2) In the zones of care model, a "care under fire" situation where the medic is in the heart of a violent scene. The care in this zone of operation is simple: scoop and run.

Human stampede Compressive forces that result when people are trampled by a closely pushed together mass of people.

Hydraulic current Water flowing over a dam and being pulled back into the dam face, creating a rolling boil of water.

Hydrogels Transparent membrane dressings, like the film dressings, that are also absorbent, like the foam dressings. These dressings also absorb heat, making them ideal for use as a burn dressing (superficial and partial thickness burns).

Hymenoptera An animal classification that includes the Apis species (bees), vespids (wasps, yellow jackets, hornets), and Formicidae (ants).

Hyperemia In Jackson's thermal burn theory, the outermost ring of a burn, which is generally superficial. This results in dilation of capillary beds and is manifest by reddened skin.

Hyperkalemia A condition of elevated levels of electrolyte potassium.

Hyperpyrexia An abnormally high fever.

Hypertrophic scar Raised prominent scars that tend to fade over time as the wound regresses, which may take years. Hypertrophic scars more often occur with healing by secondary intention.

Hyphema Blood that collects in the anterior chamber of the eye between the cornea and the iris.

Hyponatremia A low level of sodium in the blood.

Hypothermia A suboptimal body temperature, one that—if allowed to persist—is incompatible with life.

Ice awls Simple tools that mostly consist of two ice picks attached to the rescuer or to each other with a leash. The ice awls are used to stab the ice and provide grip when a rescuer falls through the ice and needs to pull himself up.

Iced gastric lavage/gavage A method used for heat reduction in which 10 cc/kg of ice water is instilled into the stomach for one minute, then suctioned out of the stomach for one minute. A lavage/gavage system, using an orogastric tube, can lower the core body temperature 0.3°F (0.15°C)/min.

Ice water immersion Placing the body in very cold water, which is viewed as the gold standard for treatment of heatstroke. Ice water immersion can reduce the body's core temperature in 20 to 40 minutes.

Immediate category In the START triage system, the classification for patients who have potentially life-threatening injuries affecting the airway, breathing, or circulation with an alteration of mental status or other clinical signs of shock.

Immediately Dangerous to Life and Health (IDLH) A system that defines concentration levels that cause unconsciousness, incapacitation (and an inability to self-rescue), or adverse health effects during a 30-minute exposure.

Immersion pulmonary edema (IPE) A noncardiogenic pulmonary edema caused by significant increase in vascular resistance when the patient is immersed in cold water that puts strain on the heart and causes a backwards failure.

Incident Command System (ICS) A flexible organizational structure that integrates personnel, facilities, procedures, and equipment to develop an effective response to emergencies.

Incident Management Assist Team (IMAT) A group sent to incident sites to assess the situation and determine immediate federal requirements. The IMAT contains subject matter experts and identifies facilities for potential federal field sites such as the Joint Field Office or Joint Information Center.

Incident support teams (ISTs) The three 21-person teams of highly qualified specialists that support and coordinate the USAR teams in the United States.

Index case The first reported case of an illness or outbreak, which may go unrecognized for some time before a response is even initiated.

Indirect search tactics Actions that do not take place in the search area itself, but focus on fact finding, attraction, and containment.

Inflatable boats Light boats that can be filled with air. They have shorter gunwales, or sides, than wooden boats, which can make it easier for a patient or rescuer to be parbuckled or retrieved into the boat, and also make it easier to deploy rescuers into the water.

Infrared thermal imaging cameras Devices that create pictures based on heat radiation rather than exposure to light.

Infratentorial herniations Herniations that occur in the area below the tentorium.

Instrument flight rules (IFR) A situation in which an aircraft pilot relies upon the aircraft's instruments for navigation, with additional instruction from air traffic control (ATC).

Intelligent transportation systems (ITS) A number of new technologies that are currently available to enhance safety and collision avoidance. These technologies pertain to driver behavior modification, intelligent vehicle design, and other roadside safety technologies.

Interfacility transports The process of moving a patient from one facility to another.

Internal pneumatic splint Positive pressure ventilation used to stop the paradoxical motion of the flail segment while supporting the patient's ventilation.

International Association of Flight Paramedics (IAFP) A group, founded in 1986 (originally named the National Flight Paramedics Association), that aims to support and coordinate educational and research activities relating to the Paramedic industry, and establish standard levels of training and performance.

International terrorism Violent acts to human life that occur outside the United States and are violations of U.S. criminal laws. As the FBI states, they are acts that "occur outside the United States or transcend national boundaries in terms of the means by which they are accomplished, the persons they appear intended to coerce or to intimidate, or the locale in which their perpetrators operate or seek asylum."

Intracerebral hemorrhage Sometimes called intraparenchymal bleeding, bleeding that occurs within the brain's soft tissues (i.e., the cerebral cortex).

In-vehicle telematics technology Computer systems that electronically offer real time driver monitoring and immediate auditory feedback to gauge a driver's performance.

Isolation The physical separation of individuals with a communicable disease from others, as opposed to quarantine where susceptible but not necessarily infected individuals are separated from others.

Israeli trauma bandage Sometimes simply called an Israeli bandage, a sterile inner gauze pad applied directly to the wound. Unlike the standard pressure dressing, the trauma dressing has an elastic wrap and a locking mechanism. This elastic wrap serves to help slow bleeding while keeping the dressing in place, whereas the locking device prevents the bandage from slipping.

Jackson's thermal burn theory and zones of injury A description of the various area and severities of a burn. The zones, from least severe to most severe, are hyperemia, stasis, and coagulation.

John-boats Rescue boats often made from aluminum that can range from 10 feet to upward of 16 or 18 feet, and are fairly easy to move with rescuers through tough terrain. Since aluminum is naturally light, they are also easy to slide, both on land and over ice.

Joint Field Office (JFO) A shared command where two or more organizations pool their resources to put together an emergency response.

Joint Information Center (JIC) The area at an emergency site where media representatives gather for press conferences and important messages. Public affairs/public information officers (PA/PIO) meet at the JIC to provide official information and support to the media.

JumpSTART triage tool A triage system developed in 1995 by Dr. Lou Romig that aimed to incorporate pediatric physiologic parameters into triage decisions.

Keloids Lesions that can develop up to one year after an injury and are thought to be due to genetic influences, which are the result of an overgrowth of scar tissue. Keloids are different than hypertrophic scars because the keloid formation extends past the confines of the original scar and they tend to be more permanent.

Kernmantle The type of rope used in most rescues, consisting of a nylon core with a fabric sheath often made of polyester.

Khumbu cough A dry, persistent, and sometimes debilitating cough that can be the precursor to HAPE.

Kinetic energy Energy associated with an object's movement that is equal to one-half the object's mass multiplied by the velocity squared.

KKK specifications Federal purchase specifications for a General Services Administration (GSA) Star of Life ambulance. These are purchase specifications, not safety performance standards.

Knee supplemental restraint system A supplemental restraint system that deploys an airbag from the lower section of the vehicle's dashboard during a frontal crash. The device is designed to protect the front seat occupant's legs and protects the occupants from "submarining" and going under the vehicle's dash during a high-speed impact.

Kocher's method One of the oldest leverage technique used for shoulder reduction. With the arm adducted, and stabilizing the elbow in the palm of the hand, the Paramedic grasps the wrist, forms a 90-degree bend at the elbow, and rotates the arm externally until resistance is felt. Then, lifting the limb until the shoulder is reduced, the Paramedic ends by rolling the forearm into the body to a splintable position.

Kraissl's line Tension that exists along the body's planes of movement, in which the underlying muscle creates the tension. An example of Kraissl's lines is when wrinkles appear on a person's forehead during a frown.

Laceration An injury that develops when traumatic force tears, cuts, or rends the flesh, leaving a jagged wound.

Landing zone (LZ) An area intended for the purpose of landing and taking off in the helicopter.

Land navigation (landnav) Techniques, including use of a map and compass, used for maneuvering and finding directions when traveling on land.

Langer's lines Static tension lines that appear in the skin's folds.

LAST A mnemonic that sums up the goal of all search and rescue operations: Locate, Access, Stabilize, Transport.

Last known position (LKP) The last area where evidence exists showing the person was there, which helps to narrow the search perimeters, increasing the probability of detection in the process.

Latrodectus facies A pattern of facial swelling and symptoms manifest by ptosis of the eyelids, with rhinitis, conjunctivitis, and facial spasms.

Law enforcement officers (LEO) Sworn officers who may be members of the special operations team. It is ideal for them to acquire and maintain some degree of emergency medical training as well when they are part of a special operations team. The primary advantage of this model is that a medical care provider is present who is also a member of the tactical unit.

Lethal concentration 50% Abbreviated LC50, the concentration of a chemical in the air that is lethal to 50% of those exposed.

Lethal dose 50% Abbreviated as LD50, a chemical exposure that is lethal to 50% of the patients exposed.

Level A protective suit A protective outfit that should be worn where the type of airborne agent, dissemination method, duration of dissemination, or exposure concentration is unknown.

Level B protective suit A protective outfit that should be worn when the biological aerosol is no longer being generated and where conditions may present a splash hazard.

Level I rescuers People who are generally trained to use, deploy, and support surface-based or shore-based rescues, using some specific tools that are key to the mission being undertaken.

Level II rescuers People who use specific equipment and wear specific PPE that will protect them from a particular environment, who also receive training on how to extricate a patient from the hazard.

Life safety ropes Ropes designed to support a life load during an emergency. Only these ropes should be used in rescue. For example, escape ropes or throwlines are not considered life safety ropes by the NFPA 1983 standards.

Ligamentum teres hepatis Sometimes called the falciform ligament, the ligament that attaches the liver to the anterior body wall, dividing the liver into a right and left lobe.

Light construction Structures, generally wood and brick construction, built to withstand vertical load forces.

Line-of-duty deaths (LODDs) Fatalities that occur among emergency responders while in the act of providing service.

Liquefaction necrosis An injury that results from saponification, protein binding, and dessication that literally melts the skin as it proceeds and allows for deeper penetration of the alkali into the deeper tissue, similar to the way a hot knife runs through butter.

Litigation profile The chance that the organizers of a mass-gathering event will be sued.

Load-distributing anchor A configuration that spreads the climber's load during a technical rescue (i.e., the patient's weight) over multiple anchors simultaneously for increased safety.

Local Emergency Planning Committee (LEPC) A local group that includes representatives from emergency services (fire, police, and EMS), as well as local industry. The LEPC maintains copies of the MSDS sheets for known hazardous materials within the area, which are made available during an emergency.

Locked-in syndrome A patient presentation that can occur in trauma in which the entire body is paralyzed with the exception of the eyes. The patient with locked-in syndrome may be conscious and alert but unable to move or speak.

Lock off A technique in which the technical rescue climber's rope is wrapped securely around the descent control device, thus allowing the rescuer's hands to be free to assess the patient, render aid, use a radio, and so on.

Loose grid searches A search done in teams of no more than seven search and rescue Technicians (three searchers is the ideal number) who quickly cover an area. Searchers deployed for a loose grid type search form up on a search baseline and are widely spaced. They take random paths in the same general direction and visually scan between themselves and their adjacent searchers.

Lost person behavior Unique behavioral characteristics different individuals possess, leading to differences in the search tactics needed to find them.

Lost Person Questionnaire A tool recommended by NASAR and other organizations as a way to focus rescue personnel on important information that will speed the potential rescue of the subject. The information gathered in the Lost Person Questionnaire includes the person's name, age, detailed physical description, and past medical history. The questionnaire also includes what the person was last seen wearing and items the person possessed or carried.

Low angle Sometimes called slope rescue, rescue from terrain that includes inclines up to 30 degrees. In this first level of terrain, the majority of the Paramedic's weight is on his feet during a rescue, although the terrain is uneven and presents a fall hazard to rescuers.

Lower explosive limit (LEL) A concentration that has too little vapor in the fuel-air mixture (the mixture is too lean), in which case ignition will not occur.

Lowering system A descent control device to lower patient care supplies and rescue equipment to the Paramedic at the patient's side in a technical rescue.

Low-head dam A simple wall across a waterway, usually less than 12 feet tall, with no way of controlling the flow over it. Results in creation of an undertow at the base of the dam.

Low water Reduced water levels that occur when an area experiences a drought. Since areas with normally navigable water might not be so easy to maneuver through in periods of extreme drought, this makes getting to a patient via water difficult.

Lucid interval A situation that occurs when a patient is rendered unconscious, then regains consciousness, only to deteriorate into unconsciousness again. This momentary consciousness is thought to be due to intracranial compensatory mechanisms that temporarily mitigate the effects of rising intracranial pressure.

Lymphangitis An infection that has taken a tract through the lymphatic system.

Malgaigne fracture A pelvic vertical shear injury that occurs when a force is applied from the direction of the feet toward the head, such as what occurs in a fall from a height when the patient lands on one foot first, fracturing the pelvis. This pelvic fracture typically involves one-half of the pelvis.

Mallet fracture A common distal phalangeal injury that occurs when something, like a baseball or basketball, strikes the end of the patient's finger, the distal finger is pushed beyond its normal range of motion (hyperflexed), and the extensor tendon is damaged.

Manes method A form of shoulder reduction in which the patient is seated. The Paramedic stands behind the patient and inserts her flexed forearm into the axilla of the patient's affected arm. Then, the Paramedic places her other hand on the patient's forearm and applies gentle traction. This technique is effective for those with little muscle mass (i.e., elderly, children, and some women).

Mass-casualty incident (MCI) A situation involving several potential patients and a large emergency response.

Mass effect Situation that occurs when pressure builds up in one compartment, due to an expanding hematoma or other space-occupying lesion, causing that compartment to compress the other compartments.

Mass evacuation An organized effort to remove all individuals from a certain area, like a stadium or concert hall, if a credible threat exists to its occupants (i.e., WMD).

Mass gathering A group of more than 1,000 people. However, the potential for medical emergencies and the ability of local EMS to respond to those emergencies dictates the use of the descriptor "mass gathering" more than a specific number.

Material safety data sheets (MSDS) A document that accompanies any potentially hazardous chemical that identifies its properties and safety measures to use around it.

Maximum use concentration (MUC) The largest concentration of a chemical in the atmosphere that a rescuer is protected from when wearing the appropriate respirator.

MC306 (DOT406) Oval tankers that carry approximately 9,000 gallons of liquids, in one or two internal compartments, that are not under pressure. These tankers are single-shell aluminum construction. They typically carry motor fuels or nonvolatile materials such as milk or water.

MC307 (DOT 407) Rounded tankers that have double-hulled, low-pressure chemical tanks. The flattened ends of these tankers give rise to their nickname, "blunties."

MC312 (DOT 412) A tanker that carries approximately 5,000 to 6,000 gallons of corrosive liquids under low pressures (35 to 50 pounds per square inch). Because of the dangerous nature of these chemicals, the tank is typically constructed of stainless steel or carbon steel and has reinforcing outer rings.

MC331 A high-pressure tanker that carries liquefied gasses such as propane or anhydrous ammonia.

MC332 A tanker with elaborate relief valves that vent the gas to the environment rather than risk an explosion, specifically a boiling liquid expanding vapor explosion (BLEVE).

MC338 A tanker with the classic "thermos bottle" construction (i.e., double-walled construction with insulation and relief valves). The MC338 is used to transport liquid oxygen, liquid nitrogen, liquid hydrogen, and liquefied natural gas.

Mechanical advantage The result of a simple machine like a pulley or lever that multiplies the force put into it. The formula is length of arm divided by length of resistance arm.

Mechanism of injury (MOI) The study of how specific forms of energy transferred to a patient can create predictable injury patterns (PIP). The term "mechanism of injury" describes a group of principles that can be applied to predict the presence of life-threatening injuries, even when the injuries are not apparent externally.

Medevac Medical evacuation of patients, either by ground EMS or air medical transport.

Medical monitoring The observation of emergency responders for adverse health effects of firefighting, special operations, etc., from the effects of heat or cold stress, physical and psychological stress, and environmental stress.

Medical Reserve Corps (MRC) A volunteer program for medical professionals that organizes public health, medical, and other volunteers who want to donate their time and expertise to prepare for, and respond to, emergencies.

Medical specialists Paramedics who work on a USAR medical team.

Medical surveillance A plan for evaluating rescuers at a chemical exposure for health effects, which typically has three elements: baseline, exposure specific, and on-scene rehabilitation.

Medical team Physicians and Paramedics trained for situations and medical conditions encountered in the field during structural collapse search and rescue.

Medical team managers Physicians who work on a USAR medical team.

Medical threat assessment An overview of the potential for combat-related injuries to SWAT technical operators, perpetrators, and civilians, as well as the chances of accidental injury during a mission. The threat assessment also considers potential environmental, chemical, biological, or animal (i.e., dog bites) exposure, and a listing of the nearest hospitals and trauma centers, possible helicopter landing zones, and other important information.

Melting point The point at which a solid becomes a liquid.

Minimum breaking strength The force needed to break the ropes and hardware used in a technical rescue. It is essential that this point not be reached for safety purposes.

Minor category In the START triage system, those patients injured in the event, but who do not have any life-threatening or life-altering injuries.

Mission critique A review of the search process that is best done shortly after the incident. This affords the best recollection of events and the best opportunity for searchers to express factual information regarding improvement of the process or review of something that worked particularly well during the incident.

Mobile Emergency and Response Support (MERS) The basis for maintaining federal communications in the field during a disaster response. MERS is equipped with self-sustaining telecommunications, logistics, and operations support elements that can be driven or airlifted to the disaster location from six strategic locations.

Moderate altitude Any elevation between 8,000 and 12,000 feet.

Modified dash roll An extrication technique in which, after stabilizing the vehicle, the rescuer cuts the seat belt at the point closest to the door. Using a short ram or spreaders, the rescuer then rolls the dash forward after making several strategic cuts in the dashboard.

Modified Glasgow Coma Score for Children An objective measure that can be used to gauge the severity of a child's head injury. The range is between 3 for a comatose child up to 15 for a neurologically intact child.

Monteggia's fracture An ulnar fracture associated with a dislocation of the radioulnar joint. This fracture/dislocation is seen in cases in which the patient falls forward onto a pronated outstretched hand.

Mountain Rescue Association (MRA) A critical mountain search and rescue organization that is among the oldest SAR associations in the United States.

Myocardial contusion A bruising of the heart muscle that can lead to a period of abnormal heart contraction, often caused by a blunt force trauma such as a fall, motor-vehicle accident, or cardiopulmonary resuscitation.

Myocardial rupture A collapse of the heart after a rapid deceleration when it may be displaced rapidly into the sternum or the spine.

National Association for Search and Rescue (NASAR) A nonprofit association dedicated to advancing professional, literary, and scientific knowledge in fields related to search and rescue.

National Association of Flight Paramedics A regulatory organization that also outlines minimum guidelines for flight Paramedic education.

National Emergency Medical Services Information System (NEMSIS) An organization that establishes standards for EMS data collection to maintain a national EMS dataset collected from all states on a limited number of data elements.

National Fire Protection Association (NFPA) An organization that brings together key players in the fire and public safety industries to develop consensus on standards and guidelines. However, NFPA has no enforcement authority or ability to test, certify, or inspect for compliance with published standards and guidelines.

National Incident Management System (NIMS) A system that coordinates emergency preparedness and responses between the local, state, and federal level.

National Institute for Occupational Safety and Health (NIOSH) An organization that is historically geared toward epidemiology, biohazards, and ergonomic research.

National Nurse Response Team (NNRT) An asset of the National Disaster Management System that provides hundreds of nurses to assist in chemoprophylaxis, a mass vaccination program, or a scenario that overwhelms the nation's supply of nurses when responding to a disaster or terrorist event.

National Pharmacy Response Teams (NPRT) Groups composed of pharmacists, pharmacy technicians, pharmacy students, and support personnel located in each of the 10 federal regions that assists with drug administration, such as vaccinations or antitoxins.

National Preparedness Guidelines National planning scenarios intended to focus local, state, and federal emergency managers on planning for incidents with potentially catastrophic consequences. The scenarios include both terrorist acts and natural disasters.

National Response Framework Sometimes called the National Response Plan, the organization, concept of operations, and responsibilities of federal departments and agencies tasked to respond to a disaster.

National Response Plan The federal all-hazards response guide that integrates local, state, and federal disaster management and response concepts.

National Search and Rescue Committee (NSARC) A government agency that includes the Department of Transportation, the Department of Defense (DOD), the Department of Commerce, the Federal Communications Commission (FCC), the National Aeronautics and Space Administration (NASA), and the Department of the Interior.

Necrotic arachnidism The formation of a necrotic lesion from a spider's venom. These necrotic lesions tend to become evident over 24 to 48 hours after envenomation.

Necrotizing fasciitis A life-threatening soft-tissue infection that starts as a small abscess following a puncture wound from a nail or needle. During its spread, the enzymes from the infection literally liquefy the fascia as it spreads.

Needle thoracostomy An emergent treatment for a tension pneumothorax where a long, large bore needle is inserted through the chest wall and into the pleural cavity to allow relief of the built up thoracic pressure.

Needs assessment A review of human resources as well as equipment. This needs assessment should address personnel needs for training as well as equipment needs.

Negatively buoyant A condition in which an object sinks.

Nematocyst Microscopic structures found on the tentacles and around the mouth of most Cnidaria that are used for stinging. Each nematocyst contains a coiled threaded tube-like structure that contains venom. If these are disturbed, or if the creature feels threatened or is hunting prey, the tubule uncoils and fires.

Neovascularization The development of new blood vessels to provide nutrients to the growing skin.

Neurogenic shock A systemic manifestation of spinal cord injury. The classic triad of hypotension, bradycardia, and peripheral vasodilation is suggestive of neurogenic shock.

Neuropraxia A condition in which a nerve no longer transmits impulses after an injury. Neuropraxia is often a temporary condition.

Newton's laws of motion Three statements developed by Sir Isaac Newton describing the movement of objects. His first law of motion, called the law of inertia, states that *all objects remain in their state of rest, or in motion in a straight line, unless acted upon by an outside force*. Newton's second law of motion states that *force is equal to the product of mass and acceleration*. Newton's third law of motion states that *for each action there is an equal and opposite reaction*.

NFPA 471 A hazardous materials standard that establishes competency standards for each level of responder.

NFPA 472 A hazardous materials standard that expands on the previous OSHA standards.

NFPA 473 A hazardous materials standard that relates to EMS response and describes two levels, EMS/HM1 and EMS/HM2.

NFPA 704 standard A standard that describes the four-diamond hazard placard warning system used for fixed storage tanks and buildings.

NFPA 1006 Titled *Standard for Technical Rescuer Professional Qualifications*, a technical rescue standard that calls for a tiered training format, classified as Awareness, Operations, and Technician.

NFPA 1582 A national firefighter standard designed to assist departments in maintaining a staff of medically qualified firefighters.

NFPA 1583 Titled *Standard on Health-Related Fitness Programs for Fire Fighters*, a national firefighter standard that provides guidelines for departments to create fitness programs that optimize the physical condition of firefighters to the degree necessary for performing their very strenuous duties.

NFPA 1584 Titled *Standard on the Rehabilitation Process for Members During Emergency Operations and Training Exercises*, a national firefighter standard that provides data regarding rehabilitation and incentives to encourage compliance.

NFPA 1670 Titled *Standard on Operations and Training for Technical Search and Rescue Incidents*, a national standard that stresses the need for the agency having jurisdiction (AHJ) to preplan and break preplanning down into three steps.

NFPA 1983 A technical rescue standard titled *Standard on Life Safety Rope and Equipment for Emergency Services*.

Night vision goggles Technology that amplifies available light from the moon or stars to enhance an image, allowing the user wearing specialized eyewear to distinguish between different objects in the dark.

Nitrogen narcosis Sometimes called "rapture of the deep," increased nitrogen dissolved in the blood which alters the electrical properties of nervous tissues, creating an anesthetic effect.

Nonexertional heatstroke (classic heatstroke) A heat illness; an abnormally elevated body temperature with accompanying physical and neurological symptoms, usually seen in elderly patients who, because of medical conditions or age, are unable to compensate for a change in temperature and/or humidity.

North American Emergency Response Guidebook (NAERG) A publication that provides recommendations for working with and treating particular chemicals and the proper PPE to wear when exposed to them. Also called the *Emergency Response Guidebook*.

Off-gas The process where a chemical leaves the body through exhalation.

Ohms The unit used for measuring electrical resistance.

On rappel A command commonly used with technical rescue, meaning "Are you ready for me to rappel?"

Open pelvic fracture A disruption of the bony structure of the pelvis.

Open pneumothorax A lung injury in which the air accumulating in the pleural space escapes through an open wound upon exhalation.

Operations responder (Hazmat) The second level of training, which is primarily tasked to take defensive actions such as containment and control of the scene. These responders are also expected to understand basic decontamination procedures.

Orbital blowout fractures A break in the facial bones caused by force creating an inferior and medial displacement of the orbital walls, or a "blowing out" of the orbit, without fracturing the stronger and thicker orbital rim.

Organophosphate compounds Nerve agents often found in farming communities and pesticides that attack the nervous system by impairing nerve impulse transmission through inhibition of acetylcholinesterase and preventing the re-uptake of excess acetylcholine.

Orthopaedics The study of musculoskeletal injuries, including injuries to the bones, joints, ligaments, tendons, and muscles.

Osborne wave A positive deflection on an EKG occurring at the junction between the QRS complex and ST segment, and is pathomnemonic in patients with hypothermia.

Osteogenesis imperfecta A rare condition in which a genetic defect causes abnormal collagen secretion and brittle bones. Osteogenesis imperfecta leads to pathologic fractures in children, which may lead to an incorrect suspicion of child abuse.

Osteomalacia A disorder of bone formation secondary to a lack of calcium and/or phosphorus.

Otorrhea Leakage of cerebrospinal fluid from the ear.

Overtriage Overestimating the seriousness of a patient's injuries, which results in patients with non-life-threatening injuries being treated before those with more serious conditions, leading to depletion of trauma resources, emergency department overcrowding, and delays in patient care.

Oxidizers Chemicals that can support combustion although they do not create heat. These chemicals release oxygen that in turn supports combustion, increasing the potential for a small fire to rapidly expand.

Oxyhemoglobin dissociation curve The relationship between available oxygen and oxygen carried by hemoglobin that is effected by temperature and pH.

Packaged A term that describes a technical rescue patient being transferred and secured into a rescue basket.

Paget's disease A chronic and progressive disease that is more common in patients over age 50 and increases in frequency with the patient's age. Its medical name, osteitis deformans, speaks to a major effect of Paget's disease: deformity of the bones.

Painful distracting injury A circumstance in which a person is not able to participate in a reliable exam because a painful (although possibly minor) injury takes attention away from what might be more serious conditions, such as cervical spine injury. These injuries or circumstances might include a broken limb, trouble breathing, or a significant laceration.

Paradoxical motion Motion opposite the rest of the rib cage. When inhalation occurs, the chest wall cavity normally expands to accommodate the increased lung volume. However, the flail chest segment is unable to expand adequately, leading to this motion, which alters the mechanics of breathing.

Paradoxical undressing A condition associated with hypothermia in which patients state they have an overwhelming feeling of warmth and take off their clothes just before losing consciousness.

Paraplegia A thoracic or lumbar spinal cord injury that limits or eliminates motor control and/or sensation in the lower extremities.

Partial thickness burns Painful tissue damage that extends into the dermis, a reticular layer of specialized cells and blood vessels below the epidermis, which is also referred to as the true skin.

Passive cooling techniques Methods to relieve firefighters of excess heat during rehabilitation that often involve "common sense" activities such as removal of PPE, evaporation of sweat, and moving to a cooler environment.

Passive rewarming A technique wherein the patient's own body heat is used to rewarm the patient with a reduced body core temperature.

Passive search measures Procedures designed to find clues pertaining to a possible lost patient, rather than an active search for a patient who was actually observed in an area.

Patellofemoral joint syndrome A number of patellofemoral joint complaints, characterized by knee pain that often involves athleticism, such as sports, hiking, or even repetitive deep knee bends.

Patent foramen ovale An opening in the heart's septal wall that incompletely closes upon birth, often giving rise to an "innocent" murmur. It is estimated that 10% to 20% of the population have a patent foramen ovale, many without being aware of it.

Patient load The number of patients expected at a mass gathering based on the type of event and size of the crowd.

Pediatric Trauma Score A tool used to gauge the severity of a pediatric patient's injury, which is computed by adding the scores for the individual categories. Scores may range from +12 to −6; a score less than 8 indicates severe injury.

Pelvic binder A device used to immobilize a fractured pelvis. One method of creating one is to use a draw sheet folded approximately 20 cm wide that can be slid under the small of the patient's back and moved down over the anterior superior iliac spine (ASIA) and over the ischial tuberosity. The Paramedic then creates a square knot with the sheet anteriorly and places a dowel in the middle of knot, and turns the dowel like a corkscrew to tighten the sheet, creating a form of Spanish windlass.

Pelvic sling An immobilization device similar to a pelvic binder that uses an approximately 20-cm circumferential belt with an anterior ratchet device. The pelvic sling allows access to the anterior pelvis for central venous cannulation and urinary catheterization, permits use of the traction splint, and has a self-limiting locking device to prevent overtightening of the pelvic sling.

Penetrating trauma An injury in which the skin is disrupted by entry of a penetrating object into, or passage through, underlying tissue. Penetrating injuries are frequently caused by firearms, knives, or projectiles from malfunctioning machinery, shrapnel due to an explosion, and impalements.

Permissible exposure limits (PEL) The level of exposure to a chemical a rescuer can tolerate during an average 40 hour work week.

Permissive hypotension An approach to fluid resuscitation that suggests offering more controlled fluid resuscitation using physiologic measures to determine the need for administration of additional fluid. Permissive hypotension supporters argue that hypotension is protective, as it lowers the blood pressure enough to allow the coagulation system to work at stabilizing any clots that have formed.

Personal flotation devices (PFDs) Items that, when properly used and worn, allow the wearer to float in the water with no effort.

Personal throw bag A small bag with a length of rope inside used as a rescue device that can fit in a pocket or a hip belt.

Pick off A rescue technique in which the patient is taken off her rope system after she has been clipped into the rescuer's rope system.

Pillows A phenomenon that forms on the water when water piles up against a submerged object, making the water appear to be a raised area. These pillows may signal a shallow object that can injure someone striking it.

Plague A bacterial disease, *Yersinia pestis*, which is transmittable from human to human if the *Yersinia pestis* bacterium is aerosolized, released, and inhaled. Patient symptoms may include fever, cough, weakness, shortness of breath, chest pain, and hemoptysis, as well as gastrointestinal signs and symptoms such as nausea, vomiting, and abdominal pain.

Platysma The sheet-like muscle that superficially covers the anterior portion of the neck from the floor of the mouth to the clavicle.

Plunging waves Associated in most people's minds with the sport of surfing, waves that pass over the bottom ground much faster, forcing the wave up and over onto itself so fast that the crest collapses on the wave.

Pneumatic tourniquet A device developed by Henry Cushing in 1904 that inserts compressed gas into a cylindrical bladder to constrict blood flow and prevent bleeding.

Pointer The rescue searcher with the sign cutting stick who moves forward along the assumed direction of the subject's travel, with the flankers slightly behind and off to each side. The pointer looks for each successive step based on the subject's stride length.

Point last seen (PLS) The exact location the person needing assistance was last observed.

Point-of-dispensing (POD) site An area where people may go to receive post exposure prophylaxis. Within the POD site itself, patients will be moved through the process of being screened, examined, and treated, and Paramedics may be involved in any of these tasks.

Polymerization A violent reaction that occurs as two chemicals' molecules combine to become one larger molecule. If this reaction occurs in a closed container or a small space, the result can be explosive.

Positively buoyant Having the ability to float, as air remains in the lungs.

Post-concussive seizures Seizures that occur after a head injury, primarily in children, and generally resolve on their own within a few minutes.

Posterior gutter splint Sometimes known as an ulnar gutter splint, an immobilization device used for midshaft radial or ulnar fractures. The Paramedic measures a malleable splinting material for a length from the distal palmar crease to the midshaft humerus, ensuring joints above and below the fracture are immobilized. The splinting material is then formed into a gutter and held in place with an Ace® wrap.

Posterior leg splint An immobilization device used to stabilize distal leg and ankle injuries. Using a malleable splinting material, the Paramedic measures from the head of the metatarsal to the mid-calf and forms a gutter splint.

Post-Katrina Emergency Management Reform Act (PKEMRA) A core federal authority that requires FEMA to coordinate precautionary evacuations of people with disabilities, children, pets, and service animals in the event of an impending crisis.

Posse Comitatus Act A military authority (18 U.S.C.) that prevents the Army or Air Force from being used in a law enforcement capacity within the United States.

Potential energy Energy stored within a mechanical system ready to become kinetic energy.

Pralidoxime chloride (2-PAM) An auto-injector approved for civilian medical use that is packaged in the Mark 1 kits.

Pressure sores An ulceration of the skin that occurs because of prolonged pressure along bony prominences such as the sacrum, elbows, knees, and ankles.

Priapism A painful sustained erection without apparent stimulation, which may be an indication of sacral nerve injury.

Primary blast injuries Wounds caused by the direct effects immediately after an explosion.

Primary brain injury Damage that occurs to the brain at the time of a trauma. Primary brain injury can further be divided into soft-tissue injuries, those involving the gray and white matter, and vascular injury that results in intracranial hemorrhage.

Primary wound healing Healing by first intention, which occurs within hours of an incision. These wounds, which are usually clean wounds, heal with good cosmetic result and little scar formation, because of the close approximation of the wound edges.

Probability of area (POA) An area in which to begin a search, determined by knowledge of the subject and the statistical probability that the subject is within an area.

Probability of detection (POD) The chance that the lost subject is in the area that will be searched.

Probability of success (POS) The chance of finding the lost subject.

Procedural pain Pain occurring while a burn patient's procedures are being performed, which is the result of mechanical manipulation and pressure, such as occurs during the application or reinforcement of dressings.

Process Safety Management Federal regulations that require a site action plan for fixed facilities in the event of an accidental spill, including emergency shutdown procedures and failure mode analysis.

Proliferative phase The second stage of wound healing, which starts on about day two and may last three weeks. During this stage, fibroblasts start to form a bed of collagen and rudimentary tissue.

Protect-in-place A technique in which the tactical medic and patient remain under cover at the violent scene while care is provided, rather than evacuating the patient to a hospital or trauma center.

Protective envelope A layer of PPE used by the Paramedic to shield himself from injury in dangerous environments.

Prusik A small diameter (usually 7, 8, or 9 mm) rope that is knotted, forms a loop, and is then wrapped around a larger diameter rope. When a force is applied to the prusik, it binds up and locks the device being used.

Public health The practice and discipline of maintaining and improving the health of communities. This occurs through assessment of the population's health, assurance of health care including prevention services for all, and promotion of public policy designed to protect the public's health.

Public health emergencies Incidents that are typically large, poorly demarcated, potentially escalating events that involve humans. These include large foodborne illness outbreaks, bioterrorism, chemical and radiation release, and pandemic infections.

Public information officer (PIO) A person at a mass gathering who distributes relevant data about an event to the media.

Pulleys A device frequently used to change the direction of a rope or, like a block and tackle, to provide a mechanical advantage.

Pulmonary barotrauma A condition that occurs during a rapid underwater ascent. As the diver ascends, lung expansion is limited by the rib cage. As a result of subsequent increased intrathoracic pressures and pulmonary overinflation, a pneumothorax occurs and/or the pulmonary vein ruptures, which leads to arterial gas embolism.

Pulmonary contusion An injury to the lung, which is the most common injury in blunt thoracic trauma. There are three impacts of trauma directly to the lungs: swelling, bleeding, and atelectasis.

Pulmonary decompression sickness Sometimes called the "chokes," a condition that occurs when multiple pulmonary gas emboli form bubbles in the blood, disrupting circulation.

Puncture wound A wound that penetrates through the skin, which can be either superficial or full thickness.

Purulent A classification of exudates that is opaque, tan, or yellow. If the exudate has an offensive odor, suggestive of infection, then it is called foul purulent.

Pyrophorics Chemicals with flammable vapors that will self-ignite when exposed to air (i.e., these chemicals do not need an ignition source).

Quaternary blast injuries Injuries and illnesses that follow an explosion which are not due to the primary, secondary, or tertiary injuries. Quaternary blast injuries include burns, crush injuries due to prolonged entrapment, hypoxic brain injury, and complications of asthma and COPD due to inhalation of fumes, dust, and toxins.

Quinary blast injuries A relatively new classification of blast injuries describing a hyperinflammatory state some patients develop with an excessive and unusual rise in body temperature, sweating, decreased central venous pressure, and a significant positive fluid balance during treatment. Quinary injuries are thought to be caused by additives to bombs such as bacteria, radiation, and chemicals.

Rappel A technique wherein the technical rescuer descends to the patient, using a friction device to slow and control the descent.

Rappel on A command commonly used with technical rescue that means the belayer is ready for the rescuer to rappel and she may proceed to rappel.

Rattlesnakes Snakes that have the longest fangs of the pit vipers, with some reaching 3 to 4 cm in length. These needle-like structures are able to retract into the snake's mouth on a hinge-like mechanism and then extend to bite and inject venom.

Recovery The search for deceased patients. This is usually a less pressured situation than rescue, in which considerations like evidence preservation, resource conservation, the need for rest, and even finances take a more prominent role.

Rehabilitation An intervention designed to mitigate the impact of the stressors of firefighting activities, restore the rescuers' work capacity, improve performance, and decrease risks for injury and death.

Remodeling phase The final stage of wound healing during which the body's skin starts to return to a more normal condition. Within six weeks, the new skin covering the wound (scar) will have 80% to 90% of its wound "bursting" strength. Within 6 to 12 months, the wound will change its texture, color, and thickness to match the surrounding skin.

Reperfusion injury A condition that occurs when a limb that has been compressed under a heavy weight is released, restoring blood flow to the limb. As the blood flow returns, the potassium-laden, acidotic blood trapped within the limb is released into the general circulation, which can serve as the catalyst for ventricular fibrillation and sudden cardiac death.

Rescue Efforts to save living or presumed living patients. It is the driving force behind every member's participation in USAR and, as such, is a powerful motivator, driving people to work 24 hours a day in all kinds of weather and safety conditions.

Rescue specialist People who use powerful breaching tools such as diamond chain saws, core drills, exothermic torches, and breakers to safely create a safe ingress to and egress from the entrapped patient.

Rescue tube A small foam tube that not only holds a patient up, but can also be used under a backboard to keep the patient floating.

Resistor An object that opposes the passage of an electrical current.

Retinal detachment A condition that may occur when a tear develops in the retina, allowing the vitreous fluid in the globe to leak behind and displace the retina. The retina lifts up from the posterior portion of the globe, interrupting its blood supply and causing ischemia. Unless repaired within 24 hours, visual deficits can be permanent.

Retroperitoneal hematoma Internal bleeding posterior to the peritoneum.

Rewarming shock A body reaction that can occur when the body is rewarmed. In this reaction, vasoconstriction is reversed and a normal vascular space returns. The patient, who is volume contracted, will develop hypoperfusion that can even lead to cardiac arrest.

Rhabdomyolysis The rapid breakdown of muscle tissue.

Rhinorrhea Leakage of cerebrospinal fluid from the nose.

Rigging plate A piece of rescue hardware that permits multiple carabiners to be attached to a single solid plate of metal.

Ring buoys A donut-shaped flotation device that can be attached to throw bags or lines and used in a throw rescue. The added weight can give the rescuer some better distance with the throw and the device provides better flotation assistance for the patient.

Ring vaccination Large-scale vaccination and/or medication dispensing instituted in an area to prevent the spread of disease.

Rip currents The result of waves or currents pushing water up the shore. The water must go somewhere, and a rip current involves this water draining back to the open water from which it came.

Risk manager A person who represents the insurance company that is providing coverage for a mass-gathering event. These risk managers have a wealth of knowledge and experience from insuring similar events and can be an invaluable asset to the preparation efforts.

River ice Ice located in rivers, which is especially dangerous if it is exposed to strong currents. As the river rises, the ice will be stressed as it moves upward, and as the water recedes it may leave dead air space in between the river water and the remaining ice.

Robert Jones bandage A bulky compression bandage used for knee injuries. Starting with a shell of bulky dressing, such as cotton wool or foam, around the knee from midshaft femur to mid-calf, the Paramedic winds a layer of recurrent bandage around the entire length of the dressing.

Rollover protection systems (ROPS) A fixed device contained in most convertibles, usually mounted as a pair in the rear of the occupant area. The device is designed to deploy if the vehicle is potentially going to go on to its side or "roll over."

Rope bag A storage container for nylon rope to prevent its breakdown from environmental conditions.

Rope free A command commonly used with technical rescue that tells the belayer that the rescuer is safe.

Rostered three deep A policy of having three people available to handle each station or post on a rescue team to guarantee availability and facilitate rapid deployment.

Rotator cuff tear A sprain in the muscles of the rotator cuff, which leads to destabilization of the shoulder joint and pain.

Rotor wash The wind created by a helicopter's rotor blades.

Rotor wing Helicopters, which make up the majority of aircraft dedicated to emergency air medical transport.

Rotten ice Ice that has been thawed slowly, refrozen, and is very weak. It has a milky or opaque look, can fail without warning, and can be a very difficult surface to operate on. Most ice rescues involve this type of ice.

Sacco Triage and Resource Methodology (STM) A triage system designed to maximize the number of expected survivors of a traumatic event through use of an objective, measurable, interoperable, and reproducible method. In contrast to an algorithm, STM determines a score based on the patient's respiratory rate, pulse rate, and best motor response.

Safety officer A person at a mass gathering who oversees the well-being of attendees and may be part of the venue's risk management team.

Saliva osmolarity monitoring device A method of testing hydration that analyzes saliva collected on an oral sampling stick that is inserted into a companion machine, much like a portable glucose monitor. The analysis provides reliable hydration values.

Salt depletion heat exhaustion A condition that usually occurs in non-acclimatized patients and can also occur during prolonged periods of strenuous exercise in even temperate temperatures. The salinity of the sweat secreted is high, leading to systemic hyponatremia.

Salter–Harris fractures Physeal fractures that are divided into five classifications according to the fracture's location. A type I Salter-Harris fracture is a transverse fracture between the metaphysis and epiphysis. A type II Salter-Harris fracture includes a type I fracture as well as a fracture of the metaphysis, whereas a type III fracture includes a type I fracture and a fracture of the epiphysis. A Salter-Harris type IV fracture includes types I, II, and III (i.e., complete separation of the metaphysis from the epiphysis) and fractures of both the metaphysis and epiphysis of the bone. A type V is actually a compression fracture of the growth plate secondary to axial loading.

Saponification The process through which alkali dissolve fats.

Scant A measure of the amount of exudate present if the wound is dry or moist in appearance, but not enough to be absorbed through a thickness of gauze dressing.

Scent dogs Animals that track by following the human scent through the air. Tracking/trailing dogs are exposed to an object that contains the subject's scent and, while on the lead, follow the scent at ground level and on vegetation.

Scope of practice The extent to which a healthcare provider is permitted to perform medical procedures. This is defined differently from state to state and might be based upon the educational curriculum, protocols, or a stand-alone document detailing the procedures allowed.

Scorpions Arthropods that envenom humans not by biting, but by stinging with a specialized apparatus called a telson.

Seabather's eruption A cutaneous, pruritic reaction to the larvae of the thimble jellyfish (*Linuche* unguiculata). The eruption typically occurs underneath the bathing suit, which is believed to trap the jellyfish larvae against the skin. Skin lesions usually develop after severe pruritus begins and are made up of vesicles, pustules, and urticarial lesions.

Search and rescue Technician A person capable of executing a search and rescue. The search and rescue Technician must also be trained to the Technician level for rope rescue and to the Awareness level for water rescue.

Searcher rehabilitation Techniques used to physically refresh rescuers who work long hours, sometimes in extreme temperatures and harsh weather, carrying heavy equipment.

Search theory A mathematical approach to determining the best way to find something one is seeking. The principles of search theory apply to any situation where the objective is to find, in the most efficient manner, a person or object contained in some geographic area.

Search width A measure of the effectiveness with which a particular sensor (person or dog) can detect a particular object under specific environmental conditions.

Seat belt pretensioners Powered devices that remove slack from the seat belt, ensuring that the occupant is seated properly when the airbag systems deploy.

Secondary Assessment of Victim Endpoint (SAVE) A triage method that focuses on treatment more than transport. Patients are triaged and divided into categories, then reassessed and divided into three categories based upon the resources needed, the resources available, and the prognosis given the injury and the time expected to elapse until definitive care.

Secondary blast injuries Also called fragmentation injuries, wounds caused as the patient is struck by debris propelled by the blast wind, causing lacerations, penetrating wounds, and fractures.

Secondary brain injury Damage to the brain secondary to extracranial etiology that impairs the brain's function.

Secondary device A weapon intended to attack those responders who arrive to assist the patients from the primary explosion or event.

Secondary exposure Indirect exposure to hazardous material as a result of contact with a contaminated patient.

Second impact syndrome (SIS) A condition caused when a patient suffers a second concussion following an initial concussion, within days or weeks, which can be a deadly situation. This syndrome is thought to occur because the brain loses its ability to autoregulate cerebral perfusion. The second concussion triggers a cascade of events that include cerebral edema, increased intracranial pressure, and, eventually, herniation.

Self-care first aid kit A basic collection of medical supplies, such as gloves, tourniquet, trauma dressings, and rolls of gauze.

Shaken baby syndrome A brain injury that occurs in young children when violently shaken to and fro. These rotational forces can cause diffuse axonal injury as well as the creation of subdural hematoma, literally causing the brain to slush within the skull.

Shallow water blackout (SWB) A condition in which people pass out while free diving and snorkeling. This condition is due to hyperventilation and subsequent hypocapnia prior to swimming.

Sheppard's crooks Large hooks used to actually sweep a water rescue patient toward shore. The half-circle design will hold a patient in the hook when being pulled.

Shin splints Sometimes known as medial tibial stress syndrome, a condition that results from inflammation of the peroneal tendon that creates pain over the lower half of the anterior shin. A cause of shin splints is pes planus (flat feet), which cause the posterior tibialis to become overstretched and inflamed.

Shivering The rhythmic contraction of muscle at a rate of 10 to 20 contractions per second, which is used to generate body heat.

Short arm volar splint An immobilization device used for distal fractures of the radius or ulna, as well as the wrist (volar means palmar surface). The malleable splinting material is made into a sugar tong splint. The Paramedic should note the position of the hand. To preserve the "position of function," some Paramedics have the patient grasp a roller bandage. The splint is then held in place with a bandage.

Shoulder impingement syndrome An injury associated with the rotator cuff, sometimes called outlet impingement. A patient with shoulder impingement syndrome experiences severe pain in the narrow space between the acromion and the humeral head whenever the humerus is internally rotated or elevated.

Side-curtain supplemental restraint system As opposed to the side-impact supplemental restraint system, a safety system that usually deploys downward from the roof edge along the interior of the vehicle's sides.

Side-impact supplemental restraint system A supplemental restraint system designed to protect vehicle occupants from a side impact. These SRSs are mounted either in the sides of the seat facing toward the vehicle's exterior or mounted in the door facing toward the occupants.

Sign Visual evidence, such as broken twigs on a limb of a tree, scuff marks in vegetation, trampled vegetation, a stone pushed into the soil, or anything else, that does not look natural or looks out of place compared to the surrounding environment.

Sign cutting The actual search for evidence that a subject has been in an area, thereby establishing a point from which to track.

Sign cutting stick An approximately 40-inch stick that is used to determine the length of a person's stride. The searcher uses this stick to measure the distance between tracks, and then establishes a radius for finding the next track based on that length.

Silver dressings A pad of gauze that contains silver cream as a topical antibiotic. Previously used in burn care, in the form of silver sulfadiazine cream, silver is broad spectrum and inactivates all bacteria. Silver dressings are particularly useful for burns and wide area abrasions such as those that occur in motorcycle crashes.

Simple pneumothorax A collection of air between the lung and the chest wall that causes the lung on the injured side to partially collapse. With a simple pneumothorax, the air is trapped in the pleural space but does not compromise circulation.

Simple Triage and Rapid Transport (START) A triage technique promoted as a way to reduce the chaos at the scene of a disaster and thus increase prehospital scene effectiveness. START has become the de facto triage protocol across the United States and in many places around the world.

Singed vibrissae Stiff nasal hairs that provide evidence of facial burns that may involve smoke inhalation.

Sinus squeeze Pressure within the sinuses, which can lead to headaches. Sinus squeeze is worsened by an infection or pre-existing polyps.

Situational awareness Awareness of the Paramedic's surroundings and the potential dangers in those surroundings.

Slack A command commonly used with technical rescue that refers to the looseness or tightness of the rope.

Sling Loops of webbing that can be attached to the rescue basket with a hitch to help the litter bearers balance the load over their shoulders.

Slope analysis A review of the geographic terrain and its inclines to determine the degree of hazard in the jurisdiction and the need for specialized rope rescue teams.

Smallpox An extremely contagious viral illness that has no cure, but has been nearly eradicated in the general public by vaccination programs at the end of the last century. The trademark signs of smallpox are small, raised bumps that appear on the infected person's body and face similar to chickenpox.

Smith fracture A "reverse Colles" fracture that occurs if the patient falls onto a flexed hand. With volar displacement of the hand, there is an obvious intra-articular "step off" at the wrist.

Snow blindness Sometimes called ultraviolet keratitis, a very painful eye condition caused by exposure to extreme solar ultraviolet radiation that typically occurs from wearing no protection or inadequate eye protection in high glare conditions.

Snow ice Ice with a layer of frozen snow on top of it. Melting snow can degrade the ice layer, and may insulate the ice enough to cause melting from underneath. It can also trap air in the mix, weakening the ice.

Social distancing Efforts to stop the spread of disease by closing areas where people naturally congregate, such as schools, businesses or government offices, and religious buildings.

Soft body armor Apparel made of Kevlar or some other fabric that is worn for protection during routine activities due to its increased flexibility and decreased weight in comparison to hard body armor. As a force is applied to the armor, the energy from the force transfers horizontally and vertically due to the armor's weave pattern, dispersing energy across and away from the point of impact.

Sort–Assess–Lifesaving interventions–Treat/ transport (SALT) triage system A triage system developed by a task force commissioned by the U.S. Centers for Disease Control in an effort to develop a standardized triage algorithm that can be used across the country.

Space making The process of creating a larger space around the patient for access, care, and egress.

Specialist level A hazardous materials responder who supports the Technician. This person is familiar with the local emergency response plan as well as the state's emergency response plan. The Specialist may also be capable of implementing decontamination procedures and may be responsible for contributing to the site safety plan by working closely with the safety officer.

Specialty care Paramedic Education beyond the Paramedic curriculum to specifically enable the Paramedic to care for critically ill patients during interfacility transport.

Specialty care transport (SCT) A separate category of reimbursement for interfacility transport patients requiring specialized interventions beyond the Paramedic's scope of practice, provided by professionals with appropriate training such as emergency or cardiovascular physicians, nurses, respiratory technicians, or Paramedics with additional training.

Special Weapons and Tactics (SWAT) Certain police operations that involve skills beyond typical law enforcement practices and often have a high life hazard.

Specific gravity A comparison of the mass of a liquid or solid to an equal amount of distilled water. Water has a specific gravity of one. Any substance with a specific gravity of less than one (e.g., flaming gasoline) will float and be carried on the surface. Any liquid with a specific gravity of greater than one (e.g., mercury, which has a specific gravity of 13.56), will sink.

Spilling waves Waves that flow up and onto a gently sloping, mostly unobstructed surface, such as a beach that gradually gets shallower as the waves travel inshore.

Spinal cord injury without obvious radiographic abnormality (SCIWORA) A condition in which the patient exhibits signs and symptoms that are typical of a spinal cord injury although X-rays or CT scans performed in the emergency department are normal.

Spinal shock The loss of both sensation and motor function (paralysis) below the level of the spinal cord transection.

Spinal transection A severing of the spinal cord, causing nerve conduction and communication to cease at the injury site.

Spinothalamic tract Ascending sensory nerve tract (from the spine to the thalamus) that transmits sensations such as touch or proprioception to the thalamus.

Sprain An injury to the ligaments that connect bone to bone, which tends to make a joint unstable.

Stafford Act The Robert T. Stafford Disaster Relief and Emergency Assistance Act of 1974, which, as amended, covers all hazards and defines the processes for federal provisions of disaster assistance.

Standard operating guidelines (SOGs) A systematic approach for how EMS organizations intend to provide rehabilitation for their own members at incidents and certain training exercises.

Standard pressure dressing Sometimes called a battle dressing, a piece of sterile material used to stop the flow of blood, consisting of a pad of gauze attached to a cotton cravat.

Stasis A zone in Jackson's thermal burn theory where edema and blisters form because of microvascular injury.

State Emergency Response Commission (SERC) A statewide group that includes representatives from various LEPC groups that establishes a comprehensive response network for the state.

Static rope Rope that does not stretch. A true static rope has less than 6% elongation with a load. For those conditions when a little stretch is desirable, there is low-stretch rope (rope with more than 6% but less than 10% elongation when a load is placed on it).

Static tension The constant tension that the skin always maintains as it hangs on the skeleton.

Steep angle Rescue on any terrain with an incline of 30 degrees or greater that requires the use of both the rescuer's hands and feet to ascend. It can range from a scramble over scree (loose rock covering a slope) to talus (loose rock at the base of a cliff) to a more traditional rock climb.

Step off An indication of either dislocation or displaced fracture. Its location should be carefully noted using anatomical terms before swelling obscures the defect.

Sternoclavicular (SC) sprain An injury to the freely movable synovial joint, which rolls the shoulder backward and the clavicle forward. This may occur due to a blow to the anterior shoulder, such as occurs during a football tackle.

Stimson maneuver A hip dislocation reduction technique in which the patient is prone with the leg hanging over the edge of the stretcher. The Paramedic applies downward pressure to the pelvis to stabilize the hip and downward traction on the back of the knee. Rotation of the ankle reduces the hip.

Stimson method A shoulder reduction technique, sometimes called the hanging arm technique, in which the patient lies prone on a stretcher, with a sandbag (or similar weight) placed under the clavicle. With the hanging arm in forward flexion, a 10-pound counterweight pulls traction. This method is most effective when the patient has received analgesia.

Stinger A transient neurologic symptom that occurs at the time of injury due to the stretching of nerves. It resolves after a short period of time, often before the patient's arrival at the emergency department.

Stirrup splint An immobilization device used for ankle fracture/dislocation that provides lateral and medial support to prevent eversion/inversion of the ankle.

Stokes basket The classic basket used in technical rescue, made of wire, that has been in use since before World War II.

Straddle injury A special type of soft-tissue injury that involves the perineum. A straddle injury occurs when the genitals (in particular) and the perineum (in general) strike an object.

Strain An injury to a tendon caused by the tearing, twisting, or pulling of a muscle.

Strainers Items in a body of water, such as trees, cars, bridge pilings, and many other items, that water can flow through. Rescuers and patients alike can end up in, under, or on top of these strainers.

Strategic ice packing A method of temperature reduction in which ice packs are placed strategically at pulse points on the patient's body.

Strategic National Stockpile (SNS) A supply of antibiotics, chemical antidotes, antitoxins, life-support medications, IV and airway maintenance supplies, and other medical/surgical items designed to supplement and resupply state and local public health agencies in the event of a national emergency.

Stress fracture A bone break caused by repetitive loading of the musculoskeletal interface, which is an overuse injury. It starts as an incomplete fracture that, if untreated, can evolve into a complete fracture. A combination of poor conditioning, short adaptation time for bone remodeling to stress, and general poor bone health, secondary to insufficient diet, can lead to stress fractures.

Stridor An abnormal high-pitched musical sound typically caused by a partial airflow obstruction in the upper airway.

Structural specialists Engineers who evaluate both intact and damaged structures for active and potential collapse threats.

Subcapsular hematomas Collections of blood that form between the surface of the organ and the inner face of the capsule surrounding the solid organ.

Subcapsular hematomas can form from an adjacent laceration or from a leak in the vascular supply to the organ.

Subconjunctival hemorrhage Bleeding that occurs due to capillary leaking within the conjunctiva over the sclera. This benign condition is similar to developing ecchymosis on the skin.

Subdural hematoma (SDH) A rapidly expanding collection of blood into an organized clot following a sudden force that exerts downward pressure onto the already damaged cerebral cortex and increases intracranial pressure in the process.

Subdural hygroma A form of hydrocephalus (water on the brain) caused by a buildup of cerebrospinal fluid. The localized mass effect of this fluid collection can cause neurological deficits that mimic a stroke.

Subluxation Sometimes called a partial dislocation, a misalignment of bones in a joint that results in the joint's instability.

Sucking chest wound Sometimes called an open pneumothorax, an injury that occurs when a penetrating wound communicates with the pleural cavity and the outside air. Air enters through the injury but is then able to escape through the same wounds during exhalation. It gets its name because of the sound that the air makes going through the wound.

Sugar tong splint An immobilization device used for fractures of the humerus, or the elbow, above and below the suspected fracture. Forming malleable splinting material into a pincer shape, measured from the axilla to the elbow and the elbow to the acromion process, the upper arm is immobilized laterally and medially. Then a recurrent bandage is used to hold the splint in place.

Superficial burns Tissue damage that affects the epidermis, the outermost layer of the skin.

Superficial fascia A layer of loose connective tissue that constitutes the subcutaneous layer of skin and encloses the fatty tissues that insulate and cushion the skin.

Superfund Amendment and Reauthorization Act (SARA) An update to CERCLA which provided more details about hazardous materials operations including the "community right to know." It also established the State Emergency Response Commissions (SERC) and Local Emergency Planning Committees (LEPC).

Supplemental restraint systems (SRS) Equipment within a vehicle, such as airbags, seat belts, and so on, designed to minimize passenger injuries in the event of a collision.

Suppressive fire Gunfire from the SWAT team that provides a deterrent for assailants who might attack the provider at a violent scene.

Supratentorial herniation A condition in which the tentorium separates the cerebrum from the cerebellum. As a result, any expanding hematoma exerts a downward pressure and essentially funnels the cerebrum into the foramen magnum or exerts horizontal pressure across the brain from one hemisphere to another. There are three types: central, uncal, and cingulated.

Surface water A catchall term for any flat, calm water found in a lake, pond, or waterway.

Surf areas Water areas that are showing wave action.

Surge capacity Supplemental resources that can be called upon in cases of sudden and unexpected numbers of casualties that exceed the site's ability to care for them.

Surging waves Waves that do not break on shore, but instead are pushed into rocks, cliffs, seawalls, or other large objects. The energy of the wave does not dissipate on a beach, but rather gets bounced into other waves and objects, making the seas very choppy and rough.

Surrounding area The area above and around the touchdown area, which should be free of any obstacles that may get tangled with the helicopter.

Sustained medical operations Ongoing response efforts that can be broken up into two broad categories. Short-term missions are those lasting approximately one week, whereas long-term missions are any missions lasting longer than one week.

Sweep width A specific field of view, which generally extends half way between the searcher and adjacent searchers, for the search area.

Swift water Any water moving faster than one knot, or 1.15 miles per hour.

System safety factor A ratio of the projected load that various rescue elements, such as rescuers, equipment, and the patient, will have on the system, including ropes and hardware.

Tactical Emergency Medical Support (TEMS) The medical support tailored for tactical law enforcement operations. It is further described as a non-military EMS system designed to provide and maintain medical services for all law enforcement special operations.

Tactical medic Medical provider specifically trained for the tactical environment who should be able to provide any and all emergency medical care to the members of the tactical team (i.e., tactical operators) prior to, during, and immediately after a law enforcement operation.

Tactical medical aid packs An advanced first aid kit including supplies for assessment, airway management, breathing control, and bleeding control.

Tactical medicine Treatment provided to people in a hostile environment, either patients, law enforcement, or the perpetrator.

Technical rescue The use of ropes and rigging by specially trained personnel to effect a rescue. It encompasses rope rescue, confined space rescue, cave rescue, trench rescue, tower rescue, and structural collapse rescue.

Technical search operators Specially trained rescuers who use specialized computer equipment, microphones, listening devices, fiberoptic cameras, and vibration detectors to search for and locate entrapped patients in areas where they cannot see with direct line of sight, such as around inaccessible corners or through layers of concrete.

Technical team A collection of specialists in USAR whose primary goal is evaluating the safety of a confined space environment in order to ensure the safety of the rescuers and the patient. The team is comprised of the following specialists: hazardous materials, structural, and heavy equipment and rigging.

Technician level (Hazmat) Those hazardous materials workers who are trained to respond to the scene of a hazardous materials incident, don special protective clothing, and enter the hot zone to stop the release of hazardous materials.

Techniques for effective alcohol management (TEAM) An educational program that teaches a concessionaire, or a Paramedic, the skills needed to identify an intoxicated individual and to intervene in a "non-confrontational way" to ensure the safety of the attendee and the staff.

Tension A command commonly used with technical rescue that refers to the looseness or tightness of the rope.

Tension diagonal A line stretched across moving water that is used to direct an object's movement to one side or the other.

Tensionless hitch The simplest anchor technique, which involves wrapping the rope around a tree or post. This anchor depends on the strength of the rope to hold the load.

Tension pneumothorax A situation that arises during an injury when air enters the lung and escapes into the pleural cavity through the damaged section and compresses the heart, lung, and great vessels. The air accumulates in the chest wall and increases pressure in the chest cavity, causing mediastinal compression, movement of the PMI and tracheal shifts in severe cases.

Terminal burrowing A condition associated with hypothermia wherein the patient enters into a confined space.

Terrorism Violent acts, directed against one or more persons, intended to intimidate an individual or group in order to bring about, or draw attention to, one's agenda.

Tertiary blast injuries Wounds that occur when patients are thrown to the ground or against objects following an explosion.

Tetanus prophylaxis Techniques used to prevent the painful disease caused from neurotoxins in clostridium tetani. Prophylaxis is more a function of the number of previous doses received for tetanus immunization than the length of time that has elapsed from previous vaccinations.

Tetraplegia Loss of sensation and motor control in the arms and legs as well as the torso after an injury in the cervical spine region.

Therapeutic hyperventilation Providing a patient with faster and deeper respirations than needed to help oxygenate the blood.

Thermogenesis Processes the body uses to generate heat.

Thermolysis The process through which sweat reaches the skin surface and it evaporates into the atmosphere, taking heat with it. The dissipated heat lowers the body's internal core temperature.

Thermoneutral A body temperature between 97.7°F and 99.5°F (36.5°C and 37.5°C). When the internal, or core, body temperature is within this range, the body's metabolic reactions can best occur.

3:1 Z rig A variation of mechanical advantage in which the rope forms a Z pattern as it winds between two pulleys that are pulled closer together. Thus, a moderately efficient pulley can make lifting 200 pounds feel like lifting 91 pounds.

Threshold limit A system developed by the federal government, toxicologists, and occupational medicine and industry experts to balance a philosophy of zero tolerance to exposure with one of acceptable risk provided proper PPE is worn. This way of thinking shows an understanding that dangers exist and exposure can occur.

Threshold limit value–concentration (TLV-C) The concentration of chemical exposure that should not be exceeded in any situation.

Threshold limit value–short-term exposure limit (TLV-STEL) The maximum acceptable exposure a person can tolerate, without apparent ill effects, for 15 minutes of exposure.

Throw bags A water rescue device comprised of a length of rope stuffed into a bag that is thrown. Some bags are equipped with a small float in the bottom of the bag that allows the bag to stay at the surface.

Thumb spica splint An immobilization device used for suspected gamekeeper's thumb/skier's thumb or suspected scaphoid fractures. Like the radial gutter splint, the thumb spica splint starts at the mid-forearm, wraps the thumb to the distal interphalangeal (DIP) joint, and keeps the hand in the wine glass position.

Tight grid searches Very slow, methodical, and thorough searches, yielding high coverage of the search area.

Timeline A determination of when the incident occurred and whether rescue actions can be taken. Most traumas are treated under what EMS terms the "Golden Hour" (60 minutes).

Tonsillar herniation A herniation that results from expanding hematoma formation proximal to the cerebellum.

Tooth squeeze A syndrome in which air under a tooth's filling, especially older or temporary fillings, leads to pressure-induced toothache or barodontalgia.

Touchdown area The actual site where a rotorcraft will land, which should be between 75 square feet and 100 square feet. The preference is 100 square feet.

Tourniquet pain A sensation that may occur 45 minutes to an hour after application of the tourniquet. It generally starts with a dull ache and progresses to severe pain.

TRACEM An acronym used to identify the different types of harm a Paramedic may encounter on the scene of a WMD: **T**hermal, **R**adiological, **A**sphyxiation, **C**hemical, **E**tiological, and **M**echanical hazards.

Tracheobronchial disruption Injuries to the trachea or bronchi, which can cause a pneumothorax, simple or tension, from air leaking into the chest cavity.

Tracking Looking for evidence that a subject has been in a given area, rather than looking for the subject himself. Tracking is performed by both humans and dogs.

Transcalvarial herniation Herniation of the brain through an open fracture. Any time gray matter leaves the skull, the impact can be devastating and may lead to meningitis, encephalitis, and permanent brain damage.

Transport area The location where patients are prepared for routing to a hospital or trauma center.

Trauma An injury caused by exposure to excessive physical forces such as mechanical forces, heat and cold, electricity, chemicals, and ionizing radiation. Trauma also occurs when essential substances are withheld from the body.

Trauma center An area designated for a certain level of patient care. The ACS has defined criteria for trauma center designation in four center levels— Levels I-IV. Level I Trauma Centers provide 24-hour in-house general surgical intervention as well as specialty care and serve as teaching hospitals. Level II Trauma Centers also include 24-hour immediate care by trauma surgeons, as well as specialty care, but their role in providing education and research as a teaching hospital may be more limited. Level III Trauma Centers must have 24-hour coverage by emergency medicine physicians with prompt availability of general surgeons and anesthesiology (30-minute surgical response). Level IV Trauma Centers provide 24-hour emergency department facilities with the ability to implement Advanced Trauma Life Support (ATLS) protocols and 24-hour laboratory coverage.

Trauma registries Databases that provide trauma-related data from prehospital care records and hospital trauma data. Through the use of data captured by the trauma registries, continuous quality improvement processes and clinical research occur that will allow for refinements of, and improvements in, the field triage process.

Trauma system Organizational structure that integrates local, regional, and state resources for preventing injury, treating trauma patients, providing rehabilitation services, collecting data on trauma for research, and improving quality.

Traumatic aortic disruptions An condition typically seen in rapid deceleration injuries. A speed gradient is established across the arch that pulls on the ligamentum arteriosum, the remnants of fetal circulation, which leads to shearing of the vessel. Between 85% and 95% of these patents die instantaneously.

Traumatic asphyxia A rare condition that occurs when a massive crushing force causes trauma due to a lack of oxygenation. This occurs in events such as a landslide or when a vehicle falls off of a jack and onto the patient's chest.

Traumatic brain injury (TBI) A traumatic insult to the brain capable of producing intellectual, emotional, social, and vocational changes.

Traumatic iritis A condition that occurs in the setting of blunt trauma to the eye in which the iris is contused and has difficulty contracting.

Traumatic rhabdomyolysis Rapid breakdown of skeletal muscle.

Traumatic subarachnoid hemorrhage (SAH) An extracerebral hemorrhage of the small corticomeningeal blood vessels within the arachnoid space. The blood often mixes with the cerebral spinal fluid (CSF) that is present and quickly spreads over the brain's surface.

Trench foot Localized tissue damage that occurs from prolonged exposure to moisture that is below body temperature.

Triage The process of sorting patients to prioritize their need for care when resources are limited. During the triage process, patients are not treated on a "first come first serve" basis, but instead in the order determined to be most appropriate based on available resources.

Triangulation Using different lines of sight to narrow down a location, which is very effective if multiple witnesses are interviewed from where they saw events.

Triggered devices Explosives that allow the terrorist to be distant from the scene at the point of ignition. Triggers may be made using a chemical reaction such as an inside burning fuse.

Tularemia A serious illness that naturally occurs in the United States through exposure to animals (rodents, rabbits, and hares) infected with the *Francisella tularensis* bacterium. Signs and symptoms of exposure include a sudden onset of fever, chills, headaches, diarrhea, muscle aches, joint pain, nonproductive cough, and progressive weakness.

Two-line taglines A method to deploy and control a flotation object from each side of moving water. A line is deployed and operated on each side of the current, and each line is connected to the flotation device, which will be moving in the water flow.

Tympanic membrane perforation An ear injury that may occur either from direct penetrating trauma to the tympanic membrane (for example, from a projectile or cotton-tipped swab) or can occur from barotraumas, which is often seen with blast injuries.

Type 1 PFDs Horse-collar life jackets that fasten to the wearer by hanging around the neck. Type 1 PFDs are used primarily on commercial and offshore craft (for example, cruise ships) and are used in heavy seas when rescue may not arrive quickly. They should turn an unconscious patient face up while floating, and must deliver a minimum of 22 pounds of buoyancy.

Type 2 PFDs Flotation devices with the same basic design as a Type 1 PFD, but which only provide 15 pounds of buoyancy for an adult. These smaller, more common PFDs are used on smaller, noncommercial pleasure craft.

Type 3 PFDs The typical "ski-vest" style PFDs found on many EMS, fire, and law enforcement vehicles. The Type 3 PFD does not necessarily turn unconscious wearers face up, but they are comfortable to wear, and provide the same 15-pound buoyancy as Type 2 PFDs.

Type 4 PFDs Devices that are not actually worn, but are meant to be thrown to a patient in distress in order to assist flotation until a very quick rescue is performed. They include throw ring buoys, seat cushions, and the like.

Type 5 PFDs Specialized, job-functional PFDs that can include float coats, work vests, paddling PFDs, and swift water rescue PFDs.

Type I response A USAR team response that deploys the full 70-person team, four canines, and a full equipment cache. This type of team is typically deployed for structural collapse scenarios, such as the Murrah federal building bombing in Oklahoma City in 1995.

Type I searchers Skilled searchers who are often trained to the Awareness and/or Operations level. Their searches are conducted by local resources.

Type II searchers Searchers who cover more specifically defined areas, with searchers organized into search lines with specific boundaries, which are usually drawn on a map.

Type III response A USAR team response that deploys a team of 28 personnel, two canines, and a limited equipment cache. These teams are typically deployed to natural disasters not involving structural collapse, such as the floods after Hurricane Katrina in 2005 when all 28 teams were deployed to the Gulf Coast.

Type III searchers Searchers for a lost individual aligned in a parallel or echelon formation of equal spacing as the terrain allows. Each searcher has a specific field of view for the search area between himself and other searchers.

Uncal herniation A supratentorial herniation in which lateral forces created by the expanding space-occupying lesion created by a blood clot compress the brain in the opposite hemisphere. The expanding lesion obliterates the cerebral ventricles within the core of the cerebral cortex. As a result, the patient may experience contralateral motor signs along with unilateral papillary changes on the ipsilateral side during the early phases of the herniation.

Undertriage Underestimating the severity of trauma patients, which causes seriously injured trauma patients not to receive vital trauma care services in a timely fashion.

Unified Command Shared authority for an emergency response due to an incident that crosses political boundaries and involves more than one agency with the authority to respond.

Up-and-over pathway A condition in which, during a motor vehicle collision, the patient's head leads as the body travels toward the windshield, steering column, and dashboard.

Upstream V An indication of an object in the water which the water is flowing around, with wake disturbances found on each side. The V, pointing upstream, marks the hazard.

Urban Search and Rescue (USAR) The science of locating, reaching, medically treating, and safely extricating deeply entombed survivors of collapsed structures and confined spaces.

Vapor density The concentration of a gas when compared to air.

Velocity The distance an object travels over time in a specified direction. Acceleration is the rate of change in velocity.

Velpeau bandage An alternative to the sling and swathe, which is sometimes preferred by patients with a dislocated shoulder as it allows the arm's weight to be supported.

Veterinary Medical Assistance Team (VMAT) A group including veterinarians, veterinary pathologists, animal health technicians, disease specialists, epidemiologists, toxicologists, and support personnel that provides local emergency personnel with services unique to the effects of disasters on animals. In addition to the treatment of animals, VMATs conduct surveillance for animal disease outbreaks, assist with food and water inspections, and assist with animal decontamination.

Viperidae An animal classification that contains most of the venomous snakes, such as rattlesnakes (Crotalus and Sistrurus), cottonmouths (also called water moccasins), and copperheads (Agkistrodon).

Viral hemorrhagic fevers (VHF) Zoonotic diseases that are generally spread from contact with infected animals and affect the body on a multisystem level. These diseases impair the body's ability to self-regulate, damage the vascular system, and sometimes cause non-life-threatening hemorrhages. There are four distinct families of these viruses, but the ones of greatest concern are filoviruses and arenaviruses.

Visual flight rules (VFR) Aviation regulations that essentially permit a pilot to fly only when environmental conditions allow him to actually see with his own eyes well enough to safely navigate the aircraft.

Volkmann's contracture A compartment syndrome, first described by Volkmann in 1872, which results from a too tight bandage on an elbow fracture.

Voltage (V) Named in honor of the Italian physicist Volta, a common unit of measurement which measures the difference between the two electrical poles in an electrical pathway or circuit, as well as the strength of the current.

Walking wounded A term sometimes used to describe patients in the Minor category of START triage classifications as they are usually ambulatory to some degree and may be able to assist in the care of other, more severely injured patients.

Warm zone (1) The area of a chemical spill immediately outside of the hot zone. This area contains staging and support for the hazmat team within the hot zone. (2) In the zones of care model, the area where tactical field care occurs. This is a zone where the provider may be relatively exposed to gunfire.

Water depletion heat exhaustion A condition that occurs when the person fails, either voluntarily or involuntarily, to replace fluid losses when exposed to intense heat. These patients present as hyperthermic, tachycardiac, and hyperventilating.

Water moccasin Snakes that have a white mouth which gives rise to another of its common names, the cottonmouth. These snakes are known to be somewhat more aggressive than other pit vipers and can bite underwater.

Water-reactive materials A chemical that may react, sometimes violently, upon contact with water.

Water rescue helmets Light protective head gear that has minimal foam padding inside so water is not absorbed.

Wave-off Vigorous crossing and uncrossing of the landing zone officer's arms over his head to signal immediate danger to the helicopter pilot. This will cause the pilot to quickly abort the landing.

Webbing Flat woven rope that has great strength and durability. Webbing is used for anchors, slings, and any number of uses where a short rope is helpful.

Wet drowning A medical emergency in which the patient's lungs contain at least some liquid. Wet drowning accounts for approximately 80% to 90% of recorded drowning.

Wilderness medicine Medical care rendered to patients who are at least one hour or more from definitive (medical facility) care and who are generally found in frontier or backwoods environments.

Woods shock The sudden onset of overwhelming panic and confusion a person may feel after initially realizing he is lost. It is responsible for bizarre behaviors in otherwise rational people.

Worker Visibility Act An initiative requiring emergency personnel (among others) in highway zones to wear high-visibility garments and reflective bands to aid others in observing them.

Worst first A triage technique in which the most seriously injured are the first to receive treatment.

Wound contraction The process during which granulation starts on the inside of a wound and pushes the scab up and out.

Wrap three, pull two anchor A common anchor technique that uses a loop of webbing wrapped around the anchor three times. Two loops are then pulled out. A carabiner is connected to the loops and the rope is clipped in. Usually a figure eight knot is tied on the end of the rope and a carabiner can be attached.

Zones of care A concept developed by the Committee on Tactical Combat Casualty Care (TCCC) that essentially means care of the wounded occurs in three separate zones: green (cool), yellow (warm), and red (hot).

INDEX